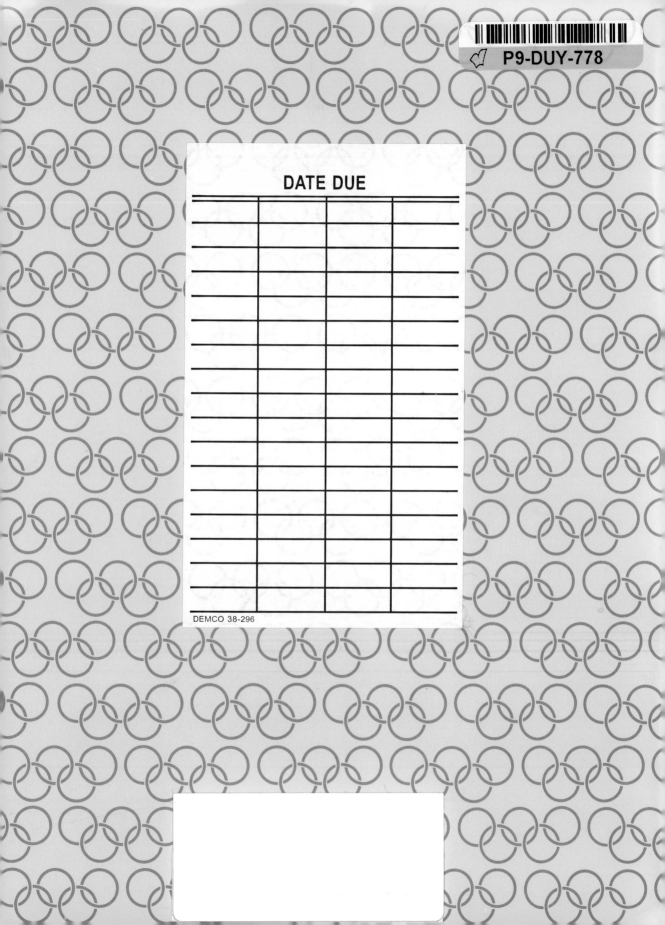

DATE DUE

THE CHILD AND
ADOLESCENT ATHLETE

The Child and Adolescent Athlete

VOLUME VI OF THE ENCYCLOPAEDIA OF SPORTS MEDICINE

AN IOC MEDICAL COMMISSION PUBLICATION

IN COLLABORATION WITH THE

INTERNATIONAL FEDERATION OF SPORTS MEDICINE

EDITED BY

ODED BAR-OR

**Blackwell
Science**

The child and adolescent athlete

© 1996 International Olympic Committee
Published by
Blackwell Science Ltd
Editorial Offices:
Osney Mead, Oxford OX2 OEL
25 John Street, London WC1N 2BL
23 Ainslie Place, Edinburgh EH3 6AJ
238 Main Street, Cambridge
   Massachusetts 02142, USA
54 University Street, Carlton
   Victoria 3053, Australia

Other Editorial Offices:
Arnette Blackwell SA
  1, rue de Lille, 75007 Paris
  France

Blackwell Wissenschafts-Verlag GmbH
  Kurfürstendamm 57
  10707 Berlin, Germany

  Feldgasse 13, A-1238 Wien
  Austria

First published 1996

Set by Setrite Typesetters, Hong Kong
Printed and bound in Great Britain
at the University Press, Cambridge

Part title illustrations by Grahame Baker

DISTRIBUTORS

  Marston Book Services Ltd
  PO Box 87
  Oxford OX2 ODT
  (*Orders*: Tel: 01865 791155
          Fax: 01865 791927
          Telex: 837515)

USA
  Human Kinetics Books
  Human Kinetics Publishers, Inc.
  Box 5075, Champaign
  Illinois 61825-5076
  (*Orders*: Tel: 1-800-747-4457)

Canada
  Human Kinetics Publishers, Inc.
  PO Box 24040
  Windsor, Ontario N8Y 4Y9
  (*Orders*: Tel: 1-800-465-7301)

Australia
  Blackwell Science Pty Ltd
  54 University Street
  Carlton, Victoria 3053
  (*Orders*: Tel: 03 9347-0300
          Fax: 03 9349-3016)

A catalogue record for this title
is available from the British Library

ISBN 0-86542-904-9

Library of Congress
Cataloging-in-Publication Data

The child and adolescent athlete/
edited by Oded Bar-Or.
       p.   cm. — (Encyclopaedia of
  sports medicine; v. 6)
    'An IOC Medical Commission publication
  in collaboration with the
  International Federation of Sports Medicine.'
    Includes bibliographical references and index.
    ISBN 0-86542-904-9
    1. Pediatric sports medicine. I. Bar-Or, Oded.
    II. IOC Medical Commission.   III. International
  Federation of Sports Medicine.   IV. Series.
    [DNLM: 1. Sports Medicine.
    2. Sports — physiology. 3. Pediatrics.
  QT 13 E527 1988 v.6]
  RC1218.C45C45   1995
  617.1'027'083 — dc20
  DNLM/DLC for Library of Congress

Contents

List of Contributors

F.J.G. BACKX MD, PhD, *The Netherlands Institute for Sports and Health, PO Box 302, 6800 AH Arnhem, the Netherlands*

O. BAR-OR MD, *Department of Pediatrics, McMaster University, Hamilton, Ontario L8N 3Z5, Canada*

D.A. BAILEY BA, MSc, PED, *College of Physical Education, University of Saskatchewan, Saskatoon S7N 0W0, Canada*

G. BEUNEN PhD, *Faculty of Physical Education and Physiotherapy, Katholieke Universiteit Lueven, B-3001 Leuven (Heverlee), Belgium*

C.J.R. BLIMKIE PhD, *Department of Kinesiology, McMaster University, Hamilton, Ontario L8P 4N9, Canada*

R.A. BOILEAU PhD, *Departments of Kinesiology, Nutritional Sciences and Internal Medicine, University of Illinois, Urbana, Illinois 61801, USA*

M.J. BURGESS-MILLIRON MS, *Biomechanics Laboratory, Converse Inc., 1 Fordham Road, North Reading, Massachusetts 01864, USA*

J. COAKLEY PhD, *Department of Sociology, University of Colorado at Colorado Springs, Colorado Springs, Colorado 80933-7150, USA*

D.M. COOPER MD, *Division of Respiratory and Critical Care, Department of Pediatrics, Harbor-UCLA Medical Center, Torrance, California 90509, USA*

R.A. DLIN MD, *Links Clinic, Professional Centre on 11th, 11910-111 Avenue, Edmonton, Alberta T5G 3G6, Canada*

D. DOCHERTY PhD, *School of Physical Education, University of Victoria, PO Box 3015, Victoria, British Columbia V8W 3P1, Canada*

H. DORCHY MD, PhD, *Clinique de Pédiatrie Ambulatoire et de Diabétologie, Hôpital Universitaire des Enfants Reine Fabiola, Université Libre de Bruxelles, B-1020 Brussels, Belgium*

P.G. DYMENT MD, *Department of Pediatrics and the Student Health Center, Tulane University, New Orleans, Louisiana 70118, USA*

V. EBBECK PhD, *Department of Exercise and Sport Science, Oregon State University, Corvallis, Oregon 97331, USA*

R.C. EKLUND PhD, *Department of Health, Physical Education and Recreation, University of North Dakota, Box 8235, Grand Forks, North Dakota 58202, USA*

J. FAGARD PhD, *Laboratoire de Psycho-Biologie du Développement, EPHE-CNRS (URA 315), 41 rue Gay-Lussac, 75005 Paris, France*

B. FALK PhD, *Ribstein Center for Research and Sport Medicine Sciences, Wingate Institute, Netanya 42902, Israel*

K. FROBERG MSc, *Department of Physical Education, Faculty of Health Sciences, Odense University, DK 5230 Odense M, Denmark*

E. GERON PhD, *Zinman College of Physical Education, Wingate Institute, PO Box 23027, Jerusalem 97725, Israel*

D. GOULD PhD, *Department of Exercise and Sport Science, University of North Carolina at Greensboro, Greensboro, North Carolina 27412-5001, USA*

O. INBAR EdD, *Zinman College, Wingate Institute, Netanya 42902, Israel*

H.C.G. KEMPER PhD, *Department of Health Science, Faculty of Human Movement Sciences, Vrije Universiteit, 1081 BT Amsterdam, the Netherlands*

O. LAMMERT PhD, *Department of Physical Education, Faculty of Health Sciences, Odense University, DK 5230 Odense M, Denmark*

R.M. MALINA PhD, *Institute for the Study of Youth Sports, 213 IM Sports Circle, Michigan State University, East Lansing, Michigan 48824-1049, USA*

V.K.R. MATSUDO MD, *Center of Studies of the Physical Fitness Research Laboratory from São Caetano do Sul (CELAFISCS), Avenue Goiás 1400, São Caetano do Sul, São Paulo 09521-300, Brazil*

L.J. MICHELI MD, *Division of Sports Medicine, Children's Hospital, Boston, Massachusetts 02115, USA*

S.B. MURPHY MS, *Biomechanics Laboratory, Converse Inc., 1 Fordham Road, North Reading, Massachusetts 01864, USA*

M.A. NELSON MD, *University of New Mexico Medical School, 4100 High Resort Building, Rio Rancho, New Mexico 87124, USA*

S. NELSON STEEN DSc, RD, *Weight and Eating Disorders Program, Department of Psychiatry, University of Pennsylvania School of Medicine, Philadelphia, Pennsylvania 19104, USA*

D.M. ORENSTEIN MD, *Department of Pediatrics, University of Pittsburgh and the Children's Hospital of Pittsburgh, Pittsburgh, Pennsylvania 15213, USA*

R.R. PATE PhD, *Department of Exercise Science, School of Public Health, University of South Carolina, Columbia, South Carolina 29208, USA*

L.M. PETLICHKOFF PhD, *Department of Health, Physical Education and Recreation, Boise State University, Boise, Idaho 83725, USA*

J.R. POORTMANS PhD, *Chimie Physiologique, Institut Supérieur d'Education Physique et de Kinésitherapie, Université Libre de Bruxelles, B-1050 Brussels, Belgium*

A.D. ROGOL MD, PhD, *Department of Pediatrics, the University of Virginia Health Sciences Center, Box 386, Charlottesville, Virginia 22908, USA*

W.D. ROSS PhD, *Rosscraft, 14732 16-A Avenue, Surrey, British Columbia V4A 5M7, Canada*

T.W. ROWLAND MD, *Department of Pediatrics, Baystate Medical Center, Springfield, Massachusetts 01199, USA*

W.H.M. SARIS MD, PhD, *Nutrition and Toxicology Research Institute Maastricht (NUTRIM), University of Limburg, 6200 MD Maastricht, the Netherlands*

A.D. SMITH MD, *Department of Orthopaedics, Case Western Reserve University School of Medicine, Cleveland, Ohio 44106, USA*

R.D. STEADWARD BPE, MSc, PhD, *Rick Hansen Centre, W1-67 Van Vliet Centre, University of Alberta, Edmonton, Alberta T6G 2H9, Canada*

E. VAN PRAAGH PhD, *Department of Exercise Physiology, Faculty of Sport Science, Université Blaise Pascal, 63172 Aubière, France*

D.S. WARD EdD, *Department of Exercise Science, School of Public Health, University of South Carolina, Columbia, South Carolina 29208, USA*

R.L. WASHINGTON MD, *Rocky Mountain Pediatric Cardiology, Suite 5600, 1601 E. 19th Avenue, Denver, Colorado 80218, USA*

M.R. WEISS PhD, *Department of Exercise and Movement Science, University of Oregon, Eugene, Oregon 97403-1240, USA*

G.D. WHEELER BEd, MEd, MSc, PhD, *Rick Hansen Centre, W1-67 Van Vliet Centre, University of Alberta, Edmonton, Alberta T6G 2H9, Canada*

J.H. WILMORE PhD, *Department of Kinesiology and Health Education, the University of Texas at Austin, Austin, Texas 78712, USA*

E.M. WINTER BEd, MSc, PhD, *Department of Physical Education, Sport and Leisure, De Montfort University, Bedford MK40 2BZ, UK*

Forewords

As President of the International Olympic Committee I welcome the new IOC Medical Commission's publication, the VIth volume of the Encyclopaedia of Sports Medicine series addressing the specific issue of the child and adolescent athlete.

On behalf of the International Olympic Committee I should like to thank all those involved in the preparation of this volume whose work is highly respected and appreciated by the whole Olympic Family.

JUAN ANTONIO SAMARANCH
Marqués de Samaranch

The International Olympic Committee's Medical Commission takes this opportunity to present the new volume of our encyclopaedia series: *The Child and Adolescent Athlete*. Our gratitude goes to the IOC Medical Commission's Publications Advisory Sub-Committee, with a special mention for the effort of the editor, Professor Oded Bar-Or, and the 46 contributing authors.

On behalf of the IOC Medical Commission I should like to extend our sincere appreciation to Blackwell Science, who have made the publication of this book possible.

PRINCE ALEXANDRE DE MERODE
IOC Vice-President
Chairman, IOC Medical Commission

The International Olympic Committee would like to inform its readership that all revenue obtained from sale of IOC Medical Commission publications goes towards future Commission publications and the distribution of these free of charge in less developed countries.

xiii

Preface

The five previous volumes of the Encyclopaedia of Sports Medicine have focused either on general issues within sports medicine (Volumes I, IV and V) or on specific components of fitness and performance (Volumes II and III). The current volume on *The Child and Adolescent Athlete* is the first to focus on a demographic portion of the population. I congratulate the Medical Commission of the International Olympic Committee on their decision to dedicate a whole encyclopaedia volume to children and adolescents. This reflects the growing importance of paediatric sports medicine and paediatric exercise medicine within the science and practice of sports medicine.

In general, knowledge regarding physiological, psychosocial and medical aspects of paediatric exercise has lagged behind that generated for adults. This reflects ethical and methodological constraints in studying children and, to a lesser extent, adolescents.

For ethical reasons, studies with children should not include procedures that cause pain or embarrassment or that may compromise the child's health. This limits an investigator's ability to obtain biopsies, insert catheters, use radioactive isotopes or other imaging techniques that require radiation, or to expose the child to 'hostile' climates. Furthermore, intervention programmes that are designed to cause physical or emotional damage to the subjects (e.g. the effect of extreme training and dietary regimens on the incidence of anorexia nervosa) should not be used with children, even if their parents formally consent.

Methodological constraints include, for example, a need to modify apparatus (e.g. ergometers) or to create protocols compatible with differences in body size, maturational stage, temperament or cognitive ability. Another challenge is to properly equate training dosages among subjects who markedly differ in age or in body size.

In spite of the above constraints, much information has been generated in recent years on the responses of children to exercise and training. This information is reviewed in 40 chapters by authors who have been recognized worldwide as leaders in their respective fields. Even though the title of this, Volume VI, is *The Child and Adolescent Athlete*, some chapters do not limit their focus to athletes, but expand the scope to the effects of exercise and sports on the general child and adolescent population.

The book is subdivided into seven parts. Part 1 addresses the physiological effects of growth and maturation on several body systems and on physical performance. It also includes a chapter on the prediction of athletic excellence. The effects of training on morphological and physiological characteristics, as well as on present and future performance, are discussed in Part 2. Part 3 focuses on epidemiological, biomechanical, orthopaedic and rehabilitative aspects of injuries induced by sports participation. It also addresses means of preventing such injuries. Health-related issues in sports participation are not limited to trauma. Nutritional deficiencies, eating disorders, delayed puberty, cardiological concerns and responses to hot or cold climates are discussed in Part 4. Psychosocial issues such as socialization, self-esteem, perceptions of competence, emotional stress, anxiety, intelligence of young athletes and the drop-out dilemma are summarized in Part 5. With proper management, children and adolescents with a chronic disease can participate, and even excel, in sports. Part 6 focuses on exertion-related issues of such young athletes with asthma, diabetes mellitus, hypertension or a motor disability. Finally, Part 7 comprises eight chapters that review recommended methods for assessing morphological and physiological characteristics of the young athlete.

This volume should provide valuable reference material for professionals who are interested in the effects of exercise and sports on children and adolescents. Specifically, it would be useful to sports physicians, general practitioners, paediatricians, physiotherapists, dietitians, coaches, students and researchers in the exercise sciences. I am indeed grateful and honoured to have been selected as editor for this volume.

ODED BAR-OR
Hamilton
1995

PART 1

GROWTH, MATURATION AND PHYSICAL PERFORMANCE

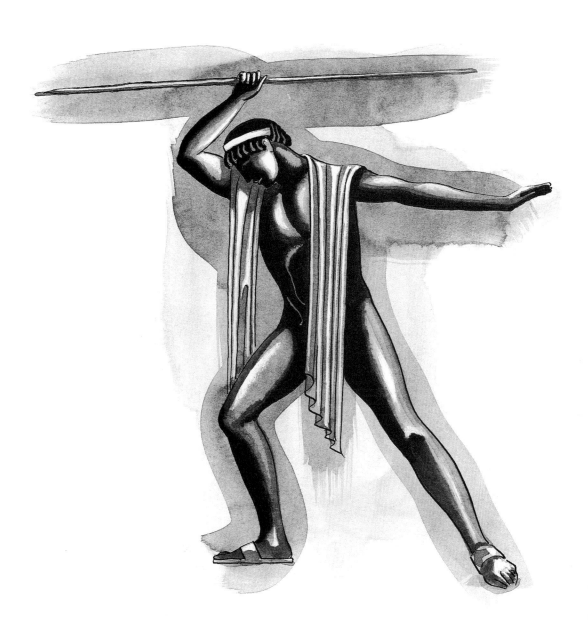

Chapter 1

Growth and Biological Maturation: Relevance to Athletic Performance

GASTON BEUNEN AND ROBERT M. MALINA

Introduction

Growth refers to measurable changes in size, physique and body composition and various systems of the body, whereas maturation refers to progress towards the mature state. Maturation varies not only among the systems, but also in timing and tempo (rate) of progress. Chronological age (CA) has limited utility as an indicator of individual maturity status. There is considerable variability in physical characteristics among individuals of the same CA, especially during the pubertal years. The processes of growth and biological maturation are related, and both influence physical performance.

Those engaged in education or coaching of youths are certainly familiar with the following scenario: boy A who is 13.5 years old, has a stature of 171 cm, weight 60 kg and a static strength score of 65 kg on an arm pull test, while boy B who is also 13.5 years old, has a stature of 150 cm, weight 40 kg and a strength score of 32 kg. These boys of exactly the same CA are often required to compete against each other in a variety of team and individual sports, and often on fitness tests.

One of the main reasons for the size and strength gap between the two boys is their difference in biological maturity status. Boy A is advanced and has a skeletal age (SA) of 15.5 years and boy B, who is a slow maturer, has an SA of 11.5 years. There is, however, the possibility that boy B will catch up and eventually outperform boy A in late adolescence and adulthood.

This chapter considers the interrelationships among growth, maturation and performance with four objectives.
1 Age- and sex-associated variation in physical performance are briefly described.
2 Maturity-associated variation in performance is discussed.
3 Growth and maturation of young athletes is briefly outlined.
4 Effects of training on growth and maturation are briefly considered.

Growth and physical performance

The development of gross motor functions are analysed in the context of growth in somatic dimensions. Adolescent spurts in performance relative to the timing of the growth spurt in stature are also considered.

Overview of somatic growth

When viewed as size attained, growth in stature is rapid in infancy and early childhood, rather steady during middle childhood, rapid once again during the adolescent spurt, and then gradually slows as adult stature is attained. This pattern of rate and size attained is generally similar for body weight and other dimensions except subcutaneous fat and fat distribution (Malina & Bouchard, 1991). The growth rate of stature is highest during the first year of life, gradually declines until the onset (take-off) of the adolescent growth spurt (about 10 years in girls and 12 years in boys). With the spurt, growth rate increases, reaching peak velocity at about 12 years in girls and 14 years in boys, and then gradually declines and eventually ceases with the attainment of adult stature (Tanner, 1962, 1978; Malina & Bouchard, 1991). There is evidence for a small mid-growth spurt in childhood in stature and probably in other dimensions in many, but not all, children (see Chapter 14).

Changes in physical performance during growth

Physical performance is an important component of the behavioural repertoire of children and adolescents, perhaps more so for boys than for girls, although the recent acceptance of girls and women in the role of élite athletes may influence the views of and values attached to physical performance in girls. Motor performance is most often measured in a variety of gross motor tasks which require abilities such as speed, balance, flexibility, explosive strength and local muscular endurance, while muscular strength is traditionally measured by static dynamometric tests such as gripping, pulling and pushing.

In boys, isometric strength increases linearly with age from early childhood to approximately the age of 13 years, when there is a clear adolescent spurt, i.e. an acceleration in strength development. In girls, strength increases linearly until 15 years in several studies though there is less evidence of a clear adolescent spurt (Jones, 1949; Asmussen, 1962; Malina & Bouchard, 1991). However, in a large cross-sectional population study of Flemish girls an acceleration was observed in arm pull strength between 12 and 14.5 years (Fig. 1.1). The sex difference in strength is consistent, though small, through childhood. Thereafter, the differences become increasingly larger so that at the age of 16 years and later, only a few girls perform as high as the average boy. In Belgian

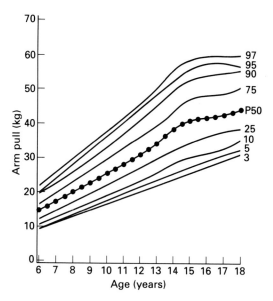

Fig. 1.1 Median performances in static strength (arm pull) in Flemish girls at chronological ages 6–18 years. Redrawn with permission from Beunen and Simons (1990).

youths, for example, the median arm pull score of 17-year-old girls falls below the 3rd percentile of the scores of 17-year-old boys (Beunen *et al.*, 1989).

Strength is related to body size and muscle mass, so that the sex difference might relate to a size advantage in boys. During childhood and adolescence boys tend to have greater strength per unit body size, especially in the upper body and trunk, than girls. From 7 years of age there are, however, negligible sex differences in lower extremity strength when body size is controlled. Isometric strength in boys and girls increases more than predicted from height alone (Asmussen & Heeboll-Nielsen, 1955). The disproportionate strength increase is most apparent during male adolescence, and is greater in the upper extremities than in the trunk or lower extremities (Asmussen, 1962; Carron & Bailey, 1974).

Performance in a variety of motor tasks such as speed, explosive strength, local muscular endurance, flexibility and balance also show improvement, on average, from childhood through adolescence in boys. The performances in girls increase until the age of 13 or 14 years, with little subsequent improvement (Branta *et al.*, 1984; Malina & Bouchard, 1991). Some evidence suggests that the plateau of performances of adolescent girls in a number of motor tasks has shifted to a slightly older age in more recent studies (Haubenstricker & Seefeldt, 1986; Beunen & Simons, 1990). This is apparent in the distance curves for explosive strength, muscular endurance, running speed and speed of limb movement in Flemish girls (Fig. 1.2).

In early adolescence, motor performances of

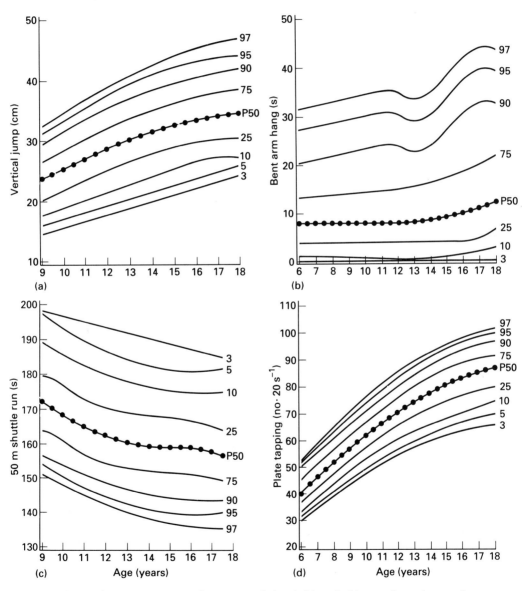

Fig. 1.2 Median performances in: (a) explosive strength (vertical jump), (b) muscular endurance (bent arm hang), (c) running speed (50 m shuttle run), and (d) speed of limb movement (plate tapping) in Flemish girls at chronological ages 6–18 and 9–18 years. Redrawn with permission from Beunen and Simons (1990).

girls fall, on average, within 1 SD below average performances of boys, with the exception of softball throw for distance. However, after 14 years of age, average performances of girls are consistently beyond the bounds of 1 SD below the means of boys in most tasks (Beunen *et al.*, 1989; Malina & Bouchard, 1991). An exception is flexibility; girls show greater levels of flexibility at virtually all ages (Merni *et al.*, 1981; Haubenstricker & Seefeldt, 1986; Beunen *et al.*, 1989; Malina & Bouchard, 1991). Mean scores in the sit-and-reach are stable or decline slightly during childhood, increase during adolescence and reach a plateau at about 14–15 years of age. In boys the scores decline through mid-adolescence and then increase.

Correlations between somatic dimensions and motor tasks during childhood are generally low (0 to about 0.35). Tasks in which the body is projected (jumps and dashes) correlate negatively and tasks in which an object is projected (throws) correlate positively. Correlations during adolescence are of the same magnitude and in the same direction as during childhood (Malina, 1975; Malina & Bouchard, 1991).

Most fitness test batteries include a direct or indirect estimate of aerobic power. Absolute ($\dot{V}O_{2\,max}$, $l \cdot min^{-1}$) aerobic power increases from childhood through adolescence in boys, but reaches a plateau at 13–14 years of age in girls. Before 10–12 years of age, $\dot{V}O_{2\,max}$ of girls reaches about 85–90% of mean values of boys, but after the adolescent spurt average $\dot{V}O_{2\,max}$ in girls reaches only 70% of mean scores in boys (Krahenbuhl *et al.*, 1985; Malina & Bouchard, 1991).

The dependence of aerobic power on body size during growth is indicated in the growth curve of relative aerobic power, i.e. per unit body mass ($ml \cdot kg^{-1} \cdot min^{-1}$). The values are rather stable throughout the growth period in cross-sectional samples of boys (Krahenbuhl *et al.*, 1985), but trends in longitudinal samples suggest a decline throughout adolescence (Mirwald & Bailey, 1986). On the other hand, relative $\dot{V}O_{2\,max}$ decreases systematically with

age in girls (Krahenbuhl *et al.*, 1985; Mirwald & Bailey, 1986). Sex differences in relative $\dot{V}O_{2\,max}$ are generally smaller, 80–95%, than in absolute $\dot{V}O_{2\,max}$.

Adolescent spurts in performance

Individual variation in the timing and tempo of the adolescent growth spurt in stature is described in Chapter 14. 'Timing' refers to the CA at which the spurt occurs, while 'tempo' refers to the rate at which an individual goes through the spurt. Cross-sectional studies are not appropriate for quantifying the timing and tempo of the growth spurt. Individuals pass through adolescence at their own pace and consequently have their growth spurts over a wide range of CAs, the so-called time-spreading effect (Tanner, 1962). Cross-sectional studies or cross-sectional analysis of longitudinal data present smooth growth curves resulting in the absorption of individual differences in the timing and tempo of the spurt. Only longitudinal or mixed-longitudinal data properly analysed provide adequate information about tempo and timing of spurts in a variety of characteristics.

In addition to documenting the occurrence of adolescent spurts in performance, the timing of the spurts is ordinarily viewed relative to the timing of peak height velocity (PHV), i.e. relative to a biological milestone, rather than to CA. By doing so, the time spread along the CA axis is reduced considerably and better information is obtained about the timing and magnitude of adolescent spurts in performance. This concept was first realized by Boas (1892).

In such analyses, individual velocities are estimated for each performance item using one of the models for stature described in Chapter 39. These individual velocities are then aligned on the individual's PHV. In this procedure, growth rates in performance are viewed in terms of years before and after the individual child's PHV regardless of the age at which PHV occurred. A mean constant velocity curve is obtained from these individual values in which the aligned individual values are combined. When mathematical functions are used, the mean-constant curve is obtained by fitting the function to each individual, estimating the constants for each individual, and then averaging the constants to yield the curve.

Longitudinal data show well-defined adolescent spurts in the strength, motor performance and absolute aerobic power of boys. Corresponding data for girls are less extensive and show a spurt in absolute aerobic power, while data for strength are variable.

The male adolescent spurt in static strength occurs about 0.5−1 year after PHV and is more coincident with peak weight velocity (PWV) (Stolz & Stolz, 1951; Carron & Bailey, 1974; Kemper & Verschuur, 1985; Beunen et al., 1988). The strength spurt (arm pull) of Dutch girls occurs at about the same time as in boys, 0.5 years after PHV. Peak strength gain in boys is

$12\,kg\cdot year^{-1}$ compared to $6\,kg\cdot year^{-1}$ in girls. Among Californian girls, however, a composite strength score of four different tests shows an inconsistent pattern: the spurt in strength preceded PHV in about 40% of the girls, coincided with PHV in 11%, and followed PHV in 49% (Faust, 1977).

Half-yearly velocities for six performance tasks in Belgian boys are summarized in Fig. 1.3. On the average, peak velocities in static strength (arm pull), explosive strength (vertical jump) and muscular endurance (bent arm hang) occur after PHV. The adolescent spurt in these characteristics appears to begin about 1.5 years prior to PHV and reach a peak 0.5−1 year after PHV. In contrast, maximum velocities in speed tests (shuttle run and plate tapping) and flexibility (sit-and-reach) occur before PHV. The lower age limit in the Leuven growth study of Belgian boys, 12 years of age, does not permit

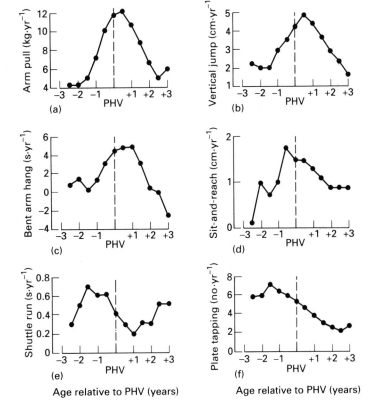

Fig. 1.3 Median velocities of several tests of strength and motor performance aligned on peak height velocity (PHV) in the Leuven growth study of Belgian boys. (a) Arm pull, (b) vertical jump, (c) bent arm hang, (d) sit-and-reach, (e) shuttle run, and (f) plate tapping. Velocities for the performance items are plotted as years before and after PHV. Drawn from data reported by Beunen et al. (1988).

an accurate estimate of the onset of the spurts in flexibility and speed.

It is of interest that during the years of rapid increase in stature none of these gross motor functions show a negative velocity which would indicate a decline in performance. Such a period of 'adolescent awkwardness' has often been suggested in the general child development literature but is not shown in longitudinal studies of gross motor performance (Beunen & Malina, 1988).

An overview of the timing in strength and motor performance relative to PHV, PWV and peak strength velocity (PSV) is given in Table 1.1. Since PWV and PSV follow PHV, it is obvious that maximum velocities in running speed (shuttle run), speed of limb movement (plate tapping) and flexibility (sit-and-reach) also precede PWV and PSV. Maximum velocities in strength and muscular endurance follow PWV and coincide with PSV. The evidence thus indicates that during adolescence boys are first stretched (spurt in stature) and then filled-out (spurt in muscle mass, weight and strength).

Data relating motor performance to PHV for girls are not available. However, when performance is related to age at menarche, which generally occurs after PHV, there is no tendency for motor performance to peak before, at or after menarche (Espenschade, 1940).

Absolute $\dot{V}o_{2\,max}$ $(l \cdot min^{-1})$ shows a clear

adolescent spurt in both sexes in a sample of Canadian children (Mirwald & Bailey, 1986). Estimated peak velocities are greater in boys $(0.41 l \cdot min^{-1})$ than in girls $(0.28 l \cdot min^{-1})$. Corresponding data for Dutch (Kemper, 1985), German and Norwegian (Rutenfranz et al., 1982) adolescents, though not analysed in the same manner, suggest a similar trend. Absolute $\dot{V}o_{2\,max}$ begins to increase several years before PHV and continues to increase after PHV. $\dot{V}o_{2\,max}$ per unit body mass $(ml\,O_2 \cdot kg^{-1} \cdot min^{-1})$, conversely, generally begins to decline 1 year before PHV and continues to decline after PHV. The decline reflects the rapid changes in stature and body mass, so that per unit body mass, oxygen uptake declines during the growth spurt. The significance of relative aerobic power as expressed per body weight or other body dimensions can be questioned. The relationships between aerobic power and several body dimensions and systemic functions during growth are complex. Relative aerobic power masks the sex-specific changes in body composition, size and function. Changes in relative aerobic power during adolescence probably reflect changes in body composition and not changes in aerobic function, which increases at this time. There is thus a need for new approaches to the assessment of changes in aerobic function during growth.

Table 1.1 Timing of maximum observed velocities of motor performance relative to adolescent spurts in stature, body weight and arm pull strength. The X indicates whether the maximum observed velocities for each performance characteristic precedes, coincides with or follows either peak height velocity, peak weight velocity or peak arm pull velocity (static strength). Data from the Leuven growth study of Belgian boys (Beunen et al., 1988).

Physical fitness test	Height spurt			Weight spurt			Arm pull spurt		
	Precedes	Coincides	Follows	Precedes	Coincides	Follows	Precedes	Coincides	Follows
Arm pull			X			X			
Vertical jump			X			X		X	
Plate tapping	X			X			X		
Shuttle run	X			X			X		
Sit-and-reach	X			X			X		
Bent arm hang			X			X	X		

Maturity-associated variation in physical performance

Athletes, and especially élite athletes, represent a very small percentage of the general population. Quite often they show, already at a rather young age, distinct morphological and performance characteristics. It is thus reasonable to review maturity-associated variation in performance in the general population and then to discuss the associations in athletes.

Maturity-associated variation in the general population

SOMATIC CHARACTERISTICS

Maturation and body dimensions, composition and proportions are confounded in their effect on performance (Malina, 1975). The association between maturity status and somatic characteristics is generally approached in two ways: (i) by correlational analysis; and (ii) by contrasting groups of the same CA but different maturity status.

Skeletal maturity is strongly related to the percentage of adult stature attained (Beunen, 1989). Age at menarche is also related to stature and stature increments, which has led some authors to predict age at menarche from stature and weight (Frisch, 1974) or from stature increments (Ellison, 1981). In boys, correlations between skeletal maturity and anthropometric dimensions in three longitudinal studies show strikingly similar trends (Bayley, 1943a,b; Clarke, 1971; Beunen et al., 1978b). Correlations increase until 14 years of age and then gradually decrease for all body dimensions. At the age of 14 years, correlations for stature and sitting height vary between 0.59 and 0.89. For limb circumferences, correlations vary between 0.50 and 0.61 at the same age. Correlations in girls are similar; stature is most closely related to skeletal maturity, followed by weight, widths and circumferences. However, correlations reach a maximum at about 11 years of age in girls. Thus, in both sexes the highest corre-

lations between skeletal maturity and anthropometric dimensions occur around the time of most rapid growth during the adolescent spurt. Muscle size and mass are also associated with skeletal maturity. The relationship is weak during childhood, but moderately strong during adolescence, especially in boys (Reynolds, 1946; Malina & Johnston, 1967).

Since skeletal maturation is reasonably well correlated with indicators of sexual and somatic maturity (see Chapter 14), it may be expected that the associations between skeletal maturity and somatic characteristics also hold for the other maturity criteria. As long ago as the 1930s, Richey (1937) demonstrated that girls who attained menarche early are already taller and heavier than later maturing girls at 6 years of age, long before menarche occurs. These differences between early and late maturing girls are also apparent for chest width and bi-iliac diameter (Shuttleworth, 1937). Corresponding trends in body size are also apparent in boys of contrasting maturity status during childhood and adolescence (Malina & Bouchard, 1991).

Much discussion in the past 20 years or so has centred around a proposed association between a critical body weight and the timing of menarche (Frisch & Revelle, 1970). This notion has been replaced by a critical level of fatness (Frisch et al., 1973). Frisch (1987) emphasizes that the associations are causal; too little fat (less than 17%) 'causes' delay in menarche and perhaps primary amenorrhoea. These hypotheses have been severely criticized in terms of research design, statistical analysis and techniques for the estimation of body fat. Bronson and Manning (1991), in a recent review of human and animal evidence, including a number of experimental studies with animals, concluded that there is no doubt that ovulation can be regulated in relation to whole-body energy balance and that fat stores are an important component of energy balance, but that there is no reason to accord body fat a direct causal role in regulating ovulation.

Children with a high level of fatness are not

only fatter than age and sex peers but are also taller and have increased skeletal size, fat-free mass and muscle size. In contrast, lean children are correspondingly smaller and later in maturity status (Wolff, 1955; Garn & Haskell, 1959; Seltzer & Mayer, 1964; Cheek *et al.*, 1970; Parizkova, 1977; Beunen *et al.*, 1982).

Differences in stature, weight and body composition between early and late maturing children can be translated into physique differences. In boys, endomorphs tend to be early maturers while ectomorphs tend to be late maturers. Correlations between skeletal age and somatotype components in boys confirm this trend and suggest that mesomorphy is also associated with early maturation (Fig. 1.4). However, results are not consistent for mesomorphy, although boys with an early age at PHV have higher mesomorphy ratings from 15 to 18 years of age (Beunen *et al.*, 1987).

Relationships between maturity status and physique in girls have not been extensively investigated. However, late maturation is associated with linearity of physique in girls

(McNeill & Livson, 1963). It should be stressed, however, that the chronology of pubertal changes shows considerable independence of somatotype in boys (Barton & Hunt, 1962). Corresponding data are lacking for girls.

Several studies suggest associations between subcutaneous fat distribution and biological maturation. Advanced maturation is associated with a centripetal (truncal) distribution of subcutaneous fat (Malina & Bouchard, 1988). The associations are only moderate (0.20−0.40) and seem to be stronger in boys than in girls (Frisancho & Flegel, 1982; Xi *et al.*, 1989; Beunen *et al.*, 1992a). The associations, however, may be influenced by the skinfolds used to estimate relative fat distribution.

PHYSICAL PERFORMANCE

Skeletal maturation and absolute aerobic power are significantly related. The correlations are higher (0.89) when a broad age range (8−18 years) is considered (Hollman & Bouchard, 1970), compared to a narrower range of 8−14

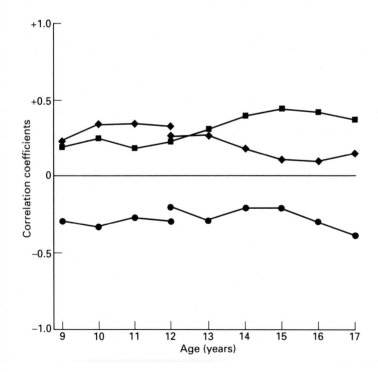

Fig. 1.4 Correlations between somatotype components and skeletal age in two longitudinal samples of boys at chronological ages 9−12 years and 12−17 years from the Medford boys' growth study. ◆, endomorphy; ■, mesomorphy; ●, ectomorphy. Drawn from data reported by Clarke (1971).

years (0.55−0.68; Labitzke, 1971). When $\dot{V}O_{2\,max}$ is expressed per kilogram body mass, correlations are not significant (Hollman & Bouchard, 1970; Labitzke, 1971; Savov, 1978; Shephard *et al.*, 1978). Non-significant and generally lower associations are apparent between several indices of submaximal performance capacity and maturity status, except around the growth spurt in boys when higher correlations are observed (Hebbelinck *et al.*, 1971; Kemper *et al.*, 1975; Bouchard *et al.*, 1976, 1978). In a national sample of Belgian girls, skeletal maturation is significantly correlated with submaximal power output (physical working capacity, PWC) at heart rates of 130, 150 and 170 beats·min^{-1}. The correlations generally increased with age, reaching a maximum between 11 and 13 years of age. The highest correlation (0.59) was noted between SA and PWC170 in 13-year-old girls (Beunen, 1989).

Early maturing boys have, on average, a higher absolute $\dot{V}O_{2\,max}$ than late maturing boys except in later adolescence. A similar trend is evident for early and late maturing girls, but the differences are smaller than in boys. Conversely, relative $\dot{V}O_{2\,max}$ is higher in late maturers of both sexes (Kemper *et al.*, 1986). This observation most probably reflects the higher absolute and relative fatness of early maturing girls. However, among boys, early maturers have an absolutely larger fat-free mass and relatively less fat than late maturers. The better relative $\dot{V}O_{2\,max}$ of late maturers more probably reflects the rapid growth of body mass, so that oxygen uptake per unit body mass becomes progressively less.

In an early study, Espenschade (1940) demonstrated different associations between maturation and motor performance in adolescent girls and boys. With increasing skeletal maturity, motor performance reached a plateau or declined in girls, but continued to improve in boys. In a longitudinal analysis of muscular strength of boys and girls of contrasting maturity status (Jones, 1949; see also Malina & Bouchard, 1991), early maturing boys performed better than late maturing boys at all

ages between 11 and 17 years of age, while early maturing girls performed only slightly better than late maturing girls only in early adolescence (aged 11−13 years). Subsequently, there were no differences in strength among girls of contrasting maturity status. The association between various maturity indicators and static or isometric strength has been consistently documented, and indicates a positive relationship between maturity status and strength in boys and girls (Clarke, 1971; Carron & Bailey, 1974; Beunen *et al.*, 1981b; Bastos & Hegg, 1986).

Correlations between different gross motor performances and SA are summarized in Tables 1.2−1.4. When only age-specific correlations are considered, static strength is associated with SA at all ages in preadolescent boys and girls. Static strength is positively correlated, while muscular endurance (functional strength or dynamic strength) is negatively correlated to SA in adolescent girls 11−13 years of age. In boys, static strength is positively related to SA, but from 14 years onwards all gross motor abilities are positively associated with SA. However, muscular endurance of the lower trunk and upper body are negatively related to SA in 12−13-year-old boys. This reflects the negative influence of body weight at this time. The greater strength that accompanies male adolescence compensates for the higher body weight so that from 14 years on positive associations are apparent between SA and muscular endurance.

The association between performance and skeletal maturity declines considerably when stature and weight are considered (Seils, 1951; Rarick & Oyster, 1964; Carron & Bailey, 1974; Shephard *et al.*, 1978), leading to the conclusion that in preadolescents SA is not an important predictor of physical performance. Among adolescent boys, however, correlations between SA and flexibility (sit-and-reach), speed of limb movement (plate tapping), explosive strength (vertical jump) and static strength (arm pull) were significant at all CA between 13 and 17 years, even when CA, stature and weight were

Table 1.2 Correlation between skeletal age and motor performances of preadolescent boys (B) and girls (G). From Beunen (1989) which contains the primary references.

	Grades			7–11 year olds		6 year olds		Girls (age in years)				
	1–3	1–3	2					6	7	8	9	10
	B	G	B	B	G	B	G					
Static strength												
flexion–extension			0.35–0.60									
hand grip						0.35	0.30					
arm pull								0.26	0.21	0.25	0.31	0.39
Explosive strength												
standing long jump	0.27	0.58	0.25	0.54	0.62	0.16	NS	NS	NS	NS	NS	NS
softball throw	0.42	0.38	0.48			NS	NS					
Muscular endurance												
bent arm hang				0.17	NS			NS	NS	−0.11	−0.19	−0.18
sit-ups				0.36	0.17	NS	NS					
Running speed												
dash	0.51	0.46	0.32	0.61	0.71	0.23	NS	0.19				
shuttle run				0.48	0.56				NS	NS	NS	NS
Speed of limb movement												
plate tapping								NS	NS	−0.11	NS	+0.10
Flexibility												
sit-and-reach								NS	NS	−0.09	−0.10	NS

NS, non-significant correlation ($P > 0.05$).

Table 1.3 Correlations between skeletal age and motor performances of 11–16-year-old girls. From Beunen (1989) which contains the primary references.

Factor	Test	Age (years)					
		11	12	13	14	15	16
Static strength	Arm pull		0.36	0.33	0.28	0.28	NS
	Arm pull	0.39	0.35	0.39	0.26	0.17	0.23
Explosive strength	Vertical jump		NS	NS	NS	NS	NS
	Vertical jump	NS	0.11	0.08	0.07	NS	NS
Muscular endurance	Bent arm hang		−0.42	−0.20	NS	NS	NS
	Bent arm hang	−0.26	−0.19	−0.18	NS	NS	NS
	Leg lifts		NS	NS	NS	NS	NS
	Leg lifts	−0.21	NS	NS	NS	NS	NS
Running speed	Dodge run		NS	NS	NS	NS	NS
	Shuttle run	0.08	NS	NS	NS	NS	NS
Speed of limb movement	Plate tapping		NS	NS	NS	NS	NS
	Plate tapping	NS	0.06	0.09	NS	NS	NS
Flexibility	Sit-and-reach		NS	NS	NS	NS	NS
	Sit-and-reach	NS	NS	NS	NS	NS	NS

NS, non-significant correlation ($P > 0.05$).

Table 1.4 Correlations between skeletal age and motor performances of 12–16-year-old boys. From Beunen (1989) which contains the primary references.

Factor	Test	Age (years)				
		12	13	14	15	16
Static strength	Extension–flexion	NS	NS	0.28	0.29	NS
	Extension–flexion	0.44	0.68	0.81	0.67	0.54
	Arm pull	0.43	0.55	0.65	0.63	0.51
Explosive strength	Standing long jump	NS	NS	0.39	0.40	NS
	Vertical jump	NS	0.20	0.32	0.38	0.32
Muscular endurance	Bent arm hang	−0.19	−0.14	NS	NS	NS
	Leg lifts	−0.15	−0.12	0.04	0.13	0.19
Running speed	Shuttle run	NS	NS	0.13	0.12	0.09
Speed of limb movement	Plate tapping	NS	0.15	0.12	0.18	0.17
Flexibility	Sit-and-reach	NS	0.06	0.16	0.19	0.14

NS, non-significant correlation ($P > 0.05$).

statistically controlled (Beunen *et al.*, 1981b). Third-order partial correlations for these motor tasks were lower than the zero-order correlations. However, corresponding correlations were higher for muscular endurance tests (bent arm hang and trunk strength). In the same data set, differences in performance between early and late maturing boys were somewhat smaller but significant when stature and weight were statistically controlled (Beunen *et al.*, 1979). The interaction between CA and SA *per se*, or in combination with stature and/or weight, explained a larger percentage of the performance variance than each of the predictor variables independently (Beunen *et al.*, 1981b). The explained variance in performance using CA, SA, stature, weight and their first, second and third interaction terms ranged from 0 to 17%, which indicates a low to moderate association. However, for static strength the explained variance varied between 33 and 58%, and the predictive value was highest at 14–15 years of age.

It should also be noted that CA by itself explains only a small percentage of the variance in motor performance. First-order partial correlations between CA and performance of different motor tests, with SA partialled-out, range from 0.05 for static strength (arm pull) to 0.26

for speed of limb movement (plate tapping) in 13-year-old Belgian boys. The small but positive association between CA and performance in early adolescent boys probably reflects improved neuromotor control that occurs with age (Beunen *et al.*, 1978a).

Finally, there is good evidence that, at least in boys, the performance advantage of early maturers disappears at adult age (Lefevre *et al.*, 1990). Performances of 30-year-old men grouped on the basis of their age at PHV do not significantly differ for static strength (arm pull), muscular endurance of the lower trunk (leg lifts), running speed (shuttle run) and flexibility (sit-and-reach). Early maturers still perform better at 30 years for speed of limb movement (plate tapping), but late maturers perform better in muscular endurance of the upper body (bent arm hang). The results also indicate that late maturing males improve significantly in performance between 18 and 30 years more so than early or average maturing males (Lefevre *et al.*, 1990).

Maturity status of élite young athletes

The biological maturity status of athletes has been studied quite extensively, especially age at menarche. The subject has been reviewed most recently by Beunen (1989), Malina (1983, 1986, 1988, 1994b) and Malina and Bouchard (1991). In considering the maturity status of athletes it should be kept in mind that the analyses are beset with a number of difficulties. First, the definition of an athlete is vague and a wide variety of skill and competitive levels exist. Second, young athletes are a highly selected group not only with regard to skill and performance level but also with regard to size and physique. The selection may be made by the individual, parents, coach, influential others or some combination of these. Further, earlier maturation is intrinsically related to growth in size and both are associated with performance. Finally, athletic performance is influenced by many factors other than those of a biological nature.

Figure 1.5 summarizes available evidence on ages at menarche of athletes in different sports. Mean ages were calculated from 46 samples, representing 1820 athletes competing at the high school, university, national or international levels. From this meta-analysis, it is clear that gymnasts and figure skaters are, on average, the latest maturing athletes. Age at menarche is later in athletes than in the general population, varies among athletes in different sports, and tends to be later in athletes who are at a higher competitive level. Note, however, that these trends are based upon

means, and there are in fact many athletes who attain menarche at an average or early age (Fig. 1.6).

The difference between ages at menarche in younger and older athletes in a given sport should receive more attention. The data in Fig. 1.5 suggest that swimmers reach menarche within the bounds of variation of reference populations. This is apparently so for age group swimmers and the swimming population of 15–20 years ago. Percentages of age group swimmers ($n = 268$), junior Olympic divers ($n = 161$) and world class gymnasts ($n = 113$) who have attained menarche at each CA compared to a national sample of Flemish girls are shown in Fig. 1.7. Estimated median ages at menarche for the four samples, based on probit analysis, are 13.1, 13.6 and 15.6 years for the three samples of athletes compared to 13.2 for the reference sample. Note that the sample of world class gymnasts did not include girls less than 13 years of age so that the estimate may be slightly biased towards an older age. The distribution of age group swimmers is very similar to the reference sample. Recent mean retrospective estimates for élite university level swimmers are considerably later, at 14.3 and 14.4 years (Malina & Bouchard, 1991), than estimates for age group swimmers and retrospective estimates of 15–20 years ago (Malina, 1983). With the increased opportunity for swimmers to compete at the university level associ-

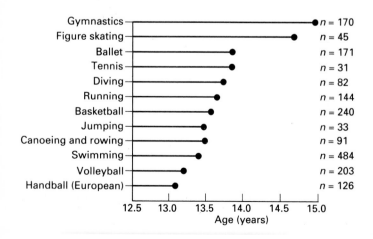

Gymnastics — $n = 170$
Figure skating — $n = 45$
Ballet — $n = 171$
Tennis — $n = 31$
Diving — $n = 82$
Running — $n = 144$
Basketball — $n = 240$
Jumping — $n = 33$
Canoeing and rowing — $n = 91$
Swimming — $n = 484$
Volleyball — $n = 203$
Handball (European) — $n = 126$

12.5 13.0 13.5 14.0 14.5 15.0
Age (years)

Fig. 1.5 Mean ages at menarche in athletes grouped by sport. Mean ages are recalculated for each sport from data reported by Beunen (1989), Claessens *et al.* (1991), Malina (1983) and Malina and Bouchard (1991). Reference means or medians for the populations from which the athletes originate range from 12.8 to 13.4 years.

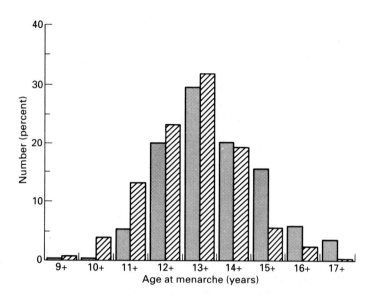

Fig. 1.6 Relative frequencies of ages at menarche in white university student athletes (*n* = 265) and non-athlete students at the same university (*n* = 350). The athletes represent seven sports: swimming, diving, tennis, golf, track and field, basketball and volleyball. The data are limited to white athletes as black athletes (track and field, basketball, volleyball) attain menarche at a significantly earlier age than white athletes. ▣, athletes; ▨, non-athletes. From R.M. Malina, unpublished data.

ated with Title IX legislation in the USA (which provided for equal opportunities in education, including sport, and went into effect in 1975), the composition of the swimming population has apparently changed.

In contrast to menarche, there are much less data for other maturity indicators in female athletes (Beunen, 1989). Local level age group athletes and non-athletes do not differ in the distributions of stages 2–4 of breast and pubic hair development (Plowman *et al.*, 1991). Gymnasts are not as advanced in both breast and pubic hair development compared to swimmers or control subjects of the same age, who do not differ from each other (Bernink *et al.*, 1983; Peltenburg *et al.*, 1984). Among 113 gymnasts competing at the 1987 World Championships in Rotterdam, the SA−CA

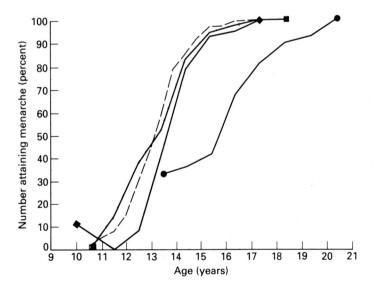

Fig. 1.7 Percentages of age group swimmers (■) (*n* = 268, provided by J. Stager), junior Olympic divers (◆) (*n* = 161, R.M. Malina, unpublished data) and world class gymnasts (●) (*n* = 118, Claessens *et al.*, 1992) in each chronological age group who have attained menarche compared to a national sample of Flemish girls (– – –) (Wellens & Malina, 1990).

difference was −1.9 years, indicating late maturation (Claessens *et al.*, 1991). These observations are consistent with earlier reports documenting slower maturation in female gymnasts (Novotny & Taftlova, 1979; Beunen *et al.*, 1981a). In a small sample of ballet dancers (*n* = 15) followed from 12 to 15 years, breast development occurs at later ages, while pubic hair develops at expected ages (Warren, 1980). In contrast, among 30 girls training in rowing and light athletics in Polish sport schools (about 8−12 h·week^{-1}) and followed longitudinally from 11 to 14 years of age, breast and pubic hair development, age at menarche (prospectively obtained), and estimated growth velocities do not differ from reference data for the general population (Malina *et al.*, 1990).

With few exceptions, male athletes of different competitive levels in various sports are characterized by average or advanced biological maturity status. Whatever the biological maturity indicator is used or the competitive level observed, studies point to the same direction (Malina, 1986, 1988; Beunen, 1989; Malina & Bouchard, 1991). There is some indication that in boys, the most marked advancement in maturity status is observed in adolescence, which is probably due to the size, physique, fat-free mass and performance (strength, power, speed) advantages of the early maturers. This advantage is reduced as boys approach late adolescence/early adulthood, when late maturers catch up or even tend to outperform the early maturers (Lefevre *et al.*, 1990). In a nationally selected sample of Belgian male track athletes, all 15−16 year olds except one had an SA in advance of CA. Among 17−18-year-old athletes, about two-thirds had an SA equal to or in advance of that expected for CA, while one-third had an SA that was less than their CA (Malina *et al.*, 1986). The statures of 16-year-old athletes advanced in SA, of 17−18-year-old athletes who had already attained skeletal maturity, and of 17−18-year-old athletes who had reached skeletal maturity did not differ, although athletes who were 16−18

years advanced in skeletal maturity were heavier. Although the data are cross-sectional, the trend suggests catch-up in stature of those late in skeletal maturation, but persistent differences in body weight.

At least two formal hypotheses have been offered to explain the later maturation in female athletes: (i) training 'delays' menarche (Frisch *et al.*, 1981); and (ii) a two-part, biocultural hypothesis that the characteristics of physique associated with later maturation are more suitable for successful athletic performance, and that early maturing girls are socialized away from sport or, in contrast, late maturing girls are socialized into sport (Malina, 1983). The first hypothesis (Frisch *et al.*, 1981) is commonly accepted in the popular literature. This hypothesis relates to the critical weight and critical fat hypothesis, which has been severely criticized on the basis of methodological, statistical and experimental considerations. The training hypothesis has also received much criticism (see Malina, 1991). Stager *et al.* (1984, 1990) clearly demonstrated the inadequacy of the initial research design and logic of the Frisch hypothesis. Using a simulation model, Stager *et al.* (1990) demonstrated that the design leads to inherently biased results.

Hormonal data for active prepubertal or pubertal girls are limited. The data are not consistent across studies, are based on small samples, and can be characterized as weak. The results are often based on single samples of hormones whose temporal sequence is markedly pulsatile. Further, the effects of regular training on basal levels of hormones in children and adolescents are not certain (see Malina, 1991).

Sexual maturation of gymnasts and ballet dancers has received more attention than young athletes in other sports. Selective criteria for gymnasts, for example, include physical characteristics associated with later maturation (Bajin, 1987; Hartley, 1988). Diet is a potentially confounding factor as indicated in young gymnasts from the former German Democratic Republic who were on a dietary regime '...intended to maintain the optimal body weight, i.e. a slightly negative energy balance, and thus a limited energy depot over a long period' (Jahreis *et al.*, 1991, p. 98). Similar selective criteria and dietary restrictions are apparent among ballet dancers (Hamilton, 1986; Hamilton *et al.*, 1988). Ages at menarche in ballet dancers, however, are not as late as reported for gymnasts (see Fig. 1.5).

Recent research has focused more on energy balance and eating problems as factors in the pathogenesis of primary and secondary amenorrhoea (Brooks-Gunn *et al.*, 1987; Myerson *et al.*, 1991). Note, of course, that the two major causes of primary amenorrhoea are constitutional delay and congenital factors (Shangold, 1988; see also Chapter 21). There is no doubt that suppressive food restriction and excessive exercise has an effect on the pulsatile release of gonadotrophin-releasing hormone (GnRH) and hence on luteinizing hormone (LH) in postmenarcheal women and animal models. In contrast, the potential links between body fat and the GnRH pulse generator that have been postulated so far seem too subtle to account for such robust effects (Bronson & Manning, 1991). Thus, although menarche occurs later in female athletes than in non-athletes, it has yet to be shown that training 'delays' menarche in anyone (Loucks *et al.*, 1992).

Malina's (1983) two-part hypothesis combines selective biological (i.e. size, physique and skill) and social factors. Data on the socialization of girls into sports or into the role of an athlete are not extensive. Most information comes from studies on white, male, high school and college athletes or top level amateurs (Coakley, 1987). For boys, sports participation is viewed as directly linked to the development of masculinity. In the case of girls, sports participation is seldom associated with femininity. For factors such as size, physique or skill, conversely, evidence from twin and family studies gives support to the hypothesis. Although estimates of heritability vary with age, sex, population and methodology of the studies, they are high for skeletal lengths and breadths followed by circumferences, muscle diameters and skinfolds (Bouchard & Malina, 1983). This has more recently been confirmed in a large family and twin study including measures of size and physique, strength and motor skill, and skeletal maturation (Maes *et al.*, 1992). Estimates of heritability for skeletal maturation are very high, explaining 94% of the variance, while additive genetic factors explain between 41% (for balance) and 75% (for functional strength) of the variance in eight motor fitness components. It has also been shown that in the general population, as well as in athletes, age at menarche in mothers and sisters (many of whom are involved in sport) correlate quite well with age at menarche in the athlete, which also indicates the genetic determination of this maturity indicator (Brooks-Gunn & Warren, 1988; Stager & Hatler, 1988; Malina *et al.*, 1994). Further, support for this hypothesis is also found in the association between size, physique and body composition in female adolescents (see pp. 9–10). Nevertheless, in order to obtain direct evidence for the hypothesis suggested by Malina (1983), longitudinal and mixed-longitudinal studies need to be designed in which a large number of biological, familial, psychological, social and cultural factors are considered and in which non-athletes as well as athletes, preferably in a variety of sports, are included.

Based on observations on Japanese athletes, Hata and Aoki (1990) proposed a somewhat modified two-part hypothesis: (i) the ascending trend of age at menarche with increasing level of athletic competition is mostly produced by selection in the socialization process into (or away from) sports participation; and (ii) the diversity of mean age at menarche by sport at a given competitive level is mainly a reflection of diversity of suitable physiques by sport. At first glance, this specification seems logical but needs, of course, further evaluation.

Effects of training on the growth and maturation of young athletes

The influence of training on the sexual maturation of young girls, and more specifically, on the age at menarche, is discussed in the preceding section. The limited data are variable and inconclusive (Malina, 1991, 1994b; Loucks *et al.*, 1992). The effects of training on the sexual maturation of boys has not received much attention given the advanced maturity status that is characteristic of young male athletes. It is somewhat puzzling why one would expect training to influence the sexual maturation of girls and not of boys. Underlying neuroendocrine processes that trigger sexual maturation are generally similar, and other environmental stresses related to sport, such as anxiety and sleep, undoubtedly affect boys as well as girls. However, with the exception of wrestling and perhaps judo and karate, emphasis on extreme weight regulation is not characteristic of sports for boys.

The literature dealing with the effects of regular training or physical activity on growth has a relatively long history. Early experimental studies (Beyer, 1896; Schwartz *et al.*, 1928) suggest a stimulatory effect of regular training on growth. Interindividual variation in biological maturity status was, however, not considered and consequently the value of these observations is limited. Conversely, Rowe (1933) expressed concern about the negative influence of regular physical activity, especially sport competition on statural growth. The less rapid gain in stature of the participants, however, was probably due to their advanced biological maturity status.

Longitudinal data are needed to address the effects of training on growth and maturation. Data from two longitudinal studies of boys indicate no differences in the statures (Fig. 1.8), ages at PHV and PHVs of active and inactive boys, although inactive boys tend to be slightly heavier. SAs of active and inactive Belgian boys also do not differ (Beunen *et al.*, 1992b). Conversely, Polish and Czech boys regularly active

in sport are consistently taller than respective reference data for each country, and also attain PHV at an earlier age (Fig. 1.8). Polish boys active in sport are also advanced in SA during adolescence. The data for Polish and Czech boys active in sport, primarily team sports, show a pattern of early maturation, which is consistent with data for cross-sectional samples of young male athletes.

Longitudinal data for girls are less available than for boys. Retrospective longitudinal data for the statures of Dutch gymnasts and Swedish swimmers, and prospective data for Polish girls attending a sport school (rowing and athletics), are expressed as SD scores in Fig. 1.9. The data indicate smaller statures than average for gymnasts and taller statures for swimmers and sports school participants. Differences between gymnasts and swimmers are already apparent in early childhood, before formal training for sport had begun. Further, the statures of the three groups tend to maintain their position relative to reference data, suggesting no effect of regular training. The available evidence thus suggests that regular physical activity and sport training/participation does not affect statural growth, the timing and magnitude of PHV, and skeletal maturation (Malina, 1994a,b). These conclusions are consistent with those addressed for sexual maturation in the preceding section.

Challenges for future research

• There is a need for information about individual patterns (attained levels, velocity and/or acceleration) in the strength, motor, aerobic and anaerobic performance in adolescent girls. Longitudinal or mixed-longitudinal studies incorporating these characteristics on sufficiently large samples of female adolescents are needed. Mixed-longitudinal studies are recommended because information can be collected over a shorter period. Such studies need to be carefully planned, including cohorts that are followed over a short period but are selected so that they overlap in time (Goldstein, 1979); moreover, control cohorts can be used for the

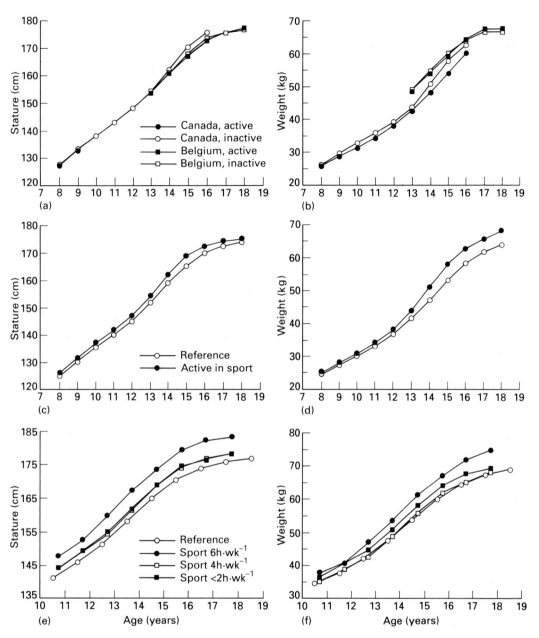

Fig. 1.8 (a) Stature of active and inactive Belgian and Canadian boys, (b) weight of active and inactive Belgian and Canadian boys (key as in (a)), (c) stature of active Polish boys, (d) weight of active Polish boys (key as in (c)), (e) stature of active Czech boys, and (f) weight of Czech boys active in sport (key as in (d)). Redrawn from Malina (1994a).

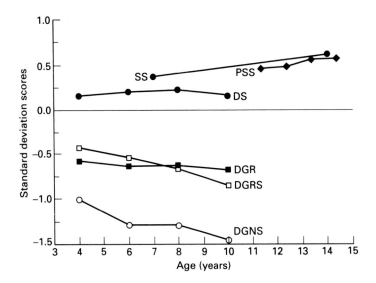

Fig. 1.9 SD scores for statures of longitudinal samples of Dutch gymnasts, Swedish swimmers and Polish sports school participants in athletics and rowing. DGNS, Dutch gymnasts, national selection; DGR, Dutch gymnasts, recreational; DGRS, Dutch gymnasts, regional selection; DS, Dutch swimmers; PSS, Polish school participants; SS, Swedish swimmers. Redrawn from Malina (1994a).

control of certain factors such as test or learning effects (see van't Hof *et al.*, 1976).

• Muscular strength, endurance and aerobic power show well-defined adolescent spurts in boys. Can performance be enhanced by training during the spurts? This question implies that knowledge about somatic growth and maturation be incorporated into the experimental studies of the effects of various training programmes. Further, it would be interesting to see if the ultimate adult performance is influenced by training programmes initiated earlier in life.

• There is a need for prospective longitudinal studies following youngsters training for different sports from the prepubertal years through puberty. Such studies should include a variety of somatic, maturity and performance characteristics together with information about physical activity, nutrition and hormonal secretions. Given the pulsatile nature of hormonal secretions, it is of importance that the hormonal levels are monitored at regular intervals over a 24-h period.

• For studies in which human subjects are inappropriate animal models need to be developed that closely replicate the human situation and allow experimental control of intervening or disturbing variables. It is probably advisable

to launch multicentre studies in order to set up projects that have enough power to give valid answers to the questions raised in this chapter.

• More information is required about the genetic determination of physical performance capacities of children and youth, and about genotype−environment (training, physical activity) interactions.

References

Asmussen, E. (1962) Muscular performance. In K. Rodahl & S.M. Horvath (eds) *Muscle as a Tissue*, pp. 161−75. McGraw Hill, New York.

Asmussen, E. & Heebøll-Nielsen, K. (1955) A dimensional analysis of performance and growth in boys. *J. Appl. Physiol.* **7**, 593−603.

Bajin, B. (1987) Talent identification program for Canadian female gymnasts. In B. Petiot, J.H. Salmela & T.B. Hoshizaki (eds) *World Identification for Gymnastic Talent*, pp. 34−44. Sports Psyche Editions, Montreal.

Barton, W.H. & Hunt, E.E. (1962) Somatotype and adolescence in boys. *Hum. Biol.* **34**, 254−70.

Bastos, F.V. & Hegg, R.V. (1986) The relationship of chronological age, body build, and sexual maturation to handgrip strength in schoolboys ages 10 through 17 years. In J.A.P. Day (ed.) *Perspectives in Kinanthropometry*, pp. 45−9. Human Kinetics, Champaign, IL.

Bayley, N. (1943a) Size and body build of adolescents

in relation to rate of skeletal maturity. *Child Dev.* **14**, 47−90.

Bayley, N. (1943b) Skeletal maturity in adolescence as basis for determining percentage of completed growth. *Child Dev.* **14**, 1−46.

Bernink, M.J.E., Erich, W.B.M., Peltenburg, A.L., Zonderland, M.L. & Huisveld, I.A. (1983) Height, body composition, biological maturation and training in relation to socio-economic status in girl gymnasts, swimmers, and controls. *Growth* **47**, 1−12.

Beunen, G. (1989) Biological age in pediatric exercise research. In O. Bar-Or (ed.) *Advances in Pediatric Sport Sciences*, Vol. 3. *Biological Issues*, pp. 1−39. Human Kinetics, Champaign, IL.

Beunen, G., Claessens, A., Lefevre, J., Ostyn, M., Renson, R. & Simons, J. (1987) Somatotype as related to age at peak velocity and to peak velocity in height, weight and static strength in boys. *Hum. Biol.* **59**, 641−55.

Beunen, G., Claessens, A. & Van Esser, M. (1981a) Somatic and motor characteristics of female gymnasts. *Med. Sport* **15**, 176−85.

Beunen, G., Colla, R., Simons, J. *et al.* (1989) Sexual dimorphism in somatic and motor characteristics. In S. Oseid & K.-H. Carlsen (eds) *Children and Exercise XIII*, pp. 83−90. Human Kinetics, Champaign, IL.

Beunen, G., Lefevre, J., Claessens, A. *et al.* (1992a) Association between skeletal maturity and adipose tissue distribution during growth. *Am. J. Phys. Anthropol.* **14** (Suppl.), 49 (abstract).

Beunen, G. & Malina, R.M. (1988) Growth and physical performance relative to the timing of the adolescent spurt. *Exerc. Sport Sci. Rev.* **16**, 503−40.

Beunen, G., Malina, R.M., Ostyn, M., Renson, R., Simons, J. & Van Gerven, D. (1982) Fatness and skeletal maturity of Belgian boys 12 through 20 years of age. *Am. J. Phys. Anthropol.* **59**, 387−92.

Beunen, G., Malina, R.M., Ostyn, M., Renson, R., Simons, J. & Van Gerven, D. (1983) Fatness, growth and motor fitness of Belgian boys 12 through 20 years of age. *Hum. Biol.* **55**, 599−613.

Beunen, G.P., Malina, R.M., Renson, R., Simons, J., Ostyn, M. & Lefevre, J. (1992b) Physical activity and growth, maturation and performance: a longitudinal study. *Med. Sci. Sports Exerc.* **24**, 576−85.

Beunen, G.P., Malina, R.M., Van't Hof, M.A. *et al.* (1988) *Adolescent Growth and Motor Performance: A Longitudinal Study of Belgian Boys*. Human Kinetics, Champaign, IL.

Beunen, G., Ostyn, M., Renson, R., Simons, J. & Van Gerven, D. (1976) Skeletal maturity and physical fitness of girls aged 12 through 16. *Hermes* (Leuven) **10**, 445−57.

Beunen, G., Ostyn, M., Renson, R., Simons, J. & Van Gerven, D. (1978a) Motor performance as related to chronological age and maturation. In R.J. Shephard & H. Lavallée (eds) *Physical Fitness Assessment: Principles, Practice and Application*, pp. 229−36. C.C. Thomas, Springfield, IL.

Beunen, G., Ostyn, M., Renson, R., Simons, J. & Van Gerven, D. (1979) Growth and maturity as related to motor ability. *S. Afr. J. Res. Sports, Phys. Educ. Recr.* **3**, 9−15.

Beunen, G., Ostyn, M., Simons, J., Renson, R. & Van Gerven, D. (1981b) Chronological and biological age as related to physical fitness in boys 12 to 19 years. *Ann. Hum. Biol.* **8**, 321−31.

Beunen, G., Ostyn, M., Simons, J., Van Gerven, D., Swalus, P. & De Beul, G. (1978b) A correlational analysis of skeletal maturity, anthropometric measures and motor fitness of boys 12 through 16. In F. Landry & W.A.R. Orban (eds) *Biomechanics of Sports and Kinanthropometry*, pp. 343−9. Symposia Specialists, Miami.

Beunen, G.P. & Simons, J. (1990) Physical growth, maturation and performance. In J. Simons, G.P. Beunen, R. Renson, A.L.M. Claesens, B. Vanreusel & J.A.V. Lefevre (eds) *Growth and Fitness of Flemish Girls: The Leuven Growth Study*, pp. 69−118. Human Kinetics, Champaign, IL.

Beyer, H.G. (1896) The influence of exercise on growth. *J. Exp. Med.* **1**, 546−58.

Boas, F. (1892) The growth of children. *Science* **19/20**, 256−7, 281−2, 351−2.

Bouchard, C., Leblanc, C., Malina, R.M. & Hollmann, W. (1978) Skeletal age and submaximal working capacity in boys. *Ann. Hum. Biol.* **5**, 75−8.

Bouchard, C. & Malina, R.M. (1983) Genetics of physiological fitness and motor performance. *Exerc. Sport Sci. Rev.* **11**, 306−39.

Bouchard, C., Malina, R.M., Hollmann, W. & Leblanc, C. (1976) Relationship between skeletal maturity and submaximal working capacity in boys 8 to 18 years. *Med. Sci. Sports* **8**, 186−90.

Branta, C., Haubenstricker, J. & Seefeldt, V. (1984) Age changes in motor skills during childhood and adolescence. *Exerc. Sport Sci. Rev.* **12**, 467−520.

Bronson, F.H. & Manning, J.M. (1991) Mini-review: the energetic regulation of ovulation: a realistic role for body fat. *Biol. Reprod.* **44**, 945−950.

Brooks-Gunn, J. & Warren, M.P. (1988) Mother-daughter differences in menarcheal age in adolescent girls attending national dance company schools and non-dancers. *Ann. Hum. Biol.* **15**, 35−44.

Brooks-Gunn, J., Warren, M.P. & Hamilton, L.H. (1987) The relation of eating problems and amenorrhea in ballet dancers. *Med. Sci. Sports Exerc.* **19**, 41−4.

Carron, A.V. & Bailey, D.A. (1974) Strength development in boys from 10 through 16 years. *Monogr. Soc. Res. Child Dev.* **39** (Serial No. 157).

Cheek, D.B., Schulz, R.B., Parra, A. & Reba, R.C. (1970) Overgrowth of lean adipose tissues in adolescent obesity. *Pediatr. Res.* **4**, 268–9.

Claessens, A.L., Malina, R.M., Lefevre, J. *et al.* (1992) Growth and menarcheal status of élite female gymnasts. *Med. Sci. Sports Exerc.* **24**, 755–63.

Claessens, A.L., Veer, F.M., Stijnen, V. *et al.* (1991) Anthropometric characteristics of outstanding male and female gymnasts. *J. Sports Sci.* **9**, 53–74.

Clarke, H.H. (1971) *Physical and Motor Tests in the Medford Boys' Growth Study.* Prentice-Hall, Englewood Cliffs, NJ.

Coakley, J.J. (1987) Children and sport socialization process. In D. Gould & M.R. Weiss (eds) *Advances in Pediatric Sport Sciences*, Vol. 2. *Behavioral Issues*, pp. 43–60. Human Kinetics, Champaign, IL.

Ellison, P.T. (1981) Prediction of age at menarche from annual height increments. *Am. J. Phys. Anthropol.* **56**, 71–5.

Espenschade, A. (1940) Motor performance in adolescence, including the study of relationships with measures of physical growth and maturity. *Monogr. Soc. Res. Child Dev.* **5** (Serial No. 24).

Faust, M.S. (1977) Somatic development of adolescent girls. *Monogr. Soc. Res. Child Dev.* **42** (Serial No. 169).

Frisancho, A.R. & Flegel, R.N. (1982) Advanced maturation associated with centripetal fat pattern. *Hum. Biol.* **54**, 717–27.

Frisch, R.E. (1974) A method of prediction of age of menarche from height and weight at ages 9 through 13 years. *Pediatrics* **53**, 384–90.

Frisch, R.E. (1987) Body fat, menarche, fitness and fertility. *Hum. Reprod.* **2**, 521–33.

Frisch, R.E., Gotz-Welbergen, A.V., McArthur, J.W. *et al.* (1981) Delayed menarche and amenorrhea of college athletes in relation to age of onset of training. *JAMA* **246**, 1559–63.

Frisch, R.E. & Revelle, R. (1970) Height and weight at menarche and a hypothesis of critical body weights and adolescent events. *Science* **169**, 397–9.

Frisch, R.E., Revelle, R. & Cook, S. (1973) Components of weight at menarche and the initiation of the adolescent growth spurt in girls: estimated total water, lean body weight and fat. *Hum. Biol.* **45**, 469–83.

Garn, S.M. & Haskell, J.A. (1959) Fat and growth during childhood. *Science* **130**, 1711–12.

Goldstein, H. (1979) *The Design and Analysis of Longitudinal Studies.* Academic Press, London.

Hamilton, L.H., Brooks-Gunn, J., Warren, M.P. & Hamilton, W.G. (1988) The role of selectivity in the pathogenesis of eating problems in ballet dancers. *Med. Sci. Sports Exerc.* **20**, 560–5.

Hamilton, W.G. (1986) Physical prerequisites for ballet dancers: selectivity that can enhance (or nullify) a career. *J. Musculoskel. Med.* **3**, 61–6.

Hartley, G.A. (1988) A comparative view of talent selection for sport in two socialist states — the USSR and the GDR — with particular reference to gymnastics. In *The Growing Child in Competitive Sport*, pp. 50–60. The National Coaching Foundation, Leeds.

Hata, E. & Aoki, K. (1990) Age at menarche and selected menstrual characteristics in young Japanese athletes. *Res. Q. Exerc. Sport* **61**, 178–83.

Haubenstricker, J.L. & Seefeldt, V.D. (1986) Acquisition of motor skills during childhood. In V. Seefeldt (ed.) *Physical Activity and Well-being*, pp. 41–102. American Alliance for Health, Physical Education, Recreation and Dance, Reston, VA.

Hebbelinck, M., Borms, J. & Clarys, J. (1971) La variabilité de l'âge squelettique et les corrélations avec la capacité de travail chez des garçons de 5me année primaire (Variability in skeleton age and correlation with physical work capacity in 5th grade boys). *Kinanthropologie* **3**, 125–35.

Hollmann, W. & Bouchard, C. (1970) Untersuchungen über die Beziehungen zwischen chronologischem und biologischem Alter zu spiroergometrischen Messgrössen, Herzvolumen, anthropometrischen Daten und Skelettmuskelkraft bei 8–18 jährigen Jungen (Study of the relationship between chronological and biological ages and spiroergometric values, heart volume, anthropometric data and muscular strength in youths of 8–18 years). *Zeitschr. Kreislaufforsch.* **59**, 160–76.

Jahreis, G., Kauf, E., Frohner, G. & Schmidt, H.E. (1991) Influence of intensive exercise on insulin-like growth factor I, thyroid and steroid hormones in female gymnasts. *Growth Reg.* **1**, 95–9.

Jones, H.E. (1949) *Motor Performance and Growth: A Developmental Study of Static Dynamometric Strength.* University of California Press, Berkeley.

Kemper, H.C.G. (ed.) (1985) *Growth, Health and Fitness of Teenagers.* Karger, Basel.

Kemper, H.C.G. & Verschuur, R. (1985) Motor performance fitness tests. In H.C.G. Kemper (ed.) *Growth, Health and Fitness of Teenagers*, pp. 96–106. Karger, Basel.

Kemper, H.C.G., Verschuur, R., Ras, K.G.A. *et al.* (1975) Biological age and habitual physical activity in relation to physical fitness in 12- and 13-year old schoolboys. *Zeitschr. Kinderheilk.* **119**, 169–79.

Kemper, H.C.G., Verschuur, R. & Ritmeester, J.W. (1986) Maximal aerobic power in early and late maturing teenagers. In J. Rutenfranz, R. Mocellin & F. Klimt (eds) *Children and Exercise XII*, pp. 220–221. Human Kinetics, Champaign, IL.

Krahenbuhl, G.S., Skinner, J.S. & Kohrt, W.M. (1985)

Developmental aspects of maximal aerobic power in children. *Exerc. Sports Sci. Rev.* **13**, 503–38.

Labitzke, H. (1971) Über Beziehungen zwischen biologischen Alter (Ossifikationsalter) und der Körperlänge, den Körpergewicht und der Körperoberfläche sowie der maximalen Sauerstoffaufnahme (Concerning relations between biological age (skeletal age) and stature, weight, body surface and maximal oxygen uptake). *Mediz. Sport* **11**, 82–6.

Lefevre, J., Beunen, G., Steens, G., Claessens, A. & Renson, R. (1990) Motor performance during adolescence and age thirty as related to age at peak height velocity. *Ann. Hum. Biol.* **17**, 423–34.

Loucks, A.B., Vaitukaitis, J., Cameron, J.L. *et al.* (1992) The reproductive system and exercise in women. *Med. Sci. Sports Exerc.* **24** (Suppl. 6), S288–9.

McNeill, D. & Livson, N. (1963) Maturation rate and body build of women. *Child Dev.* **34**, 25–32.

Maes, H., Beunen, G., Vlietinck, R. *et al.* (1992) Univariate genetic analysis of physical characteristics of 10-year-old twins and their parents. In J. Coudert & E. Van Praagh (eds) *Children and Exercise*, Vol. XVI. *Pediatric Work Physiology. Methodological, Physiological and Pathological Aspects*, pp. 205–7. Masson, Paris.

Malina, R.M. (1975) Anthropometric correlates of strength and motor performance. *Exerc. Sport Sci. Rev.* **3**, 249–74.

Malina, R.M. (1983) Menarche in athletes: a synthesis and hypothesis. *Ann. Hum. Biol.* **10**, 1–24.

Malina, R.M. (1986) Maturational considerations in élite young athletes. In J. Day (ed.) *Perspectives in Kinanthropometry*, pp. 29–43. Human Kinetics, Champaign, IL.

Malina, R.M. (1988) Biological maturity status of young athletes. In R.M. Malina (ed.) *Young Athletes: Biological, Psychological and Educational Perspectives*, pp. 121–140. Human Kinetics, Champaign, IL.

Malina, R.M. (1991) Darwinian fitness, physical fitness and physical activity. In C.G.N. Mascie-Taylor & G.W. Lasker (eds) *Applications of Biological Anthropology to Human Affairs*, pp. 143–84. Cambridge University Press, Cambridge.

Malina, R.M. (1994a) Effects of physical activity on growth in stature and adolescent growth spurt. *Med. Sci. Sports Exerc.* **26**, 759–66.

Malina, R.M. (1994b) Physical growth and biological maturation of young athletes. *Exerc. Sport Sci. Rev.* **22**, 389–433.

Malina, R.M., Beunen, G., Wellens, R. & Claessens, A. (1986) Skeletal maturity and body size of teenage Belgian track and field athletes. *Ann. Hum. Biol.* **13**, 331–9.

Malina, R.M. & Bouchard, C. (1988) Subcutaneous fat distribution during growth. In C. Bouchard & F.E.

Johnston (eds) *Fat Distribution during Growth and Later Health Outcomes*, pp. 63–84. Alan R. Liss, New York.

Malina, R.M. & Bouchard, C. (1991) *Growth, Maturation and Physical Activity*. Human Kinetics, Champaign, IL.

Malina, R.M., Eveld, D.J. & Woynarowska, B. (1990) Growth and sexual maturation of active Polish children 11–14 years of age. *Hermes* (Leuven) **21**, 341–53.

Malina, R.M. & Johnston, F.E. (1967) Significance of age, sex and maturity differences in upper arm composition. *Res. Q.* **38**, 219–30.

Malina, R.M., Ryan, R.C. & Bonci, C.M. (1994) Age at menarche in athletes and their mothers and sisters. *Ann. Hum. Biol.* **21**, 417–22.

Merni, F., Balboni, M., Bargellini, S. & Menegatti, G. (1981) Differences in males and females in joint movement range during growth. In J. Borms, M. Hebbelinck & A. Venerando (eds) *The Female Athlete*, pp. 167–175. Karger, Basel.

Mirwald, R.L. & Bailey, D.A. (1986) *Maximal Aerobic Power: A Longitudinal Analysis*. Sports Dynamics, London, Ontario.

Myerson, M., Gutin, B., Warren, M.P. *et al.* (1991) Resting metabolic rate and energy balance in amenorrheic and eumenorrheic runners. *Med. Sci. Sports Exerc.* **23**, 15–22.

Novotny, V.V. & Taftlova, R. (1971) Biological age and sport fitness of young gymnast women. In V.V. Novotny (ed.) *Anthropological Congress Dedicated to Ales Hrdlicka*, pp. 123–30. Academia, Prague.

Parizkova, J. (1977) *Body Fat and Physical Fitness*. Martinus Nijhoff, The Hague.

Peltenburg, A.L., Erich, W.B.M., Berninck, M.J.E., Zonderland, M.L. & Huisveld, I.A. (1984) Biological maturation, body composition, and growth of female gymnasts and control group of schoolgirls and girls swimmers aged 8 to 14 years: a cross-sectional survey of 1064 girls. *Int. J. Sports Med.* **5**, 36–42.

Plowman, S.A., Liu, N.Y. & Wells, C.L. (1991) Body composition and sexual maturation in premenarcheal athletes and non-athletes. *Med. Sci. Sports Exerc.* **23**, 23–9.

Rarick, G.L. & Oyster, N. (1964) Physical maturity, muscular strength, and motor performance of young school-age boys. *Res. Q.* **35**, 523–31.

Reynolds, E.L. (1946) Sexual maturation and the growth of fat, muscle and bone in girls. *Child Dev.* **17**, 121–49.

Richey, H.G. (1937) The relation of accelerated, normal and retarded puberty to the height and weight of school children. *Monogr. Soc. Res. Child Dev.* **2**, (Serial No. 8).

Rowe, F.A. (1933) Growth comparisons of athletes and non-athletes. *Res. Q.* **4**, 108–16.

Rutenfranz, J., Andersen, K., Seliger, V. *et al.* (1982) Maximal aerobic power affected by maturation and body growth during childhood and adolescence. *Eur. J. Pediatr.* **139**, 106–12.

Savov, S.G. (1978) Physical fitness and skeletal maturity in girls and boys 11 years of age. In R.J. Shephard & H. Lavallée (eds) *Physical Fitness Assessment: Practice and Application*, pp. 222–8. C.C. Thomas, Springfield, IL.

Schwartz, L., Britten, E.H. & Thompson, L.R. (1928) Studies in physical development and posture. I. The effect of exercise in the physical condition and development of adolescent boys. *Publ. Health Bull.* **179**, 1–38.

Seils, L.R.G. (1951) The relationship between measurements of physical growth and gross motor performance of primary-grade school children. *Res. Q.* **22**, 244–60.

Seltzer, C.C. & Mayer, J. (1964) Body build and obesity. Who are the obese? *JAMA* **190**, 103–10.

Shangold, M.M. (1988) Menstruation. In M.M. Shangold & G. Mirkin (eds) *Women and Exercise: Physiology and Sports Medicine*, pp. 129–44. F.A. Davis, Philadelphia.

Shephard, R.J., Lavallée, H., Rajic, K.M., Jéquier, J.C., Brisson, G. & Beaucage, C. (1978) Radiographic age in the interpretation of physiological and anthropological data. In J. Borms & M. Hebbelinck (eds) *Pediatric Work Physiology*, pp. 124–33. Karger, Basel.

Shuttleworth, F.K. (1937) Sexual maturation and the physical growth of girls aged six to nineteen. *Monogr. Soc. Res. Child Dev.* **2** (Serial No. 12).

Stager, J.M. & Hatler, L.K. (1988) Menarche in athletes: the influence of genetics and prepubertal training. *Med. Sci. Sports Exerc.* **20**, 369–73.

Stager, J.M., Robertshaw, D. & Miescher, E. (1984) Delayed menarche in swimmers in relation to age at onset of training and athletic performance. *Med. Sci. Sports Exerc.* **16**, 550–5.

Stager, J.M., Wigglesworth, J.K. & Hatler, L.K. (1990) Interpreting the relationship between age of menarche and prepubertal training. *Med. Sci. Sports Exerc.* **22**, 54–8.

Stolz, H.R. & Stolz, L.M. (1951) *Somatic Development of Adolescent Boys*. Macmillan, New York.

Tanner, J.M. (1962) *Growth at Adolescence*, 2nd edn. Blackwell Scientific Publications, Oxford.

Tanner, J.M. (1978) *Foetus into Man: Physical Growth from Conception to Maturity*. Open Books, London.

Van't Hof, M.A., Roede, M.J. & Kowalski, C.J. (1976) Estimation of growth velocities from individual longitudinal data. *Growth* **40**, 217–40.

Warren, M.P. (1980) The effects of exercise on pubertal progression and reproductive function in girls. *J. Clin. Endocrinol. Metab.* **51**, 1150–6.

Wellens, R. & Malina, R.M. (1990) The age at menarche. In J. Simons, G.P. Beunen, R. Renson, A.L.M. Claessens & J.A.V. Lefevre (eds) *Growth and Fitness of Flemish Girls: The Leuven Growth Study*, pp. 119–25. Human Kinetics, Champaign, IL.

Wolff, O.H. (1955) Obesity in children: a study of the birth weight, the height, and the onset of puberty. *Q. J. Med.* **24**, 109–23.

Xi, H., Roche, A.F. & Baumgartner, R.N. (1989) Association between adipose tissue distribution with relative skeletal age in boys: the Fels Longitudinal Study. *Am. J. Hum. Biol.* **1**, 589–96.

Chapter 2

Development of Muscle Strength during Childhood

KARSTEN FROBERG AND OLE LAMMERT

Introduction

Muscular strength is the integrated expression of conditions in the neural system, endocrine system and muscles together with external conditions such as age, sex and environment. Strength is required for movements, and the level of strength determines, in part, the ease and effectiveness of performance in many day-to-day, occupational, recreational and sport activities. Increasing size and strength of skeletal muscle is an important feature of childhood and adolescence. Since the rate of anatomical growth, maturation and changes in the internal milieu may vary independently, their combined influence on strength cannot be expected to correlate in a simple way with chronological age (CA). There is a lack of information about the factors that initiate and control the process of increasing muscle size and strength.

It is important that physiologists, physicians, coaches and teachers in physical education are familiar with the healthy age- and sex-associated variations in muscle strength and with the various factors known to influence strength. This chapter will only deal with the topic of muscle strength and not with muscle power or endurance. Strength is discussed in terms of the force or torque development during (i) maximal voluntary isometric contractions; (ii) electrically evoked single twitch isometric muscle contractions; (iii) electrically evoked tetanic isometric muscle contractions; and (iv) maximal voluntary isokinetic muscle

contractions. A brief description of the key characteristics of these contractions is presented in Appendix 2.1.

This chapter is limited to the discussion of muscle strength development in normal healthy children. The aim is to describe and discuss changes in skeletal muscle strength during childhood and adolescence in normal healthy children, and relate the changes to biological, anthropometric, morphological, neurological, endocrinological and genetic factors. The reader is referred to earlier excellent reviews by Asmussen (1973), Malina (1975, 1986b), Beunen and Malina (1988) and Blimkie (1989).

Methodological constraints

There are two kinds of growth and development studies: cross-sectional and longitudinal. When discussing development in muscle strength in children and adolescents, it is necessary to take individual variations in development into account. Individual variations are well documented in relation to the rate and tempo of the adolescent growth spurt (Tanner, 1962). There are fewer reports about individual variations in relation to the development of muscle strength, one of the reasons being a lack of longitudinal studies where the measurements can be compared.

Cross-sectional studies are descriptions of the present status and can only be used as a description of what may be expected when younger groups grow older. If used to predict changes over time, cross-sectional studies can provide a rough approximation, but one must interpret such predictions with caution. Cross-sectional studies of changes in body size, body composition and muscle strength during adolescence, normally present smooth growth curves. The well-known wide range of individual differences both in the initiation and the duration of the adolescent spurt therefore disappears when cross-sectional data are gathered.

Longitudinal studies are characterized by repeated measurements on the same subjects at regular intervals over a longer period of time. Data from longitudinal studies permit analysis of individual growth and development patterns. Observed changes in such patterns can also be analysed in relation to different conditions in the internal or environmental conditions. Sample size in longitudinal studies is often quite small, and sampling bias then becomes a serious problem. Sample size as well as sample representativeness is often not discussed in this area regardless of the research designs. Unfortunately, this makes it very difficult when comparisons between studies are made to draw more general conclusions.

When analysing results of the development of muscle strength both in cross-sectional and longitudinal studies, testing procedures must minimize skill or learning by the subject.

Discussion of the development of muscle strength in this chapter is based on results from both cross-sectional and longitudinal studies, which yield complementary information. This chapter primarily discusses the development of isometric muscle strength in well-defined muscle groups, though isokinetic data is also briefly discussed.

Strength measured as isometric or dynamic force reflects the same relative strength between individuals regardless of the type of test method. There is a well-defined relationship between force and velocity. Isometric strength is force measured at zero velocity. This was first shown in adults by Asmussen *et al.* (1965) and has lately been confirmed by Hortobágyi *et al.* (1989, 1990), where evidence for a general strength component was investigated.

Measurements of strength in hand grip, knee flexion, elbow flexion and extension, abdominal flexion and back extension — and therefore also in composite strength (e.g. muscle strength measured in several of the major muscle groups) — are often used in studies of muscle strength, but it is important to note that hand grip strength is correlated to the strength in the other muscle groups with a low correlation coefficient of 0.25–0.51 (Asmussen, 1973). No studies of a possible general strength component have so far been conducted in children or young adolescents.

Dominant versus non-dominant sides. There are differences between strength in the left and right side in the same individual's muscle groups, as shown in Table 2.1. Muscle strength in the right side is often 3–5% higher (Asmussen, 1973).

Reproducibility of strength measurements. The reproducibility of the maximal voluntary isometric strength was assessed by Asmussen *et al.* (1959), Edwards *et al.* (1987) and Blimkie

Table 2.1 Correlation coefficients from strength measurements in different muscle groups on the left and right side in a group of late adolescents and adult males and females combined. From Asmussen & Hohwü-Christensen (1973).

	Hand grip left	Arm pull left	Back extension	Abdominal flexion	Leg extension left
Hand grip right	0.78	0.51	0.30	0.25	0.40
Arm pull right		0.82	0.36	0.34	0.44
Back extension				0.57	0.39
Abdominal flexion					0.47
Leg extension right					0.81

(1989). The reported test—retest variability for maximal voluntary isometric muscle strength in well-defined muscle groups of children from 10 to 18 years of age ranged from 3.7 to 11%. Based on a few subjects, Molnar and Alexander (1973) and Molnar *et al.* (1979) found the test—retest variability in maximal isokinetic torque a little higher than in maximal voluntary isometric muscle strength. This indicates that if design and measuring devices are carefully controlled, then it is possible to perform repeated measurements on children with an acceptable degree of reproducibility.

Development of muscle strength in relation to age and sex

Cross-sectional studies

Cross-sectional analyses of a variety of isometric strength measurements suggest several trends. Muscular strength increases fairly linearly with CA from early childhood until approximately 13 or 14 years of age (mid-puberty) in boys. It is then followed by a marked acceleration through the late teenage period, whether expressed as individual strength measurements or as composite strength (total of strength scores) from several muscle groups (Jones, 1949; Asmussen, 1973; Malina, 1975; Faust, 1977; Parker *et al.*, 1990). Conversely, in girls strength improves fairly linearly with age up until about 15 years of age, but there is no clear evidence of an adolescent spurt (Asmussen, 1973; Malina, 1986b; Parker *et al.*, 1990).

The marked acceleration in strength development during male adolescence amplifies the relatively small preadolescent sex difference. The result is that after 16—17 years of age, only a few girls perform as well as boys in strength tests (Jones, 1949; Asmussen, 1973). This is illustrated in Fig. 2.1, where the relationship between CA and the maximal voluntary isometric elbow flexion strength is shown in 92 girls and 131 boys aged 9—17 years (O. Lammert *et al.*, 1982 unpublished data).

Based on studies by Alexander and Molnar (1973), Molnar and Alexander (1973) and Gilliam *et al.* (1979) it appears that isokinetic elbow and knee extensor and flexor strength develop in the same manner in boys and girls until the age of 10—11 years. Thereafter the isokinetic strength increase in boys is consistently greater than in girls. Extensor torques are always higher than flexor torques, and the ratio between them increases with age.

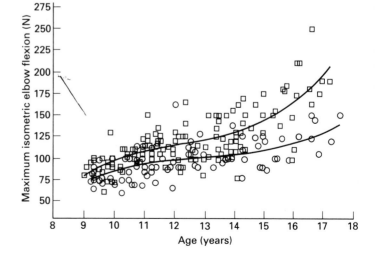

Fig. 2.1 The relationship between the maximal voluntary isometric elbow flexion strength and chronological age in 92 girls (○) and 131 boys (□) aged 9—18 years. Unpublished data from the study of O. Lammert *et al.* (1982).

Longitudinal studies

Results from longitudinal studies by Stolz and Stolz (1951), Faust (1977) and unpublished data from the study of K. Froberg *et al.* (1989) demonstrate that the relative isometric strength normalized for body mass varies only slightly during childhood and adolescence in most strength measurements, especially in girls. However, inspection of data from both cross-sectional and longitudinal studies also shows that two phases of growth can be registered in boys. The first phase is the prepubertal years until mid-puberty or the age of peak height velocity (PHV). The second phase is from the age of PHV until the end of the postpubertal period. This is shown in Figs 2.2−2.4. Strength normalized for body mass (relative strength) is constant or increases very slightly in both sexes until the age of PHV. In contrast to girls, there is an increase in relative strength in boys after the age of PHV and during adolescence. Figures 2.2 and 2.3 also show that in these muscle groups at all ages boys are consistently stronger in isometric strength than girls, even after adjusting for body mass. This was also found by Asmussen (1962) in the upper extremity and trunk in boys and girls from 7 to 17 years of age

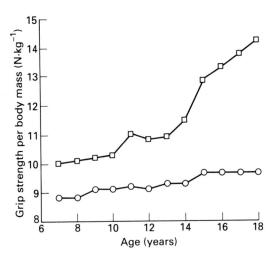

Fig. 2.2 Grip strength (N) normalized for body mass (kg) in relation to age and sex. Values are derived from the Canada Fitness Survey (1985) (cross-sectional data). Data points are based on age-specific 50th percentile scores for hand grip strength and mass; ○, girls; □, boys. Redrawn from Blimkie (1989).

after adjusting for body mass, but not in the lower extremity. Gilliam *et al.* (1979) measured isokinetic muscle strength in both knee and elbow extensors in a group of 28 boys and 28 girls of 7−15 years of age. They found that,

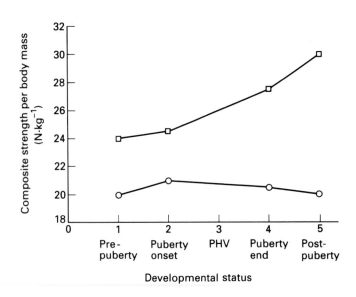

Fig. 2.3 Composite isometric strength normalized for body mass ($N \cdot kg^{-1}$), in relation to age, sex and developmental status with the age of peak height velocity (PHV) (years). Values are derived from Stolz and Stolz (1951) and Faust (1977) (longitudinal) and are based on the total of four strength measures: right-hand grip, left-hand grip, shoulder pull and shoulder thrust. The mean ages of the girls (○) and boys (□) measured were: prepuberty, 8.8 and 11.5; onset of puberty, 10.1 and 12.7; end of puberty, 12.9 and 15.6; and postpuberty, 14.2 and 16.8, respectively. Redrawn from Blimkie (1989).

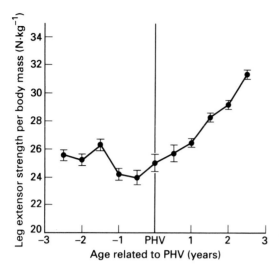

Fig. 2.4 Maximal voluntary isometric strength in leg extensors normalized for body mass ± SE (N·kg⁻¹), in relation to the age of peak height velocity (PHV) (years) in 14 moderately active boys. The boys were measured twice a year from 11 to 17 years of age. Thereafter data are rearranged according to PHV. Unpublished data from the longitudinal study of K. Froberg et al. (1989).

or biomechanical differences or differences in the level of physical activity in boys and girls (Blimkie, 1989).

Peak strength

Data from longitudinal studies (Stolz & Stolz, 1951; Carron & Bailey, 1974; Faust, 1977; Kemper & Veschur, 1985; Beunen et al., 1988; K. Froberg et al., 1989, unpublished data) make it possible to relate changes in static strength to the timing of the adolescent growth spurt. Data from the studies in boys are rather consistent. The peak in strength development occurs about 1–1.5 years after the age of PHV, thus, the strength spurt could also be considered as a maturity indicator.

Results from Canadian boys (Carron & Bailey, 1974) are summarized in Fig. 2.5; those for Belgian boys (Beunen et al., 1988), Dutch boys and girls (Kemper & Veschur, 1985) and Danish boys (K. Froberg et al., unpublished data) are summarized in Fig. 2.6. In the sample of 99 Canadian boys, upper body strength (the aver-

when the values were adjusted for height differences, there were no sex differences in relation to isokinetic knee extension strength, while sex differences were still present in the elbow extensor strength measurement.

Sex differences before puberty in strength, normalized for body mass in trunk and upper extremity, are at least in part related to the higher proportion of body fat and lower proportion of lean tissue in females from midchildhood onwards (Faust, 1977; Kemper, 1986; Malina, 1986b; Saris, 1986). The differences between the sexes during puberty and adolescence may be caused in part by a continued increase in subcutaneous fat in females (Faust, 1977; Canada Fitness Survey, 1985; Kemper, 1986) and by a greater increase in muscle size and lean body mass in males (Malina & Johnston, 1967; Cheek, 1975; Malina, 1986b). There could be other factors than body composition involved which could influence sex differences, such as hormonal, neuromuscular

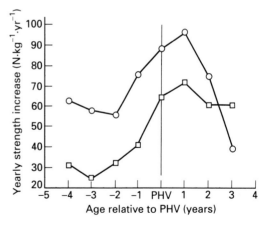

Fig. 2.5 Strength increase in upper and lower body per year (N·kg⁻¹·yr⁻¹). The isometric strength was measured in the upper body (□) as well as lower body strength (○) and aligned on the age of peak height velocity (PHV) (years) in boys from the Saskatchewan study. Data from Carron and Bailey (1984) and Beunen and Malina (1988).

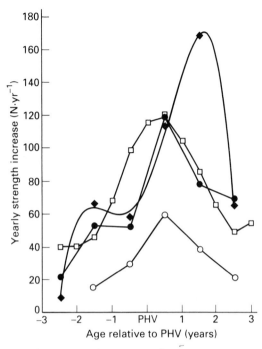

Fig. 2.6 The yearly increase of the static arm pull strength aligned on the age of peak height velocity (N·yr⁻¹). Measurements are from Belgian boys (□) (median half-yearly increases), Dutch boys (●) and girls (○) (mean yearly increases) and Danish boys (◆) (mean yearly increases). Data for Belgian boys and Dutch adolescents are redrawn from Beunen and Malina (1988).

about 1.5 years before the age of PHV and reaches a peak about 6 months after the age of PHV. The spurt lasts for about 2 years, followed by a gradual slowing in the rate of increase in strength. Results from 14 Danish boys measured longitudinally with half-yearly intervals are consistent with the above-mentioned results except for the peak in strength gain which occurred about 1.5 years after the age of PHV.

Results from Belgium (Beunen *et al.*, 1988), the USA (Faust, 1977) and Canada (Carron & Bailey, 1974) show that the maximal gain in strength actually coincides more with the age of peak body weight velocity (PWV) than with the age of PHV, but the data also suggest that there were individual differences in the development of peak strength in boys in relation to PHV or PWV (Beunen *et al.*, 1988). The adolescent peak in dynamic strength coincides with the peak in static strength (Beunen *et al.*, 1988). In absolute values, peak strength development in girls was only half that of boys. The peak appears about 6 months after the age of PHV, but there are considerable individual variations (Faust, 1977).

Development of muscle strength in relation to body mass and height

In the cross-sectional study of Lammert *et al.* (1982), discussed in Fig. 2.1, the maximal voluntary strength in the elbow flexors was also related to height, body mass, bone age (BA) (using the method of Greulich & Pyle, 1959) and predicted peak height velocity (PPHV) age (using the method of Helm *et al.*, 1971). The positive correlation values between strength and CA, height, body mass and also with BA and PPHV age, are shown in Table 2.2. In boys there was a moderate to strong correlation — and in girls a moderate correlation — between strength measurements, height, mass and the different age and maturity markers. These moderate to strong relationships were also found by Clarke and Degutis (1962), when using an age range from before puberty to several years after puberty.

age of shoulder extension, wrist extension and flexion, elbow extension and flexion) and lower body strength (average of hip flexion and knee extension) reach a peak 1 year after the age of PHV. These samples also show that when strength increments are expressed as a percentage of the level of strength attained, the relative increase is greater for upper than for lower body strength.

Data on Dutch and Belgian adolescents were based on arm pull tests and on Danish adolescents on the maximal isometric strength in the elbow flexors. The increase in strength for 96 Dutch boys (measured yearly) and for 219 Belgian boys (measured half-yearly) are generally similar. The spurt in arm strength begins

Table 2.2 Correlation coefficients between muscle strength — maximal voluntary isometric (MVI) elbow flexion strength — and chronological age, bone age, the age of predicted peak height velocity (PPHV), height and weight. The data are from cross-sectional measurements of 92 girls (G) and 131 boys (B) aged 9−17 years. Unpublished data from the study of O. Lammert *et al.* (1982).

	Chronological age		Bone age		PPHV age		Height		Weight	
	G	B	G	B	G	B	G	B	G	B
MVI elbow flexion	0.62	0.78	0.61	0.80	0.55	0.74	0.64	0.77	0.71	0.79
MVI elbow flexion		0.95*					0.69	0.71†		

* Data from Blimkie, 1989.
† Data from Parker *et al.*, 1990.

The variability in the correlation values are quite small in boys. The same variability is somewhat larger in girls, with body mass as the marker with the highest correlation to strength. The similarity in the correlation values is not surprising when the very high inter-relationships between the different markers are considered (Table 2.3). Analysed separately, the correlations indicate that 40−80% of the variation in children's strength is associated with differences in age, height or body mass. This was also found by Clarke (1971), Stolz and Stolz (1951), Carron and Bailey (1974), Beunen *et al.* (1988) and Parker *et al.* (1990). Using a stepwise regression approach to the above-mentioned cross-sectional data, sex, body mass and CA in combination accounted for as much as 67% of the variation in strength in boys and girls aged 9−17 years. In boys body mass and CA accounted for as much as 69% of the variation in the strength measurement; body mass alone for 62%. In girls, no other parameter than body mass was associated with strength in the stepwise regression approach, and it accounted for 52% of the variation.

Rarick and Oyster (1964) found in two independent groups of primary school-aged children (6−9 years of age) that CA, skeletal age, height and body mass in combination accounted for as much as 65% of the variation in muscle strength. No other studies have dealt with a multiple regression approach in children.

Muscle strength and body mass

When relating muscle strength to different growth periods, it has been found that the age-specific correlations between strength and body mass for males are generally low to moderate during the mid-childhood years, tend to increase and then peak during puberty, and decrease during adolescence (Jones, 1949; Clarke, 1971; Carron & Bailey, 1974; Parker *et al.*, 1990).

In girls, Faust (1977) and Parker *et al.* (1990) reported moderate positive correlations between strength and body mass for females

Table 2.3 Matrix of the correlations between height, body mass, chronological age, bone age and the age of predicted peak height velocity (PPHV) in 92 girls and 131 boys aged 9−17 years. Data from Lammert *et al.* (1982).

	Height	Weight	Chronological age	Bone age
Weight	0.917			
Chronological age	0.829	0.795		
Bone age	0.855	0.841	0.911	
PPHV age	0.735	0.740	0.785	0.852

during the prepubertal years and at the onset of puberty, and only low correlations at the end of puberty and during adolescence.

Muscle strength and height

Correlations between strength and height seem to vary with age for both females and males during childhood and adolescence in the same manner as between strength and body mass, though the correlations are somewhat weaker (Canada Fitness Survey, 1985).

Asmussen and Heebøll-Nielsen (1955, 1956) and Asmussen et al. (1959) measured maximal voluntary isometric strength in different muscle groups in the upper body, trunk and lower body in 300 boys and 300 girls aged 6–16 years. One of the purposes of the studies was to analyse the manner in which muscle strength developed compared to the development of height. They found that little and tall children and adults are geometrically similar. Theoretically, one should therefore expect that muscle strength is proportional to the physiological cross-sectional area (CSA) of the muscle, according to the work of Hill (1950). Their assumption, therefore was that muscle strength must vary as height squared.

Table 2.4 shows the actual values of the single exponential function to the relationship between muscle strength in different muscle groups and height in children. Power functions relating muscle strength and height from a few other studies are also shown (Lammert et al., 1982; Parker et al., 1990; and K. Froberg et al., 1989 unpublished data). The exponents in these power functions vary with the site of the strength measurements (elbow flexion versus leg extension), showing differences between the sexes.

During growth, the strength of both boys and girls in most muscle groups increases more than the theoretically expected value of 2 if strength increase is based on the increase in height alone. The exponents related to height for the different strength measurements shown are close to the exponent of three. Height to

Table 2.4 Muscle strength (S) in boys and girls can be related to height (H) with a power function as in the following equation: ($S = bH^a$). From theoretical considerations the exponent (a) relating muscle strength to height should derive a value of 2. The a values are derived from linear regression of log-transformed data.

Dependent variable	Boys (a)	Girls (a)
Elbow flexors*	2.091	1.649
Elbow flexors†	1.99	1.93
Leg extensors‡	2.891	2.742
Leg extensors†	3.02	2.98
Leg extensors§	3.625	
Finger flexors‡	3.274	3.585
Back muscles‡		2.36
Back muscles§	2.902	
Abdominal muscles‡		2.33
Body mass‡	2.684	2.876
Body mass†	2.908	2.919

* Unpublished data in the study of O. Lammert et al. (1982).
† Data from Parker et al. (1990).
‡ Data from Asmussen and Hebøll-Nielsen (1955, 1956) and Asmussen (1973).
§ Unpublished data in the study of K. Froberg et al. (1989).

power of 3 is proportional to body mass. Exceptions are the exponents of the back muscles strength and the arm flexor strength in girls. These are more in agreement with the theoretical predicted height squared.

The composite strength in boys from 10 to 16 years had an average yearly increase of 22.7% (data from a longitudinal study by Carron & Bailey, 1974). This is approximately twofold higher than expected from a theoretical viewpoint which would predict a change of only 12.1%. The discrepancy in most muscle groups between actual strength measurements and those predicted on the basis of height has been ascribed both to quantitative differences (greater relative increase in muscle mass and CSA of muscles compared to height) and qualitative differences (neural or biochemical changes within motor units) as well as differences between sexes and changes across ages within the neuromuscular system (Asmussen &

Heebøll-Nielsen, 1955; Asmussen, 1973; Carron & Bailey, 1974).

Summary

Predominantly based on cross-sectional studies it can be stated that the development of strength in relation to age is characterized by a growth curve very similar to the curves in body mass and height. Based on longitudinal studies, maximal gain in muscle strength occurs after the age of PHV and coincides approximately with the age of PWV.

Both in absolute values and when normalized for body mass there are sex differences in most muscle groups both in isometric and dynamic strength measurements. There are moderate to strong correlations between strength and body mass or height when analysed over the age spectrum from mid-childhood to late adolescence. When related to shorter periods of growth (mid-childhood, puberty, etc.), the correlations become weaker with the period of puberty as the most predictive period, especially in boys. In most muscle groups muscle strength in children does not vary as height squared but as height to the power of 3.

Other correlates and determinants of strength

As mentioned, there are other factors than age, sex, growth in height and body mass which influence and differentiate strength performance. Maturation and neurological factors, muscle size, fibre type and contractile characteristics, endocrinological influences, genetic influences and physical activity are factors thought to be interrelated and thus may influence strength development through common or shared variance. In this section each of the factors are discussed independently.

Maturation

Rarick and Oyster (1964) found in primary school-aged boys, when they were divided into skeletally mature and immature groups, that the former were stronger, taller and heavier. Thus, they concluded that strength differences among young boys primarily reflect size differences. Data from Clarke (1971), Espenschade (1940), Jones (1949) and Beunen et al. (1976, 1978) indicate that during adolescence, maturity relationships to strength are more apparent for boys than for girls. Data from 224 Danish boys and girls O. Lammert et al., 1982, unpublished data) registered in relation to BA and PPHV age indicated moderate positive correlations to strength in both boys and girls, though strongest in the boys, as shown in Table 2.2.

Early maturing boys have a larger muscle strength at each age than their average and later maturing peers. The strength differences between contrasting maturity groups are most marked among 13 and 16 year olds. The higher strength for the early maturing boys reflects their larger body size and muscle mass. When the effect of body mass is removed in comparing early and late maturing boys, strength differences between the contrasting groups are reduced, though not entirely eliminated (Carron & Bailey, 1974; Beunen et al., 1980). In later adolescence strength differences are reduced with the catch-up of the late maturing boys (Espenschade, 1940; Jones, 1949; Clarke, 1971).

During the early period of female adolescence, early maturing girls are stronger than late maturers, differences being most apparent in girls aged 11−15 years. However, they do not maintain the strength superiority. In late adolescence, differences between contrasting maturity groups of girls are not as great as those between contrasting maturity groups of boys (Jones, 1949; Beunen et al., 1976; Carron et al., 1977).

Neurological factors

Maturity might exert an independent influence on maximal voluntary strength, possibly through mechanisms of enhanced neurological maturation and control. Less mature boys and girls are perhaps not able to maximally activate their muscles because the degree of motor unit activation, which is dependent upon both the level of voluntary neural drive and the level of activation of recruited motor units, is diminished in comparison with older or more mature boys and girls.

Asmussen and Heebøll-Nielsen (1955) divided 300 boys into 10 cm height groups and then into two age groups, an older and a younger. The average difference in age turned out to be approximately 1.5 years. Strength measurements in arms and legs showed that at corresponding heights the older subgroups were stronger than the younger by 5−10%.

Using a technique where supramaximal electrical stimulation is applied during the peak of a maximal voluntary isometric contraction, the degree of motor unit activation can be more directly assessed. The increment in force above that obtained voluntarily provides a measure of the degree of motor unit activation during voluntary contractions. Blimkie (1989) has recently applied this technique to both the elbow flexor and knee extensor muscle groups in 10−16-year-old males. In relation to the elbow flexors there was no difference between age groups for percentage motor unit activation (89.4% versus 89.9%, for 10−16 year olds, respectively). However, there was a substantial age difference in degree of motor unit activation of the knee extensors (77.7% versus 95.3%, for 10−16 year olds, respectively). The variability in the ability to activate motor units appears to be lower in older boys.

Based on the observations of Asmussen and Heebøll-Nielsen (1955) and Blimkie (1989) it is clear that differences in the ability to activate the muscles contribute to the age- and sex-associated variation in voluntary strength during childhood, though further investigations are needed.

Muscle size

The relationship between muscle size and strength has been examined by measuring muscle widths, lean body mass or CSA of muscle and these results have been correlated with the measured muscle strength. Malina (1975) has carefully reviewed the relationship between width and maximal isometric muscle strength in different upper and lower body muscle groups in both boys and girls in mid-childhood (age approximately 7 years). The correlations found were weak to moderate, with a tendency for boys at this age to be slightly stronger per unit of muscle area than girls. It was not apparent from the data whether the observation reflects a real biological difference or motivational differences between boys and girls. Parker et al. (1990) found in a cross-sectional study in 267 boys and 284 girls aged 5−18 years, that the changes in strength were very similar to changes in radiographically determined widths of muscles in boys and girls from the Harpenden growth study reported by Tanner et al. (1981). Muscle widths at maximum calf diameter and half-way down the upper arm were similar in boys and girls up to the onset of puberty, with greater increase in boys after this time. The increase in elbow flexor strength of 20% in girls and of 95% in boys from 12 to 18 years of age could be explained fully by the changes in muscle widths in both boys and girls. Apart from this, there are surprisingly few studies which relate muscle width and strength during growth.

Forbes (1965) measured lean body mass by the potassium 40 technique and correlated the data with grip strength in boys. He demonstrated a very strong positive correlation ($r = 0.908$). No comparable result could be found describing a similar relationship in girls.

The relationship between strength and muscle CSA has been studied for various muscle groups under both maximal voluntary contractions (Ikai & Funaga, 1968; Chapman et al., 1984; Davies, 1985; Blimkie, 1989) and electrically evoked contractions (Davies et al., 1983; Davies, 1985; Blimkie, 1989). In a study of two boys, 10 and 12 years of age and 20 adults from 22 to 35 years of age, Chapman et al. (1984) studied the relationship between the CSA of the quadriceps muscle (determined by computerized tomography) and isometric knee extensor strength and they found a strong positive correlation ($r = 0.87$) between muscle size and strength. Ikai and Fukunuga (1968) studied the relationship between voluntary isometric elbow flexion strength and ultrasonically determined CSA of the arm flexors in a large number of males and females from 12 to 20 years of age. The data indicated a positive correlation in boys and girls between muscle CSA and strength. Normalized for CSA, there were no strength differences between sexes, and the ratio of strength to CSA was $62 \, \text{N} \cdot \text{cm}^{-2} \pm 8$ and fairly constant from 12 to 20 years of age. The CSA of the muscles was measured in the fully extended position of the forearm. When the strength per unit area was calculated at the 90° flexed position of the forearm it was found to be $46 \, \text{N} \cdot \text{cm}^{-2}$. Davies et al. (1983) and Davies (1985) studied the strength and mechanical properties of the triceps surae muscle in children and young adults of both sexes ranging from 9 to 21 years of age. They related both maximal voluntary and evoked strength to the muscle CSA determined by anthropometry. The strength of the triceps surae was the same in 9- and 11-year-old boys and girls, but it then increased with age. Adolescent children were significantly stronger than their younger counterparts, but weaker than young adults. However, when standardizations were made for muscle (plus bone) CSA, the differences in muscle strength between the sexes and with respect to age disappeared. In both boys and girls and in a group of adult subjects the absolute value of electrically evoked and voluntary maximal strength was linearly related to CSA and the correlations were very strong, $r = 0.86$ ($n = 42$) and 0.92 ($n = 91$), respectively.

When normalized for muscle CSA, the mean specific tension of the muscle was $33 \, \text{N} \cdot \text{cm}^{-2}$ for the children and young adults irrespective of age and sex. This value is lower than that found by Ikai and Fukunuga (1968). The discrepancy is not discussed by Davies. Ikai and Fukunuga measured strength in the arm flexors and Davies the triceps surae muscle. The discrepancy may be due to this, and/or to methodological differences in the assessment of either maximal voluntary force or CSA of the muscles involved.

Davies (1985) concluded that differences in strength in children and young adults appeared to be a function of muscle bulk, and reflect the different extent to which muscles hypertrophy with respect to age and sex. Thus, neither age nor gender appear to be important factors governing specific tension of young human muscles.

Blimkie (1989) measured the relationship between muscle CSA (via computerized tomography) and both maximal voluntary isometric strength and evoked twitch torque in the elbow flexors of 46 males aged between 9 and 18 years. Furthermore, the relationship between muscle CSA and both maximal voluntary isometric strength and evoked twitch torque in the knee extensors of 35 males aged between 9 and 18 years of age was investigated. He found a strong correlation between CSA and strength both in the elbow flexor (voluntary and evoked, $r = 0.86$ and 0.71, respectively) and in the knee extensors (voluntary and evoked, $r = 0.86$ and 0.87, respectively).

The data from Davies (1985) however, also showed a decreased ratio between peak tension of maximal electrically evoked twitch to maximal voluntary strength in males aged between 11 and 21 years. These observations indicate that the age-associated increase in voluntary strength in males may also be due in part to changes in the degree of voluntary activation of muscles; the latter increases between childhood and adulthood. The physiological background for this change still remains undetermined.

A part of the variability in the relationship between maximum voluntary isometric force and CSA in adults has been suggested to reflect biomechanical factors (Maughan, 1984), such as individual differences in the internal muscle architecture (differences in the angle of pennation to the long axis of the muscle, leading to a smaller force acting on the tendon), and in limb length and joint structure (mechanical advantage of the lever system). The age-associated relationships between these factors have until now not been investigated in children.

Muscle fibre composition and contractile characteristics

It could also be argued that muscle strength in children and adolescents is influenced by muscle fibre composition, because most muscles are made up of muscle fibres with different mechanical and contractile properties. In adults, the maximal isometric force is found to depend on the CSA of the muscle, irrespective of the fibre distribution, possibly with the exception of a very fast contraction where type II fibres may be superior (Coyle *et al.*, 1979; Nygaard *et al.*, 1983; Maughan, 1984). It has been found that, at a velocity of $180° \cdot s^{-1}$ or larger, type II fibres may be able to produce greater force than type I fibres during isokinetic contractions. However, there are no available studies of the relationship between muscle fibre type distribution, fibre diameter or area, and either voluntary or evoked absolute strength or specific tension in children.

Endocrinological influences

Gender differences in hormone levels and activity affect the development of the adolescent, the differences in muscularity and therefore differences in muscle strength between girls and boys. Based on a longitudinal study in boys where height velocity was related to testosterone concentration, Preece (1986) added strong credence to the belief that in boys it is the testosterone secretion which has the dominant effect on the adolescent growth spurt. There is also an increase in testosterone concentration in girls, but it is of a lower magnitude. Testosterone is believed to be the most active stimulator of the anabolic processes in the muscles, but it is not the only hormone which affects muscle growth. Growth hormone, the somatomedins, insulin and the thyroid

hormones are also known to be important effectors of normal somatic and muscle growth (Florini, 1987). Muscle growth and strength performance may not be determined by the sex steroids alone but perhaps by the balance between hormonally regulated anabolic and catabolic processes (Blimkie, 1989). The relative importance of both the anabolic and catabolic hormones and the balance between them in the age- and sex-associated differentiation of muscle size and strength development during childhood remain to be elucidated.

Genetic influences

The influence of the genotype component of variance in the development of isometric muscle strength is reviewed by Bouchard and Malina (1983) and Malina (1986a). Most of the data reviewed are derived from twins. The results show a wide variability in the heritability estimates for isometric muscle strength, but most of the data indicate a low to moderate genetic effect in most of the muscle groups studied, and a higher heritability for males than females. Sibling data suggest a similar trend, where brothers tend to resemble each other more than sisters in strength. These results therefore suggest sex influence in the estimated heritabilities of muscle strength, but it could also be an environmental covariation that differs with respect to sex.

There are no available studies of the heritability of isokinetic muscle strength. Kovar (1975) and Jones and Klissouras (1986) reported a very high heritability of the force−velocity relationship and thus for dynamic strength and muscle power. It was 85% for the dynamic strength and 97% for the power production measured in the elbow flexors. Komi and Karlsson (1979) reported a heritability estimate of 98% for leg muscle power in a combined sample of children and young adults.

Based on the existing literature regarding the influence of the genotype component of variance in the development of muscle strength, it is difficult to provide a reliable statement about the differentiation of strength performance during childhood. As is the case for most biological characteristics, data indicate a low to moderate heritability for muscle strength or performance, except perhaps for dynamic muscle strength and power in specific muscle groups. There is a need for studies which quantify the specific environmental factors that influence muscle strength and performance as for example, training, level of habitual physical activity, and the shared sibling and familial environment.

Physical activity

Until now, no controlled study covering both sexes over the entire childhood period have measured the influences of different physical activity levels on the relationship between age- and sex-associated differences and development of muscle strength. One reason could be the extreme difficulty in quantifying the intensity of different physical activities (Saris, 1986).

Little is known about the extent of children's physical activity levels, though it appears that children exhibit little vigorous physical activity (Simons-Morton et al., 1987) and that a higher energy expenditure and intake can be found in boys compared to girls (Saris, 1986). Both surveys of the Canadian and Danish youth, 10–19 years of age, show that there was a slightly higher participation rate in self-reported physical activity for boys compared to girls up to 13 years of age (Canadian Fitness Survey, 1983; Holstein et al., 1990). From 14 years of age, there was a progressive drop in participation rates for females in the Canadian children. In the Danish children, this drop was registered from 15 years of age and equal in boys and girls. Such a drop was not seen in the Canadian boys and adults. In both studies it was shown that boys prefer activities requiring a higher degree of muscular strength and power.

Engström (1989) reported a drop in self-reported physical activity levels in Swedish boys and girls over the last two decades.

Heebøll-Nielsen (1982) reported less maximal isometric muscle strength in most muscle groups but especially in the back muscles (10–15%) in Danish children, when compared to measurements taken in Danish children in the 1950s (Asmussen & Heebøll-Nielsen, 1955, 1956).

There appear to be differences in participation rates and in the nature and intensity of habitual physical activity between the sexes. With increasing age there is a decrease in overall activity in both sexes. The extent to which these patterns influence age- and sex-associated differences in strength performance during childhood, and perhaps over years, remains to be determined.

Challenges for future research

• There are inconsistencies in the results discussed in this chapter. Until more extensive studies are published one may speculate on the reasons for these and caution researchers to both carefully select their groups and thoroughly construct their designs so that more light can be cast on these inconsistencies.

• In the studies used as background for this chapter it is impossible to know whether the different results occur as a consequence of selection and/or (i) training; (ii) differences in development; (iii) differences in lean body mass; (iv) differences in muscle mass. Muscle strength is known to be proportional to height squared in some muscle groups and related to height to the power of 3 in other muscle groups. The ratio of the dynamic torque measured in extensors and flexors is known to change with age, as well as differ between normal and active children. These observations indicate that in general normal children are not equally trained in different muscle groups, but this remains to be investigated, as does the possible existence of a general strength factor in children.

• Peak strength growth spurt is evident in both sexes, but not clearly related to either PHV or PWV; this calls for studies to determine exactly when this strength spurt occurs and what kinds of biological processes it is related to. It is also unknown whether it is similar in boys and girls.

• There is a lack of knowledge on children's muscle strength in relation to muscle fibre composition and/or the CSA of different fibres. In relation to this, both static and dynamic strength development should be investigated. In relation to dynamic strength it should be investigated over a speed range as wide as possible. In isokinetic studies the effects of learning should be taken into account, especially at high velocity tests.

• The longitudinal influence of the child's daily and recreational activities on the development of muscle strength and on the occurrence of the peak strength gain in puberty is at present unknown. With the double labelled water technique (Schoeller, 1983) and reliable heart rate monitors, the tools are now available for such an analysis.

• The relationship between development of strength on the one hand and muscle mass and anabolic and catabolic hormonal changes on the other is at present unknown.

Appendix 2.1 Force and torque during different types of muscle contractions

Muscle contractions can either be *static* or *dynamic*. Static contractions are muscle force applied while the muscle length is unchanged (*isometric*). Dynamic contractions are muscle force applied while muscle length is either shortened (*concentric* contractions) or extended (*eccentric* contractions). A special case of dynamic contractions are movements performed with a constant speed over the whole range of the movement. Such contractions are called *isokinetic* contractions.

Force. Peak tension (measured externally by a strain gauge or dynamometer) developed during voluntary or involuntary (electrically evoked) activation of muscle. Because of the mechanical construction of the muscle–tendon–skeletal system, the measured external force is less than that developed within the muscle. Force is expressed in newtons (N) (in the older literature it is often expressed in kp (kilopond) or kg (force)).

Torque. Peak force (tension) developed around a joint. Torque is the product of force applied at the point of contact with the dynamometer and the moment arm. Thus torque is proportional to the force the muscle applies times the distance between the point of force application on the bone and the centre of the joint axis. Torque is expressed in $N \cdot m^{-1}$ (earlier kilopond metre, kpm).

Maximal isometric contraction. Isometric means equal (iso) length (metric). Thus maximal force produced with no change in muscle length either voluntary or electrically evoked and activated against an immovable resistance is termed MVI or maximal voluntary isometric strength and is expressed in N.

Maximal isokinetic contraction. Muscle force produced against a movable resistance, resulting in maximal force development throughout the joint's full range of motion. The force is applied with a constant speed (isokinetic). Often only the peak force is published. In that case it is measured in N at a certain (constant) speed, or at a certain angular velocity. The angular velocity is either measured in degrees $\cdot s^{-1}$ or rad $\cdot s^{-1}$. The speed of the movement can also be normalized by relating the speed to the subjects limb length. Then it is expressed in per cent limb length $\cdot s^{-1}$.

Evoked twitch contraction. A single isometric contraction lasting a few milliseconds and activated by a single percutaneous supramaximal electrical stimulation. It is expressed in N.

Evoked tetanic contraction. A fused isometric contraction usually lasting a few seconds and activated by repetitive percutaneous electrical stimulations. It is expressed in N.

Maximal voluntary contraction. An all-out voluntary isometric or dynamic muscle contraction. Maximal voluntary isometric contractions usually last a few seconds, whereas the duration of dynamic contractions will vary from less than 1 s to a few seconds, depending on the speed and range of movement.

References

Alexander, J. & Molnar, G.E. (1973) Muscular strength in children: preliminary report on objective standards. *Arch. Phys. Med. Rehab.* **54**, 424–7.

Asmussen, E. (1962) Muscular performance. In K. Rodahl & S.M. Horvath (eds) *Muscle as a Tissue*, pp. 161–75. McGraw-Hill, New York.

Asmussen, E. (1973) Growth in muscular strength and power. In G.L. Rarick (ed.) *Physical Activity*

Human Growth and Development, pp. 60–79. Academic Press, New York.

Asmussen, E., Hansen, O. & Lammert, O. (1965) The relation between isometric and dynamic muscle strength in man. *Communication from the Testing and Observation Institute of the Danish National Association for Infantile Paralysis*, Report No. 20, pp. 1–12.

Asmussen, E. & Heebøll-Nielsen K. (1955) A dimensional analysis of physical performance and growth in boys. *J. Appl. Physiol.* **7**, 593–603.

Asmussen, E. & Heebøll-Nielsen, K. (1956) Physical performance and growth in children. Influence of sex, age and intelligence. *J. Appl. Physiol.* **8**, 371–80.

Asmussen, E., Heebøll-Nielsen, K. & Molbech, S.V. (1959) Methods for evaluation of muscle strength. *Communication from the Testing and Observation Institute of the Danish National Association for Infantile Paralysis*, Report No. 5, pp. 3–13.

Asmussen, E. & Hohwü-Christensen E. (1973) *Legemsøvelsernes Specielle Teori*, p. 32. Akademisk Forlag, Copenhagen.

Beunen, G. & Malina, R.M. (1988) Growth and physical performance relative to the timing of the adolescent spurt. *Exerc. Sport Sci. Rev.* **16**, 503–40.

Beunen, G., Malina, R.M., Van't Hof, M.A. *et al.* (1988) *Adolescent Growth and Motor Performance: A Longitudinal Study of Belgian Boys.* Human Kinetics, Champaign, IL.

Beunen, G., Ostyn, M., Renson, R., Simons, J. & Van Gerven, D. (1976) Skeletal maturation and physical fitness of girls aged 12 through 16. *Hermes* (Leuven) **10**, 445.

Beunen, G., Ostyn, M., Simons, J. & Van Gerven, D. (1978) A correlational analysis on skeletal maturity, anthropometric measures and motor fitness of boys 12 through 16. In F. Landry & W.A.R. Orban (eds) *Biomechanics of Sports and Kinanthropometry*, pp. 343–9. Symposia Specialists, Miami, FL.

Beunen, G., Simons, J., Ostyn, M., Renson, R. & Van Gerven, D. (1980) Learning effects in repeated measurements designs. In K. Berg & B.O. Eriksson (eds) *Children and Exercise*, Vol. IX, pp. 41–8, University Park Press, Baltimore.

Blimkie, C.J.R. (1989) Age- and sex-associated variation in strength during childhood: anthropometric, morphologic, neurologic, biomechanical, endocrinologic, genetic, and physical activity correlates. In C.V. Gisolfi & D.R. Lamb (eds) *Perspectives in Exercise Science and Sports Medicine*, Vol. 2. *Youth, Exercise, and Sport*, pp. 99–163. Benchmark Press, Indiana, PA.

Bouchard, C. & Malina, R.M. (1983) Genetics of physiological fitness and motor performance. *Exerc. Sport Sci. Rev.* **11**, 306–39.

Canada Fitness Survey (1985) Physical fitness and Canadian youth. *Fitness and Amateur Sport.* Ottawa.

Carron, A.V., Aitken, E.J. & Bailey, D.A. (1977) In H. Lavallee & R.J. Shephard (eds) *Frontiers of Activity and Child Health*, pp. 139–43. Pelican, Ottawa.

Carron, A.V. & Bailey, D.A. (1974) Strength development in boys from 10 through 16 years. *Monogr. Soc. Res. Child Dev.* **39**, 1–37.

Chapman, S.J., Grindrod, S.R. & Jones, D.A. (1984) Cross-sectional area and force production of the quadriceps muscle. *J. Physiol.* **353**, 53P.

Cheek, D.B. (1975) Growth and body composition. In D.B. Cheek (ed.) *Fetal and Postnatal Cellular Growth: Hormones and Nutrition*, pp. 389–408. Wiley, New York.

Clarke, H.H. (1971) *Physical and Motor Tests in the Medford Boy's Growth Study.* Prentice-Hall, Englewood Cliffs, NJ.

Clarke, H.H. & Degutis, E.W. (1962) Comparison of skeletal age and various physical and motor factors with the pubescent development of 10-, 13-, and 16-year-old boys. *Res. Q.* **33**, 356–68.

Coyle, E.F., Costill, D.L. & Lesmes, G.R. (1979) Leg extension power and muscle fibre composition. *Med. Sci. Sports Exerc.* **11**, 12–15.

Davies, C.T.M. (1985) Strength and mechanical properties of muscle in children and young adults. *Scand. J. Sports Sci.* **7**, 11–15.

Davies, C.T.M., White, M.J. & Young, K. (1983) Muscle function in children. *Eur. J. Appl. Physiol.* **52**, 111–14.

Edwards, R.H.T., Chapman, S.J., Newham, D.J. & Jones, D.A. (1987) Practical analysis of variability of muscle function measurements in Duchenne muscular dystrophy. *Muscle Nerve* **10**, 6–14.

Engström, L.M. (1989) *Idrottsvaner i förändring* (in Swedish). Gotab, Stockholm.

Espenschade, A. (1940) Motor performance in adolescence including the study of relationships with measures of physical growth and maturity. *Monogr. Soc. Res. Child Dev.* **5** (Serial No. 24).

Faust, M.S. (1977) Somatic development of adolescent girls. *Monogr. Soc. Res. Child Dev.* **42**, 1–90.

Florini, J.R. (1987) Hormonal control of muscle growth. *Muscle Nerve* **10**, 577–98.

Forbes, G.B. (1965) Toward a new dimension in human growth. *Pediatrics* **36**, 825–35.

Froberg, K., Andersen, B. & Lammert, O. (1991) Maximal oxygen uptake and respiratory function during puberty in boy groups of different physical activity. In R. Frenkl & I. Szmodis (eds) *Children and Exercise: Pediatric Work Physiology*, Vol. XV, pp. 265–80. National Institute for Health Promotion, Budapest, Hungary.

Gilliam, T.B., Villanacci, J.F., Freedson, P.S. & Sady, S.P. (1979) Isokinetic torque in boys and girls ages

7 to 13: effect of age, height, and weight. *Res. Q.* **50**, 599–609.

Greulich, W.W. & Pyle, S.I. (1959) *Radiographic Atlas of Skeletal Development of the Hand and Wrist*, 2nd edn. Standford University Press, Stanford.

Heebøll-Nielsen, K. (1982) Muscle strength in boys and girls, 1981 compared to 1956. *Scand. J. Sport Sci.* **4**, 37–43.

Helm, S., Siersbæk-Nielsen, S., Skieller, V. & Björk, A. (1971) Skeletal maturation of the hand in relation to maximal puberal growth in body height. *Danish Dental J.* **75**, 1223–35.

Hill, A.V. (1950) The dimensions of animals and their muscular dynamics. *Proc. Roy. Instit. GB* **34**, 450–71.

Holstein, B.E., Hirobumi, I. & Due, P. (1990) Physical exercise in Danish school children. *J. Danish Med. Ass.* **152**, 2721–7.

Hortobágyi, T., Katch, F.I., Katch, V.L., LaChance, P.F. & Behnke, A.R. (1990) Relationships of body size, segmental dimensions, and ponderal equivalents to muscular strength in high-strength and low-strength subjects. *Int. J. Sports Med.* **11**, 349–56.

Hortobágyi, T., Katch, F.I. & LaChance, P.F. (1989) Interrelationships among various measures of upper body strength assessed by different contraction modes. *Eur. J. Appl. Physiol.* **58**, 749–55.

Ikai, M. & Fukunaga, T. (1968) Calculations of muscle strength per unit cross-sectional area of human muscle by means of ultrasonic measurement. *Int. Zeitschr Angewandte Physiol. Einschliess. Arbeitsphysiol.* **26**, 26–32.

Jones, B. & Klissouras, V. (1986) Genetic variation in the force–velocity relation of human muscle. In R.M. Malina & C. Bouchard (eds) *Sports and Human Genetics*, pp. 155–63. Human Kinetics, Champaign IL.

Jones, H.E. (1949) *Motor Performance and Growth*. University of California Press, Berkley.

Kemper, H.C.G. (1986) Health and fitness of Dutch teenagers: a review. In J.A.P. Day (ed.) *Perspectives in Kinanthropometry*, pp. 61–80. Human Kinetics, Champaign, IL.

Kemper, H.C.G. & Verschuur, R. (1985) Maximal aerobic power. In H.C.G. Kemper (ed.) *Growth Health and Fitness of Teenagers*, pp. 107–26. Karger, Basel.

Komi, P.V. & Karlsson, J. (1979) Physical performance, skeletal muscle enzyme activities, and fiber types in monozygous and dizygous twins of both sexes. *Acta Physiol. Scand.* 462, (Suppl.) 1–28.

Kovar, R. (1975) Motor performance in twins. *Acta Genet. Med. Geme Illolog.* **24**, 174.

Lammert, O., Andersen, B. & Froberg, K. (1982) The effect of training in relation to chronological age

and development in children 9 to 17 years. In P. Russo (ed.) *Human Adaptation. A Workshop on Growth and Physical Activity*, pp. 17–29. Cumberland College of Health Sciences, Sydney.

Malina, R.M. (1975) Anthropometric correlates of performance. *Exerc. Sport Sci. Rev.* **3**, 249–74.

Malina, R.M. (1986a) Genetics of motor development and performance. In R.M. Malina & C. Bouchard (eds) *Sport and Human Genetics*, pp. 23–58. Human Kinetics, Champaign, IL.

Malina, R.M. (1986b) Growth of muscle tissue and muscle mass. In F. Falkner & J.M. Tanner (eds) *Human Growth. A Comprehensive Treatise*, Vol. 2. *Postnatal Growth Neurobiology*, pp. 77–99. Plenum Press, New York.

Malina, R.M. & Johnston, F.E. (1967) Relations between bone, muscle and fat widths in the upper arms and calves of boys and girls studied cross-sectionally at ages 6 to 16 years. *Hum. Biol.* **39**, 211–23.

Maughan, R.J. (1984) Relationship between muscle strength and muscle cross-sectional area. Implications for training. *Sports Med.* **1**, 263–9.

Molnar, G.E. & Alexander, J. (1973) Objective, quantitative muscle testing in children: a pilot study. *Arch. Phys. Med. Rehabil.* **54**, 224–8.

Molnar, G.E., Alexander, J. & Gutfield, N. (1979) Rehability of quantitative strength measurements in children. *Arch. Phys. Med. Rehabil.* **60**, 218–21.

Nygaard, E., Houston, M., Suzuki, Y., Jørgensen, K. & Saltin, B. (1983) Morphology of the brachial biceps muscle and elbow flexion in man. *Acta Physiol. Scand.* **117**, 287–92.

Parker, D.F., Round, J.M., Sacco, P. & Jones, D.A. (1990) A cross-sectional survey of upper and lower limb strength in boys and girls during childhood and adolescence. *Ann. Hum. Biol.* **17**, 199–211.

Preece, M.A. (1986) Prepubertal and pubertal endocrinology. In F. Falkner & J.M. Tanner (eds) *Human Growth*, Vol. 2, *Postnatal Growth Neurobiology*, pp. 211–24. New York, Plenum Press.

Rarick, G.L. & Oyster, N. (1964) Physical maturity, muscular strength, and motor performance of young school-age boys. *Res. Q.* **35**, 523–31.

Saris, W.H.M. (1986) Habitual physical activity in children: methodology and findings in health and disease. *Med. Sci. Sports Exerc.* **18**, 253–63.

Simons-Morton, B.G., O'Hara, N.M., Simons-Morton, D.G. & Parcel, G.S. (1987) Children and fitness: a public health perspective. *Res. Q. Exerc. Sport* **58**, 295–302.

Schoeller, D.A. (1983) Energy expenditure from double labeled water: some fundamental considerations in humans. *Am. J. Clin. Nutr.* **38**, 999–1005.

Stolz, H.R. & Stolz, L.M. (1951) *Somatic Development*

of Adolescent Boys. Macmillan, New York.

Tanner, J.M. (1962) *Growth at Adolescence*, 2nd edn. Blackwell Scientific Publications, Oxford.

Tanner, J.M., Hughes, P.C.R. & Whitehouse, R.H. (1981) Radiographically determined widths of bone, muscle and fat in the upper arm and calf from age 3–18 years. *Ann. Hum. Biol.* 8, 495–517.

Chapter 3

Development of Anaerobic Power and Local Muscular Endurance

OMRI INBAR

Introduction

Anaerobic energy production is important for the growing child because many of the activities of children involve bursts of energy expenditure (or sprints) rather than activities of moderate intensity for extended periods of time. The energy needs of the exercising child thus cannot always be met by the oxidative properties of the working skeletal muscles. Anaerobic energy production mechanisms must come into play to permit such activities.

Until the mid-1960s, exercise-related research focused on the young adult or the middle-aged individual. Recent years have witnessed a surge of interest among exercise scientists in the child and young adolescent. A major impetus for such interest has been the increasing involvement of children in advanced level athletics. In the 1990s, preadolescent athletes are often exposed to training regimens which only a decade ago were considered too demanding even for adult athletes. As a result, in such sports as gymnastics, ice-skating, tennis and swimming, champions and record-holders are younger than ever before.

The contribution of the alactacid and lactacid systems to physical performance has received much deserved attention in recent years. Many tests have been devised to assess anaerobic power and endurance for the evaluation of anaerobic fitness levels and to examine anaerobic training effects. Tests have measured both physiological and performance variables.

Physiological parameters examined have included oxygen debt, and postexercise blood and muscle lactate and substrate levels. However, these tests are invasive and/or require sophisticated equipment and therefore are not feasible for mass testing. Performance tests, on the other hand, are non-invasive, simple and inexpensive to administer, and although providing no direct physiological data, are assumed to reflect the maximal anaerobic ability of the subject (Margaria *et al.*, 1966; Di Prampero & Cerretelli, 1969; Thorstensson & Karlsson, 1976; Inbar & Bar-Or, 1977b; Bar-Or & Inbar, 1978; Bar-Or *et al.*, 1980; Inbar *et al.*, 1981; Sargent *et al.*, 1984; Inbar, 1985; Mackova *et al.*, 1985; Watson & Sargent, 1986; Denis *et al.*, 1992).

A widely used measure of anaerobic power is provided by the peak power (PP) output generated during the first or second $2.5-5$-s interval of the all-out 30-s cycle ride of the Wingate anaerobic test (WAnT) (Inbar & Bar-Or, 1977a,b, 1986; Kurowski, 1977; Bar-Or, 1983; Tharp *et al.*, 1985; Maud & Shultz, 1989; Denis *et al.*, 1992). Performance during such a task (5 s), depends predominantly on the adenosine triphosphate (ATP)−creatine phosphate system, with creatine kinase being the rate-limiting enzyme, or the capacity to replenish ATP by means of the immediately available muscle sources of energy. A commonly used measure of local (legs or arms) muscular endurance is the WAnT 30-s mean power (MP) output or total work. Maximal performance of such a duration (30 s), depends predominantly on the anaerobic glycolytic system. Control of glycolysis is determined largely by the catalytic and regulatory properties of two enzymes, phosphofructokinase (PFK) and phosphorylase. (For more details about tests of anaerobic performance see Chapter 36.)

The following discussion is based predominantly, but not exclusively, on data obtained from various studies using WAnT which has proved to be both valid and reliable (Inbar, 1985; Inbar & Bar-Or, 1986; Blimkie et al., 1988; Saavedra et al., 1991).

In order to assess reliably the stability (or instability) of anaerobic performance across age during childhood and adolescence, longitudinal data are necessary. There are, nevertheless, very few studies from which such data are available (Parizkova, 1974; Verschuur, 1987; Beunen et al., 1992). These studies, however, have all used field-type performance tests for the measurement of anaerobic power and/or muscular endurance.

This chapter, while attempting to compare the anaerobic characteristics during childhood, adolescence and young adulthood, will be limited, therefore, to cross-sectional data. Furthermore, some morphological determinants of anaerobic performance change during growth. Muscle mass, for example, increases with age, particularly during and after the adolescent growth spurt in males. This may have a direct consequence on the absolute anaerobic power output that can be generated. Metabolic and biomechanical performance parameters are also influenced by age. These factors, in turn, contribute to the differences in energy cost, work and efficiency during exercise. Children are typically smaller, have shorter legs, causing their stride frequency during walking or running to be greater and their stride length to be shorter than in adults. However, the ratio of stride length to leg length may be similar at any given age. Maximum flexion angle and total range of motion of the knee joint are also significantly different between children and adults and, therefore, may be responsible, at least

partially, for the age-related differences in running as well as in cycling and other leg-generated power and endurance activities (Inbar et al., 1983; Sargent & Dolan, 1986; Ebbeling et al., 1992).

There is ample evidence to show that work efficiency during aerobic-type activities increases with age, ranging between 15 and 22% in children and 25 and 35% in adults (Bar-Or, 1983; Ebbeling et al., 1992). Although no published data are available, it is reasonable to assume that such, and probably even greater, differences in work efficiency exist during anaerobic-type work between children and adults. Thus, we should not expect a 6-year-old child to run or cycle as fast or as far as a teenager who, in turn, is slower and weaker than a young adult. Similarly, a child cannot share the same absolute muscle strength as the more mature individual. Therefore, part of the differences between children and adults in anaerobic performance may result from geometrical (quantitative) differences which must be taken into consideration when comparing populations of different sizes.

Logically, normalization of anaerobic power should be based on the size of the effective muscle mass involved in power generation. However, such a measurement (volume of active muscle mass) requires specialized facilities and is time-consuming. Other scaling criteria such as total body mass (kg) and fat-free mass (FFM) have been employed to analyse and interpret anaerobic data when growth- or age-related trends are sought. Obviously, relating power output values to overall body mass instead of the muscle mass that is involved in the actual production of power output implies an accountable error. However, it is attractive in terms of feasibility and simplicity. The incorporated error of such a crude reference unit, especially if trend analysis is at stake, has been reported to be relatively small (Inbar & Bar-Or, 1980; Blimkie et al., 1988; Saavedra et al., 1991).

The purpose of this chapter is to examine the relationship between anaerobic performance and growth. An attempt will be made to compare anaerobic-type data among various age groups, in both absolute (growth dependent) and relative (growth independent) terms, in order to isolate the true quantitative (size related) and the qualitative (size independent), factors which affect the changes in anaerobic performance during the growth period in females and males.

Age differences

Figure 3.1 illustrates changes in absolute and relative (to body mass) leg power output for the highest 5-s measurement (PP) and for the total work generated (MP) during the 30-s WAnT for measuring anaerobic power and muscle endurance in a cross-sectional sample of 150 untrained boys aged 8–18 years (Inbar, 1985; Inbar & Bar-Or, 1986). To allow for intra- and interstudy comparisons despite differences in testing procedures, protocols and populations, a common scale is used where values are shown as a percentage, taking the value at 18 (or 19) years as 100%.

Absolute as well as relative (to body mass)

PP output increase with age throughout the entire growth period. However, while absolute anaerobic power at ages 8 and 16 is only 30–40% and 75–85% of that at age 18, respectively, relative (body mass independent) anaerobic power in the respective ages is already 70–80% and 85–90% of that at age 18, indicating the important role of body mass (and thus muscle mass) in the age-associated increase in anaerobic power. The same trend is evident for the total work output in 30 s (muscle endurance), namely, linear and relatively steep increase of absolute muscle endurance and continuous yet much slower increase of relative (to body mass) muscle endurance (MP · kg^{-1}).

Figure 3.2 illustrates the same age-related progression but for the arms (85 boys performing the WAnT) (Inbar, 1985; Inbar & Bar-Or, 1986). A very similar pattern of arm muscle anaerobic power and endurance development to that of the legs is apparent, suggesting parallel developmental growth pattern of anaerobic performance in various muscle groups. Thus, the short-term anaerobic power (PP) and local muscle endurance capacity (MP) of boys

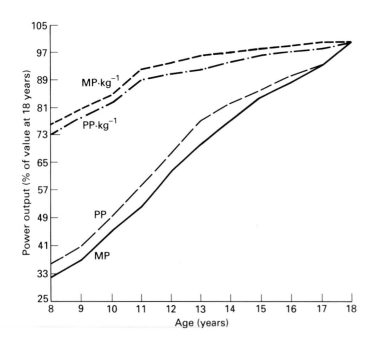

Fig. 3.1 Age-related differences in absolute and relative (to body mass) leg anaerobic power in 150 males aged 8–18 years old, presented as percentage of value at age 18. MP, mean power; PP, peak power. Data from Inbar (1985) and Inbar and Bar-Or (1986).

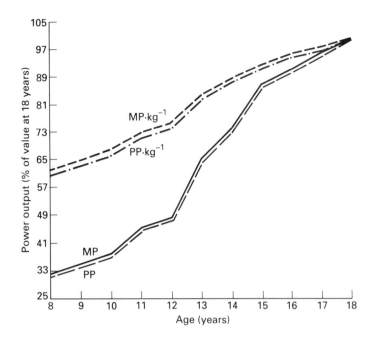

Fig. 3.2 Age-related differences in absolute and relative (to body mass) arm anaerobic power in 85 males aged 8−18 years old, presented as percentage of value at age 18. MP, mean power; PP, peak power. Data from Inbar (1985) and Inbar and Bar-Or (1986).

are less than those of young adults, even after adjustment for body mass (though to a much lesser degree). A similar age-related progression in anaerobic-type activities has been reported by other authors using not only the WAnT, but other anaerobic tests as well (Morse *et al.*, 1949; Di Prampero & Cerretelli, 1969; Davies *et al.*, 1972; Parizkova, 1974; Kindermann *et al.*, 1975; Kurowski, 1977; Paterson *et al.*, 1981; Berger, 1982; Verschuur, 1987; Matsudo, 1988; Weijiang & Juxiang, 1988; Barabas & Eiben, 1991; Beunen *et al.*, 1992). It seems therefore, that the adult− child differences in anaerobic power and muscle endurance persist even after controlling for muscle mass, height squared, lean body mass or active muscle cross-sectional area (Davies *et al.*, 1972; Komi & Karlsson, 1979; Berger, 1982; Inbar & Bar-Or, 1986; Blimkie *et al.*, 1988; Malina & Bouchard, 1991; Saavedra *et al.*, 1991).

Figure 3.3 illustrates age-related changes in leg anaerobic power and endurance in a cross-sectional sample of 84 untrained girls 9−19 years old, performing a repetitive one-legged maximal knee flexion and extensions on a modified Hydra-Gym dynamometer (Saavedra *et al.*, 1991). Unlike males, both absolute and relative values in females increase only from age 9 to around age 15 with no further increase in anaerobic performance thereafter. The absol- ute total work output in 10 and 30 s (anaerobic power and endurance, respectively) of 9-year- old preadolescent girls was about one-third of the performance of the 15- or 19-year-old females. On average, the maximal anaerobic performance relative to body mass during both the 10- and 30-s knee extension tests at the age of 9 years was about two-thirds that observed at age 15 or 19 years.

Maximal anaerobic performance, whether expressed as absolute values or per kilogram of body weight, per kilogram of FFM or per square centimetre of lean cross-sectional area of the thigh increases with age until 15 years. This suggests, like in males, that at least until that age, factors other than just the muscle mass must be involved in the observed age-related differences in maximal muscle endurance between girls and women.

Group values for arm power and endurance of 80 9−19-year-old females who performed the arm WAnT (Inbar, 1985 for ages 9−13 years; Blimkie *et al.*, 1988 for ages 14−19 years), are

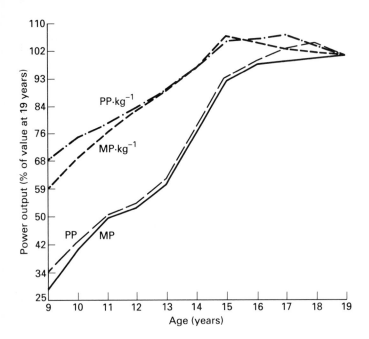

Fig. 3.3 Age-related differences in absolute and relative (to body mass) leg anaerobic power in 84 females aged 9−19 years old, presented as percentage of value at age 19. MP, mean power; PP, peak power. Data from Saavedra *et al.* (1991).

shown in Fig. 3.4. Here too, data are presented in percentage, taking values at age 19 as 100%.

Absolute PP and MP increased sharply between 9 and 14−16 years of age with no further increase thereafter. Relative values (PP·kg^{-1} and MP·kg^{-1}) follow a similar trend but, again, at a much slower rate. While both absolute arm PP and MP at the age of 9 years were on average some 45−55% of those at age 15−19 years, relative arm power and endurance at the age of 9 were already 80−90% those of 15 or 19 year olds. Hence, it seems that in females, as in males, arm and leg anaerobic performance is also predominantly, but not solely, growth (muscle mass?) related.

Unlike for maximal aerobic power in which children are on a par with adults (in relative terms (Robinson, 1938; Åstrand, 1952; Davies, 1971; Davies *et al.*, 1972; Bar-Or, 1983), anaerobic performance is lower in the child in absolute and relative terms alike, whether scaled to body weight, height squared, lean body mass or limb lean volume (Davies *et al.*, 1972; Berger, 1982; Murphy *et al.*, 1984; Inbar, 1985; Inbar & Bar-Or, 1986; Blimkie *et al.*, 1988; Malina & Bouchard, 1991; Saavedra *et al.*, 1991).

However, and as shown above, some of the observed age-associated variation in anaerobic performance is most likely related to variation in muscle mass rather than to any other factors (as indicated by the much slower rate of increase in relative than in absolute anaerobic performance). Nevertheless, these trends suggest that age-related differences in anaerobic performance cannot be explained merely by differences in body size or in the active muscle mass (as indicated by the continuous, although slower, increase in the weight-adjusted anaerobic power and endurance). Therefore, qualitative rather than quantitative characteristics of the muscle, or the nature of its motor unit activation must be responsible for the remaining age-related differences in the body mass independent anaerobic performance capacity in females and males alike.

Gender differences

As demonstrated above, it is apparent that, in males, anaerobic power as well as muscular endurance increase with age when expressed in absolute terms or per kilogram of body

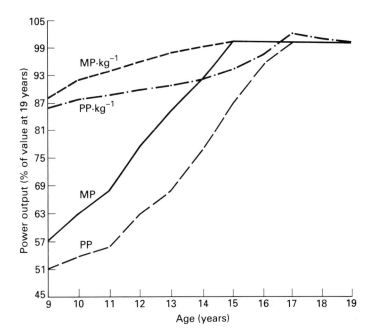

Fig. 3.4 Age-related differences in absolute and relative (to body mass) arm anaerobic power in 80 females aged 9–19 years old, presented as percentage of value at age 19. MP, mean power; PP, peak power. Data from Inbar (1985 for ages 9–13) and Blimkie *et al.* (1988 for ages 14–19 years).

mass, throughout the entire growth period. In girls, on the other hand, anaerobic performance improves only until just after puberty and then remains constant or even slightly reduced. On average, and based on the actual power output data reported in the above-mentioned original studies (Blimkie *et al.*, 1988; Inbar, 1985; Inbar & Bar-Or, 1986; Saavedra *et al.*, 1991), no meaningful differences are observed in absolute leg anaerobic power or endurance between girls and boys at 9–11 years of age. However, significant differences appear between genders from 13 years of age on. For these older age groups, leg PP and MP of girls represent about 75% those of boys. When expressed per kilogram of body mass, leg PP of girls is significantly lower than in boys, already from the age of 11. For these age groups, leg $PP \cdot kg^{-1}$ represents about 85% that of boys at age 12 and about 70% at the age of 18 years. Similar gender-related differences have been reported using other test protocols (Wirth *et al.*, 1978; Gregor *et al.*, 1979; Berger, 1982; Bar-Or, 1983; Simoneau *et al.*, 1983; Sargent *et al.*, 1984; Verschuur, 1987; Matsudo, 1988; Barabas & Eiben, 1991; Bouchard, 1991; Beunen *et al.*,

1992) and/or other relevant reference measures (FFM or thigh cross-sectional area) (Berger, 1982; Murphy *et al.*, 1984; Verschuur, 1987; Weijiang & Juxiang, 1988; Serresse *et al.*, 1989; Simoneau & Bouchard, 1989; Barabas & Eiben, 1991; Malina & Bouchard, 1991; Beunen *et al.*, 1992).

As for the arm anaerobic performance, boys have significantly larger absolute PP and MP than girls at each age. From age 9 to 12, arm PP and MP of girls represent about 85% those of boys. These gender differences in absolute arm anaerobic power and endurance increase with age, with girls reaching only 50% those of boys at the age of 19 years. When normalized for body mass and/or arm volume, arm PP and MP are still about 13% lower in girls already at the age of 9 years, with the gender-related differences increasing steadily and reaching 25% at age 19 (Inbar, 1985; Inbar & Bar-Or 1986; Blimkie *et al.*, 1988). These findings are also concordant with previous cross-sectional or longitudinal studies that have used other arm testing procedures in children and adolescents (Parizkova, 1974; Berger, 1982; Verschuur, 1987; Bouchard, 1991; Beunen *et al.*, 1992).

It seems that gender differences in both

absolute and relative anaerobic performance appear before the onset of male puberty and continue to widen throughout the growth period.

As in the case of age-related differences, these observations suggest that even when divided by total body mass, FFM of muscle or even muscle cross-sectional area, gender-related differences in anaerobic performance cannot be explained merely by differences in body size or in the volume of the active muscle. If this is indeed so, then gender-related differences in anaerobic performance must also be explained in part by qualitative factors such as hormonal variation, qualitative characteristics of the muscle, or the nature of the activation of the motor units.

Possible underlying mechanisms

Hormonal mechanisms

Male hormones are important regulators of protein synthesis. Adult males have about 10 times the activity level of androgens, compared with prepubertal children or adult women (Florini, 1987). Assuming all other factors being equal, maximal strength and strength-gaining potential is not possible until adult levels of androgens are achieved. Therefore, physical performance in children and adolescents must always be assessed in the light of the growth process. Growth involves a series of developmental stages that are remarkably similar in all people. Individual differences in diet, exercise and health may affect these stages to a certain extent, but the basic pattern remains the same. Each stage has a profound influence on individual capability for physical performance.

During the pubertal growth spurt in height (peak height velocity, PHV), muscle grows at a rapid rate, particularly in boys. The increase in muscle tissue typically occurs slightly after the PHV (Florini, 1987; Malina & Bouchard, 1991). Such an increase in muscle size is related, especially in boys, to a significant elevation in male hormone production (principally tes-

tosterone). Logically, if the observed body mass independent increase in anaerobic performance is influenced predominantly by hormonal changes that occur primarily during the growth spurt period, peak power velocity (PPV) should coincide with PHV. In a recent study on boys of various developmental stages (Falk & Bar-Or, 1993), it was found that peak and mean anaerobic power (in $W \cdot kg^{-1}$) differ among maturation groups, suggesting hormonal (maturation) influence on muscle power and endurance.

One way of probing such possibilities would be to establish an age-associated rate of increase in anaerobic power and verify matching (or mismatching) between PPV and PHV. Figure 3.5 illustrates the half-yearly rate of change in leg and arm muscular endurance based on the above reported cross-sectional data. In males, leg muscle endurance increases by about 10% per year from age 6 to 8, with PPV ($20\% \cdot year^{-1}$) reached between ages 10 and 12 years. Thereafter, there is a continuous decline in the rate of increase, reaching $4\% \cdot year^{-1}$ between 16 and 18 years. Arm muscle endurance improvement rate shows a similar pattern, reaching peak velocity ($15\% \cdot year^{-1}$) between ages 12 and 14 years. It seems therefore, that in males leg PPV is reached just before the growth spurt (Fig. 3.5), while arm PPV is reached around the PHV. It should be noted that the year at PHV was not individually measured in our subjects, but taken from the literature (Tanner, 1962).

In females (Fig. 3.6) the rate of increase in leg and arm anaerobic performance is $8-10\% \cdot year^{-1}$ between 7 and 9 years of age, reaching PPV ($22-25\% \cdot year^{-1}$) at age $9-11$ years in both legs and arms. Thereafter, there is a steady decline in the rate of increase until age $17-19$ years were we see an actual decrease in muscle endurance (-7% and $-3\% \cdot year^{-1}$ in legs and arms, respectively). Thus, in females PPV of both arms and legs occurs prior to their assumed growth spurt.

In the light of the present information it appears that changes in muscle endurance are not solely dependent on direct hormonal

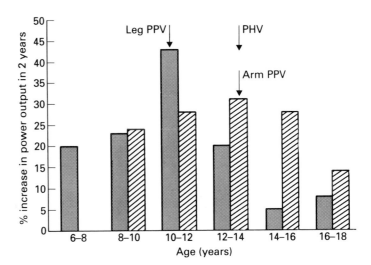

Fig. 3.5 Rate increase (per kg) in leg (□) and arm (▨) muscle endurance in males aged 6–18 years old. Data from Inbar (1985) and Inbar and Bar-Or (1986) for legs; Inbar (1985) and Blimkie *et al.* (1988) for arms. Peak height velocity (PHV) is assumed, based on the liturature (Tanner, 1962). PPV, peak power velocity.

influence, as indicated by the lack of time synchronization between PPV and PHV in both genders (Figs 3.5 & 3.6). This contention is further supported by the significant inter-gender differences in muscle endurance found already prior to their respective growth spurts (even when normalized for body or muscle mass). Thus, exclusive hormonal or sexual maturation influence on both age- and gender-related differences in anaerobic performance seems unlikely.

Biochemical mechanisms

Several studies have suggested that the bio-chemical correlates of anaerobic performance may be age or maturation dependent (Åstrand, 1952; Eriksson *et al.*, 1971, 1973; Eriksson, 1980; Matejkova *et al.*, 1980; Bar-Or, 1983; Mackova *et al.*, 1985; Inbar & Bar-Or, 1986; Blimkie *et al.*, 1988; Malina & Bouchard, 1991; Denis *et al.*, 1992). Indeed, some of the biochemical deter-minants of anaerobic performance change

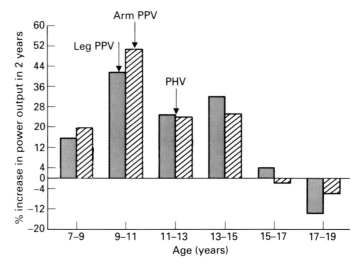

Fig. 3.6 Rate increase (per kg) in leg (□) and arm (▨) muscle endurance in females aged 7–19 years old. Data from Saavedra *et al.* (1991) for legs; Inbar (1985) and Blimkie *et al.* (1988) for arms. Peak height velocity (PHV) is assumed, based on the liturature (Tanner, 1962). PPV, peak power velocity.

during growth. The ATP and creatine phosphate concentrations in muscle tissue are about 30% less in early postnatal life than at maturity (Malina & Bouchard, 1991). Children are not able to attain high blood and muscle lactate concentrations during maximal exercise, compared to adults (Åstrand, 1952; Eriksson *et al.*, 1971; Eriksson, 1980). However, maximal blood lactate concentration increases with age during growth (Åstrand, 1952; Eriksson *et al.*, 1971, 1973; Eriksson, 1980). Muscle lactate concentration during submaximal exercise is also lower in children and adolescents, compared to adults (Åstrand, 1952; Bar-Or, 1983; Moritani *et al.*, 1989). These observations suggest that growing individuals rely less than adults on the glycogen to lactate metabolic pathway to replenish ATP during both aerobic and anaerobic exercise.

Consistent with these observations is the fact that the activity of the enzyme PFK, a major regulator of glycolysis, is lower in children and adolescents than in adults (Eriksson *et al.*, 1973; Eriksson, 1980). In addition, children and adolescents are not able to generate or sustain levels of acidosis (as indicated by blood pH or base excess) as high as those reported in adults (Kindermann *et al.*, 1975; Metejkova *et al.*, 1980; Bar-Or, 1985).

Regarding the observed lean tissue mass independent gender differences throughout the growing period, a lower glycolytic potential in female skeletal muscle as compared to male muscle has been suggested (Komi & Karlsson, 1979; Nygaard, 1981; Jacobs *et al.*, 1982; Simoneau & Bouchard, 1989; Malina & Bouchard, 1991). As in boys, this difference in glycolytic potential is thought to be a function of lower activities of key enzymes such as PFK and phosphorylase (Komi & Karlsson, 1979; Nygaard, 1981; Simoneau & Bouchard, 1989; Malina & Bouchard, 1991).

It is suggested, therefore, that the biological mechanisms associated with the production of anaerobic work and the tolerance to the related acidosis are not fully mature until some time after the adolescent growth spurt and are

inherently lower in females than in males. This translates into improvement in anaerobic performance during growth and sexual maturation in both sexes, into considerable gender differences in anaerobic performance, even when calculated per kilogram of muscle mass, at all ages, and into differences in the growth patterns of anaerobic performance.

Neurological mechanisms

Considering that a similar amount of muscle mass involved in running, cycling or knee extension tasks can generate different work outputs during maximal efforts of short duration, the pattern and percentage of muscle fibre activation as well as the angle of muscle pennation, must also be taken into account as possible contributing factors to the age-related increments in anaerobic performance (Sale, 1989). In addition, it has been shown that adult males have a greater capacity to utilize stored elastic energy of muscle, known to be produced during such activities (running, cycling, jumping), than prepubertal boys (Moritani *et al.*, 1989). If the capacity to utilize stored elastic energy in the muscles is limited in children and improves from prepubertal ages to adulthood, or is less in females than in males, differences between children and adults and between males and females in the anaerobic-type maximal performance, could also, at least partially, be explained by such mechanisms.

Conclusion

Despite some methodological limitations, the available data suggest that anaerobic performance, irrespective of gender, is closely related to body mass, and probably more so to lean tissue mass, of the growing individual. These relationships could be regarded as causal since it is likely that these variables could vary independently of each other under certain conditions, e.g. intense anaerobic training, loss or gain in FFM through diet and resistance training (Eriksson *et al.*, 1973; Inbar & Bar-Or, 1980;

Serresse *et al.*, 1989; Denis *et al.*, 1992). However it is apparent, that during growth, many modifications occur at the cellular, biochemical and physiological levels that sustain the developmental changes in anaerobic performance beyond those obtained by physical growth alone. Whether and how these modifications can explain all or parts of the remaining age- and sex-dependent characteristics of anaerobic power and endurance remain to be proved.

Challenges for future research

With the availability of newly developed technologies, it is now possible and feasible to approach scientifically the issue of anaerobic metabolism and performance (and the interaction between them) in a more profound and detailed manner than ever before (for details, see Chapter 36).

• A major effort should be directed toward tackling the prominent question of the relative contribution of growth *per se* versus other physiological and/or biochemical (including hormones) factors, to the development of anaerobic power and improved performance.

• Another issue that needs further clarification is the net effects of physical training on the overall gain in anaerobic power during the growth period. Within this line of investigation we need to identify the most effective training protocols as well as the time (age) of training commencement (for both safety and effectiveness), for optimal development of the anaerobic power and performance (for more details see Chapter 7).

• The influence of heredity on anaerobic power should also be at the front line of the scientific agenda for those interested in human performance in general and anaerobic performance in particular.

• Yet another challenging and highly important mission is the creation of large and standardized database of anaerobic performance indices, including ratios between aerobic and anaerobic indices and leg and arm anaerobic power, out of which normative values for various populations (age groups, genders, sports, diseases) could be established. Such reference values are desperately needed if an objective and accurate interpretation of anaerobic characteristics for any individual is sought.

References

Åstrand, P.O. (1952) *Experimental Studies of Physical Working Capacity in Relation to Sex and Age*, pp. 94–117. Munksgaard, Copenhagen.

Barabas, A. & Eiben, O.G. (1991) Changes in physical performance related to age and biological development. In R. Frenkl & I. Szmodis (eds) *Children and Exercise Paediatric Work Physiology*, Vol. XV, pp. 100–6. National Institute for Health Promotion, Budapest.

Bar-Or, O. (1983) *Paediatric Sports Medicine for the Practitioner: From Physiological Principles to Clinical Application*. Springer-Verlag, New York.

Bar-Or, O., Dotan, R., Inbar, O. *et al.* (1980) Anaerobic capacity and muscle fiber distribution in man. *Int. J. Sports Med.* **1**, 82–5.

Bar-Or, O. & Inbar, O. (1978) Relationship among anaerobic capacity, sprint, and middle distance running of school children. In R.J. Shephard & H. Lavallee (eds) *Physical Fitness Assessment*, pp. 142–7. C.C. Thomas, Springfield, IL.

Berger, R.A. (1982) *Applied Exercise Physiology*, pp. 15–26. Lea & Febiger, Philadelphia.

Beunen, G.P., Malina, R.M., Renson, R., Simons, J., Ostyn, M. & Lefever, J. (1992) Physical activity and growth, maturation and performance: a longitudinal study. *Med. Sci. Sports Exerc.* **24**, 576–85.

Blimkie, C.R., Roche, P., Hay, J.T. & Bar-Or, O. (1988) Anaerobic power of arms in teenage boys and girls: relationship to lean tissue. *Eur. J. Appl. Physiol.* **57**, 677–83.

Davies, C.T.M. (1971) Body composition in children: a reference standard for maximal aerobic power output on a stationary bicycle ergometer. *Acta Paediatr. Scand.* **217** (Suppl.), 136–37.

Davies, C.T.M., Barnes, C. & Godfrey, S. (1972) Body composition and maximal exercise performance in children. *Hum. Biol.* **44**, 195–214.

Denis, C., Linossier, M.T., Dormois, D., Padilla, S., Lacour, J.R. & Inbar, O. (1992) Power and metabolic responses during supramaximal exercise in 100-m and 800-m runners. *Scand. J. Med. Sci. Sports* **2**, 62–9.

Di Prampero, P.E. & Cerretelli, P. (1969) Maximal muscular power (aerobic and anaerobic) in African natives. *Ergonomics*, **12**, 51–9.

Ebbeling, C.J., Hamill, J., Freedson, P.S. & Rowland, T.W. (1992) An examination of efficiency during

walking in children and adults. *Paediatr. Exerc. Sci.*
4, 36−49.

Eriksson, B.O. (1980) Muscle metabolism in children:
a review. *Acta Paediatr. Scand.* **283** (Suppl.), 20−7.

Eriksson, B.O., Gollnick, P.D. & Saltin, B. (1973)
Muscle metabolism and enzyme activities after
training in boys 11−13 years old. *Acta Physiol.
Scand.* **87**, 485−97.

Eriksson, B.O., Karlsson, J. & Saltin, B. (1971) Muscle
metabolites during exercise in pubertal boys. *Acta
Paediatr. Scand.* **217** (Suppl.), 154−57.

Falk, B. & Bar-Or, O. (1993) Longitudinal changes in
peak aerobic and anaerobic mechanical power of
circumpubertal boys. *Paediatr. Exerc. Sci.* **5**, 318−31.

Florini, J.R. (1987) Hormonal control of muscle
growth. *Muscle Nerve* **10**, 577−98.

Gregor, R.J., Edgerton, V.R., Perrine, J.J., Campion,
D.S. & Debus, C. (1979) Torque−velocity relationships and muscle fiber composition in male and
female athletes. *J. Appl. Physiol.* **47**, 388−92.

Inbar, O. (1985) *The Wingate Anaerobic Test −
Characteristics, Applications, and Norms* (in Hebrew).
Wingate Press, Netania Israel.

Inbar, O. & Bar-Or, O. (1977a) Anaerobic capacity
and running performance of children. *Isr. J. Med.
Sci.* **13**, 1141 (abstract).

Inbar, O. & Bar-Or, O. (1977b) Relationships of
anaerobic and aerobic arm and leg capacities to
swimming performance of 8−12-year-old children.
In R.J. Shephard & H. Lavallee (eds) *Frontiers of
Activity and Child Health*, pp. 283−92. Pelican,
Quebec.

Inbar, O. & Bar-Or, O. (1980) Changes in arm and leg
performance in laboratory and field tests, following vigorous physical training. In U. Simri (ed.)
*Proceedings: International Seminar on Art and Science
in Coaching*, pp. 38−48. Wingate Institute, Netania.

Inbar, O. & Bar-Or, O. (1986) Anaerobic characteristics in male children and adolescents. *Med. Sci.
Sports Exerc.* **18**, 264−9.

Inbar, O., Dotan, R., Trousil, T. & Dvir, Z. (1983) The
effect of bicycle crank-length variation upon power
performance. *Ergonomics* **26**, 1139−46.

Inbar, O., Kaiser, P. & Tesch, P. (1981) Relationships
between leg muscle fiber-type distribution and leg
exercise performance. *Int. J. Sports Med.* **3**, 154−9.

Jacobs, I., Bar-Or, O., Karlsson, J. *et al.* (1982) Changes
in muscle metabolites in females with 30-s exhaustive exercise. *Med. Sci. Sports Exerc.* **14**, 457−60.

Kindermann, V.W., Huber, G. & Keul, J. (1975)
Anaerobic capacity in children and adolescents in
comparison with adults (in German). *Sportarzt
Sportmed.* **6**, 112−15.

Komi, P. & Karlsson, J. (1979) Physical performance,
skeletal muscle enzyme activities and fiber types in
monozygous and dizygous twins of both sexes.
Acta Physiol. Scand. **462** (Suppl.), 1−28.

Kurowski, T.T. (1977) *Anaerobic power of children from
ages 9 through 15 years*, pp. 18−43. MSc thesis,
Florida State University.

Mackova, E.V., Melichna, J., Vondra, K., Jurimae, T.,
Poul, T. & Novak, J. (1985) The relationship between
anaerobic performance and muscle metabolic
capacity and fiber distribution. *Eur. J. Appl. Physiol.*
54, 413−15.

Malina, R.M. & Bouchard, C. (1991) *Growth, Maturation, and Physical Activity*, pp. 187−235. Human
Kinetics, Champaign, IL.

Margaria, R., Aghemo, P. & Rovelli, E. (1966)
Measurement of muscular power (anaerobic) in
man. *J. Appl. Physiol.* **21**, 1662−4.

Matejkova, J., Koprivova, Z. & Placheta, Z. (1980)
Changes in acid−base balance after maximal
exercise. In Z. Placheta (ed.) *Youth and Physical
Activity*, pp. 191−9. J.E. Purkyne University, Brno.

Matsudo, V.K.R. (1988) Forty seconds run test:
perspective of a decade. *Human Biology* (Budapest)
18, 127−31.

Maud, P.J. & Shultz, B.B. (1989) Norms for the Wingate
anaerobic test with comparison to another similar
test. *Res. Q.* **60**, 144−51.

Moritani, T., Oddsson, L., Thorstensson, A. &
Astrand, P.O. (1989) Neural and biomechanical
differences between men and young boys during a
variety of motor tasks. *Acta Physiol. Scand.* **137**,
347−55.

Morse, M., Schultz, F.W. & Cassels, D.E. (1949)
Relation of age to physiological responses of the
older boy (10 to 17 years) to exercise. *J. Appl.
Physiol.* **1**, 683−709.

Murphy, M.M., Patton, J.F. & Frederick, F.A. (1984) A
comparison of anaerobic power capacity in males
and females accounting for differences in thigh
volume, body weight, and lean body mass. *Med.
Sci. Sports Exerc.* **16**, 108 (abstract).

Nygaard, E. (1981) Skeletal muscle fiber characteristics
in young women. *Acta Physiol. Scand.* **112**, 299−304.

Parizkova, J. (1974) Particularities of lean body mass
and fat development in growing boys to their
motor activity. *Acta Paediatr. Belg.* **28** (Suppl.),
232−42.

Paterson, D.H., Cunningham, D.A. & Bumstead, L.A.
(1981) Development of anaerobic capacity in boys
aged 11 to 15 years. *Can. J. Appl. Sport Sci.* **6**, 134.

Robinson, S. (1938) Experimental studies of physical
fitness in relation to age. *Arbeitsphysiology* **10**,
251−23.

Saavedra, C., Lagasse, P., Bouchard, C. & Simoneau,
J.A. (1991) Maximal anaerobic performance of the
knee extensor muscles during growth. *Med. Sci.
Sports Exerc.* **23**, 1083−9.

Sale, D.G. (1989) Strength training in children.
In C.V. Gisolfi & D.R. Lamb (eds) *Perspectives
in Exercise and Sports Medicine*, pp. 165−222.

Benchmark Press, Carmel.

Sargent, A.J. & Dolan, P. (1986) Optimal velocity of muscle contraction for short-term (anaerobic) power output in children and adults. In J. Rutenfranz, R. Mocellin & F. Klint (eds) *Children and Exercise*, Vol. XII, pp. 39–42. Human Kinetics, Champaign, IL.

Sargent, A.J., Dolan, P. & Thorn, A. (1984) Isokinetic measurement of maximal leg force and anaerobic power output in children. In J. Ilmarinen & I. Valaimaki (eds) *Children and Sports*, pp. 93–8. Springer-Verlag, Berlin.

Serresse, O., Ama, P., Simoneau, J.A., Lortie, G., Bouchard, C. & Boulay, M.R. (1989) Anaerobic performances of sedentary and trained subjects. *Can. J. Sport Sci.* **14**, 46–52.

Simoneau, J.A. & Bouchard, C. (1989) Human variation in skeletal muscle fiber type proportion and enzyme activities. *Am. J. Physiol.* **257**, E567–72.

Simoneau, J.A., Lortie, G., Boulay, M. & Bouchard, C. (1983) Tests of anaerobic alactacid and lactacid capacities: description and reliability. *Can. J. Appl. Sport Sci.* **8**, 266–70.

Tanner, J.M. (1962) *Growth at Adolescence*. Blackwell Scientific Publications, Oxford.

Tharp, G.D., Newhouse, R.K., Uffelman, L., Thorland, W.G. & Johnson, G.O. (1985) Comparison of sprint and run times with performance on the Wingate anaerobic test. *Res. Q. Exerc. Sport* **56**, 73–6.

Thorstensson, A. & Karlsson, J. (1976) Fatiguability and fiber composition of human skeletal muscle. *Acta Physiol. Scand.* **98**, 318–22.

Verschuur, R. (1987) *Daily Physical Activity and Health. Longitudinal Changes During the Teenage Period*, pp. 21–157. De Vrieseborch, Haarlem.

Watson, R.C. & Sargent, T.L.C. (1986) Laboratory and on-ice comparisons of anaerobic power of ice hockey players. *Can. J. Appl. Sport Sci.* **11**, 218–24.

Weijiang, D. & Juxiang, Q. (1988) Anaerobic performance of Chinese untrained and trained 11–18-year-old boys and girls. *Med. Sport Sci.* **28**, 52–6.

Wirth, A., Trager, E., Scheele, K. *et al.* (1978) Cardiopulmonary adjustment and metabolic response to maximal and submaximal physical exercise of boys and girls at different stages of maturity. *Eur. J. Appl. Physiol.* **39**, 229–40.

Chapter 4

Cardiorespiratory and Metabolic Responses to Exercise: Maturation and Growth

DAN M. COOPER

Introduction

Exercise and the physical activity of daily living represent critical and frequently occurring tests of the child's ability to maintain cellular homeostasis. Even seemingly simple activities such as walking result in increased cellular demand for energy by 10- or 20-fold. The sudden activation of aerobic and anaerobic metabolic pathways to replenish high-energy phosphates consumed as muscles do physical work is accompanied by increased cellular carbon dioxide (CO_2) production. Muscular work is possible because of elaborate systems of intracellular buffering, regulation of substrate metabolism, and oxygen (O_2) and CO_2 transport. The ways in which energy metabolism at the cellular level is linked to respiratory and cardiac function are not yet fully understood.

When considering the regulation of metabolic and cardiorespiratory activity during exercise in the growing child, additional factors become important. Maturational or growth-related changes in the pattern of daily physical activity, control of breathing, CO_2 storage, neuroendocrine control of substrate utilization, and enzymatic profile of muscle tissue can each influence the linkage between cellular activity and cardiopulmonary response. Moreover, there is mounting evidence that the vigorous and frequent bouts of exercise universally observed in children can themselves play a role in the process of growth and development. The observation that exercise is one of the major physiological stimuli of growth hormone (GH) release (Hunter *et al.*, 1965), along with current understanding of growth factors (e.g. insulin-like growth factor-1, IGF-1) suggest specific ways in which the physiological importance of the physical activity of daily life can be viewed in the child. This chapter will review a number of fundamental aspects of the regulation of metabolism during exercise and how metabolic and cardiorespiratory responses are linked. In particular, the focus will be on maturation of cardiorespiratory responses to exercise and on the underlying mechanisms that may be responsible for growth-related changes in the exercise response.

High- and low-intensity exercise

The hormonal and metabolic responses to exercise are not linearly related to the work rate input. For example, one of the earliest observations made of the metabolic responses to exercise was that lactate concentrations become elevated in the blood only when exercise is performed above a certain level. This observation eventually led to the concept of the anaerobic or lactate threshold (AT or LT) denoting a specific metabolic rate during exercise above which lactic acid concentration in the blood increases (Wasserman *et al.*, 1973). The concept of the threshold has engendered a great deal of research and a modicum of controversy (Katz & Sahlin, 1988). Identifying the AT by measuring gas exchange is possible because the predominate intracellular buffer is bicarbonate. When lactic acid is produced during anaerobic metabolism, the accompanying hydrogen ion is buffered and additional CO_2 is produced. Using breath-to-breath measurements of gas exchange, the point at which CO_2 production increases out of proportion to the O_2 uptake, indicates the AT (Wasserman et al., 1981). The AT or LT are discussed in greater detail in Shephard (1992).

We have found it useful to consider low-intensity exercise as work performed below the subject's AT and high-intensity exercise as above AT work. High-intensity exercise is accompanied by non-linear increases in catecholamines, GH responses, and blood glucose turnover when compared with low-intensity work (Cooper et al., 1989). These observations form a practical and physiological basis for this relatively simple division of exercise intensity.

Maturation of oxygen uptake responses to exercise

Previous studies of the $\dot{V}O_2$ response to constant work rate, low-intensity exercise have demonstrated that the steady-state $\dot{V}O_2$ is achieved by 3 min (approximately six time constants) (Lamarra, 1982). But when adults perform constant work rate, cycle ergometer, exercise in the high-intensity range the difference between the $\dot{V}O_2$ at 6 and 3 min is positive; indicating that the attainment of a steady-state is delayed if ever achieved (Roston et al., 1987; Casaburi et al., 1989). The high correlation between lactate concentration and the magnitude of the O_2 drift in adults (as indicated by the slope in the $\dot{V}O_2$ response between 3 and 6 min of exercise) prompted speculation that the O_2 drift was in fact related to lactate metabolism (Roston et al., 1987; Casaburi et al., 1989).

Children reach lower lactate concentrations and are less able to sustain exercise in the high-intensity range compared with adults (Bar-Or, 1983). These observations suggest that the magnitude of the O_2 drift would likely be lower in children. This hypothesis was tested in our laboratory (Armon et al., 1991a) by examining the dynamic $\dot{V}O_2$ response to exercise in a group of adults and children. Studies were done over a range of work rates from below to above the AT of the subject. The results are shown in Fig. 4.1. The data demonstrate that the pattern of the $\dot{V}O_2$ response to high-intensity exercise is both qualitatively and quantitatively different in children. Fewer children than adults develop an O_2 drift during high-intensity exercise. And in children, the magnitude of the drift both in absolute terms and when normalized to body weight is smaller and not correlated with work intensity.

Current theory holds that the rate of adenosine

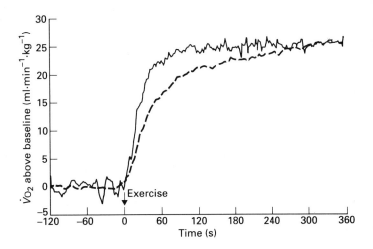

Fig. 4.1 Group mean $\dot{V}O_2$ response (normalized to body weight, above baseline) to the same above lactate threshold (LT) work rate exercise ($2\,W \cdot kg^{-1}$) in children (solid line) and adults (dashed line). Note the lack of a $\dot{V}O_2$ slope in children compared with adults. In addition, note the slower $\dot{V}O_2$ kinetics in adults compared with children. By contrast, $\dot{V}O_2$ kinetics at the onset of low-intensity (below LT) exercise are the same in children and young adults. From Armon et al. (1991).

triphosphate (ATP) degradation with increasing concentration of adenosine diphosphate (ADP) in contracting muscle cells stimulates mitochondrial oxidative phosphorylation (Chance et al., 1985). For low-intensity exercise, O_2 is sufficiently available so that ATP regeneration is supplied solely by oxidative phosphorylation. Consequently, $\dot{V}O_2$ and concentrations of ADP, phosphocreatine (PCr), inorganic phosphate (Pi) and O_2 at the cellular level all reach new steady-states relatively quickly. But during heavy exercise, insufficient availability of cellular O_2 leads to anaerobic regeneration of ATP and net lactate release. Increasing lactate concentrations could stimulate metabolism of lactate to glucose via the Cori cycle (an O_2-dependent process) or the oxidation of lactate in muscle cells (McGilvery, 1983; Wasserman, 1986). Additionally, the acidification of the blood in the muscle circulation may progressively shift the oxyhaemoglobin dissociation curve to the right. This would facilitate unbinding of O_2 and increase local and, perhaps, total body $\dot{V}O_2$ (Wasserman et al., 1991). As noted, lactate levels are known to be lower at comparable levels of work intensity in children

compared with adults (Eriksson et al., 1971; Paterson et al., 1986). Thus, our finding of smaller O_2 drifts in children is consistent with the hypothesis that the O_2 drift reflects metabolism of lactic acid.

Maturation of $\dot{V}O_2$ responses to exercise was also examined in our laboratory by using experimental protocols which would, to some extent, mimic patterns of exercise found in the daily life of children (Zanconato et al., 1991). We found that the response to, and recovery from 1-min bursts of exercise reveal much about the integrated cardiorespiratory adjustment to changes in metabolic rate (Fig. 4.2). The data from these kinds of experiments can be analysed in several ways. First, the total, O_2 cost of exercise can be determined by integrating the $\dot{V}O_2$ with respect to time from the onset of exercise to the return of the $\dot{V}O_2$ to pre-exercise values. Moreover, since cycle ergometry permits a precise assessment of the actual work being performed, the O_2 cost can be normalized to the external work performed (e.g. ml $O_2 \cdot J^{-1}$). This allows the investigator to compare O_2 costs in children and adults.

Second, the time course of the exercise

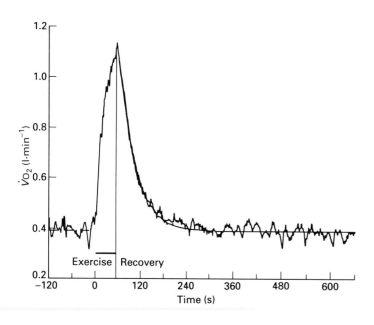

Fig. 4.2 O_2 uptake response to 1 min of high-intensity exercise (125% of the maximal work rate) in an 8-year-old girl. The cumulative O_2 cost was normalized to the external work performed (ml $O_2 \cdot J^{-1}$) in order to compare adults to children and to determine the effect of different work intensities. In addition, the time constant for $\dot{V}O_2$ recovery can be calculated. From Zanconato et al. (1991).

response (e.g. $\dot{V}o_2$) can be determined. In our laboratory, we used a single exponential model for the recovery kinetics with the equation:

$$\Delta\dot{V}o_{2(t)} = \Delta\dot{V}o_{2(\text{end exercise})} \cdot e^{-t/\tau}$$

where $\Delta\dot{V}o_2$ is the difference between pre-exercise $\dot{V}o_2$ and either the $\dot{V}o_2$ at time t into recovery or the $\dot{V}o_2$ at end-exercise; and τ is the time constant and corresponds to the time required to achieve about 63% of the response.

It is noteworthy that in both adults and children over 50% of the total O_2 used for 1-min exercise occurred during the recovery period. The significantly greater cumulative O_2 cost in children at virtually all work rates was the major difference between the groups (Fig. 4.3). In addition, the $\dot{V}o_2$ recovery time was prolonged in adults at the highest work rate. (These observations were corroborated recently by Hebestreit et al., 1993, who studied children at even higher work rates than those used in our studies.) Surprisingly, we found that the

$\dot{V}o_2$ recovery times and cumulative O_2 cost were minimally affected by work rate in both adults and children. The data suggest that the mechanisms responsible for the $\dot{V}o_2$ adaptation to short bursts of exercise are robust across work intensities in both adults and children and that there are identifiable ways in which these processes mature in healthy humans.

There are several possible mechanisms for the higher total O_2 costs in children. Substrate utilization itself can modify the relationship between $\dot{V}o_2$ and work rate because the P:O (high-energy phosphate to O_2) ratio is 2.82 for fats and 3 for glucose (McGilvery, 1983). If children metabolized solely fat and adults only glucose (which is highly unlikely), then the difference in O_2 cost could be no more than 6%. But the difference we observed was, on average, almost 40% greater in children, and, therefore, inconsistent with a growth-related difference in substrate utilization.

The larger O_2 cost in children could reflect a greater influence of O_2-requiring processes, such as thermoregulation, that accompany muscular work (Kleiber, 1975). But heat loss during exercise in children is likely to be facilitated by their larger ratio of surface area to body mass, and this would tend to reduce rather than increase any additional O_2 requirement for the maintenance of temperature homeostasis. Other O_2-dependent processes like cardiac or respiratory work are small in magnitude and unlikely to account for the differences in cumulative O_2 cost that we observed between adults and children (Casaburi et al., 1989).

There is a particularly intriguing (albeit hypothetical) explanation for the greater O_2 cost in children. Bessman (1987) theorized that the creatine phosphate shuttle which, during exercise, acts primarily to transport high-energy phosphate between the mitochondrion and the myofibril might also act to increase energy supply to the microsome and thereby stimulate protein synthesis. Perhaps, the increased O_2 cost of exercise observed in children represents a growth-related

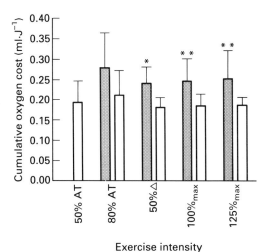

Fig. 4.3 Cumulative O_2 cost $\cdot J^{-1}$ at different work intensities in adults (□) and children (▨). Values are given as mean ± SD. The cumulative O_2 cost was not affected by increasing work intensity in children and adults. However, the cost was significantly higher in children compared to adults at 50%△ (*$P < 0.001$), 100%$_{max}$ and 125%$_{max}$ (**$P < 0.01$). AT, anaerobic threshold. From Zanconato et al. (1991).

phenomenon whereby exercise itself induces O_2-dependent, growth-related processes to a greater extent in children compared with adults.

Do higher values of $\dot{V}_{O_2} \cdot W^{-1}$ indicate a more effective cardiorespiratory response to exercise in children, or, alternatively, do the higher values result from a less developed ability of children to support anaerobic ('O_2 sparing') mechanisms of ATP metabolism? Bar-Or and others have suggested that children are less able than adults to sustain exercise in supramaximal range, indicating a reduced anaerobic 'potential' in children (Eriksson, 1980; Bar-Or, 1983; Paterson et al., 1986). Lower lactate levels found during exercise in children are consistent with their relatively reduced ability to utilize anaerobic, glycolytic processes for ATP turnover. In one investigation of glycolytic enzymes in children during exercise (Eriksson et al., 1971), lower levels of phosphofructokinase (PFK) were found in 11–13-year-old children compared with young adults. In addition, studies in rats showed a 17-fold increase in total PFK activity occurring during the first 2 months or age (equivalent to the period of birth to puberty in humans). This was accompanied by a dramatic decrease in C-type PFK subunit and increase in M-type subunit, the isozyme best suited for glycolysis (Dunaway et al., 1990).

Maturation of the muscle metabolic response to exercise might be related to the hormonal changes (increases in testosterone, oestradiol, GH and IGF-1) occurring during puberty (Marshall & Tanner, 1986). To date, little is known about the effect of these hormones on functional and structural muscle growth. Testosterone has been shown to increase sarcotubular and mitochondrial enzymes in mature male subjects (Saborido et al., 1991). In addition, Kelly et al. (1983) demonstrated that testosterone administration stimulated the transition from type IIa (fast oxidative glycolytic) to type IIb (fast glycolytic) fibres in guinea pig temporalis muscles.

The finding of lower blood lactate levels during exercise in children (either in the blood, as noted above, or in the muscle; Eriksson et al., 1971) might be used to support the idea of a reduced anaerobic potential in children. But lactate levels alone cannot be used to determine overall lactate metabolism since blood or tissue lactate concentration is determined by the balance between production and removal. Children may metabolize lactate more quickly than adults. The latter mechanism is not inconsistent with our results. The higher $\dot{V}_{O_2} \cdot W^{-1}$ seen in children at all work intensities could indicate a greater ability to oxidize the lactate produced during exercise. In this context, it is noteworthy that the neonatal heart muscle is less sensitive to hypoxia than the adult myocardium, specifically because of the greater capacity of the neonate for anaerobic glycolysis and more rapid removal of lactate (Su & Friedman, 1973; Chiu & Bindon, 1987).

Although the recovery $\tau\dot{V}_{O_2}$ in children tended to be smaller (i.e. faster recovery) in children at all work intensities, $\tau\dot{V}_{O_2}$ was significantly faster than adults only at $125\%_{max}$ (children 35 s; adults 46 s). We also found that the $\tau\dot{V}_{O_2}$ at the onset of exercise was the same in children and teenagers for low-intensity exercise (Cooper et al., 1985; Springer et al., 1989). Thus, the developmental changes in exercise O_2 transport reflect mechanisms primarily involved in the adjustment to high-intensity exercise. As noted, the metabolism of lactate produced during above AT exercise may explain the slower $\dot{V}_{O_2}$ responses, thus, the slower $\dot{V}_{O_2}$ kinetics at the highest work rate in the adults suggest greater anaerobic metabolism under these conditions in older compared with younger subjects.

Magnetic resonance spectroscopy studies of muscles during exercise in children

The difficulty in determining whether children have reduced anaerobic capacity or increased aerobic efficiency may be lessened with the use of phosphorus nuclear magnetic resonance spectroscopy (^{31}P MRS). This technique provides non-invasive means of monitoring Pi, PCr and pH (Chance *et al.*, 1986), that are acceptable for studies in children. These variables, in turn, allow the assessment of muscle oxidative metabolism and intramuscular glycolytic activity (Chance *et al.*, 1986). We hypothesized that the growth-related changes in whole-body O$_2$ uptake and O$_2$ cost of exercise observed during high-intensity exercise reflect a maturation of the kinetics of high-energy phosphate metabolites in muscle tissue. This hypothesis was tested by examining Pi, PCr, β-ATP and pH kinetics in calf muscles during progressive incremental exercise (Zanconato *et al.*, 1993). Results obtained from 10 children (age range, 7–10 years) were compared with eight adults (20–42 years).

^{31}P MRS spectra from the calf muscles during single leg, treadle exercise in a representative child is shown in Fig. 4.4. Examples of Pi:PCr and pH changes during exercise in one adult and one child are shown in Fig. 4.5 and 4.6. The study showed that during high-intensity exercise muscle Pi:PCr ratio increases to a smaller extent in children compared with adults even when the data are scaled appropriately for body size. In addition, children show a smaller drop in intramuscular pH. A slow and fast phase of Pi:PCr increase and pH decrease

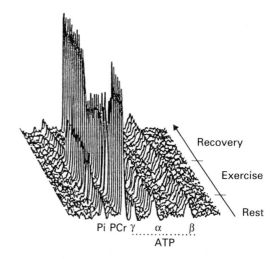

Fig. 4.4 ^{31}P MRS spectra from the right calf of an 8-year-old boy at rest, during incremental exercise, and recovery. ATP, adenosine triphosphate; PCr, phosphocreatine; Pi, inorganic phosphate. From Zanconato *et al.* (1993).

were noted in 75% of the adults and 50% of the children. We speculate that the transition between the slow and fast phases of the Pi:PCr slope represents the cellular mechanisms ultimately responsible for the gas exchange correlates of the AT. And similar to the AT, the transition of the Pi:PCr slopes occurred at a higher percentage of the overall work done in

Fig. 4.5 Pi:PCr (□) and pH (■) at rest and during incremental exercise in a 33-year-old man. The arrows indicate the transition points between the slow and fast phases of Pi:PCr increase and pH reduction. Exercise intensity was regulated by a pneumatic device and normalized to body weight. From Zanconato *et al.* (1993).

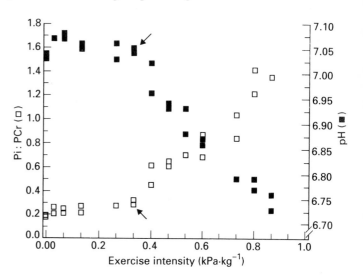

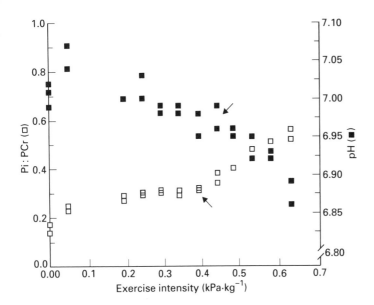

Fig. 4.6 Pi : PCr (□) and pH (■) at rest and during incremental exercise in a 9-year-old girl. The arrows indicate the transition points between the slow and fast phases of Pi : PCr and pH changes. From Zanconato *et al.* (1993).

children compared with adults (Cooper *et al.*, 1984).

As leg muscle work rate increases, ADP and Pi are released from the breakdown of ATP and PCr. Current theory holds that ADP and Pi regulate the rate of oxidative phosphorylation precisely so that homeostasis of the ATP concentration is obtained (Chance *et al.*, 1986). As the rate of ATP hydrolysis approaches the maximal rate of tissue oxidative phosphorylation, glycolysis (similarly activated by ADP and Pi) assumes an increasing proportion of the metabolic burden (Chance *et al.*, 1986). In healthy adult subjects, the relationship between Pi : PCr and work rate is characterized by an initial linear portion. The slope of Pi : PCr to work rate is directly proportional to the rate of mitochondrial oxidative metabolism. This is followed by a second steeper slope that is associated with disproportionate activation of glycolytic processes (Chance *et al.*, 1986), resulting in net production of lactic acid and increased [H+]. Therefore, ^{31}P MRS can indirectly monitor glycolytic activity by measuring intracellular pH. The initial linear slope was the same in children and adults suggesting a similar rate of mitochondrial oxidative metabolism during low-intensity

exercise. But the different responses in Pi : PCr ratio and pH during high-intensity exercise indicate growth-related differences in energy metabolism in the high-intensity exercise range.

Our data might suggest that children have a higher rate of muscle oxidative phosphorylation during heavy exercise than adults. A greater, O_2 utilization could result from factors that influence mitochondrial oxidative ATP resynthesis: (i) delivery of O_2 from the capillary blood; (ii) delivery of substrates; or (iii) greater density of mitochondrial population. Each of these factors might be responsible for a greater O_2-dependent ATP generation, lower Pi : PCr ratio and higher pH during exercise in children.

But a more efficient oxidative metabolism in children alone should not inhibit the glycolytic capability. As work rate increases, the children, like the adults, would eventually require glycolysis, and its accompanying lactate production, as an additional mechanism of ATP rephosphorylation. This phenomenon is observed after physical training in adults: although anaerobic metabolism occurs at higher work rates than pretraining, peak lactate levels ultimately achieved are significantly higher (Katz *et al.*, 1984).

Alternatively, there could be less functional glycolytic capability in children, so that the rate of glycolysis may not be sufficient to meet muscle energy requirements and result in early muscle exhaustion. The minimal drop in pH seen in children with heavy exercise demonstrates that even after the transition point, i.e. when further energy sources appear to be required, the glycolytic processes play less of a role. Moreover, the children achieved an end-exercise Pi:PCr value of 0.54 ± 0.12 (only 27% of adult values). This indicates that soon after the threshold, when the oxidative rate has presumably reached its maximum, children can no longer sustain muscular contraction.

A maturation of skeletal muscle fibre-type pattern might also account for growth-related differences in the metabolic response to high-intensity exercise. In particular, the children studied may have had a higher proportion of slow fibres. However, to date there have been only a few small studies in children where biopsies of human diaphragm (Keens et al., 1978) and lower limb muscles (Bell et al., 1980) have been examined. These works demonstrated that fibre-type differentiation occurs relatively early in life and by 6 years of age the skeletal muscle histochemical profile is similar to that of a young adult.

In conclusion, muscle high-energy phosphate kinetics during high-intensity exercise are different in children and adults. In this range of work children seem to rely less on anaerobic glycolytic metabolism than do adults. Our results suggest that ^{31}P MRS during exercise may prove useful in identifying abnormal muscle metabolism and in assessing the value of therapeutic approaches designed to improve exercise tolerance in children with a variety of diseases.

Maturation of heart rate responses

The recovery time for heart rate (HR) was found to be greater for high-intensity compared to low-intensity exercise in both children and adults in our studies of 1-min exercise (Baraldi et al., 1991), but the magnitude of the difference in children (e.g. τHR at 125%$_{max}$ was 27 ± 9s compared to 16 ± 7s at 80% AT) was substantially less than in adults (e.g. τHR at 125%$_{max}$ was 83 ± 20s compared to 23 ± 8s at 80% AT). Moreover, HR recovered significantly faster in children compared to adults for each of the high-intensity exercise protocols (but not low-intensity exercise). The maturation of the HR response reveals regulatory mechanisms associated with both metabolic rate per se and neuroendocrine modulation of physiological function.

Indeed, previous work (done in adults) demonstrated that HR during dynamic exercise is regulated by a combination of neural, hormonal and intrinsic mechanisms (Savin et al., 1982; Darr et al., 1988). Immediately after exercise, accelerating influences from higher brain centres and peripheral nerve reflexes diminish, and HR is thought to be primarily regulated by restoration of vagal inhibitory tone and by prevailing levels of circulating catecholamines (Savin et al., 1982; Blomqvist & Saltin, 1983). The role of neural control of HR response was also recently demonstrated in exercise studies of patients who had undergone heart transplants (Degre et al., 1987; Cerretelli et al., 1988), an in vivo model of a virtually denervated heart. In these individuals, treadmill exercise revealed a drastically slowed HR increase at the onset of exercise (HR increased only after the first 60–90 s) as well as a slowed decrease at the end of exercise (HR did not begin to slow for 1–2 min after exercise stopped). Moreover, there was a strong correlation between the HR response in these patients and plasma catecholamines. These observations indicate that sympathetic–parasympathetic factors are responsible for the rapid HR response while circulating catecholamines modulate HR responses more slowly.

Thus, the growth-related differences in the HR response could be attributable either to maturation of sympathetic–parasympathetic neural regulation or to differences in the levels or effects of circulating modulators. Indirect evidence for the latter mechanism is provided by our data, and this may explain the prolongation of HR recovery with increasing exercise intensity in adults and children, as well as the large differences between the groups. As noted above, low-intensity exercise revealed virtually no differences in the HR recovery between adults and children. It is noteworthy that there is very little change in levels of circulating catecholamines during low-intensity exercise (Cooper *et al.*, 1989). This, therefore, suggests that the purely neural control (i.e. sympathetic versus parasympathetic) of the HR response to exercise is similar between the children and adults tested.

By contrast, the largest differences in recovery τHR occurred following high-intensity exercise, and it is the above AT range where increases in hydrogen ion, lactate and catecholamines are known to be smaller in children compared with adults (Eriksson *et al.*, 1971; Matejkova *et al.*, 1980; Lehmann *et al.*, 1981). Thus, we hypothesize that the growth-related changes in HR response to work intensity are a reflection of substantially different hormonal and metabolic responses to high-intensity exercise in adults compared with children. The mechanisms of the different lactate, catecholamine and hydrogen ion responses to high-intensity exercise have not been fully elucidated, nor are there data which specifically address the clearance of lactate, hydrogen ion and catecholamines following exercise in children compared with adults.

Maturation of carbon dioxide output and ventilatory responses

The ability to increase rapidly the metabolic rate (as happens frequently, e.g. with physical activity or thermoregulation) can occur only if substantial cellular accumulation of metabolically produced CO_2 is prevented. Redistribution of CO_2 from cells is facilitated by several mechanisms including: (i) dissolution in body fluids and tissues; (ii) binding with haemoglobin; and (iii) most importantly, rapid conversion to HCO_3^- with haemoglobin serving as

a buffer for increased H^+. There is evidence suggesting that the linkage between CO_2 production ($\dot{V}CO_2$) and ventilation ($\dot{V}E$) undergoes a process of maturation during growth, i.e. there is a difference between children and adults in the ventilatory response to changes in metabolic rate. The magnitude and mechanisms of these differences have not been fully elucidated, most likely because studying gas exchange in ways that are acceptable to children is difficult and because there are no uniform approaches to normalize physiological responses in subjects of widely different sizes. Again, we found 1-min exercise bouts to be very useful in examining the dynamic $\dot{V}CO_2$ and $\dot{V}E$ responses in children.

Our data demonstrate substantial differences between children and adults in the kinetics of $\dot{V}CO_2$ and $\dot{V}E$ in responses to, and recovery from, high-intensity exercise (Fig. 4.7). Both the CO_2 and ventilatory costs of exercise increased from low to high-intensity exercise in adults, but these costs were largely independent of work intensity in children (only the ventilatory cost at $125\%_{max}$ was significantly greater than the cost at $80\%AT$). Adults took longer than children to recover from exercise, and τ$\dot{V}CO_2$ and τ$\dot{V}E$ increased with work intensity in adults but not in children. These results are consistent with the hypothesis of a reduced anaerobic capability in children. If high-intensity exercise in children results in a smaller increase in lactic acid concentrations, then, *pari pasu*, less CO_2 will be produced from bicarbonate buffering of hydrogen ion.

There is a remarkably closer coupling of $\dot{V}CO_2$ and $\dot{V}E$ in children compared with adults. The rise in end-tidal CO_2 concentration ($PetCO_2$) that we commonly see with exercise seen in both children and adults indicates that $\dot{V}CO_2$ increased more rapidly than $\dot{V}E$, but the exercise-induced jump in $PetCO_2$ was much smaller in children (from 37.8 ± 0.4 to 40.1 ± 0.3 mmHg) compared with adults (from 40.5 ± 0.2 to 49.9 ± 0.4) suggesting that $\dot{V}E$ kept pace with $\dot{V}CO_2$ better in children than in adults during exercise and early in recovery. Qualitatively similar observations

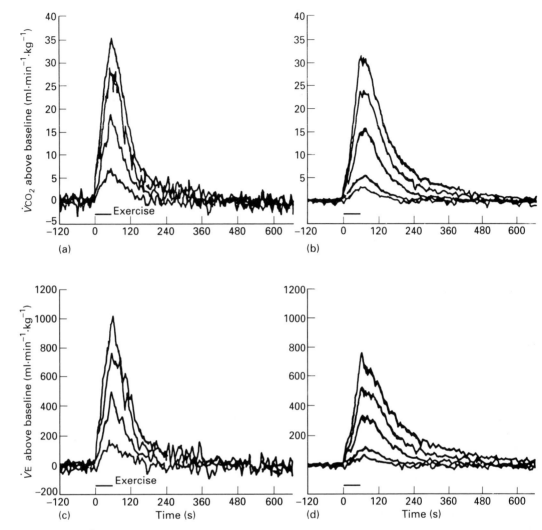

Fig. 4.7 (a, b) $\dot{V}co_2$ responses (above a baseline of 0 W pedalling) to a 1-min burst of exercise in children (a) and adults (b). The data are normalized to body weight and can be distinguished in order of work intensity, i.e. 50%AT, 80%AT, 50%△, 100%max, 125%max (in children the 50%AT exercise was excluded from the study). Note the generally faster recovery in children. (c, d) $\dot{V}E$ responses (above a baseline of 0 W pedalling) to a 1-min burst of exercise in children (c) and adults (d). The data are normalized to body weight and can be distinguished in order of work intensity, i.e. 50%AT, 80%AT, 50%△, 100%max, 125%max (in children the 50%AT exercise was excluded from the study). Note the faster recovery in children. AT, anaerobic threshold. From Armon *et al.* (1991).

have been made during recovery from exercise. While recovery $\tau\dot{V}E$ was significantly longer than $\tau\dot{V}co_2$ in adults following 1 min of high-intensity exercise, the recovery times for $\dot{V}E$ and $\dot{V}co_2$ were indistinguishable in the children. Although $Petco_2$ is only an indirect estimate of alveolar or arterial Pco_2, the patterns in $Petco_2$ appropriately reflected the disparity in the time constants of $\dot{V}E$ and $\dot{V}co_2$ in high-intensity exercise: in children, end-recovery $Petco_2$ was virtually the same as pre-exercise rates, while in adults, a persistent hyperventilation manifested itself as significantly lower $Petco_2$. Both breathing frequency and tidal volume are determinants of the $Petco_2$, but our experience with these variables in children during exercise is that the great variability in these signals precludes much useful data analysis from them.

There are additional possible mechanisms for the differences in all $\dot{V}E$ and $\dot{V}co_2$ recovery times observed between adults and children. One explanation is related to the distribution dynamics of CO_2–bicarbonate in the body. It has been suggested that at least three kinetically distinct compartments exist with rate constants ranging from several minutes to close to 1 h (Kornberg et al., 1951; Barstow et al., 1990). Although tracer estimates of CO_2–bicarbonate stores are similar in adults compared with children at rest (Armon et al., 1990), it appears that children store less CO_2 during exercise than adults (Cooper et al., 1987). We postulate that more CO_2 was stored in the slower exchanging 'compartments' (e.g. adipose tissue) during high-intensity exercise in adults compared with children. In other words, the metabolically produced CO_2 is stored intramuscularly or in adjacent adipose tissue (note that CO_2 is quite soluble in lipids) and slowly released to the central circulation. Consistent with this notion is our finding (shown in Fig. 4.7) that the time constants for $\dot{V}co_2$ (and $\dot{V}E$ which had not returned to baseline by 10 min after the highest intensity exercise) were significantly longer in the adults.

One can estimate the size of CO_2–bicarbonate stores and their dynamics using labelled bicarbonate. While the original investigations (Kornberg et al., 1951) relied on intravenous injections of the radioactive tracer ^{14}C, more recent work in our laboratory has focused on oral administration of the stable isotope tracer ^{13}C (Armon et al., 1990). By using nonradioactive labels and oral administration of tracer, studies in children become much more feasible.

From the washout curve for $^{13}CO_2$ in the breath following a bolus intravenous or oral administration of ^{13}C-labelled bicarbonate, the following variable can be estimated (Landaw & DiStefano, 1984; Landaw et al., 1984).

1 The area under the washout curve (AUC) and the area under the moment curve AUMC — the moment curve is (tracer concentration time) as a function of time.

2 The mean residence time (MRT), which is a measure of the average time spent by a labelled CO_2 molecule in the whole system after oral administration.

3 The steady-state mass of unlabelled CO_2 in which the tracer is distributed.

It is common practice in tracer kinetic studies to perform experiments under steady-state conditions. But our experience suggested that the 2 or 3 h of continuous exercise used for analysis of CO_2 and HCO_3^- turnover (Slanger et al., 1970; Barstow et al., 1990) would be unfeasible for younger children. We devised a protocol using 5-min periods of intermittent exercise that lasted a total of 3 h. While this may have added complexity to the analysis, short intervals of exercise more closely mimic the patterns of physical activity actually encountered in the daily lives of children. An example of $^{13}CO_2$ washout during rest and exercise in a child is shown in Fig. 4.8.

Our study showed that the magnitude of CO_2 stores in children was the same under both resting and intermittent exercise conditions. In contrast, the exercise protocol consistently increased the CO_2 stores in adults by an average of $31 \pm 18\%$. Similar to our previous results (Armon et al., 1990), resting estimates of CO_2 stores did not differ between adults and children; the changes in CO_2 stores occurred as a result of exercise. In addition, the ^{13}C MRT was strongly correlated to the metabolic rate, and the tracer estimate of CO_2 production was reasonably accurate (particularly when corrected for recovery of tracer). While not identical, the relationship between mean metabolic rate and MRT in intermittent exercise was qualitatively similar to previous studies using constant exercise protocols (Barstow et al., 1990).

Thus, growth-related changes in factors like body composition can influence CO_2 transport

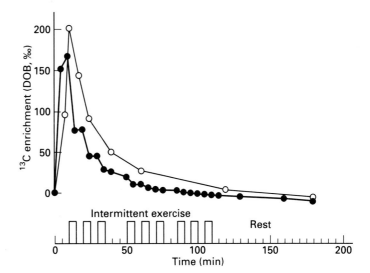

Fig. 4.8 Typical washout pattern of $^{13}CO_2$ in the breath following an oral bolus of [^{13}C] bicarbonate in an 8-year-old during rest ($\circ$) and exercise ($\bullet$). DOB, data over baseline. From Zanconato *et al.* (1992).

dynamics and, consequently, the ventilatory response to exercise. Our findings are consistent with previous studies focused on the time course of gas exchange response at the onset and cessation of exercise (Cooper *et al.*, 1987; Armon *et al.*, 1991b). Since very little O_2 is stored in the body, $\tau\dot{V}O_2$ measured at the mouth closely tracks changes in cellular metabolism over time (Barstow & Mole, 1987). In contrast, a significant amount of CO_2 produced by cells is stored. This delays CO_2 transport and $\tau\dot{V}CO_2$ measured at the mouth is slowed. The difference between $\tau\dot{V}O_2$ (an estimate of changes in cellular metabolic rate) and $\tau\dot{V}CO_2$ can be used to estimate the increase in CO_2 stores accompanying exercise (Hughson & Inman, 1985; Springer *et al.*, 1989). The response dynamics of $\dot{V}O_2$ are quite similar in children and adults (Cooper *et al.*, 1985; Zanconato *et al.*, 1991), but $\tau\dot{V}CO_2$ is faster in children. We also found in separate studies slower kinetics of $\dot{V}CO_2$ at the onset of exercise in obese children compared with normal controls (Cooper *et al.*, 1990). In the obese subjects, CO_2 transport from cell to lungs is, perhaps, delayed by CO_2 solubility in adipose tissue.

Storage of a significant amount of CO_2 is facilitated by haemoglobin, either as dissolved bicarbonate or bound as carbamate, and chil-dren have lower haemoglobin than adults (Kornberg *et al.*, 1951). In the presence of smaller CO_2 storage capacity, CO_2 originating in the exercising muscle cells may saturate the tissue stores more quickly and reach the central and pulmonary circulation faster, accounting for the more rapid $\dot{V}CO_2$ kinetics observed in children (Cooper *et al.*, 1987; Armon *et al.*, 1991b).

Finally, growth-related changes in the control of ventilation may explain the observed differences in stored CO_2. As noted ventilation and CO_2 production are more closely coupled in children compared with adults resulting in smaller accumulation of CO_2 at the onset of exercise. And the sensitivity of the carotid body to hypoxia during exercise was shown in our laboratory to be different in children compared with adults (Springer *et al.*, 1988).

Exercise modulation of growth

Naturally occurring physical activity in humans plays a profound role in tissue anabolism (i.e. constructive metabolic processes involved in tissue adaptation to the environment), growth and development. Yet, little is understood about the mechanisms which link patterns of exercise with muscle hypertrophy (Pearson, 1990), increased capillarization and mitochondrial capacity (Blomqvist & Saltin, 1983), stronger bones (Kelly et al., 1990), changes in body composition (Åstrand & Rodahl, 1977; Ballor et al., 1990), and modulation of puberty and menarche (Nicklas et al., 1989). The interaction between physical activity and growth is not limited to individuals engaged in competitive sports and athletics. Disuse atrophy — the reduction in muscle mass and bone density that accompanies bedrest, limb immobilization or neural injury — occurs even in sedentary individuals (Booth & Gollnick, 1983). This implies that a sizeable anabolic stimulus arises from the relatively modest physical activity of daily living. Moreover, the existence of the 'training effect' — the ability to improve performance with repeated exercise — suggests a 'dose–response' relationship between activity and anabolic effect. Thus, it is not surprising that many of the therapeutic uses of exercise (e.g. respiratory muscle training, treatment of obesity and rehabilitation following a variety of illnesses) depend on these anabolic effects.

In 1969 when Johnson and O'Shea reported in Science (Johnson & O'Shea, 1969) that the combination of high protein diet, weight training and methandrostenolone improved muscle strength and the maximal $\dot{V}o_2$, a vigorous scientific and ethical controversy erupted which has yet to be resolved. But beyond focusing on the specific goal of optimizing athletic achievement, Johnson and O'Shea's observation raised the more fundamental question of what mediates and regulates the anabolic effects of physical activity. And while the use of anabolic agents in athletes represents a non-physiological phenomenon, it is striking that naturally occurring levels of physical activity, energy expenditure and muscle strength exhibit some of their most rapid increases during childhood and puberty. This particular combination of rapid growth and development, high levels of naturally occurring physical activity, and spontaneous, puberty-related increases in anabolic hormones (GH, testosterone and oestradiol) suggest the possibility of integrated mechanisms linking exercise with a variety of anabolic responses.

Little is known about the specific biological role of exercise during childhood, but observations of children under field conditions suggest several possibilities. Most children, even those not involved in sports or training programmes probably pass through phases where the physical activity of daily life far exceeds that of adults, and that some biologically essential, minimal threshold of activity is reached by the vast majority of healthy children. Thus, the effects of exercise on somatic growth (height, weight) per se become important only if the child's level of activity falls below this biological threshold. This may occur as a result of social or psychological factors or from chronic disease when cardiorespiratory or metabolic impairment prevents normal vigorous activity.

Thus, exercise modulation of growth need not imply that increasing levels of physical activity will increase somatic growth in healthy children. Conflicting results have been obtained from studies performed to test the effect of training on growth rates in children. Although some investigators have concluded that training increases growth velocity by a small but significant degree (Åstrand et al., 1963; Milicer & Denisuk, 1964), their studies were not carefully controlled for onset of maturity (Bailey et al., 1986). Other workers could find no such activity-related growth effect despite a significant effect of training on $\dot{V}o_{2\,max}$ and lung function (Mirwald et al., 1981; Sprynarova, 1987). Unfortunately, detailed analyses of energy expenditure were provided in none of these studies.

It may be more useful to focus on exercise anabolic effects in terms of cardiorespiratory adaptation rather than somatic growth per se. There is evidence that integrated cardiorespiratory and muscular response to exercise may be modulated by childhood patterns of physical activity. An intriguing example of this was demonstrated by Maloiy et al. (1986) who investigated the ability of women of the Leo and Kikuyu tribes in East Africa to carry up to 80% of their body weight. The job of carrying large loads throughout the village is assumed by girls at a relatively young age. $\dot{V}o_2$ during treadmill walking was measured in village women, and the investigators were surprised to find that their subjects could carry loads of up to 20% of their body weight before an increase in $\dot{V}o_2$ was detected. This was in marked contrast to control subjects whose $\dot{V}o_2$ increased in proportion with the increasing load. One can hypothesize that the habitual load-bearing had influenced the development of elastic properties of tendons and muscles in the tribal women, and they had become physiologically more efficient in the complex energy metabolism of walking.

Patterns of physical activity during childhood may affect the incidence and morbidity of disease later in life. For example, Freeman et al. (1990) recently studied potential risk factors among children who lived in neighbourhoods in the UK where adults had a high incidence of coronary artery disease. Lack of physical activity was more predominate in children living in the high-risk neighbourhoods. These observations may prove to be clinically important, but the mechanism of these effects remains unknown.

A conceptual model is presented which includes what might be termed 'central' and 'peripheral' mechanisms of exercise modulation of growth (Fig. 4.9). The peripheral pathways involve direct effects of exercise on tissue anabolism. Physical stretching, or changes in cellular pH, $P\text{CO}_2$ may directly stimulate cellular growth factors and, ultimately, tissue growth. Central mechanisms include possible hormonal modifications which act synergistically with the local effects. One intriguing possibility is that GH, which is released following exercise of sufficient intensity, might mediate local anabolic effects either directly or through the actions of GH on IgFs.

Peripheral mechanisms include processes in which energy generated by exercise is transformed into signals that stimulate cellular anabolism at the site of the exercise. For example, current understanding of vascular growth, an important component of exercise anabolism, includes the activation of both intrinsic and extrinsic growth factors (by stimuli such as local hypoxia) as well as cell–cell interaction (D'Amore, 1992). Moreover, physical stretch itself profoundly influences endothelial cell orientation and actin cytoskeleton organization in cell cultures grown on silicon membranes (Shirinsky et al., 1989). Vandenburgh et al. (1989) also demonstrated this phenomenon using avian skeletal myoblasts grown on collagen-coated medium. Mechanical stretch led to an increase in protein production. It is noteworthy that muscle cell growth was significantly reduced in basal medium without

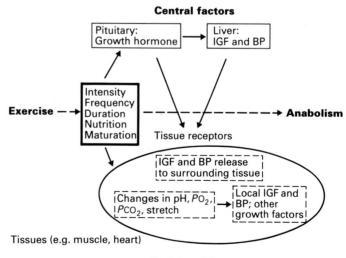

Fig. 4.9 A model of exercise modulation of growth. BP, binding protein; IGF, insulin-like growth factor.

growth factors prompting the authors to comment that mechanically stimulated cell growth was dependent on these growth factors.

In exercising muscle, Po_2 and pH are low and lactate concentrations are high. Similar conditions can be found in the interior milieu of wounds. The healing wound is characterized by new capillary and collagen formation, and a number of investigators have focused on possible growth-promoting effects of the changes in pH and respiratory gas concentrations. Might there be common mechanisms at the tissue level linking wound healing with exercise-induced anabolism?

At least two independent studies of healthy humans have demonstrated significant correlations between physical fitness (determined by the maximal $\dot{V}o_2$ of the subject) and blood levels of IGF-1 (Kelly et al., 1990; Poehlman & Copeland, 1990). Presumably, the increased levels of IGF-1 (which is now known to stimulate growth in almost all tissues; LeRoith, 1991) reflect the increased anabolism associated with physical fitness. But the mechanisms linking exercise and increased IGF-1 are unknown. Since the observations of Hunter et al. (1965), it is well recognized that physical activity is a naturally occurring stimulator of GH release into the circulation (Felsing et al., 1992). Moreover, GH induces tissue production of IGF-1 and elevations in serum IGF-1 (Maiter et al., 1988). Thus, the intriguing hypothesis exists that exercise-induced GH release is responsible — directly or indirectly — for anabolic effects of exercise.

There are studies in animals supporting the idea that exercise-induced growth is modulated in part by hypothalamic–pituitary (i.e. central) hormonal activity. Dr Katarina Borer has pioneered research into exercise-modulated growth. Borer et al. (1986) found that in the hamster — an animal that continues somatic growth throughout its life and one in which vigorous physical activity (e.g. running) is spontaneous — GH is reduced and somatic growth rate falls when exercise is prevented. Voluntary running reinstates rapid somatic and

skeletal growth and induces oversecretion of GH. In addition, preliminary data from studies in detrained, hypophysectomized rats indicate that GH is required in combination with exercise to bring about a retraining of atrophied muscles.

While the role of GH as a powerful tissue growth factor has been recognized for many years, current understanding of growth regulation holds that the GH effect on tissue growth is mediated, in part, by a variety of polypeptides, such as IGF-1 and IGF-2 (Balk et al., 1984). (Note that it has been theorized that GH acts to promote cell differentiation rendering cells sensitive to IGF-1 actions; Green et al., 1987.) In vitro IGF-1 stimulates DNA synthesis and induces cellular growth phase progression from the G1 to S phase. IGF-1 promotes anabolism in almost all tissues studied, ranging from haematopoietic to bone and cartilage. Originally, the liver was considered the only source of IGF-1, but it is now known that most, if not all, tissues of the body produce IGF-1 and IGF-2 (LeRoith et al., 1990; LeRoith & Roberts, 1991). These findings suggest that IGFs are not only classic endocrine growth factors, but can also function in a paracrine (i.e. stimulating surrounding tissues) and/or an autocrine (i.e. self-stimulatory) mode.

GH clearly plays an important role in anabolic effects of exercise, but the mechanism of this regulation is not known. At the simplest level, GH pulses caused by frequent, individual exercise bouts may have an additive effect, increase tissue IGF production and synergistically promote tissue anabolism. In this context, the role of the pattern or tempo of physical activity in the adult or developing child may prove to be particularly important. Maiter et al. (1988), for example, used the hypophysectomized rat to demonstrate that when exogenous GH was administered in pulses, the resulting serum IGF-1 and growth rates were significantly greater than when equivalent doses of GH were given continuously. It is intriguing that activity patterns in children are characterized by short bursts of exercise; perhaps this pattern optimizes the anabolic effects of exercise in the growing child.

Alternatively, it is possible that the correlation between physical fitness and IGF-1 noted above (Kelly *et al.*, 1990; Poehlman & Copeland, 1990) may result from an exercise effect on the overall pattern of GH secretion, rather than from the GH effects of single exercise bouts. Recently, for example, Weltman *et al.* (1992) noted a significant increase in the amplitude of spontaneously occurring GH pulses in women following 1 year of training at above LT work intensities. The mechanism of this effect is not known.

Finally, it is noteworthy that exercise-associated increases in IGF-1 mRNA can occur in the absence of GH. For example, we recently examined the response to endurance training in young rats (Cooper *et al.*, 1994; Zanconato *et al.*, 1994). We suppressed GH in these animals using anti-GH releasing hormone antibodies (Wehrenberg *et al.*, 1984), thereby, avoiding the surgical and metabolic complications often encountered with hypophysectomy. Growth was substantially suppressed in these rats, but there was a marked training effect in both the control and GH-suppressed rats (Fig. 4.10). In addition, IGF-1 mRNA was increased in the hind limb muscles of the trained, GH-suppressed rats (Fig. 4.11). Thus, both

GH-dependent and GH-independent pathways probably exist that link exercise with tissue anabolism.

Challenges for future research

● This is an exciting time for developmental biologists and paediatric exercise physiologists. New methodologies are now available to focus on mechanisms of maturation of the cardiorespiratory response to exercise in children. For example, MRI and ^{31}P MRS allow non-invasive assessments of growth and development of both anatomic and functional importance. The changes in muscle size can be accurately gauged as cross-sectional area or volume, perhaps the critical dimensions in assessing muscle power, and studies can now be done which specifically focus on the developmental aspects of a child's response to programmes of physical training. Dynamic responses of muscle pH, PCr and Pi during exercise are feasible with MRS. These tools should open important new insights into the effects of exercise on cardiorespiratory and muscle function not only in healthy children, but in those suffering from chronic diseases of the heart or lungs.

● Recent new understanding of growth factors and their physiology is also very compelling. If

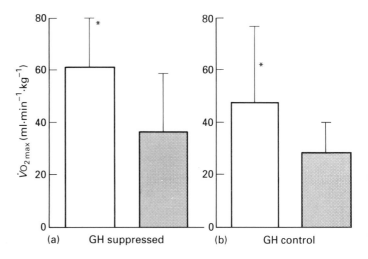

Fig. 4.10 Effect of treadmill training on $\dot{V}o_{2\,max}$ in (a) growth hormone (GH) suppressed and (b) GH control rats (mean ± SD). Training increased $\dot{V}o_{2\,max}$ in both the GH-suppressed and GH control groups (*$P < 0.05$). Body weight in the GH-suppressed rats was reduced by about 40%. □, trained ▨, untrained. From Cooper *et al.* (1994).

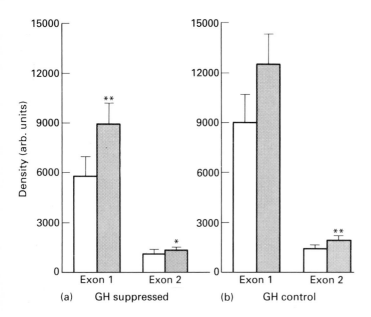

Fig. 4.11 Effect of treatment with anti-growth hormone (GH) releasing hormone antibodies and training on IGF-1 mRNA levels in hind limb muscle. Exon 2 mRNA was significantly reduced by GH suppression in the trained animals (▨) (*$P < 0.01$), while in the untrained rats (▢), no significant changes were observed in either exon 1 or 2 mRNAs. In the GH control rats (b), training induced a significant increase in exon 2 transcripts (**$P < 0.05$), while in the GH-suppressed animals (a), a significant increase was observed for exon 1 mRNA (**$P < 0.05$). From Zanconato et al. (1994).

the pathways which link physical exercise with anabolic effects of particular tissues can be identified, then the concept of the 'exercise prescription' can advance from empirical observation to an optimized and precise therapeutic tool for rehabilitation in both adults and children. Particularly intriguing is the possibility that IGF-1 represents a common regulatory pathway between nutrition and physical activity. In much of the world, marginal nutrition (Spurr et al., 1986) inhibits both growth and physical performance. Perhaps studies focused on the mechanisms of anabolic adaptations to exercise can allow us to develop the most efficient approach to combine programmes of physical activity and nutrition for children in the developing world.

Acknowledgements

This work was supported by United States Public Health Service National Institutes of Health Grants HD26939 and HL11907, and NIH General Clinical Research Grant RR00425. Dr Cooper is a recipient of the Career Investigator Award of the American Lung Association.

References

Armon, Y., Cooper, D.M., Flores, R., Zanconato, S. & Barstow, T.J. (1991a) Oxygen uptake dynamics during high-intensity exercise in children and adults. *J. Appl. Physiol.* **70**, 841–8.

Armon, Y., Cooper, D.M., Springer, C. et al. (1990) Oral ^{13}C-bicarbonate measurement of CO_2 stores and dynamics in children and adults. *J. Appl. Physiol.* **69**, 1754–60.

Armon, Y., Cooper, D.M. & Zanconato, S. (1991b) Maturation of ventilatory responses to one-minute exercise. *Pediatr. Res.* **29**, 362–8.

Åstrand, P.-O., Engstrom, L., Eriksson, B. et al. (1963) Girls swimmers (with special reference to respiratory and circulatory adaptation). *Acta Paediatr. Scand.* **147**, (Suppl.) 1–75.

Åstrand, P.-O. & Rodahl, K. (1977) *Textbook of Work Physiology*, 2nd edn. McGraw-Hill, New York.

Bailey, D.A., Malina, R.M. & Mirwald, R.L. (1986) Physical activity and growth of the child. In R. Falkner & J.M. Tanner (eds) *Human Growth*, Vol. 2, 2nd edn, pp. 147–79. Plenum Press, New York.

Balk, S.D., Morisi, A., Gunther, H.S. et al. (1984) Somatomedins (insulin-like growth factors), but not growth hormone, are mitogenic for chicken heart mesenchymal cells and act synergistically with epidermal growth factor and brain fibroblast growth factor. *Life Sci.* **35**, 335–46.

Ballor, D.L., Tommerup, L.J., Smith, D.B. & Thomas, D.P. (1990) Body composition, muscle and fat pad changes following two levels of dietary restriction and/or exercise training in male rats. *Int. J. Obes.* **14**, 711−22.

Baraldi, E., Cooper, D.M., Zanconato, S. & Armon, Y. (1991) Heart rate recovery from 1 minute of exercise in children and adults. *Pediatr. Res.* **29**, 575−9.

Bar-Or, O. (1983) *Pediatric Sports Medicine for the Practitioner.* Springer-Verlag, New York.

Barstow, T.J., Cooper, D.M., Sobel, E., Landaw, E. & Epstein, S. (1990) Influence of increased metabolic rate of ^{13}C-bicarbonate washout kinetics. *Am. J. Physiol.* **259**, R163−71.

Barstow, T.J. & Mole, P.A. (1987) Simulation of pulmonary O_2 uptake during exercise transients in humans. *J. Appl. Physiol.* **63**, 2253−61.

Bell, R.D., MacDougall, J.D., Billeter, R. & Howald, H. (1980) Muscle fiber types and morphometric analis of skeletal muscle in six-year-old children. *Med. Sci. Sports Exerc.* **12**, 28−31.

Bessman, S.P. (1987) The creatine phosphate energy shuttle — the molecular asymmetry of a 'pool'. *Anal. Biochem.* **161**, 519−23.

Blomqvist, C.G. & Saltin, B. (1983) Cardiovascular adaptations to physical training. *Ann. Rev. Physiol.* **45**, 169−89.

Booth, F.W. & Gollnick, P.D. (1983) Effects of disuse on the structure and function of skeletal muscle. *Med. Sci. Sports Exerc.* **15**, 415−20.

Borer, K.T., Nicoski, D.R. & Owens, V. (1986) Alteration of pulsatile growth hormone secretion by growth-inducing exercise: involvement of endogenous opiates and somatostatin. *Endocrinology* **118**, 844−50.

Brady, J.P. & Ceruti, E. (1966) Chemoreceptor reflexes in the newborn infant: effect of varying degrees of hypoxia on heart rate and ventilation in a warm environment. *J. Physiol.* (London) **184**, 631−45.

Brady, J.P., Cotton, E.C. & Tooley, W.H. (1964) Chemoreflexes in the newborn infant: effect of 100% oxygen on heart rate and ventilation. *J. Physiol.* (London) **172**, 332−4.

Casaburi, R., Barstow, T.J., Robinson, T. & Wasserman, K. (1989) Influence of work rate on ventilatory and gas exchange kinetics. *J. Appl. Physiol.* **67**, 547−55.

Cerretelli, P., Grassi, B., Colombini, A., Caru, B. & Marconi, C. (1988) Gas exchange and metabolic transients in heart transplant recipients. *Respir. Physiol.* **74**, 355−71.

Chance, B., Leigh, J.S., Clark, B.J. *et al.* (1985) Control of oxidative metabolism and oxygen delivery in human skeletal muscle: A steady-state analysis of the work/energy cost transfer function. *Proc. Natl. Acad. Sci.* **82**, 8384−8.

Chance, B., Leigh, J.S., Kent, J. & McCully, K. (1986) Metabolic control principles and ^{31}P NMR *Fed.* *Proc.* **45**, 2915−20.

Chiu, R.C.-J. & Bindon, W. (1987) Why are newborn hearts vulnerable to global ischemia? The lactate hypothesis. *Circulation* **76** (Suppl. V), V146−9.

Cooper, D.M., Barstow, T.J., Bergner, A. & Lee, W.-N.P. (1989) Blood glucose turnover during high- and low-intensity exercise. *Am. J. Physiol.* **257**, 405−12.

Cooper, D.M., Berry, C., Lamarra, N. & Wasserman, K. (1985) Kinetics of oxygen uptake and heart rate at onset of exercise in children. *J. Appl. Physiol.* **59**, 211−17.

Cooper, D.M., Kaplan, M., Baumgarten, L., Weiler-Ravell, D., Whipp, B.J. & Wasserman, K. (1987) Coupling of ventilation and CO_2 production during exercise in children. *Pediatr. Res.* **21**, 568−72.

Cooper, D.M., Moromisato, D.Y., Zanconato, S., Moromisato, M., Jensen, S. & Brasel, J.A. (1994) Effect of growth hormone suppression on exercise training and growth responses in young rats. *Pediatr. Res.* **35**, 223−7.

Cooper, D.M., Poage, J., Barstow, T.J. & Springer, C. (1990) Are obese children truly unfit? Minimizing the confounding effect of body size on the exercise response. *J. Pediatr.* **116**, 223−30.

Cooper, D.M., Weiler-Ravell, D., Whipp, B.J. & Wasserman, K. (1984) Aerobic parameters of exercise as a function of body size during growth in children. *J. Appl. Physiol.* **56**, 628−34.

D'Amore, P.A. (1992) Mechanisms of endothelial growth control. *Am. J. Respir. Cell. Mol. Biol.* **6**, 1−8.

Darr, K., Basset, D., Morgan, B. & Thomas, D.P. (1988) Effects of age and training status of heart rate recovery after peak exercise. *Am. J. Physiol.* **254**, H340−3.

Degre, S.G., Niset, G.L., De Smet, J.M. *et al.* (1987) Cardiorespiratory response to early exercise testing after orthotopic cardiac transplantation. *Am. J. Cardiol.* **60**, 926−8.

Dunaway, G.A., Kasten, T.P., Crabtree, S. & Mhaskar, Y. (1990) Age-related changes in subunit composition and regulation of hepatic 6-phosphofructo-1-kinase. *Biochem. J.* **266**, 823−7.

Eriksson, B.O. (1980) Muscle metabolism in children — a review. *Acta Paediatr. Scand.* **283**(Suppl.), 20−8.

Eriksson, B.O., Karlsson, J. & Saltin, B. (1971) Muscle metabolites during exercise in pubertal boys. *Acta Paediatr. Scand.* **217**(Suppl.), 154−7.

Felsing, N.E., Brasel, J. & Cooper, D.M. (1992) Effect of low- and high-intensity exercise on circulating growth hormone in men. *J. Clin. Endocrinol. Metab.* **75**, 157−62.

Freeman, W., Weir, D.C., Whitehead, J.E. *et al.* (1990) Association between risk factors for coronary heart disease in schoolboys and adult mortality rates in the same localities. *Arch. Dis. Child.* **65**, 78–83.

Green, H., Zezulak, K. & Djian, P. (1987) On the action of growth hormone as revealed by the study of adipose conversion. In O. Isaksson, C. Binder, K. Hall & B. Hokfelt (eds) *Growth Hormone Basic and Clinical Aspects*, pp. 289–93. Elsevier, New York.

Hebestreit, H., Mimura, K. & Bar-Or, O. (1993) Recovery of muscle power after high-intensity short-term exercise: comparing boys and men. *J. Appl. Physiol.* **74**, 2875–80.

Hughson, R.L. & Inman, M.D. (1985) Gas exchange analysis of immediate CO_2 storage at onset of exercise. *Respir. Physiol.* **59**, 265–78.

Hunter, W.M., Fonseka, C.C. & Passmore, R. (1965) Growth hormone: important role in muscular exercise in adults. *Science* **150**, 1051–3.

Johnson, L.C. & O'Shea, J.P. (1969) Anabolic steroid: effects on strength development. *Science* **164**, 957–9.

Katz, A. & Sahlin, K. (1988) Regulation of lactic acid production during exercise. *J. Appl. Physiol.* **65**, 509–18.

Katz, A., Sharp, R.L., King, D.S., Costill, D.L. & Fink, W.J. (1984) Effect of high intensity interval training on 2,3-diphosphoglycerate at rest and after maximal exercise. *Eur. J. Appl. Physiol.* **52**, 331–5.

Keens, T.G., Bryan, A.C., Levison, H. & Ianuzzo, C.D. (1978) Developmental pattern of muscle fiber types in human ventilatory muscles. *J. Appl. Physiol.* **44**, 909–13.

Kelly, A., Lyons, G., Gambki, B. & Rubinstein, N. (1983) Influence of testosterone on contractile proteins of the guinea pig temporalis muscle. *Adv. Exp. Med. Biol.* **182**, 155–68.

Kelly, P.J., Eisman, J.A., Stuart, M.C., Pocock, N.A., Sambrook, P.N. & Gwinn, T.H. (1990) Somatomedin-C, physical fitness, and bone density. *J. Clin. Endocrinol. Metab.* **70**, 718–23.

Kleiber, M. (1975) *The Fire of Life.* Krieger, New York.

Kornberg, H.L., Davies, R.E. & Wood, D.R. (1951) The metabolism of ^{14}C-labelled bicarbonate in the cat. *Biochem. J.* **51**, 351–7.

Lamarra, N. (1982) *Ventilatory control, cardiac output, and gas exchange dynamics during exercise transients in man.* PhD thesis, UCLA, Los Angeles.

Landaw, E.M., Chen, B.C. & DiStefano, J.J. (1984) An algorithm for the idenifiable parameters combinations of the general mammillary compartmental model. *Math. Biosci.* **72**, 199–212.

Landaw, E.M. & DiStefano, J.J. (1984) Multiexponential, multicompartmental, and noncompartmental modelling. II. Data analysis and statistical considerations. *Am. J. Physiol.* **246**; R665–77.

Lehmann, M., Keul, J. & Korsten-Reck, U. (1981) The influence of graduated treadmill exercise on plasma catecholamines, aerobic and anaerobic capacity in boys and adults. *Eur. J. Appl. Physiol.* **47**, 301–11.

LeRoith, D. (1991) *Insulin-Like Growth Factors: Molecular and Cellular Aspects.* CRC Press, Boca Raton.

LeRoith, D., Adamo, M. & Roberts, C.T. Jr (1990) Regulation of insulin-like growth factor-1 gene expreession. In V.R. Sara, K. Hall & H. Low (eds) *Growth Factors from Genes to Clinical Applications*, pp. 11–24. Raven Press, New York.

LeRoith, D. & Roberts, C.T. Jr (1991) Insulin-like growth factor 1: a molecular basis for endocrine versus local action? *Mol. Cell. Endocrinol.* **77**, C57–61.

Maiter, D., Underwood, L.E., Maes, M., Davenport, M.L. & Ketelslegers, J.M. (1988) Different effects of intermittent and continuous growth hormone (GH) administration on serum somatomedin-C/insulin-like growth factor 1 and liver GH receptors in hypophysectomized rats. *Endocrinology* **123**, 1053–9.

Maloiy, G.M.O., Heglund, N.C., Prager, L.M., Cavagna, G.A. & Taylor, C.R. (1986). Energetic cost of carrying loads: have African women discovered an economic way? *Nature* **319**, 668–9.

Marshall, W.A. & Tanner, J.M. (1986) Puberty. In F. Falkner & J.M. Tanner (eds) *Human Growth*, 2nd edn, pp. 171–210. Plenum Press, New York.

Matejkova, J., Kiprivova, Z. & Placheta, Z. (1980) Changes in acid–base balance after maximal exercise. In Z. Placheta (ed.) *Youth and Physical Activity*, pp. 191–9. Purkyne University, Brno.

McGilvery, R.W. (1983) *Biochemistry: a Functional Approach*, 3rd edn. W.B. Saunders, Philadelphia.

Milicer, H. & Denisuk, L. (1964) The physical development of youth. In E. Jokl & E. Simon (eds) *International Research in Sport and Physical Education.* pp. 262–85. C.C. Thomas, Springfield.

Mirwald, R.L., Bailey, D.A., Cameron, N. & Rasmussen, R.L. (1981) Longitudinal comparison of aerobic power on active and inactive boys aged 7–17 years. *Ann. Hum. Biol.* **8**, 405–14.

Nicklas, B.J., Hackney, A.C. & Sharp, R.L. (1989) The menstrual cycle and exercise: performance, muscle glycogen, and substrate responses. *Int. J. Sports Med.* **10**, 264–9.

Paterson, D.H., Cunningham, D.A. & Bumstead, L.A. (1986) Recovery O_2 and blood lactic acid: longitudinal analysis in boys aged 11 to 15 years. *Eur. J. Appl. Physiol.* **55**, 93–9.

Pearson, A.M. (1990) Muscle growth and exercise. *Crit. Rev. Food Sci. Nutr.* **29**, 167–96.

Poehlman, E.T. & Copeland, K.C. (1990) Influence of physical activity on insulin-like growth factor-1 in healthy younger and older men. *J. Clin. Endocrinol. Metab.* **71**, 1468–73.

Roston, W.L., Whipp, B.J., Davis, J.A., Cunningham, D.A., Effros, R.M. & Wasserman, K. (1987) Oxygen uptake kinetics and lactate concentrations during exercise in humans. *Am. Rev. Respir. Dis.* **135**, 1080–4.

Saborido, A., Vila, J., Molano, F. & Megias, A. (1991) Effect of anabolic steroids on mitochondria and sarcotubular system of skeletal muscle. *J. Appl. Physiol.* **70**, 1038–43.

Savin, W., Davidson, D. & Haskell, W.L. (1982) Autonomic contribution to heart rate recovery from exercise in humans. *J. Appl. Physiol.* **53**, 1572–5.

Shephard, R.J. (1992) Muscular endurance and blood lactate. In R.J. Shephard & P.-O. Åstrand (eds) *Endurance in Sport*, pp. 215–25. Blackwell Scientific Publications, Oxford.

Shirinsky, V.P., Antonov, A.S., Birukov, K.G. *et al.* (1989) Mechano-chemical control of human endothelium orientation and size. *J. Cell. Biol.* **109**, 331–9.

Slanger, B.H., Kusubov, N. & Winchell, H.S. (1970) Effect of exercise on human $CO_2–HCO_3$ kinetics. *J. Nucl. Med.* **11**, 716–18.

Springer, C., Barstow, T.J. & Cooper, D.M. (1989) Effect of hypoxia on ventilatory control during exercise in children and adults. *Pediatr. Res.* **25**, 285–90.

Springer, C., Cooper, D.M. & Wasserman, K. (1988) Evidence that maturation of the peripheral chemoreceptors is not complete in childhood. *Respir. Physiol.* **74**, 55–64.

Sprynarova, S. (1987) The influence of training on physical and functional growth before, during, and after puberty. *Eur. J. Appl. Physiol.* **56**, 719–24.

Spurr, G.B., Reina, J.C. & Barac Nieto, M. (1986) Marginal malnutrition in school-aged Colombian boys: metabolic rate and estimated daily energy expenditure. *Am. J. Clin. Nutr.* **44**, 113–26.

Su, J.Y. & Friedman, W.F. (1973) Comparison of the responses of fetal and adult cardiac muscle to hypoxia. *Am. J. Physiol.* **224**, 1249–53.

Vandenburgh, H.H., Hatfaludy, S., Karlisch, P. & Shansky, J. (1989) Skeletal muscle growth is stimulated by intermittent stretch–relaxation in tissue culture. *Am. J. Physiol.* **256**, C674–82.

Wasserman, K. (1986) Anaerobiosis, lactate, and gas exchange during exercise: the issues. *Fed. Proc.* **45**, 2904–9.

Wasserman, K., Hansen, J.E. & Sue, D.Y. (1991) Facilitation of oxygen consumption by lactic acidosis during exercise. *News Physiol. Sci.* **6**, 29–34.

Wasserman, K., Whipp, B.J. & Davis, J.A. (1981) Respiratory physiology of exercise: metabolism, gas exchange, and ventilatory control. In J.G. Widdicombe (ed.) *Respiratory Physiology*, Part III, Vol. 23. *International Review of Physiology Series*. University Park Press, Baltimore.

Wasserman, K., Whipp, B.J., Koyal, S.N. & Beaver, W.L. (1973) Anaerobic threshold and respiratory gas exchange during exercise. *J. Appl. Physiol.* **35**, 236–43.

Wehrenberg, W.B., Bloch, B. & Phillips, B.J. (1984) Antibodies to growth hormone-releasing factor inhibit somatic growth. *Endocrinology* **115**, 1218–20.

Weltman, A., Weltman, J.Y., Schurrer, R., Evans, W.S., Veldhuis, J.D. & Rogol, A.D. (1992) Endurance training amplifies the pulsatile release of growth hormone: effects of training intensity. *J. Appl. Physiol.* **72**, 2188–96.

Zanconato, S., Buchthal, S., Barstow, T.J. & Cooper, D.M. (1993) ^{31}P-magnetic resonance spectroscopy of leg muscle metabolism during exercise in children and adults. *J. Appl. Physiol.* **74**, 2214–18.

Zanconato, S., Cooper, D.M. & Armon, Y. (1991) Oxygen cost and oxygen uptake dynamics and recovery with one minute of exercise in children and adults. *J. Appl. Physiol.* **71**, 993–8.

Zanconato, S., Cooper, D.M., Barstow, T.J. & Landaw, E. (1992) $^{13}CO_2$ washout dynamics during intermittent exercise in children and adults. *J. Appl. Physiol.* **73**, 2476–82.

Zanconato, S., Moromisato, D.Y., Moromisato, M.Y. *et al.* (1994) Effect of training and growth hormone suppression on insulin-like growth factor-1 mRNA in young rats. *J. Appl. Physiol.* **76**, 2204–9.

Chapter 5

Skill Acquisition in Children: a Historical Perspective

JACQUELINE FAGARD

Introduction

Skill refers to the proficiency with which an integrated activity is carried out. The concept of skill covers a wide range of behaviours that allow mastery and control over our environment. This chapter will be exclusively concerned with the development and acquisition of motor and perceptual-motor skills.

Skill acquisition can be described at several levels. Going from descriptive to explanatory levels, one can distinguish: (i) age of skill onset; (ii) qualitative differences in achievement within a skill and in the motor patterns used to perform it (performance steps); and (iii) underlying processes leading to a new acquisition or to significant changes in mastering a skill.

The tremendous changes in the study of motor skill development over the course of this century reflect changing analytical emphases. Studies during the 1930s to 1950s were descriptive and established norms for *when* to expect a normal infant to achieve any given skill. They provided age-related data on the acquisition of a wide range of common motor skills such as reaching, walking, and so on. With the description of steps within a skill, through longitudinal studies, and with precise descriptions of the movements themselves, some of these early studies documented the qualitative changes leading to the mature form of a skill. Such studies raised the question of *what* changes occur over time during skill acquisition (Halverson, 1931; Shirley, 1931; McGraw, 1941).

Early motor development was then considered to be mostly driven by maturation. Some authors, however, recognized the reciprocal interweaving of the different areas of development (McCaskill & Wellman, 1938; Gesell, 1954), thereby anticipating the current idea that development is non-linear and driven by the interaction of many subsystems.

After a temporary decline in the study of motor development, the topic regained interest in the 1960s and 1970s with more process-oriented analyses. In particular, the current approach viewing the operator as an engineering system (Craik, 1947) or an information-processing system (Hick, 1952), led to experimental research on motor control in children (Davol et al., 1965; Connolly et al., 1968; Connolly, 1970; Pew & Rupp, 1971; Fairweather & Hutt, 1978). This research raised the question of the underlying mechanisms accounting for changes in motor control with age and practice. It evaluated *how* change occurs.

Also in the 1960s, interest was growing in the initial state of the motor repertoire in newborns and fetuses. This was due to technological advances such as ultrasound recording. Understanding the early antecedents of skill behaviour became particularly relevant after the pioneering work of Bernstein (1967), who stimulated interest in synergies and motor coordination. During the last 20 years, the technical progress in computerized movement analysis devices, in addition to the theoretical breakthrough of the dynamic system approach, focused motor skills studies on the issue of spatiotemporal invariants and reinforced the shift of focus from motor control to motor coordination.

The origin of complex skills can be traced back to early childhood as fundamental skills develop, such as grasping, walking, catching, throwing, and so on. This chapter briefly describes the state of the motor repertoire at birth and its development during infancy, then analyses how skills develop with practice or training during childhood. Finally, a brief review is given of the different theoretical points of view accounting for processes underlying skill acquisition.

Skills present at birth

Any exteroceptive stimulus, whether tactile, visual, auditory or olfactory, can induce responses from the newborn, within the limits given by the constraints of his or her limited motor repertoire, lack of postural support for the movement and low attentional capacity. These responses to external stimuli, in which we distinguish reflexes from early sensorimotor patterns, are only part of the motor repertoire of the newborn which also comprises the so-called spontaneous movements.

Spontaneous motor patterns and rhythmical stereotypies

Movement of the human fetus can be observed by 7–8 weeks of gestational age without apparent external stimulation (Fig. 5.1). Much evidence exists that developmentally, integrated spontaneous movements precede reactive movements (Fentress & Mcleod, 1986). Thus, early movement patterns could, to a large extent, be accounted for by endogenous central pattern generators which become secondarily available for selection and direction by sensory influences.

Spontaneous movement patterns, such as mouthing, can be observed in neonates in a drowsy state (Wolff, 1966). They are often rhythmical, in which case they are called rhythmical stereotypies. During their first year, infants perform a great variety of stereotypies, such as kicking, waving, banging, rocking, bouncing, and so on (Wolff, 1968; Thelen, 1981). The different stereotypies appear and peak at different ages. The number of patterns increases while the actual frequency of expression declines toward the end of the first year. It has been proposed that these stereotypies are manifestations of immature sensorimotor integration of inherent motor patterns and that they provide the temporal substrata for coordinated movements. Kicking, for example, provides temporal substrata for the development of walking (Thelen, 1983).

Reflexes

Reflexes form an important part of the infant's motor repertoire at birth. Reflexes are distinguished from more elaborate sensorimotor patterns because (i) they can be elicited easily with a short latency following specific stimulus onset; (ii) they tend to resist habituation; (iii) they do not require attention; and (iv) they generally disappear during the first year. Many different reflexes have been described (Dennis, 1934; André-Thomas & Saint-Anne Dargassies, 1952; Peiper, 1962; Illingworth, 1975). Reflexes that can be elicited at birth or during the first weeks of life and normally disappear were often called primitive. Some postural reflexes also disappear during the first year. For instance the asymmetrical tonic neck reflex (ATNR) declines at around 2 or 3 months of age. However, most postural reflexes do not decline, instead becoming integrated into mature motor behaviours. These postural reflexes have a particular importance for the development of skills in that they 'provide a behavioral background upon which voluntary behavior can be projected' (McDonnell & Corkum, 1991).

The question of how reflexes decline and give way to voluntary behaviours has received considerable attention. One widely shared position holds that reflexes are the building

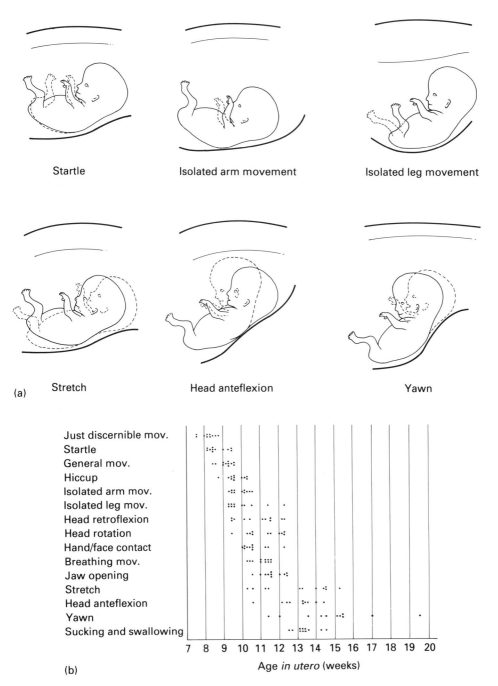

Fig. 5.1 Fetal movement patterns: (a) drawings from video monitor — initial (——) and end (– – –) positions; (b) first occurrence of specific fetal movement pattern: each dot represents an individual. Redrawn with permission from de Vries *et al.* (1982).

blocks on which skills develop (Piaget, 1936; Easton, 1972). Others suggest that reflexes must be inhibited for voluntary behaviour to emerge (Bruner & Bruner, 1968). Finally, some consider that reflexes disappear because increasingly elaborated and adapted motor patterns are available, leaving no need for the low level controlled reflexes (Connolly, 1981; see McDonnell & Corkum, 1991 for a review). Newborns exhibit other early motor responses to stimuli, as discussed in the next section.

Early sensorimotor patterns of higher order

Early sensorimotor patterns, such as visual tracking of a moving object, represent a particular category of motor integration, not reflexive albeit usually in response to stimulation. They are more flexible and more difficult to elicit than reflexes, and require attention or a particular state to appear. They are sometimes called 'instrumental' (McDonnell & Corkum, 1991) to distinguish them from reflexive and involuntary movements. Early sensorimotor patterns provide the best example of early skill development. Interestingly, they usually differ qualitatively from their functional equivalent observed a few months later, thereby providing insights for developmental processes. For

instance, when experimentally provided with postural support and stimulation of attention, newborns exhibit reaching movements toward an object (Bower, 1974; Grenier, 1981; von Hofsten, 1982; Fig. 5.2). These so-called pre-reaching movements consist in one straight-line, ballistic, not very well-coordinated movement; infants withdraw their hand after reaching. They differ from the visually guided reaching movements that develop a few weeks later, as discussed in the next section. Newborns can also visually track a moving object if the object is placed at the right distance from them or they can react to an auditory stimulus, and so on.

Hand–mouth coordination is a precocious example of motor coordination. This behaviour, observable in the fetus (Humphrey, 1970), occurs with a high frequency at birth (Korner & Beason, 1972; Butterworth, 1986) or soon after (Piaget, 1936; Rochat et al., 1988). Although there is no universal agreement on the underlying control of this behaviour (Michel, 1991), it seems that hand–mouth coordination is from the beginning associated with the feeding system, and can be facilitated by the delivery of sucrose into the mouth (Rochat et al., 1988; Blass et al., 1989).

All these early behaviours progressively give

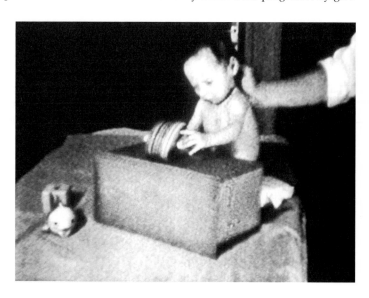

Fig. 5.2 Newborn infant reaching for an object after being provided with postural support and stimulation of attention. Reprinted with permission from Grenier (1981).

way to a wide range of functional, goal-directed and intentional activities which develop at a tremendous pace during infancy.

Skill development during infancy

Many skills are acquired during the first year of life. At 12 months of age, babies can sit, crawl, stand, walk, grasp objects, perform manipulations requiring bimanual coordination and use a spoon to feed themselves. Skill development follows a series of general rules.

General principles for motor skill acquisition

It is traditional to dichotomize motor development into gross and fine motor development. For instance Gesell (1954), one of the pioneers of the detailed study of infant motor development, distinguished between postural and locomotive behaviour (gross motor) versus prehensive skills (fine motor behaviour). This distinction is useful here for the sake of clarity, but it must be remembered that fine motor skill is only the last part of a chain where the whole body is involved in achieving a goal: postural development allows the emergence of reaching and grasping skills which in turn are the forerunners of the development of the coordinated bimanual patterns required for exploring and manipulating objects. Development occurs following a cephalocaudal direction (head control is achieved before trunk control, which in turn is achieved before leg control) and a proximodistal direction (arm control is achieved before hand control which precedes finger control) (Gesell, 1954). The proximodistal tendency partly explains another developmental principle frequently referred to as the mass to specific tendency: infants tend to respond by global body reactions before being able to restrict the response to specific motor patterns. Unskilled movements are mass movements whereas skilled movements are restricted to fewer synergies. For instance, early grasping movements involve more participation of shoulder

and elbow than mature grasping which is more restricted to hand and finger movements (Halverson, 1931), ball throwing first involves whole body movements, and so on.

Development of postural and locomotor control

Postural and locomotor stages are directly related to the development of axial muscle tone, newborn posture being characterized by axial hypotonia. During the first months, labyrinthine postural reflexes develop, helping control the head against gravity (Peiper, 1962). The control of the upright position starts with the capacity to hold the head up at around 3 months of age. The sitting posture is acquired at around 6–7 months, and infants are able to stand up around 8.5 months of age.

Before infants can walk, they usually develop primitive means to move around. Early patterns of prone progression preceding walking were first described by Burnside (1927) as the following: (i) crude forms of locomotion such as rolling or hitching (locomotion in a sitting posture); (ii) crawling (any type of locomotion in which the body is prone on the floor); and (iii) creeping (locomotion in which the body is raised from the floor but remains roughly parallel with it, with cross coordination and rhythm developing). Other descriptions of prone progression have been presented since by McGraw (1941) and Touwen (1976).

Early studies of locomotion identified grossly defined distinct phases for achieving independent walking. More recent sophisticated biomechanical techniques allow a clearer description of change in the characteristics of walking from early independent walking to mature walking. The initial form of independent walking is characterized by steps with a wide base, hyperflexion of hips and knees, arms held in abduction and elbows in extension (Connolly, 1981). Despite these immature characteristics of early walking, biomechanical studies of locomotion have shown that temporal organization of the infant gait, such as interlimb coordination, is similar to that of adults as early as 3 months after onset of independent walking (Clark *et al.*, 1988). Some temporal parameters however, such as the relative duration of the double-support phase, were found to change with walking experience (Bril & Brenière, 1991).

The development of postural control provides a background against which voluntary manual control can emerge. Postural control remains part of the voluntary movements even in adults. For instance, it has been shown that postural muscles are activated prior to the prime mover muscles in voluntary tasks, whether the focal movements are triggered by visual stimuli (Belen'kii *et al.*, 1967) or self-initiated, untriggered voluntary movements (Cordo & Nashner, 1982).

Development of reaching and grasping

As already mentioned, when provided with adequate postural support, newborns respond to the visual presentation of an object with a sweeping movement toward the object. During the first postnatal weeks, visually elicited pre-reaching movements decrease (von Hofsten, 1984), to reappear around 7 weeks of age in a more mature form. Reaching becomes less ballistic; there are more corrective segments during action. Thus vision both elicits and guides reaching towards an object. At 2–3 months of age, responses to object presentation are usually unilateral, and they are more likely to occur if the object is presented on the side of the commonly viewed hand, which is the hand extended in the favoured tonic neck reflex position (White *et al.*, 1964). As the ATNR declines and posture becomes more symmetrical at around 3 months of age, unilateral arm approaches decrease in favour of bilateral patterns such as hands clasping to the midline. Bilateral arm activity in response to object presentation becomes more frequent up to 4–4.5 months but, as the object begins to be crudely

grasped, unilateral responses reappear. These predominate at 5 months in what White *et al.* (1964) term 'top level reaching' which consists in a rapid lifting of one hand to the object (Table 5.1).

Since the detailed descriptions of Halverson (1931) of the changes in approach components of reaching (from backhand to circuitous to straight) and of the progressive development of grasping (from a primitive squeeze to palm grasp to finger–thumb opposition which allows the precise mature grip), many studies have shown the changes in the trajectory of the reaching movement and in the shape of grasping from onset to mature form (Twitchell, 1965; McDonnell, 1975; von Hofsten, 1979; von Hofsten & Rönnqvist, 1988). As soon as infants can grasp an object, they start to explore and thus manipulate it, a gain of the second part of the first year of life.

Object manipulation

The 7–12 month age span is a time of substantial development with object manipulations becoming increasingly complex (Piaget, 1936; McCall, 1974; Lézine, 1978). Mouthing, fingering, shifting an object from hand to hand, rotating an object while looking at it, banging objects at the midline, and so on are behaviours commonly observed in this period. At 6 months of age infants have some difficulty in shifting objects from hand to hand, an activity which becomes more common at 7 months (Lézine, 1978). Mouthing peaks at around 6–7 months of age and decreases in frequency after that (McCall, 1974; Lézine, 1978; Ruff, 1984). At 7 months of age the manipulative repertoire of the infant also includes banging objects at the midline (Fenson *et al.*, 1976; Ramsay, 1985), and scratching with the finger of one hand the object held in the other (Lézine, 1978; Ruff, 1984). After 7 months of age, infants manipulate objects in increasingly long and better organized sequences (Lézine, 1978).

These motor schemes, which clearly have an

Table 5.1 Reaching and grasping development: parameters whose increasing (↑) or decreasing (↓) value is likely to play a role in changes in movement patterns from onset to mature form.

	At birth	2 months	3 months	4–4.5 months	5–6 months	8–9 months
Parameters likely to exert a controlling influence	Visually triggered	Antagonist inhibition ↑; dissociation of prestructured patterns	Maturation of proximal motor system; ATNR ↓	Maturation of distal motor system; visual guidance ↑	Postural control of upper body ↑	Inter-hemisphere maturation, visual guidance ↓
Arm movement pattern response to object presentation	Sweeping movement toward object (with postural support and attention stimulation)	Decline of prereaching	Reaching movements awkward (zig-zag, difficulty in counter-balancing gravity)	Bilateral reaching	Unilateral reaching (arm transport stabilized)	Bimanual coordination during manipulation
Hand movement pattern response to object presentation	Hand opened during arm extension; tactually elicited grasp reflex	Hand fisted during arm extension	Hand often fisted	Hand oriented; object crudely grasped	Anticipatory opening; smooth grasping	Grasping with thumb–index pincer

ATNR, asymmetrical tonic neck reflex.

exploratory function, are determined from the outset in form and duration as a function of object characteristics and familiarity. Infants vary their action with the physical properties of the object as soon as they start exploring them (McCall, 1974; Lézine, 1978; Ruff, 1984; Palmer, 1989).

Piaget first showed that around the eighth month, during what he called stage 4 of sensori-motor development, the capacity to use known schemes to solve new problems in means–ends behaviours emerges. After 8 months of age infants can succeed at means–ends behaviour using a bimanual strategy where both hands play a complementary role (Fig. 5.3). They can pull a cloth to retrieve an object too far away to be grasped directly (Casati & Lézine, 1968; Willatts, 1987), pull a box near to them with one hand while reaching for the toy inside with the other hand (Diamond, 1991), pull a string to get a toy attached at its end, or raise a transparent cover to get a small figure under it (Fagard,

1994). After 10 months of age, they can succeed at means–ends behaviour requiring not only successive two-step actions, but more difficult spatiotemporal coordination between the two hands. For instance they can hold the lid of a box open while reaching inside for a toy (Bruner et al., 1969; Ramsay & Weber, 1986; Fagard, 1994), hold and orient an object to pick up something from inside (Flament, 1975; Fagard & Jacquet, 1989; see Fagard, 1994 for a review). This kind of complementary bimanual co-ordination forms the basis of most skills which will gradually form the repertoire of the child, as he or she learns many new skills during childhood.

Skill acquisition during childhood

During the first years of their life, children exhibit most basic skills, such as throwing, jumping, catching, as well as skills of social value such as feeding, dressing, and so on. By

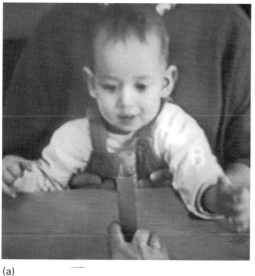

(a)

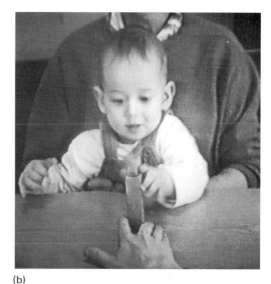

(b)

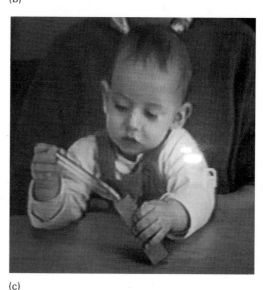

(c)

Fig. 5.3 Means–ends behaviour: example of the first successful complex manipulations in a 10-month-old infant.

the age of 6, i.e. by the time the child enters primary school, most fundamental skills are mastered by the child who then often starts refining more sophisticated skills such as music, sport and dance. There have been fewer extensive studies on skill acquisition in children, as compared with infants, especially in the last 20 years. Most of these studies focused on information processing.

Information processing in fine motor skills: reaction time, movement time and practice effects

Age-related improvements in speed and accuracy have been observed for a variety of fine motor skills such as target aiming, rotary pursuit, manipulatory tasks or tapping tasks. Developing from the theoretical debate in the 1960s and 1970s on the relative role of the central versus peripheral system in controlling movement, the questions raised by most of these studies concerned the age changes in the regulation of action by proprioceptive and exteroceptive afferents. According to some models, the different stages at which information processing may regulate the action are (i) prior to action (during stimulus identification, response selection or response programming); (ii) during action (feedback processing); or (iii) upon its completion (through knowledge of results). Age-related changes in information processing were observed at all stages of development, as attested by the improvements observed in reaction time and movement time, and in speed and accuracy with practice.

Reaction time decreases with age, with a more abrupt decrease around certain age periods, depending on the task. When not related to goal-directed movement, reaction time decreases abruptly between early age and about 8–9 years, and more progressively between 8 and 16–17 years of age. When preceding target aiming movements, reaction time decreases more between 2 and 5 years of age than after (Brown et al., 1986; see Hay, 1989 for a review). Developmental change in information processing prior to action have been documented to reduce reaction time during the early stage of stimulus identification (Wickens, 1974), as well as during the later stages of response selection (Fairwheather & Hutt, 1978; Clark, 1982), and response programming (Reilly & Spirduso, 1991).

Speed of movement improves with age, although not always linearly. Speed of finger tapping, for instance, increases exponentially from 2.5 to 6 years, and more linearly from 6 to 16 years of age (Schulman et al., 1969). Comparing 6-, 8- and 10-year-old children on a task which required them to alternate dot circles (reciprocal tapping), Connolly et al. (1968) found no age difference in accuracy, but older children performed the task faster than younger ones (Fig. 5.4). According to the authors, the differences reflected the fact that the older children treated the task as a whole, as opposed to the

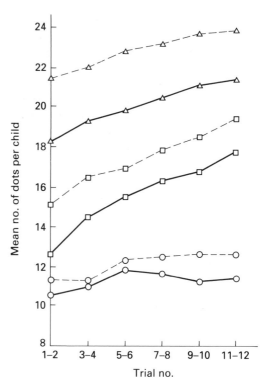

Fig. 5.4 Mean number of dots made by boys and girls in the three age groups over the 12 trials. Trials one and two are combined, and so on. − − −, Girls; —, boys; △, 10-year-old group; □, 8-year-old group; ○, 6-year-old group. Redrawn with permission from Connolly et al. (1968).

younger ones who treated it as a series of discrete movements. Similar conclusions were drawn by Burton (1987) who compared 7-, 9- and 11-year-old children, and adults on a button-pushing task involving one, three or five sequences, and found that the younger subjects require more processing time than the older subjects or the adults at the later components positions. Burton's interpretation of this was that the younger children require more processing time to integrate discrete movements into a coordinated sequence. Speed of movement is dependent on the use of feedback during action, whose importance varies with the kind of skill, precision required and degree of practice. The capacity to process feedback information during motor skill acquisition increases with age (Thomas, 1980), as well as the capacity to integrate feedback from different modalities (Connolly & Jones, 1970). Age changes in use of feedback are not always linear. In her study of target pointing while wearing prisms, Hay (1978) reported that 7-year-old children use feedback during the movement itself more than both 5- and 9-year-old subjects. As their efficiency in using feedback during movement increases, children become temporarily more dependent on it. These age-related changes in basic perceptual-motor capacities may explain why older children profit more from practice than younger ones.

Practice effects increase with age. In their reciprocal tapping task, Connolly et al. (1968) found that the performance of 6-year-old children improves less across a fixed number of trials than in 8- and 10-year-old children, indicating that the younger children benefit less from a given practice episode than older ones (Fig. 5.4). According to McCracken (1983), who used a task similar to that of Connolly et al., faster tapping of older subjects is due to less visual direct monitoring of the hand. That younger children show less efficiency in the use of feedback was also demonstrated in a positioning task providing knowledge of results (Thomas, 1980), and in other studies showing an age × practice effect. In a rotary pursuit task for instance, Davol et al. (1965) found that time on target increases with age from kindergarten to third grade and with practice (across five trials), but that practice magnified the age effect. Similarly, in a bimanual rotary task, we found that adults improve earlier than children in resisting the strong tendency to turn two cranks at the same velocity (Fagard et al., 1985). When the subjects were told to turn one crank twice as fast as the other, the 5- and 7-year-old children did not improve across the six trials, whereas the 9-year-old children did (Fagard, 1987). Changes in the capacity to integrate feedback during learning, which accounts for age-related differences in practice effect, may be of central (processing capacities) or more peripheral (motivation, strategies) origins.

Although mostly investigated on fine motor tasks, these age-related progresses in sensorimotor capacities also play a role in the extensive acquisition of gross motor skills during childhood.

Developmental sequences during gross motor skills acquisition

Children acquire many skills during childhood. First performances are usually awkward, energy-consuming and not very well coordinated.

More interesting than an off/on categorization for skill acquisition is the analysis of the qualitative changes in movement patterns from the first occurrences that may be considered as an expression of a skill, to the mature pattern of the same skill (Fig. 5.5). For instance at 18 months of age, children can throw an object when standing up, but only with many postural compensations. At the age of 4 years, they can throw an object with proper vertical standing and balance, but the support leg is still on the right, whereas the leg support of the 5-year-old child is on the left, which is the mature pattern for the balance component of the skill. On other components however (actions of the humerus, forearm, pelvis—spine or trunk), the overarm throw was not found to be fully developed even in seventh graders (Halverson et al., 1982). Such a 'component approach' of developmental sequence was promoted by Roberton (1978) and used by many researchers to study fundamental motor skills. It showed that skill development corresponds to sequential changes in some of the body components over time and with practice. Observations of clear sequences has often led to the delimitation of particular stages of skill acquisition. For instance Strohmeyer et al. (1991) described four components for the two-handed catch (arm preparation, arm reception, hand and body action; Fig. 5.6). Two components (hand and body action) were found to be age related.

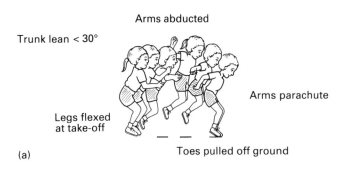

Trunk lean < 30°

Arms abducted

Arms parachute

Legs flexed
at take-off

Toes pulled off ground

(a)

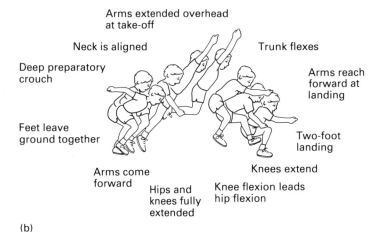

Arms extended overhead
at take-off

Neck is aligned

Trunk flexes

Deep preparatory
crouch

Arms reach
forward at
landing

Feet leave
ground together

Two-foot
landing

Arms come
forward

Knees extend

Hips and
knees fully
extended

Knee flexion leads
hip flexion

(b)

Fig. 5.5 Qualitative changes from an early to a more mature pattern of a skill: long jump by (a) a beginner, and (b) an advanced long jumper. Redrawn with permission from Haywood (1993).

Clear developmental ordering has also been observed for arm and leg sequences in the standing long jump between 3 and 7 years of age (Clark & Phillips, 1985), jumping with both feet together which becomes possible after 29 months (Vaivre-Douret, 1994), hopping (Halverson & Williams, 1985; Roberton, 1987; Roberton & Halverson, 1988) and forward roll between 5 and 9 years of age (Williams, 1987). A component approach was also used to study more complex motor skills such as the overhead serve in tennis (Messik, 1991).

Training

Several factors influence the age at which a child benefits from skill training. Task constraints is one and must be considered as an important factor for the efficacy of training. For instance young children can catch a ball

provided that the trajectory is not too high (DuRandt, 1985), that the ball is of an optimum size (McCaskill & Wellman, 1938; Isaacs, 1980), and thrown against a contrasted background (Morris, 1976). Another example of the influence of task constraints is given by 'jump-and-reach'. Whereas early investigators suggested that 4–6-year-old children could not successfully perform a vertical jump, Poe (1976) found that 2-year-old children could do it when an overhead target was provided. The role of task demands decreases as children grow and become more likely to change patterns as task demands increase (Strohmeyer et al., 1991).

Although, in general, specific training results in gains in the practised skill, training effects have not always been found to exceed gains produced by structural growth and general practice (Hicks, 1930; Dusenberry, 1952; Dohrmann, 1964). When training a child in a

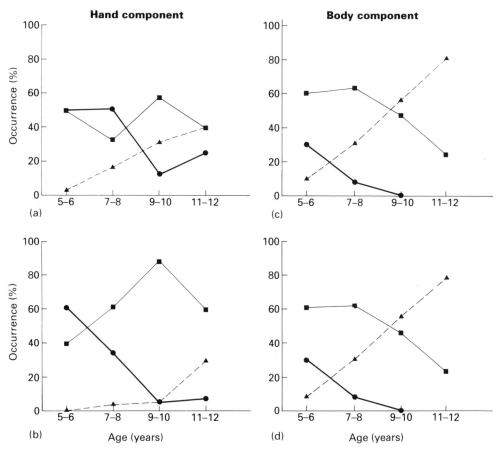

Fig. 5.6 Example of the component approach to study skill acquisition: hand and body component percentages of occurrence during catching. Hand component: (a) throws to body, (b) throws to various locations. Step 1 (●): the palms of the hands face upward. Step 2 (■): the palms of the hands face each other. Step 3 (▲): the palms of the hands are adjusted to the flight and size of the oncoming object. Thumbs or little fingers are placed close together, depending on the height of the flight path. Body component: (c) throws to body, (d) throws to various locations. Step 1: no adjustment of the body occurs in response to the flight path of the ball. Step 2: the arms and trunk begin to move in relation to the ball flight path but the head remains erect, creating an 'awkward' movement to the ball. The catcher seems to be fighting to remain balanced. Step 3: the feet, trunk and arms all move to adjust to the path of the oncoming ball. Redrawn with permission from Strohmeyer *et al.* (1991).

particular skill, one must take into account the specific constraints associated with age, the immaturity of the nervous system, cognitive limitations in terms of information processing and the limited performance capacities of the motor system itself. For more details about training of skills, see Chapter 6.

Gender differences

Gender differences were found in perceptual-motor and in gross motor skills. These differences can either be observed early, or appear only after a certain age, depending on the causes. Gender differences may be the result of early sexual differentiation of the brain. At a later age, they may result from hormonal effects upon the more mature brain and musculature, as well as cultural differences triggering different levels of motivation, exposure to skill and differing opportunities to practice.

When gender differences result from a different developmental rate, they appear very early in life. Studies on neuromotor repetitive tasks (such as touching each finger in succession as fast as possible, or heel–toe alternation) indicate that girls have an earlier lateralization and skill asymmetry toward the right than boys (Denckla, 1973). Girls are often better than boys at fine movement tasks. For instance on a simple perceptual-motor skill such as a serial choice response task, girls had a shorter response time than boys (Fairwheather & Hutt, 1978). Girls were also faster at alternate dot circle (Connolly et al., 1968; see Fig. 5.4), tapping, bead stringing (Silva et al., 1984) and at copying letters (Broadhead & Church, 1985). On a visual pursuit tracking task, boys were found to be better, with gender difference increasing from grade 9 to 12, during which performance in boys kept improving with age, whereas performance in girls decreased (Ammons et al., 1955). Gender differences were not always found however (Davol et al., 1965), and they depend on the nature of the task, being more evident when the task is simple and when considering speed rather than accuracy, thus mainly reflecting the faster rate of maturation in girls (Tanner, 1961).

On gross motor tasks, boys often perform better than girls. In addition, the difference, although sometimes present even during the early preschool or elementary school years, tends to increase with age. For instance, after 8 years of age boys were found to be better than girls at keeping an arm flexed while hanging on a bar with no support, or at jump-and-reach, whereas no or only slight gender differences were found in 5–8-year-old children. Concerning running, gender differences in favour of boys were found as of kindergarten age (Milne et al., 1976; Morris et al., 1982) or at age 7 years (Silva et al., 1984), and increased after the age of 13 or 14 (Branta et al., 1986). Boys were found to be better than girls at throwing (McCaskill & Wellman, 1938; Dohrmann, 1964;

Morris et al., 1982, Silva et al., 1984; however, see also Broadhead & Church, 1985), and the gap between the sexes increases throughout elementary school (Halverson et al., 1982). Boys were also found to be better at jumping (Milne et al., 1976; Silva et al., 1984), kicking a ball (Dohrmann, 1964) and ball catching (McCaskill & Wellman, 1938; Isaacs, 1980).

In contrast, girls were found to be better than boys at hopping, skipping or rope skipping (McCaskill & Wellman, 1938; Broadhead & Church, 1985) and balancing (Morris et al., 1982). Girls also show superior flexibility at all ages (Phillips et al., 1955; Branta et al., 1986), although the results of Milne et al. (1976) differ on this aspect. Most of the skills for which gender differences were found are gender-oriented activities, for instance ball throwing and kicking are associated with male-dominated games such as soccer, whereas jumping or hopping are typical games of girls in a social surrounding. Therefore cultural expectations and practice may reinforce gender differences. This does not imply, however, that biological factors had no influence on gender-related preference for some physical activities.

Processes of skill acquisition

Understanding skill acquisition requires a knowledge of how the motor system is controlled as well as the processes underlying change from immature or unskilled to skilled performance. The last two decades have seen a theoretical shift in the concept of motor control and coordination. A traditional view considered that activation of the motor sequence was determined by a centrally represented programme or schema with, when possible and necessary, the help of feedback loops which allowed flexibility of movement as a function of the subject's knowledge of results and/or changes in the environment. In 1967, Bernstein recognized that central command could not bear on each single effector, given the huge numbers of muscles and articulations, but rather that control must bear on synergies or collectives of muscles. Bernstein's work, together with theoretical developments in non-linear physics, contributed to the building of the dynamic view that motor coordination is an emergent property and a posteriori consequence of the organization of the motor system. Structural or temporal regularity results from the assembly of the system under certain energy constraints, and one must find the basic laws which explain some of the coordination at the lower level.

This prescriptive/dynamic opposition generates the same contradiction regarding skill development, where the traditional constructivist approach is competing with the dynamic system approach. In both perspectives, the main questions bear on (i) what can be considered the inherent basic units on which motor coordination develops; and (ii) what explains change. Concerning the first question, the idea that the new synergies are built on pre-existing basic patterns, is common to most points of views: 'Acts are synthesized from a set of coordinative structure for which the reflexes constitute a basis' (Turvey, 1977). As already mentioned, however, there is no agreement on the process by which these basic patterns give way to voluntary movements. It is mainly on point (ii) above that the theoretical perspectives diverge.

In the traditional and prescriptive conceptions of motor development, emergence of skills and change in proficiency are either considered to be due to maturation of the central nervous system as an endogenously controlled process (Gesell, 1954) or to the progressive construction of schemes through the processes of assimilation and accommodation (Piaget, 1936). Other models stress the role of the processes of differentiation–integration (Fentress, 1984), made possible by the construction of representations (Mounoud, 1983). Another possible explanation of change during skill acquisition is modularization of action (Bruner, 1970; Connolly, 1973). In this theory, skill development consists of successive levels of organization of components. When a component is mastered, it is modularized and can be combined into more complex integrated sequences of action. No more feedback processing is then necessary for this component, allowing the child to draw his or her attention to new components.

The maturation and constructivist theories are like the prescriptive view in that infants are believed to build an increasing number of motor patterns, represented and stored in the central nervous system, whether this progressive building of a motor repertoire is due to maturation and/or learning processes. Within the dynamic system theory, a new spatiotemporal order emerges not from centrally prescribed programmes but from system dynamics, not from rule or prescription but from general laws which govern non-linear systems with large numbers of fluctuating components. Complex systems autonomously 'prefer' certain patterns of behaviour as a result of the cooperativeness of the participating elements. As the infant grows, change in some parameters induces instability of early forms, until change in one parameter past a critical value, induces the emergence of a new more stable form of behaviour (Thelen *et al.*, 1987). The parameter whose critical value induces a new organization is called the control parameter and can have various origins (body growth, environmental changes, and so on).

Conclusion

Skill performance reflects the capacity of individuals to adapt known motor schemes in order to solve new problems as they are perceived in the environment. This brings the topic of skill acquisition to the fore in the consideration of motor, cognitive and perceptual processes. Searching for a single framework to explain skill acquisition is Utopian as no single process can possibly explain the acquisition of the many different skills. Decades of research on skill acquisition have pointed to some of the main topics with which research on skill acquisition could fruitfully deal.

Challenges for future research

• Maturation of the central nervous system, no longer considered as the only event responsible for the unfolding of intrinsic capacities, obviously imposes several constraints on skill development, particularly during early childhood. For instance, the order of skill development is rather invariable, despite the variability of age at which each skill is reached depending on practice. However, maturational constraints are themselves influenced by the intertwinement of different skills, for instance grasping cannot occur before reaching is successful, manipulation is not afforded before grasping is mastered, and so on. The reciprocal interweaving between maturation and function has been fully exemplified in animal research, but further research is needed in humans.

• At a more peripheral level, skeletal-muscular growth remains an important factor of change during childhood and adolescence. The awkwardness that adolescents frequently display is probably due to the fast rate of growth of their body. So far not much research has been devoted to this aspect which needs further investigation.

• Change in information processing and integration of the sensorimotor system are particularly relevant during stages of skill acquisition. The signature of skillfulness is the smoothness in the spatiotemporal relationship between segments involved as well as between component actions. At a late stage of acquisition, little peripheral feedback is necessary for action, although unexpected changes in environment are quickly responded to. Before such a stage is reached, feedback must be continuously integrated for the correction of errors. The magnifying effect of practice over age differences probably reflects cognitive and perceptual progress. More peripheral factors such as attention or motivation have sometimes been evoked to explain age differences in sensorimotor integration, but these have received little investigation.

• Non-linearity in development is a long-standing topic of interest. The more recent component approach to study skill acquisition offers a means for describing developmental steps within a skill.

• Finally, gender differences are seldom made central to research, and are often treated as peripheral topics. Although they can arise from various origins, including speed of maturation, hormonal effects or cultural factors, little research has been devoted so far to disentangle the different factors.

Acknowledgements

I am grateful to Eliott Blass for his critical reading of the manuscript. I also thank Anna Pezé for her invaluable help during its preparation.

References

Ammons, R.B., Alprin, S.I. & Ammons, C.H. (1955) Rotary pursuit performance as related to sex and age of pre-adult subjects. *J. Exp. Psychol.* **49**(2).

André-Thomas, A.S. & Saint-Anne Dargassies, A. (1952) *Etudes Neurologiques sur le Nouveau-né et le Jeune Nourisson* (Neurological Studies of Newborns and Infants). Masson, Paris.

Belen'kii, V.Y., Gurfinkel, V.S. & Pal'tsev, Y.I. (1967) On the elements of control of voluntary movements. *Biophysics* **12**, 154–60.

Bernstein, N. (1967) *The Coordination and Regulation of Movements*. Pergamon Press, Oxford.

Blass, E.M., Fillion, T.J., Rochat, P., Hoffmeyer, L.B. & Metzger, M.A. (1989) Sensorimotor and motivational determinants of hand–mouth coordination in 1–3 day-old human infants. *Dev. Psychol.* **25**(6), 963–75.

Bower, T.G.R. (1974) *Development in Infancy*. Atkinson, Freeman & Thomson, San Francisco.

Branta, C., Haubenstricker, J. & Seefeldt, V. (1986) Age changes in motor skills during childhood and adolescence. *Exerc. Sport Sci. Rev.* **12**, 467–520.

Bril, B. & Brenière, Y. (1991) Timing invariances in toddlers' gait. In J. Fagard & P.H. Wolff, (eds) *The Development of Timing Control and Temporal Organization in Coordinated Action*. Elsevier/North Holland, Amsterdam.

Broadhead, G.D. & Church, G.E. (1985) Movement characteristics of preschool children. *Res. Q. Exerc. Sport* **56**(3), 208–14.

Brown, J.V., Sepher, M.M., Ettlinger, G. & Skreczek,

W. (1986) The accuracy of aimed movements to visual targets during development: the role of visual information. *J. Exp. Child Psychol.* **41**, 443–60.

Bruner, J.S. (1970) The growth and structure of skill. In K.J. Connolly (ed.) *Mechanisms of Motor Skill Development*, pp. 63–94. Academic Press, New York.

Bruner, J.S. & Bruner, B.M. (1968) On voluntary action and its hierarchical structure. *Int. J. Psychol.* **3**, 239–55.

Bruner, J.S., Kaye, K. & Lyons, K. (1969) *The growth of human manual intelligence. II. Acquisition of complementary two-handedness.* Unpublished manuscript, Center for Cognitive Studies, Harvard University, Harvard.

Burnside, L.H. (1927) Coordination in the locomotion of infants. *Gen. Psychol. Monogr.* **2**(5), 283–372.

Burton, A.W. (1987) The effect of number of movement components on response time in children. *J. Hum. Move. Stud.* **13**, 231–47.

Butterworth, G. (1986) Some problems in explaining the origins of movement control. In M.G. Wade & H.T.A. Whiting (eds) *Motor Development in Children: Problems of Coordination and Control*, pp. 23–32. Martinus Nijhoff, Dordrecht.

Casati, I. & Lézine, I. (1968) *Les Étapes de l'Intelligence Sensori-motrice: Épreuves Adaptées de J. Piaget.* Centre de Psychologie Appliquée, Paris.

Clark, J.E. (1982) The role of response mechanisms in motor skill development. In J.A.S. Kelso & J.E. Clark (eds) *The Development of Motor Control and Coordination*. Wiley, New York.

Clark, J.E. & Phillips, S.J. (1985) A developmental sequence of the standing long jump. In J. Clark & J. Humphrey (eds) *Motor Development: Current Selected Research*, vol. 1. Princeton Book Co., Princeton, NJ.

Clark, J.E., Whitall, J. & Phillips, S.J. (1988) Human interlimb coordination: the first 6 months of independent walking. *Dev. Psychobiol.* **21**, 445–56.

Connolly, K.J. (1970) Skill development: problems and plans. In K.J. Connolly (ed.) *Mechanisms of Motor Skill Development*. Academic Press, London.

Connolly, K.J. (1973) Factors influencing the learning of manual skills by young children. In R.A. Hinde & J.S. Hinde (eds) *Constraints on Learning*, pp. 337–65. Academic Press, London.

Connolly, K.J. (1981) Maturation and the ontogeny of motor skills. In K.J. Connolly & H.F.R. Prechtl (eds) *Maturation and Development: Biological and Psychological Perspectives*, pp. 216–30. Spastics International Medical Publications/Heinemann Medical, London.

Connolly, K.J., Brown, K. & Basset, E. (1968) Developmental changes in some components of a motor

skill. *Br. J. Psychol.* **59**(3), 305–14.

Connolly, K.J. & Jones, B. (1970) A developmental study of afferent–reafferent integration. *Br. J. Psychol.* **61**, 259–66.

Cordo, P.J. & Nashner, L.M. (1982) Properties of postural adjustments associated with rapid arm movements. *J. Neurophysiol.* **47**(2), 287–302.

Craik, K.J.W. (1947) Theory of the human operator in control systems. *Br. J. Psychol.* **38**, 56–61.

Davol, S.H., Hastings, M.L. & Klein, D.A. (1965) Effect of age, sex, and speed of rotation on rotary pursuit performance by young children. *Percept. Motor Skill* **21**, 351–7.

Denckla, M. (1973) Development of speed in repetitive and successive finger movements in normal children. *Dev. Med. Child Neurol.* **15**, 635–45.

Dennis, W. (1934) A description and classification of the responses of the newborn infant. *Psychol. Bull.* **31**, 5.

de Vries, J.E.P., Visser, G.H.A. & Prechtl, H.F.R. (1982) The emergence of fetal behavior. I. Qualitative aspects. *Early Hum. Dev.* **7**, 301–22.

Diamond, A. (1991) Neuropsychological insights into the meaning of object concept development. In S. Carey & R. Gelman (eds) *Biology and Knowledge: Structural Constraints on Development*, pp. 37–80. Lawrence Erlbaum, Hillsdale, NJ.

Dohrmann, P. (1964) Throwing and kicking ability of 8-year-old boys and girls. *Res. Q.* **35**, 464–71.

DuRandt, R. (1985) Ball catching proficiency among 4-, 6- and 8-year-old girls. In J. Clark & J. Humphrey (eds) *Motor Development: Current Selected Research*, pp. 35–44. Princeton Book Co., Princeton, NJ.

Dusenberry, L. (1952) A study of the effects of training in ball throwing by children ages three to seven. *Res. Q.* **23**, 9–14.

Easton, T.A. (1972) On the normal use of reflexes. *Am. Sci.* **60**, 591–9.

Fagard, J. (1987) Bimanual stereotypes: bimanual coordination in children as a function of movements and relative velocity. *J. Motor Behav.* **19**(3), 355–66.

Fagard, J. (1994) Manual strategies and interlimb coordination during reaching, grasping, and manipulating throughout the first year of life. In S.P. Swinnen, H. Heuer, J. Massion & P. Casaer (eds) *Interlimb Coordination: Neural, Dynamical and Cognitive Constraints*, pp. 439–60. Academic Press, New York.

Fagard, J. & Jacquet, A.Y. (1989) Onset of bimanual coordination and symmetry versus asymmetry of movement. *Infant Behav. Dev.* **12**, 229–36.

Fagard, J., Morioka, M. & Wolff, P.H. (1985) Early stages in the acquisition of a bimanual motor skill. *Neuropsychologia* **23**, 535–43.

Fairweather, H. & Hutt, S.J. (1978) On the rate

of gain of information in children. *J. Exp. Child Psychol.* **26**, 216–19.

Fenson, L., Kagan, J., Kearsley, R.B. & Zelazo, P.R. (1976) The developmental progression of manipulative play in the first two years. *Child Dev.* **47**, 232–6.

Fentress, J.C. (1984) The development of coordination. *J. Motor Behav.* **16**(2), 99–134.

Fentress, J.C. & McLeod, P.J. (1986) Motor patterns in development. In E.M. Blass (ed.) *Handbook of Behavioral Neurology: Developmental Processes in Psychobiology and Neurobiology*, pp. 35–97. Plenum Press, New York.

Flament, F. (1975) *Coordination et Prévalence Manuelle chez le Nourisson* (Coordination and Hand Preference in Infants). Editions du Centre National de la Recherche Scientifique, Paris.

Gesell, A. (1954) The ontogenesis of infant behavior. In L. Carmichael (ed.) *Manual of Child Psychology*, pp. 335–73. Wiley, New York.

Grenier, A. (1981) 'Motricité libérée' par fixation manuelle de la nuque au cours des premières semainès de la vie ('Liberated motricity' by manual fixation of the neck in the course of the first weeks of life). *Arch. Franç. Pédiatr.* **38**, 557–61.

Halverson, H.M. (1931) An experimental study of prehension in infants by means of systematic cinema records. *Gen. Psychol. Monogr.* **10**, 107–286.

Halverson, L.E., Roberton, M.A. & Langendorfer, S. (1982) Development of the over arm throw: movement and ball velocity changes by seventh grade. *Res. Q. Exerc. Sport* **53**(3), 198–205.

Halverson, L.E. & Williams, K. (1985) Developmental sequences for hopping over distance: a prelongitudinal screening. *Res. Q. Exerc. Sport* **56**, 37–44.

Hay, L. (1978) Visual guidance of movements with displaced vision in children. *Exp. Brain Res.* **32**, R18–R19.

Hay, L. (1989) Developmental changes in eye–hand coordination behaviors: programming versus feedback control. In C. Bard, M. Fleury & L. Hay (eds) *Development of Eye–Hand Coordination*. University of South Carolina Press, Columbia.

Haywood, K.M. (1993) *Life Span Motor Development*. Human Kinetics, Champaign, IL.

Hick, W.E. (1952) On the rate of gain of information. *Q. J. Exp. Psychol.* **4**, 11–26.

Hicks, J.A. (1930) The acquisition of motor skill in young children. *Child Dev.* **1**, 90–105.

Humphrey, T. (1970) The development of human fetal activity and its relation to postnatal behavior. In H.W. Reese & L.P. Lipsitt (eds) *Advances in Child Development and Behavior*, Vol. 5, pp. 1–57. Academic Press, New York.

Illingworth, R.S. (1975) *The Development of the Infant and Young Child*. Churchill Livingstone, Edinburgh.

Isaacs, L.D. (1980) Effects of ball size, ball color, and preferred color on catching by young children. *Percept. Motor Skills* **51**, 583–6.

Korner, A.F. & Beason, L.M. (1972) Association of two congenitally organized behavior patterns in the newborn: hand–mouth coordination and looking. *Percept. Motor Skills* **35**, 115–18.

Lézine, I. (1978) Premières organisations des activités manipulatoires chez des enfants de 5 à 9 mois (First organization of manipulatory actions in 5–9 month old infants). *Arch. Psychol.* **XLVI**, 177.

McCall, R.B. (1974) Exploratory manipulation and play in the human infant. *Monogr. Soc. Res. Child Dev.* **39**(2) (Serial No. 155).

McCaskill, C.L. & Wellman, B.L. (1938) A study of common motor achievements at the preschool ages. *Child Dev.* **9**(2), 141–50.

McCracken, H.D. (1983) Movement control in a reciprocal tapping task: a developmental study. *J. Motor Behav.* **15**(3), 262–79.

McDonnell, P. (1975) The development of visually guided reaching. *Percept. Psychophys.* **18**, 181–5.

McDonnell, P.M. & Corkum, V.L. (1991) The role of reflexes in the patterning of limb movements in the first six months of life. In J. Fagard & P.H. Wolff (eds) *The Development of Timing Control and Temporal Organization in Coordinated Action*. Elsevier, Amsterdam.

McGraw, M.B. (1941) Development of neuromuscular mechanisms as reflected in the crawling and creeping behavior in the human infant. *J. Gen. Psychol.* **58**, 83–111.

Messick, J.A. (1991) Prelongitudinal screening of hypothesized developmental sequences for the overhead tennis serve in experienced tennis players 9–19 years of age. *Res. Q. Exerc. Sport* **62**(3), 249–56.

Michel, G.F. (1991) Development of infant manual skills: motor programs, schemata, or dynamic systems? In J. Fagard & P.H. Wolff (eds) *The Development of Timing Control and Temporal Organization in Coordinated Action*. Elsevier, Amsterdam.

Milne, C., Seefeldt, V. & Reuschlein, P. (1976) Relationship between grade, sex, race, and motor performance in young children. *Res. Q.* **47**, 726–30.

Morris, A.M., Williams, J.M., Atwater, A.E. & Wilmore, J.H. (1982) Age and sex differences in motor performance of 3 through 6 year old children. *Res. Q. Exerc. Sport* **53**(3), 214–21.

Morris, G. (1976) Effects ball and background color have upon the catching performances of elementary school children. *Res. Q.* **47**, 409–16.

Mounoud, P. (1983) L'évolution des conduites de préhension comme illustration d'un modèle de développement (Changes in prehension as an illustration of a model of development). In S. de Schonen (ed.) *Le Développement dans la Première Année*. PUF, Paris.

Palmer, C.F. (1989) The discriminating nature of infants' exploratory actions. *Dev. Psychol.* **25**(6), 885–93.

Peiper, A. (1962) Réflexes de posture et de mouvements chez le nourisson (Infant's postural and movement reflexes). *Rev. Neuropsychiatr. Infant.* **10**(11–12), 511–30.

Pew, R.W. & Rupp, G.L. (1971) Two quantitative measures of skill development. *J. Exp. Psychol.* **90**(1), 1–7.

Phillips, M., Bookwalter, C., Denman, C. *et al.* (1955) Analysis of results from the Kraus–Weber test of minimum muscular fitness in children. *Res. Q.* **26**, 314–23.

Piaget, J. (1936) *La Naissance de l'Intelligence chez l'Enfant* (*The Origins of Intelligence in the Child*). Routledge, New York (English translation 1952).

Poe, A. (1976) Description of the movements characteristics of two-year-old children performing the jump and reach. *Res. Q.* **47**, 260–8.

Ramsay, D.S. (1985) Infants' block banging at the midline: evidence for Gesell's principle of 'reciprocal interweaving' in development. *Br. J. Dev. Psychol.* **3**, 335–43.

Ramsay, D.S. & Weber, S.L. (1986) Infants' hand preference in a task involving complementary roles for the two hands. *Child Dev.* **57**(2), 300–7.

Reilly, M.A. & Spirduso, W.W. (1991) Age-related differences in response programming. *Res. Q. Exerc. Sport* **62**(2), 178–86.

Roberton, M.A. (1978) Longitudinal evidence of developmental stages in the forceful overarm throw. *J. Hum. Move. Stud.* **4**, 167–75.

Roberton, M.A. (1987) Developmental changes in the relative timing of locomotion. In M. Wade & H.T.A. Whiting (eds) *Themes in Motor Development*. Martinus Nijhoff, Dordrecht.

Roberton, M.A. & Halverson, L.E. (1988) The development of locomotor coordination: longitudinal change and invariance. *J. Motor Behav.* **20**(3), 197–241.

Rochat, P., Blass, E.M. & Hoffmeyer, L.B. (1988) Oropharyngeal control of hand–mouth coordination in newborn infants. *Dev. Psychol.* **24**(4), 459–63.

Ruff, H.A. (1984) Infants' manipulative exploration of objects: effects of age and object characteristics. *Dev. Psychol.* **20**(1), 9–20.

Schulman, J.L., Buist, C., Kasper, J.C., Child, D. & Fackler, E. (1969) An objective test of speed of fine motor function. *Percept. Motor Skills* **29**, 243–55.

Shirley, M.M. (1931) *The First Two Years: Postural and Locomotor Development*. University of Minnesota Press, Minneapolis.

Silva, P.A., Birkbeck, J., Russell, D.G. & Wilson, J. (1984) Some biological, developmental, and social correlates of gross and fine motor performance in Dunedin seven year olds. *J. Hum. Move. Stud.* **10**, 35–51.

Strohmeyer, H.S., Williams, K. & Schaub-George, D. (1991) Developmental sequences for catching a small ball: a prelongitudinal screening. *Res. Q. Exerc. Sport* **62**(3), 257–66.

Tanner, J.M. (1961) *Education and Physical Growth*. University of London Press, London.

Thelen, E. (1981) Rhythmical behavior in infancy: an ethological perspective. *Dev. Psychol.* **17**, 237–57.

Thelen, E., Kelso, J.A.S. & Fogel, A. (1987) Self-organizing systems and infant motor development. *Dev. Rev.* **7**, 39–65.

Thomas, J.R. (1980) Acquisition of motor skills: information processing differences between children and adults. *Res. Q. Exerc. Sport* **51**(1), 156–73.

Touwen, B.C.L. (1976) Neurological development in infancy. In *Clinics in Developmental Medicine*, Vol. 58. National Spastics Society, London.

Turvey, M.T. (1977) Preliminaries to a theory of action with reference to vision. In R. Shaw & J. Bradford (eds) *Perceiving, Acting and Knowing*, pp. 211–65. Lawrence Erlbaum, Hillsdale, NJ.

Twitchell, T.E. (1965) The automatic grasping responses in infants. *Neuropsychologia* **3**, 247–59.

Vaivre-Douret, L. (1994) Postural constraints at the emergence of jumping in young children. *Infant Behav. Dev.* **17**, 987.

von Hofsten, C. (1979) Development of visually guided reaching: the approach phase. *J. Hum. Move. Stud.* **5**, 160–78.

von Hofsten, C. (1982) Eye–hand coordination in the newborn. *Dev. Psychol.* **18**(3), 450–61.

von Hofsten, C. (1984) Developmental changes in the organization of prereaching movements. *Dev. Psychol.* **20**, 378–88.

von Hofsten, C. & Rönqvist, L. (1988) Preparation for grasping an object: a developmental study. *J. Exp. Psychol. Hum. Percept. Perf.* **14**, 610–21.

White, B.L., Castle, P. & Held, R. (1964) Observations on the development of visually directed reaching. *Child Dev.* **35**, 349–64.

Wickens, C.D. (1974) Temporal limits on information processing: a developmental study. *Psychol. Bull.* **11**, 739–55.

Willatts, P. (1987) Development of problem-solving. In A. Slater & J.G. Bremner (eds) *Infant Development*. Lawrence Erlbaum, Hillsdale, NJ.

Williams, K. (1987) The temporal structure of the forward roll: inter- and intra-limb coordination. *Hum. Move. Sci.* **6**, 373–87.

Wolff, P.H. (1966) The causes, controls, and organization of behavior in the neonate. *Psychol. Issues* **5**(1) (Monograph 17).

Wolff, P.H. (1968) Stereotypic behavior and development. *Canad. Psychol.* **9**(4), 474–84.

Chapter 6

Prediction of Future Athletic Excellence

VICTOR K.R. MATSUDO

Introduction

The search for talent is one of the most demanding challenges faced by sports scientists. One of the difficulties is that the sport coach, who is in direct contact with the young athlete, seldom has the appropriate background to apply a scientific approach to this subject. Conversely, most sport scientists who generate the scientific know-how, do not have the practical experience to develop the more applicable programmes. Another aspect is that in those societies where there was a good interaction between the 'practitioners' and 'theoreticians', publications have often been adulterated and classified as national security. Indeed, there are very few authoritative publications that deal with talent identification in detail.

In recent years the challenge of predicting the future in the field of science and movement has received the attention of researchers such as Åstrand (1993), Bento (1989), Bloom (1985), Bloomfield (1991), Hebbelinck (1990) and Malina (1986, 1994). Their contribution might be considered modest in the light of the immensity of the theme but it was a beginning that further encouraged more challenging approaches.

The initiatives of the International Council of Sports Sciences and Physical Education (ICSSPE) have been a major step in this direction. In a study sponsored by the International Olympic Committee, it analysed the up-to-date approaches to talent identification. Their effort was summarized in a manual of recommendations (Fisher & Borms, 1990).

International perspective

In spite of the lack of scientific approach, there have been attempts, and even actual programmes, of talent detection in many countries including Germany (schools in Köln and Leipzig), the USA (Colorado Springs Olympic Center), Cuba-INDER (Alonso & Pila, 1985), Portugal (Bento, 1989; Maia, 1993; Marques, 1993), Czechoslovakia (Ejam et al., 1988; Ejam, 1988), Japan (Matsuura, 1988), Australia (Bloomfield, 1991), Brazil (Matsudo, 1987a) and India (Sodhi, 1985).

Among such programmes, the former German Democratic Republic offered the best system which consisted of an annual evaluation of approximately 200 000 pupils. Out of these, 20 000 were selected by simple tests and then attended a basic sports programme. From these, 2000 underwent an advanced programme, out of which emerged the top 20 athletes (Bauersfeld, 1990).

An analysis of the different programmes for talent detection offers the following classification.

1 Systematic governmental. The state coordinates and sponsors the systematic application of tests and appraisals in the population handling the exceptional individuals (e.g. Cuba).

2 Systematic non-governmental. The programme follows the above pattern, but is sponsored by schools, universities and corporations, rather than by governments (e.g. the USA, Japan).

3 Non-systematic. In this case, search for

talents is made on an irregular basis. The state, company, club or even the family try to support an individual. In this system, an international winner may appear at random with a lucky combination of genetic background and supportive environment.

Limitations and difficulties

There are many difficulties to be faced in the attempt to create a perfect model for talent detection caused by many intervening variables that may hamper a good model or benefit a weak one. These include political priorities, cultural characteristics, socioeconomic level, nutritional status of the athlete, ethnic pattern, premature reliance on sport performance, and family and peer group influences.

There is a lack of an efficient and practical statistical model for talent identification (Tanaka & Matsuura, 1982; Tatsuoka, 1988; Maia *et al.*, 1992). The literature generally assumes parametric models, but it is well known that top athletes often constitute a very special group of exceptional individuals, where non-parametric models may contribute more efficiently.

Another limitation is the lack of specific tests that can reproduce the real conditions of a given performance. As a result, much of what is predicted today is based on general physical fitness, which limits the chances of a valid prediction.

One of the most common mistakes is made in predicting future performance based on a single variable. Such predictions may have a low validity even when the test is performed by sophisticated equipment. An example is the direct measure of $\dot{V}o_{2\,max}$ or the determination of anaerobic threshold. Even though the assessment of those variables is of utmost importance, they correspond to only one element in a multifactorial phenomenon.

Another important factor is that a given model may not be equally applicable to individual and team sports nor will it be applicable to both cyclic tasks such as running and noncyclic tasks such as gymnastics. Sometimes, a

detection approach is useful, but its efficacy may be masked by a training programme of very high physical and mental loads that may induce early drop-outs or damage the participants. Another factor that may mask the efficiency of a talent detection approach is the use of performance-enhancing drugs in the young athlete.

Genetic variability

Genetic variability is responsible for the development of exceptional individuals, i.e. those who are gifted with a characteristic that makes them different from the majority of the population (Malinowski, 1986). Those talented in sports are a good example of this variation (De Garay *et al.*, 1974).

Genetic variability is thus responsible for the appearance of exceptionally gifted athletes (Jacquard, 1989), particularly because such athletes often possess more than one exceptional trait, which demands extremely rare genetic combinations. Variables such as height, weight, adiposity, muscular strength, speed, aerobic and anaerobic power seem to be strongly linked to genetic background.

Some studies have suggested (Bouchard, 1988; Bouchard *et al.*, 1986, 1992) that the outcome of a training programme (phenotype) is not only genotype and environment dependent but also related to the sensitivity of that genotype to the environment (training). Alternatively, sensitivity to training is dependent on mitochondrial DNA. Therefore, since the Y chromosome lacks mitochondrial DNA, the training sensitivity of a boy who has XY chromosomes is probably inherited from his mother.

It is important to realize that heredity can determine the pattern of response to training, e.g. high or low response, and a late or early response. These four different patterns must always be taken into consideration when observing an athlete who has started a training regimen. This will help to avoid the underestimation of individuals with a high but late response or overestimate those with an early response but with a low subsequent progression.

Recent years have seen an increase in our understanding of the role of heredity in high level performance (Bouchard *et al.*, 1988). Heredity can affect performance during the detection time and also during the follow-up period. Monozygotic (MZ) twin pairs have shown $r = 0.86-0.95$ concordance for body height; and $0.35-0.89$ for body weight in children ranging from 1 to 9 years old (Wilson & Poster, 1985). In dizygotic (DZ) twins, concordance for peak height velocity and peak weight velocity was 0.43 and 0.48, respectively (Fischbein, 1977). MZ twins had a 0.80 concordance in age of menarche, compared with $r = 0.60$ in DZ twins.

Values for aerobic power were 0.70 ($\dot{V}o_{2\,max}$ per body weight) and 0.61 ($\dot{V}o_{2\,max}$ per fat-free mass) in MZ twins and 0.51 and 0.57 for DZ twins (Lesage *et al.*, 1985; Bouchard *et al.*, 1986).

Heredity seems to contribute about 70% to long-term anaerobic performance (90 s high-intensity exercise) (Simoneau *et al.*, 1986) and 77% to the magnitude of response to maximum aerobic power to endurance training (Prud'homme, 1984).

Performance indicators

Even though biological, psychological and social indicators are all of importance, there are more data about the biological factors.

In spite of methodological limitations and criticisms, the measurement of specific and general physical fitness has gained most attention. Among the anthropometric variables, the ones used as predictors are: body weight, height, fat-free mass, fat mass, length of legs, arms, feet, hands and relations among these variables. Among those, the somatotype has been the most useful. Metabolic indices used include: physical capacity of work, maximum oxygen uptake, anaerobic power (lactic and alactic) and more recently the anaerobic threshold or the onset of blood lactate accumulation (OBLA). The neuromotor variables used as performance predictors include muscular strength of the lower limbs, upper limbs and trunk, speed, reaction time, agility, flexibility, balance and running economy.

In detecting talent in children and adolescents, the biological maturation must be assessed because the results obtained in the variables mentioned above are much more biological-age than chronological-age dependent. Even though bone age may be the best indicator of biological age, sexual maturation has been used more often because of safety considerations, greater practicality and lower costs. The assessment of age at menarche (retrospective or status quo method), pubic hair (boys and girls), external genitalia (boys) and breast development (girls) have been more frequently used. The Tanner protocol for assessment by an investigator (Tanner & Whitehouse, 1969) and more recently by means of the self-evaluation procedure (Matsudo & Matsudo, 1994) allow for an accurate analysis. For more details about the assessment of biological maturation see Chapter 39.

Each of the above-mentioned indicators has a distinct maturational curve, the functional maturational curve, that is calculated by taking the mean score at 18 years of age as being the adult value (100%) and the mean for each one of the other ages as a percentage of this value. There are variables which present an earlier maturation, such as agility and speed (Matsudo, 1987a); others such as aerobic power (Matsudo, 1989) and anaerobic alactic power, that mature later. Anaerobic lactic power (Matsudo, 1989) and muscular strength (Matsudo, 1987a) seem to take the longest to mature.

Individuals with a nutritional compromise tend to have a late anthropometric (Santos *et al.*, 1991), metabolic (Santos *et al.*, 1989), neuromotor (Santos *et al.*, 1991) and sexual (Campos *et al.*, 1990) maturation. It is thus of fundamental importance to perform a nutritional appraisal of each candidate.

Among the specific indicators of physical fitness, natural and acquired abilities are among the more extensively studied though knowledge of this topic is still scanty (Caicedo *et al.*, 1993). Natural ability in some sports modalities is considered genetically dependent. The acquired ability depends on the response to training and is partially genetically dependent, but environmental factors such as technique and strategy are also of importance.

Less studied but equally relevant are the psychological and social indicators (Nunnally, 1978; Cavasini *et al.*, 1978, 1980; Israel *et al.*, 1988; Samulski, 1991). The important psychological traits include: (i) personality traits, such as concentration, aggressiveness, self-confidence and anxiety (Hemery, 1986); (ii) self-concept, which would differentiate non-athletes from athletes, and among the latter those with greater or lesser success (Cazelatti *et al.*, 1980); and (iii) the response to exercise assessed by the Borg (1973) and Cavasini and Matsudo (1983) perceived exertion scales.

A low socioeconomic level can be a negative indicator because of the constitutional and nutritional implications (Matsudo, 1992). Alternatively, it can act as a positive indicator when considering that for these groups, achievement in high level sports may be the only avenue for socioeconomic mobility, ensuring maximum effort (Cavasini, 1984). Children of various socioeconomic groups attempt to join training programmes, which causes a large range of genetic variability among candidates. This is an extremely important phenomenon in developing countries and in those minority groups from postindustrialized countries. Even early in their athletic career, talented young athletes must deal with their peer group, coach, sports manager, family members, audience and journalists, among others. To be successful in such interactions, the young athlete must have good social skills. In that sense, sociometric assessments have been extremely useful in predicting the star athletes, the positive or negative leader, as well as drop-outs from sports (Cazelatti *et al.*, 1977). The method has shown high indices of objectivity and reproducibility (Osse *et al.*, 1981).

Interrelationship of variables

The biological, psychological and social variables discussed above have different degrees of predictive importance depending on the sports modality. Scientists have been trying to set limits to the diverse variables to determine a sports modality profile. In general, an athlete's profile is obtained through a comparison of his or her results to standard reference values that represent the population mean.

The types of profiles which are most widely used are: (i) team or modality profile as a whole; (ii) functional roles within a team (e.g. forwards, guards and centres in basketball) or events within individual sports (e.g. sprinters, marathon runners); and (iii) profile of the individual athlete. The variables that score farthest from the population mean are those considered the most important. A variable that yields the highest differentiation from the population mean is considered the critical variable. For instance, the maximal oxygen uptake in a marathon runner or the lower limb strength among jumpers.

These variables are fundamental to success in such events and so deserve more attention in the detection and tracking of the sports talent through appropriate tests and training programmes. However, in an international competition such as the Olympic Games, most top athletes show high levels in such critical variables with very small differences among them. In this situation, those variables that appear next in line to the critical variables assume a very important influence on the final outcome and have been termed the relevant variables (second, third and sometimes fourth in the list of variables). For instance, because $\dot{V}o_{2\,max}$ is extremely high, but often similar among élite distance runners, their anaerobic power and speed become the variables that may have a stronger influence on the final outcome of a race.

Because these variables are manifested in the same individual, they have to interact in an integrated pattern and not in isolation from one another. The implication of interaction among variables has been investigated, particularly between structure and function (which is the aim of kinanthropometry), but its applicability to talent detection needs further validation.

The effects of the integration of prediction indicators can be classified as compensation, potentiation and suppression. The interaction between such variables as body height and vertical jump in basketball players presents a good example of compensation, whenever smaller players score higher in vertical jump than the taller ones, and of suppression when centres, in spite of having a better stature, do not have a same level of vertical jump scores. Potentiation effect is observed for example, in weight-lifters, whose high scores in upper limb strength are positively influenced by the high values of arm circumference.

Test batteries

Success in sport is not only a function of one variable. It is therefore essential during the detection phase to assess a large number of variables (often referred to as a test battery). Such batteries include measurements that do not need sophisticated apparatus or complex methods, but they should have high coefficients of validity, reproducibility and objectivity and, whenever possible, normative tables.

Although not constructed for talent detection, the most commonly used batteries are those introduced by the American Association of Health, Physical Education, Recreation and Dance (AAHPERD, 1976), the International Council for Standardization of Physical Fitness Tests (ICSPFT) (Larson, 1974), the Canadian Association of Health, Physical Education and Recreation (CAHPER, 1966), the International Biological Program (IBP) (Weiner & Lourie, 1969), Eurofit (Conseil De L'Europe, 1983), the Center of Studies of the Physical Fitness Research Laboratory from São Caetano do Sul (CELAFISCS) in Latin America (Matsudo, 1987b) and in former socialist countries the routine that follows the Leipzig protocol (Bauersfeld, 1990).

As a general rule, all batteries should include athletic and health histories. A summarized physical examination with special attention to the cardiopulmonary and musculoskeletal system and the assessment of sexual maturation are always desirable. Some of these require laboratory examinations such as blood, stool and urine analysis. An electrocardiogram is required less often. All batteries include anthropometric measurements such as body weight, height, limb diameters and circumferences. Adiposity has been assessed through skinfolds and less often through the hydrostatic weight. For more details about anthropometry see Chapter 34.

In these batteries, the aerobic power is estimated by means of performance tests, such as 1000- or 2000-m run, or the 12- or 15-min run; and in some cases by a step or cycle ergometer test. The anaerobic power is estimated through short-term performance tests like jumps, 50 m or 40 s (Matsudo, 1987b), speed and the Wingate test (Bar-Or *et al.*, 1977). The tests of motor performance used in those batteries are summarized in Table 6.1.

Test batteries specifically designed for talent selection have been suggested (Lehman, 1988; Bauersfeld, 1990; Sodhi, 1990; Stork, 1990; Thorland, 1990). These are similar to those previously cited (Table 6.1) including various general physical fitness tests and other specific elements. Bauersfeld (1990) and Lehman (1988) reported that in the former German Democratic Republic the battery consisted of the measurement of weight, height, biological age, 800- or 1500-m running velocity, triple hop, shot put and the number of weekly training sessions. Such selection was done for the specific sport groups of distance running, jumping, sport running, throwing and mixed events. For each group of events there were a number of tests considered more important (for instance, for sprinting — 60-m velocity, triple hop and body weight) and among these, one was considered a major criterion (for instance, 60-m velocity). Thorland (1985) reported that in the United States Olympic Center the battery consisted of: (i) endurance assessment, using physical work

Table 6.1 Test batteries: motor performance items (see text for abbreviations).

	CAHPER	AAHPERD	ICSPFT	IBP	CELAFISCS	Total
Long jump	+	+	+	+	+	5
Vertical jump	−	−	−	−	+	1
Hand grip	−	−	+	+	+	3
Sit-ups	+	+	+	+	−	4
Shuttle run (9.14 m)	+	+	(10 m) +	+	+	5
50-m dash	+	+	+	+	+	5
273-m (300-yard) run	+	−	−	−	−	1
546-m (600-yard) run	−	+	+	+	−	3
1000-m run	−	−	+	−	+	2
40-s run	−	−	−	−	+	1
Pull-ups						
number	−	+	+	+	+	5
time	+	+	+		+	4
Sit-and-reach	−	−	−	−	−	1
Ball throw	−	−	−	+	−	1

capacity (PWC)170, $\dot{V}o_{2\,max}$, OBLA or mechanical efficiency using a cycle ergometer treadmill or running; (ii) anaerobic response using the Wingate test, Margaria stair running and a vertical jump; (iii) strength measurements, using isometric, isotonic or isokinetic tests by dynamometers, strength machines or Cybex; and (iv) body composition measurement using skinfolds, hydrostatic weighing or Health-Carter somatotype (Carter, 1980).

Stability

One of the basic questions in sports talent detection is to what extent the good performance of a 10–12-year-old child can be maintained into adult life. The capacity of an individual to maintain the same position in a group with the passing of time or to stay in a certain percentile position is called stability (Malina, 1989). To establish the degree of stability longitudinal studies are necessary as is determination of the intertest correlation coefficients. The level of stability is the more practical way to track the athlete once selected.

Kovar (1981) points out that when a variable presents a high degree of stability, the possibility of influencing its behaviour is low but its predictive power is high. Bloom (1964) considers a minimal intertest correlation value of 0.50 as being an indicator of significant stability. When the result of a variable is a good predictor of adult performance, it is called good tunnelling (Waddington, 1957).

For a long time it was thought that scores during childhood would not predict adult performance. Nevertheless, there are authors that reported optimistic results. Among the anthropometric variables, body height has stability coefficients of 0.65−0.80, when first measured at age the age of 3 years. Because of timing variables, intensity and duration in early puberty, the stability coefficients decrease, but after puberty they increase significantly (Beunen & Malina, 1988; Malina & Bouchard, 1991; Malina 1994).

High stability has been reported for the somatotype characteristics in Belgian boys (Claessens et al., 1986) and Czech girls and boys (Parizkova & Carter, 1976). Adiposity has shown stability correlations of up to 0.65 between the ages of 12 and 18 years (Lefevre et al., 1989), up to 0.50 in males and females from 4 to 14 years of age (Baumgartner & Roche, 1988; Roche & Baumgartner, 1988) and up to 0.56 in swimmers from ages 10 to 17 years

(Boulgakova, 1990). Parizkova (1977) found high correlations (0.50−0.86) for fat-free mass in boys aged between 11 and 18 years.

Tracking of aerobic power from age 11 to 14 has yielded correlation coefficients of 0.70 in boys and 0.60 in girls while in boys ranging from 11 to 18 years it was 0.30 (Sprynarova & Parizkova, 1977). Alternatively, in 30 boys ranging from 10 to 12 years of age who were tested yearly for 8 years, the aerobic power remained constant throughout (Vanden Eynde *et al.*, 1988). The stability correlations of swimmers between the ages of 11 and 16 changed year by year (from 0.08 to 0.92) (Boulgakova, 1990).

Stability of several neuromotor variables has been analysed extensively. Rarick and Smoll (1967) were the first to report low correlations (0.50 or less) in dynamometer tests between the ages of 4 and 9 years. Nevertheless, higher coefficients were found (Rarick, 1981) in the same boys (0.70) and girls (0.80) for vertical jump. Kovar (1981) reported coefficients of 0.70−0.80 for hand grip, knee extension and elbow flexion. Isokinetic flexion and extension elbow strength assessed on three different occasions in 27 wrestlers showed correlation from 0.58 to 0.94 (Housh *et al.*, 1986). A strong stability was found in the jumping power of boys followed from 14 to 18 years of age even after intense training (Szabo, 1989).

Correlation coefficients for reaction time and displacement speed were statistically significant although of low magnitude ($r < 0.50$) in 146 young boys followed from ages 7 to 13 years. In 30-, 50-, 60-, 100- and 300-m running tests the annual tracking coefficients ranged from 0.51 to 0.91 (Kovar, 1981). It was higher for 30-m dash in girls (0.56−0.77) than in boys (0.07−0.18) between ages 7 and 17 years (Rarick & Smoll, 1967).

A great part of the tracking instability is due to the timing, intensity and duration of puberty (Malina, 1994). Body dimensions can have a positive influence on the yearly tracing value of motor variables, but they can have a negative influence on longer tracking intervals. One

should realize that the above results are based on parametric statistical procedures that may not be precise for individual assessment. Furthermore, in those fundamental and critical variables the talented subject is often not near the population mean, where the stability is lower and the tracking is poorer, but at the extremes of the distribution curve, where the stability is higher and tracking is better.

This latter consideration shows that the eventually low tracking values of some studies and the scepticism and criticism of some authors (Maia, 1993) can be overcome in the near future when more tracking studies based on the extremes of the population curves are available.

The CELAFISCS experience — Z strategy

The detection of a gifted young athlete requires a high level of perception of the 'uncommon'. Therefore, it is of fundamental importance to know precisely the 'normal' or what is more common. In our laboratory (CELAFISCS), research into the normative values of different physical fitness variables of our population has been carried out in order to better know their behaviour, central point and distribution.

Based on more than 20000 evaluated individuals of a databank, we have developed standard criteria reference (Soares *et al.*, 1981; Duarte & Matsudo, 1986; Oliveira *et al.*, 1986; Sessa *et al.*, 1986; Matsudo, 1987a, 1988; Franca *et al.*, 1988; Duarte & Duarte, 1989) based on 5200 school children (2600 of each gender) and of approximately 3000 athletes from different sports modalities. All of them performed the CELAFISCS test battery as described above (Matsudo, 1987b).

Various degrees of habitual physical activity were established:
- Level I: students involved in 2−3 week physical education (PE) classes.
- Level II: students who took PE and were involved in intramural sports programmes.
- Level III: students who took PE, sports pro-

grammes and were involved in interschool or local club competition.
- Level IV: athletes who took part in intercity team competition.
- Level V: athletes who took part in state team and national competition.
- Level VI: athletes from national teams who took part in international competition (Matsudo et al., 1987).

The assessment of team results was made through the comparison of reference standard values in terms of absolute values, percentage difference and the position of an individual related to the sample mean, using standard deviation units (Z score), as follows:

$$Z = \frac{X - u}{\sigma} \quad \text{or} \quad Z = \frac{x - u}{\sigma}$$

where Z = distance from population mean or standard criteria reference; X = individual score; x = sport team mean; u = population mean or standard criterion reference for the individual's age and gender; and σ = population standard deviation for the individual's age and gender.

The strategy is based on the comparison of the Z profile of a potentially talented individual to the Z profile of the corresponding national team (level VI) that has an outstanding international performance (Fig. 6.1).

Applying the Z strategy, one can address questions such as whether a 14-year-old boy with a vertical jump score of 48 cm will be on the national volleyball team at the age of 21. To answer this, the mean vertical jump score of the national volleyball team is determined (72 cm). By comparing this value to the population mean for that age (60 cm) and dividing by the standard deviation (3 cm) we obtain a Z value of 4. The same procedure is taken with the 14-year-old boy, who jumps 48 cm. The standard criterion of reference for his age is 40 cm and standard deviation is 2 cm, giving a Z value of 4. This result is a positive indication for potential talent, since although the boy is 14 years old, he already presents the 'ideal' profile for that variable. Of course, one cannot give this diagnosis based upon one single variable, but only on several variables. These Z values held for the Brazilian national volleyball men's team, who obtained a gold medal at the 1992 Olympic Games.

In our study, the Z profile was initially assessed only on national teams showing extraordinary international performance, in those modalities in which Brazil has a successful tradition. The men's volleyball team was the silver medal winner at Los Angeles (1984) and Olympic champion in Barcelona (1992). The women's volleyball team has twice become

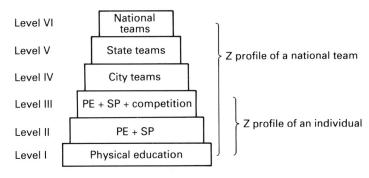

Fig. 6.1 Pyramid model, indicating levels of sports involvement. Level I, students involved in curricular physical education (PE) classes; level II, students who take PE and are involved in intramural sports programmes (SP); level III, students who take PE, SP and are involved in interscholastic or local club competitions; level IV, athletes who take part in intercity team competitions; level V, athletes who take part in state teams and national competitions; level VI, athletes, who are on national teams and take part in international competitions. Adapted from Matsudo et al. (1987).

world juvenile champion and took fourth place at the Barcelona Olympic Games. The male basketball team was the champion in the Pan American Games at Indianapolis (1987) and silver medallist at the Pan American Games in Havana (1991). The women's basketball team won the World Championship in Australia (1994) and the Pan American Games in Havana (1991). The Z profile of these teams are described in Table 6.2 (Matsudo *et al.*, 1987).

The establishment of the gold standard for these modalities should be on the basis of the best international performance. We have to take care in using the so-called 'top athletes' who sometimes only correspond to athletes at college or university level. This fact can lead to bias in the analysis of a more serious detection programme.

In our procedure, the first step is the comparison of the subject's Z profile to the team profile. In those modalities where athletes play a specific position (or role) as in volleyball or basketball, the Z profile is assessed for each functional subgroup. Table 6.3 shows the Z profile of guards, forwards and centres from the men's basketball team (Matsudo *et al.*, 1986b). Table 6.4 shows the Z profile of setters, central and forward attackers from a men's

Table 6.3 Physical fitness Z values from the Brazilian basketball national team (men), as related to game function. Forwards (FA), guards (G) and centres (C).

	FA	G	C
Body weight	4.1	2.2	5.5
Body height	4.4	2.5	6.0
$\dot{V}O_{2\,max}$ (l·min^{-1})	3.0	3.7	3.9
$\dot{V}O_{2\,max}$ (ml·kg^{-1}·min^{-1})	0.8	2.3	0.8
Vertical jump (without arm assistance)	3.6	3.7	2.4
Vertical jump (with arm assistance)	5.2	4.1	2.9
Shuttle run	−1.5	−2.0	−0.8

(Silva & Rivet, 1988) and women's volleyball team (Figueira & Matsudo, 1992).

We have also assessed the Z profile sensitivity in order to differentiate among top athletes. For this purpose, we made a comparison of Z profiles of athletes selected to the male national volleyball team, and also to the Z profile of the best setter and best attacker. Table 6.5 shows a positive relationship between Z scores and the quality of the top athletes in metabolic and neuromotor variables that cannot be explained merely in terms of body structure advantages since there were no differences among the

Table 6.2 Percentage △ and Z score values from Brazilian national basketball and volleyball teams (men and women).

	Basketball				Volleyball			
	Men		Women		Men		Women	
	△%	Z	△%	Z	△%	Z	△%	Z
Body weight	44	4.0	35	3.0	32	2.9	28	2.4
Body height	15	3.8	12	2.9	12	3.4	12	2.0
Skinfolds	−18	−0.4	−21	−0.4	−16	−0.4	−21	−0.5
$\dot{V}O_{2\,max}$ (l·min^{-1})	73	3.9	53	2.7	35	1.9	38	1.6
$\dot{V}O_{2\,max}$ (ml·kg^{-1}·min^{-1})	30	1.3	33	1.7	13	0.7	21	1.1
50-m dash	−0.7	−1.3	−12	−2.8	−0.6	−1.0	−0.9	−1.5
40-s run	0.5	0.7	24	2.4	0.7	1.1	—	—
Vertical jump (without arm assistance)	39	2.8	37	2.8	63	4.5	51	3.3
Vertical jump (with arm assistance)	40	3.7	51	3.8	59	5.4	56	4.1
Long jump	26	2.8	35	3.7	30	3.2	37	3.9
Shuttle run	−0.8	−1.4	−11	−2.1	−12	−2.2	−0.8	−1.5

Table 6.4 Physical fitness Z profile from the Brazilian national volleyball team (men) as related to game function: forwards (FA), central attackers (CA) and setters (S).

	FA	CA	S
Weight	3.9	3.1	2.8
Height	3.3	4.1	2.5
Skinfolds	−0.2	−0.7	0.0
$\dot{V}O_{2\,max}$ (l·min^{-1})	2.6	2.4	2.2
$\dot{V}O_{2\,max}$ (ml·kg^{-1}·min^{-1})	0.6	0.8	0.9
40-s run	1.5	1.4	1.8
50-m dash	−2.4	−1.6	−2.1
Vertical jump (without arm assistance)	5.2	3.7	4.8
Vertical jump (with arm assistance)	6.1	4.4	5.2
Long jump	4.3	3.1	3.1
Shuttle run	−3.1	−1.7	−2.8
Hand grip	2.1	1.9	1.5

Table 6.5 Physical fitness Z values from the athletes selected to the national team (NT), the main team (MT), best setter (S) and best attacker (A).

	NT	MT	S	A
Body weight	2.9	3.3	2.9	3.8
Body height	3.4	3.3	2.5	2.9
Skinfolds	−0.4	−0.5	−0.7	−0.7
$\dot{V}O_2$ (l·min^{-1})	1.9	3.1	3.1	4.0
$\dot{V}O_2$ (l·ml^{-1}·kg^{-1})	−0.7	1.2	1.5	1.8
40-s run	1.0	1.5	2.6	2.0
50-m dash	−1.1	−2.0	−2.4	−2.5
Shuttle run	−2.2	−2.9	−3.1	−3.9
Vertical jump	5.4	6.3	5.9	7.0
Long jump	3.2	3.9	4.0	4.8
Hand grip	1.3	2.0	1.4	2.7

body weight and height indices (Matsudo *et al.*, 1986a).

The track-and-field Z profile analysis gave interesting results (Nascimento *et al.*, 1989). It was observed (Fig. 6.2) that in the Brazilian sprinters (level VI) the variables which were farthest from the mean were 50-m dash (Z = 2.44), vertical and horizontal jump and 40-s dash (Z = 3.28). The same critical or fundamental variables were found for the Brazilian

100-m South American champion. As shown in Fig. 6.2, his Z scores farthest from the mean were 50-m dash (2.78) vertical jump (5.5), long jump (4.4) and 40-s dash (3.27).

The Z profile of middle- and long-distance runners (Fig. 6.3) clearly shows that the critical variable was maximal aerobic power in absolute (1·min^{-1}) and relative (ml·kg^{-1}·min^{-1}) values. The anaerobic power (40-s dash) assumed significant position among the fundamental variables, followed by leg strength (vertical and long jump). When the Z profile of the 800- and 1500-m Pan American champion (who also finished fourth in the Moscow Olympic Games) was taken for evaluation (Fig. 6.3), the following variables had the most extraordinary Z indices: $\dot{V}O_{2\,max}$ (3.98), 40-s dash (4.21) and vertical jump (4.21). Alternatively, the Brazilian 5000- and 10 000-m champion showed a Z profile that represents a good balance of aerobic, anaerobic and leg power capacities (Fig. 6.3). In the same way, when we compared the triple jump record holder to the Z profile of the national jumpers (Fig. 6.4), it became clear that although the jumping strength of the national jumpers was above the population mean (Z = 3.6), the world record holder presented a Z score of 6.15 for that particular critical variable.

This information shows the practicality, sensitivity and accuracy of the Z profile in distinguishing the extraordinary athletes from the others, and those from the general population. It also demonstrates that those record holders and world champions were not only somewhat above the mean in the critical and relevant variables, but extraordinarily above it.

In our centre many gifted boys and girls have been followed longitudinally who have subsequently become international sports stars. We have verified that the Z scores obtained at the first physical fitness measurements, although of smaller magnitude than the adult scores, were relatively constant. This was particularly true when the Z score of a critical variable was far from the population mean or standard criterion reference.

In Table 6.2 it is evident that for national

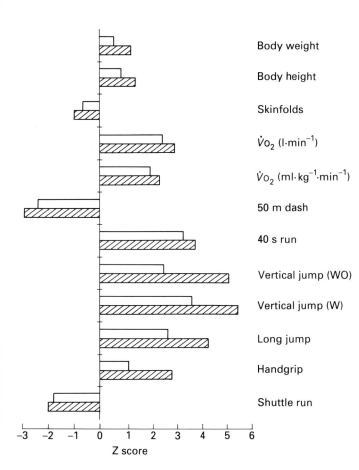

Body weight

Body height

Skinfolds

$\dot{V}O_2$ (l·min^{-1})

$\dot{V}O_2$ (ml·kg^{-1}·min^{-1})

50 m dash

40 s run

Vertical jump (WO)

Vertical jump (W)

Long jump

Handgrip

Shuttle run

Z score

Fig. 6.2 Z profile of Brazilian national sprinters (□) and a South American sprinting champion (▨). W, with arm assistance; WO, without arm assistance. Adapted from Nascimento *et al.* (1989).

level basketball players body height and vertical jump were farthest from the reference standard criteria. These are compared with the scores of an athlete who had been selected as one of the best 10 athletes in various world and Pan American basketball championships during the 1980s and 1990s. His Z profile (Fig. 6.5) shows that he had already presented excellent Z scores in the critical variables (height and vertical jump) since he was first measured in our centre in 1976, and those indices remained constant until adult life (1983).

In analysing the Z profile of female guards and forwards (basketball) vertical jump, speed and agility emerged as critical or relevant variables. However, Hortencia Marcari, considered the best basketball player in the world during the last decade, had extraordinarily high Z scores in variables such as agility (3.5), velocity (4.3) and vertical jump (8.3) (Fig. 6.5).

In addition to the Z profile analysis, according to the CELAFISCS strategy for detecting talent, the following factors should be taken into account: (i) functional maturation curve; (ii) sexual maturation status; (iii) nutritional level; and (iv) sports activity level. These items allow a better trainability prognosis of the critical or fundamental variables. This particular topic has attracted the attention of different sport scientists (Bar-Or, 1989; Rowland, 1992) and is discussed in other chapters.

Functional maturation curves have been developed in the author's laboratory taking the value at age 18 as 100% and calculating a proportional maturation value for each age (Matsudo, 1987a, 1989). Variables like agility

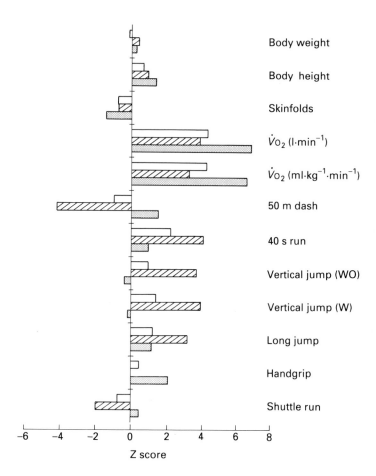

Fig. 6.3 Z profile of Brazilian middle- and long-distance runners (□), the Pan American middle-distance champion (▨) and the Brazilian long-distance champion (▧). W, with arm assistance; WO, without arm assistance. Adapted from Nascimento *et al.* (1989).

and velocity were found to have an earlier maturation (prepuberty), anaerobic alactic power and aerobic power presented an intermediate maturation (at puberty) and anaerobic lactic power and strength showed a late maturation pattern (postpuberty). Therefore, for a determined Z value, prediction of future performance will be better if that variable has a late functional maturation curve (e.g. strength). It would be worse if the variable has an early maturation curve (e.g. agility).

Sexual maturation has a significant impact upon physical fitness (see also Chapter 1). In general, in any given age group, individuals with advanced sexual maturation tend to perform better (Franca, 1992; Matsudo, 1992b). Thus, for the same Z value and functional maturation level, the future performance prog-

nosis will be better for the subject who is at an earlier sexual maturation level (Tanner stage I–II) and worse for the more advanced ones (Tanner stage IV–V).

Nutritional level can negatively influence physical fitness results, especially in developing countries. It has been shown that populations at nutritional risk presented lower values as well as a maturational delay in characteristics such as metabolic, neuromotor and anthropometric (Santos *et al.*, 1991; Matsudo & Matsudo, 1993), psychological (Matsudo, 1992; Matsudo *et al.*, 1992a; Matsudo & Matsudo, 1993) and sexual development (Campos *et al.*, 1990). Thus, for any given Z score or functional and sexual maturation level, the prognosis will be better for the well-nourished subject and worse for the undernourished.

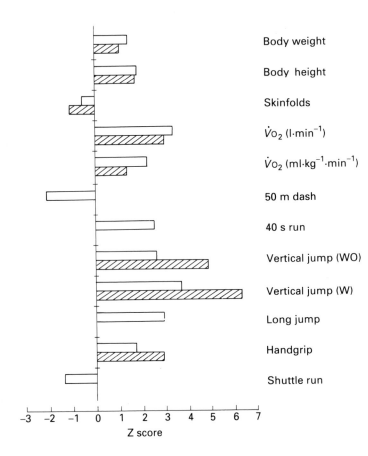

Fig. 6.4 Z profile of Brazilian national triple jumpers (□) and the world record holder in triple jump (▨). W, with arm assistance; WO, without arm assistance. Adapted from Nascimento *et al.* (1989).

It is also important to consider the level of sport experience. If a talented candidate has not been involved in a systematic training programme, the first screening test results would better reflect his or her genetic profile. However, if the candidate has already taken part in an organized training programme, then the performance on those initial tests would represent the sum of genotype, training and sensitivity to training. In a case where two boys present similar physical fitness Z values, functional and sexual maturation, and nutritional levels, the prognosis will tend to be better for the boy who has never trained before.

The limitations of our model include: (i) variables which do not have a normal distribution; and (ii) the absence of normative data or standard criteria of references in many countries. At present, some proposals have been studied to improve this model. These include the use of Z values corrected for the variance of each variable and the establishment of critical Z values for the relevant and critical variables in different sports.

In summary, the CELAFISCS strategy for talent detection includes the following steps:

1 Use of a physical fitness battery of tests, with specific items if possible.

2 Comparison to normative values and standard reference criteria.

3 Developing the Z profile, with special attention to the critical and relevant variables.

4 Analysis of functional maturational pattern of the critical variable.

5 Evaluation of sexual maturation status.

6 Determination of nutritional level.

7 Verification of sports experience level.

The present model is based on biological cri-

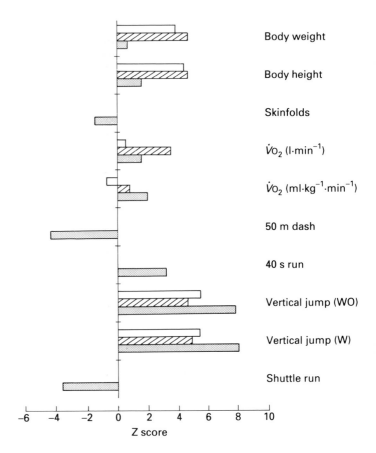

Fig. 6.5 Z profile of international basketball stars: a male at ages 14 (□) and 21 (▨) years, and a woman (▣). W, with arm assistance; WO, without arm assistance. Adapted from Matsudo *et al.* (1987).

teria but it is clear that the inclusion of psycho-social aspects will expand its applicability.

Challenges for future research

The following topics should receive priority amongst researchers:

• A better knowledge of the 'normal' which permits better accuracy in the perception and detection of the well-gifted youth.

• Creation of a databank at regional, national, continental and world levels as well as of ethnic groups.

• Development of specific physical fitness test batteries for each sport modality.

• Development of an international system of information about the progress reached in the area, for research and applied purposes.

• Improvement of training models which permit the monitoring of progress and decline, including indices of 'burn-out'.

• Development of statistical models that could concurrently offer high accuracy and practical application.

• Integration of 'practitioners' and 'theoreticians' by means of promoting scientific events, publications and field research programmes.

• Determination of the critical and more relevant variables linked to excellence in performance, as well as the integration among them.

• Longitudinal projects to determine the natural development of the gifted athlete, and then implement intervention or experimental programmes.

References

AAHPERD (1976) *Youth Fitness Test Manual.* AAHPERD Publications, Washington.

Alonso, A.F. & Pila, H. (1985) *Experiences on a Method for Athlete Preparation.* Ciências Médicas, Habana.

Åstrand, P.O. (1993) Children and adolescents: performance, measurements, education. *Braz. J. Sci. Move.* 7(1), 11–14.

Bar-Or, O. (1989) Trainability of the prepubescent child. *Phys. Sports Med.* 17(5), 64–82.

Bar-Or, O., Dotan, R. & Inbar, O. (1977) A 30 sec all out ergometric test its reability and validity for anaerobic capacity. *Isr. J. Med. Sci.* 13, 126.

Bauersfeld, K.H. (1990) The selection of top class athletes. In R.J. Fisher & J. Borms (eds) *The Search for Sporting Excellence*, pp. 40–4. Hofmann Verlag, Schorndorf.

Baumgartner, R.N. & Roche, A.F. (1988) Tracking of fat pattern indices in childhood: the Melbourne growth study. *Hum. Biol.* 60, 549–67.

Bento, J.O. (1989) Detecção e fomento de talentos (Detection and muturing of talent). *Braz. J. Sci. Move.* 3(3), 84–93.

Beunen, G. & Malina, R. (1988) Growth and physical performance relative to the timing of the adolescent spurt. *Exerc. Sport Sci. Rev.* 16, 503–40.

Bloom, B.S. (1964) *Stability and Change in Human Characteristics.* John Wiley, New York.

Bloom, B.S. (1985) *Developing Talent in Young People.* Ballantine, New York.

Bloomfield, J. (1991) Physical education and sports: an international perspective. *Sports Excell.* (Hong Kong) 3, 8–16.

Borg, G.A.V. (1973) Perceived exertion: a note on 'history' and methods. *Med. Sci. Sports* 5(2), 90–3.

Bouchard, C. (1988) Genetics and adaptation to training. In *New Horizons of Human Movement*, pp. 84–90. Seoul Olympic Scientific Congress, Cheonan.

Bouchard, C., Dionne, F.T., Simoneau, J.A. & Boulay, M.R. (1992) Genetics of aerobic and anaerobic performances. *Exerc. Sport Sci. Rev.* 20, 27–58.

Bouchard, C., Lesage, R., Lortie, G. *et al.* (1986) Aerobic performance in brothers, dizygotic and monozygotic twins. *Med. Sci. Sports Exerc.* 18, 639–46.

Bouchard, C., Perusse, L., Leblanc, C., Tremblay, A. & Theriault (1988) Inheritance of the amount and distribution of human body fat. *Int. J. Obes.* 12, 205–15.

Boulgakova, N. (1990) *Sélection et Preparation des Jeunes Nageurs* (Selection and Preparation of Young Talent). Vigor, Paris.

CAHPER (1966) *Le Manual d'Instructions di Test d'Efficience Physique de la CAHPER à la Usage des Garçons et Filles de 7 a 17 ans* (Instruction Manual of the CAHPER Physical Fitness Tests for Boys and Girls aged 7–17 years). CAHPER, Toronto.

Caicedo, J.G., Matsudo, S.M.M. & Matsudo, V.K.R. (1993) Measurement of agility among soccer players through a specific test and its correlation to pass performance in a real game situation. *Braz. J. Sci. Move.* 1(2), 7–15.

Campos, M.A.Z., França, N.M. & Matsudo, V.K.R. (1990) Age of menarche from Ilhabela students. In *Annals from XXVII International Symposium on Sports Sciences*, p. 85.

Carter, J.E.L. (1980) *The Heath–Carter Somatotype Method.* San Diego State University Syllabus Service, San Diego.

Cavasini, S.M. (1984) Social influences upon Brazilian children participation in physical activities and sports. In *New Horizons of Human Movement.* Olympic Scientific Congress. Eugene.

Cavasini, S.M. & Matsudo, V.K.R. (1983) The development of a Brazilian perceived exertion scale. *Braz. J. Sports Sci.* 5(3).

Cavasini, S.M., Matsudo, V.K.R. & Cazelatti, S. (1980) Personality of the athlete: a literature review. *Braz. J. Sports Sci.* 2(1), 9–13.

Cavasini, S.M., Matsudo, V.K.R. & Soeiro, A.C. (1978) The influence of positive and negative audience as selected by sociometry on motor performance. In *XXI World Congress in Sports Medicine, Brazil.*

Cazelatti, S., Cavasini, S.M. & Matsudo, V.K.R. (1977) Applicability of sociometric measurements in sports. *Braz. J. Sports Med.* 4(3–4), 95–9.

Cazelatti, S., Matsudo, V.K.R. & Cavasini, S.M. (1980) Self-concept and participation in physical activities. *Braz. J. Sports. Sci.* 2(1), 32–5.

Claessens, A., Beunen, G. & Simons, J. (1986) Stability of anthroposcopic and anthropometric estimates of physique in Belgian boys followed longitudinally from 13 to 18 years of age. *Ann. Hum. Biol.* 13, 235–44.

Conseil de l'Europe (1988) *Eurofit: Manual Pour les Tests Eurofit d'Aptitude Physique.* Comite Pour Development du Sport, Rome.

de Garay, A.L., Levine, L. & Carter, J.E. (1974) *Genetic and Anthropological Studies of Olympic Athletes.* Academic Press, New York.

Duarte, C.R. & Duarte, M.F.S. (1989) Aerobic capacity among students from 10 to 18 years old. *Braz. J. Sci. Move.* 3(3), 17–25.

Duarte, C.R. & Matsudo, V.K.R. (1986) Velocity in the 50 m dash: results in students from 7 to 18 years. In *CELAFISCS, Ten Years of Contribution to Sports Sciences*, p. 257. CELAFISCS, São Caetano do Sul.

Ejem, M. (1988) Study of relationships among parameters of performance in volleyball and selected anthropometric and motoric measures. In *New Horizons of Human Movement*, p. 82. Seoul Olympic Scientific Congress, Cheonan.

Ejem, M., Bunc, V., Tlapak, P., Moraveo, P. & Kucera, V. (1988) The determination of special motor abilities under field conditions. In *New Horizons of Human Movement*. Seoul Olympic Scientific Congress, Cheonan.

Figueira Jr A.J. & Matsudo, V.K.R. (1992) Determination of physical performance of Brazilian volleyball players through Z index (abstract). In J. Coudert & E. van Praagh (eds) *Pediatric Work Physiology*, p. 164. Masson, Paris.

Fischbein, S. (1977) Onset of puberty in MZ and DZ twins. *Acta Gen. Med. Gemellol.* **26**, 151–8.

Fisher, R.J. & Borms, J. (1990) *The Search for Sporting Excellence*. Hofmann Verlag, Schorndorf.

França, N.M., Matsudo, V.K.R. & Brandao, M.R.F. (1992) Impact of menarche on velocity and ability performance among girls at the same chronological age. In J. Coudert & E. van Praagh (eds) *Pediatric Work Physiology*, pp. 229–31. Masson, Paris.

França, N.M., Matsudo, V.K.R. & Sessa, M. (1988) Skinfolds in students from 7 to 18 years old. *Braz. J. Sci. Move.* **2**(4), 7–16.

Hebbelinck, M. (1990) Talent identification and development in sport: kinanthropometric issues. *Braz. J. Sci. Move.* **4**(1), 46–62.

Hemery, D. (1986) *Sporting Excellence. A Study of Sport's Highest Achievers*. Willow Books, London.

Housh, T.J., Thorland, W.G., Johnson, G.O., Hughes, R.A. & Cisar, C.J. (1986) Body composition and body build variables as predictor of middle distance running performance. *J. Sports. Med. Phys. Fitness* **26**(3), 258–62.

Israel, S., Kunath, P. & Kunat, H. (1988) On the athletic activity and physical perfection in view of the bio-psycho-social entity of human beings. In *ICSSPE Executive Board Meeting*. CSSPE, Leipzig.

Jacquard, A. (1989) *Elogio da Diferença: A Genética e os Homens*. Publicações Europa-América, São Paulo.

Kovar, R. (1981) *Human Variation in Motor Abilities and its Genetic Analysis*. Charles University, Prague.

Larson, L.A. (1974) *Fitness, Health and Work Capacity. International Standards for Assessment*. Macmillan, New York.

Léfevre, J., Beunen, G., Claessens, A. *et al.* (1989) Stability in level of subcutaneous fat between adolescence and adulthood. In G. Beunen, J. Guesquière, T. Reybrouck & A. Claessens (eds) *Children and Exercise*, pp. 45–51. Ferdinand Enke Verlag, Stuttgart.

Lehman, G. (1988) Talent determination and talent promotion in sports. In *New Horizons in Human Movement*, p. 24. Seoul Olympic Scientific Congress, Cheonan.

Lesage, R., Simoneau, J.A., Jobin, J., Leblanc, C. & Bouchard, C. (1985) Familiar resemblance in maximal heart rate, blood lactate and aerobic power. *Hum. Hered.* **35**, 182–9.

Maia, J.A.R. (1993) *Anthropobiological approach on selection in sports*. Doctoral thesis, University of O'Porto.

Maia, J., Silva, R., Janeira, M. & Vicente, C. (1992) Somatotype and motor performance: a discriminant study in young female volleyball players. In A.L. Claessens, J. Lefevre & B.V. Eynde (eds) *Worldwide Variation in Physical Fitness*, p. 93. Katholieke Universiteit Leuven, Leuven.

Malina, R. (1986) Readiness for competitive sport. In M.R. Weiss & D.M. Gould (eds) *Sport for Children and Youths: The 1984 Olympic Scientific Congress Proceedings*, Vol. 10. Human Kinetics, Champaign, IL.

Malina, R.M. (1989) Tracking of physical fitness and performance during growth. In *XIV International Seminar on Pediatric Work Physiology*. Leuven.

Malina R.M. (1994) Physical growth and biological maturation of young athletes. *Exerc. Sport Sci. Rev.* **22**, 389–434.

Malina, R.M. & Bouchard, C. (1991) *Growth, Maturation and Physical Activity*. Human Kinetics, Champaign, IL.

Malinowski, A. (1986) Conceptions of norm and normality in biology of manuals medicine. In N. Wolanski & M. Szemir (eds) *Studies in Human Ecology, Growth and Socio-Economic Conditions*. Polish Academy of Sciences, Varsow.

Marques, A. (1993) Basis for developing a model to detect and select sport talents in Portugal. *Espaço* **1**(1), 47–58.

Matsudo, S.M.M., Henao, S.M. & Matsudo, K.R. (1992a) The perceived exertion among undernourished girls. In *Olympic Scientific Congress, Malaga*, p. KIN-38.

Matsudo, S.M.M. & Matsudo, V.K.R. (1993) The perceived exertion among undernourished girls and boys. *Med. Sci. Sports Exerc.* **25**(5).

Matsudo, S.M.M. & Matsudo, V.K.R. (1994) Self-assessment and physician assessment of sexual maturation in Brazilian boys and girls: concordance and reproducibility. *Am. J. Hum. Biol.* **6**, 451–5.

Matsudo, V.K.R. (1987a) Motor characteristics of Brazilian boys and girls from 7 to 18 years of age. *Sport Sci. Rev.* **10**, 55–61.

Matsudo, V.K.R. (1987b) *Tests in Sports Sciences*, 4th edn, p. 34. CELAFISCS, São Caetano do Sul.

Matsudo, V.K.R. (1988) Forty seconds run test: perspectives of a decade. *Hum. Biol.* (Budapest), **18**, 127–31.

Matsudo, V.K.R. (1989) Aerobic and anaerobic maturational indices among peripubertal boys and girls. *Med. Sci. Sports Exerc.* **21**(4), S83 (abstract).

Matsudo, V.K.R. (1992) Physical fitness in developing countries. In A.L. Claessens, J. Lefevre, B.V. Eynde (eds) *World-wide Variation in Physical Fitness*, pp. 111–25. Katholieke Universiteit Leuven, Leuven.

Matsudo, V.K.R., França, N.M. & Matsudo, S.M.M. (1992b) Quantitative and qualitative differences in motor performance in adolescent Brazilian girls. In T.J. Couder & E. van Praagh (eds) *Pediatric Work Physiology*, pp. 225–7. Masson, Paris.

Matsudo, V.K.R. & Matsudo, S.M.M. (1993) Structural and neuromotor changes in undernourished boys and girls. *Med. Sci. Sports Exerc.* **25**(5), S92.

Matsudo, V.K.R., Pereira, M.H.N. & Rivet, R.E. (1986a) Z-indices migration in athletes from the Brazilian national men team, as related to evolution in technical level (abstract). In *Annals of the XIV Symposium on Sports Sciences*, p. 69. CELAFISCS, São Caetano do Sul.

Matsudo, V.K.R., Rivet, R.E. & Pereira, M.H.N. (1987) Standards score assessment on physique and performance of Brazilian athletes in a six tiered competitive sports model. *J. Sports Sci.* **5**, 49–53.

Matsudo, V.K.R., Soares, J. & Duarte, C.R. (1986b) Brazilian basketball men team Z-profile centers, guards and forwards (abstract). In *Annals of the XIV Symposium on Sports Sciences*, p. 57. CELAFISCS, São Caetano do Sul.

Matsuura, Y. (1988) Prediction of future status of physical fitness of Japanese youth using the annual data from 1964 through 1985. In *New Horizons of Human Movement*, p. 28. Seoul Olympic Scientific Congress, Cheonan.

Nascimento, M.B., Duarte, C.R. & Santos, A.R.B. (1989) Physical fitness Z-profile from track and field top athletes. *Braz. J. Sci. Move.* **3**(3), 26–34.

Nunnally, J.C. (1978) *Psychometric Theory*. McGraw-Hill, New York.

Oliveira, A.J., França, N.M. & Duarte, M.F.S. (1986) Diameter and circumferences in students from 7 to 18 years old. In *CELAFISCS Ten Years of Contribution to Sports Sciences*, p. 139. CELAFISCS, São Caetano do Sul.

Osse, C.M.C., Cavasini, S.M. & Matsudo, V.K.R. (1981) Objectivity and reproductibility of sociometric measurements applied in sports. *Braz. J. Sports Sci.* **2**(3), 28–31.

Parizkova, J. (1977) *Body Fat and Physical Fitness*. Martinus Nijhoff, The Hague.

Parizkova, J. & Carter, J.E.L. (1976) Influence of physical activity on stability of somatotype in boys. *Am. J. Phys. Anthropol.* **44**, 327–40.

Prud'homme, D., Bouchard, C., Leblanc, C., Landry, F. & Fontaine, E. (1984) Sensitivity of maximal aerobic power to training is genotype dependent. *Med. Sci. Sports Exerc.* **16**, 489–93.

Rarick, G.L. (1981) The emergence of the study of human development. In G.A. Brooks (ed.) *Perspectives on the Academic Discipline of Physical Education — a Tribute to Lawrence Rarick*. Human Kinetics, Champaign, IL.

Rarick, L.G. & Smoll, F.L. (1967) Stability of growth in strength and motor performance from childhood to adolescence. *Hum. Biol.* **39**(3), 295–306.

Roche, A.F. & Baumgartner, R.N. (1988) Tracking in fat distribution during growth. In C. Bouchard & F.E. Johnston (eds) *Fat Distribution during Growth and Later Health Outcomes*. Alan R. Liss, New York.

Rowland, T.W. (1992) Aerobic responses to physical training in children. In R.S. Shephard & P.-O. Åstrand *Endurance in Sport*, pp. 377–84. Blackwell Scientific Publications, Oxford.

Samulski, D. (1991) Sport and personality development. *Braz. J. Sci. Move.* **5**(3), 24–8.

Santos, G., França, N.M. & Matsudo, V.K.R. (1989) Impact of undernutrition on aerobic and anaerobic characteristics of boys and girls. *Braz. J. Sports Sci.* **11**(1), 93.

Santos, V.C., Figueira Jr. A.J. & Matsudo, V.K.R. (1991) Percentage of maturation and growth velocity of anthropometric and neuromotor variables of two different regions. *Braz. J. Sci. Move.* **5**(2), 52–60.

Sessa, M., Matsudo, V.K.R., Vivolo, M.A. & Tarapanoff, A.M.P.A. (1986) Development of lower limb strength in students from 7 to 18 years old as related to sex, age, weight, height and physical activity. In *CELAFISCS, Ten Years of Contribution to Sports Sciences*, pp. 214–20. CELAFISCS, São Caetano do Sul.

Silva, R.C. & Rivet, R.E. (1988) Physical fitness variables from the 1986 national men volleyball team as related to game function. *Braz. J. Sci. Move.* **2**(3), 28–32.

Simoneau, J.A., Lortie, G., Boulay, M.R., Margotte, M., Thilbault, M.C. & Bouchard, C. (1986) Inheritance of human skeletal muscle and anaerobic capacity adaptation to high-intensity intermittent training. *Int. J. Sports Med.* **7**, 167–71.

Soares, J., Miguel, M.C. & Matsudo, V.K.R. (1981) Development of handgrip strength as related to age, sex, weight, and height in students from 7 to 18 years old. *Braz. J. Sports Sci.* **2**(2), 20–4.

Sodhi, H.S. (1990) Scouting for future top class athletes. In R.J. Fisher & J. Borms (eds) *The Search for Sporting Excellence*, p. 70. Hofmann Verlag, Schorndorf.

Sprynarova, S. & Parizkova, J. (1977) The influence of training on physical and function growth bones before, during and after puberty. *Eur. J. Appl. Physiol.* **56**, 719–24.

Stork, H.M. (1990) Strategies of talent scouting and talent development based on model projects in track and field athletics in the Federal Republic of Germany. In R.J. Fisher & J. Borms (eds) *The Search for Sporting Excellence*, pp. 44–5. Hofmann Verlag, Schorndorf.

Szabo, T. (1989) Pattern stability of power jumps in young males (abstract). In *XIV International Seminar on Pediatric Work Physiology*. Leuven.

Tanaka, K. & Matsuura, Y. (1982) A multivariate analysis of the role of certain anthropometric and physiological attributes in distance running. *Ann. Hum. Biol.* **9**, 473–82.

Tanner, J.M. & Whithehouse, R.M. (1969) *Atlas of Children's Growth. Normal Variation and Growth Disorders*. Academic Press, New York.

Tatsuoka, M.M. (1988) *Multivariate Analysis. Techniques for Education and Psychological Research*. Macmillan, New York.

Thorland, W. (1990) Selected physiological and struc-tural characteristics of élite adult athletes and younger competitors. In R.J. Fisher & J. Borms (eds) *The Search for Sporting Excellence*, pp. 71–3. Hofmann Verlag, Schorndorf.

Vanden Eynde, B., Vienne, D., Vuylsteke-Wauters, M. & Van Gerven, D. (1988) Aerobic power and pubertal peak height velocity in Belgian boys. *Eur. J. Appl. Physiol.* **57**, 430–4.

Waddington, C.H. (1957) *The Strategy of the Genes*. Allen & Unwin, London.

Weiner, J.S. & Lourie, J.A. (1969) *Human Biology. A Guide to Field Methods*. IBP Handbook 9. Blackwell Scientific Publications, Oxford.

Wilson, J.P. & Poster, D.W. (eds) (1985) *Williams Textbook of Endocrinology*, 7th edn. W.B. Saunders, Philadelphia.

PART 2

TRAINING: PRINCIPLES AND TRAINABILITY

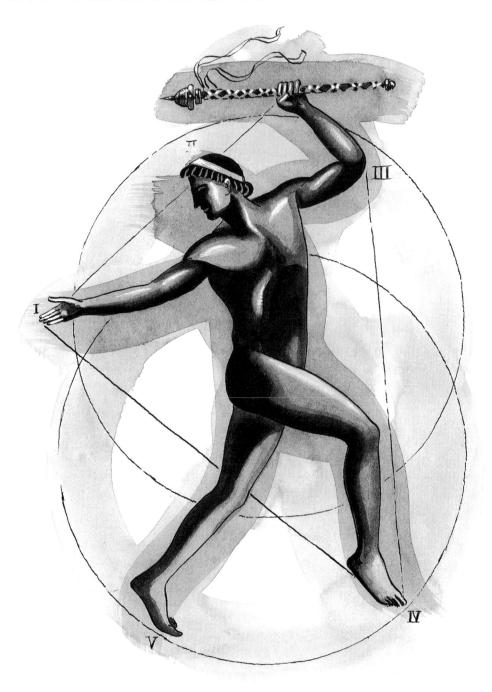

Chapter 7

Trainability of Muscle Strength, Power and Endurance during Childhood

CAMERON J.R. BLIMKIE AND ODED BAR-OR

Trainability of muscle strength

Strength is defined as the peak force or torque developed during a maximal voluntary effort, whereas power is defined as the rate at which mechanical work is performed within a given period of time (Sale, 1991). The two are inextricably linked as depicted in the well-known force–velocity–power relationship (Fig. 7.1). Strength and power are important prerequisites for activities of daily living and success in sport during childhood; the relative importance of the two may vary, however, depending on the nature of the activity or sport, and the health status of the child. There is substantial information about the factors which determine strength and power, and the trainability of these capacities in adults (Green, 1991; Komi, 1992). By comparison, little is known about the determinants of strength and power or their trainability during childhood. This chapter focuses on the trainability of muscle strength, power and endurance at different stages of development during childhood. Because of the paucity of information about the trainability of muscle power and endurance in children, most of the chapter is devoted to the trainability of strength.

Skeletal muscle strength

There is considerable public and scientific interest in strength training during childhood. The key areas of interest relate to the risk of injury, the effectiveness of training to increase strength especially during the pre- and early pubertal years, and the mechanisms underlying training-induced strength gains and changes in strength during detraining. These topics have been recently and thoroughly reviewed (Kraemer *et al.*, 1989; Sale, 1989; Weltman, 1989; Freedson *et al.*, 1990; Webb, 1990; Blimkie, 1992, 1993a,b). The following sections address the trainability of strength, the mechanisms underlying training-induced strength gains, and changes in strength during detraining at different developmental stages during childhood.

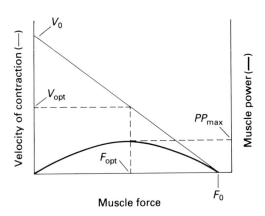

Fig. 7.1 Theoretical relationship among muscle force, velocity of muscle contraction and muscle power. F_0: peak force during an isometric contraction at 0 velocity; V_0: peak rate of muscle contraction; PP_{max}: maximum peak power; V_{opt}: rate of contraction which elicits PP_{max}; F_{opt}: muscle force which elicits PP_{max} at V_{opt}.

Childhood encompasses several developmental periods, and in this chapter will be arbitrarily divided into two stages: (i) preadolescence which includes pre- and early pubertal girls and boys 11 and 13 years of age or younger, respectively; and (ii) adolescence which includes girls and boys in the mid- and late stages of puberty who are 12 and 14 years of age or older, respectively. Division by chronological age is problematic since it does not take into consideration the influence of individual rates of maturation on pubertal status (for more detail see Chapter 14). Nevertheless, at these age divisions, the majority of children either have not yet experienced their peak growth spurt in stature or are in the midst or past their peak growth spurts, and this seems a rationale point of division from which to consider the issue of trainability of strength.

In this chapter, resistance training refers to the use of progressive resistance training methods to exert or resist force (Cahill, 1988); this term will be used interchangeably with strength training. Resistance training methods vary in design, training mode, and relative strain or intensity of applied resistance. Resistance training studies involving children have incorporated a variety of training methods, and these differences have confounded interpretation of resistance training studies in this population.

Effectiveness of resistance training

A number of earlier studies (Kirsten, 1963; Ainsworth, 1970; Vrijens, 1978; Docherty et al., 1987b) failed to demonstrate any significant effect of resistance training on strength in prepubertal children. Despite their design limitations (Blimkie, 1992, 1993b), these studies suggested that strength training would be ineffective prior to puberty. Additionally, it was thought that strength gains were not possible with training until circulating testosterone levels increased substantially during mid- to late puberty.

Studies which have controlled for the con-founding effects of growth and motor skill acquisition, and which have incorporated moderate to high training loads provide rather convincing evidence that strength training can result in substantial and significant increases in strength during preadolescence (Nielsen et al., 1980; Pfeiffer & Francis, 1986; Sewall & Micheli, 1986; Weltman et al., 1986; Sailors & Berg, 1987; Hakkinen et al., 1989; Mersch & Stoboy, 1989; Hassan, 1991; Ozmun et al., 1994; Fukunga et al., 1992).

The results of one of the longest and most strenuous strength training studies to date involving preadolescents (Ramsay et al., 1990) also support this view. In this study, healthy, normoactive prepubertal (9–11 years of age) boys participated in 20 weeks of dynamic resistance training which emphasized the elbow flexor and knee extensor muscle groups. The training involved progressive resistance loading (resistance was increased as subjects became stronger), a similar frequency (three times per week) and intensity (75–85% of the one repetition maximum — 1 RM — loads) of training as commonly used in strength training programmes for adults (Fleck & Kraemer, 1987). Strength testing was both training mode-specific (1 RM lifts) and non-specific (isometric and isokinetic testing), and the effects of skill acquisition or motor learning were controlled by performing interim testing, and including a control group. Training resulted in significant increases (Fig. 7.2) in the 1 RM bench press (35%), the 1 RM double leg press (22%), maximal voluntary isometric elbow flexion (37%) and knee extension (25%) strength, and maximal voluntary isokinetic elbow flexion (26%) and knee extension (21%) strength.

It appears from these later studies that strength training can effectively increase strength during the preadolescent period. The effectiveness of training appears, as it does also in adults, to be dependent primarily on the provision of a sufficient training intensity and volume, and to a lesser degree on training duration. Strength improvements have been reported using isometric, isotonic and iso-

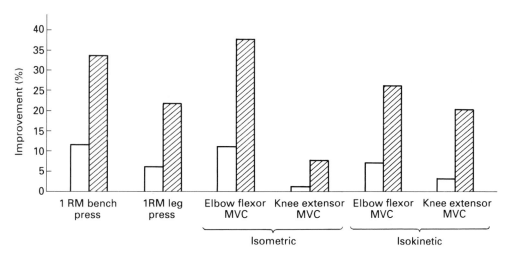

Fig. 7.2 Effects of 20 weeks of heavy resistance training on various measures of strength in preadolescent boys (Ramsey *et al.*, 1990). □, control; ▨, trained; MVC, maximum voluntary contraction.

kinetic training methods involving high-intensity loading. The optimal combination of training method, mode, intensity, volume and duration of training for maximal strength gain during preadolescence however, has yet to be determined.

The trainability of strength during adolescence is a less contentious issue. Significant strength gains have resulted from isometric training (Wolbers & Sills, 1956; Rarick & Larsen, 1958; Kirsten, 1963; Fukunaga, 1976; Komi *et al.*, 1978; Nielsen *et al.*, 1980; DeKoning *et al.*, 1984), dynamic or isotonic weight training (Gallagher & DeLorme, 1949; DeLorme *et al.*, 1952; Kusinitz & Keeney, 1958; Vrijens, 1978; Westcott 1979, 1991; Gillam, 1981; Munson *et al.*, 1985; Pfeiffer & Francis, 1986), isokinetic (McCubbin & Shasby 1985) and hydraulic resistance training (Blimkie *et al.*, 1993). With dynamic or isotonic training, strength gains appear to be directly related to the frequency of training (Gillam, 1981) nevertheless, as for the preadolescent population, the optimal combination of training mode, intensity, volume and duration of resistance training for strength increases during adolescence has yet to be established.

Trainability at different maturational stages

How effective is strength training during preadolescence compared to training during adolescence, and adulthood? Results from a number of earlier studies suggested that preadolescent children had either the same or lower relative (per cent improvement) trainability, but lower absolute (actual gains in lifting capacity in pounds, kilograms or newton metres) trainability than adolescents and young adults (Hettinger, 1958; Kirsten, 1963; Vrijens, 1978). The conclusions from these studies are questionable however, given the relatively low training loads and the failure in some cases to clearly formulate groups on the basis of distinct maturity levels.

Studies which used similar training programmes across developmental stages, which incorporated moderate to high training intensities and volumes, and which used distinct maturity groups, have consistently reported comparable, and sometimes greater relative strength trainability in preadolescents, compared to adolescents and adults (Westcott, 1979; Nielsen *et al.*, 1980; Pfeiffer & Francis, 1986; Sailors & Berg, 1987; Sale, 1989). A summary of the results from the study of Pfeiffer and Francis

(1986) is provided in Fig. 7.3. A recent study (Hakkinen *et al.*, 1989), likewise, reported greater relative squat extension strength gains in preadolescent boys, compared to a group of élite junior weight-lifters following 1 year of weight-training. The results from this study cannot be taken as support of greater relative strength trainability of preadolescents since there were differences in initial level of training experience, and the training programmes differed considerably between groups. There is less information about the trainability of absolute strength; four studies have reported lower absolute strength trainability in preadolescents compared to adolescents (Hakkinen *et al.*, 1989) and adults (Sailors & Berg, 1987; Sale, 1989; Fukunaga *et al.*, 1992), whereas a fifth study, which may be criticized because of its small sample size (Westcott, 1979), reported greater absolute strength gains in preadolescent girls compared to adolescent and adult females.

It appears that preadolescents are probably less trainable in terms of absolute strength gains, but equally, if not more trainable in a relative (percentage improvement) sense compared to adolescents and young adults.

Additional studies which include distinct maturity groups, identical training programmes across levels of maturity, and which also control for age- and gender-associated differences in background level of physical activity and training are required however, before the question of comparative strength trainability is unequivocally resolved.

Persistence of strength gains

Will training-induced strength gains be maintained or lost during periods of partial or complete withdrawal (detraining) from training? The answer to this question is not as straightforward as it first appears, since any loss in strength due to a reduction in training may be partially or wholly offset by a concomitant growth-related increase in strength (Blimkie, 1989; see Chapter 2). A simple model of the potential interactions between growth and training/detraining during childhood is presented in Fig. 7.4.

In this model, if strength gains are permanent, one would expect strength for a previously trained group to increase by the same magni-

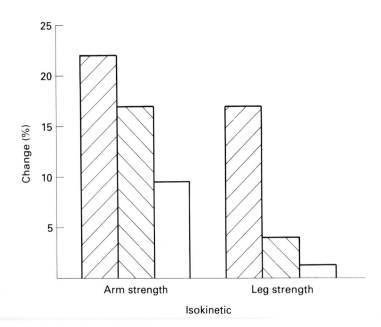

Fig. 7.3 Comparative (relative) strength changes in torque per kilogram of body weight in preadolescent (▨), adolescent (▧), and adult (□) males in response to 9 weeks of resistance training. Drawn from data in Pfeiffer and Francis (1986).

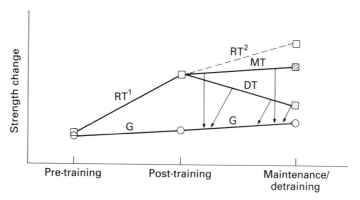

Fig. 7.4 Model of expected strength changes with growth (G), resistance training (RT), maintenance training (MT) and detraining (DT) during childhood. Section G: strength increases due to growth and maturation — serves as a control for growth and maturation in training studies during childhood. Rates may vary depending on developmental stage. Section RT^1: strength increases rapidly during the initial stage of training due to growth and training effects — assumes that learning effects are controlled; RT^2: strength increases more slowly during the later stages of training and is due to growth and a dampened training effect; MT: strength increases beyond the post-training level due solely to growth — the post-training difference in strength is sustained during this period as indicated by the equal length long arrows; DT: strength decreases below the post-training level due to the complete withdrawal of training — the post-training strength difference is lost progressively with time and may converge with the control level (G) as indicated by the diagonal arrows of diminishing length.

tude as the change in a control group (simple additive effect of the growth-related increase in strength) during the detraining period, and persistence of the strength difference that had been established at the end of training. If strength gains are not permanent, and there is a loss in strength due to detraining, then there will be a gradual regression in the strength curve of the previously trained group, and a convergence with the strength curve for the control group at a level below the peak strength achieved at the end of training.

Only two studies, both of which have design limitations, have investigated this question in preadolescents (Sewall & Micheli, 1986; Blimkie *et al.*, 1989a). In the only study which included a requisite control group (Blimkie *et al.*, 1989a), the majority of strength measures in the previously trained group converged toward the control values, suggesting that training-induced strength gains during preadolescence are probably impermanent. Whether the strength gains will revert fully to the growth-adjusted

control levels will probably depend upon both the magnitude of the initial strength gains as well as the duration of the detraining period.

If prior strength gains are lost during detraining, how much maintenance training is required to preserve these gains? In the only study (Blimkie *et al.*, 1989a) to investigate this question, a single, weekly, high-intensity strength training session was not sufficient to preserve prior training-induced strength gains in a group of preadolescent boys. The training-induced strength gains regressed toward the growth-adjusted control level in a manner identical to that for a totally detrained group.

Based on rather limited information, it appears that training-induced strength gains are probably impermanent, and that one high-intensity training session per week is probably insufficient for maintenance training at least during preadolescence. No firm guidelines can be provided at this time regarding the requirements for maintenance training during either preadolescence or adolescence.

Mechanisms underlying strength changes

What are the physiological adaptations, and the mechanisms underlying training- and detraining-induced strength changes during childhood?

MORPHOLOGICAL ADAPTATIONS
DURING TRAINING

Training-induced changes in gross limb morphology, and by inference, changes in muscle size, have been assessed using indirect anthropometric techniques. With these techniques, there is no evidence of training-induced muscle hypertrophy in any of the studies which reported significant increases in strength during preadolescence (Sailors & Berg, 1987; McGovern, 1984; Weltman et al., 1986; Blimkie et al., 1989b; Hakkinen et al., 1989; Siegel et al., 1989; Ramsay et al., 1990; Hassan, 1991; Ozmun et al., 1994).

More sensitive imaging techniques, including soft tissue roentgenography, ultrasound, computerized tomography and magnetic resonance imaging have also been used to investigate the effects of strength training on muscle size in children (Vrijens, 1978; Mersch & Stoboy, 1989; Ramsay et al., 1990; Fukunaga et al., 1992). Two of these studies (Vrijens, 1978; Blimkie et al., 1990), of which only the former resulted in a significant increase in strength, found no evidence of muscle hypertrophy in preadolescent boys. Two other recent studies, however, have reported resistance training-induced muscle hypertrophy in preadolescents. Mersch and Stoboy (1989) reported significant strength training-induced increases in both knee extension isometric strength and quadriceps muscle cross-sectional area determined by magnetic resonance imaging in two preadolescent twin boys. This is the first study to report muscle hypertrophy resulting from strength training in preadolescents. Likewise, Fukunaga et al. (1992) reported significant increases in upper arm isometric and isokinetic strength and lean (muscle and bone) cross-sectional area determined by ultrasound in preadolescent Japanese girls and boys. The absolute increase in muscle size, however, was only half of the typical change observed in adults in response to similar training. It is difficult given the small sample and other peculiarities in the data of Mersch and Stoboy (1989), and the imprecision inherent in the ultrasound technique employed by Fukunaga et al. (1992) to totally discount the largely negative results from all the other studies in this area. Nevertheless, these results leave open the possibility of strength training-induced muscle hypertrophy even during preadolescence. Whether resistance training in the context of recreational, fitness or sport-based programmes provides sufficient additional mechanical strain beyond normal levels of generally high background muscular activity to induce muscle hypertrophy in otherwise healthy preadolescent children remains to be unequivocally established.

For adolescent boys, strength training-induced increases in muscle size have been inferred both from indirect anthropometric measures of increased arm and thigh girths (Delorme et al., 1952; Kusinitz & Keeney, 1958; Hakkinen et al., 1989) and from roentgeno-graphically determined increases in arm and thigh muscle cross-sectional areas (Vrijens, 1978). An increase (8.3%) in upper arm lean area (bone and muscle) determined by ultrasound was reported by Von Fukunaga (1976) for a group of 13-year-old Japanese girls following a 3-month programme of isometric training which elicited a 93.4% increase in absolute isometric strength. However, in a recent study involving adolescent females (C.J.R. Blimkie et al., unpublished results), 26 weeks of heavy resistance training which resulted in significant strength increases failed to cause any increase in anthropometrically determined upper arm girth or quadriceps muscle cross-sectional area determined by computerized tomography.

It appears that training-induced muscle hypertrophy may be possible, but is probably unlikely during preadolescence. Muscle hypertrophy appears to be a more consistent outcome of strength or resistance training during adolescence, especially for males; the hypertrophy response may be more variable and of a smaller (absolute) magnitude in adolescent females. There are no studies to date, however, which permit a valid comparison between sexes of the relative hypertrophy responses to identical training programmes during adolescence, or between adolescents and adults. Whatever the hypertrophy response, the magnitude of this morphological adaptation is small in comparison to the reported strength gains. Other factors besides changes in muscle size must also contribute to the strength gains.

NEUROLOGICAL ADAPTATIONS
DURING TRAINING

By inference, and based solely on the lack of evidence for muscle hypertrophy, training-induced strength increases in preadolescent boys have been attributed to undefined neurological and neuromotor adaptations (Weltman *et al.*, 1986; Hakkinen *et al.*, 1989; Hassan, 1991). These studies provide only weak indirect support for unspecified neurological and motor coordination contributions to strength training-induced strength gains in preadolescents.

A more direct means of neurological assessment, the twitch interpolation technique (Belanger & McComas, 1981), has recently been used by Blimkie *et al.* (1989b) and Ramsay *et al.* (1990), to assess the contribution of changes in motor unit activation (MUA) to training-induced strength increases in preadolescent boys. MUA of the elbow flexors and knee extensors increased by 9 and 12%, respectively, after 10 weeks of training, and an additional 10 weeks of training resulted in much smaller increases of only 3 and 2%, respectively. The percentage increases in MUA were less than the increases in strength for both muscle groups. Recently, Ozmun *et al.* (1994) used electromyography (EMG) to measure strength training-induced changes in neuromuscular activation of the elbow flexors in preadolescent boys and

girls: 8 weeks of training resulted in significant increases in both integrated EMG (IEMG) amplitude (16.8%) and maximal isokinetic strength (27.8%). Results from these studies suggest that training-induced strength gains in preadolescents, especially during the early stages of strength training, are attributable at least in part to increases in neuromuscular activation.

During adolescence, concomitant increases in isometric strength and maximum IEMG activity, an indirect measure of maximal voluntary neural activation, have been reported for the vastus lateralis and vastus medialis muscles in males (Hakkinen *et al.*, 1989) and the rectus femoris muscle (Komi *et al.*, 1978) in both males and females. In both studies, the increase in IEMG activity was greater than the observed strength increase (8.9 versus 5.2%, Hakkinen *et al.*, Kauhanen 1989; 38 versus 20%, Komi *et al.*, 1978). In a recent study of adolescent females, training-induced knee extensor strength gains (23.3%) were accompanied by a smaller increase (9.5% in knee extensor MUA (C.J.R. Blimkie *et al.*, unpublished results).

Resistance training-induced strength gains both during preadolescence and adolescence appear to be achieved in part by increased voluntary neuromuscular activation. The magnitude of the changes in neuromuscular activation is generally smaller than the observed increases in strength during preadolescence, but appear to be more proportional to strength gains, at least in males, during adolescence. These findings suggest differences in the relative importance of neurological adaptations in relation to strength gains between preadolescents and adolescents. Alternatively, these observations may simply reflect differences in measurement techniques and muscle groups used to assess neuromuscular activation between studies, and differences in the nature and intensity of the resistance training programmes.

Other factors besides increased neuromuscular drive may also play an important role in the determination of training-induced strength gains. It is likely that part of the strength gain may simply reflect improved motor coordination. This is probably a more important contributor to strength gains in more complex, multijoint exercises, e.g. the 1 RM arm curl or leg press exercises, than in less complex and more isolated actions such as those involved in isometric strength assessment of the elbow flexors or knee extensors. Results from the studies by Blimkie et al. (1989b) and Ramsay et al. (1990) indirectly support this contention, since training resulted in larger per cent improvements in 1 RM arm curl and leg press strength (specific exercises performed during training), than in non-specific isometric elbow flexion and knee extension strength. Improved motor coordination may also contribute to increased strength gains in adolescent females, since gains measured on training devices were larger than gains assessed with non-specific strength testing dynamometers (C.J.R. Blimkie et al., unpublished results).

INTRINSIC ADAPTATIONS DURING TRAINING

Training-induced changes in the intrinsic contractile characteristics of muscle could also account for part of the observed increase in strength in preadolescents following strength training. In the only study to investigate this issue in preadolescents (Ramsay et al., 1990), twitch torque, a measure of intrinsic muscle strength, increased significantly for both the elbow flexors and knee extensors after 20 weeks of strength training. Since there were no corresponding increases in muscle size, these results indicate an improvement in twitch-specific tension (strength per cross-sectional area). If this adaptation in twitch-specific tension persists and transfers to maximal voluntary efforts, it may account for some of the unexplained increase in training-induced maximal voluntary strength gains evident in preadolescents. These undefined qualitative adaptations in muscle may account in part for the training-induced strength gains evident during preadolescence. Whether resistance or strength training induces intrinsic muscle adaptations during adolescence remains to be determined.

ADAPTATIONS DURING DETRAINING

In adults, strength training-induced increases in muscle size and neural drive decay during detraining at about the same rate as they increase during training (Narici et al., 1989). Detraining in adults is apparently characterized by a relatively rapid reduction in neuromuscular activation, and a more gradual reduction in muscle size (Narici et al., 1989). Since strength training appears to have little if any effect on muscle size during preadolescence, it is probable that the decrement in training-induced strength gains in this group during detraining is attributable predominantly to changes in level of neuromuscular activation and motor coordination.

In the only study (Blimkie et al., 1989a) to investigate this issue to date, 8 weeks of detraining had no significant effect on the magnitude of change in estimated (by anthropometry) lean upper arm or thigh cross-sectional areas among groups of maintenance trained, detrained and control preadolescent boys. The maintenance trained and detrained groups had completed 20 weeks of heavy strength training prior to detraining. The lack of change in muscle size with detraining in this study was not surprising, however, since there was no evidence of muscle hypertrophy at the end of the training programme. Results from this study suggest, however, that any loss in strength during reduced training or total detraining in preadolescents is probably not attributable to a reduction in muscle size.

In the same study (Blimkie et al., 1989a), there was a trend towards reduced neuromuscular drive (reduced MUA) in both the maintenance trained and totally detrained groups; the reductions were considerably larger in the totally detrained than in the maintenance trained group. These results suggest that the loss of strength gains during detraining in preadolescents is attributable in part to a reduction in neuromuscular activation. Although it has never been assessed directly, it is likely that part of the decrement in strength during detraining, especially for more complex, multijoint strength manoeuvres, may also be attributed to a loss in motor coordination. There are no studies of the detraining response to resistance or strength training involving adolescents. Clearly, more information is required about detraining, and the physiological adaptations which accompany this process during both preadolescence and adolescence. Table 7.1 and Fig. 7.5 provide a summaries of the probable physiological adaptations underlying strength training- and detraining-induced strength changes during childhood.

Potential benefits and safety considerations

Strength training has the potential of improving sports performance, enhancing body composition, and reducing sports injury rate and rehabilitation time following injury. These potential beneficial effects of strength training remains, however, largely unproven for both the preadolescent (Blimkie, 1993a,b) and, with the exception of the potential positive impact on injury rate and rehabilitation time, the adolescent. Strength training is also a potentially risky activity in that it may induce temporary or permanent musculoskeletal injury, and may have detrimental effects on cardiorespiratory fitness and cardiovascular function. With appropriate technique instruction, and proper exercise prescription and supervision, strength training does not appear to be a particularly risky activity for either preadolescents or adolescents in terms of injury, and it seems to have no detrimental effect on either cardiorespiratory fitness or blood pressure (Blimkie, 1993a,b).

Whereas it may be an effective and relatively low risk activity for most healthy children, strength training should be recommended cautiously, and then only under close medical supervision and monitoring for children with physical, mental and medical handicaps.

Table 7.1 Probable physiological adaptations underlying strength changes with resistance training and detraining during preadolescence and adolescence — relative responses.

	Relative response
Training phase	
Absolute strength	Greater gains in the adolescent compared to the preadolescent
Relative strength	Equal or greater gains in the preadolescent compared to the adolescent
Muscle hypertrophy	Smaller gains in muscle size in the preadolescent compared to the adolescent
Neuromuscular activation	Possible greater potential for increased activation in the preadolescent compared to the adolescent due to a lower lifetime exposure to different types of activities
Motor skill	Possible greater potential for improvement in skill in the preadolescent compared to the adolescent due to lower lifetime exposure to skilled activities
Detraining phase	
Absolute strength	Probably a smaller loss in strength in the preadolescent compared to the adolescent due to a greater degree of compensation from growth
Relative strength	Same as for absolute strength
Muscle hypertrophy	Muscle size will probably continue to increase during preadolescence due to growth, but may decrease or remain unchanged in the adolescent depending on the magnitude of the weaker (compared to preadolescence) but still present growth effect
Neuromuscular activation	Will probably decrease in both the preadolescent and adolescent stages by an equal magnitude
Motor skill	Will probably decrease more in the preadolescents than in the adolescent due to relative inexperience with related types of skilled activities which may transfer to strength

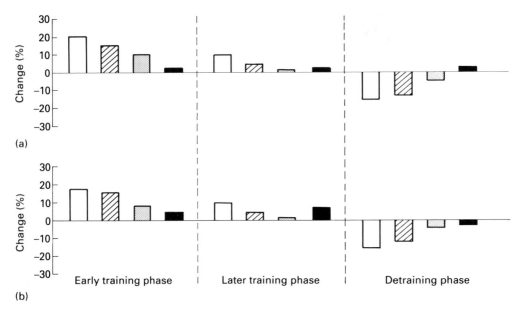

Fig. 7.5 Model of the probable physiological adaptations underlying resistance training- and detraining-induced changes in strength during (a) preadolescence, and (b) adolescence. □, strength; ▨, neuromuscular adaptation; ▨, motor skills; ■, muscle hypertrophy.

Additionally, because it is such a highly specialized type of exercise, strength training should be recommended as only one of a variety of physical activity and sport pursuits for the child.

Lastly, a distinction must be made between strength training and participation in the sports of competitive and Olympic weight-lifting and power-lifting. Strength training if done under supervision and with appropriate technique instruction and prescription of loads can be an enjoyable and relatively low risk activity for most children. Competitive and Olympic weight-lifting, power-lifting and body building however, may prove riskier activities for children, and according to some professional bodies should not be recommended for preadolescents (American Academy of Pediatrics, 1990; American Orthopaedic Society for Sports Medicine — see Cahill, 1988).

General guidelines for resistance training

The following guidelines are provided to ensure the safety, effectiveness and enjoyment of strength training in a non-competitive recreational, fitness or sport context for children.

1 Preclude physical and medical contraindications.

2 Provide instruction in, and demand, proper technique.

3 Warm-up with calisthenics and stretches.

4 Begin with exercises that use body weight as resistance before progressing to free weights or weight-training machines.

5 Individualize training loads when using free weights and training machines.

6 Train all major muscle groups, and both flexors and extensors.

7 Exercise muscles through their entire range of motion.

8 Alternate days of training with rest days, and do not train more than three times per week.

9 When using free weights or machines, progress gradually from light loads, high repetitions (> 15), and few sets (two to three), to heavier loads, fewer repetitions (six to eight),

and moderate numbers of sets (three to four).

10 Cool-down after training with stretching exercises for major joints and muscle groups.

11 When selecting equipment, check for durability, stability, sturdiness and safety.

12 Heed sharp or persistent pain as a warning, and seek medical advice.

Developmental considerations

1 Encourage resistance training as only one of a variety of normal recreational and sport activities, especially during preadolescence.

2 Encourage using a variety of different training modalities, e.g. free weights, springs, machines and body weight.

3 Discourage interindividual competition, and stress the importance of personal improvement, especially during preadolescence.

4 Discourage extremely high-intensity (loading) efforts, e.g. maximal or near-maximal lifts with free weights or weight machines, especially during preadolescence.

5 Avoid isolated eccentric training until the latter stages of adolescence.

6 Encourage a circuit system approach to capitalize on possible cardiorespiratory benefits.

7 If using weight-training machines, select those which have either been designed for children, or those for which the loads and levers can be easily adjusted to accommodate the reduced strength capacity and size of the child.

8 Ensure experienced supervision, preferably by an adult when free weights or training machines are used in training.

Trainability of muscle power and local muscle endurance

In this section, muscle power denotes the peak mechanical power generated by one or more muscle groups over a brief period (e.g. 1–5 s), whereas muscle endurance denotes the ability to sustain high mechanical power over time (e.g. 30–60 s).

Much less information is available on the trainability of muscle power and endurance in children and adolescents, compared with trainability of their muscle strength. One reason for such a paucity of information is that the equipment and protocols needed for testing power and changes in power are more complex than those available for strength testing. While the latter requires measurement of force only, the former calls for the simultaneous measurement of force and velocity over time (see Fig. 7.1). For details about methods used for testing muscle power and muscle endurance see Inbar et al. (1995) and Chapter 36.

Another difference between the study of muscle strength on the one hand and muscle power and endurance on the other is that the latter must include the analysis of anaerobic energy turnover, in addition to mechanical and neurological considerations.

Effectiveness of training programmes

In adults, numerous intervention studies have demonstrated trainability of muscle power and endurance, as reviewed by Skinner and Morgan (1985) and by Inbar et al. (1995). Training regimens have spanned various approaches, but the common denominator has been the use of repetitions of short-term (e.g. 5–30 s) activities such as cycling or running at maximal or near-maximal intensity.

Cross-sectional comparisons among children and adolescents have demonstrated higher muscle power and muscle endurance among trained individuals than among untrained controls. An example is a study of Chinese 13–16-year-old girls and boys (Weijiang & Juxiang, 1988), which compared performance in the Wingate anaerobic test (for description see Chapter 36) of track-and-field athletes ($n = 47$) with that of non-athletes ($n = 126$). When expressed per kilogram of body mass, peak power and mean power of the girl athletes were, respectively, 21 and 28% higher than in the non-athletes. Somewhat lower differences (14 and 15%, respectively) were observed among the boys. A similar pattern emerged when performance was calculated per kilogram of lean body mass. While the above differences could, in part, reflect a training effect, they could also result from preselection.

Very few intervention studies assessed the trainability of muscle power and endurance (see Bar-Or, 1989 for a review). Clarke and Vaccaro (1979) tested 9–11-year-old American girls and boys before and after a 7-month intense four per week swimming programme. Fifteen girls and boys served as controls. A combined score of pull-ups and push-ups served as an index of arm and shoulder girdle muscle endurance. As shown in Fig. 7.6, muscle endurance increased by more than 100% in the swimmers, but not in the controls. Grodjinovsky et al. (1980), in a 6-week, three per week programme, compared the effects of sprint running (40 and 150 m) and sprint cycling (8- and 30-s all-out bouts) on 11–13-year-old Israeli boys. Using the Wingate test, peak power and the mean power over 30 s (taken as muscle endurance) increased by about 3–5% in the two

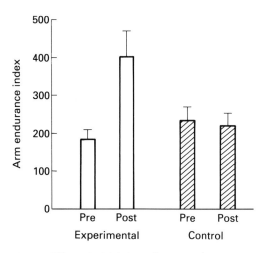

Fig. 7.6 Effect of a high-intensity 7-month swimming programme on muscle endurance of 15 9–11-year-old girls and boys. A combined index (mean and SEM) of push-ups, pull-ups and body mass was taken to represent the endurance of the arm and shoulder girdle muscles. Both the training and the control groups included 13 girls and two boys. Adapted from Clarke and Vaccaro (1979).

training groups, but not in the controls (Fig. 7.7). Such a small training effect may reflect the mild nature of the intervention, which was held during a 10–15-min segment of regular physical education classes.

Indeed, a greater training effect was observed when the programme was more intense and prolonged: 10.2–11.6-year-old Israeli boys underwent a 9-week (three 45-min sessions per week) interval running programme. Distances ranged from 150 to 600 m per interval. As determined by the Wingate test, the programme induced a 14% increase in peak power and 10% increase in mean power. There were no changes in muscle performance of a control group of boys, matched for age and initial activity level. This programme was not specific for muscle power and endurance, because it also yielded an increase in maximal oxygen uptake and in 1200-m running velocity. Such non-specificity may have resulted from the relatively long duration (approximately 2 min) of the 600-m intervals.

Grodjinovsky and Bar-Or (1984) compared the responses of 12–13-year-old Israeli girls and boys to a 7-month programme of six physical education classes per week, plus three per week practices of European handball. As seen in Fig. 7.8, this non-specific programme was accompanied by similar increases in the anaerobic performance of both genders. Control girls and boys, attending two physical education classes per week, also had an increase in performance, but less than the experimental groups.

As is true for other fitness components (Katch, 1983), muscle power and endurance trainability in children seems to depend on the fitness level prior to the start of the training programme. Docherty et al. (1987) administered a three per week, 4-week programme to 12-year-old Canadian boys who had just completed a competitive ice hockey or soccer season. The programme comprised all-out repetitions of 20-s bouts of isokinetic activities with various muscle groups, including 20-s cycling at high intensity. Using a modified Wingate test, the authors found no training-

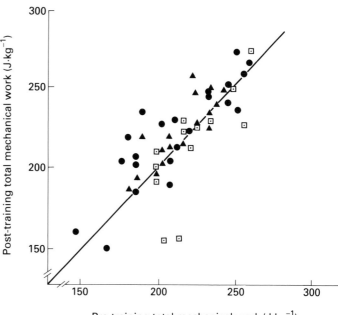

Fig. 7.7 Effect of moderately intense 6-week sprint running and sprint cycling programmes on the leg muscle endurance of 11–13-year-old boys. Total mechanical work per kilogram of body mass during the 30-s Wingate anaerobic test was taken as muscle endurance. Individual data of 50 boys were divided into sprint cycling (▲), sprint running (●) and control (▢) groups, each representing a whole six grade class. The diagonal line denotes identity. Adapted from Grodjinovsky *et al.* (1980).

induced difference in performance. There are no data to tell whether a similar regimen would have been more effective for children who were not trained athletes.

Mechanisms for trainability of muscle power and endurance

Conceptually, neurological changes as described above for muscle strength trainability can also explain improvement in peak power and, possibly, muscle endurance. However, there are no studies that have analysed associations between the improvement in the latter functions on the one hand, and EMG or MUA on the other, in children or adolescents.

Some data link the improvement in anaerobic power and muscle endurance to morphological and histochemical changes. In a longitudinal study of 11–13-year-old Swedish boys who participated in a 4-year sprint training programme (Jacobs *et al.*, 1982), the improvement in muscle endurance (50 all-out repetitions of isokinetic knee extensions) was associated with an increase in muscle cross-sectional area, but

without changes in muscle fibre-type composition. This study did not include a control group to tease out the effects of growth *per se*. In another, uncontrolled intervention study, Spanish 15–17-year-old girls and boys were tested before and after a year of intense sprint, power and strength training. Biopsies of the vastus lateralis muscle revealed an increase in the diameter of both type I and II fibres, the proportion of type I fibres, the contents of glycogen, as well as the activity of glycolytic (phosphofructokinase and primarily pyruvate kinase) and oxidative (succinate dehydrogenase and amino acid transferases) enzymes. Again, the lack of controls does not allow to determine the extent to which the above changes resulted from growth *per se* and from training. However, similar changes in some muscle enzymes, as well as in muscle lactate, have been shown in young adult Swedish men and women following a 6-week 'supramaximal' controlled training programme (Jacobs *et al.*, 1987). This suggests that an increase in glycolytic enzymes can result directly from high-intensity power training. An increase in 'anaerobic' substrates (creatine

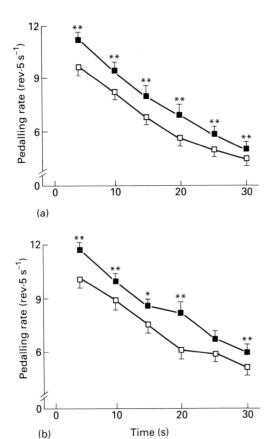

(a)

(b)

Time (s)

Fig. 7.8 Trainability of muscle power and muscle endurance of 12–13-year-old girls ($n = 18$) (a) and boys ($n = 14$) (b), who took part in a 7-month enhanced physical education programme. The programme included six periods per week, plus three European handball training sessions per week. The highest 5-s pedalling rate represents peak power, whereas the area under the curve reflects muscle endurance. □, pretraining; ■, post-training. *, $P < 0.05$; **, $P < 0.01$. Redrawn with permission from Grodjinovsky and Bar-Or (1984).

phosphate, adenosine triphosphate and glycogen), as well as in phosphofructokinase, may result also from a non-specific mix of aerobic and anaerobic training, as shown for 11–13-year-old Swedish boys (Eriksson et al., 1973).

In summary, there is some, but inconclusive, evidence that an increase in glycolytic flux is one factor that may contribute to training-induced changes in peak muscle power and

muscle endurance of children and adolescents. More research is needed regarding the respective contribution of enhanced muscle contractility and other neurological factors.

Challenges for future research

- Establish the minimal effective training load (intensity, volume, frequency) required for significant strength, power and endurance gains at different stages of development.
- Establish the minimal effective training loads for maintenance of strength, power and endurance gains at different developmental stages.
- Determine whether it is possible to induce muscle hypertrophy with tolerable (without injury and pain) resistance training programmes during preadolescence.
- Clarify the neurological adaptations and establish their relative importance and temporal sequence in relation to strength, power and endurance changes with training and detraining at different stages of development.
- Determine the degree, nature and relative importance of intrinsic muscle adaptations to strength, power and endurance changes with training and detraining at different stages of development.
- Compare the effectiveness and safety of different resistance training modes (e.g. free weights, isokinetic, accommodating) and methods (e.g. Berger, DeLorme, pyramid, etc.) on strength gains and other physiological outcomes at different stages of development.
- Determine the importance of neuroendocrine adaptations for training-induced strength, power and endurance, and muscle morphological adaptations at different stages of development and between the sexes.
- Determine the optimal training regimen for specific improvement of strength, power and endurance in children and adolescents.

References

Ainsworth, J.L. (1970) *The effect of isometric-resistive exercises with the Exer-Genie on strength and speed in swimming*. Unpublished doctoral thesis, University of Arkansas, Arkansas.

American Academy of Pediatrics (1990) Strength training, weight and power lifting, and body building by children and adolescents. *Pediatrics* **86**, 801–3.

Bar-Or, O. (1989) Trainability of the prepubescent child. *Phys. Sports Med.* **17**, 65–82.

Belanger, A.Y. & McComas, A.J. (1981) Extent of motor unit activation during effort. *J. Appl. Physiol.* **51**, 1131–5.

Blimkie, C.J.R. (1989) Age- and sex-associated variation in strength during childhood: anthropometric, morphologic, neurologic, and biomechanical correlates. In C.V. Gisolfi & D.R. Lamb (eds) *Perspectives in Exercise Science and Sports Medicine*. Vol. 2. *Youth, Exercise and Sport*, pp. 99–163. Benchmark Press, Indianapolis.

Blimkie, C.J.R. (1992) Resistance training during pre- and early puberty: efficacy, trainability, mechanisms, and persistance. *Canad. J. Sport Sci.* **17**, 264–79.

Blimkie, C.J.R. (1993a) Benefits and risks of resistance training in children. In B.R. Cahill & A.J. Pearl (eds) *Intensive Participation in Children's Sports*, pp. 133–65. Human Kinetics, Champaign, IL.

Blimkie, C.J.R. (1993b) Resistance training during preadolescence. Issues and controversies. *Sports Med.* **15**, 1–18.

Blimkie, C.J.R., Martin, J., Ramsay, J., Sale, D. & MacDougall, D. (1989a) The effects of detraining and maintenance weight training on strength development in prepubertal boys *Canad. J. Sport Sci.* **14**, 102P (abstract).

Blimkie, C.J.R., Ramsay, J., Sale, D., MacDougall, D., Smith, K. & Garner, S. (1989b) Effects of 10 weeks of resistance training on strength development in prepubertal boys. In S. Oseid & K.-H. Carlsen (eds) *Children and Exercise XIII*, pp. 183–97. Human Kinetics, Champaign, IL.

Blimkie, C.J.R., Rice, S., Webber, C.E., Martin, J., Levy, D. & Gordon, C.L. (1993) Effects of resistance training on bone mass and density in adolescent females. *Med. Sci. Sports Exerc.* **25**(5) (Suppl.), S48 (abstract).

Cadefau, J., Casademont, J., Grau, J.M. *et al.* (1990) Biochemical and histochemical adaptation to sprint training in young athletes. *Acta Physiol. Scand.* **140**, 341–51.

Cahill, B.R. (ed.) (1988) *Proceedings of the Conference on Strength Training and the Prepubescent*. American Orthopaedic Society for Sports Medicine, Chicago.

Clarke, D.H. & Vaccaro, P. (1979) The effect of swimming training on muscular performance and body composition in children. *Res. Q.* **50**, 9–17.

DeKoning, F.L., Binkhorst, R.A., Vissers, A.C.A. &

Vos, J.A. (1984) The influence of static strength training on the force–velocity relationship of the arm flexors of 16-year-old boys. In J. Ilamarian & I. Vilimaki (eds) *Pediatric Work Physiology*, pp. 201–5. Springer-Verlag, New York.

DeLorme, T.L., Ferris, B.G. & Gallagher, J.R. (1952) Effect of progressive resistance exercise on muscle contraction time. *Arch. Phys. Med. Rehab.* **33**, 86–92.

Docherty, D., Wenger, H.A. & Collis, M.L. (1987a) The effects of resistance training on aerobic and anaerobic power of young boys. *Med. Sci. Sports Exerc.* **19**, 389–92.

Docherty, D., Wenger, H.A., Collis, M.L. & Quinney, H.A. (1987b) The effects of variable speed resistance training on strength development in prepubertal boys. *J. Hum. Move. Stud.* **13**, 377–82.

Fleck, S.J. & Kraemer, W.J. (1987) *Designing Resistance Training Programs*. Human Kinetics, Champaign, IL.

Freedson, P.S., Ward, A. & Rippe, J.M. (1990) Resistance training for youth. *Adv. Sport Med. Fitness* **3**, 57–65.

Fukunaga, T. (1976) Die absolute muskelkraft und das muskelkrafttraining (Absolute strength and strength training). *Sport. Sportmediz.* **11**, 255–66.

Fukunaga, T., Funato, K. & Ikegawa, S. (1992) The effects of resistance training on muscle area and strength in prepubescent age. *Ann. Physiol. Anthropol.* **11**, 357–64.

Gallagher, J.R. & DeLorme, T.L. (1949) The use of the technique of progressive-resistance exercise in adolescence. *J. Bone Joint Surg.* **31**A, 847–58.

Gillam, G.M. (1981) Effects of frequency of weight training on muscle strength enhancement. *J. Sports Med.* **21**, 432–6.

Green, H.J. (1991) What do tests measure? In J.D. MacDougall, H.A. Wenger & H.J. Green (eds) *Physiological Testing of the High-Performance Athlete*, 2nd edn, pp. 7–19. Human Kinetics, Champaign, IL.

Grodjinovsky, A. & Bar-Or, O. (1984) Influence of added physical education hours upon anaerobic capacity, adiposity and grip strength in 12- to 13-year-old children enrolled in a sports class. In J. Ilmarinen & I. Valimaki (eds) *Children and Sport*, pp. 162–9. Springer-Verlag, New York.

Grodjinovsky, A., Inbar, O., Dotan, R. & Bar-Or, O. (1980) Training effect on the anaerobic performance of children as measured by the Wingate anaerobic test. In K. Berg & B.G. Eriksson (eds) *Children and Exercise IX*. University Park Press, Baltimore.

Hakkinen, K., Mero, A. & Kauhanen, H. (1989) Specificity of endurance, sprint and strength training on physical performance capacity in young athletes.

J. Sports Med. **29**, 27–35.

Hassan, S.E.A. (1991) Die trainierbarkeit der maximalkraft bei 7-bis 13 jahrigen kindern (Trainability of muscle strength in 7–13 year old children). *Leistungssport* 5, 17–24.

Hettinger, T.H. (1958) Die Trainierbarkeit menschlicher Muskeln in Abhängigkeit vom Alter und Geschlecht (The trainability of human muscles depending on age and sex). *Int. Zeitschr. Angewandte Physiol. Einschliess. Arbeitsphysiol.* **17**, 371–7.

Inbar, O., Bar-Or, O. & Skinner, J.S. (1995) *The Wingate Anaerobic Test: Development, Characteristics and Applications.* Human Kinetics, Champaign, IL.

Jacobs, I., Esbjornsson, M., Sylven, C., Holm, I. & Jansson, E. (1987) Sprint training effects on muscle myoglobin enzymes, fiber types, and blood lactate. *Med. Sci. Sports Exerc.* **19**, 368–74.

Jacobs, I., Sjodin, B. & Svane, B. (1982) Muscle fiber type, cross-sectional area and strength in boys after 4 years' endurance training. *Med. Sci. Sports Exerc.* **14**, 123.

Katch, V.L. (1983) Physical conditioning of children. *J. Adolsc. Health Care* 3, 241–6.

Kirsten, G. (1963) Der Einflub isometrischen muskeltrainings auf die entwicklung der Muskelkraft Jugendlicher (The influence of muscle training on the development of muscle strength in juveniles). *Int. Zeitschr. Angewandte Physiol. Einschliess. Arbeitsphysiol.* **19**, 387–402.

Komi, P.V. (ed.) (1992) *Strength and Power in Sport.* III. The Encyclopedia of Sports Medicine, Vol. 3. Blackwell Scientific Publications, Oxford.

Komi, P.V., Viitasalo, J.T., Rauramaa, R. & Vihko, V. (1978) Effect of isometric strength training on mechanical, electrical, and metabolic aspects of muscle function. *Eur. J. Appl. Physiol.* **40**, 45–55.

Kraemer, W.J., Fry, A.C., Frykman, P.N., Conroy, B. & Hoffman, J. (1989) Resistance training and youth. *Pediatr. Exerc. Sci.* **1**, 336–50.

Kusinitz, I. & Keeney, C.E. (1958) Effects of progressive weight training on health and physical fitness of adolescent boys. *Res. Q.* **29**, 294–301.

McCubbin, J.A. & Shasby, G.B. (1985) Effects of isokinetic exercise on adolescents with cerebral palsy. *Adapt. Phys. Act. Q.* **2**, 56–64.

McGovern, M.B. (1984) Effects of circuit weight training on the physical fitness of prepubescent children. *Dissertation Asbtr. Int.* 45(2), 452A–3 (abstract).

Mersch, F. & Stoboy, H. (1989) Strength training and muscle hypertrophy in children. In S. Oseid & K.-H. Carlsen (eds) *Children and Exercise XIII*, pp. 165–82. Human Kinetics, Champaign, IL.

Munson, W.W., Baker, S.B. & Lundegren, H.M. (1985) strength training and leisure counselling as treatments for institutionalized juvenile delinquents. *Adapt. Phys. Act. Q.* **2**, 65–75.

Narici, M.V., Roi, G.S., Landoni, L., Minetti, A.E. & Cerretteli, P. (1989) Changes in force, cross-sectional area and neural activation during strength training and detraining of the human quadriceps. *Eur. J. Appl. Physiol.* **59**, 310–19.

Nielsen, B., Nielsen, K., Behrendt-Hansen, M. & Asmussen, E. (1980) Training of 'functional muscular strength' in girls 7–19 years old. In K. Berg & B.D. Eriksson (eds) *Children and Exercise IX*, pp. 69–78. Human Kinetics, Champaign, IL.

Ozmun, J.C., Mikesky, A.E. & Surburg, P.R. (1994) Neuromuscular adaptations following prepubescent strength training. *Med. Sci. Sports Exerc.* **26**, 510–14.

Pfeiffer, R.D. & Francis, R.S. (1986) Effects of strength training on muscle development in prepubescent, pubescent, and postpubescent males. *Phys. Sportsmed.* **14**, 134–43.

Ramsay, J.A., Blimkie, C.J.R., Smith, K., Garner, S., MacDougall, J.D. & Sale, D.G. (1990) Strength training effects in prepubescent boys. *Med. Sci. Sports Exerc.* **22**(5), 605–14.

Rarick, G.L. & Larsen, G.L. (1958) Observations on frequency and intensity of isometric muscular effort in developing static muscular strength in postpubescent males. *Res. Q.* **29**, 333–41.

Rotstein, A., Dotan, R., Bar-Or, O. & Tenenbaum, G. (1986) Effect of training on anaerobic threshold, maximal aerobic power and anaerobic performance of preadolescent boys. *Int. J. Sports Med.* **7**, 281–6.

Sailors, M. & Berg, K. (1987) Comparison of responses to weight training in pubescent boys and men. *J. Sports Med.* **27**, 30–6.

Sale, D.G. (1989) Strength training in children. In C.V. Gisolfi & D.R. Lamb (eds) *Perspectives in Exercise Science and Sports Medicine*, Vol. 2. *Youth, Exercise and Sport*, pp. 165–222. Benchmark Press, Indianapolis.

Sale, D.G. (1991) Testing strength and power. In J.D. MacDougall, H.A. Wenger & H.J. Green (eds) *Physiological Testing of the High-Performance Athelete*, 2nd edn, pp. 21–106. Human Kinetics, Champaign, IL.

Sewall, L. & Micheli, L.J. (1986) Strength training for children. *J. Pediatr. Orthoped.* **6**, 143–6.

Siegel, J.A., Camaione, D.N. & Manfredi, T.G. (1989) The effects of upper body resistance training on prepubescent children. *Pediatr. Exerc. Sci.* **1**, 145–54.

Skinner, J.S. & Morgan, D. (1985) Aspects of anaerobic performance. In D. Clarke & H. Eckert (eds) *Limits of Human Performance*, pp. 31–44. Human Kinetics, Champaign, IL.

Vrijens, J. (1978) Muscle strength development in the pre- and post-pubescent age. *Med. Sport* **11**, 152–8.

Webb, D.R. (1990) Strength training in children and

adolescents. *Pediatr. Clin. N. Am.* **37**, 1187–210.

Weijang, D. & Juxiang, Q. (1988) Anaerobic performance of Chinese untrained and trained 11–18-year old boys and girls. *Med. Sports Sci.* **28**, 52–60.

Weltman, A. (1989) Weight training in prepubertal children: physiologic benefit and potential damage. In O. Bar-Or (ed.) *Advances in Pediatric Sport Sciences*, Vol. 3, pp. 101–29. Human Kinetics, Champaign, IL.

Weltman, A., Janny, C., Rians, C.B. *et al.* (1986) The effects of hydraulic resistance strength training in pre-pubertal males. *Med. Sci. Sports Exerc.* **18**, 629–38.

Westcott, W.L. (1979) Female response to weight training. *J. Phys. Educ.* **77**, 31–3.

Westcott, W.L. (1991) Safe and sane strength training for teenagers. *Scholastic Coach* **Oct**, 42–4.

Wolbers, C.P. & Sills, F.S. (1956) Development of strength in high school boys by static muscle contractions. *Res. Q.* **27**, 446–50.

Chapter 8

Endurance Trainability of Children and Youths

RUSSELL R. PATE AND DIANNE S. WARD

Introduction

Regular participation in moderate to vigorous physical activity is now widely accepted as a key component of a healthy lifestyle. Nonetheless, physical inactivity is highly prevalent among adults in the industrialized nations of the world. While physical activity levels tend to be higher in children and adolescents than in adults, numerous authorities have expressed concern that a great many youths are less active than recommended (Centers for Disease Control, 1992). In addition, it has been demonstrated that many children and youths fail to meet health-related standards for physical fitness (Corbin & Pangrazi, 1992).

Because many children and youths are less physically active and fit than desirable, a consensus has developed that systematic exercise intervention programmes should be provided for children (Simons-Morton *et al.*, 1988). In general, experts have indicated that these programmes should be designed to accomplish two major goals: (i) exercise programmes for youths should, in the short term, enhance physical fitness; and (ii) programmes should promote long-term adoption of a physically active lifestyle, which in turn can be expected to maintain physical fitness into and throughout adulthood.

In addition, in recent decades organized sport programmes for children and youths have become increasingly common. Such programmes also have become increasingly competitive. Endurance sport programmes (e.g. swimming, distance running) for youths have become quite popular, and often involve long-term exposure to heavy training. Some experts have raised concerns about the health consequences of this, and some have suggested that youngsters at certain developmental stages may be minimally adaptive to endurance training (Bar-Or, 1983).

Because endurance exercise training is frequently used with children and youths for the purpose of promoting health-related physical fitness and for enhancement of sport performance, paediatric exercise scientists have been interested in the physiological adaptations that result from the training process. In particular, there has been interest in 'trainability' — that is, the extent to which the physiological markers of endurance fitness change with regular participation in endurance exercise. Accordingly, the major purpose of this chapter is to review the scientific literature pertinent to trainability in children and youths. Secondary purposes are to compare prepubescent, pubescent and postpubescent youths in terms of trainability and to present important directions for future research on this issue.

Physiology of endurance exercise performance

In the sport setting, exercise training is designed to enhance exercise tolerance and ultimately to improve sport performance. If a training programme succeeds in enhancing performance, it is likely that it will do so largely by enhancing one or more of the key physiological factors that are known to limit tolerance for endurance exercise. Therefore, it is logical to begin a discussion of trainability with a brief review of the physiological determinants of endurance performance.

Three physiological variables, operating in combination, are thought to determine endurance exercise performance (Sjodin & Svedenhag, 1990; Pate & Branch, 1992). Maximal aerobic power, also described as maximal oxygen consumption ($\dot{V}O_{2\,max}$), is the greatest rate at which the individual can use oxygen in the aerobic metabolic process. This is a key determinant of endurance performance because endurance exercise must depend primarily on aerobic metabolism. Hence the individual with the higher $\dot{V}O_{2\,max}$ is capable of a higher maximal rate of aerobic energy expenditure (though it should be noted that this maximal rate typically can be sustained for no more than a few minutes).

The ability to sustain a high rate of aerobic energy expenditure for a prolonged period of time is a function of $\dot{V}O_{2\,max}$ and a second important physiological variable — lactate threshold. Lactate threshold is the rate of aerobic expenditure at which the fatiguing byproduct of anaerobic metabolism, lactic acid, begins to accumulate in the blood. Often lactate threshold is expressed as the percentage of the $\dot{V}O_{2\,max}$ at which it is observed, and this percentage varies markedly across individuals, even among endurance-trained athletes. Athletes typically perform long duration sport events at intensities approximating the lactate threshold. Therefore, ability to sustain a high rate of aerobic energy expenditure can be enhanced by increasing either or both of $\dot{V}O_{2\,max}$ and lactate threshold.

A third important physiological variable, economy, sets the ratio between the rate of aerobic energy expenditure and the pace of endurance exercise. Economy is typically quantified as the rate of oxygen consumption observed at a specified movement pace (e.g. running, cycling or swimming speed). The more economical individual is able to perform at a given speed with a lower rate of oxygen consumption (and hence lower rate of energy expenditure) than a less economical counterpart.

Based on this discussion it would be anticipated that training would enhance endurance performance by increasing maximal aerobic power, lactate threshold and/or economy. Of these three variables, by far the most information is available for maximal aerobic power. This is the case because the relationship between this variable and endurance performance has been recognized longer than for the other two variables. Accordingly, much of the following discussion will be based on the changes in maximal aerobic power that have been shown to result from endurance training in children and youths. Nonetheless, it should be remembered that training could enhance endurance performance in at least some individuals by increasing lactate threshold and economy. For more details about the development of maximal aerobic power during childhood and adolescence, see Chapter 4.

Trainability of youths

Exercise scientists have been interested in the effects of physical training on the functional capacity of children and youth for over 60 years (Schwartz et al., 1928). In recent years, interest in the exercise trainability of youngsters has been fuelled by the publication of several scientific reviews on this issue (Cunningham et al., 1984; Krahenbuhl et al., 1985; Rowland, 1985; Sady, 1986; Vaccaro & Mahon, 1987; Bar-Or, 1989; Pate & Ward, 1990). In general, the conclusions have been similar — children and youths are physiologically adaptive to endurance exercise training, if the training stimulus is adequate. However, the authors also agree that the pertinent scientific literature is scant and there are a number of unresolved issues.

An examination of these reviews indicates that the following major issues are of particular interest. First, questions have been raised concerning the trainability of prepubescent children. It has been hypothesized that pre-pubescent children may be less adaptive to endurance exercise training than older youths and adults. An increase in $\dot{V}o_{2\,max}$ requires an increase in maximal cardiac output and/or maximal arteriovenous oxygen difference. It has been noted that maximal arteriovenous oxygen difference tends to be high in pre-pubescent children in the absence of training (Bar-Or, 1983). This observation has led investi-gators to theorize that the overall adaptation to endurance training could be limited by a 'ceiling effect' in maximal arteriovenous oxygen difference.

Second, it is well known that maximal aerobic power tends to be relatively high in youngsters as compared with adults (Rowland, 1990). This may be related to genetic factors, i.e. the genetic programme promotes a high level of function. However, it may also be explained, at least in part, by the fact that youngsters tend to be more physically active than adults (Siegel *et al.*, 1991). Regardless of the explanation, the typical youngster's relatively high baseline fitness level may tend to limit his or her functional adap-tation to training.

Third, youngsters, particularly at certain critical periods, experience rapid growth and development. These phenomena certainly operate as complicating factors for scientists studying the physiology of exercise in paedi-atric populations. This is because some of the changes associated with growth and develop-ment are also associated with exercise training. However, beyond this effect, it is possible that trainability in youngsters may vary with devel-opmental status (Malina & Bouchard, 1991). As discussed above, it has been suggested that prepubescent children may be less adaptive to training than the older population. It is also possible that during certain developmental periods youngsters are highly adaptive to training. In any case, both growth and develop-ment are factors to consider whenever exercise training is studied in children and youths.

In these previously published reviews of endurance trainability in children and youths, varying numbers of primary research articles were included. This indicates, of course, that different authors have applied different inclusion criteria. In the preparation of this chapter a total of 48 published studies were reviewed, but for various reasons most of them were excluded from the set of papers on which conclusions were based. Some of the excluded studies were limited by the failure to employ a control group — given the afore-mentioned importance of growth and development, this is a particularly critical limitation. Other studies were excluded because the dose of training was not precisely quantified or described. Many of the studies that carried this limitation used either sport participation or physical edu-cation classes as the exercise treatment. Some other studies were excluded because they used special populations of subjects (e.g. children with hypertension, asthma or mental handicap).

In a previous review article (Pate & Ward, 1990) the authors examined the trainability in children and youth by applying a stringent set of criteria for inclusion of primary research studies. These criteria included: (i) use of a control group (random or pair-matched); (ii) provision of a clear description of the training protocol; (iii) application of physiological measures as indicators of training outcomes; (iv) use of appropriate statistical procedures; and (v) publication in a peer-reviewed research journal. In that review a total of 15 papers were included, 12 of them using children of age 13 years or less and three using youths over the age of 13 years.

In this chapter our intention is to go beyond our earlier review by setting even more strin-gent inclusion criteria to promote greater con-fidence in our conclusions. In addition to the inclusion criteria listed above, the following criteria were used in this chapter: (i) use of a training protocol administered outside the physical education class setting; (ii) use of sub-jects with no known health problems; and (iii) use of endurance training without any supplementary modes of training such as weight-training.

Functional adaptations to endurance training

The 11 studies included in this review are summarized in Table 8.1. The majority of these studies used male subjects, two studies used female subjects and two studies used both males and females. Of the 11 studies 10 found a net increase in $\dot{V}O_{2\,max}$ in the training group(s) over the control group. The range of net increases in $\dot{V}O_{2\,max}$ was large extending from a high of 16% (Eisenman & Golding, 1975; Stransky et al., 1979) to a low of 1% (Weber et al., 1976). The average net increase in $\dot{V}O_{2\,max}$ across these 10 studies was 9.7%. In one study a larger increase in $\dot{V}O_{2\,max}$ was seen in the control group than the two training groups (Yoshida et al., 1980).

Figure 8.1 provides a graphic comparison of experimental and control groups in terms of the observed changes in $\dot{V}O_{2\,max}$ as measured before and after the training period. A total of 13 comparisons, drawn from the 11 published studies, are presented. Of these comparisons 11 fall above the line of identity, indicating that across the studies reviewed for this chapter there was a clear trend toward increased $\dot{V}O_{2\,max}$ with training. The study of Yoshida provides the one data point falling below the line of identity in Fig. 8.1, and this study is unique in that the subjects were very young (5 years of age).

Measures of functional status other than $\dot{V}O_{2\,max}$ were used in only a few of the studies included in this chapter. In two studies (Becker & Vaccaro, 1983; Mahon & Vaccaro, 1989) ventilatory measures of anaerobic threshold were used, and in both cases much larger increases were observed in the training group than the control group. Somewhat surprisingly, pure performance measures (e.g. run times or distances; time to fatigue at submaximal power outputs) have been used very rarely as outcome measures in training studies with children. We

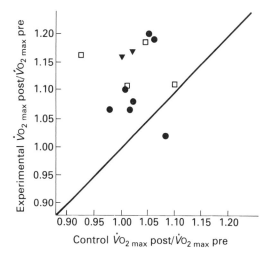

Fig. 8.1 Comparison of pre- to post-test changes in $\dot{V}O_{2\,max}$ as observed in training and control groups in selected studies of trainability in children and youths. Data points represent mean effect in each study listed in Table 8.1. Each data point is coded to indicate the age (and presumed developmental status) of the group: ●, young (prepubescent); ▼, older (postpubescent); □, mixed or middle (pubescent or mixed).

consider this to be an unfortunate deficiency because, in the most fundamental sense, the purpose of the training process is to enhance fitness (i.e. exercise performance or tolerance). While physiological measures such as $\dot{V}O_{2\,max}$ certainly are related to endurance performance, they are not synonymous with performance. In our view, it would be desirable for training studies to use both physiological and performance measures as outcome variables.

Gender and developmental age

Data were analysed separately for females in only two of the studies included in this review (Eisenman & Golding, 1975; Stransky et al., 1979). In both cases the subjects were adolescents in the 15–16-year age range, and in both studies $\dot{V}O_{2\,max}$ was observed to increase by 15–16% in the training group. Based on this very limited number of studies, the tentative conclusion is that adolescent girls appear

Table 8.1 Procedures and findings of selected studies addressing the trainability of children and youths.

Subjects	Age (years)	$\dot{V}O_{2\,max}$ (% change)	$\triangle$AT (% change)	Training stimulus	Reference
Boys ($n = 22$); random assignment	9–11	E: 20% C: 10%	E: 28% C: 13%	Cycle: 8 weeks; 3 days·week^{-1}; 40 min; 85% HR$_{max}$	Becker & Vaccaro (1983)
Boys ($n = 11$)	11	E: 10.2% C: 0.6%		Run (interval): 26 weeks; 2 days·week^{-1}	Ekblom (1969)
Girls ($n = 16$); women ($n = 16$)	12–14; adult	*Girls* E: 16.2%* C: <0% *Women* E: 17.6%* C < 0		Run, bench step: 14 weeks; 3 days·week^{-1}	Eisenman & Golding (1975)
Boys and girls ($n = 26$)	8–12	E: 6.8%* C: 1.5%		Cycle: 12 weeks; 4 days·week^{-1}	Lussier & Buskirk (1977)
Boys ($n = 16$)	10–14	E: 7.6%* C: 1.1%	E: 19%* C: 5%	Run and interval: 8 weeks; 4 days·week^{-1}; 30 min; 90% HR$_{max}$	Mahon & Vaccaro (1989)
Boys ($n = 36$); randomized block design	11–13	E1: 10.9%* E2: 1% E3: 3% C: <0		Cycle: 6 weeks; 3 days·week^{-1}; E1: 91%, E2: 78%; HR$_{max}$, 12 min	Massicotte & McNab (1979)
Boys ($n = 28$); matched	10–11.6	E: 8%* C: 2%		Run and interval: 9 weeks; 3 days·week^{-1}; 45 min	Rotstein *et al.* (1986)
Boys ($n = 34$); men ($n = 34$); random assignment	8–9; adults	*Boys* E1: 6.7%* E2: 4.0 C: <0 *Men* E1: 7.9%* E2: 2.7% C: <0		Run: 11 weeks; 3 days·week^{-1}; E1: 85%; E2: 68%; HR$_{max}$	Savage *et al.* (1986)
Girls ($n = 24$)	15	E: 16.1%* C: 0		Swim: 7 weeks; 4 days·week^{-1}	Stransky *et al.* (1979)
Boys ($n = 26$); twin pairs	10, 13 & 16	*10 year old* E: 19%* C: 6% *13 year old* E: 11% C: 10% *16 year old* E: 17% C: 2%		Run, bench step and cycle — interval: 10 weeks; 4 days·week^{-1}	Weber *et al.* (1976)
Boys and girls ($n = 30$)	5	E1: 2% E2: 2% C: 8%		Run: 28 weeks; 1–3 or 1 days·week^{-1}	Yoshida *et al.* (1980)

* Statistically significant difference from the control group.

AT, anaerobic threshold; C, control group; E, experimental group (E1–E3 denote sequential testing of the experimental group); HR, heart rate.

to be at least as adaptive to endurance training as are boys. Clearly there is a need for studies on younger girls.

As mentioned above, developmental age has often been hypothesized as a factor that could affect endurance exercise trainability. Child development is typically divided into three periods: (i) prepubescence; (ii) pubescence (circumpubertal stage); and (iii) postpubescence (adolescence). The period of most rapid linear growth (peak height velocity) is considered the best marker of pubescence, with pre- and post-pubescence falling before and after this period. Unfortunately, few exercise training studies have been designed to examine comprehensively trainability in youngsters in the three developmental stages. Also, most of the relevant studies have used chronological age, not developmental status, as the basis for categorizing the subjects. For more details about the relevance of developmental age to fitness, see Chapters 1 and 14.

Of the available studies, Weber *et al.* (1976) has most directly addressed the impact of developmental stage on trainability. Subjects were twin pairs randomly assigned to either training or control groups. Pairs were categorized as prepubescent, pubescent or postpubescent. Net increases in $\dot{V}O_{2\,max}$ of 13 and 15%, respectively, were observed in the prepubescent and post-pubescent groups. Interestingly, in the pubescent developmental category both training and control groups showed 10–11% increases in $\dot{V}O_{2\,max}$. This observation suggests that pubescence may be a unique developmental period with regard to the adaptations to endurance training. Unfortunately, pubescent youths have rarely been included in exercise training studies.

Applications

The overall conclusion of this chapter is that children and youths are physiologically adaptive to endurance exercise training. This is typically manifested by increases in $\dot{V}O_{2\,max}$ of approximately 10%. This conclusion must be tempered by noting that it is based on a scientific literature that is very limited in terms of both volume and depth. However, within those limitations, it appears that both male and female, prepubescent and postpubescent youths are trainable. The available literature on pubescent youths is so scant as to preclude drawing even a tentative conclusion.

As noted above, youngsters are often exposed to endurance exercise training for the purpose of promoting their health and fitness. This can occur in the context of school-based physical education classes or many other settings. The conclusion that youths are trainable indicates that, if the exercise programme meets the criteria for intensity, frequency and duration as applied in the available studies, improvements in physiological function and performance should be attained. However, a word of caution should be added. In settings such as physical education classes, as noted above, a goal is to promote long-term development of an active lifestyle while providing for short-term enhancement of physical fitness. Dealing effectively with both of these goals is a challenge because, with some youngsters, it is difficult to provide the relatively heavy dose of exercise needed to generate a training effect in a manner that is enjoyable and psychologically reinforcing.

An increasing number of children and youths participate in endurance sport competitions. The conclusion of this review, when applied in the youth sport setting, is that young athletes are trainable and should manifest improved performance with regular participation in endurance exercise. These improvements would be above and beyond those that are expected to occur with normal growth and development. Unfortunately, few of the controlled exercise training studies in children and youths have used pure performance measures (e.g. run, swim or cycling time) as outcome variables. Consequently, based on the available studies, it is not possible to characterize the expected levels of improvement in endurance performance than should be expected with endurance training.

Challenges for future research

Since the existing literature includes so few studies that meet the criteria established for this chapter, it is clear that much more research is needed. Virtually all of the pertinent issues require further investigation.

• Among the high priorities should be replication of the studies that have been examined, in a precise and well-controlled manner, the effects of endurance training on $\dot{V}_{O_2 max}$ in prepubescent, pubescent and postpubescent boys and girls. Furthermore, it would be desirable that these include measures of lactate (or ventilatory anaerobic) threshold and economy. Also, these studies should include pure performance measures such as distance run times. Such studies would provide an enhanced understanding of the effects of developmetal status and gender on endurance trainability.

• In addition, research should provide a better understanding of the extent to which endurance performance and its various physiological determinants can be expected to improve with training.

References

Bar-Or, O. (1983) *Pediatric Sports Medicine for the Practitioner*. Springer-Verlag, New York.

Bar-Or, O. (1989) Trainability of the prepubescent child. *Phys. Sports Med.* **17**, 65–83.

Becker, D.M. & Vaccaro, P. (1983) Anaerobic threshold alterations caused by endurance training in young children. *J. Sports Med.* **23**, 445–9.

Centers for Disease Control (1992) Vigorous physical activity among high school students – United States, 1990. *Morbid. Mortal. Weekly Rep.* **41**, 33–5.

Corbin, C.B. & Pangrazi, R.P. (1992) Are American children and youth fit? *Res. Q. Exerc. Sport* **63**, 96–106.

Cunningham, D.A., Paterson, D.H. & Blimkie, C.J.R. (1984) The development of the cardiorespiratory system with growth and physical activity. In R.A. Boileau (ed.) *Advances in Pediatric Sport Sciences*, Vol. 1, pp. 85–116, Human Kinetics, Champaign, IL.

Eisenman, P.A. & Golding, L.A. (1975) Comparison of effects of training on $\dot{V}_{O_2 max}$ in girls and young women. *Med. Sci. Sports Exerc.* **7**, 136–8.

Ekblom, B. (1969) Effect of physical training in adolescent boys. *J. Appl. Physiol.* **27**, 350–5.

Kranhenbuhl, G.S., Skinner, J.S. & Kohrt, W.M. (1985) Developmental aspects of maximal aerobic power in children. *Exerc. Sports Sci. Rev.* **13**, 503–38.

Lussier, L. & Buskirk, E. (1977) Effects of an endurance training regimen on assessment of work capacity in prepubertal children. *Ann. N. York Acad. Sci.* **301**, 734–47.

Mahon, A.D. & Vaccaro, P. (1989) Ventilatory threshold and $\dot{V}_{O_2 max}$ changes in children following endurance training. *Med. Sci. Sports Exerc.* **21**, 425–31.

Malina, R.M. & Bouchard, C. (1991) *Growth, Maturation and Physical Activity*. Human Kinetics, Champaign, IL.

Massicotte, D.R. & MacNab, R.B. (1979) Cardiorespiratory adaptation to training at specified intensities in children. *Med. Sci. Sports Exerc.* **6**, 242–6.

Pate, R.R. & Branch, J.D. (1992) Training for endurance sport. *Med. Sci. Sport Exerc.* **24**, s340–3.

Pate, R.R. & Ward, D.S. (1990) Endurance exercise trainability in children and youth. In W.A. Grana, J.A. Lombardo, B.J. Sharkey & J.A. Stone (eds) *Advances in Sports Medicine and Fitness*, Vol. 3, pp. 37–55. Year Book Medical Publishers, Littleton, MA.

Rotstein, A., Dotan, R., Bar-Or, O. & Tenenbaum, G. (1986) Effects of training on anaerobic threshold, maximal aerobic power and anaerobic performance of pre-adolescent boys. *Int. J. Sports Med.* **7**, 281–6.

Rowland, T.W. (1985) Aerobic response to endurance training in prepubescent children: a critical analysis. *Med. Sci. Sports Exerc.* **17**, 493–7.

Rowland, T.W. (1990) *Exercise and Children's Health*. Human Kinetics, Champaign, IL.

Sady, S.P. (1986) Cardiorespiratory exercise, training in children. *Clin. Sports Med.* **5**, 493–514.

Savage, M.P., Petratis, M.M., Thomson, W.H., Berg, K., Smith, J.L. & Sady, S.P. (1986) Exercise training effects on serum lipids of prepubescent boys and adult men. *Med. Sci. Sports Exerc.* **18**, 197–204.

Schwartz, L., Britten, R.H. & Thompson, L.R. (1928) Studies in physical development and posture. I. The effect of exercise on the physical condition and development of adolescent boys. *Publ. Health Bull.* **179**, 1–124.

Siegel, P.Z., Brackbill, R.M., Frazier, E.L., Mariolis, P., Sanderson, L.M. & Waller, M.N. (1991) Behavioral risk surveillance, 1986–1990. *Morbid. Mortal. Weekly Rep.* **40**, 1–22.

Simons-Morton, B.G., Parcel, G.S., O'Hara, N.M., Blair, S.N. & Pate, R.R. (1988) Health-related physical fitness in childhood: status and recommendations. *Ann. Rev. Publ. Health* **9**, 403–25.

Sjodin, B. & Svedenhag, J. (1990) Applied physiology of marathon running. *Sports Med.* **2**, 83–99.

Stransky, A.W., Mickelson, R.J., Van Fleet, C. & Davis, R. (1979) Effects of a swimming training regimen on hematological, cardiorespiratory and body composition changes in young females. *J. Sports Med.* **19**, 347–54.

Vaccaro, P. & Mahon, A. (1987) Cardiorespiratory response to endurance training in children. *Sports Med.* **4**, 352–63.

Weber, G., Kartodihardjo, W. & Klissouras, V. (1976) Growth and physical training with reference to heredity. *J. Appl. Physiol.* **40**, 211–15.

Yoshida, T., Ishiko, I. & Muraoka, I. (1980) Effect of endurance training on cardiorespiratory function of 5 year old children. *Int. J. Sports Med.* **1**, 91–4.

Chapter 9

The Role of Physical Activity in the Regulation of Bone Mass during Growth

DONALD A. BAILEY

Introduction

The human skeleton consists of 206 bones assembled to form a framework for the body which provides support against gravity, protection for vulnerable organs and tissues, and a rigid lever system for muscular action to enable locomotion and other movements. Bones also have an essential role to play in terms of a number of vital body functions related to calcium and phosphate homeostasis, the immune system and blood formation. Contrary to previous thought, bone is not an inert, unchanging tissue. In its structural and metabolic roles, bone is capable of remarkable adaptation in response to many factors including mechanical stress, endocrine status, nutritional patterns and exposure to certain drugs and toxins.

From an engineering point of view, bone is a remarkable structural material. It is stronger than the hardest wood, brick or concrete (Koch, 1971) and yet light enough to allow movement and solid enough to provide support. It is also flexible, which allows it to bend and absorb sudden impacts without shattering. Bone composition is primarily the combination of a protein (collagen), a mineral (hydroxyapatite) and water, with each constituent contributing about one-third by volume (Bouvier, 1989).

The compression-resisting hydroxyapatite crystals have a relatively high strength but relatively low elasticity, while the tension-resisting collagen fibres have a relatively low strength but high elasticity. The composite material is stronger than either constituent by itself (Evans, 1973). Bone has a tensile strength equal to cast iron, although it is three times lighter and very much more flexible (Ascenzi & Bell, 1971). This flexibility helps bone, unlike brick or concrete, to respond to strong forces by bending and changing shape rather than breaking. Bone remains elastic up to about three-quarters of its breaking stress.

The collagen in bone is mineralized in an ordered fashion to form two types of skeletal tissue: cortical and trabecular. The cortical component is the densely compacted tissue forming the outer surface of all bones and the shafts of the long bones. The trabecular component forms a meshwork of thin, bony plates or scaffolding found inside the cortical shell in the vertebral bodies, the small bones and the metaphyses of long bones. The trabecular plates arrange themselves in response to lines of force. Both of these constituent parts contribute to the strength of bone (Carter & Hayes, 1977). Both bone types may be influenced by similar factors but probably to a different degree (Mora et al., 1991). Trabecular bone which has a relatively greater surface area than cortical bone is thought to be more susceptible to the influences of mediating factors like nutrition and activity (Gallagher, 1990). Different bones or parts of bone have different proportions of each component. In an adult human the ratio of cortical to trabecular bone is approximately 4:1 (Marcus & Carter, 1988).

Bone-shaping processes

Skeletal tissue is in a constant state of change throughout life. Three processes are involved in this dynamic condition: growth, modelling and remodelling. A single process may dominate at different times during the lifespan or the three processes may function concurrently at other times. Each process appears to have a different function (Schultheis, 1991).

Growth is the expression of the genetically programmed process of enlargement of the entire skeleton under the control of the endocrine system. There is no selective enlargement of individual bones or specific regions within a single bone. Growth involves the entire skeleton and longitudinal growth ceases with the closure of the epiphyses of the long bones.

Modelling is the process that alters the shape and mass in specific bones in response to local factors. It occurs mainly during the growing years and is distinguished from growth by the fact that it is a regional response to a specific influencing factor. Modelling increases bone strength by adding mass and improving geometric architecture where mechanical loading is greatest. The modelling response to weight-bearing physical activity in the young results in a reserve of bone beyond that needed for normal activity (Frost, 1989a). Thus, the high school student who finds recreation in weight-lifting may be less vulnerable to fractures later in life than a comparable piano player with a smaller bone bank (Schultheis, 1991).

Remodelling, although present in young individuals, is the predominant bone process modifying shape and mass in adults. Unlike modelling, remodelling does not make a contribution to the 'bone bank'. The primary function of remodelling is to repair micro-fractures that occur with normal everyday stress (Frost, 1989b). In normal remodelling, the bone resorbing osteoclast cells and the bone-forming osteoblast cells are coupled so that formation follows resorption. This process provides a mechanism for the maintenance of calcium homeostasis and allows the skeleton to maintain its mechanical integrity through the renewal of bone (Eriksen *et al.*, 1989). Remodelling results in net resorption and is responsible for the bone losses that accompany ageing. In middle-aged pre-menopausal women there is an estimated 1% annual bone loss as a result of remodelling (Riggs *et al.*, 1982).

It is important to note that only modelling can significantly increase the amount of bone beyond the genetic expression of growth. Remodelling results in a net loss of bone. Thus, the processes of modelling and remodelling have opposite effects in terms of regional bone mass (Frost, 1989a). These two processes are essentially under the control of mechanical strain.

Strain is the slight deformation of bone induced by a mechanical load. Strain below a lower threshold will result in adaptive remodelling to reduce bone mass. Unopposed remodelling will result in thinner, lighter bones Physical activity producing strain above an upper limit will induce modelling to increase bone mass in response to increasing load requirements (Schultheis, 1991). Since bone mass is increased by the modelling process which occurs mainly before middle age, the importance of promoting load-bearing activity in children and young adults becomes apparent.

Peak bone mass

The establishment of an optimum level of bone mass during the growing years when modelling is superimposed upon growth is a crucial consideration in terms of lifelong skeletal adequacy. Since bone loss is a normal consequence of ageing, those who acquire a greater bone mass in early years should be at reduced risk for the health risks associated with skeletal fragility in later life. This has led some researchers to study factors that may enhance bone gain during the growing years, and is the genesis of the concept of peak bone mass.

Peak bone mass is a simple concept that is still in need of clarification. Theoretically, it is the highest bone mass that an individual attains. However, present measurement techniques do not measure bone mass *per se*. Most current measurements are of bone mineral density (BMD), typically for the hip or lumbar spine and sometimes for the whole body. This has led to some confusion in the literature. For instance, women on average have a smaller peak bone mass than men because their skeletons are physically smaller, but a gender difference in BMD is not nearly as clear-cut and probably varies from site to site (Bonjour *et al.*, 1991). Also, peak BMD values for different skeletal sites are likely to occur at different ages.

Early studies suggested that peak bone mass was attained after a 10–15 year period of bone consolidation following skeletal maturation. During this presumed consolidation period skeletal mass could increase by 10–15% (Avioli, 1984). With improved instrumentation, recent studies have questioned this contention. The prevailing opinion now is that peak bone density, and perhaps bone mass, is achieved at an earlier age than previously thought, probably shortly after the cessation of linear growth (Gilsanz *et al.*, 1988a; Stevenson *et al.*, 1989; Bonjour *et al.*, 1991). Bone loss is also now thought to begin earlier in most people, sometime during the third decade (Fujii *et al.*, 1989; Riggs & Melton, 1990).

The current interest in skeletal fragility in elderly people has resulted in considerable research to identify factors underlying bone loss. Osteoporosis (the thinning of bones with age) represents a tremendous public health problem in certain societies. Three determinants have been advanced to explain the cause of dangerously reduced bone mass in the older population.
1 Failure to attain a sufficiently high peak bone mass during the growing years.
2 Failure to maintain peak bone mass for a sufficient period of time during the early adult years.

3 Accelerated bone loss in later years.
It is probable that reduced bone mass in elderly people results from some combination of these factors.

Most research to date has been directed at understanding the mechanisms of, and providing strategies for, reducing the rate of bone loss in the adult and elderly populations. As a result we know much more about bone loss in adults than we do about bone gain in children and adolescents when skeletal modelling can be stimulated by load-bearing physical activity (Bailey & McCulloch, 1992). Failure to attain a sufficient level of bone mass during the growing years may be a significant contributing cause of the dangerously low bone mass status in older populations (Recker, 1987). From a purely biological perspective, entering senescence with a strong dense skeleton as a result of the development of a high peak bone mass attained during growth should confer a level of protection against skeletal fragility. The attainment of an optimal level of peak bone mass is probably more effective in preventing osteoporosis than measures taken to preserve bone in later years (Burckhardt & Michel, 1989).

While there are still unanswered questions regarding peak bone mass (the age of attaining peak bone mass is still not precisely defined and may be site specific) a number of determinants of peak bone mass can be identified (Fig. 9.1). In addition to mechanical loading, hormonal milieu, nutrition and environmental factors all act upon the genetically programmed skeletal template. These factors are at play throughout life but are probably more important during the growth period when developing bones are highly responsive to mediating influences (Angus & Eisman, 1988; Gilsanz *et al.*, 1988b).

Lifestyle factors and peak bone mass

Although skeletal development is under genetic and endocrine control, the peak bone mass attained by an individual is also a reflection of the loading history on the skeleton induced by

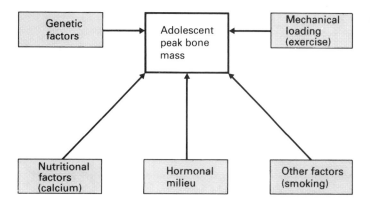

Fig. 9.1 Determinants of peak bone mass during adolescence.

physical activity (Lanyon, 1984). In addition, nutritional factors affecting calcium absorption play an important role in bone mass accumulation during growth (Heaney, 1991a). These lifestyle factors, physical activity and nutrition, are the two exogenous influences of pre-eminent importance in terms of skeletal development. There is a synergistic relationship between these energy factors. Calcium supplementation in the absence of weight-bearing is ineffective in terms of bone maintenance (Kanis, 1991) while adequate lifetime calcium intake augments the bone-building effects of exercise (Kanders *et al.*, 1988; Halioua & Anderson, 1989). Shangold *et al.* (1990) have stated that the beneficial effects of exercise on bone cannot be realized if dietary calcium is inadequate.

Physical activity

Gravity and muscular contraction are the two primary mechanical forces applied to bone. Mechanical loading in the form of weight-bearing activity against the force of gravity influences bone mass. This was recognized by Galileo in 1638 who discussed the relationship between body weight and skeletal mass in his *Discorsi e Dimostrazioni Matematiche Intorno a due Nuone Scienze* (Galileo, 1638). (English translation: Crew & de Salvio, 1933.) This work points out the importance of gravity in establishing the dimensions and mechanical charac-

teristics of bones in animals of different sizes. The loading of bone through the muscular contractions involved in physical activity provides another stimulus to bone in addition to weight-bearing. This was understood by Darwin in 1859 who noticed the functional adaptation of bone in the domestic duck, whose 'bones of the wing weigh less and bones of the leg more, in proportion to the whole skeleton, than do the same bones in the wild duck, and the change may be safely attributed to the domestic duck flying less and walking more than its wild parents' (Darwin, 1872). A Berlin anatomist, Julius Wolff in 1892 is given credit for first articulating a proposition to explain the changes in bone mass that accompany changes in mechanical loading. He noted that bone tissue reorganizes when mechanical forces change (Wolff, 1892). His seminal work in German, *Das Gesetz der Transformation der Knochen*, has been translated into English (Maquet & Furlong, 1986) and Wolff's law, as it has come to be known, can be restated as follows: the general form of bone being given, alterations to the internal architecture and external form occur as a consequence of primary changes in mechanical stressors.

Wolff's observation that bone alters its shape and architecture to withstand external mechanical forces has prompted numerous studies over the years which have investigated the effects of physical activity and levels of loading on bone-shaping processes. Animal studies have shown that bone mass, density and shape all change in response to weight-bearing physical activity (Woo *et al.*, 1981). One of the best experimental examples of this has been provided by Goodship *et al.* (1979). These workers measured the strain on the radius bone in the foreleg of a pig before partial removal of the complementary ulna bone. After 3 months of walking on the single weight-bearing radius, this bone had changed its shape and conformation to meet the altered load requirement and the strain level had returned close to baseline (Fig. 9.2).

Another example of Wolff's law, this time with a human model, has been documented by Houston (1978) in a case study of a boy born with only one instead of two bones in the lower leg (congenital absence of the tibia). Orthopaedic surgeons operated on this handicapped infant when he was 2 years old and moved the fibula, which is normally a thin strut bone, centrally beneath the femur so that it could bear weight. When this boy was 3.5 years old, after 18 months of weight-bearing, the fibula which was doing the work of the tibia assumed essentially the size, shape and strength of the missing tibia. In this case the initial absence of the tibia was genetic, but the

later development of the fibula was due to weight-bearing stress (Fig. 9.3).

Wolff's law also applies to the density of bone. Numerous studies have observed higher BMD values in athletes compared to non-athletes (Nilsson & Westlin, 1971; Bailey *et al.*, 1986). Lifetime tennis players have significantly greater bone mineral content in the dominant arm in contrast to the non-dominant arm (Huddleston *et al.*, 1980; Pirnay *et al.*, 1987). Cross-sectional studies examining active and sedentary populations indicate a positive relationship between physical activity and BMD (Snow-Harter & Marcus, 1991).

The potential of weight-bearing physical activity to increase BMD in the growing years and retard bone loss in later life is an area of considerable current interest in view of the high correlation between BMD status and fracture risk in the elderly population. Fracture frequency increases as bone mass and density decreases (Melton *et al.*, 1986, 1990) thus low BMD is a major determinant of fracture (Johnston & Slemenda, 1991). In adults, cross-sectional studies have shown that less active individuals have a lower BMD than athletes and physically active individuals (Jacobson *et al.*, 1984; Lane *et al.*, 1986; Stillman *et al.*,

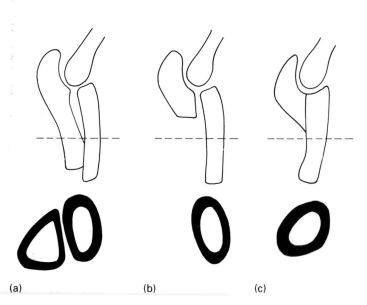

(a)   (b)   (c)

Fig. 9.2 Experimental demonstration of Wolff's law. (a) Normal forelimb of pig with the ulna present. The strain on the radius in walking is 100%. (b) The same forelimb with the ulna partially removed. The strain on the radius in walking is 210%. (c) After 3 months, the radius has changed shape and conformation. The strain on the radius is restored to 110%. From Goodship *et al.* (1979) in Curry (1984).

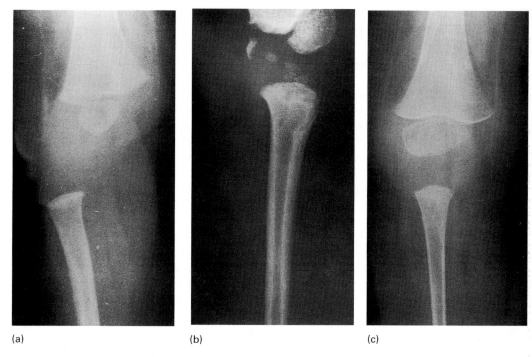

(a)   (b)   (c)

Fig. 9.3 The case of the transformed fibula. (a) Congenital absence of the tibia, fibula at 4.5 months. (b) At 2 years following surgical centring. (c) At 3.5 years after 18 months of weight-bearing. The fibula has assumed the size, shape and cortical thickness of a normal tibia. From Houston (1978) with permission.

1986). Results from prospective studies on adults range from equivocal to generally positive, indicating that reductions in BMD loss in older adults and perhaps even modest increases in bone density are possible following an exercise regime (Chow *et al.*, 1987; Dalsky *et al.*, 1988; Rikli & McManus, 1990). Overall, the evidence suggests that the positive effect of exercise on adult bone is modest in the short term, but may be quite powerful in the long term (Eisman, 1991).

In children, our knowledge about the long-term effects of physical activity on BMD accretion is incomplete, and studies on paediatric populations have only recently been undertaken. The results of prospective studies suggest that physical activity must be vigorous if BMD is to be enhanced in young individuals (Margulies *et al.*, 1986; Snow-Harter *et al.*, 1992). In studies that have used physical activity questionnaires to classify subjects into levels of

activity, most have reported a significant but modest association between activity as a youth and BMD at certain skeletal sites (Slemenda *et al.*, 1991; Kroger *et al.*, 1992). Childhood activities that preferentially stress one side of the body over the other provide the strongest evidence that physical activity can modulate BMD during the growing years above genetic considerations (Watson, 1974; Bailey *et al.*, 1992; Faulkner *et al.*, 1993). Animal studies provide incontrovertible evidence that the bones of growing animals, in comparison to the bones of adult animals, have a greater capacity to respond to exercise by adding bone (Forwood & Burr, 1993). Furthermore, one study has shown that the benefits of exercise begun before skeletal maturation are maintained into and throughout adulthood (Silberman *et al.*, 1991). The results of these studies suggest that important increments in skeletal mass may result from increased physical activity levels during the growing years. Any advantage derived from optimizing the level of BMD at maturity is likely to persist through adult life and provide some protection against skeletal fragility in later years.

A number of studies investigating the effects of physical activity on bone mass in children and young adults have been carried out by the Bone Density Study Group at the University of Saskatchewan. An early study investigated the trabecular bone density of the weight-bearing os calcis bone by quantitative computed tomography (QCT) in 51 normally menstruating female university students aged 18–29 years (Bailey et al., 1986). Four activity groups were represented in the study, 24 élite athletes who had had a long background throughout childhood and adolescence in basketball, volleyball or athletics; 13 high level recreation women ($>5\,h\cdot week^{-1}$); nine low level recreation women ($1-3\,h\cdot week^{-1}$); and five controls ($<1\,h\cdot week^{-1}$). There was a significant relationship between trabecular bone density and levels of activity with the athletic group having the highest values and the control group the lowest (Fig. 9.4).

Another study considered current and past lifestyle factors and BMD at the same weight-bearing site, the os calcis measured by QCT, in 101 healthy female hospital workers aged 20–35 years (McCulloch et al., 1990). The only lifestyle factor, out of 25, that was significantly related to trabecular BMD was childhood activity. Those women who had engaged in sport and activity programmes in their youth had significantly higher calcaneal BMD as adults (Fig. 9.5).

To control for self-selection and genetic differences inherent in the studies listed above, the BMDs in specific regions of the proximal femur were measured by dual energy X-ray absorptiometry (DXA) in 17 children with unilateral Legg–Calvé–Perthes disease (LCPD) (Bailey et al., in press). Comparisons were made between the affected and non-affected hips with each child acting as his or her own control. In three regions of interest in the proximal femur the BMD on the non-affected side significantly exceeded the density on the painful affected side. In addition, density values on the non-affected side, which had become the major weight-bearing side, were greater than age-and sex-specific normative values. This was in contrast to values on the affected side which were less than normative values for children of the same age and sex. While it is generally agreed that LCPD represents a general disorder of skeletal growth, it is clear from the results of this study that compromised weight-bearing resulted in a differential BMD response in the proximal femur in children with unilateral involvement (Fig. 9.6). Obviously, mechanical loading during childhood had an impact on skeletal modelling and bone mass in these children.

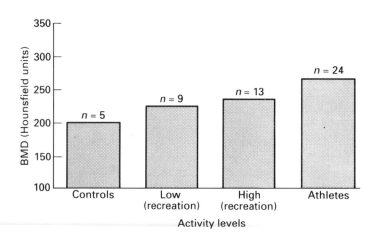

Fig. 9.4 Trabecular bone mineral density (BMD) in the os calcis in 51 young women aged 18–25 years categorized according to physical activity patterns. From Bailey et al. (1986).

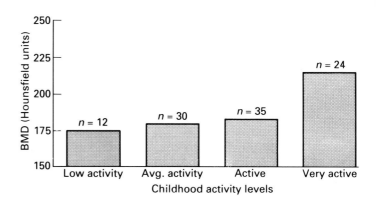

Fig. 9.5 Trabecular bone mineral density (BMD) in the os calcis in 101 young premenopausal women aged 20–35 years categorized according to self-reported childhood physical activity. From McCulloch *et al.* (1990).

The influence of different types of loading through physical activity (i.e. weight-bearing versus non-weight bearing) is an area of current interest. In children, it has been suggested that activities that do not involve weight-bearing will not be associated with higher levels of bone density (Slemenda *et al.*, 1991). For instance, there is speculation that the buoyant environment of a pool during swimming training may have a dampening effect on BMD accretion in weight-bearing bones in a manner similar to the problems of zero gravity encountered by astronauts (Arnaud *et al.*, 1986; Stillman, 1987). Risser *et al.* (1990) found significantly lower BMD in the lumbar spine and os calcis in university aged female swimmers compared to age-matched control subjects, volleyball and basketball players. In a study of 11 competitive gymnasts aged 10–16 years who were matched for gender, stage of maturity and weight with competitive swimmers, lumbar

spine and femoral neck BMD was significantly greater in the gymnasts in comparison to the swimmers (Grimston *et al.*, 1993). In our own laboratory we found a similar trend in os calcis BMD in a study involving 14–16-year-old swimmers and soccer players as shown in Fig. 9.7 (McCulloch *et al.*, 1992).

The need to distinguish between various types of physical activities and their effect on bone has been recognized (Ott, 1990). Aerobic exercises and swimming do not appear to increase bone mass to the same extent as training with weights or specific compressive exercises. A number of cross-sectional investigations on young adults (Westfall *et al.*, 1989; Davee *et al.*, 1990; Heinrich *et al.*, 1990; Risser *et al.*, 1990) have reported a positive effect on BMD from weight-training or specific loading programmes, but to date there have been no studies in children.

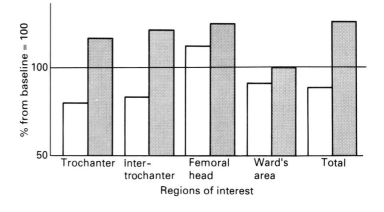

Fig. 9.6 Bone mineral density in regions of the affected (□) and non-affected (▨) proximal femur in 18 children with unilateral Legg–Calvé–Perthes disease compared with normal values (based on $n = 696$). From Bailey *et al.* (in press).

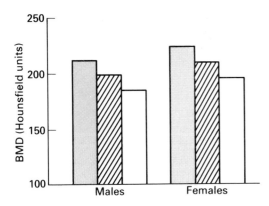

Fig. 9.7 Trabecular bone mineral density (BMD) in the os calcis in 68 young boys and girls aged 13–17 years categorized according to élite athletic participation. □, Control; (12 M, 13 F); ▨, soccer (11 M, 12 F); ▨, swimming (10 M, 10 F). From McCulloch *et al.* (1992).

Calcium

Adequate calcium intake is an essential prerequisite for bone development and maintenance. However, it should be stressed that calcium is not the cause of skeletal integrity, rather it is a necessary condition for it (Heaney, 1991a). It is mechanical loading through physical activity that is of primary importance for bone (Schultheis, 1991). Potentially, the childhood and adolescent years are the most important in terms of the influence of calcium on bone status (Eisman, 1991). The skeleton of a newborn contains about 25 g of calcium, for a normal healthy adult this figure is over 1000 g. This difference has to come from dietary sources (Heaney, 1991a). Calcium alone cannot prevent bone loss in later life or make up for an earlier skeletal deficit (Heaney, 1991b), but evidence does support the importance of dietary calcium over the long term (Dawson-Hughes *et al.*, 1990) and its influence on the attainment of peak bone mass (Cumming, 1990).

There have been few prospective trials investigating calcium-induced bone accretion in growing children, hence, the exact nature of the relationship between calcium intake, calcium absorption and BMD during the critical growth period is not well understood, but preliminary evidence suggests a positive effect. In a double-blind placebo-controlled study of 22 prepubertal identical twin pairs, whose average dietary intake of 900 mg of calcium approximated the recommended dietary allowance, one twin per pair was given a daily calcium supplement of 700 mg. After 3 years it was clear that the calcium-supplemented group had an enhanced rate of increase in BMD at the radius and lumbar spine site (Johnston *et al.*, 1992). Among the 23 pairs who were postpubertal or who had passed through puberty during the course of the study, the twins receiving the supplement derived no benefit. The authors concluded that BMD accretion was enhanced by calcium supplementation in prepubertal children and if the gain persisted peak bone mass would be increased and the risk of future fracture reduced.

In an earlier study, Sandler *et al.* (1985) reported a relationship between BMD of the radius in a group of postmenopausal women and self-reported consumption of milk during childhood and adolescence. No relationship between present milk or calcium intake was found. It was concluded that milk consumption in childhood may be needed not only for skeletal growth and development but also to assure, within genetic limits, optimal bone mass.

While the evidence is not all in, an adequate intake of calcium during the growing years is clearly an essential requirement if one is to build an optimal level of skeletal mass within genetic bounds. What constitutes an adequate intake is still being debated. It is well known that a low calcium intake during growth can limit the attainment of skeletal potential (Heaney, 1991b). Chan (1991) studied 164 healthy white children, aged 2–16 years, and found that those children ingesting more than 1000 mg of calcium daily had a higher BMD than those ingesting less. A recent study by Matkovic *et al.* (1990) suggests that calcium requirements during adolescence, when skeletal growth is accelerating, are quite high. Augmenting the calcium intake of adolescent females from 250 to 1600 mg · day^{-1} did not produce a significant increase in urinary calcium. This suggests that even at 1600 mg · day^{-1}, well above recommended levels in most countries, the capacity of the growing skeleton to utilize calcium has not been saturated. Peacock (1991), on the basis of known values for calcium absorption, skeletal accretion rates and obligatory losses in children and adolescents, suggests that it is unlikely that an optimal level of peak bone mass can be achieved by children with average daily intakes of calcium below 1000 (males) and 850 mg (females). Heaney (1991a), taking into consideration the same factors as Peacock, recommends a dietary intake of calcium of 1500 mg · day^{-1} to ensure the achievement of the genetically programmed level of peak bone mass.

This is an important consideration in view of the recent trends towards declining milk consumption and increasing soft drink and coffee utilization among adolescent girls (Guenther, 1986; Recker, 1987). The health and nutrition surveys in the USA, Hanes I (Abraham et al., 1977) and Hanes II (Carroll et al., 1983), obtained calcium intake values by 24-h dietary recall on a representative probability sample of over 28 000 people. By the age of 10, average calcium intake in females had fallen well below the recommended dietary allowance of 1200 mg in the Hanes I data. In the Hanes II survey some 7 years later, the average values had dropped a further 10% below the recommended dietary allowance to a value of 800 mg. Obviously, the majority of adolescent females in the USA are not meeting the recommended dietary allowance for calcium and it is probably reasonable to assume that a calcium deficiency exists in the majority of adolescent females, most likely throughout the world (Chesnut, 1991).

Lifestyle changes and bone mass

In addition to the changes in the nutritional habits of children, noted above, current research indicates a pattern of change in the way children use their leisure time (Bailey, 1981). These child-

hood nutritional and physical activity trends may have implications in terms of long-term skeletal health.

Current activity trends

Over the last several decades, there appears to have been a significant decline in the amount of time children are involved in self-generated, free time spontaneous play involving weight-bearing physical activity. There are probably a number of reasons for this including the world-wide trend towards urbanization, where crowded cities, traffic congestion, apartment living and concrete jungles mitigate against natural forms of childhood physical activity. In the technologically developed and developing countries, television is another enemy of human movement. In most Western countries children spend in excess of 24 h · week^{-1} watching television. This is probably a conservative estimate. In many countries home entertainment systems are becoming increasingly popular. Video games and home movies add to television viewing time. Twenty-four or more hours per week, over and above normal sleeping time and sitting time at school, represents a substantial amount of non-movement time that is now part of the lifestyle of the present generation of many children. In addition to this, the automobile and school bus have substantially reduced walking time for many children. This situation does not bode well for future skeletal health. And, of course, this reality is insignificant compared to the problems faced by many children in the Third World where malnutrition, disease and famine rob surviving children of any chance of realizing their skeletal potential.

An evolutionary perspective

It has been suggested that the genetic make-up of humans remains adapted for circumstances as they existed thousands of years ago and that the physical activity and nutritional patterns of humans living in the late palaeolithic era can be considered the natural paradigm (Eaton & Nelson, 1991). These workers postulate that there has been little alteration in genetic constitution since the emergence of agriculture some 10000 years ago, but living conditions have changed almost beyond belief. Thus, our present day lives may be out of step with our bodies which carry genetic requirements adapted for another age.

Past and present diets and physical exertion requirements differ significantly in many respects. Past lifestyles demanded levels of exertion far exceeding those of today (Eaton *et al.*, 1988) and dietary calcium intakes were probably double what they are today (Eaton & Nelson, 1991). The sources of calcium were also different, coming from vegetable rather than dairy origin. Taking these lifestyle differences into consideration one would expect early humans to have denser skeletons than modern day people, and anthropological studies have confirmed this (Smith *et al.*, 1984; Larsen, 1987). While it is unrealistic to try and turn back the clock, a return to increased levels of physical activity and the restoration of a high calcium nutritional environment would appear to be prudent in terms of the development of skeletal mass during youth and young adulthood.

Lifestyle recommendations for bone health

Taking into account the fact that our knowledge of the complicated mechanisms controlling BMD accretion is still incomplete, there are still some sound lifestyle guidelines that can be offered to young people and their parents (Bailey & McCulloch, 1992).
1 Avoid long periods of immobilization.
2 Develop a lifelong enthusiasm for physical activity.
3 Eat a well-balanced diet that meets or exceeds current recommended allowances for calcium.
4 Girls should be alert to the fact that menstrual dysfunction and amenorrhoea associated with nutritional deficits, or exercise excesses, will have deleterious effects on bone.

Unfortunately, the lifestyles and habits of many young people are self-destructive in respect to the skeleton and it will take the concerted efforts of health professionals and educators, as well as parents, to change the lifestyle of adolescents in the hope of avoiding many of the problems associated with skeletal fragility in later years.

Challenges for future research

- Studies are needed to ascertain the best types of exercise and activity to achieve an optimal peak bone mass. What is the upper threshold of strain needed to induce skeletal modelling, and conversely, what is the lower level of strain below which bone mass is lost through adaptive remodelling? These and other questions related to exercise frequency, duration and intensity for maximum skeletal benefit need to be answered.
- Additional studies are required to determine the optimal conditions, such as hormonal milieu and dietary calcium intake, needed to facilitate a bone response to exercise. In spite of some conflicting data, the hypothesis that increased calcium levels will have a positive effect on the acquisition of peak bone mass remains tenable. What the level should be is still an open question.
- During the growth period, there may be a critical age when bone is more responsive to the mechanical load imposed by activity. Or, conversely, there may be vulnerable periods when immobilization is to be particularly avoided. These hypotheses need to be investigated.
- The timing of adolescence related to bone status is another area needing study. We have recently demonstrated an increase in fracture incidence in boys and girls accompanying the state of high bone turnover at the time of peak height velocity during adolescence (Bailey *et al.*, 1989) and in another study the timing of the growth spurt has been identified as an important determinant of peak bone mass in men (Finkelstein *et al.*, 1992). Clearly, we need

more information on the relationship between maturational status and bone mass acquisition.

• The interpretation of BMD changes during growth when assessed by projectional methods like single or dual photon absorptiometry or by DXA techniques is complicated and needs to be studied. These methods provide an areal measure of density in $g \cdot cm^{-2}$ which can be confounded by size changes that accompany growth. Larger bones resulting from growth will yield a higher areal density measurement than smaller bones of the same volumetric density because bone thickness is not taken into consideration (Katzman et al., 1991; Carter et al., 1992; Bailey et al., 1993). This needs further investigation.

• Clearly there are more questions than answers. From a practical health standpoint, perhaps the most important question of all is this. If the failure to attain a sufficient bone mass at the time of skeletal maturity is related to bone fragility in the late adult years, how do you relate a disease of elderly people to a teenage population that will not be at risk for 50 or 60 years? Promoting an awareness of the importance of physical activity and good nutrition during the growing years will be a challenge for all health professionals.

Acknowledgements

The author acknowledges the support of the National Health Research and Development Program of Health and Welfare, Canada for grant support to study bone dynamics in growing children; Dean Robert Mirwald and colleagues in the College of Physical Education at the University of Saskatchewan and Dr Stuart Houston, Professor of Diagnostic Radiology in the College of Medicine at the University of Saskatchewan for encouraging and supporting interdisciplinary research endeavours; and to those graduate students working in the bone area for their many contributions over the years.

References

Abraham, S., Carroll, M.D., Dresser, C.M. & Johnson, C.L. (1977) *Dietary Intake Findings, United States 1971–1974 (Hanes I)*. National Center for Health Statistics, Hyattsville, MD.

Angus, R. & Eisman, J. (1988) Osteoporosis: the role of calcium intake and supplementation. *Med. J. Austral.* **148**, 630–3.

Arnaud, S.B., Schneider, V.S. & Morey-Holton, E. (1986) Effects of inactivity on bone and calcium metabolism. In H. Sandler & J. Vernikos (eds) *Inactivity: Physiological Effects*, pp. 49–76. Academic Press, Orlando, FL.

Ascenzi, A. & Bell, G.H. (1971) Bone as a mechanical engineering problem. In G.H. Bourne (ed.) *The Biochemistry and Physiology of Bone*, 2nd edn, pp. 311–46. Academic Press, New York.

Avioli, L.V. (1984) Calcium and osteoporosis. *Am. J. Nutr.* **4**, 471–91.

Bailey, D.A. (1981) Inactivity and the Canadian child. *Recr. Can.* **81**, 14–18.

Bailey, D.A., Daniels, K., Dzus, A. et al. (in press) Bone mineral density in the proximal femur of children with Legg–Calvé–Perthes disease.

Bailey, D.A., Drinkwater, D., Faulkner, R., McKay, H., McCulloch, R. & Houston, S. (1993) Longitudinal bone mineral changes in the femoral neck in growing children: dimensional considerations. *J. Bone Mineral Res.* **8**, S266.

Bailey, D.A. & McCulloch, R. (1992) Osteoporosis: are there childhood antecedents for an adult health problem? *Can. J. Pediatr.* **4**, 130–4.

Bailey, D.A., Martin, A.D., Howie, J.L. et al. (1986) Bone density and physical activity in young women. In P. Russo & G. Gass (eds) *Exercise, Nutrition, and Performance*, pp. 127–37. Cumberland College of Science, Sydney.

Bailey, D.A., Wedge, J.H., McCulloch, R.G., Martin, A.D. & Bernhardson, S.C. (1989) Epidemiology of fractures of the distal end of the radius in children as associated with growth. *J. Bone Joint Surg.* **71A**, 1225–31.

Bonjour, J.P., Theintz, G., Buchs, B., Slosman, D. & Rizzoli, R. (1991) Critical years and stages of puberty for spinal and femoral bone mass accumulation during adolescence. *J. Clin. Endocrinol. Metab.* **73**, 555–63.

Bouvier, M. (1989) The biology and composition of bone. In S.C. Cowin (ed.) *Bone Mechanics*, pp. 1–14. CRC Press, Boca Raton, FL.

Burckhardt, P. & Michel, C. (1989) The peak bone mass concept. *Clin. Rheumatol.* **8**, 16–21.

Carroll, M.D., Abraham, S. Dresser, C.M. (1983) *Dietary Intake Source Data: United States 1976–1980*

(Hanes II). National Center for Health Statistics, Hyattsville, MD.

Carter, D.R., Bouxsein, M.L. & Marcus, R. (1992) New approaches for interpreting projected bone densitometry data. *J. Bone Mineral Res.* **7**, 137–45.

Carter, D.R. & Hayes, W.C. (1977) The compressive behaviour of bone as a two-phase porous structure. *J. Bone Joint Surg.* **59A**, 954–62.

Chan, G.M. (1991) Dietary calcium and bone mineral status of children and adolescents. *Am. J. Dis. Child.* **145**, 631–4.

Chesnut, C. (1991) Theoretical overview: bone development, peak bone mass, bone loss, and fracture risk. *Am. J. Med.* **91**, 2S–4.

Chow, R., Harrison, J.E. & Notarius, C. (1987) Effect of two randomized exercise programmes on bone mass of healthy postmenopausal women. *Br. Med. J.* **295**, 1441–4.

Crew, H. & de Salvio, A. (1933) *Dialogues Concerning Two New Sciences*. Macmillan, New York.

Cumming, R.G. (1990) Calcium intake and bone mass: a quantitative review of the evidence. *Calc. Tiss. Int.* **47**, 194–201.

Curry, J.D. (1984) *The Mechanical Adaptations of Bone*, p. 247. Princeton University Press, Princeton.

Dalsky, G.P., Stocke, K.S., Ehsani, A.A., Slatopolsky, E., Lee, W.E. & Birge, S.J. (1988) Weight bearing exercise training and lumbar bone mineral content in postmenopausal women. *Ann. Int. Med.* **108**, 824–8.

Darwin C. (1872) *The Origin of Species*, 6th edn. New American Library, New York.

Davee, A.M., Rosen, C.J. & Adler, R.A. (1990) Exercise patterns and trabecular bone density in college women. *J. Bone Mineral Res.* **5**, 245–50.

Dawson-Hughes, B., Dallal, G.E., Krall, E.A., Sadowski, L., Sahyown, N. & Tannenbaum, S. (1990) A controlled trial of the effect of calcium supplementation on bone density in postmenopausal women. *New Engl. J. Med.* **323**, 878–83.

Eaton, S., Konner, M. & Shostak, M. (1988) Stone agers in the fast lane: chronic degenerative diseases in evolutionary perspective. *Am. J. Med.* **84**, 739–49.

Eaton, S. & Nelson, D. (1991) Calcium in evolutionary perspective. *Am. J. Clin. Nutr.* **54**(28), 1S–7S.

Eisman, J. (1991) Osteoporosis – prevention. *Austral. New Z. J. Med.* **21**, 205–9.

Eriksen, E.F., Steiniche, T., Mosekilde, L. & Melsen, F. (1989) Histomorphometric analysis of bone in metabolic bone disease. In R.D. Tiegs (ed.) *Metabolic Bone Disease*, Part I. *Endocrinology and Metabolism Clinics of North America*, pp. 919–54. W.B. Saunders, Philadelphia.

Evans, F.G. (1973) *Mechanical Properties of Bone*, pp. 219–310. C.C. Thomas, Springfield, IL.

Faulkner, R., Houston, C., Bailey, D., Drinkwater, D., McKay, H. & Wilkinson, A. (1993) Comparison of bone mineral content and bone mineral density between dominant and non-dominant limbs in children 8–16 years of age. *Am. J. Hum. Biol.* **5**, 491–9.

Finkelstein, J.L., Neer, R.M., Biller, B.M.K., Crawford, J.D. & Klibanski, A. (1992) Osteopenia in men with a history of delayed puberty. *New Engl. J. Med.* **326**, 600–4.

Forwood, M. & Burr, D. (1993) Physical activity and bone mass: exercise in futility? *Bone Mineral*, **21**, 89–112.

Frost, H. (1989a) Mechanical usage, bone mass, bone fragility: a brief overview. In M. Kleerekoper & S. Krane (eds) *Clinical Disorders of Bone and Mineral Metabolism*, pp. 15–40. Mary Ann Liebert, New York.

Frost, H. (1989b) Transient steady state phenomena in microdamage physiology: a proposed algorithm for lamellar bone. *Calc. Tiss. Int.* **44**, 367–81.

Fujii, Y., Tsutsumi, M., Tsunenari, T. *et al.* (1989) Quantitative computed tomography of lumbar vertebrae in Japanese patients with osteoporosis. *Bone Mineral* **6**, 87–94.

Galileo, G. (1638) *Discorsi e Dimonstrzioni Matematiche in Torno a due Nuone Scienze*. Appreffo gli Elfevirri, Leida.

Gallagher, J.C. (1990) The pathogenesis of osteoporosis. *Bone Mineral* **9**, 215–27.

Gilsanz, V., Gibbens, D.T., Carlson, M., Boechat, M.I., Cann, C.E. & Schulz, E.E. (1988a) Peak trabecular vertebral density: a comparison of adolescent and adult females. *Calc. Tiss. Int.* **43**, 260–2.

Gilsanz, V., Gibbens, D.T., Roe, T.F. *et al.* (1988b) Vertebral bone density in children: effect of puberty. *Radiology* **166**, 847–50.

Goodship, A.E., Lanyon, L.E. & McFie, H. (1979) Functional adaptations of bone to increased stress. *J. Bone Joint Surg.* **61A**, 539–46.

Grimston, S., Willows, N. & Hanley, D. (1993) Mechanical loading regime and its relationship to bone mineral density in children. *Med. Sci. Sports Exerc.* **25**, 1098–102.

Guenther, P.M. (1986) Beverages in the diets of American teenagers. *J. Am. Diet. Ass.* **86**, 493–9.

Halioua, L. & Anderson, J. (1989) Lifetime calcium intake and physical activity habits: independent and combined effects on the radial bone of healthy premenopausal Caucasian women. *Am. J. Clin. Nutr.* **49**, 534–51.

Heaney, R.P. (1991a) The effect of calcium on skeletal development, bone loss, and risk of fractures. *Am. J. Med.* **91**, 23S–8.

Heaney, R.P. (1991b) Lifelong calcium intake and prevention of bone fragility in the aged. *Calc. Tiss.*

Int. **49S**, S42−5.

Heinrich, C.H., Going, S.B., Pamenter, R.W., Perry, C.D., Boyden, T.W. & Lohman, T.G. (1990) Bone mineral content of cyclically menstruating female resistance and endurance trained athletes. *Med. Sci. Sports Exerc.* **22**, 558−63.

Houston, C.S. (1978) The radiologists' opportunity to teach bone dynamics. *J. Can. Ass. Radiol.* **29**, 232−8.

Huddleston, A., Rockwell, D. & Kulund, D. (1980) Bone mass in lifetime tennis players. *JAMA* **244**, 1107−9.

Jacobson, P.C., Beaver, W., Grubb, S.A., Taft, T.N. & Talmage, B.V. (1984) Bone density in women: college athletes and older athletic women. *J. Orthop. Res.* **2**, 328−32.

Johnston, C., Miller, J., Slemenda, C. *et al.* (1992) Calcium supplementation and increases in bone mineral density in children. *New Engl. J. Med.* **327**, 82−7.

Johnston, C. & Slemenda, C. (1991) Risk prediction in osteoporosis: A theoretical overview. *Am. J. Med.* **91**, 47S−9.

Kanders, B., Dempster, D.W. & Lindsay, R. (1988) Interaction of calcium nutrition and physical activity on bone mass in young women. *J. Bone Mineral Res.* **3**, 145−9.

Kanis, J.A. (1991) Calcium requirements for optimal skeletal health in women. *Calc. Tiss. Int.* **149S**, S33−41.

Katzman, D.K., Bachrach, L.K., Carter, D.R. & Marcus, R. (1991) Clinical and anthropometric correlates of bone mineral acquisition in healthy adolescent girls. *J. Clin. Endocrinol. Metab.* **73**, 1332−9.

Koch, J.C. (1971) The laws of bone architecture. *Am. J. Anat.* **21**, 211−98.

Kroger, H., Kotaniemi, A., Vainio, P. & Alhava, E. (1992) Bone densitometry of the spine and femur in children by dual-energy X-ray absorptiometry. *Bone Mineral* **17**, 75−85.

Lane, N.E., Bloch, D.A., Jones, H.H., Marshall, H.W. Jr, Wood, P.D. & Fries, J.F. (1986) Long-distance running, bone density and osteoarthritis. *JAMA* **255**, 1147−51.

Lanyon, L.E. (1984) Functional strain as a determinant for bone remodelling. *Calc. Tiss. Int.* **36**, 556−61.

Larsen, C. (1987) Bioarchaeological interpretations of subsistence economy and behavior from human skeletal remains. *Adv. Archaeol. Methodol. Theory* **10**, 339−445.

McCulloch, R.G., Bailey, D.A., Houston, C.S. & Dodd, B.L. (1990) Effects of physical activity, dietary calcium intake and selected lifestyle factors on bone density in young women. *Can. Med. Ass. J.* **142**, 221−7.

McCulloch, R.G., Bailey, D.A., Whalen, R., Houston, C.S. & Craven, B. (1992) Bone density and bone

mineral content of adolescent soccer athletes and competitive swimmers. *Pediatr. Exerc. Sci.* **4**, 319−30.

Maquet, P. & Furlong, R. (trans.) (1986) *The Laws of Bone Remodelling.* Springer-Verlag, Berlin.

Margulies, J.Y., Simkin, A. Leichter, I. *et al.* (1986) Effect of intense physical activity on the bone-mineral content in the lower limbs of young adults. *J. Bone Joint Surg.* **68A**, 1090−3.

Matkovic, V., Fonatana, D., Tominac, C., Goel, P. & Chesnut, C.H. (1990) Factors which influence peak bone mass formation: a study of calcium balance and the inheritance of bone mass in adolescent females. *Am. J. Clin. Nutr.* **52**, 878−88.

Melton, L., Eddy, D. & Johnston, C. (1990) Screening for osteoporosis. *Ann. Int. Med.* **112**, 516−28.

Melton, L., Wahner, H., Richelson, L., O'Fallon, W. & Riggs, B. (1986) Osteoporosis and the risk of hip fracture. *Am. J. Epidemiol.* **124**, 254−61.

Mora, S., Schulz, E., Roe, T., Sith, B. & Gilsanz, V. (1991) Gains in cancellous and cortical bone during growth are determined by different factors. *J. Bone Mineral Res.* **6**, S307.

Nilsson, B. & Westlin, N. (1971) Bone density in athletes. *Clin. Orthop.* **77**, 179−82.

Ott, S. (1990) Attainment of peak bone mass. *J. Clin. Endocrinol. Metab.* **71**, 1082A−C.

Peacock, M. (1991) Calcium absorption efficiency and calcium requirements in children and adolescents. *Am. J. Clin. Nutr.* **54**, 251S−65.

Pirnay, F., Bodeau, M. & Crielaard, J. (1987) Bone mineral content and physical activity. *Int. J. Sport Med.* **8**, 331−5.

Recker, R. (1987) Bone mass and calcium nutrition. *Nutr. Res.* **11**, 19−21.

Riggs, B.L. & Melton III, L.J. (1990) Clinical heterogeneity of involutional osteoporosis: implications for preventive therapy. *J. Clin. Endocrinol. Metab.* **70**, 1229−32.

Riggs, B.L., Wahner, H., Seeman, E. *et al.* (1982) Changes in bone mineral density of the proximal femur and spine with aging. *J. Clin. Invest.* **70**, 716−23.

Rikli, R.E. & McManus, B.G. (1990) Effects of exercise on bone mineral content in postmenopausal women. *Res. Q.* **61**, 243−9.

Risser, W.L., Lee, E.J., Leblanc, A., Poindexter, H.B., Risser, J.M.H. & Scneider, V. (1990) Bone density in eumenorrheic female college athletes. *Med. Sci. Sports Exerc.* **22**, 570−4.

Sandler, R.B., Slemenda, C.W., LaPorte, R.E. *et al.* (1985) Postmenopausal bone density and milk consumption in childhood and adolescence. *Am. J. Clin. Nutr.* **42**, 270−4.

Schultheis, L. (1991) The mechanical control system of bone in weightless space flight and in aging.

Exp. Gerontol. **46**, 203–14.

Shangold, M., Rebar, R.W., Colston Wentz, A. & Schiff, I. (1990) Evaluation and management of menstrual dysfunction in athletes. *JAMA* 263, 1665–9.

Silberman, M., Schapira, D., Leichter, J. & Steinberg, R. (1991) Moderate physical exercise throughout adulthood increases peak bone mass at middle age and maintains higher trabecular bone density in vertebrae of senescent female rats. *Cells Materials* **1** (Suppl.), 151–8.

Slemenda, C.W., Christian, J.C., Williams, C.J. & Johnston Jr, C.C. (1990) The changing relative importance of genetics and environment in adult women. In D.V. Cohn, F.H. Glorieux & T.J. Martin (eds) *Calcium Regulation and Bone and Metabolism*, pp. 491–6. Elsevier Science, Montreal.

Slemenda, C.W., Millder, J.Z., Hui, S.L., Reister, T.K. & Johnston, C.C. (1991) Role of physical activity in the development of skeletal mass in children. *J. Bone Mineral Res.* **6**, 1227–33.

Smith, P., Bloom, R. & Berkowitz, J. (1984) Diachronic trends in humeral cortical thickness of near eastern populations. *J. Hum. Evol.* **13**, 603–11.

Snow-Harter, C., Bouxsein, M., Lewis, B., Carter, D. & Marcus, R. (1992) Effects of resistance and endurance exercise on bone mineral status of young women: A randomized exercise intervention trial. *J. Bone Mineral Res.* **7**, 761–9.

Snow-Harter, C. & Marcus, R. (1991) Exercise, bone mineral density and osteoporosis. *Exerc. Sport Sci. Rev.* **19**, 351–88.

Stevenson, J.C., Lees, B., Devenport, M., Cust, M.S. & Ganger, K.F. (1989) Determinant of bone density in normal women: risk factors for future osteoporosis? *Br. Med. J.* **298**, 924–8.

Stillman, R.J. (1987) Physical activity and skeletal health: a brief survey. *Med. Sports Sci.* **24**, 1–12.

Stillman, R.J., Lohman, T.H., Slaughter, M.H. & Massey, B.H. (1986) Physical activity and bone mineral content in women aged 30 to 85 years. *Med. Sci. Sports Exerc.* **18**, 576–80.

Watson, R. (1974) Bone growth and physical activity in young males. In Mazess, R. (ed.) *International Conference on Bone Mineral Measurements*, pp. 380–5. DHEW Publication NIH 75–683. Department of Health, Education and Welfare, Washington.

Westfall, C., Going, S., Parmenter, R., Perry, C., Boyden, T. & Lohman, T. (1989) Femur and spine bone mineral of eumenorrheic female body builders, swimmers, runners and controls. *Med. Sci. Sports Exerc.* **19**, S60.

Wolff, J. (1892) *Das Gesetz der Transformation der Knochen*. A. Hirschwald, Berlin.

Wood, S. II, Kuei, S., Amiel, D. *et al.* (1981) The effect of prolonged physical training on the properties of long bone: a study of Wolff's law. *J. Bone Joint Surg.* **63A**, 780–6.

Chapter 10

Athleticism, Physical Activity and Health in the Early Years: a Question of Persistence

THOMAS W. ROWLAND

Introduction

Recorded history is replete with the theme that regular exercise is important for health. As early as 300 BC Aristotle's admonition that 'a man falls into ill health as a result of not caring for exercise' was evidence that the maintenance of well-being was considered linked to physical activity. The virtues of exercise in the treatment of disease have been extolled since antiquity, as has the role of physical activity in normal psychosocial development and emotional well-being. Indeed, throughout history, physical fitness, athleticism and a physically active lifestyle have been placed on an equal plane with the moral and intellectual contributions to the human 'total being' (Ryan, 1984).

It is of interest, then, that only during the past 30 years has sufficient research accumulated to begin to document scientifically the salutary effect of exercise on health. This has been particularly true in the area of preventive medicine. Indeed, in 1995 one can construct a list of a broad variety of chronic diseases that research information indicates may be favourably influenced by the protective effect of regular physical activity (Table 10.1).

On reviewing this list several features become apparent. First, these illnesses collectively are responsible for the great majority of deaths and disability in contemporary society. The importance of regular physical activity may be significant, then, in its potential for reducing morbidity and mortality within the population.

Second, this list is composed almost exclusively of diseases that affect the physical well-being of adults, rather than children. Even obesity, conspicuously common in the paediatric age group, rarely causes medical complications until the adult years. And third, these diseases for the most part involve lifelong processes that have their genesis in childhood and only surface clinically in later adult life.

It is this latter observation that has drawn those involved in the health care of children into the promotion of physical activity and athleticism for youngsters in the growing years (Rowland, 1990). If physical activity has an ameliorating effect on blood lipid profile, for instance, would it not make sense to begin regular exercise habits during childhood, when the atherosclerotic processes begins, as the best means of preventing coronary artery disease in adults? This rationale for the early promotion of exercise in children is consistent with similar preventive medicine strategies in the paediatric

Table 10.1 Disease processes which may be ameliorated by physical activity and/or fitness.

Back disease
Coronary artery disease
Debility of ageing
Diabetes mellitus
Emotional disorders
Injury prevention
Obesity
Osteoporosis
Systemic hypertension

age group such as advocating proper diet, advising against smoking and avoiding obesity. The possible benefit of activity during childhood as it relates to peak bone mass and reduced severity of osteoporosis in adult years is addressed in Chapter 9.

Despite this commonsense approach, many questions remain unanswered. Which is more important to good health, physical activity or physical fitness? Despite a tendency to lump them together in considering health outcomes, the two are very different. Habitual physical activity concerns the amount of movement an individual engages in on a daily basis, measured in terms of caloric output. Physical fitness, on the other hand, indicates how well one performs on motor tasks. Its measurement depends on the activity involved (time on a 45-m sprint, distance throwing a baseball, number of sit-ups, etc.). Probably both are important to different health outcomes (Rowland, 1990). Prevention of obesity is clearly related to caloric expenditure (physical activity), while chronic back disease might be forestalled by good muscle tone and strength (physical fitness).

The threshold amounts of physical activity and/or fitness for beneficial health outcomes are unknown. Also unclear is the current status of activity and fitness levels in children and youth. The best means of both measuring and improving activity and fitness in youngsters remain equally uncertain.

Among the issues that deserve attention is determining the most likely mechanism for the relationship of exercise and health which justifies the promotion of physical activity and athleticism during the paediatric years. Blair et al. (1989) outlined three possibilities:

1 Physical fitness and activity directly improve the health of children and youth during the growing years.

2 Exercise during childhood produces physical or biochemical changes which will have a later beneficial influence on health during adulthood.

3 Participation in sports and exercise in the paediatric years will carry over to regular physical activity in adulthood, and this long-term habitual activity will have salutary effects.

This chapter will address these possibilities, with particular attention to the possibility that early sports training may have a 'carry-over' effect on adult fitness. It is important to examine these possible mechanisms critically, since appropriate strategies for promoting exercise and sport for children hinge on the most likely means by which activity in children and health outcomes can be linked.

Influence of exercise or athleticism on the health of children

There is little evidence for this. Rehabilitative exercise programmes offer potential benefit for children with chronic cardiopulmonary and musculoskeletal diseases (Bar-Or, 1990), but regular exercise and sports participation should not be expected to improve the well-being of the general population of children and adolescents. During the preteen years, accidents are overwhelmingly the major mortality risk, along with cancer, congenital malformations and infections (US Department of Health and Human Services, 1988). And in adolescence, accidents, suicide and homicide are the major causes of death (Blum, 1987). Regular exercise habits would not reduce the incidence of these tragedies. Likewise, as Blair et al. (1989) pointed out, activity should not influence the morbidities of adolescence, such as unwanted pregnancy, substance abuse and physical or sexual abuse.

Indeed, sports participation itself adds to the morbidity and mortality statistics during the growing years. Mueller and Cantu (1990) reported that 148 deaths occurred in high school and college sports in the USA between 1982 and 1988, as well as 87 non-fatal catastrophic injuries. For detailed epidemiological data on sports injuries, see Chapter 11.

There is no evidence to suggest that activity or athletic participation should have a favourable impact on the rate or severity of infectious diseases, the major cause of illness days during the paediatric years. Osterback and Qvarnberg

(1987) evaluated a group of 12-year-old swimmers, hockey players and gymnasts for incidence of respiratory infections, antimicrobial treatment, days of fever and absences from school. No significant differences could be found in any of these measures between the athletes and a non-athletic control group. In fact, Douglas and Hanson (1978) reported that members of a college rowing team had a higher frequency and greater severity of viral upper respiratory infections than their non-athletic peers.

An argument can be made that regular physical activity and sports participation can provide direct benefits to emotional health during the childhood years (Rowland, 1990). The obese adolescent who uses exercise to lose weight may improve in self-esteem and social confidence. It is possible, based on adult models, that physical activity can help relieve feelings of stress, anxiety and depression, major problems for the teenage population. Participation in sports has been variously promoted as a means of improving self-concept, teaching cooperation and self-discipline, preventing juvenile delinquency, and improving academic performance (Segrave, 1983; Sonstroem, 1984; Kirkendall, 1986).

Influence of exercise and athleticism during childhood on adult health

In 1969, Ekblom suggested that athletic training during the growing years might serve to 'fix' increased cardiovascular dimensions and high levels of physical fitness that would persist through adulthood. This idea was inspired by the observation that physical training of a previously sedentary adult could raise $\dot{V}o_2$ by 15–20%, but not to a level characteristic of the lifelong athlete, which might be 50% higher. Assuming health outcomes can be related to physical fitness, this concept bears importance not simply from the standpoint of athletic performance. If Ekblom is correct, programmes to improve physical fitness through increased activity or sports participation during child-

hood could be justified by a carry-over affect on the fitness and health of adults.

Do training effects during childhood and adolescence persist through the adult years, even if involvement in athletics is not continued? Likewise, if a highly active youth becomes a sedentary adult, will there be some carry-over benefit in health outcomes such as decreased risk of coronary artery disease? The current research literature provides limited insights into these questions.

Persistence of physical fitness

A steady decline of aerobic fitness (as indicated by $\dot{V}o_{2\,max}$) is observed throughout the entirety of the adult years, a fact ascribed variously to decline in cardiac function, fall in habitual activity, shrinking skeletal muscle mass and age-related drop in maximal heart rate (Shephard, 1989). Several authors have presented data suggesting that adult athletes who maintain their training have less decline in $\dot{V}o_{2\,max}$ with increasing age. In reviewing these data, Shephard (1989) concluded that while maximum oxygen uptake does diminish with time in training adult athletes (5–6%· $decade^{-1}$), this fall appears to be 'somewhat less' than that of the general population in most cross-sectional studies.

Individuals who had participated on scholastic athletic teams earlier in their lives have consistently shown greater levels of physical fitness in their adult years than non-athletes. These former athletes have greater lung function, larger heart volumes, higher $\dot{V}o_{2\,max}$, lower blood pressure and better heart muscle function than non-athletic peers (Fardy et al., 1978).

Pertinent to the question of persistence of fitness, studies indicate that these characteristics are evident even if the former athletes failed to continue training in the adult years. Pyorala et al. (1967) investigated cardiovascular findings in 38 healthy former élite Finnish endurance athletes at the mean age of 51.4 years. Competitive training had ceased at an average of 37 years. Age of onset of training was not determined, but considering the competitive levels of these athletes (nine had won Olympic gold medals), an early age might be assumed. Compared to a group of sedentary men, the former athletes had lower blood pressures, greater heart volume and higher estimated maximal oxygen uptake.

Saltin and Grimby (1968) found that athletes who were still training in older years had approximately 20% higher maximal oxygen uptake than those athletes who had ceased training. Importantly, however, the latter group demonstrated a 20% greater $\dot{V}O_{2\,max}$ than non-athletes of the same age.

These studies in adults can be compared with two investigations that have prospectively examined changes in fitness in school-aged athletes who discontinue training. Murase et al. (1981) followed measurements of maximal aerobic power longitudinally in a small group of highly trained Japanese runners. In the six who maintained training from age 14 to 21 years, mean $\dot{V}O_{2\,max}$ rose from 65.4 to 75.5 ml $\cdot$ kg$^{-1} \cdot$ min^{-1}, an improvement consistent with other studies of training adolescent runners (Elovainio & Sundberg, 1983). Five runners discontinued training after the age of 17 years. In these subjects, $\dot{V}O_{2\,max}$ had increased from 64.8 to 70.8 ml $\cdot$ kg$^{-1} \cdot$ min^{-1} with training at age 17, but at age 21, after they had stopped training, $\dot{V}O_{2\,max}$ fell to 62.9 ml $\cdot$ kg$^{-1} \cdot$ min^{-1}. In non-athletes average $\dot{V}O_{2\,max}$ at this age was 51.8 ml $\cdot$ kg$^{-1} \cdot$ min^{-1}.

These findings indicate that (i) training is effective in improving $\dot{V}O_{2\,max}$ in adolescent runners; and (ii) these athletes demonstrate a greater degree of aerobic fitness than non-athletes even when training is discontinued. The girl swimmers reported by Eriksson et al. (1978) did not support the latter conclusion, however. Thirty girls were initially studied at age 12–16 years after 2.5 years of swim training. The group was then reinvestigated 10 years later, when all the girls had stopped training. Heart volumes which were significantly greater than normal initially had decreased, but values were still greater than in the non-athletic population. Mean $\dot{V}O_{2\,max}$ fell from 51.4 ml $\cdot$ kg$^{-1} \cdot$ min^{-1} during the training years to 36.4 ml $\cdot$ kg^{-1} on follow-up, a level not different from that expected in the non-athlete population.

The girl swimmers notwithstanding, most data indicate that aerobic fitness can be improved from early sports participation, and these athletes can be expected to show greater levels of aerobic function in later adult years even if training is discontinued (Fig. 10.1). Whether similar effects can be expected from non-aerobic activities (speed, strength) is unknown.

While these observations are consistent with the concept of early training 'fixing' fitness levels for adult years, they can also be accounted for by alternative explanations. Greater levels of fitness in athletes who have stopped training may simply represent genetic traits which have allowed them previously to excel in sports. That is, the same high levels of adult fitness might be observed even if the athletes had never participated in sports during adolescence. Alternatively, the enjoyment of sports participation might foster a greater interest in increased daily physical activity in the ex-athletes. The influence of environment, particularly the association of athletes with exercise-oriented family and friends, cannot be discounted either.

Early physical activity and coronary heart disease

While no conclusions can be drawn regarding the 'fixing' of fitness by early sports participation, the data regarding the influence of early physical activity on coronary artery disease risk in adulthood are less equivocal. Studies addressing this issue have indicated that sports participation and physical activity in childhood and adolescence which is not carried into adulthood has no ameliorating effect on coronary disease risk. The findings are disappointing, since cross-sectional studies of young athletes have indicated favourable serum lipoprotein profiles (Rowland, 1990).

In their landmark study of Harvard alumni,

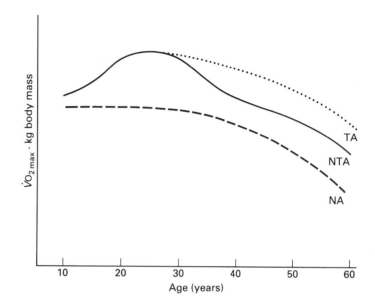

Fig. 10.1 Effect of age on aerobic fitness ($\dot{V}O_{2\,max}$) in consistently training athletes (TA), athletes who discontinue training (NTA) and non-athletes (NA). Data from Murase *et al.* (1981) and Saltin and Grimby (1968).

Paffenbarger *et al.* (1978) reported coronary heart disease rates which were inversely related in a continuous manner with current adult daily caloric expenditure. No such association was observed, however, in those who had been college athletes but were no longer involved in an active lifestyle. Indeed, those individuals tended to have an even greater risk for coronary heart disease than those who had not been involved in athletics as students. Conversely, sedentary students who became active adults demonstrated a decreased risk. These findings indicate that vigorous physical activities must persist from college into adult years if a protective effect against coronary heart disease is to be expected.

Brill *et al.* (1989) studied 345 men aged 25–60 years who had participated in competitive sports teams in high school or college. Level of regular physical activity during adult years was not different in the former athletes when compared to 75 non-athlete control subjects. Most coronary risk factors (body mass index, serum lipid profile and blood pressure) were similar in the two groups. Prevalence of smoking was greater in the ex-athletes (22%), who had longer treadmill endurance times than the non-athletes.

Physical activity during childhood as a factor in creating lifetime exercise habits

The link between exercise and health outcomes has been documented almost entirely in adults. It follows logically then that physical activity and athleticism during childhood might be primarily of importance by creating lifetime exercise habits with positive health outcomes in the adult years. If so, promotion of exercise in children is predicated on the assumption that exercise habits and fitness levels persist, or 'track', into the adult years. Unfortunately, there are very little data at present to support or refute this concept.

Tracking of habitual physical activity

No longitudinal study has yet been performed to determine if levels of daily physical activity track from childhood into the adult years. This critical piece of information is lacking from want of an accurate, practical means of measuring caloric expenditure, a difficult problem at all ages, but particularly in children (Freedson, 1989). Lacking this technology, researchers have approached the question of persistence of exercise through questionnaire studies of adults, trying to link a history of exercise and/ or sports participation during childhood with adult physical activity patterns. Many of these reports have, in fact, observed such an association. This does not mean, of course, that childhood activity and/or athleticism is necessarily a determinant of adult levels of habitual activity. Alternatively, these results may be simply reflecting 'those that can, do'; that is, individuals who have the abilities for physical activities may be more likely to participate — at all ages.

A survey of 3875 adults by the President's Council on Physical Fitness and Sports in 1972 indicated a relationship between participation in organized sports teams during youth and adult activity levels (Bucher, 1974). Those who had participated in two or more school sports were two to five times as likely to be involved in a list of activities such as cycling, swimming, calisthenics, jogging and weight-lifting than those who had not been members of school sports teams. Paffenbarger *et al.* (1978) also showed a relationship in their evaluation of Harvard alumni between daily caloric expenditure during adulthood and participation in sports during college.

In a longitudinal study, Kuh and Cooper (1992) related physical activity patterns in British adults to characteristics of the same individuals during adolescence. In 1982, when they were 36 years old, subjects were divided into three levels of daily activity based on their involvement in sports and recreational activities, heavy gardening and do-it-yourself activities. Evaluations by teachers of the same individuals when they were 13 years old indicated that above average ability at school games, high energy level and an extrovert personality were positive predictors of high adult levels of physical activity.

Dishman (1988) felt that previously reported relationships between youth sports and adult activity failed to consider subject selection bias, the validity of activity recall and degree of supervision of the exercise environment. He studied the association of past participation in school sports with adult physical activity in 265 men, controlling for these variables. In cross-sectional and prospective analysis of free-living and supervised settings, no significant association was observed between adult activity and athleticism during youth.

Montoye *et al.* (1959) reported the interesting finding that the relationship between adult physical activity and earlier athleticism held up only when the adults were participating in team sport activities. They compared physical activity patterns in adulthood by questionnaire between men who were varsity collegiate athletes before 1938 and their non-athletic peers. Adult activity was assessed as time spent per day in 'vigorous', 'moderate' or 'mild' activities at different times following graduation. The athletes were more likely to engage in physical activities before the age of 45 years, but the reverse was true afterwards. This change occurred because of decreased participation in team sports by the ex-athletes. In almost every age group the non-athletes reported higher levels of daily non-sports activities. The authors were suspicious that these findings resulted from athletes underestimating the intensity of their daily activities.

In a short-term follow-up study, Dennison *et al.* (1988) examined whether results in physical fitness tests during childhood could predict exercise habits in adulthood. They studied the relationship between adult physical activity (by a 7-day activity recall method) at age 23−25 years with the fitness test scores of the same 453 men during their school years (10−11 and 15−18 years of age). The active and inactive adult groups did not differ significantly in obesity, participation in high school sports or medical illness. The more physically active adults had scored significantly better on the 548-m run, sit-ups, 40-m dash and shuttle run than the more sedentary adults. When adult physical inactivity was plotted against distance run performance, the only significant risk for a sedentary lifestyle was observed for those who had finished in less than the 20th percentile for run score.

In summary, lacking an effective tool for

measuring physical activity, the tendency for habitual daily activity levels to track through life is unknown. The limitations of retrospective questionnaire studies, which have shown conflicting results, are substantial.

Tracking of physical fitness

In contrast to activity levels, physical fitness is readily measured, but longitudinal data examining tracking tendencies for fitness from the paediatric to adult years are scant. Kemper *et al.* (1990) conducted a follow-up study of 93 males and 107 females with serial maximal treadmill tests over an 8-year period from age 13 to 21 years. Correlation coefficients for maximal aerobic power at the beginning and end of the study period were 0.36 for males and 0.46 for females. Sixty-five per cent of males and 71% of females who were above the 75th percentile for $\dot{V}_{O_2 max}$ at age 13 were still there at age 21.

Conclusion

The body of research information available to analyse the possible exercise—health link for the paediatric population is clearly limited. Still, it is critical for those organizing strategies for promotion of physical activity, sports and fitness in children to assess probabilities based on the data reviewed above. Advocating exercise as a means of directly influencing children's health appears ill-founded. Likewise, there are no good data to suggest that exercise in children *per se* has any effect on adult health outcomes. As Blair *et al.* (1989) emphasized, if exercise in children is to affect health beneficially, the most likely means is by initiating habits which will be maintained throughout life.The research studies to support such a concept, however, have not yet been performed.

If creation of a lifestyle pattern of regular activity were the primary goal during childhood, current strategies might need to be realigned. A behavioural approach to advocating exercise in children (What 'turns them on' to activity? How can exercise be made most enjoyable?) would be paramount. Testing for levels of physical fitness and concern over means of improving performance measures in children would become of secondary importance. Physical education curricula would be designed primarily to create an interest and pleasure in physical activities rather than concentrating on improving exercise abilities. High risk children for physical inactivity (such as those with obesity or chronic disease) would be identified for special counselling.

Challenges for future research

Large gaps clearly exist in our understanding of how exercise in children might affect health. There is no lack of opportunity for a research focus on this issue to solve many of its unanswered questions.

• Especially needed are long-term longitudinal studies to determine if physically active children become physically active adults. If so, is there truly a health 'pay-off' from this kind of lifetime investment? What threshold amounts of activity are necessary? What kinds of activity are best? What is the role of fitness and athletic participation?

• Both physical activity and fitness are prominently influenced by genetic factors. Heritability of physical activity, for instance, has been estimated from 0.29 to 0.62 (Perusse *et al.*, 1989). A demonstration that physical activity tracks significantly from child to adult years would need to take this into account; i.e. this finding would not necessarily imply that *induced* physical activity in children would also track into adulthood.

• Given adequate information to understand how exercise in children is beneficial to health, research will be needed to plan proper strategies for its promotion. As noted above, this is most likely to be initially in the realm of the behavioural scientist rather than the exercise physiologist. The appropriate roles of the family, school, community and medical profession as child exercise advocates will need to be identified based on these strategies.

References

Bar-Or, O. (1990) Disease-specific benefits of training in the child with a chronic disease. What is the evidence? *Pediatr. Exerc. Sci.* **2**, 384−94.

Blair, S.N., Clark, D.G., Cureton, K.J. & Powell, K.E. (1989) Exercise and fitness in childhood: implications for a lifetime of health. In C.V. Gisolfi & D.R. Lamb (eds) *Perspectives in Exercise Science and Sports Medicine*, Vol. 2, pp. 401−30. *Youth, Exercise, and Sport*. Benchmark Press, Indianapolis, IN.

Blum, R. (1987) Contemporary threats to adolescent health in the United States. *JAMA* **257**, 3390−5.

Brill, P.A., Burkhalter, H.E., Kohl, H.W., Blair, S.N. & Goodyear, N.N. (1989) The impact of previous athleticism on exercise habits, physical fitness, and coronary heart disease risk factors in middle-aged men. *Res. Q. Exerc. Sport* **60**, 209−15.

Bucher, C.A. (1974) National adult physical fitness survey: some implications. *J. Phys. Educ. Recr. Dance* **45**, 25−8.

Dennison, B.A., Straus, J.H., Mellits, E.D. & Charney E. (1988) Childhood physical fitness tests: predictor of adult physical activity levels? *Pediatrics* **82**, 324−30.

Dishman, R.K. (1988) Supervised and free-living physical activity: no differences in former athletes and non-athletes. *Am. J. Prevent. Med.* **4**, 153−60.

Douglas, D.J. & Hanson, P.G. (1978) Upper respiratory infection in the conditioned athlete. *Med. Sci. Sports* **10**, 55 (abstract).

Ekblom, B. (1969) Effect of physical training in adolescent boys. *J. Appl. Physiol.* **27**, 350−5.

Elovainio, R. & Sundberg, S. (1983) A five-year follow-up study on cardiorespiratory function in adolescent élite endurance runners. *Acta Pediatr. Scand.* **72**, 351−6.

Eriksson, B.O., Engstrom, I., Karlberg, P., Lundin, A., Saltin, B. & Thoren, C. (1978) Long-term effect of previous swim training in girls. A 10-year follow-up of the 'girls swimmers'. *Acta Pediatr. Scand.* **67**, 285−92.

Fardy, P.S., Maresh, C.M., Abbott, R. & Kristiansen, T. (1978) A comparison of habitual lifestyle, aerobic power, and systolic time intervals in former athletes and non-athletes *J. Sports Med.* **18**, 287−99.

Freedson, P. (1989) Field monitoring of physical activity in children. *Pediatr. Exerc. Sci.* **1**, 8−18.

Kemper, H.C.G., Snel, J., Verschuur, R. & Storm-van Essen, L. (1990) Tracking of health and risk indicators of cardiovascular diseases from teenager to adult: Amsterdam Growth and Health Study. *Prevent. Med.* **19**, 642−55.

Kirkendall, D.R. (1986) Effects of physical activity on intellectual development and academic performance. In G.A. Stull & H.M. Eckert (eds) *Effects of Physical Activity on Children*, pp. 49−63. Human Kinetics, Champaign, IL.

Kuh, D.J.L. & Cooper, C. (1992) Physical activity at 36 years: patterns and childhood predictors in a longitudinal study. *J. Epidemiol. Comm. Health* **46**, 114−19.

Montoye, H.J., Van Huss, W. & Zuidema, M. (1959) Sports activities of athletes and nonathletes in later life. *Phys. Educ.* **16**, 48−51.

Mueller, F.O. & Cantu, R.C. (1990) Catastrophic injuries and fatalities in high school and college sports, fall 1982 to spring 1988. *Med. Sci. Sports Exerc.* **22**, 737−41.

Murase, Y., Kobayashi, K., Kamei, S. & Matsui, H. (1981) Longitudinal study of aerobic power in superior junior athletes. *Med. Sci. Sports Exerc.* **13**, 180−4.

Osterback, L. & Qvarnberg, Y. (1987) A prospective study of respiratory infections in 12 year old children actively engaged in sports. *Acta Pediatr. Scand.* **76**, 944−9.

Paffenbarger, R.S., Wing, A.L. & Hyde, R.T. (1978) Physical activity as an index of heart attack risk in college alumni. *Am. J. Epidemiol.* **108**, 161−75.

Perusse, L., Tremblay, A., LeBlanc, C. & Bouchard, C. (1989) Genetic and environmental influence on habitual physical activity and exercise participation. *Am. J. Epidemiol.* **129**, 1012−22.

Pyorala, K., Karvonen, M.J., Taskinen, P., Takkunen, J., Kyronseppa, H. & Peltokallio, P. (1967) Cardiovascular studies on former endurance athletes. *Am. J. Cardiol.* **20**, 191−205.

Rowland, T.W. (1990) *Exercise and Children's Health*. Human Kinetics, Champaign, IL.

Ryan, A.J. (1984) Exercise and health: lessons from the past. In H.M. Eckert & H.J. Montoye (eds) *Exercise and Health*, pp. 3−13. Human Kinetics, Champaign, IL.

Saltin, B. & Grimby, G. (1968) Physiological analysis of middle-aged and old former athletes. *Circulation* **38**, 1104−15.

Segrave, J.O. (1983) Sports and juvenile delinquency. *Exerc. Sport Sci. Rev.* **11**, 181−209.

Shephard, R.J. (1989) Effects of exercise on biological features of aging. In R.S. Williams & A.G. Wallace (eds) *Biological Effects of Physical Activity*, pp. 55−62. Human Kinetics, Champaign, IL.

Sonstroem, R.J. (1984) Exercise and self-esteem. *Exerc. Sport Sci. Rev.* **12**, 123−55.

US Department of Health and Human Services (1988) *Vital Statistics of the United States*. US Department of Health and Human Services, Hyattsville, MD.

PART 3

INJURIES: EPIDEMIOLOGY, PREVENTION, TREATMENT AND REHABILITATION

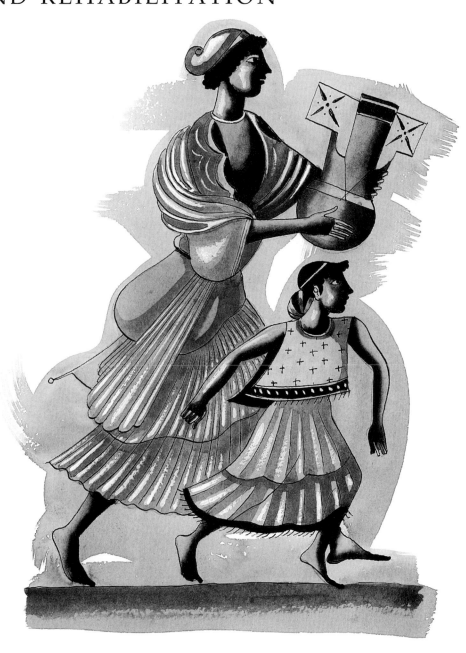

Chapter 11

Epidemiology of Paediatric Sports-related Injuries

FRANK J.G. BACKX

Introduction

Sports injuries are the unwanted side-effects of sports participation. To understand the phenomenon of sports injuries in childhood and adolescence, there is a need for epidemiological evidence (Chan *et al.*, 1984). Many publications have confirmed that epidemiological methods can be useful in the investigation of sports injuries (Mueller & Blyth, 1982; Walter *et al.*, 1985; Wallace, 1988; Landry, 1992).

Research into the causes of sports injuries creates the opportunity for finding some starting points for preventive measures (van Mechelen *et al.*, 1987). Prevention of sports injuries in young individuals is important in order to reduce the short- and long-term effects of injuries in terms of their social and economic consequences (Tursz & Crost, 1986).

First, the need for an epidemiological approach in sports injury research will be outlined. Second, the incidence, type and severity of sports injuries in childhood will be presented. Third, the aetiology of internal and external factors will be described. Based upon those aetiological factors, measures likely to reduce the risk and/or severity of sports injuries will be summarized.

The value of an epidemiological approach

Published injury studies on children and adolescents vary enormously in extent and depth.

The scope of datasets depends strongly on the methods of data acquisition, particularly on the locus of measurement. Most studies have been based on records from out-patient clinics or casualty departments (Hammer *et al.*, 1981; Sahlin, 1990). Others have been based on the reports of physical education (PE) teachers (Medved & Pavisic-Medved, 1973; Backx *et al.*, 1989). Seldom do the injury records have a population-based design. Another problem arises when young athletes themselves have to fill out registration forms. Retrospective study designs in particular introduce a recall bias which results in under- or overrecording.

Because data on sports injuries traditionally have been acquired from clinical case series (Walter *et al.*, 1985), it is not surprising that most of the studies on the number and severity of sports injuries are of poor quality and suffer from a lack of comparability. This is due to:
1 A lack of uniform definitions of sports participation and sports injury.
2 Limited reliability of collected data.
3 Insufficient information on the population at risk and/or on the exposure time (Tursz & Crost, 1986; van Mechelen *et al.*, 1987).
If research into the epidemiology of sports injuries is to produce valid and reliable results and conclusions, a number of conditions must be taken into account.

Uniform definition of sports-related injury. This is imperative. The Council of Europe proposed the following definition:

A sports injury is a result of participation in sport with one or more of the following consequences:
1 a reduction in amount or level of sports activity,
2 a need for advice or treatment, and
3 adverse social or economic aspects (van Vulpen, 1989).

This definition includes both acute and over-use injuries. It does not limit management to medical care and covers factors such as loss for the team of an injured child or absence from school or study.

Most studies are not as broadly based as the Council's definition suggests. Several reasons can be given for the non-uniformity in injury definitions. For example, each country has its own unique system of health care which to a large degree determines methods of research. Another reason why the proposed injury definitions have not been adhered to is because researchers in this field, due to pragmatic considerations, regularly have to make concessions regarding their intended research design, depending on the target group, the locus of measurement and financial factors (Backx, 1991).

Reliable participation data. There must be reliable estimates both of the number of people engaging in sport and of the numbers engaging in particular activities or belonging to particular levels of sports participation. The true population at risk defines the denominator and allows injury events to be understood as a rate rather than a number (Hunter & Levy, 1988). Reliable participation data subdivided on the basis of factors such as age and gender are needed if potential differences between groups are to be identified (van Vulpen, 1989).

Reliable research methodology. The research methodology requires a representative sample and reliable methods to produce injury statistics. Obviously, diagnosis by medical staff or assessment by PE teachers and school-aged children themselves can affect results on

paediatric sports injuries considerably. It is clear that the medical system is aware of only a small and distorted segment of the total injury problem. In this context, reference is made to the well-known 'tip of the iceberg' phenomenon. Therefore, the population approach to injury is preferable, as it allows considerable insight into the rate of occurrence, the causes of injury and the identification of high risk groups (Walter *et al.*, 1985). The severity of sports injuries also needs to be described in an efficient and practical manner. The consequence of the epidemiological approach is the registration of a lot of minor injuries.

Accurate measurement of exposure time. The incidence per exposure time must be measured to estimate the risk of a sports injury and to draw distinctions between different types of sports or activities. Furthermore, it is important to distinguish organized versus non-organized activities, and competitive versus non-competitive sport, and the frequency and intensity of the sports activity.

The relevance of this point is clearly demonstrated by several investigators who identified major differences in incidence according to gender, age and category of sports (Watson, 1984; Yde & Nielsen, 1990; Backx *et al.*, 1991). It has been suggested that the definition of incidence of sports injuries should be further sharpened by using 'actual' exposure time (Lindenfeld *et al.*, 1988).

Incidence rates

In general, the amount of sports participation and consequently the number of sports injuries in young people have increased considerably in the last two decades. From several countries, studies have reported the incidence and types of paediatric sports-related injuries. As a result of the variability in the definitions of injury, locus of measurement, characteristics and level of sporting activities it is not surprising that incidence rates of injuries in, for instance, club gymnastics vary between 2.4 (Pettrone &

Ricciardelli, 1987) and 39.9 per 100 school-children $\cdot$ year^{-1} (Backx et al., 1991).

Clearly, the ranking of sports according to their injury rate depends on the participation rate and the extent of involvement. For instance in the USA, American football and baseball are very popular, but they are less so in Europe. Two prospective studies performed in American high schools were compared by Landry (1992) (Table 11.1). Football, girl's gymnastics and wrestling showed the highest injury rates.

Surprisingly, there is no consensus about the role of gender. On the one hand, authors claim that girls in mixed team sports are not more injury prone (Garrick, 1982; Watson, 1984: Backx et al., 1991). Evidence from the mixed team sport of korfball bears out the claim in adults that females are not more liable to injury (Diederiks et al., 1984). On the other hand, retrospective studies in youth soccer (Maehlum et al., 1986; Backous et al., 1988) and also a prospective study in young European handball

Table 11.1 Injury rates in high school sports. From Landry (1992).

Sport	Sex	Duration of study	
		2 years	1 year
Football	M + F	81	61
Gymnastics	M	28	40
	F	40	46
Wrestling	M + F	75	40
Basketball	M	31	37
	F	25	31
Volleyball	M + F	10	17
Baseball	M + F	18	15
Cross-country	M	29	13
	F	35	7
Soccer	M	30	13
	F	—	17
Softball	M + F	44	13
Track	M	33	10
	F	35	18
Badminton	M + F	6	7
Field hockey	M + F	—	6
Tennis	M	3	0
	F	7	3
Swimming	M	1	0
	F	9	0

players (Yde & Nielsen, 1990) showed higher incidence rates in girls compared to boys.

Comparison of the incidence per 1000 h of training with 1000 h of competition shows an overall incidence rate in children that was three times higher in competition than in training (Table 11.2). However, in several specific sports, e.g. volleyball, martial arts and club gymnastics, incidence rates in training were considerably higher than in game activities. The incidence rate during games was very high, especially in basketball, but also in handball, korfball, soccer and field hockey (Backx et al., 1991).

Comparison of incidence rates is difficult not only because of differences in injury definition, but also because of the very wide variety of activities within a single sport. Because each kind of activity has its own characteristics, important differences in risk factors emerge.

Location of injury

The distribution of injuries among body sites is substantially determined by the type of sport. As each country has its own favourite sports, the distribution of injuries by body site can differ considerably. In very young children (aged 5–9 years), most of the sports injuries are localized to the head (Kvist et al., 1989; van Galen & Diederiks, 1990). In adolescents the head and fingers are the most frequently injured parts, followed by ankles and knees (Zaricznyj et al., 1980).

Based on the popularity of ball games in school, the ball is considered to be an important factor in causing finger injuries. Finger injuries are dominant with younger children, while ankle joint injuries occur more in older pupils (Rümmele, 1987). This is in accordance with an injury registration in an Austrian hospital in which hand and finger injuries were most frequently treated (Schmidt & Höllwarth, 1989). A population-based study on children aged 8–17 years revealed that most of the injuries (73%) involved the lower extremity (Backx et al., 1989). The ankle, accounting for 26.5% of all injuries, proved to be the most affected part

Table 11.2 Incidence rates per 1000 h of practice and per 1000 h of games in organized sports with more than 15 participants. From Backx *et al.* (1991).

	Practice		Games
Volleyball	6.7	Basketball	23
Handball	4.3	Handball	14
Martial arts	3.8	Korfball	12
Club gymnastics	3.6	Soccer	8
Korfball	3.4	Field hockey	7
Baseball	3.0	Baseball	3
Horse riding	1.7	Ballet*	
Soccer	1.6	Track and field*	
Tennis	1.5	Martial arts*	
Swimming	1.2	Volleyball*	
Field hockey	1.2	Badminton*	
Track and field	1.0	Tennis*	
Basketball*		Swimming*	
Table-tennis*		Table-tennis*	
Badminton*		Horse riding*	
Ice-skating*		Ice-skating*	
Ballet*		Club gymnastics*	
Dance*		Dance*	

* The incidence rate was not calculated for types of sport in which fewer than five sports injuries were registered in practice or games.

of the body, followed by the knee (21.9%), followed by the distal parts of the upper and lower limbs (Fig. 11.1).

Type of injury

In epidemiological studies using a broad injury definition, the fracture rate is low (Backx *et al.*, 1989). However, hospital records have shown a rather different picture. Depending on the type of sport, the fracture rate varies between 15 and 60% of acute sports trauma (Schmidt & Höllwarth, 1989; Sahlin, 1990). In young athletes, fractures of the upper extremity are the most common types of fracture (Schmidt-Olsen *et al.*, 1985; Sahlin, 1990).

Soft tissue injuries predominate among acute injuries in athletes between the ages of 10 and 18 years. The most common soft tissue injuries encountered with exercise are sprains and contusions (Sahlin, 1990; Yde & Nielsen, 1990; Backx, 1991). Girls especially have a high risk of ankle and finger sprains (Nielsen & Yde, 1988; Kvist *et al.*, 1989).

Besides acute macrotrauma, the importance of microtrauma and overuse injuries in children is still growing. It is certain that injury registrations by insurance companies or hospitals

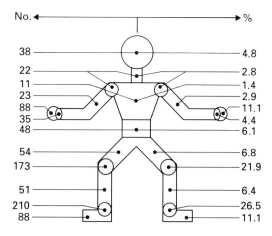

Fig. 11.1 Absolute and per cent distribution of sports injuries over the body area in school-aged children aged 8–17 years. Redrawn from Backx *et al.* (1989).

reflect relatively serious sports accidents, which means implicitly that the more chronic injuries are ignored. Most chronic or overuse injuries to the musculoskeletal system in adults are soft tissue injuries affecting the bursa, tendons, muscles and ligaments (Jones *et al.*, 1988). Other frequently encountered overuse injuries are stress fractures, chondromalacia patellae and back pain syndrome. In fact, young athletes with overuse injuries have come dangerously close to exceeding the strength limit of their body tissues.

In particular, children are prone to overuse during periods of growth. Injuries incurred as a result of the growth process have been referred to as overgrowth injuries. One-third of the so-called exertion injuries were growth disturbances or osteochondroses (Orava & Puranen, 1978). Children with osteochondroses, e.g. Osgood−Schlatter disease, Scheuermann's disease, Panner's disease and Legg−Calvé−Perthes disease, may have different reasons for seeking health care. One symptom can be pain associated with sports activity (Pappas, 1989). In such circumstances, sports activities are presumably not the cause but, rather, the provocative factor.

With a view to prevention it is very important to realize that a substantial number of the injured children (32%) had experienced the injury before at the same site within the past year (Nielsen & Yde, 1988). Girls had the highest risk of reinjury. Ankle sprain and chondromalacia of the patella reoccurred most frequently (DeHaven & Lintner, 1986; Backx, 1991).

Severity of injuries

To understand the phenomenon of sports injuries a good definition of sports injury and incidence are needed as well as a description of severity. Therefore, van Mechelen *et al.* (1987) have distinguished six indicators of importance to define the severity of injuries in an efficient and practical manner. Using these indicators, the following can be formulated concerning young athletes.

Nature of sports injury. In case of sport, one of the main reasons for consultation with a medical doctor is the nature of the sports injury. In 75% of all cases medical treatment is considered to be unnecessary, since the most common injuries are abrasions, or other less severe injuries diagnosed as minor sprains, strains and contusions (Backx *et al.*, 1991). It is important to realize that injuries treated in a casualty department constitute a highly selected group being of a more serious nature (van Mechelen *et al.*, 1987).

Very serious sports accidents in youth, e.g. brain or spinal cord damage, or lesions of the heart or submersion, leading to invalidity or death, are exceptional (Tursz & Crost, 1986). It was reported recently that blunt chest trauma can induce commotio cordis which causes two to three deaths in Little League baseball each year (Abrunzo, 1991).

Nature and duration of treatment. The type and duration of treatment of injuries in school-aged children have not been well analysed, although there are indications that the demand on the time of health-care professionals seems to be less than in adults.

From an epidemiological point of view, only 25% of all injuries registered called for medical attention by a general practitioner or a medical specialist. Pupils who were injured in PE classes had to consult a doctor more frequently compared with other sports activities (Backx *et al.*, 1991).

The most severe injuries in sports leading to hospital admission occur during horse riding, skating, tobogganing, cycle riding or racing, and skiing (Schmidt & Höllwarth, 1989; Sahlin, 1990). Surprisingly, there is a serious lack of research concerning the type and duration of therapies used in young athletes in the post-injury phase.

Time lost from sport. The actual number of days elapsing until the athlete returns to sports activity is often reported as a measure of injury severity (Noyes *et al.*, 1988). A well-known, often used, measure was introduced by Ekstrand and Gillquist (1983) who classified the absence from sports activity due to injury into three grades — minor, moderate and major — according to absence of less than 1 week, more than 1 week but less than 1 month, and more than 1 month respectively. In general, these three grades correspond with the codes 1, 2 and 3 in the abbreviated injury scale (AIS). The highest AIS severity codes (4, 5, 6), ranging from life-threatening to fatal injuries, seems to be exceptional in sports for young athletes (Nathorst Westfelt, 1982; de Loës & Goldie, 1988).

The most striking data concerning time lost from sport in youngsters were registered in Ireland and Denmark. Nearly half of the injuries in Irish secondary schools resulted in at least 10 days off sport (Watson, 1986). Loss of participation in Danish soccer, handball and basketball was 2 weeks for half of the injured adolescents (Yde & Nielsen, 1990). Defining the severity of injury by time lost from sport raises the issue of subjectivity. One player will participate in sports with a sports injury while another is more anxious and returns much later (Noyes et al., 1988). Although van Mechelen et al. (1987) stated that the length of sports absenteeism provides the most precise indication of the consequences of a sports injury to an athlete, this claim is questionable in regard to young athletes. Bias can easily develop, induced by factors such as an individual's pain tolerance, type of treatment, parents and coach. The time-loss definition of injury is not useful in studies which include non-organized sports.

School absenteeism. Similar to days off work, defining the severity of an injury by the amount of time lost in school is highly subjective, as it is with time lost from sports. Those estimates of injury severity are more practical than reliable. In general, most injuries are neither severe nor long lasting and resulted in little loss of time from PE classes or school (Backx, 1991). In contrast with research on adults, this form of absenteeism is seldom used in school-aged children and adolescents.

Permanent damage. Children's sports accidents very rarely cause permanent disabilities. For example, Zaricznyj et al. (1980) recorded in schoolchildren participating in sports and PE that 1.2% of those injured had sustained a permanent injury, such as a compression fracture of the spine or a ruptured spleen. Actually, the permanent damage resulting from sports injuries is usually mild. However, it seems reasonable to be cautious about long-term prognoses, particularly since some investigators found such injuries as angulation of limbs, shortening of limbs and limited joint mobility (Tursz & Crost, 1986). The prevailing opinion is that it is too early to grade the degree of permanent disability that results from growth disturbance or epiphyseal fractures (Sahlin, 1990).

Costs. Severity in terms of cost has to include the direct costs resulting from (para)medical treatment and also the indirect social costs (in particular sick leave of family members) to the injured pupil, his or her family and school (Watson, 1986). The financial costs stemming from sports injuries in youth are not explored as a single category, so the known calculations are usually derived from figures concerning adults. A slight exception to this can be made for a prospective study of acute injuries in Sweden (de Loës, 1990). Nearly 70% of the sports injuries registered in the total population of a municipality occurred in the age group under 20 years. The overall mean cost per injury was $US335. In particular, motorcycling, downhill skiing and horse riding created by far the most costly injuries.

Aetiology

The epidemiological studies on children and adolescents do mention the causes, primarily as reported by the subject himself or herself or reconstructed by the coach or physician. For example, retrospective data from a population-based study revealed that most reported causes of sports injuries were falling/stumbling (24%), misstep/twist (22%) and kick/push (18%) induced by the injured athletes themselves rather than other pupils (Backx *et al.*, 1991).

In the 1990s, it has become widely accepted that a sports injury occurs as the result of the interaction of variables at a given point in time (Taimela *et al.*, 1990). The variables affecting the aetiology of sports injuries in children and adolescents can be divided into two main categories: internal (athlete-related) and external (environmental) risk factors. In the last decade more investigations have focused their attention on the internal risk factors, which are possibly more responsible for the majority of sports injuries than external factors (Lysens *et al.*, 1989). Most risk factors that have been accounted for in various international publications focus primarily on the adult athlete.

The most important internal factors in the predisposition to injury are: (i) age; (ii) gender; (iii) physical build; (iv) physical fitness; (v) physical defect; and (vi) psychological factors. The main external factors involved in the occurrence of injuries are: (i) sport-related factors; (ii) playing surface; (iii) equipment; (iv) weather conditions; (v) trainer/coach; and (vi) conduct of the match (van Mechelen *et al.*, 1987).

In the literature, aetiological factors are often reported erroneously, emphasizing the circumstances at the specific moment of injury. Actually, the preventative measures resulting from these descriptive studies, while well intended, can result in the wrong conclusions. Only the monitoring of all athlete-related and environmental factors can provide a truly reliable picture of the multicausal origins of sports injuries. The monitoring of all possible causes, however, will always remain impractical (Backx, 1991). The most important risk indicators with relation to the occurrence of injuries with youth in sports are shown in Fig. 11.2. Although this scheme cannot be complete it is a clear though rather artificial categorization.

The origin of a sports injury is most frequently a matter of complicated interactions between risk indicators which are athlete-related, situational (environmental-bound), load-dependent and those related to equipment. For instance, intensive training resulting in repetitive microtrauma is an external risk factor in the occurrence of overuse injuries in children's sports. In particular, the adolescent growth spurt is correlated with an increased incidence of overuse type injuries.

Prevention

Most sports injuries in childhood are not accidents and are potentially preventable (Landry, 1992). Prevention of sports injuries can be divided into primary, secondary and tertiary measures. The most applied, general measures are examples of *primary* prevention (Backx, 1991):

1 Preparticipation sports medical examination.
2 Warming up, stretching exercises, cooling down.
3 Physical fitness.
4 Training courses concerning exercise, fitness and health.
5 Safe environment (e.g. proper playing areas).
6 Adequate sports equipment: protective and instrumental.
7 Adaptation of rules.
8 Fair play.
9 Health education.

Secondary prevention includes, for instance early detection of the injury problem (reduction of patient and doctor delay) or first aid as soon as possible. Rehabilitation, e.g. muscle-strengthening exercise programmes in case of joint instability, or specific information on the prevention of injury recurrence in an athlete after a sprained ankle, can be regarded as examples of *tertiary* prevention.

In the literature so far, scientific studies directed to the application of preventive measures are scarce. Studies specifically designed for children and adolescents are lacking.

One of the strategies used against injuries is aimed at behavioural modification (Kok & Bouter, 1990). Health education as a tool in realizing behavioural change can be im-

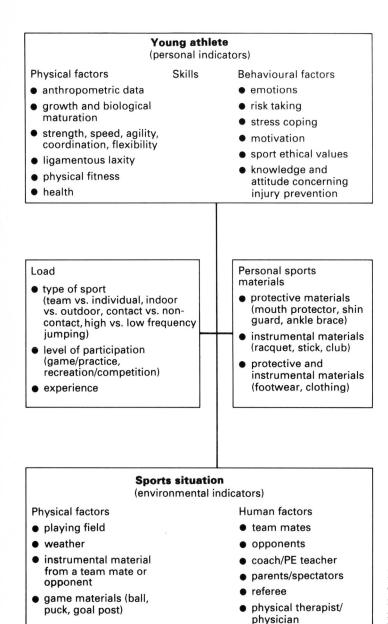

Fig. 11.2 Schematic expression of the most important risk indicators affecting sports injuries in young people. Redrawn from Backx (1991).

plemented in the school curriculum by specifically trained teachers in PE or biology (Backx, 1991).

The need for the coach of juniors to become involved in sports injury prevention may vary among countries, depending on the number of other professional groups working in the same area. The primary tasks of a coach must not be limited to the stimulating role in order to develop skills. The coach can be a message mediator by educating young athletes in practical and theoretical aspects of injury prevention. Although the effects of health education in this specific area still have to be proven, there are strong indications that in the short term this can be beneficial in reducing the number of sports injuries. The effects in the long run are only speculative.

Challenges for future research

• In future aetiological studies, three conditions need to be satisfied: (i) accurate definitions of sport and sports injury need to be developed; (ii) accurate descriptions of sports injuries are needed; and (iii) methodological homogeneity concerning characteristics such as age, gender, type of sport, sports culture, exposure time and level of play need to be agreed.

• In the near future, more prospective data acquired in observational studies must be generated to create more valuable information, which can then be translated into preventive measures.

• Because the results of health education programmes seem to be very encouraging, it would be worthwhile implementing this kind of health education within the school curriculum on a more regular basis. Thus, it would be necessary to begin courses for the teachers concerned in order to optimize their role in the prevention of sports injuries. Research into the effects of these courses and the implementation of health education would also be worthwhile.

• Because children and adolescents are increasingly involved in sports activity in a highly intensive and extensive manner, there is an increasing need to monitor overuse injuries in an accurate way.

• More well-designed intervention studies are necessary for a better understanding of injury prevention.

References

Abrunzo, T.J. (1991) Commotio cordis; the single, most common cause of traumatic death in youth baseball. *Am. J. Disabled Child* **145**, 1279–82.

Backous, D.D., Friedl, K.E., Smith, N.J., Parr, Th.J. & Carpine, W.D. (1988) Soccer injuries and their

relation to physical maturity. *Am. J. Dis. Child.* **142**, 839–42.

Backx, F.J.G. (1991) *Sports injuries in youth; etiology and prevention.* Thesis, Janus Jongbloed Research Center on Sports and Health, Utrecht, the Netherlands.

Backx, F.J.G., Beijer, H.J.M., Bol, E. & Erich, W.B.M. (1991) Injuries in persons and high-risk sports; a longitudinal study of 1,818 school children. *Am. J. Sports Med.* **19**, 124–30.

Backx, F.J.G., Erich, W.B.M., Kemper, A.B.A. & Verbeek, A.L.M. (1989) Sports injuries in school-aged children; an epidemiologic study. *Am. J. Sports Med.* **17**, 234–40.

Chan, K.M., Fu, F. & Leung L. (1984) Sports injuries survey on university students in Hong Kong. *Br. J. Sports Med.* **18**, 195–202.

DeHaven, K.E. & Lintner, D.M. (1986) Athletic injuries: comparison by age, sport and gender. *Am. J. Sports Med.* **14**, 218–24.

deLoës, M. (1990) Medical treatment and costs of sports-related injuries in a total population. *Int. J. Sports Med.* **11**, 66–72.

deLoës, M. & Goldie, K. (1988) Incidence rate of injuries during sport activity and physical exercise in a rural Swedish municipality: incidence rates in 17 sports. *Int. J. Sports Med.* **9**, 461–7.

Diederiks, J.P.M., van Galen, W.C.C. & Philipsen, H. (1984) Injuries in indoor korfball. *Int. J. Sports Med.* **5** (Suppl.), 216–17.

Ekstrand, J. & Gillquist, J. (1983) Soccer injuries and their mechanisms, a prospective study. *Med. Sci. Sports Exerc.* **15**, 267–70.

Garrick, J.G. (1982) Epidemiologic perspective. *Clin. Sports Med.* **1**, 13–18.

Hammer, A., Schwartzbach, A.L. & Paulev, P.E. (1981) Children injured during physical education lessons. *J. Sports Med.* **21**, 423–31.

Hunter, R.E. & Levy I.M. (1988) Vignettes, developed by The Research Committee. *Am. J. Sports Med.* **16** (Suppl. 1), S25–S30.

Jones, B.H., Rock, P.B. & Moore, M.P. (1988) Musculoskeletal injury: risks, prevention, and first aid. In S.N. Blair *et al.* (eds) *Resource Manual for Guidelines for Exercise Testing and Prescription.* Lea & Febiger, Philadelphia.

Kok, G.J. & Bouter, L.M. (1990) On the importance of planned health education. Prevention of ski injury as an example. *Am. J. Sports Med.* **18**, 600–5.

Kvist, M., Kujala, U.M., Heinonen, O.J. *et al.* (1989) Sports-related injuries in children. *Int. J. Sports Med.* **10**, 81–6.

Landry, G.L. (1992) Sports injuries in childhood. *Pediatr. Ann.* **21**, 165–8.

Lindenfeld, Th.N., Noyes, F.R. & Marshall, M.T. (1988) Components of injury reporting systems.

Am. J. Sports Med. **16** (Suppl. 1), S69–81.

Lysens, R.J., Ostyn, M.S., van den Auweele, Y., Lefrevre, J., Vuylsteke, M. & Renson, L. (1989) The accident-prone and overuse-prone profiles of the young athlete. *Am. J. Sports Med.* **17**, 612–19.

Maehlum, S., Dahl, E. & Daljord, D. (1986) Frequency of injuries in a youth soccer tournament. *Phys. Sportsmed.* **14**(7), 73–9.

Medved, R. & Pavisic-Medved, V. (1973) Causes of injuries during the practical classes on physical education in schools. *J. Sports Med. Phys. Fitness* **13**, 32–41.

Mueller, F. & Blyth, C. (1982) Epidemiology of sports injuries in children. *Clin. Sports Med.* **1**, 343–51.

Nathorst Westfelt, J.A.R. (1982) Environmental factors in childhood accidents; a prospective study in Götenborg, Sweden. *Acta Paediatr. Scand.* **291** (Suppl.), 6–61.

Nielsen, A.B. & Yde, J. (1988) An epidemiologic and traumatologic study of injuries in handball. *Int. J. Sports Med.* **9**, 341–4.

Noyes, F.R., Lindenfeld, Th.N. & Marshall, M.T. (1988) What determines an athletic injury (definition)? Who determines an injury (occurrence)? *Am. J. Sports Med.* **16** (Suppl. 1), S65–9.

Orava, S. & Puranen, J. (1978) Exertion injuries in adolescent athletes. *Br. J. Sports Med.* **12**, 4–10.

Pappas, A.M. (1989) Osteochondroses: diseases of growth centers. *Phys. Sporstmed.* **17**, 51–62.

Pettrone, F.A. & Ricciardelli, E. (1987) Gymnastic injuries: the Virginia experience 1982–1983. *Am. J. Sports Med.* **15**, 59–62.

Rümmele, E. (1987) Sports injuries in the Federal Republic of Germany — Part 2. In C.R. van der Togt, A.B.A. Kemper & M. Koornneef (eds) *Council of Europe: Sport for All; Sports Injuries and Their Prevention*, pp. 37–49. Proceedings of the 2nd Meeting. National Institute for Sports Health Care, Oosterbeek, The Netherlands.

Sahlin, Y. (1990) Sport accidents in childhood. *Br. J. Sports Med.* **24**, 40–4.

Schmidt, B. & Höllwarth, M.E. (1989) Sportunfälle im Kindes- und Jugendalter (Sports accidents in children and adolescents). *Zeitschr. Kinderchir.* **44**, 357–62.

Schmidt-Olsen, S., Bünemann, L.K.H., Lade, V. & Brassoe, J.O.K. (1985) Soccer injuries of youth. *Br. J. Sports Med.* **19**, 161–4.

Taimela, S., Kujala, M. & Osterman, K. (1990) Intrinsic risk factors and athletic injuries. *Sports Med.* **9**, 205–15.

Tursz, A. & Crost, M. (1986) Sports-related injuries in children; a study of their characteristics, frequency and severity, with comparison to other types of accidental injuries. *Am. J. Sports Med.* **14**, 294–9.

van Galen, W.C.C. & Diederiks, J.P.M. (1990) *Sportblessures Breed Uitgemeten* (English summary). De Vrieseborch Haarlem, The Netherlands.

van Mechelen, W., Hlobil, H. & Kemper, H.C.G. (1987) *How Can Sports Injuries be Prevented?* National Institute for Sports Health Care, Oosterbeek, The Netherlands.

van Vulpen, A.T. (1989) *Council of Europe Coordinated Research Project: Sports Injuries and Their Prevention.* National Institute for Sports Health Care, Oosterbeek, The Netherlands.

Wallace, R.B. (1988) Application of epidemiologic principles to sports injury research. *Am. J. Sports Med.* **16** (Suppl. 1), S22–5.

Walter, S.D., Sutton, J.R., McIntosh, J.M. & Connolly, C. (1985) The etiology of sports injuries: a review of methodologies. *Sports Med.* **2**, 47–58.

Watson, A.W.S. (1984) Sports injuries during one academic year in 6799 Irish school children. *Am. J. Sports Med.* **12**, 65–71.

Watson, A.W.S. (1986) *Sports Injuries in Irish Second-level Schools during the School Year 1984–1985.* Department of Education, Dublin.

Yde, J. & Nielsen, A.B. (1990) Sports injuries in adolescents' ball games: soccer, handball and basketball. *Br. J. Sports Med.* **24**, 51–4.

Zaricznyj, B., Shattuck, L.J.M., Mast, T.A., Robertson, R.V. & D'Elia, G. (1980) Sports-related injuries in school-aged children. *Am. J. Sports Med.* **8**, 318–24.

Chapter 12

Biomechanical Considerations of Youth Sports Injuries

MONICA J. BURGESS-MILLIRON AND SEAN B. MURPHY

Introduction

The participation of children in higher intensity sport programmes and the subsequent increase in injuries has recently received more attention from the sports medicine and scientific communities. Attention has been particularly focused on the re-evaluation of injury treatment protocols as well as taking a proactive approach in ways to prevent injury. A basic evaluation of any sport involves the study of the typical movements and forces made within that sport and the specific motion patterns of a given athlete. The evaluation of technique, training regimens, injuries and rehabilitation programmes in terms of the related forces, movements and anatomical structures is the objective of biomechanical studies in youth sports.

Biomechanical evaluation of sport can define movement patterns required for successful execution of a technique, identify deviation from these motions which may increase the risk of musculoskeletal injuries, and evaluate causes and long-term effects of injury. Radin (1980) suggested that biomechanics has the clearest application to the understanding of injury and the recovery of musculoskeletal problems in relation to all of the basic sciences. Application of biomechanics to injury analyses (both cause and effect) can provide a better evaluation of treatment protocols and assist in the identification of preventative approaches to sports injury. The benefits of understanding the mechanism of injury have been addressed by several authors (Alms, 1961; Kaufer, 1980; Jacobs & Ghista, 1981; Gozna, 1982; Souer, 1982; Krag *et al.*, 1986; Viano *et al.*, 1989).

Biomechanical studies have been completed to evaluate forces and movements within various sports and to investigate related injuries, but these studies have included primarily adult sport participants. The information obtained via studies on adults provides direction in the evaluation of children and adolescents in sport, but does not apply directly because children are not 'miniature adults'. The growth factor in youth creates special concerns in terms of anatomical structures, bone and muscle strength, and long-term effects of injury.

The purpose of this chapter is to provide an overview of the role which biomechanics plays in the evaluation of the forces and movement patterns in youth sports and related injuries. The evaluation of sport from a biomechanical perspective requires a fundamental knowledge of the musculoskeletal system of youth and an introduction to the basic principles used to determine forces and movements within a sport. These principles are presented in general terms as they relate to common injuries of the upper and lower extremities and the spine of young athletes. By understanding the function of the joints of the body and the biomechanical factors related to sporting activities, awareness of techniques and training protocols with respect to injury prevention and rehabilitation can be enhanced.

Special anatomical considerations in youth

In general, long bones define the segments of movement in sport biomechanics. It is important to understand the properties of these bones in young athletes during injury evaluation. Long bones have a long diaphysis (shaft) and two epiphyses (growth plates) as shown in Fig. 12.1. The slight curvature of long bones distributes forces more evenly throughout the bone providing better shock absorption and reducing the risk of fracture. Variation in anatomical alignment can influence force distribution and movement patterns. Presence of malalignment can increase the risk of injury due to modification of stress distribution and the limited ability of the body to adapt.

Epiphyseal (growth) plates

The epiphyseal plate, or growth plate, is a ring of cartilage separating the long shaft from the bulbous end of the bone. This cartilage structure contributes to the growth plate being the weakest part of the bone in youth. Growth

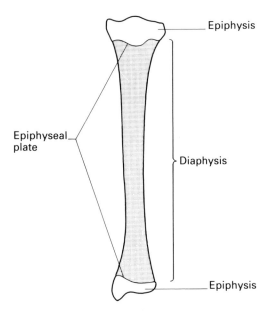

Fig. 12.1 The structure of a long bone.

cartilage is located in three primary sites in premature skeleton: (i) epiphyseal plate; (ii) joint surface; and (iii) the apophyseal insertion of major muscle tendon units. Most of the linear growth of the bone occurs at the epiphysis site. Speer and Braun (1985) described the growth plate as a contoured surface as specific as fingerprints which serves the biomechanical role of resisting or augmenting the forces imparted to the bone. These authors suggested that during bone growth, the plate unlocks making it more vulnerable to injury by shear forces. Also deserving consideration is that the epiphyseal plates throughout the body close at different times of growth. An understanding of the maturation process of bones and critical growth periods is important in preventing injuries to the growth plates throughout the skeletal system.

With regard to sport-related injuries, the physis region is involved 6–18% of the time (Pappas, 1983; Speer & Braun, 1985). Pappas (1983) reported that fewer than 5% of epiphyseal plate injuries are fractures that result in growth disturbances, though the effect of injury to this region can be complicated and long lasting. Injury to the epiphyseal plate can change the architectural structure of the region including the contour, limb lengths, angular orientation and alignment of bone. These changes can influence the biomechanical function of the body. The collagen fibres may also be disrupted which decreases the resistance of the region to tensile and shear forces (Speer & Braun, 1985). Other serious outcomes of plate damage can involve partial or complete cessation of growth. Some injuries will not present indication of long-term growth effects immediately, but will require long-term follow-up with X-rays and limb length measurements to monitor full recovery (Pappas, 1983). The extent of alteration depends on the severity and location of the injury as well as the level of activity of the individual. Minimization of aggravating factors, such as high forces, through technique evaluation and possible modification during this healing period can influence the outcome.

The result of these functional alterations can range from negligible to outcomes creating compensatory motion causing increased stress to other anatomical structures during sport activities.

Children and adolescents participating in contact sports are thought to be at higher risk for growth plate injury than other young athletes due to the high forces associated with sudden impacts. A disproportionately high incidence of epiphyseal plate injuries have been reported in athletes participating in sports with forceful collisions such as football and hockey (Benton, 1982). Due to the higher risk of growth plate injury during the rapid growth periods some questions have been raised regarding the participation of youths between the ages of 12 and 14 years in collision sports such as football (Micheli, 1988b). The maturation process of the bone is not evident by the size of the child and larger children are often placed at higher risk of injury when they are chosen based on their appearance for positions encompassing higher stress (e.g. cheerleaders serving as the base of a pyramid), without consideration of the effect on their growth plates.

Properties of bone

Bones experience loading in multiple directions and can withstand different levels of force in each direction. Injuries specific to youth often differ from those which occur to adults under similar mechanical loading. Several reasons exist for this discrepancy in injury patterns, though it centres around the unique properties of the immature musculoskeletal system (Table 12.1). The elastic property of paediatric bone is enhanced compared to adult bone due to its porous composition, but it is susceptible to failures in compression or tension. The greater elasticity in the bone structure of youth allows their bones to deform considerably more than mature bone prior to fracture (Warner & Micheli, 1991). The immature skeletal structure of children has been found to include ligaments two to five times stronger than the epiphyseal plate, making the physis the weak link

Table 12.1 Common trends in injuries of youth structures compared to adult structures.

Anatomical structure	Properties of bones in youth	Potential injury
Ligament	2–5 times stronger than bone*	Growth plate injury
Bone	More porous	More porous — can fail in compression or tension
Bone	Growth plate	Allows for small amount of displacement; can dampen forces across joints
Bone	Growth plate child versus adolescent	Prepubescent bone more resistant to shear and torsional forces
Bone	Greater potential to remodel	Increases the risk of overgrowth and angular deformity
Articular cartilage	Less resilient and increased transmission of force from bone	More susceptible to micro and macro trauma injuries†

* Caine and Lindner (1985), Collins and Evarts (1971) Micheli and Santore (1980), Tibone (1983).
† Warner and Micheli (1991)

of the musculoskeletal system (Collins & Evarts, 1971; Caine & Lindner, 1985; Micheli & Santore, 1980). Mechanical factors which usually result in a ligamentous injury in adults will often cause an epiphyseal plate injury in children and adolescents. The growth factor of immature bone allows for greater remodelling capabilities, but can also result in excessive bone restructuring causing malalignment or angular deformities which lead to altered biomechanical function. An imbalance in muscle strength can result in the bone twisting excessively under the pull of the stronger muscle group. The potential of this excessive or malaligned healing can increase the risk of injury due to altered muscle attachments, modified movement patterns, or bony protrusions creating localized high-pressure areas.

It is important to note that the body requires a minimal level of stress for normal bone growth to occur as described by Wolff's law (Weinman & Sicher, 1955). Wolff's law states that a change in the function of bone is likely to cause a change in the growth pattern which is determined by mechanical forces acting on the bone. The definition of this minimal level has not been clearly defined in terms of intensity and duration for any group (Rarick, 1960; Malina, 1972; Caine & Lindner, 1984). When the level of activity is excessive and of great intensity, bone generation is increased to the point that an irregular enlargement of the bone results. This has been seen in the radius and humerus of the dominant arm of tennis and baseball players (Jones *et al.*, 1977; Priest *et al.*, 1977), enlarged hands and feet related to loading levels in young skiers (Alekseev, 1977), and in the enlarged fibula in children with congenital absence of the tibia (Houston, 1979).

Often adolescents will experience an epiphyseal plate or avulsion fracture in which a piece of the bone fractures rather than a ligamentous injury more common in adults. Strength development of the bones lags behind that of ligaments and tendons which increases the risk for avulsion fractures especially in young athletes who experience more sudden and greater forces during sports activities. The apophysis growth centre of the bone which becomes the attachment site for tendons or ligaments is also more prone to injury at the bone rather than the tendon in the child.

Osteochondritis causes separation of abnormal ossification areas within the epiphysis. Osteochondroses are developmental disorders associated with anatomical sites undergoing transition from cartilage to bone. These disorders occur in different forms, but biomechanical factors can play a role in the course of the disorder as described by Pappas (1989). The stresses involved in training regimens can have varying effects depending on the timing with respect to the growth cycle. Repetitive trauma and muscle imbalance can aggravate osteochondrosis by disrupting the transition of a region from cartilage to bone. Effects of osteochondritis can include locking of the joints, instability, articular degeneration, compression fractures and loss of range of motion. These outcomes intensify with age as the skeleton becomes more mature, and there is less opportunity for correction towards proper growth patterns. Angular deformity and functional impairment of the limb are also possible, which may lead to leg length and angular discrepancies (as seen in Blount's disease) and the discontinuation of sporting activities (Pappas, 1982). Some precautions to take in order to minimize the effects of osteochondritis include proper technique training, properly designed footwear, and limitations on playing times in terms of practice, season length and summer camps.

Several factors related to the growth spurt can change the biomechanics of similar motions due to altered balances in muscle length and strength with respect to bone and possible changes in alignment or structural integrity. An overview of the biomechanics of the growth spurt changes in relation to injury risk is provided in Table 12.2. Speer and Braun (1985) described the effects of the growth spurt on the epiphyseal plate which included the unlocking of the plate contours resulting in the increased

Table 12.2 Effects of the growth spurt.

Characteristic	Effect
Decreased flexibility due to muscle/bone imbalance	Predisposes youth to overuse injuries (e.g. apophysitis)*
Increase in size	Higher force in collisions; more weight supported by the spine
Increase in skill	Higher level of competition
Increased speed of activity	Greater impact momentum during collisions; higher velocity requires faster muscle response
Articular cartilage structural changes	More susceptible to shear stress†
Gender differentiation more discernible	Size and strength diverge more than difference in prepubescents

* Micheli (1983)
† Micheli (1983, 1988).

susceptibility of the plate to injury at the mid-point of the growth spurt (Benton, 1982; Pappas, 1983; Speer & Braun, 1985). The effects of the growth spurt are found in the increased incidence of injuries in football players aged 14–17 years compared to a younger group. Though increased speed, strength and skill may account for this increase with regard to higher force collisions, similar trends were seen for sports with less contact such as soccer (Robey et al., 1971). The greater differential in size between competitors grouped by chronological age creates an environment with various imbalances with respect to biomechanical advantages and disadvantages (see Chapter 14).

The prepubescent athlete also has some specific patterns related to injury as compared to adolescents and adults. Younger athletes may be less susceptible to spinal cord injury compared to older children. This is possibly due to intrinsic characteristics of the immature spine supporting less weight with relatively

slower movements (Herndon, 1990). Young athletes lacking the skills necessary to participate at a certain level of play may have a higher risk of injury (Nilson & Rohas, 1978; Goldberg et al., 1979; Maroon et al., 1980; Micheli, 1988a). This risk can be associated with less strength and biomechanical factors related to incorrect technique.

Role of biomechanics in injury prevention and aetiology

The role of biomechanics with regard to injury is multifaceted. Injury can (i) reduce optimal performance; (ii) cause compensatory movements thus increasing the stress and risk of injury at other sites; and (iii) accelerate fatigue which reduces reaction time and increases injury risk. Biomechanical information on injury mechanisms can assist in understanding aetiology in addition to being used in the prevention of injury through proper training regimens and correction of poor technique. A slight modification in technique can help reduce the risk of injury by modifying the force experienced at a given joint. An example of technique modification would be the correction of posture by an athlete during bench pressing. A change in position of the arms so that the hands are in better alignment with the shoulder, would result in a reduction of shear forces at the shoulder. This modification can help reduce the risk of injury and possibly enhance the ability to lift.

Intense athletic activity influences muscle strength and flexibility. Muscle strength training can lead to decreased flexibility and muscle imbalance if asymmetrical training of a muscle group is emphasized. The result of this imbalance in muscle group strength or flexibility can be altered biomechanics or movement patterns which in turn can decrease performance and increase the risk of injury. Other potential results of a strength or flexibility imbalance are overload injuries due to incorrect technique or anatomical malalignment caused by the imbalance. In terms of growth, an increased risk of repetitive overloading injuries has been related to increased height and weight. The proposed cause has been associated with an increase in the centre of gravity and greater leverage, due to longer limbs, therefore increasing the stress on the joint structures (Bender *et al.*, 1964; Valliant, 1981; Watson, 1981; Taimela *et al.*, 1989). Permanent change in alignment due to increased strength and repetitive movement patterns are exemplified in conditions such as spondylolysis in young gymnasts due to cyclic loading of the pars interarticularis in a hyperextended posture.

Technique evaluation can play a major role in injury prevention as well as rehabilitation to minimize the risk of recurrence. Common techniques which have been evaluated include pitching (Ciccantelli, 1994), dance (Kravitz, 1986), and gymnastics (Aronen, 1985). Mechanical factors related to musculoskeletal injury involve three major aspects: (i) high levels of force or pressure resulting in acute injury or macrotrauma; (ii) smaller forces repeated over a period of time during which insufficient rest is allowed for recovery resulting in microtrauma or overuse injuries; and (iii) awkward postures that are frequent or impose high forces and increase the risk of injury. Since microtrauma injuries are less understood and more difficult to recognize in terms of biomechanical factors, these will be emphasized. A clinical view of overuse injuries is detailed in Chapter 13.

A common mechanical cause of overuse injuries can be related to training errors. A sudden change in activity level can place an overload on the musculoskeletal system — an overload to which the system is not capable of adapting. One of the most common mistakes made in training is at the start of a season where a child athlete changes from a relatively sedentary state of activity to intense practice sessions in a short period of time. This same effect is often associated with coming back from an injury too quickly or increasing mileage, number of pitches or playing time over a short period of time. Activities performed at summer camps also hold a risk of overuse injuries since the format generally includes long days of practice, drills and play concentrated into the period of the camp. The high concentration of activity provides minimal time for the musculoskeletal system to adapt and recover before the next practice or game session which increases the risk of overuse injuries or even acute injury due to fatigue and cumulative effects of forces.

Biomechanical evaluation of forces and movements indicates techniques which allow for optimal performance as well as minimizing injury risk. The involvement of the whole body in pitching a baseball will generate more power while minimizing stress to the upper extremity compared to a style where the upper body only is used in completing the pitch. The synchronization of the movements of the various joints will also play an important role in a successful pitch and potentially reduce the risk of injury.

Rehabilitation of an injury is critical to the young athlete. In addition to strengthening and flexibility exercises, other aspects such as technique modification must be considered. A gradual return to activity will minimize risk of recurrence and an evaluation of technique may provide crucial insight into the motion pattern which possibly contributed to the initial injury.

Biomechanical evaluation of injury

During rapid growth phases, which vary amongst individuals, the epiphyseal plate is vulnerable to injury (Stanitski, 1990). The epiphyseal tensile strength in infrahuman specimens has been evaluated (Malina, 1969) and these results correspond with the incidence of growth plate injury data that illustrate the predisposition of injury is greater during adolescence (Peterson & Peterson, 1972).

Hastings and Simmons (1984) reported that 34% of all fractures in young patients which occur are epiphyseal plate fractures. Caine and Lindner (1984) indicated that with regard to growth plate injuries, the highest incidence in young patients occur during adolescence and nearly 50% were sport related. Stress and compressive loads have significant influence on epiphyseal growth. Roy et al. (1985) associated intensity of training with radiological changes of the radial epiphysis in high calibre gymnasts. As the intensity of training was reduced, normal growth patterns resumed.

Though the risk of epiphyseal fractures is greater than ligamental injury in young athletes, the incidence of ligamental injuries in this population has also been increasing (Stanitski, 1990) possibly signifying even greater loading of the musculoskeletal system under current sports participation programmes. The information on the effects of training and responses of the connective tissue of the immature skeleton is not well understood. Specifically, the effects of distance running has not been determined as a contributing factor. The authors outlined three approaches to studying this topic further to extend our level of knowledge considering the concern of growth plate injuries due to potential risks of intense long-distance training in the adolescent. Repetition is a concern, but no clear evidence exists that distance running is harmful or beneficial.

In gymnastics, a correlation between intensity of activity and musculoskeletal injuries has been reported by several authors (Teitz, 1982; Carter et al., 1988; Jackson et al., 1989). Micheli (1990) reported increasing evidence that repetitive trauma in sports such as gymnastics can cause growth plate arrest. Kato and Ishiko (1984) showed stunted growth in children involved in heavy labour which extended beyond nutritional considerations.

Upper extremity

A common site of injury in young athletes, especially pitchers and gymnasts, is the elbow. The elbow is an anatomically stable joint, but in activities such as pitching and gymnastics (Aronen, 1985) the forces that are imposed on the elbow may result in hyperextension that can predispose young athletes to sport-related injuries.

Pitching in sports such as baseball has been associated with various injuries at the elbow. Potential causes of the pain can include excessive throwing, muscle imbalance, incorrect mechanics or variation in anatomical alignment with respect to specific pitching styles. In a study of 11- and 12-year-old pitchers, it was reported that between 20 and 45% of the pitchers had elbow pain. The larger portion of the group reporting pain played in a climate that allowed for a longer season (Adams, 1975; Gugenheim et al., 1976; Larson et al., 1976).

In the adolescent, the injury pattern is often an avulsion fracture through the epiphysis due to the increased muscular strength between the shoulder and elbow. In a group of 6–10-year-old prepubescent pitchers, Collins and Evarts (1971) observed fractures of the lateral condyle epiphyseal plate which was the result of varus stress in combination with an extended elbow. The forceful rapid extension of the arm may also result in posterior elbow injury or apophysitis, or non-union of the epiphysis due to the force the triceps repetitively exerts on the olecranon. Once the epiphysis partially closes around the age of 15 years avulsion fractures are more common than a complete apophysis fracture (Woods & Tullos, 1977).

One biomechanical factor associated with the high incidence of elbow pain in pitchers is the valgus force observed during the acceleration phase of the pitch. This force stretches the medial aspect of the joint and compresses the lateral side of the epicondyle. Evaluation of the young pitcher must concentrate on the type of pitch most often thrown and the pitching style the athlete adopts. Pappas (1982) found the type of pitch and alignment of the shoulder and elbow have been shown to affect the amount of force placed on the elbow. He reported that the sudden contraction of the wrist with the finger flexors of the arm, in a supinated position, increased the stress on the medial elbow when pitching a curve ball. Conversely, a fast ball pitch increased the loading on the radiocapitellar joint at the elbow.

Albright et al. (1978) evaluated delivery techniques and determined that 74% of the studied side-arm pitchers reported elbow problems compared to 27% of the pitchers with a vertical delivery. It was noted that the main difference in technique between the two styles was the improved alignment of the elbow with respect to the shoulder at the time of release in the vertical delivery.

A series of technique evaluations to determine factors which enhance the pitch, and those styles to avoid, was outlined by Ciccantelli (1994). An important point to note was that every stage of the pitch can be evaluated and suggestions made to improve the technique to help reduce the risk of injury. This evaluation also points to the importance of the full body analysis to achieve proper alignment between the elbow and shoulder as well as the positioning and movement patterns of the torso and lower extremity.

One significant way to reduce the number of overuse injuries seen in a pitcher is to minimize the exposure of the body to stresses by reducing the number of innings pitched and most importantly the number of pitches thrown in a game. This preventative measure was implemented by the Little League with positive results. Torg *et al.* (1972) reported significant decreases in elbow symptoms with these limitations. Congeni (1994) urged that excessive practice must also be avoided to benefit from the game rule.

Another athlete population in which a high incidence of elbow pain and overuse injuries have been found is gymnasts (Priest & Weise, 1981; Nocini & Silvij, 1982; Szot *et al.*, 1985). This group experiences a high incidence of elbow injury due primarily to the utilization of the upper extremity as a weight-bearing system. As in pitchers, common aetiologies at the elbow are traction injuries medially and compression-related pain laterally. Priest and Weise (1981) reported that fractures and dislocations are the most common serious injuries of the upper extremity of these athletes. One particular site of injury is the distal radial epiphysis. Roy *et al.* (1985) listed several contributing factors that are related to these injuries in

gymnasts. One such factor is the compliance of the landing mats. Mats that are too soft or compliant can contribute to injuries due to excessive dorsiflexion of the wrist. Another contributing factor is the hyperextension and ulnar deviation of the wrist which result from twisting motions as observed during vaulting activities. In beam and tumbling workouts, the hands are fixed as the forearms undergo repetitive torsional stress possibly predisposing the epiphysis, the weakest part of the bone, to excessive stress. Two final contributing factors were reported as high repetition of movements in general and practicing 'tricks' or advanced movements with incorrect technique. These authors observed that radiographical changes in the distal radial epiphysis of these 21 high-level gymnasts did not indicate a permanent effect on growth during the 6−42 month follow-up period evaluated.

The prevention of initial or recurrent injuries can be addressed by alternating between directions of twisting motions and reducing the number of movements, especially those of high force and awkward postures (excessive wrist dorsiflexion). As the levels of force and frequency of movements increase, the risk of injury increases. The resistance of the musculoskeletal system to angular deformity caused by imposed stresses is reduced due to the delayed skeletal age of this group (Ellman, 1975; Malina, 1983; Maffulli, 1989). To prevent recurrence, preventative measures should include the elimination or minimization of weight bearing following the injury. The coach or trainer should examine the strength and flexibility of the athlete and develop a programme that ensures balance. An examination of individual risk factors for each athlete in terms of anatomy and technique should be included in this evaluation.

The anatomical design of the shoulder requires muscle activity for stability. Dislocation of the shoulder joint is highly prevalent in the child and adolescent population, being reported as the most frequently dislocated joint (Meyers, 1990). A prevalent theory is that the increased elasticity of the tissue in these younger groups results in irreversible stretch. Other secondary factors include ligamentous laxity and the degree of trauma that the shoulder sustains (Rowe & Sakellaride, 1961). Unfortunately, there is a high incidence of recurrence of dislocation of the shoulder joint in young athletes. Incidence of anterior dislocation recurrence has been reported from 66% to over 90% for patients under 21 years of age (Rowe & Sakellaride, 1961; Simonet & Cofield, 1984; Hovelius, 1987).

Any increase in shoulder laxity affects the stability of the joint particularly under stressful movements. An imbalance of muscle strength modifies the function of the shoulder and can lead to asymmetrical loading. Impingement syndromes also occur due to muscle imbalance due to weak or overloaded rotator cuff muscles (Micheli, 1983). Rotation of the shoulder in a fully flexed position, as seen in swimming and pitching, increases the risk of injury. Changes in technique and training regimen are necessary to prevent recurrence of impingement.

Spine

Low back pain is one of the most common complaints in young athletes. Activities that result in hyperextension of the back have all been cited as common aggravating activities that precipitate this condition. These activities include football blocking, military press in weight-lifting, pole vaulting, diving, pitching, gymnastics and serving in tennis (Jackson, 1979). When these activities become highly repetitive, a true pars interarticularis stress fracture is usually the resulting injury (Goldberg, 1980; Stanitski, 1982). Most often the fracture is found in the L5 vertebrae, but is not limited to this location (Stanitski, 1982).

Gymnasts have been found to account for 21% of the diagnosed stress fractures, all of them in the pars interarticularis of the back, an area also commonly fractured in interior football linemen (Yngve, 1990). The incidence of stress fractures in the back of these two groups is four times that of the general population. Spondylo-

lysis is the most commonly occurring low back condition seen in the gymnast (Jackson, 1979; Goldberg, 1980; Walsh et al., 1985).

Lower extremity

One of the most common locations of lower extremity injury in children is the distal femoral epiphysis (Grana, 1990). This injury is often the result of a severe torsional stress that may be produced in a cutting movement observed in such sports as basketball and soccer or a valgus force directed at the flexed knee often seen in contact sports. The force or impact usually results in a fracture through the epiphyseal plate instead of a sprained medial collateral ligament more commonly seen in adults. As opposed to the adult sprain, an epiphyseal fracture is seen in children because the knee ligament of the child is stronger than the adjacent femoral physeal plate and articular cartilage. This imbalance can be attributed to why ligament injuries have been found to account for less than 1% of the knee injuries in the child and adolescent athlete (Grana, 1990).

Fractures of the tibia and fibula are also common and typically seen in the adolescent athlete (Collins & Evarts, 1971). In sports such as football, large forces can be imposed on the lateral aspect of the knee joint, and an epiphyseal plate injury of the proximal tibia often results. Fractures of the proximal tibial epiphysis may also involve the tibial tubercle apophysis (Nanning & Josaputra, 1987). These fractures are usually a result of a violent contraction of the quadriceps muscle during deceleration, which leads to knee extension and compression. Fractures of this nature may result from a basketball lay-up landing or a jump. In this situation, the leg is decelerated upon impact and the knee continues to extend or even hyperextend.

Fractures of the ankle usually occur prior to the closure of the tibial and fibular growth plates at approximately 15–16 years of age. Injuries involving external rotations may result in a Tillaux and triplane fracture at the distal tibia. An inversion injury may result in a Salter—Harris type I or II fracture of the distal fibular growth plate (Wong & Gregg, 1986).

In the lower extremity, apophyseal injuries most often occur on the pelvis or femur. Activities that involve large forces and sports with large forces due to contact can result in either a partial or complete separation of the apophysis from the bone (Micheli & Santore, 1980; Micheli, 1983). For example, the muscle forces produced by a child kicking a soccer ball can result in avulsion of the ischial apophysis. These injuries are particularly seen when the knee is extended and the hip is flexed (Wilkens, 1980).

Injuries resulting in avulsion fractures of the anterior superior iliac spine occur as a result of excessive contraction at the insertion of the sartorious muscle. The sartorious muscle is responsible for flexion and lateral rotation of the hip. Therefore, runners are particularly at risk of developing apophyseal fractures at this muscular insertion due to the repetitive hip flexion involved in the activity.

Apophyseal injuries can also occur due to overuse and are frequent in the lower extremity. Apophysitis of the iliac crest is an inflammation of the iliac crest growth plate that is a common site of involvement in cross-country and distance runners. The cause of this injury is thought to be due to the repetitive pull of the abdominal muscles that insert on the iliac crest (Clancy, 1991).

Osgood—Schlatter disease (non-articular or traction osteochondrosis) is another apophyseal injury and is caused by multiple small tears in the patellar tendon insertion on the tibial tubercle. The resultant tensile force developed by the quadriceps acts through the insertion of the patellar tendon which may result in a disruption of the insertional interface. It is usually the result of an overgrowth syndrome that presents an imbalanced extensor mechanism. The extensor mechanism is composed of the quadriceps tendon, the patella and patellar tendon. These structures form the primary extensors of the knee. Bone growth without muscle—tendon growth results in decreased

hamstring and quadriceps flexibility. Activities that involve the quadriceps muscles, such as running and jumping, result in painful contractions due to the pull of the patellar tendon on the tibial tubercle. Pain is usually developed at the time of rapid growth or immediately following rapid growth. The disease particularly affects children and adolescents between the ages of 10 and 15 years of age and it has been reported that 10% of the athletes in this age group will develop the disease (Wong & Gregg, 1984). The condition is more prevalent in boys than in girls and unilateral involvement is more prevalent than bilateral (Totten, 1986).

Sinding-Larsen disease is the result of multiple microtraumas to the infrapatellar tendon of the knee located on the distal pole of the patella. It is thought to be due to a repetitive traction phenomenon at the patellar tendon attachment, similar to Osgood—Schlatter disease, but on the inferior pole of the patella.

Calcaneal traction apophysitis is referred to as Sever's disease. It is typically seen in basketball and soccer players (Wong & Gregg, 1986) or in other sports that involve a great deal of running and jumping. The pull of the triceps surae and plantar fascia across the vertically oriented calcaneal apophysis results in high shearing stress and a painful heel. Micheli and Ireland (1987) reported that soccer, basketball and gymnastics were the sports most likely to present the disease. Dorsiflexion weakness and heel cord contracture were the most common conditions affecting the group of 85 children studied. Symptoms are particularly aggravated during the deceleration portion of a run or landing from a jump (Warner & Micheli, 1991). The condition is more likely to be found during a growth spurt which results in a tightened heel cord. Excessive foot pronation is also associated with Sever's disease (Warner & Micheli, 1991). The combined effects of a tightened heel cord and excessive pronation on the apophysis can place the young athlete at risk of other injuries and minimize performance due to altered force distribution and movement patterns.

Freiberg's infraction is an avascular necrosis of the metatarsal epiphysis which may result from repeated trauma. Separation of the epiphysis as well as secondary degenerative changes in the metatarsophalageal joint are often associated with this injury (Murray, 1991). Pain is usually present in the forefoot and is particularly aggravated by weight bearing. Children and adolescent runners are at greatest risk due to the repetitive nature and forces or pressures involved in the activity. Most often, the infraction affects the second metatarsal epiphysis. Binek et al. (1988) reported the second metatarsal head to be involved in 68% of the reported cases observed. The third and fourth metatarsals were involved in 27 and 5% of the cases, respectively. Children 12–15 years of age are most often afflicted, with girls having a higher incidence than boys. Since the metatarsals are vital structures in the distribution of force across the forefoot during the propulsive phase of gait, this injury can influence the child athlete's ability to participate.

Fractures of the patella are often a result of direct trauma. In the skeletally immature, the patella is composed mainly of cartilage (Ogden et al., 1982). Avulsion of the inferior pole with a sleeve of articular cartilage is a typical fracture pattern. The fracture is usually a result of an acute trauma in which the patella forcefully contacts a hard surface.

Lower extremity overuse injuries

As previously stated, injuries to the child and adolescent athlete are not always the result of a single force or impact. Loads placed on the lower extremity during running activities have been recorded at over three times body weight in an adult population (Cavangh & Lafortune, 1980). Upon impact, the inertial load must be absorbed by bone, muscle and connective tissue. The muscles are the primary mechanism for absorbing the impacting load, but may not be able to dissipate the total force under conditions of muscular fatigue or excessive force. Under these conditions, bone, tendon and articular cartilage are subjected to increased loading which may produce microtears in tendon and microfractures of bone. Injury will occur if the forces exceed the anatomical material properties.

Sports that involve repetitive activities may also result in overloading of the epiphyseal plate of the young athlete. For example, slipped femoral capital epiphysis can result from overuse in running activities (Clancy, 1991). As a result of repetitive loading, the proximal epiphyseal plate of the femur is moved from its normal perpendicular position to the load to a more compromising position in which a shear force is placed on the femoral shaft. This modification in loading can result in a displacement of the head of the femur on its neck (Speer & Braun, 1985). This potential malalignment is of particular concern due to the increase in children and adolescents participating in competitive running (Speer & Braun, 1985).

Yngve (1990) reported that 34 of 131 cases of sport-related stress fractures in young patients were related to running. Factors associated with these stress fractures were an imbalance between muscle strength and bone strength, rapid increase of training over a short period, hard surfaces and inappropriate footwear.

Running activities that are used to supplement the training regimen of sports teams should also be examined and considered as an aetiological factor of injury to the lower extremity. Godshall et al. (1981) found two cases of stress fracture through the distal femoral epiphysis in football players in which the direct cause of injury was not known by the subjects or coaches. Neither injury occurred during a football activity. In both cases, the injury was determined to occur as a result of running during a training exercise.

Excessive pronation can occur even with normal anatomical alignment but malalignment is a common aetiology for increased pronatory movement. If excessive pronation is present, full biomechanical evaluation can be extremely helpful in locating the cause (Kravitz et al., 1985).

Individuals with anatomical abnormalities may be predisposed to overuse injuries because stress may concentrate at certain anatomical locations. For example, patellofemoral stress syndrome is frequently seen in young runners who have excessive femoral anteversion. Excessive internal rotation of the hip produces overpronation of the foot at the midstance stage in the gait cycle. This results in an increase in the functional Q angle at the knee which is believed to produce an increase in the load placed on the patellofemoral joint. Excessive femoral anteversion, genu varum or valgum, increased external tibial rotation, and excessive forefoot pronation can also be contributing factors to knee pain and injury. For example, the increased genu varum of the female knee has been one of the attributions for the susceptibility of girls to develop patellofemoral pain syndrome (Warner & Micheli, 1991). This may also result in a predisposition to overuse injuries such as chondromalacia and recurrent patella dislocations.

A great deal of overuse injuries of the knee in children involve the extensor mechanism (Warner & Micheli, 1991). An imbalance between bone and muscle growth can result in the tightening of the iliotibial band which is a thick fascial layer that runs along the lateral aspect of the thigh. The tightening of this fascial band limits the range of motion or may displace skeletal structures producing altered forces and alignment. For example, the tightening of the iliotibial band often deviates the knee into valgus as well as laterally deviating the quadriceps mechanism which may result in recurrent lateral patella subluxation or dislocation.

Conclusion

Zito (1990) provided an extensive overview of the trends of musculoskeletal injuries in young athletes. Some major concerns in relation to the anatomy of young athletes relative to injury and mechanical weakness are listed in Table 12.3.

Challenges for future research

One of the most important considerations in evaluating the movement patterns and forces in youths is that they are not miniature adults. As the area of sport biomechanics has grown, the concentration on youth-specific studies has slowly increased. The growth factor in children complicates the analysis of data for youths since the subjects must be divided into small groups based on chronological age, physical activity levels or both neuromuscular and physiological stages of development (maturational age). The challenges for sports biomechanists in relation to youth sport and the rehabilitation and prevention of injuries are multifaceted. Biomechanics is an interdisciplinary area with results of studies being influenced by a multitude of factors. The following five topics are important research areas concerning sport-related injuries occurring in youth at different ages and levels of participation. As Meyers (1990) indicated, a need for recognition of age-specific, sport-specific injury patterns exists.

Table 12.3 Major biomechanical considerations of youth sport injuries. From Zito (1990).

Skeleton is immature and predisposed to breakdown

Each tissue has specific properties in terms of mechanical stress adaptation and levels

Repetitive loading of articular cartilage in the adolescent may undergo degenerative changes

Overuse injuries occur from excessive loading and can result in traction apophysitis or inflammation

Excessive tensile loading can result in injuries with considerable consequences

The epiphyseal growth plate is most vulnerable to torsional and shear forces

Injury to the epiphyseal plate can have the greatest effect on linear growth

Changes in the level of sport participation and activity will alter the effect on the musculoskeletal system

Sports booms often dictate the incidence of specific injuries

Persistent low back pain in young athletes is common and should be evaluated

- Growth patterns in children. The issues that need to be considered within this area include the variation in growth with age and gender and the timing of ossification of the growth plates. There have been limitations in the research on variation of growth with respect to gender and age including the many factors involved in the growth of bone, the large number of subjects needed for reliable data, and the antiquity of methods and populations in some of the studies. In relation to growth plate activity, Pritchett (1991) studied the growth plate activity in the upper and lower extremities of 244 children from age 7 to maturity. This study details the sites and timing of growth activity in the major bones of each extremity and indicates areas of ossification with respect to gender and age in a relatively homogeneous and healthy population of youths. A major advancement in understanding the effects on growth has been the determination that activity at the growth plates varies with age. The need exists for more studies on different populations which control for factors influencing growth.

- Changes in bone structure with participation in different sports activities. The effects of various forces on bone growth in relation to sports participation at different ages and levels are not well understood. The effects of the timing, duration and level of forces with respect to bone growth are often suggested through anecdotal or empirical data. More controlled studies of the effects of forces on immature bone would provide a better understanding of the effects of sporting activities. This challenge is twofold: (i) the forces associated with movements in various sports are not known for segments or entire youth populations in many cases; and (ii) the areas of higher incidence of injury have fortunately received the majority of interest to date (pitching, gymnastics and running), but still questions remain in these groups as well as other still relatively unexplored areas of sport.

- Anthropometric evaluation of children and adolescents. The calculation of forces based on centre of gravity and moment arm effects requires the knowledge of the lengths and body compositions of various segments of the body. Data for adult populations are in the literature (Drillis & Contini, 1966), but relatively little data exists for the spectrum of children and adolescents except for some length and girth data provided by the Product Safety Commission data (Snyder *et al.*, 1977). The procedures and sample size required for estimation equations for the centre of mass of the segments of the spectrum of ages of children is an extremely large project to undertake.

- Long-term effects of injuries in relation to the musculoskeletal systems of youth. The study of forces in sports activities would be the initial step in this area of concern. The optimal method of determining such information is to collect baseline information on young athletes and in a longitudinal study evaluate any change in techniques or training habits in relation to growth, advancement of skill and/or injuries. Documentation of the incidence and long-term effects of injury would be included. The limitations to this approach are many including: (i) differentiation of growth from skill enhancement effects; (ii) changes in technique due to growth versus compensatory motion; (iii) having baseline data which is dependent on predisposition to injury due to anatomical structure; and (iv) the need to collect data on a relatively frequent basis to document increments of changes in forces and movement patterns which occur. This project requires a large number of subjects and would probably be limited to a particular region of the body based on the sport activity chosen for analysis. The results of such studies would help to identify the forces related to injury, the long-term effect of injury to the young athlete, and the outcome of rehabilitation programmes.

- Differences between adults and children in response to physical stress. Recognition that differences exist between the mature and immature athlete encourages studies specific to youths to be conducted. As information addressing the differences between these groups becomes available, areas in which further research can be directed for the maximum benefit to all athletes can be identified.

The education of individuals involved in sports at all levels (athlete, coach, trainer and clinician) is important to help prevent and minimize the effects of injury to athletes. An important fact in the evaluation of any athlete is the effect of the many factors integrated into any performance or technique. The influences of development in terms of physical, physiological, neurological, motor control or psychological effects are key components of any analyses, particularly those of young athletes. The outcome of an extended knowledge of youth sports and related injuries can lead to improved performances, but more importantly improved health and fewer injuries in young athletes. This information could be applied during coaching and training towards the prevention of injuries as well as by the clinician treating those athletes with injuries in the most effective manner for the long-term benefit of all young athletes.

References

Adams, J.E. (1975) Injuries to the throwing arm. A study of traumatic changes in the elbow joints of boy baseball players. *Calif. Med.* **3**, 25–34.

Albright, J.A., Jokl, P., Shau, R. *et al.* (1978) Clinical studies of baseball pitchers: correlation of injury to throwing arm with method of delivery. *Am. J. Sports Med.* **6**, 15–21.

Alekseev, B.A. (1977) The influence of skiing races on the hand and foot skeleton of young sportsmen. *Arkhiv. Anatomii* (Leningrad) **72**, 35–9.

Alms, M. (1961) Fracture mechanics. *J. Bone Joint Surg.* **43B**, 162–6.

Aronen, J.G. (1985) Problems of the upper extremity in gymnasts. *Clin. Sports Med.* **4**, 61–71.

Bender, J.A., Pierson, J.K., Kaplan, H.M. & Johnson, A.J. (1964) Factors affecting the occurrence of knee injuries. *J. Assoc. Phys. Mental Rehab.* **18**, 130–5.

Benton, J. (1982) Epiphyseal fracture in sports. *Phys. Sports Med.* **10**(11), 63–71.

Binek R., Levisohn, E.M., Bersani, F. *et al.* (1988) Freiberg disease complicating unrelated trauma. *Orthopedics* **11**, 753–7.

Caine, D. & Lindner, K.J. (1984) Growth plate injury: a threat to young distance runners? *Phys. Sports Med.* **12**, 118–24.

Caine, D.J. & Lindner, K.J. (1985) Overuse injuries of growing bones: the young female gymnast at risk? *Phys. Sports Med.* **13**, 52–62.

Carter, S.R., Aldridge, M.J., Fitzgerald, R. & Davies, A.M. (1988) Stress changes of the wrist in adolescent gymnasts. *Br. J. Radiol.* **61**, 109–12.

Cavanagh, P.R. & Lafortune, M.A. (1980) Ground reaction forces in distance running. *J. Biomech.* **13**, 397–406.

Ciccantelli, P. (1994) Avoiding elbow pain. *Phys. Sports Med.* **22**(3), 65–6.

Clancy, W. Jr (1991) Running. In B. Reider (ed.) *Sports Medicine: The School Aged Athlete*, pp. 632–50. W.B. Saunders, Philadelphia.

Collins, H.R. & Evarts, C.M. (1971) Injuries to the adolescent athlete. *Postgrad. Med.* **49**, 72–8.

Congeni, J. (1994) Treating — and preventing — Little League elbow. *Phys. Sports Med.* **22**(3), 54–64.

Drillis, R. & Contini, R. (1966) *Body Segment Parameters*. Report No. 1163–03. Office of Vocational Rehabilitation, Department of Health, Education and Welfare, New York.

Ellman, H. (1975) Anterior angulation deformity of the radial head. An unusual lesion occurring in juvenile baseball players. *J. Bone Joint Surg.* **57**, 776–8.

Godshall, R.W., Hansen, C.A. & Rising, D.C. (1981) Stress fractures through the distal femoral epiphysis in athletes. *Am. J. Sports Med.* **9**, 114–16.

Goldberg, B., Whitman, P.A., Gleim, G.W. & Nicholas, J.A. (1979) Children's sports injuries: are they avoidable? *Phys. Sports Med.* **7**, 93–101.

Goldberg, M.J. (1980) Gymnastics injuries. *Orthop. Clin. N. Am.* **2**, 717–26.

Gozna, E. (1982) *Biomechanics of Musculoskeletal Injury*. Williams & Wilkins, Baltimore.

Grana, W.A. (1990) Injuries to the knee. In J.A. Sullivan & W.A. Grana (eds) *The Pediatric Athlete*, pp. 173–85. American Academy of Orthopaedic Surgeons, Park Ridge, IL.

Gugenheim, J.J. Jr Stanley, R.F., Woods, G.W. *et al.* (1976) Little League survey: the Houston study. *Am. J. Sports Med.* **4**, 189–200.

Hastings, H. & Simmons, B.P. (1984) Hand fractures in children. *Clin. Orthop.* **188**, 120–30.

Herndon, W.A. (1990) Injuries to the head, neck, and spine. In J.A. Sullivan & W.A. Grana (eds) *The Pediatric Athlete*, pp. 133–44. American Academy of Orthopaedic Surgeons, Park Ridge, IL.

Houston, S. (1979) More important than milk — the radiologists opportunity to teach bone dynamics. *Runner* (Canada) **17**, 47–54.

Hovelius, L. (1987) Anterior dislocation of the shoulder in teenagers and young adults: five year prognosis. *J. Bone Joint Surg.* **69a**, 393–9.

Jackson, D.W. (1979) Low back pain in young athletes: evaluation of stress reaction and discogenic problems. *Am. J. Sports Med.* **7**, 364–6.

Jackson, S.W., Silvino, N. & Reiman, P. (1989) Osteochondritis in the female gymnast's elbow. *Arthroscopy* **5**, 129–36.

Jacobs, R. & Ghista, D. (1981) A biomechanical basis for treatment injuries of the dorsolumber spine. In D.N. Ghista (ed.) *Osteoarthromechanics*, pp. 435–71. Hemisphere Publications, Washington.

Jones, H.H., Priest, J.D., Hayes, W.C. *et al.* (1977) Humeral hypertrophy in response to exercise. *J. Bone Joint Surg.* **59A**, 204–8.

Kato, S. & Ishiko, T. (1984) Obstructive growth of children's bone due to excess labor in remote countries. In S. Kato (ed.) *Proceedings of the International Congress of Sports Science*, Vol. 8, p. 127. University of Sports Science, Tokyo.

Kaufer, H. (1980) Mechanics of the treatment of hip injuries. *Clin. Orthop.* **146**, 53–61.

Krag, M., Pope, M. & Wilder, D. (1986) Mechanisms of spine trauma features of spinal fixation methods. Part I. 'Mechanisms' of injury. In D.N. Ghista (ed.) *Spinal Cord Injury Medical Engineering*. C.C. Thomas, Springfield, IL.

Kravitz, S.R., Murgia, C.J., Huber, S. & Saltrick, K.R. (1986) Biomechanical implications of dance injuries. In C.G. Shell (ed.) *The Dancer as an Athlete*, pp. 43–52. Human Kinetics, Champaign, IL.

Larson, R.L., Singer, K.M., Bergstrom, R. *et al.* (1976) Little League survey: the Eugene study. *Am. J. Sports Med.* **4**, 201–9.

Maffulli, N. (1989) Skeletal system: a limiting factor to sports performance? A brief review. *J. Orthop. Rheumatol.* **2**, 123–32.

Malina, R. (1969) Exercise as an influence upon growth. *Clin. Pediatr.* **8**, 16–26.

Malina, R. (1972) *Physical Education: An Interdisciplinary Approach.* Macmillan, New York.

Malina, R. (1983) Menarche in athletes: a synthesis and hypothesis. *Ann. Hum. Biol.* **10**, 1–24.

Maroon, J.C., Steele, P.B. & Berlin, A. (1980) Football head and neck injuries — an update. *Clin. Neurosurg.* **27**, 414–29.

Meyers, J.F. (1990) Injuries to the shoulder girdle and elbow. In J.A. Sullivan, W.A. Grana (eds) *The Pediatric Athlete*, pp. 145–53. American Academy of Orthopaedic Surgeons, Park Ridge, IL.

Micheli, L.J. (1979) Low back pain in the adolescent: differential diagnosis. *Am. J. Sports Med.* **7**, 362–4.

Micheli, L.J. (1983) Overuse injuries in children's sports: the growth factor. *Orthop. Clin. N. Am.* **14**, 337–60.

Micheli, L.J. (1988a) The incidence of injuries in children's sports. In E.W. Brown & C.R. Branta (eds) *Competitive Sports for Children and Youth*, pp. 279–84. Human Kinetics, Champaign, IL.

Micheli, L.J. (1988b) Strength training in the young athlete. In E.W. Brown & C.R. Branta (eds) *Competitive Sports for Children and Youth*. Human Kinetics, Champaign, IL.

Micheli, L.J. (1990) Strength training. In J.A. Sullivan & W.A. Grana (eds) *The Pediatric Athlete*, pp. 17–20. American Academy of Orthopaedic Surgeons, Park Ridge, IL.

Micheli, L.J. & Ireland, M.L. (1987) Prevention and management of calcaneal apophysitis in children: an overuse syndrome. *J. Pediatr. Orthop.* **7**, 34–8.

Micheli, L.J. & Santore, R. (1980) Epiphyseal fractures of the elbow in children. *Am. Fam. Phys.* **22**, 107–16.

Murray, R.F. Jr (1991) The role of the pediatrician and pediatric specialities in identifying disorders of the foot. In M.H. Jahss (ed.) *Disorders of the Foot and Ankle: Medical and Surgical Management*, 2nd edn, pp. 603–6. W.B. Saunders, Philadelphia.

Nanning, A.J. & Josaputra, H.A. (1987) Tibial tuberosity fractures in adolescents — report of a case and review of the literature. *Neth. J. Surg.* **39**(5), 144–6.

Nilson, S. & Rohas, A. (1978) Soccer injuries in adolescents. *Am. J. Sports Med.* **6**, 358–61.

Nocini, S. & Silvij, S. (1982) Clinical and radiological aspects of gymnast's elbow. *J. Sports Med. Phys. Fitness* **22**, 54–9.

Ogden, J.A., McCarthy, S.M. & Jokl, P. (1982) The painful bipartite patella. *J. Pediatr. Orthop.* **2**(3), 263–9.

Pappas, A.M. (1982) Elbow problems associated with baseball during childhood and adolescent. *Clin. Orthop.* **164**, 30–41.

Pappas, A.M. (1983) Epiphyseal injuries in sports. *Phys. Sports Med.* **11**(3), 140–8.

Peterson, C.A. & Peterson, H.A. (1972) Analysis of the incidence of injuries to the epiphyseal growth plate. *J. Trauma* **12**, 275–81.

Pizzutillo, P.D. (1990) Osteochondroses. In J.A. Sullivan & W.A. Grana (eds) *The Pediatric Athlete*, pp. 211–33. American Academy of Orthopaedic Surgeons, Park Ridge, IL.

Pritchett, J.W. (1991) Growth plate activity in the upper extremity. *Clin. Orthop. Rel. Res.* **268**, 235–42.

Priest, J.D., Jones, H.H., Tichenor, C.J.C. *et al.* (1977) Arm and elbow changes in expert tennis players. *Minn. Med.* **60**, 399–404.

Priest, J.D. & Weise, D.J. (1981) Elbow injury in women's gymnastics. *Am. J. Sports Med.* **9**, 288–95.

Radin, E. (1980) Relevant biomechanics in the treatment of musculoskeletal injuries and disorders. *Clin. Orthop.* **146**, 2–3.

Rarick, M.T.F. (1960) Exercise and growth. In W.R. Johnson (ed.) *Science and Medicine of Exercise and*

Sports, pp. 440–65. Harper Press, New York.

Robey, J.M., Blyth, C.S. & Mueller, F.O. (1971) Athletic injuries: application of epidemiological methods. *JAMA* **217**, 184–9.

Row, C.R. & Sakellarides, H.T. (1961) Factors related to recurrences of anterior dislocations of the shoulder. *Clin. Orthop.* **20**, 40–7.

Roy, S., Caine, D. & Singer, K.M. (1985) Stress changes of the distal radial epiphysis in young gymnasts. *Am. J. Sports Med.* **13**(5), 301–8.

Simonet, W.T. & Cofield, R.H. (1984) Prognosis in anterior shoulder dislocation. *Am. J. Sports Med.* **12**, 19–24.

Snyder, R.G., Scheider, L.W., Owings, C.L., Reynolds, H.M., Golomb, D.H. & Schork, M.A. (1977) *Anthropometry of Infants, Children, and Youths to Age 18 for Product Safety Design*. The Consumer Product Safety Commision, Contract CPSC-C-75-0068. Technical report. Highway Safety Research Institute, Ann Arbor, MI.

Souer, R. (1982) *Fractures of the Limbs: The Relationship Between Mechanism and Treatment*. C.C. Thomas, Springfield, IL.

Speer, D.P. & Braun, J.K. (1985) The biomechanical basis of growth plate injuries. *Phys. Sports Med.* **13**, 72–8.

Stanitski, C.L. (1982) Low back pain in young athletes. *Phys. Sportsmed.* **10**, 77–91.

Stanitski, C.L. (1990) Repetitive stress and connective tissue. In J.A. Sullivan & W.A. Grana (eds) *The Pediatric Athlete*, pp. 203–9. American Academy of Orthopaedic Surgeons, Park Ridge, IL.

Szot, Z., Boron, Z. & Galaj, Z. (1985) Overloading changes in the motor system occurring in élite gymnasts. *Int. J. Sports Med.* **6**, 36–40.

Taimela, S., Kujala, U.M. & Osterman, K. (1989) Individual characteristics are related to musculoskeletal injuries. *Proceedings of the Paavo Nurmi Congress*, August 28–September 1, Turku, Finland (abstract).

Teitz, C.C. (1982) Sports medicine concerns in dance and gymnastics. *Pediatr. Clin. N. Am.* **29**, 1399–421.

Tibone, J.E. (1983) Shoulder problems of adolescents. *Clin. Sports Med.* **2**, 423–6.

Torg, J.S., Pollack, H. & Sweterlisch, P. (1972) The effect of competitive pitching on the shoulders and elbows of preadolescent baseball pitchers. *Pediatrics* **49**, 267–72.

Totten, L. (1986) The prepubescent athlete: practical considerations in strengthening the prepubescent athlete. *Natl Strength Cond. Assoc. J.* **8**, 8–39.

Valliant, P.M. (1981) Personality and injury in competitive runners. *Percept. Motor Skills* **53**, 251–3.

Viano, D., King, A. & Melvin, J. (1989) Injury biomechanics research: an essential element in the prevention of trauma. *J. Biomech.* **5**, 403–17.

Walsh, W.M., Hunrman, W.W. & Shelton, G.L. (1985) Overuse injuries of the knee and spine in girls' gymnastics. *Orthop. Clin. N. Am.* **16**, 329–50.

Warner, J. & Micheli, L. (1991) Pediatric and adolescent musculoskeletal injuries. In W.A. Grana & A. Kalenak (eds) *Clinical Sports Medicine*, pp. 490–8. W.B. Saunders, Philadelphia.

Watson, A.W.S. (1981) Factors predisposing to sports injury in school boy rugby players. *J. Sports Med. Phys. Fitness* **21**, 417–22.

Weiman, J. & Sicher, H. (1955) *Bone and Bones: Fundamentals in Bone Biology*. C.V. Mosby, St Louis.

Wilkens, K.E. (1980) The uniqueness of the young athlete. Musculoskeletal injuries. *Am. J. Sports Med.* **8**, 377–85.

Williams, J.P. (1979) Wear and tear injuries in athletes, an overview. *Br. J. Sports Med.* **12**, 211–14.

Wong, J.C. & Gregg, J.R. (1984) Knee, ankle and foot problems in the preadolescent and adolescent athlete. *Clin. Pediatr. Med. Surg.* **3**, 731–46.

Wong, J.C. & Gregg, J.R. (1986) Knee, ankle and foot problems in the preadolescent and adolescent athlete. *Clin. Pediatr. Med. Surg.* **3**(4), 731–46.

Woods, G.W. & Tullos, H.S. (1977) Elbow instability and medial epicondyle fracture. *Am. J. Sports Med.* **5**, 23–30.

Yngve, D.A. (1990) Stress fractures in the pediatric athlete. In J.A. Sullivan & W.A. Grana (eds) *The Pediatric Athlete*, pp. 235–40. American Academy of Orthopaedic Surgeons, Park Ridge, IL.

Zito, M. (1990) Musculoskeletal injuries of young athletes: the new trends. In J.A. Gould III (ed.) *Orthopaedic and Sports Physical Therapy*, pp. 627–50. C.V. Mosby, St Louis.

Chapter 13

Overuse Injuries in the Young Athlete: Stress Fractures

LYLE J. MICHELI

Introduction

As children and adolescents have participated in increasing numbers in organized sport training, the occurrence of overuse injuries from repetitive microtrauma of overhand throwing or foot impact in running and jumping have been encountered.

Unfortunately, the details of the risk factors for injury are as yet not well understood. In addition, the presentation of these injuries may sometimes cause confusion with neoplastic lesions because of the abundant callous present in the child or the adolescent with stress fracture. What is presently known about risk factors for the occurrence of this overuse injury as well as typical sites of stress fracture in young athletes are reviewed.

Overuse injuries: an overview

Injuries sustained by young athletes in the course of athletic competition or training are well known to the coach, athletic administrator and sports medicine physician. Sports-related injuries occur from two different mechanisms or combinations thereof. (i) Acute macro-traumatic injuries are those which occur as a result of a single application of major force to an area of the body, such as a twisting injury of the ankle from a jump in basketball or a blow to the side of the leg in a football game. (ii) Repetitive microtrauma results in so-called overuse injuries which reflect repetitive micro-

stress to areas of the body over a prolonged period of time, typically seen in the training regimen for sports.

One of the recent and extremely healthy trends in sports medicine is to place paramount emphasis upon the prevention of injuries. Formerly, the great majority of physician attention in sport medicine was directed toward a proper diagnosis and appropriate treatment of sports-related injuries. This remains extremely important today, and the necessity for careful diagnosis and appropriate treatment cannot be overemphasized. In addition, however, the true sports medicine practitioner must assume responsibility for determining risk factors for the occurrence of injury, particularly training-related overuse injuries, as a first step in injury prevention. The prevention of sports-related injuries deserves equal emphasis in the armamentarium of the sports physician.

In recent years, we have gained more knowledge of the risk factors responsible for the occurrence of overuse injuries, particularly in young athletes (O'Neill & Micheli, 1988). Overuse injuries in this age group are being seen with increasing frequency in sports medicine clinics. There are undoubtedly a variety of reasons for this, including (i) the increased participation in organized sport by children and adolescents; (ii) the tendency towards increased specialization in one or, at the most, two sports by growing numbers of children; and (iii) the growing emphasis upon increased duration and complexity of training at younger

189

ages in a great variety of sports, particularly in the individual sports such as gymnastics, figure skating and swimming.

Overuse injuries may occur in a variety of different tissues in the young athlete. They have in common a history of repetitive training or cyclic low level forces applied to an anatomical structure with the probable association of certain anatomical or physiological susceptibilities in the affected individuals. These repetitive injuries can occur in articular cartilage, bone, muscle—tendon units or fascia.

Overuse injuries: stress fracture

The overuse injury of bone (stress fracture) has attracted particular attention in medicine and, specifically, athletic medicine. The first report of a stress fracture in the medical literature was that of the German military surgeon Breithaupt in 1855 who noted the occurrence of these lesions in young military recruits (Breithaupt, 1855). These lesions were subsequently identified as 'march fractures' because of their propensity for occurrence with military training. This entity has been identified in subsequent literature by a variety of terms, including fatigue fracture, spontaneous fracture, pseudofracture and insufficiency fracture.

Types of stress fracture

At the present time, stress fractures can be appropriately divided into two general categories: (i) insufficiency fractures; and (ii) fatigue fractures of bone. This division, first suggested by Pentecost et al. (1964), describes an insufficiency fracture as being produced by normal or physiological stresses applied to bone with deficient structural characteristics, while a fatigue fracture occurs when excessive cyclical stress is applied to bone of normal structure.

Stress fractures in children: different sites than adults

While traditionally, and certainly in adults,

stress fractures have been catalogued as those occurring in the metaphysis or diaphysis of bone and, in particular, long bones, it is appropriate at this time, particularly given additional information from the recent medical literature, to broaden the categories to include stress fractures occurring in the subchondral bone of the joint surface in children and adolescents and at the physeal plate of the child or adolescent.

It is important to note that the response of the growing skeleton to repetitive training is quite different than that of the fully mature skeleton. Stress fractures in the child or growing adolescent occur in a different pattern of injury involving different sites, both throughout the body and within the very structures of the bones involved, and also have a different clinical and radiographical presentation as well as healing response (Devas, 1963; Engh et al., 1970; Walter & Wolf, 1977). In the lower extremity, the tibia appears to be much more commonly affected than the fibula or bones of the foot as has been reported in the adult literature. In addition, fatigue fractures of the tibia in children tend to occur at the juncture of the diaphysis and metaphysis, while adult fractures more commonly in the diaphysis, in particular the distal third of the diaphysis of the tibia (Fig. 13.1).

Fibular fractures, which are much more common in the running adult, may also occur in the child. As opposed to tibial stress fractures, which are thought to be due to impact, fibular stress fractures may be related more to distraction and rotation forces occurring in the process of running or jumping.

Sports producing special risk

Additionally, there are certain trends between sports which reflect the different patterns of forces involved in these activities. Running sports characteristically involve fatigue fractures of the lower extremity but, in particular, of the tibia, fibula and foot (Devas & Sweetnam, 1956; Devas, 1958; Orava et al., 1978; Norfray et al., 1980; Orava & Hulkko, 1984; McBryde, 1985;

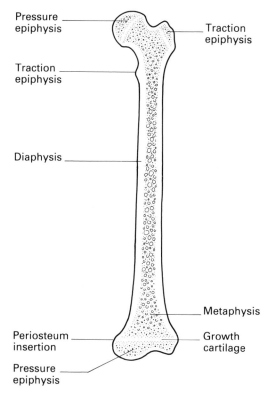

Pressure epiphysis

Traction epiphysis

Traction epiphysis

Diaphysis

Metaphysis

Periosteum insertion

Growth cartilage

Pressure epiphysis

Fig. 13.1 A schematic long bone of a child with epiphysis, metaphysis and diaphysis. Redrawn from Renström and Roux (1988).

Matheson *et al.*, 1987a,b). Certainly, stress fractures of the femur and pelvis can occur in runners, but these are less common. By contrast, the jumping sports, such as basketball, have been reported with a relatively higher incidence of stress fractures of the distal femur, pelvis and patella (Devas, 1960; Kaltsas, 1981). Overhand throwing and racquet sports are associated with stress fractures of the humerus, 1st rib and elbow (Miller, 1960; Allen, 1974; Belkin, 1980; Rettig, 1983; Lankenner & Micheli, 1985; Rettig & Beltz, 1985). Recent reports have demonstrated repetitive overuse physeal stress fractures of the distal radius and ulna in gymnasts and scaphoid stress fractures as well as articular surface osteochondral injuries of the elbow in gymnasts and throwers (Carter *et al.*, 1988; Albanese *et al.*, 1989).

Differential diagnoses

It is imperative for the sports physician dealing with a young athlete presenting with chronic pain always to include the possibility of stress fracture in the differential diagnoses. Fortunately, the clinical presentation in the child or adolescent with stress fracture may be more dramatic than that seen in the adult. In superficial bones, there may be an area of swelling or very localized tenderness and by radiographs, healing callous may be evident in response to the repetitive microfracture and subsequent partial healing at the site (Devas, 1963). This is less commonly true in the adult. A very careful history, taking into account the exact details of training and the equipment used in training, can help determine with some certainty that (i) an overuse injury is present; and (ii) what type of overuse injury and which tissue involved is most suspect. It is additionally important to remember, however, that infection or tumour may present chronically in the child or adolescent participating in organized sport competition or training. Since these entities are relatively more common in the musculoskeletal system of the child than in the adult, additional care must be taken when dealing with the young athlete presenting with extremity symptoms.

We have seen a fatigue fracture of the distal femur in a cross-country runner diagnosed unnecessarily late and initially confused with the chronic patellofemoral stress syndrome and treatment with exercise and icing to the knee. Additionally, we have seen a young athlete with pain at the knee treated again as patellofemoral stress syndrome with icing and exercise when the aetiology was actually an osteoid osteoma of the distal femur.

Risk factors

It is useful when assessing the young athlete complaining of chronic or training-related pain of gradual onset to have in mind a specific category of risk factors for overuse injuries when beginning the history and physical examination. These risk factors for overuse injuries are listed in Table 13.1 (O'Neill & Micheli, 1988).

Often two or more of these risk factors will appear to be acting in the occurrence of a given overuse injury. For example, a young athlete rapidly increases the volume of training while training in inadequately cushioned, older shoes and on surfaces which have become harder because of climatic changes such as lack of rain.

TRAINING ERROR

The most important risk factor for stress fracture is training error. It is the most frequently encountered risk factor in the development of overuse injuries in young athletes. The most important component of this appears to be an increase in the total volume and also the rate of progression of training (Nilsson & Westlin, 1971; Mustajoki et al., 1983; Swissa et al., 1989). But training error may be a risk factor in the highly skilled, élite athlete as well as the novice athlete just beginning training. We have learned empirically that most athletes should not increase their training more than 10% per week. In effect then, a young runner who is running $20 \, min \cdot day^{-1}$, 5 days$\cdot$week^{-1}, can probably safely increase to $22 \, min \cdot day^{-1}$, 5 days$\cdot$week^{-1}, the following week. Similarly, we have seen a case of an élite distance runner at college level who decreased his running training from 145

Table 13.1 Risk factors for overuse injury. Reproduced with permission from O'Neill and Micheli (1988).

Training error/error of technique
Muscle—tendon imbalance
Anatomical malalignment
Footwear
Playing surface
Associated disease state
Gender factors
Cultural deconditioning
Growth

---

to $97 \, km \cdot week^{-1}$ during a 3-week examination period. When he quickly resumed his previous training regimen of $145 \, km \cdot week^{-1}$, he developed a stress fracture of the tibia. Intensive summer sports camps specializing exclusively in one sport also increase the risk of overuse injury through training error. For example, youngsters intensely interested in soccer, who perhaps is playing a total of $8-10 \, h \cdot week^{-1}$ of soccer, may suddenly be put in a summer camp situation in which they are training in soccer $6 \, h \cdot day^{-1}$ for 5 days$\cdot$week^{-1}. This risk factor alone may be sufficient to encourage the onset of a tibial or fibular stress fracture.

MUSCLE—TENDON IMBALANCE

Muscle—tendon imbalance is perhaps the second most important risk factor in overuse injury in this age group. Growth may contribute to changes in the relative strength and flexibility of agonist or antagonist muscle groups across major joints in the young athlete and, in particular, the adolescent growth spurt in this instance (Micheli, 1983). A careful assessment of muscle—tendon characteristics should be done as a preparticipation assessment in young athletic candidates. This is particularly important with respect to the prevention of stress fractures. Matheson and Clement have proposed that muscle bulk and, in particular, the potential for muscle fatigue, may be an important contributory factor to the aetiology of stress fractures (Matheson et al., 1987b). In young athletes in particular, four different characteristics of growth should be assessed:

1 Decreases in flexibility in association with growth and, in particular, growth spurts.

2 Strength increases with growth which may not be uniform, additionally contributing to the imbalances about joints.

3 Sport-specific imbalances of muscle strength or flexibility which are related to the particular demands or training regimens of certain sports or activities.

4 Repetitive techniques, such as overhand throwing or swimming, which can actually

result in joint contractures and secondary asymmetrical stresses upon the bones and joints involved.

ANATOMICAL MALALIGNMENT

Anatomical malalignment, particularly of the spine and lower extremities, has been suggested as a contributory factor in the occurrence of overuse injuries in young athletes. The malalignments may include (i) discrepancies of leg length; (ii) abnormalities of hip rotation; (iii) coronal alignment of the femur and tibia, such as genu valgum or tibia vara; and (iv) excessive flattening of the arch or pronation of the foot. Unfortunately, no specific studies of risk factors for stress fracture in young athletes have yet been done. However, studies of military recruits have suggested a number of potential risk factors. Anatomical alignment of the hip, in particular, may contribute to the potential for stress fracture in the young athlete. Giladi et al. (1987) found that excessive external rotation of the hip in military recruits increased the risk of lower extremity stress fracture twofold compared with military recruits with less hip turnout or internal rotation. Similarly, there have been a number of clinical observations that tibia vara may increase the potential for tibial stress fracture in running athletes, particularly young female athletes (Engber, 1977; Dickson & Kichline, 1987). Excessive pronation has been discussed as a risk factor for overload of the entire lower extremity, including the potential for stress fractures (Dickson & Kichline, 1987). High-arched cavus feet, with their apparent decreased ability for impact absorption, have also been implicated in overuse injuries about the foot and lower leg in particular (Cornwell, 1984).

FOOTWEAR

Impact-absorbing qualities as well as the mechanical stabilization potential of footwear use in sports, particularly the running sports, appear to be an important component in the prevention of overuse injury (Milgrom et al., 1985). The importance of impact-absorbing materials in not only the hindfoot and heel area of the shoe, but also in the forefoot, has been noted (Cavanagh, 1980). A recent study of stress fractures of the foot in basketball players has also suggested that inadequately cushioned footwear may increase stress to these anatomical structures (Cavanagh et al., 1990).

PLAYING SURFACE

Clinical observation for a number of years has suggested that the relative hardness of the running or playing surface is a factor in the stress delivered to the lower extremities in sports. Observations of distance runners and dancers have suggested hardness of surface as a possible contributing factor in the occurrence of lower extremity stress fractures in particular (Washington, 1978; McMahon & Greene, 1979; Seals, 1983).

ASSOCIATED DISEASE STATE

In assessing the potential for overuse injury and, in particular, stress fracture, the overall health of the child, including pre-existent illnesses, particularly viral illnesses, hormonal conditions or any other factors which can affect the relative structural strength of the bones must be carefully assessed.

GENDER FACTORS

A number of recent studies have suggested deficient intake of calcium and vitamins in amenorrhoeic distance runners and ballet dancers. The combination of amenorrhoea, osteopenia and increased incidence of overuse injuries, particularly stress fractures, has been referred to as the 'female athlete triad'. Studies have shown significantly lower levels of bone mineral density in amenorrhoeic versus eumenorrhoeic female athletes matched by age, weight, sport and training regimen (Drinkwater et al., 1984; Warren et al., 1986; Warren, 1987).

Barrow and Saha (1988) found a 2:1 ratio of occurrence of stress fractures in amenorrhoeic versus menstruating runners, while another study of female athletes at Penn State University found 24% of the amenorrhoeic college athletes to have stress fractures, while the overall prevalence of stress fractures in female athletes was 9% (Cook *et al.*, 1987).

CULTURAL DECONDITIONING

At the present time, there is a great deal of debate regarding the relative level of fitness or question of declining levels of fitness in children in industrialized nations, particularly in the USA. It can be hypothesized that the child who is physically inactive will show a decline and a decreased level of fitness in its most basic sense in all the tissues of the body, particularly in the musculoskeletal tissues. The responses of the musculoskeletal system, particularly the bones, to increased levels of physiological stress are increases in bone size, density and strength. These improved physical characteristics from general physical activity would exert a protective effect on the child who begins progressive sport-specific athletic training and decrease the potential for overuse injuries in general and stress fractures in particular in the face of increased levels of sport training. Conversely, the relatively inactive and culturally deconditioned child who does an excessive amount of sitting at school, travels in cars and watches television not only has been demonstrated to have increased levels of obesity, but undoubtedly will demonstrate decreased levels of structural strength in bones and joints.

GROWTH

Growth is the telling characteristic of the child or young adolescent. With physeal closure, childhood ends; the adolescent approaches the adult stage of physical development and in turn the characteristics of the musculoskeletal system including bone changes dramatically.

Growth cartilage has been demonstrated to be more susceptible to repetitive trauma than adult cartilage, whether at the physis, articular surface or the apophyseal sites of major muscle−tendon insertions. Repetitive microtrauma to the growth plate from athletic activities has been suggested as an aetiological factor in adult-onset arthritis at both the hip and knee (Murray & Duncan, 1971; Bright *et al.*, 1974; Stulberg *et al.*, 1975).

There is a growing body of evidence demonstrating that repetitive microtrauma particularly of floor work and vaulting activities has resulted in a new overuse injury of the physeal plate in young gymnasts. The gymnast complaining of wrist pain with repetitive activities, particularly on hand impact, must be assessed very carefully for the possibility of either scaphoid stress fracture or distal radial physeal injury. This, in turn, can result in relative overgrowth of the ulna and progression of serious joint derangement at the wrist in this athletic age group.

The articular cartilage in the child is also undergoing endochondral ossification and is, in effect, a growth plate. Repetitive impact or shear stresses to the adult articular cartilage can result in mechanical disruption and the development of 'chondromalacia'. In the child, the response to similar repetitive forces appears to result in a 'stress fracture' of the subchondral bone. Osteochondritis dissecans of the capitellum in the child baseball pitcher or gymnast represents stress fractures of the subchondral bone in this age group. Similarly, osteochondritic defects at the knee, ankle and within the foot in runners, gymnasts and field sport players, as well as young dancers, may reflect similar abnormal stress fractures at the joint surface (Conway, 1937).

Osgood−Schlatter disease of the tibial tubercle is the best known apophyseal stress fracture. The general class of overuse injuries, entitled 'traction apophysitises', appears to be very similar in pattern of injury to stress fractures of long bone diaphysis and metaphysis (Ogden & Southwick, 1976; Micheli, 1987). Similar injuries occur at the heel (Sever's disease) and in the foot at the tarsal accessory navicular (Micheli & Ireland, 1987).

During periods of accelerated growth rate, particularly occurring in the summer seasons and during the adolescent growth spurt, where primary sites of growth are within the long bones, a relative tightness of the muscle–tendon units spanning these bones and joints may occur. Periods of 'growth spurt' may be followed by secondary transient increase in muscle–tendon tightness or imbalances of alignment which may increase the chance of overuse injury in general and stress fracture in particular. During these periods of rapid growth and increased susceptibility, careful attention must be given to supplemental exercises to combat these muscle imbalances as well as programmes which decrease the total volume of training.

Sites of stress fracture in young athletes

LOW BACK

Young athletes involved in sport with repetitive flexion or, in particular, repetitive extension manoeuvres of the back may have onset of back pain which ultimately is found to be due to a stress fracture through the pars intra-articularis of the lumbar spine.

These injuries were once thought to be primarily genetic or congenital in origin, but this has been largely disproved. It is now widely recognized that these are acquired lesions which result from repetitive stress to the lumbar spine. In most cases, ultimate fatigue failure occurs through the pars intra-articularis but, on occasion, this may also occur to the pedicle or facet of the spine.

Recent diagnostic techniques, including single photon emission computerized tomography (SPECT) bone scan, have greatly aided the early diagnosis of this injury, particularly before frank fracture has occurred through the pars (Fig. 13.2). In addition, however, the sports physician must be alert to the occurrence of this injury and have a very high index of suspicion for it based upon the history and physical examination. In a child involved in repetitive extension sports in particular, such as gymnastics, figure skating or dance, who complains of insidious onset of pain and who, on physical examination, is found to have pain with provocative hyperextension testing, a posterior element failure of the stress type must be presumed until proven otherwise.

If these lesions are detected early before fibrous union or non-union has occurred, there is a good potential for healing with relative rest or immobilization in spinal orthotics. Unfortunately, because the environment for fracture is that of distraction rather than compression, once the frank bone lesions have occurred, particularly if they have occurred bilaterally in the posterior elements, attainment of ultimate union can be much more difficult.

UPPER EXTREMITY

As noted above, stress fractures of the upper extremity in young athletes are relatively uncommon but certainly are to be suspected in the throwing sports or in sports involving repetitive impacting of the upper extremity. Stress fractures of the humerus and forearm occurring in the throwing sports appear to be due to repetitive torsional stress of the upper extremity. In the child athlete with open growth plates, this stress may be localized at the physeal plate and has been dubbed 'Little League shoulder' (Cahill et al., 1974). Frank rotational fractures through the humerus have occurred from throwing, and fractures of the forearm have also been reported in young athletes.

Repetitive impacting at the elbow in young athletes who have not yet reached full skeletal maturation can result in osteochondral lesions of the capitellum or partial avulsion injuries at the medial epicondyle of the elbow as a result of repetitive traction in secondary fatigue failure through the cartilage bone junction of the epicondyle. Fatigue fractures have also been reported across the olecranon from repetitive throwing in young athletes.

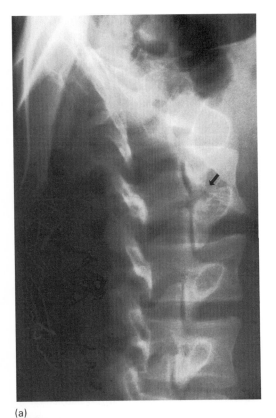

(a)

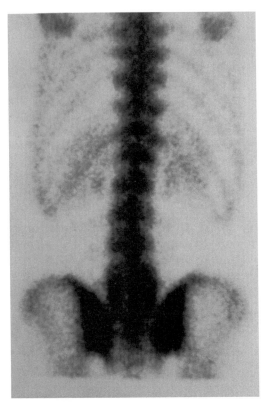

(b)

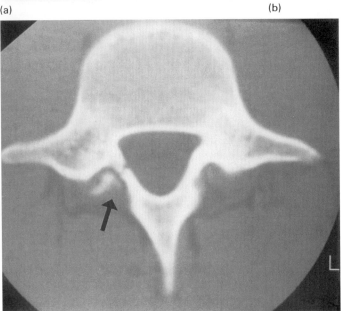

(c)

Fig. 13.2 (a) Oblique radiograph
of the lumbar spine
demonstrates fracture at the pars
intra-articularis of the 5th
lumbar vertebra (spondylolysis).
(b) Single photon emission
computerized tomography Te^{99}
bone scan demonstrating
increased radionucleotide
uptake at the site of bilateral
spondylolysis of the 5th lumbar
vertebra. (c) Computerized
tomography scan image
demonstrating a unilateral
spondylolysis of the lumbar
vertebra. Note the reactive
hypertrophy of the opposite pars
intra-articularis.

Fatigue fractures at the wrist have been reported as a result of repetitive impacting of the upper extremity in young athletes. Most notable have been the recent reports of physeal injury of the distal radius and ulna in young gymnasts. Stress fractures of the carponavicular have also been reported in this group of upper extremity athletes.

PELVIS AND HIP

Stress fractures about the pelvis and hip in young athletes are relatively unusual. These have been much more commonly reported in young female runners or athletes involved in jumping sports. Iliac crest stress injuries have been reported in young athletes as a result of repetitive training. Much more commonly in this age group, stresses about the pelvis will result in frank apophyseal avulsions (Micheli, 1990) (Fig. 13.3).

Stress fractures of the femur in young athletes have certainly been reported (Walter & Wolf, 1977). Distal stress fractures of the femur are much more common than proximal stress fractures. Occasionally, however, hip pain in the young athlete will ultimately be found to be due to a fracture of the base of the neck of the femur. Unfortunately, these stress fractures in young athletes have often been confused with the reports of stress fractures of the hip in military recruits. In military recruits, these have often been detected late with frank displacement of these fractures and a poor prognosis. In the young athlete, however, these are often compression-type stress fractures at the base of the femur and, if detected early enough, healing can be expected with relative rest and limited weight-bearing.

The stress fractures of the femur more commonly encountered in this age group are those of the distal femur. These can be encountered in the jumping sports but have also been seen in young runners. Very often the first complaint in this fracture is that of knee pain. The diagnosis may not be suspected early on. We have encountered cases of frank displacement of these fractures in this age group.

ANKLE AND FOOT

The complaint of ankle pain in young athlete undergoing repetitive training may also be due to stress fracture occurring at this site. Stress fractures of the medial malleolus have been encountered in this age group and, again, partial avulsions of the medial malleolus in younger children engaged in repetitive training activities and running have been reported (Stanitski & Micheli, 1993).

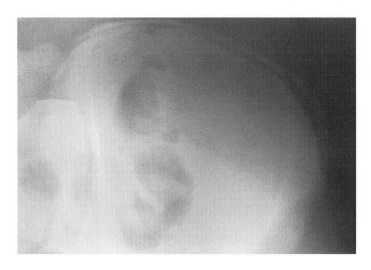

Fig. 13.3 Stress fracture of the iliac crest apophysis in a young runner resulting in pain, tenderness and limp.

Stress fractures of the foot may also occur in young athletes. While stress fractures of the body of the os calcis are relatively rare in this age group, apophyseal injury from repetitive training, such as Sever's apophysitis at the heel and painful accessory navicular in the midfoot, have been reported (Micheli, 1987; Micheli & Ireland, 1987).

Two stress fractures of the foot in young athletes bear special mention. Stress fractures of the tarsal navicular may present as low grade, aching midfoot pain (Fig. 13.4). Too often, the

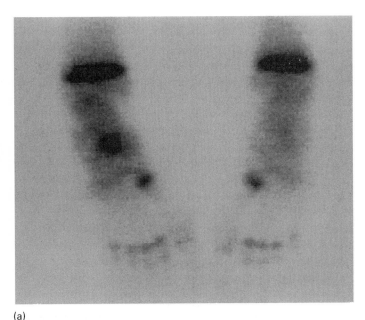

(a)

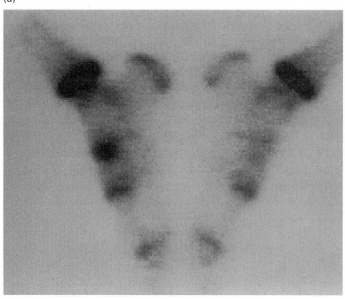

(b)

Fig. 13.4 (a) Anteroposterior and (b) lateral views of Te^{99} bone scan demonstrating increased radionucleotide uptake at the site of a right tarsal navicular stress fracture.

diagnosis is not made sufficiently early. This appears to be due to the fact that these pains are often non-specific and associated with repetitive running in particular. Often plain radiographs are unremarkable early on, and the diagnosis is not made until frank fracture has occurred through the navicular. Early detection, of course, can be made with bone scan, and dissection of the frank fracture is often possible only with computerized tomography (CT) scanning. Delayed detection of this fracture is doubly unfortunate because this is a bone with a slow rate of healing and a relatively high rate of complications develop from this fracture.

The second site of difficult stress fracture in the foot in young athletes is that of the base of the 5th metatarsal. Once again, these stress fractures are often detected late after they have become fully established. This is a slow healing bone, sometimes requiring internal fixation to attain satisfactory union of the stress fractures in the proximal third of the 5th metatarsal. Other special stress fractures have been encountered in young athletes undergoing repetitive training, including stress fractures of the proximal 2nd metatarsal, as well as the shaft of the metatarsal which is much better known.

Prevention of stress fracture in young athletes

This discussion of stress fractures in young athletes has emphasized early detection of risk factors for stress fracture in order to aid in the early diagnosis and the prevention of later complications when dealing with this entity. In most of these stress fractures, early diagnosis results in a much simpler mechanism of treatment and, in many cases, ensures satisfactory union with ability to resume progressive athletic training without problem.

In addition, however, as our understanding of the risk factors for the occurrence of this serious overuse injury increases, it will hopefully be possible to detect individuals with a special propensity for stress fractures, particularly at certain sites of the body. Steps may then be taken to prevent the occurrence of these injuries by careful management of training regimens, protective footwear or playing surfaces.

Challenges for future research

The major thrust of any repetitive or training injury in athletes of any age should be determination of risk factors for injury and steps to prevent the occurrence of these injuries. At the present time, there is growing knowledge about risk factors for the occurrence of both acute traumatic injuries and repetitive microtrauma overuse injuries in adults, particularly in such activities as military training, work activities and sports.

• All too little is known about the details of risk factors for overuse injury, particularly stress fractures in young athletes. The presence of physeal cartilage at the joint surface, epiphyseal plate and apophyseal sites of major muscle tendon insertions appears to alter the presentation and the occurrence of stress injuries to bone, but this has not been well studied or well researched in either animal models or human epidemiological studies.

• At the clinical level, much more information could be gained about these injuries by establishing a clinical registry of stress fractures in young athletes in which the occurrence of injury and the determination of associated risk factors could be recorded in addition to epidemiological data of age, gender, height and weight, and, if possible, Tanner index.

• Epidemiological studies in sport-specific environments in which the population at risk is well known would add greatly to the understanding of the particular sport activities which carry the greatest risk of the occurrence of overuse injuries and stress fractures, in particular.

• More basic research is needed in the study of response of bone to repetitive training. Little is presently known as to changes in tertiary structure, numbers of haversian systems, bone mineral density and size dimensions of long bones in response to repetitive training. The relationship of repetitive training to longitudinal transverse and circumferential bone growth in children and adolescents participating in repetitive training is now well known. Human studies of this phenomenon as well as the development of an animal model to study repetitive training and its effects upon the strength, dimensions and 'fitness' level of the musculoskeletal system remains to be developed.

References

Albanese, S.A., Plamer, A.K., Kerr, D.R., Carpenter, C.W., Lisi, D. & Levinsohn, E.M. (1989) Wrist pain and distal growth plate closure of the radius in gymnasts. *J. Pediatr. Orthop.* **9**, 23–8.

Allen, M.E. (1974) Stress fracture of the humerus: a case study. *Am. J. Sports Med.* **12**, 244–5.

Barrow, G.W. & Saha, S. (1988) Menstrual irregularity and stress fractures in collegiate female distance runners. *Am. J. Sports Med.* **16**, 209–16.

Belkin, S.C. (1980) Stress fractures in athletes. *Orthop. Clin. N. Am.* **11**, 735–42.

Breithaupt, M.D. (1855) Zur pathologie des menschlichen Fusses (The pathology of human feet). *Med. Zeitung* **24**, 169–71, 175–7.

Bright, R.W., Burstein, A.H. & Elmore, S.M. (1974) Epiphyseal plate–cartilage. A biomechanical and histological analysis and failure modes. *J. Bone Joint Surg.* **56A**, 688–703.

Cahill, B.R., Tullos, H.S. & Fain, R.H. (1974) Little League shoulder. *J. Sports Med.* **2**, 150–3.

Carter, S.R., Aldridge, M.J., Fitzgerald, R. *et al.* (1988) Stress changes of the wrist in adolescent gymnasts. *Br. J. Radiol.* **61**, 109–12.

Cavanagh, P.R. (1980) *The Running Shoe Book*. Anderson World, Mountain View, CA.

Cavanagh, P.R., Robinson, J., McClay, I.S. *et al.* (1990) *Med. Sci. Sports Exerc.* **22** (Suppl.), S104.

Conway, F.M. (1937) Osteochondritis dissecans: description of the stages of the condition and its probable traumatic etiology. *Am. J. Surg.* **38**, 691.

Cook, S.D., Harding, A.F., Thomas, K.A., Morgan, E.L., Schnurpfeil, K.M. & Haddad, R.J. (1987) Trabecular bone density and menstrual function in women runners. *Am. J. Sports Med.* **15**, 503–7.

Conrwell, G. (1984) Sports medicine and the cavus foot. *Br. Columb. Med. J.* **26**, 573–4.

Devas, M.B. (1958) Stress fractures of the tibia in athletes or 'shin soreness'. *J. Bone Joint Surg.* **40B**, 227–39.

Devas, M.B. (1960) Stress fractures of the patella. *J. Bone Joint Surg.* **42B**, 71–4.

Devas, M.B. (1963) Stress fractures in children. *J. Bone Joint Surg.* **45B**, 528–41.

Devas, M.B. & Sweetnam, R. (1956) Stress fractures of the fibula: a review of 50 cases in athletes. *J. Bone Joint Surg.* **38B**, 818–29.

Dickson, T.B. & Kichline, P.D. (1987) Functional management of stress fractures in female athletes using a pneumatic leg brace. *Am. J. Sports Med.* **15**, 86–9.

Drinkwater, B.L., Nilson, K., Chestnut, C.M. *et al.* (1984) Bone mineral content of amenorrheic and eumenorrheic athletes. *New Engl. J. Med.* **311**, 277–81.

Engber, W.D. (1977) Stress fractures of the medial tibial plateau. *J. Bone Joint Surg.* **59A**, 767–9.

Engh, C.A., Robinson, R.A. & Milgram, J. (1970) Stress fractures in children. *J. Trauma* **10**, 532–41.

Giladi, M., Milgrom C., Stein, M. *et al.* (1987) External rotation of the hip. A predictor of risk for stress fractures. *Clin. Orthop. Rel. Res.* **216**, 131–4.

Kaltsas, D.-S. (1981) Stress fractures of the femoral neck in young adults. *J. Bone Joint Surg.* **63B**, 33–7.

Lankenner, P.A. & Micheli, L.J. (1985) Stress fracture of the first rib. *J. Bone Joint Surg.* **67A**, 159–60.

McBryde, A.M. (1985) Stress fractures in runners. *Clin. Sports Med.* **4**, 737–52.

McMahon, T.A. & Greene, P.R. (1979) The influence of track compliance on running. *J. Biomech.* **12**, 893–904.

Matheson, G.O., Clement, D.B., McKenzie, D.C. *et al.* (1987a) Scintigraphic update of ^{99m}Tc at non-painful sites in athletes with stress fractures: the concept of bone strength. *Sports Med.* **4**, 65–75.

Matheson, G.O., Clement, D.B., McKenzie, D.C., Taunton, J.E., Lloyd-Smith, D.R. & MacIntyre, J.B. (1987b) Stress fractures in athletes: a study of 320 cases. *Am. J. Sports Med.* **15**, 46–58.

Micheli, L.J. (1983) Overuse injuries in children's sports: the growth factor. *Orthop. Clin. N. Am.* **14**(2), 337–60.

Micheli, L.J. (1987) The traction apophysitises. *Clin. Sports Med.* **6**(2), 389–404.

Micheli, L.J. (1990) Injuries to the hip and pelvis. In J.A. Sullivan & W.A. Grana (eds) *The Pediatric Athlete*, pp. 167–72. American Academy of Orthopaedic Surgeons, Park Ridge, IL.

Micheli, L.J. & Ireland, M.L. (1987) Prevention and management of calcaneal apophysitis in children: an overuse syndrome. *J. Pediatr. Orthop.* **7**, 34–8.

Milgrom, C., Giladi, M., Kashtan, H. *et al.* (1985) A prospective study of the effect of a shock absorbing orthotic device on the incidence of stress fractures in military recruits. *Foot Ankle* **6**, 101–4.

Miller, J.E. (1960) Javeline thrower's elbow. *J. Bone Joint Surg.* **42B**, 788–92.

Murray, R.O. & Duncan, C. (1971) Athletic activity in adolescence as an etiologic factor in degenerative hip disease. *J. Bone Joint Surg.* **53B**, 406−19.

Mustajoki, P., Laapio, H. & Meurmann, K. (1983) Calcium metabolism, physical activity, and stress fractures. *Lancet* **ii**, 797.

Nilsson, B.E. & Westlin, N.E. (1971) Bone density in athletes. *Clin. Orthop. Rel. Res.* **77**, 179−82.

Norfray, J.F., Schlacteri, L., Kernahan, W.T. *et al.* (1980) Early confirmation of stress fractures in joggers. *JAMA* **243**, 1647−9.

Ogden, J.A. & Southwick, W.O. (1976) Osgood−Schlatter disease and tibial tuberosity development. *Clin. Orthop. Rel. Res.* **116**, 180−9.

O'Neill, D.B. & Micheli, L.J. (1988) Overuse injuries in the young athlete. *Clin. Sports Med.* **7**(3), 591−610.

Orava, S. & Hulkko, A. (1984) Stress fracture of the mid-tibial shaft. *Acta Orthop. Scand.* **55**, 35−7.

Orava, S., Purenan, J. & Ala-Ketole, L. (1978) Stress fractures caused by physical exercise. *Acta Orthop. Scand.* **49**, 19−27.

Pentecost, R.L., Murray, R.A., Brindley, H.H. *et al.* (1964) Fatigue, insufficiency, and pathological fractures. *JAMA* **187**, 1001−4.

Renström, P. & Roux, C. (1988) Clinical implications of youth participation in sports. In A. Dirix, H.G. Knuttgen & K. Tittel (eds) *The Encyclopaedia of Sports Medicine*, Vol. 1. *The Olympic Book of Sports Medicine*, p. 474, Blackwell Scientific Publications, Oxford.

Rettig, A.C. (1983) Stress fracture of the ulna in an adolescent tournament tennis player. *Am. J. Sports Med.* **11**, 103−9.

Rettig, A.C. & Beltz, M.F. (1985) Stress fracture in the humerus in an adolescent tournament tennis player. *Am. J. Sports Med.* **13**, 55−8.

Seals, J.G. (1983) A study of dance surfaces. *Clin. Sports Med.* **2**, 557−61.

Stanitski, C.L. & Micheli, L.J. (1993) Observations on symptomatic medial malleolar ossification centers. *J. Pediatr. Orthop.* **13**, 164−8.

Stulberg, S.D., Cordell, L.D., Harris, W.H. *et al.* (1975) Unrecognized childhood hip disease: a main course of idiopathic osteoarthritis of the hip. In *The Hip: Proceedings of the Third Open Scientific Meeting of the Hip Society*, pp. 212−28. C.V. Mosby, St Louis.

Swissa, A., Milgrom, C., Giladi, M. *et al.* (1989) The effect of pretraining sports activity on the incidence of stress fractures among military recruits. A prospective study. *Clin. Orthop. Rel. Res.* **245**, 256−60.

Walter, N.E. & Wolf, M.D. (1977) Stress fractures in young athletes. *Am. J. Sports Med.* **5**, 165−70.

Warren, M.P. (1987) Excessive dieting and exercise. The dangers for young athletes. *J. Musculoskel. Med.* **4**, 31−40.

Warren, M.P., Brooks-Gund, J., Hamilton, L.M. *et al.* (1986) Scoliosis and fractures in young ballet dancers: relation to delayed menarche and secondary amenorrhea. *New Engl. J. Med.* **314**, 1348−53.

Washington, E.L. (1978) Musculoskeletal injuries in theatrical dancers: site, frequency, and severity. *Am. J. Sports Med.* **6**, 75−98.

Chapter 14

Matching of Opponents in Youth Sports

ROBERT M. MALINA AND GASTON BEUNEN

Introduction

Youth sports programmes are generally aimed at mass participation. Variation in size, biological maturity status, strength, skill and behavioural development in the age range with high numbers of youth sports participants (8–12 years) is considerable. Given such variability among children and youths, attempts to equalize competition, to enhance chance for success and to reduce injury associated with size and strength mismatches are often discussed and are occasionally incorporated into youth sports programmes.

Many programmes have different competitive levels based on chronological age (CA) and skill. 'Try outs' permit coaches, most of whom are volunteers, to assess the basic skills of each youngster. However, as youngsters enter the transitional years from childhood into puberty, individual differences in size, strength and skill associated with variation in biological maturity status are magnified (see Chapters 1 and 39). Size, strength and skill mismatches are rather common in many youth sports in spite of efforts to equate participants for competition. The potential competitive inequity and increased risk of injury associated with such mismatches are especially evident in contact and collision sports. Matching participants by body size and biological maturity status is often indicated as an important means of reducing size, strength and skill mismatches in youth sports (e.g. Gallagher, 1969; Seefeldt,

1981; Caine & Broekhoff, 1987). This chapter addresses several issues related to matching children and youths for sport competition with primary emphasis on contact and collision sports.

Contact and collision sports

The classification of sports recommended by the American Academy of Pediatrics (1988) is summarized in Table 14.1. In addition to contact or collision with opponents or equipment handled by an opponent, contact with the playing surface is also a significant concern. Matching children and youths is ordinarily used in the context of the former, i.e. contact with opponents or equipment handled by an opponent. Boxing is listed among the sports, though it is the view of the authors of this chapter that boxing should not be a youth sport.

Matching criteria

Matching in youth sports is viewed largely in terms of CA, sex, skill level, body size (most often body weight and then stature) and biological maturation status (almost exclusively in terms of sexual maturity). Skill, strength, size and maturity status are highly interrelated, especially in boys. Sex differences in maturational timing and in size, strength and skill, which become especially apparent about 12–14 years of age, should also be recognized.

Table 14.1 Classification of sports, adapted from the Committee on Sports Medicine, American Academy of Pediatrics (1988).

Contact/collision	Limited contact/impact
Boxing	Baseball
Field hockey	Basketball
Football	Bicycling
Ice hockey	Diving
Lacrosse	Field: high jump, pole vault
Martial arts	Gymnastics
Rodeo	Horse riding
Soccer	Skating: ice, roller
Wrestling	Skiing: cross-country, downhill, water
	Softball
	Squash, handball
	Volleyball

Chronological age

Participants in agency-sponsored youth sports are most often grouped on the basis of CA, the age of the child based on his or her date of birth. A CA category is commonly of 2 years duration. However, limited numbers of participants in some programmes, especially in smaller communities, may result in broader age categories that may span up to 4 years. Although 2 years appears to be a relatively narrow range, during the transition into puberty, 9–11 years in girls and 10–12 in boys, there is considerable variation in size, strength and skill among children of the 'same' CA. For example, two children whose ages are, respectively, 10 and 10.9 years, are classified as 10 years of age although almost 1 year separates them.

The limitation of CA for grouping youths in either child labour, school or sport was recognized early in this century. Crampton (1908, p. 142), for example, advocated the use of 'physiological age' based on the development of pubic hair rather than CA in an attempt '...to establish an age — in the child labor movement — above which a child may safely work and under which he may not'. Similarly, Rotch (1908) seriously questioned the utility of CA:

When, however, the question of age is brought to bear on our school systems, whether in classifying and grading children as to their studies, or *in pitting them against each other in athletic sports*, it becomes a very serious question as to whether chronological age is a wise decision during the formative period of life. (our italics)

Further, Rotch (1909) states that it

does not necessarily mean that...[because an individual]...is 10 or 12 chronological years of age, it should necessarily be grouped in athletics with boys or girls of that chronological age.... Anatomic age...would be a much better criterion.

In contrast to Crampton (1908) who advocated the use of 'physiological age' based on the assessment of pubic hair, Rotch (1909) advocated 'anatomic age' based on X-rays of the carpals.

An issue related to age grouping in youth sports deals with cut-off dates for a season. The selection of the cut-off point for age is somewhat arbitrary and a youngsters's fate in sport may be dictated by the calendar. An example from the highly organized sport of baseball in the USA provides evidence of this. Little League baseball has a CA limit of 12 years as of 1 August of the current season, i.e. the boy has not reached his 13th birthday by 1 August. Boys born on 1 and 2 August 1980, would thus be classified differently. The boy born on 1 August is classified as a 13 year old and is too old for Little League because he is 13 years as of 1 August 1993, while the boy born on 2 August plays as a 12 year old. The latter boy is an 'old' 12 year old, while the former is a 'young' 13 year old and must play in the older league (PONY League baseball for 13- and 14-year-old boys). The same problem is of concern to virtually all organized youth sports throughout the world.

Within a single chronological year, there is considerable variation in size, strength and skill, a good deal of which is related to individual differences in biological maturation (see below). Such variability emphasizes the need to use narrower CA categories for youth sports during the transition into puberty and during puberty. Cut-off points for a sport should be set quite close to the actual playing age.

Sex

Many youth sports are offered on a coeducational basis during middle childhood (about 6–10 years). Some sports permit coeducational participation up to about 12 years of age, but subsequently participation in the majority of youth sports is sex-limited. It is at about 12–13 years of age that sex differences in maturational timing and related sex differences in size and strength, and to a lesser extent skill, become more pronounced (Malina & Bouchard, 1991). Hence, coeducational participation in contact and collision sports should be advised with caution.

Skill and experience

Each sport has specific skill demands. Hence, level of skill and previous experience in the sport should be considered in the matching process. Many agencies which sponsor youth sports have several competitive levels aligned on the basis of proficiency in the skill demands of the sport. Initial assessment of skill levels of participants is a major concern. The majority of coaches in youth sports are volunteers, and many have personal experience in the particular sport. However, they may not have had experience with children and youths in the context of sport and in the assessment of skill. In addition, many volunteer coaches have a child of their own involved in the sport which may complicate the initial assessment process.

Ideally, assessment of skill levels of children for a specific sport should be performed by individuals who are not involved in coaching and who do not have their own children involved. Children should then be assigned to a team and then the team assigned to a coach. Drafting players, lotteries, recruiting of players,

and so on often creates extreme competitiveness, and at times ill will, among coaches and parents, and occasionally among the children.

Body size

It is misleading to match participants for sport by body size independent of CA and biological maturity status, given the close interrelationships among them. Further, as youngsters enter the transition into puberty, variability in stature and weight within a CA group is magnified. (See Tables 39.1 and 39.2 for percentiles for stature and weight.)

Matching by size, especially body weight, is common in American football, although some question the need for it as indicated in the following comment: 'Disparity of size is always a reality in football, so why not have the youngsters adapt to it at an earlier age?' (Stockwell, 1976). The potential for injury associated with size mismatches in sports which feature body contact on a regular basis, e.g. football, ice hockey and soccer, is very real and should be of concern to those involved in these sports. Age and weight limits in American youth football leagues (Pop Warner) are rather broad. For example, in the 7–9 year classification, the permitted weight range at the beginning of the season is 18.1–34 kg with an end of season maximum of 36.7 kg, i.e. the player may not be beyond the latter weight at the end of the season. The corresponding weight range for the 13–15 year olds at the beginning of the season is 54.4–72.6 kg with an end of season maximum weight of 75.3 kg. Clearly, size mismatches between runners and tacklers can be considerable.

The strength and impact force disparities between large and small boys are large. These are shown in Table 14.2 for Pee Wee ice hockey players. The CA limits for Pee Wee hockey are 12–13 years (i.e. 12–13.99). In Pee Wee hockey, 1 January is the cut-off date. If a boy is 12 years of age as of 1 January and is not 14 years of age as of 1 January of the particular season (which begins in the autumn), he is in the Pee Wee division. Thus, boys who are still 11 years of age, but who reach their 12th birthday by 1 January are eligible, and boys who are still 13 years by 1 January (i.e. have not reached their 14th birthday) are also eligible even though they will turn 14 after 1 January. Table 14.2 shows the size, strength and impact force of eight small and eight large players from the extremes in four leagues. The large ice hockey players are not only chronologically older, but, on average, they are considerably taller, have double the body mass and strength, and generate markedly greater impact force than the small players (Roy et al., 1989).

The implication of size, strength and power discrepancies for injury potential in contact sports should be obvious. Body checking is permitted in Pee Wee hockey, but some leagues do not permit it. The injury differential in leagues which permit and do not permit body checking is more than threefold (Table 14.3). About 78% of the injuries in the leagues which permitted body checking were caused by either the opponent (56%) or his stick, i.e. a part of his equipment (22%) (Roy et al., 1989).

In addition to size discrepancies *per se*, two boys of the same body weight but of different CA, e.g. a 50-kg 10-year-old boy and a 50-kg 12-year-old boy, most likely also differ in experience, stature, body composition, maturity, skill and strength.

Table 14.2 Age, body size, strength, speed and impact force of eight small and eight large Pee Wee ice hockey players. Adapted from Roy et al. (1989).

Variable	Small		Large	
	Mean	SD	Mean	SD
Age (years)	13.4	0.7	14.0	0.2
Weight (kg)	37.1	3.8	74.3	8.2
Stature (cm)	147.4	6.5	178.9	4.1
Grip strength (kg)	27.7	4.8	56.5	6.5
Maximal speed ($m \cdot s^{-1}$)	7.6	0.4	8.3	0.9
Impact force (N)	1010.0	111.0	1722.0	326.0
Speed at impact ($m \cdot s^{-1}$)	3.2	0.2	3.7	0.4

Table 14.3 Type and anatomical location of injuries in Pee Wee ice hockey games with and without body checking. Adapted from Roy et al. (1989).

	With body checking (n)	Without body checking (n)
Number of games observed	19	24
Number of injuries	54	16
Type of injury		
contusion	39	11
abrasion	4	2
strain	2	1
concussion	1	1
laceration	1	—
pain	1	—
other	6	1
Anatomical site		
lower limb	13	6
head	9	2
neck	9	1
upper limb	9	2
back	8	2
trunk	3	1
vertebral column	2	2
other	1	—

Biological maturation

The most commonly used indicators of biological maturity status for purposes of maturity matching are the secondary sex characteristics: external genitalia (G) and pubic hair (PH) in males, and breasts (B), PH and menarche in females. The criteria for each characteristic and methods of assessment are discussed in Chapter 39 (see also Malina & Bouchard, 1991). Briefly, G, B and PH development are evaluated on a five stage scale, with 1 representing absence of development, 2 initial development or appearance, 3 and 4 intermediate stages, and 5 adult status. Stage 1 refers to the prepubescent state. The appearance of stage 2 marks the onset of pubescence; individuals in stages 2, 3 and 4 are pubescent. Those in stage 5 are adult. Several issues related to matching children and youth for sport on the basis of sexual maturity status are considered subsequently.

An important logistical problem is the assessment of sexual maturity status. Ideally, this should be performed during a clinical examination. However, some have recommended self-assessment for maturity matching in young sports (Kreipe & Gewanter, 1985; Caine & Broekhoff, 1987). Self-assessment of sexual maturation is discussed in Chapter 39. An issue related to youth sports is the potential problem for a youngster to under- or overevaluate his or her maturity status for the purpose of staying with his or her friends. Or, potential pressure from parents or coaches to have an athlete underassess his or her maturity status for the sake of competitive advantage within a particular CA group.

Which specific indicators of sexual maturation status should be used in matching? Correlations between ages at attaining corresponding stages of B and PH development in girls and between stages of G and PH development in boys are moderate to high. Nevertheless, there is considerable variation so that the specific stages, e.g. B2 and PH2 in girls or G3 and PH3 in boys, are not equivalent.

VARIATION IN CRITERIA

Distributions of stages of B and PH development and of G and PH development in British and Swiss girls and boys, respectively, are shown in Tables 14.4 and 14.5. The concentration of girls and boys along the diagonal from left to right in the tables illustrates the overall relatedness of the maturation of these secondary sex characteristics; there is also considerable variation. For example, at PH3 and PH4, stages B1–B5 are represented in the British girls and stages B2–B5 are represented in the Swiss girls (Table 14.4). The same variation is apparent in the distribution of stages of PH development at B3; all five PH stages are represented.

Similar trends are evident in boys (Table 14.5). At PH2, British and Swiss boys are distributed across G1–G4. At G4, stages PH1–PH4 are represented in British boys and PH2–PH5 are represented in Swiss boys. The distributions of PH stages in the British boys are confounded to some extent by difficulties in detecting initial appearance of PH on photographs.

Table 14.4 Percentage of British and Swiss girls in each stage of breast (B) development when they reached each stage of pubic hair (PH) development (top), and in each stage of PH development when they reached each stage of B development (bottom).

PH stage	Percentage in each B stage (British)*						Percentage in each B stage (Swiss)†					
	n	B1	B2	B3	B4	B5	n	B1	B2	B3	B4	B5
PH2	88	16	49	27	8	0	103	49	46	5	0	0
PH3	93	3	23	50	24	1	114	0	36	51	12	1
PH4	102	2	4	43	45	6	106	0	4	47	33	16
PH5	80	0	1	11	49	39	99	0	1	6	34	59

B stage	Percentage in each PH stage (British)*						Percentage in each PH stage (Swiss)†					
	n	PH1	PH2	PH3	PH4	PH5	n	PH1	PH2	PH3	PH4	PH5
B2	89	61	29	8	2	0	110	16	67	16	1	0
B3	94	22	28	33	16	1	115	2	26	50	20	2
B4	97	4	10	24	51	11	80	0	4	28	43	25
B5	61	0	2	7	36	56	102	0	0	7	29	64

* Adapted from Marshall and Tanner (1969).
† Adapted from Largo and Prader (1983a).

Table 14.5 Percentage of British and Swiss boys in each stage of genital (G) development when they reached each stage of pubic hair (PH) development (top), and in each stage of PH development when they reached each stage of G development (bottom).

PH stage	Percentage in each G stage (British)*						Percentage in each G stage (Swiss)†					
	n	G1	G2	G3	G4	G5	n	G1	G2	G3	G4	G5
PH2	115	1	13	45	41	0	104	9	54	33	4	0
PH3	115	0	4	17	75	4	100	0	9	49	37	5
PH4	104	0	0	6	65	29	110	0	0	6	64	30
PH5	104	0	0	0	10	90	113	0	0	0	20	80

G stage	Percentage in each PH stage (British)*						Percentage in each PH stage (Swiss)†					
	n	PH1	PH2	PH3	PH4	PH5	n	PH1	PH2	PH3	PH4	PH5
G2	126	98	2	0	0	0	118	63	36	1	0	0
G3	109	72	17	9	2	0	116	15	50	32	3	0
G4	115	16	37	36	11	0	108	0	9	42	44	5
G5	101	0	0	8	54	38	108	0	1	10	34	55

* Adapted from Marshall and Tanner (1970).
† Adapted from Largo and Prader (1983b).

This method, however, does not consider variation in age of appearance of stages of secondary sex characteristics (timing) and the duration of each stage, i.e. how long the individual is in a particular stage (tempo).

VARIATION IN TIMING

Selected percentiles for the CA at which stages of secondary sex characteristic development are apparent in a nationally representative sample of Dutch youth have been summarized elsewhere (see Table 39.7). The 10th and 90th percentiles for B2 in Dutch girls are 9.1 and 12.3 years, respectively. Corresponding percentiles for PH2 in Dutch boys are 9.0 and 13.5 years, respectively. Thus, a small percentage of youth attain these developmental milestones quite early, while another small percentage develop them quite late.

VARIATION IN TEMPO

There is little relationship between the timing of appearance of a secondary sex characteristic and the tempo or rate at which a child progresses to the mature state. Data for British and Swiss youth are summarized in Tables 14.6 and 14.7; note that some of the differences between the two longitudinal studies are methodological. Nevertheless, mean/median intervals vary with stage and characteristic. They appear to be shorter for PH than for B and G development in British girls and boys, respectively. Differences are not as marked in Swiss adolescents. Note the extreme percentiles in the British data. A small percentage of boys pass from G2 to G5 in about 2 years and from PH2 to PH5 in about 1 year, while a small percentage of boys take almost 4 years to pass from G2 to G5 and a bit more than 2.5 years to pass from PH2 to PH5.

Such variation presents a practical problem. If biological maturity status is used in youth sports, how do you treat change in status during the course of a season? For example, Little League baseball teams in Texas are selected in March, the season starts in early April and continues into July. Or, Pee Wee hockey teams are selected in early autumn and the season continues through a good part of the spring. It

Table 14.6 Lengths of different stages (years) or genital (G), breast (B) and pubic hair (PH) development in British boys and girls. Adapted from Marshall and Tanner (1969, 1970).

Interval (boys)	Percentiles		
	2.5	50	97.5
G2−G3	0.41	1.12	2.18
G3−G4	0.24	0.81	1.64
G4−G5	0.38	1.01	1.92
G2−G5	1.86	3.05	4.72
PH2−PH3	0.11	0.44	0.87
PH3−PH4	0.31	0.42	0.54
PH4−PH5	0.20	0.72	1.45
PH2−PH5	0.82	1.59	2.67

Interval (girls)	Percentiles		
	5	50	95
B2−B3	0.21	0.86	1.03
B3−B4	0.13	0.89	2.19
B4−B5	0.12	1.96	6.82
B2−B5	1.51	4	8.99
PH2−PH3	0.16	0.62	1.27
PH3−PH4	0.18	0.51	0.93
PH4−PH5	0.57	1.30	2.37
PH2−PH5	1.39	2.49	3.10

Table 14.7 Lengths of intervals (years) between genital (G) and pubic hair (PH) stages in Swiss boys and between breast (B) and pubic hair (PH) stages and menarche (M) in Swiss girls. Adapted from Largo and Prader (1983a,b).

	Internal	n	Mean	SD
Boys	G2−G3	137	1.7	1
	G3−G5	122	1.8	0.7
	G2−G5	137	3.5	1.1
	PH2−PH3	134	1.3	0.9
	PH2−PH5	135	2.7	1
Girls	B2−B3	135	1.4	0.8
	B2−B4	140	2.3	0.9
	B2−B5	140	3.2	1.4
	B2−M	118	2.2	1.1
	PH2−PH3	134	1.8	1
	PH2−PH4	136	2.6	1
	PH2−PH5	135	3.6	1.1
	PH2−M	115	2.7	1.1

is entirely possible that some early and rapidly maturing boys will have passed through one or more stages of sexual maturation, and perhaps will have experienced their growth spurt during the course of the season. Hence, the relatively small size differences associated with variation in maturity status may now be magnified. Thus, should matching be an ongoing process during the season? This is obviously not practical.

VARIATION WITHIN CHRONOLOGICAL AGE GROUPS

As indicated earlier, children are ordinarily grouped for sport by their CA. This presents a significant problem even when sexual maturity status of the young athlete is used. How do you handle variation in maturity status within a given CA group? A similar problem occurs in research dealing with young athletes. They are often grouped by stage of sexual maturation independent of CA (e.g. Kreipe & Gewanter, 1985; Pratt, 1989; Plowman et al., 1991). Thus, a related question is: how do children of the same stage of sexual maturation but of different CA, compare in body size?

Using whole year CA categories, the distribution of stages of G and B development in a mixed-longitudinal sample of boys and girls, respectively, actively training in Polish sports schools is summarized in Table 14.8. Four of the five G/B stages are represented in 12−14-year-old boys and 11−12-year-old girls, respectively. Mean CAs, statures and weights of the boys by stage of G development within each CA group are summarized in Table 14.9. Within each CA group, boys advanced in maturity status are slightly older and especially taller and heavier. The differences in body size are more apparent at G stage 3 and higher. Also, within a specific G stage, older boys tend to be slightly taller and heavier than younger boys.

Table 14.8 Distribution of stages of genital (G) and breast (B) development within single year chronological age groups of, respectively, Polish boys and girls active in sport. Adapted from Malina *et al.* (1990).

		Stages of G development				
Age group (boys)	n	G1	G2	G3	G4	G5
11+	57	27	25	5	0	0
12+	69	11	40	14	4	0
13+	71	2	13	27	27	2
14+	65	0	5	13	40	7

		Stages of B development				
Age group (girls)	n	B1	B2	B3	B4	B5
11+	23	2	9	9	3	0
12+	34	0	3	15	15	1
13+	37	0	0	6	17	14
14+	31	0	0	0	14	17

Table 14.9 Mean chronological ages (years), stature (cm) and weight (kg) of Polish boys active in sport: variation by stage of genital (G) development within single year chronological age groups. Adapted from Malina *et al.* (1990).

		Stages of G development				
Age group		G1	G2	G3	G4	G5
Age	11+	11.4	11.6	11.6		
	12+	12.3	12.4	12.7		
	13+		13.3	13.4	13.6	
	14+			14.3	14.5	14.6
Stature	11+	148.2	152.4	155.9		
	12+	150.6	154.9	164.4		
	13+		155.7	162.9	169.3	
	14+			163.0	173.5	176.9
Weight	11+	37.8	41.5	48.4		
	12+	38.1	42.9	51.4		
	13+		43.0	48.9	57.1	
	14+			49.4	59.5	70.6

The differences are more apparent early (G1 and G2) and later (G4) in male puberty. In mid-puberty (G3), the differences in stature are especially apparent between 11-year-old boys in G3 and boys 12, 13 and 14 years old in G3. These trends may reflect the observation that serum levels of testosterone increase markedly as boys pass from G3 to G4, while levels of testosterone are only slightly higher in boys in G2 and G3 compared to those in G1 (Malina & Bouchard, 1991).

Data relating variation in stage of G development within a CA group to strength and motor performance are not available. However, boys advanced in skeletal maturation within a CA group perform better in a variety of strength, power, speed and agility tasks than boys of the same CA who are delayed in skeletal maturation (see Chapter 1). The differences between boys of the same CA but contrasting skeletal maturity status are especially marked between 13 and 15 years of age. Note also that stage of G development is highly correlated to skeletal maturation during male adolescence (Malina & Bouchard, 1991).

Since menarcheal status is often used to classify girls, mean statures and weights of a large sample of premenarcheal and postmenarcheal German schoolgirls of the same CA from Bremen are shown in Fig. 14.1. Clearly, postmenarcheal girls are taller and heavier than premenarcheal girls within each age group. The differences are more apparent at younger adolescent ages. For example, the 12-year-old postmenarcheal girl is, on average, about 9 cm taller and 10 kg heavier than the 12-year-old premenarcheal girl. The differences are only slightly less at older ages, for example, 14 years, when postmenarcheal girls are, on average, about 5 cm taller and 8 kg heavier than premenarcheal girls (Danker-Hopfe, 1984). Postmenarcheal girls also have greater static strength than premenarcheal girls of the same CA (Jones, 1949). However, within single year CA groups from 12–15 years, girls of contrasting skeletal maturity status but with the same CA do not consistently differ in tests of power (vertical jump), functional strength (bent arm hang, leg lifts), speed and agility (shuttle run) and flexibility (sit-and-reach) (Beunen *et al.*, 1976; Malina & Bouchard, 1991).

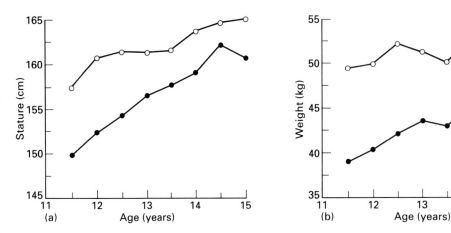

Fig. 14.1 Mean stature (a) and weight (b) of premenarcheal (●) and postmenarcheal (○) German schoolgirls of the same chronological age. Age groups are half-yearly. Drawn from data in Danker-Hopfe (1984).

More importantly for youth sports, where girls may be grouped by menarcheal status independent of CA, older premenarcheal girls are, on average, taller and heavier than younger premenarcheal girls. The differences between mean statures and weights of 12- and 14-year-old premenarcheal girls, for example, reach about 7 cm and 5 kg, respectively (Danker-Hopfe, 1984). Similarly, older premenarcheal girls are significantly stronger than younger premenarcheal girls, the difference, on average, for a composite of four static strength tests reaching about 15 kg between 12- and 14-year-old premenarcheal girls (Jones, 1949). However, among girls 12–15 years of age, differences in performances on several motor tasks (see above) between older and younger girls who are advanced or delayed in skeletal maturation are small and not consistently evident (Beunen et al., 1976; Malina & Bouchard, 1991).

Thus, strength and performance correlates of variation in biological maturity status within a CA group differ between boys and girls. There are considerable differences in the strength and motor performance of boys of the same CA but of contrasting maturity status. Static strength differs between girls of contrasting maturity status, but differences in motor performance are small and not consistently apparent.

An example of maturity matching

The selection/classification programme of the New York State Public High School Athletic Association (NYSPHSAA) is an example of a systematic and comprehensive procedure to determine the readiness of seventh and eighth grade youths (approximately 13–14 years of age) for interscholastic high school competition (Hafner et al., 1982; Willie, 1982). In addition to approval of the local board of education and the child's parents, the procedure includes assessment of the following.

1 Medical status.
2 Sexual maturation status, PH development (boys) and years past menarche (girls).
3 Stature and weight.
4 Previous experience in sports.
5 Physical fitness based on tests of agility, strength, speed and endurance.
6 A placement decision that permits the child to try out for a team.
7 The coach's rating of skill proficiency relative to the demands of the sport (Willie, 1982).

Although the selection/classification programme is still in use, it is not mandatory, due in part '...to a change in Commissioner's Regulations as well as NYSPHSAA's Modified Program Rules (junior high school) which eliminated an age requirement for participation in scholastic sports upon entry into the ninth and seventh grades respectively' (S.E. Scott, personal communication, May 1990).

Potential consequences of maturity matching

Although matching may equalize competition and reduce the risk of injury, it generally does not take into consideration individual differences in behavioural competence, i.e. the child's level of social, emotional and cognitive development. Furthermore, the child's level of behavioural development may not proceed in concert with his or her physical/physiological growth and maturation. Hence, matching may have potential behavioural consequences which influence self-concept (how the child views himself or herself) and self-esteem (value placed upon self). A late maturing 13-year-old boy may resent participating with 11-year-old boys of similar maturity status. Similarly, an early maturing 11-year-old girl may not want to participate with equally mature, but older and more experienced 13-year-old girls. Both of these extremes are the two groups who are least often represented among those who experience success in youth sports, and are quite likely good candidates for dropping out of sport. Clearly, most sports available for boys favour the larger, earlier maturing boy. On the other hand, sport opportunities may be limited for the early maturing girl so that she may be socialized away from sport participation.

Younger, early maturing boys may be threatened by having to participate and compete with chronologically older boys of the same maturity status. Conversely, older boys may not want to participate with younger boys not only due to maturity considerations, but also due to social concerns, e.g. there may be less recognition in successfully competing versus less mature individuals.

The peer group is a major force during middle childhood and early adolescence, and the team is a significant peer group. Although children and youths have several peer groups, matching by size, skill and maturity status often alters peer group structure and in turn may influence social relationships and development.

Matching sport to children and youths

Most discussions of equating for sports competition focus on the characteristics of children and youths. However, it is also important, perhaps more important, to reverse the question, i.e. how can sports be modified to match the characteristics and needs of children and youths? Sport should be ready for children and youths, and not the other way around.

The demands of a sport include objectives of the contest, rules, techniques (skills) and tactics. And, the objectives and rules of most sports have been developed by adults. Children and youths, of course, are not miniature adults. Hence, it is important to ask: how can tasks and rules of a sport be adjusted to meet the changing needs of growing, maturing and developing individuals? Clearly, eliminating body checking in ice hockey significantly reduces the number of injuries. Reducing the size of the playing area and duration of contests are other examples of modifying sports such as baseball, football and soccer to meet the characteristics of children and youths. Other modifications should also be considered, e.g. reducing the height of the basket to improve the possibility for success in basketball, perhaps granting a point if a child's shot hits the rim in basketball, enlarging the goal in soccer, and so on. There are undoubtedly many other possibilities.

Conversely, the demands of sports such as gymnastics have been altered by authorities and coaches so that 'women's' gymnastics at élite levels has essentially become a prepubertal 'girl's' sport. It has even been suggested that the rigours of training girls for élite gymnastics borders on child abuse, and there have been calls to raise the minimum age of female gymnasts at international competitions to 16 years (Press, 1992; Prieser, 1992; Todd & Hoberman, 1992).

When asked why they participate in sport,

children and youths indicate the following: to have fun, to improve skills and learn new skills, to be with friends or make new friends, for thrills and excitement, to become physically fit, and to succeed or win (Smith *et al.*, 1983). Similar motivations for participating in sport are apparent in a more recent survey: to have fun, to improve skills, to stay in shape, to do something I am good at, for the excitement of competition, to get exercise, to play as part of a team, for the challenge of competition, to learn new skills, and to win (Athletic Footwear Association, 1990). Youth sports should thus have children and youths as the primary focus. Youth sports are not and should not be the arena implied by Lurie and Kramer (1968, p. 1624) in a discussion of athletics in a paediatric textbook: '...it is only in the competitive atmosphere of sports that the civilized child is exposed to stimuli closely approximating those presented to the savage fighting for survival'.

Conclusion

Matching children to equalize competition, enhance chance for success and reduce injury in youth sports are worthwhile objectives. The incorporation of measures of biological maturity status is logistically not practical. Skill, stature and weight within relatively narrow CA groups will probably match the majority of children under 11–12 years of age. Subsequently, individual differences in biological maturation must be taken into consideration, perhaps more so for boys than for girls. Nevertheless, the consequences of matching for sport need further study and serious consideration should be given to potential modifications of sports to meet the needs and characteristics of children and youths.

Challenges for future research

• If maturity matching is viewed as essential to equalize competition and reduce the risk of injury, there is a need to develop logistically feasible and practical procedures to implement it.

• There is a need for basic information on the behavioural consequences of matching in youth sport. How does matching influence the development of behavioural competence?

• How can CA cut-off points be modified for specific sports?

• Since the majority of coaches in youth sports are volunteers, education/certification programmes for coaches should be systematically implemented. How can such programmes be implemented to improve the youth sports experiences of children and youths?

• In the context of national and international competition in sports which characteristically have an early age at entry and specialization, e.g. gymnastics, figure skating and perhaps diving, the issue of CA and biological age limits needs careful evaluation, particularly in the context of potential for child abuse in sport. Should biological age limits be imposed, e.g. skeletal age of 15 years? Such limits will undoubtedly provoke outcries from those involved in coaching and administering high level performance and competition for children. Nevertheless, such changes may be desirable for the sake of the health and well-being of the children involved.

References

American Academy of Pediatrics, Committee on Sports Medicine (1988) Recommendations for participation in competitive sports. *Pediatrics* **81**, 737–9.

Athletic Footwear Association (1990) *American Youth and Sports Participation: A Study of 10,000 Students and Their Feelings about Sports*. Athletic Footwear Association, North Palm Beach, FL.

Beunen, G., Ostyn, M., Renson, R., Simons, J. & Van Gerven, D. (1976) Skeletal maturation and physical fitness of girls aged 12 through 16. *Hermes* (Leuven) **10**, 445–57.

Caine, D.J. & Broekhoff, J. (1987) Maturity assessment: A viable preventive measure against physical and psychological insult to the young athlete? *Phys. Sports Med.* **15**, 67–80.

Crampton, C.W. (1908) Physiological age — a fundamental principle. I. *Am. Phys. Ed. Rev.* **13**, 141–54.

Danker-Hopfe, H. (1984) *Die sakulare Veranderung des Menarchealters in Europa* (The Secular Trend in Menarche in Europe). Doctoral dissertation,

University of Bremen, Germany.

Gallagher, J.R. (1969) Problems in matching competitors: adolescents, athletics and competitive sports. *Clin. Pediatr.* **8**, 434–6.

Hafner, J.K., Scott, S.E., Veras, G., Goldberg, B., Nicholas, J.A. & Shaffer, T.E. (1982) Interscholastic athletics: method for selection and classification of athletes. *N.Y. State J. Med.* **82**, 1449–59.

Jones, H.E. (1949) *Motor Performance and Growth.* University of California Press, Berkeley, CA.

Kreipe, R.E. & Gewanter, H.L. (1985) Physical maturity screening for participation in sports. *Pediatrics* **75**, 1076–80.

Largo, R.H. & Prader, A. (1983a) Pubertal development in Swiss boys. *Helv. Paediatr. Acta* **38**, 211–28.

Largo, R.H. & Prader, A. (1983b) Pubertal development in Swiss girls. *Helv. Paediatr. Acta* **38**, 229–43.

Lurie, R.L. & Kramer, J.D. (1968) Athletics. In R.E. Cooke (ed.) *The Biologic Basis of Pediatric Practice*, pp. 1622–6. McGraw-Hill, New York.

Malina, R.M. & Bouchard, C. (1991) *Growth, Maturation, and Physical Activity.* Human Kinetics, Champaign, IL.

Malina, R.M., Eveld, D.J. & Woynarowska, B. (1990) Growth and sexual maturation of active Polish children 11–14 years of age. *Hermes* (Leuven) **21**, 341–53.

Marshall, W.A. & Tanner, J.M. (1969) Variations in pattern of pubertal changes in girls. *Arch. Dis. Child.* **44**, 291–303.

Marshall, W.A. & Tanner, J.M. (1970) Variations in the pattern of pubertal changes in boys. *Arch. Dis. Child.* **45**, 13–23.

Plowman, S.A., Liu, N.A. & Wells, C.L. (1991) Body composition and sexual maturation in premenarcheal athletes and nonathletes. *Med. Sci. Sports Exerc.* **23**, 23–9.

Pratt, M. (1989) Strength, flexibility, and maturity in adolescent athletes. *Am. J. Dis. Child.* **143**, 560–3.

Press, A. (1992) Old too soon, wise too late? *Newsweek* 10 August, 22–4.

Prieser, U. (1992) Die Hochleistungskinder (High performance children). *Die Zeit*, 11 December, 22.

Rotch, T.M. (1908) Chronological and anatomical age early in life. *JAMA* **51**, 1197–205.

Rotch, T.M. (1909) A study of the development of the bones in childhood by the Roentgen method, with the view of establishing a developmental index for the grading of and the protection of early life. *Trans. Ass. Am. Phys.* **24**, 603–24.

Roy, M-A., Bernard, D., Roy, B. & Marcotte, G. (1989) Body checking in Pee Wee hockey. *Phys. Sportsmed.* **17**(March), 119–26.

Seefeldt, V. (1981) Equating children for sports competition: Some common problems and suggested solutions. *Motor Dev. Theory Prac.* **3**, 13–22.

Smith, N.J., Smith, R.E. & Smoll, R.L. (1983) *Kidsports: A Survival Guide for Parents.* Addison-Wesley, Reading, MA.

Stockwell, I.W. (1976) Height and weight vs maturity. *Phys. Sports Med.* **3**(February), 11.

Todd, T. & Hoberman, J. (1992) Tough-as-nails female athletes lost in cute wallpaper pattern. *Austin Am. Statesman* 9 August, C17.

Willie, M.C. (1982) *Revised Maturity and Physical Fitness Standards for the Selection/Classification Screening Procedures: The Selection/Classification Program Procedures for Implementation of the Regulations of the Commissioner of Education Regarding Athletic Eligibility Standards for Pupils of Advanced or Delayed Maturity.* University of the State of New York, Albany, NY.

Chapter 15

Protective Equipment

MICHAEL A. NELSON

Introduction

Many injuries in sport are unavoidable and are accepted as an inherent risk for participation in a particular sport. Conversely, other injuries are preventable by modification of a number of factors associated with sports participation. Proper conditioning and training, maintenance of the playing environment, modification of rules for young players and subsequent enforcement by coaches and referees all have potential for reducing injury rates. Protective sports equipment may also reduce the risk of injury in some sports. However, the impetus for the production of sports protective equipment is often market driven rather than research driven, leading to confusion among those in sports regarding appropriate equipment choices. Equipment issues discussed in this chapter reflect activity in the USA. Other countries may emphasize issues about equipment used in other sports. At times, it can be difficult to predict the impact of introducing protective equipment to a particular sport. Historically, sports protective equipment has been associated with both positive and negative influences on injury rates in some sports.

Coincident with the design improvement of helmets for American football during the 1960s the total number of intracranial haemorrhage and closed head injuries experienced by high school and collegiate athletes decreased dramatically. Unfortunately, the rate of cervical spine fractures and permanent quadriplegia increased (Fig. 15.1). Analysis of these unexpected trends in cervical spine injury revealed that players, when tackling, were using their helmets as weapons. Tackling using the top of the helmet against opposing players, a technique known as spearing, was associated with most cervical spine injuries (Torg et al., 1987). Consequently in 1976, rules against spearing were instituted and the rate of cervical spine injuries diminished. The number of cases of permanent quadriplegia decreased from 34 in 1976 to five in 1984 (Torg et al., 1987). However, during the 1988–90 seasons there has been a rise in the number of cervical spine injuries, apparently secondary to casual enforcement of rules and lack of training in the proper techniques of tackling (Mueller & Shindler, 1991).

In a similar fashion when the use of helmets and face guards for protection against eye and head injuries became widespread in hockey the incidence of serious cervical spine injuries and permanent quadriplegia increased. Between 1948 and 1974 one spinal injury was documented among Canadian hockey players. Subsequently, when helmet and face guard rules were implemented, 42 spinal injuries were reported between 1976 and 1983 (Tator & Edmonds, 1984).

There is controversy among those who study hockey injury rates regarding the causative factors. While helmets with heavier face masks mounted may increase torsion on the neck, the most common mechanism of injury is axial loading of the cervical spine when the helmeted

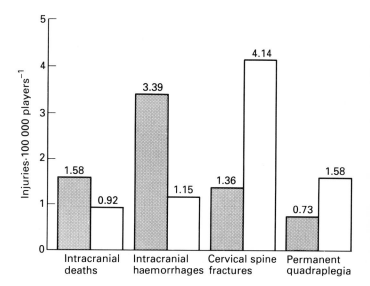

Fig. 15.1 Head and neck injuries in football before (▨) (1959–63) and after (▯) (1971–75) helmet use. Redrawn from Torg *et al.* (1987).

head strikes another object such as the boards. The most common precipitating event is a push (check) from behind. Therefore, the majority of researchers believe the additional protection of a helmet with a face mask adds to the sense of invincibility that hockey players experience and subsequently to the aggressiveness associated with the sport. While the mandatory use of helmets in youth, high school and collegiate hockey has resulted in a reduction of head injuries, the impact of the additional protection contributing to spine injuries needs to be addressed by rule changes and more importantly, enforcement of the rule changes in conjunction with coaching of proper techniques (Tator *et al.*, 1991). Despite improvements in protective equipment, youth hockey leagues that permit body checking experience as much as six times as many injuries as those which have banned body checking (Roy *et al.*, 1989).

Clearly, protective equipment can be misused resulting in unexpected increases in other injuries for which the equipment was not designed to prevent. Fortunately, the scenarios presented regarding American football and hockey are the exception to the normal use of protective equipment. What follows is a general review of principles of protective equipment use as well as more detailed information on the

use of protective equipment in baseball and utilization of protective eyewear in high risk sports. Specific information on the use of general protective equipment in other sports is available elsewhere (Ellis, 1991).

Principles of equipment use

Legal responsibility

In addition to the primary responsibility of the athlete to use equipment properly, changes in litigation law in the USA in recent years support the need for all individuals involved in sports to assume a meaningful role in decision-making regarding the selection and use of protective equipment. In the USA, during the 1970s, contributory negligence which precluded collection of any damages from a lawsuit if a plaintiff was judged to be somewhat responsible for an injury, was replaced by the doctrine of comparative negligence (Patterson, 1987). In some areas of the USA, under the doctrine of comparative liability, if a plaintiff is judged to be 75% responsible for causing the injury, the individual may still collect 25% of a judgement against a defendant. 'Strict products' liability was introduced in the 1960s holding manufacturers accountable for equipment produced for a specific purpose. Joint and several liability has been a traditional concept in determining damage awards. Under this doctrine, an individual judged to be 1% responsible for an injury to a plaintiff could still be held responsible for 100% of a damage award. Consequently, the search for 'deep pockets' (largest source of money for damage awards) should make all those involved in caring for athletes cognizant of their responsibility for selection and use of protective equipment.

The traditional concept that the coach, athletic trainer and manager for team sports have sole responsibility for selection and use of protective equipment is too limiting in today's world. Those individuals, whether administrators, physicians or other allied health professionals who interact with sports teams will need to examine their role and responsibility in providing protective equipment and education of young athletes in proper usage. When serving as a team physician, practitioners should ensure the development and use of guidelines for selection of equipment and subsequent education in the proper usage.

Selection of equipment guidelines

Equipment should be purchased that has been tested by a recognized certifying authority. Equipment that has met appropriate testing standards usually has a certifying stamp or statement on the individual item or container. The American Society for Testing and Materials (Philadelphia, Pennsylvania, USA) and the National Operating Committee on Standards for Athletic Equipment (Kansas City, Kansas, USA) are two certifying organizations for protective sports equipment in the USA. Many countries have their own certifying organizations such as the Canadian Standards Association (Rexdale, Ontario, Canada). When possible, new equipment or equipment that has been restored according to manufacturers' recommendations should be selected. In addition, only equipment that meets the guidelines or rules of the governing body of the particular sport should be utilized by the indi-

vidual athlete or members of a team. The best or safest equipment may not always be available or it may be too expensive for the financial resources of individual athletes or community-supported sport teams. However, the best equipment within the resources of the family and community should be used.

Fitting

Attention to detail is of paramount importance when fitting equipment for children and adolescents. In some instances equipment that has been designed and manufactured specifically for young athletes is not readily available. 'Hand me down' equipment in poor condition or oversized equipment previously used by older siblings are not acceptable substitutes. Guidelines are available for fitting equipment for several youth sports (Ellis, 1991). Many manufacturers provide detailed instructions regarding the proper fit of equipment. An individual who is knowledgeable or who has access to information about fitting youth sports equipment should be available for every sports programme.

Too often, an athlete or family purchases equipment based on advertising by the superstars of sports or because the item looks good or is popular. In community youth sport programmes it is not always practical for a coach or trainer to accompany a young athlete to select equipment. Sales persons in sporting goods stores may not be qualified to judge proper fit. Therefore, in team sports a coach or other individual knowledgeable about equipment should check each athlete for proper fit at the initial practice. Families with children participating in individual sports should seek out knowledgeable coaches or trainers regarding selection and fit of equipment.

Maintenance

Many equipment manufacturers have guidelines or rules regarding proper maintenance of equipment. For instance, Riddell Inc. (Chicago, IL, USA) who has specific guidelines for reconditioning football helmets, no longer rec-ommends reconditioning helmets that are older than 8 years for youth helmets. Those respon-sible for maintenance of equipment may be held accountable if they do not follow manu-facturers guidelines (Pacelli, 1990). Defective equipment should never be used. 'Hand me down' equipment should be checked for proper function and stability by a knowledgeable individual.

Compliance

All athletes need to be instructed in the use of their equipment whether of a protective nature or for general use in the sport. The historical example of the helmet being used as a weapon in American football is a classic example of misuse of protective equipment. Many school systems are developing systematic methods for counselling athletes about equipment usage and documenting the training through video-tapes or signed acknowledgements. Equipment should be used only for the purpose for which it was designed.

The rules regarding use of protective equip-ment should be applied to all venues of the sport. Some sport governing body rules for equipment apply only to competition. For in-stance, the use of protective headgear is not required for wrestling practice as it is for com-petition (Ellis, 1991). Similarly, athletes may wear protective equipment during practice, but unless mandated, avoid usage during compe-tition because it doesn't look 'cool'. Unfortu-nately, proper and consistent use of protective equipment is unlikely to occur unless mandated by governing bodies, coaches or parents.

Baseball

Epidemiology

Millions of children and adolescents around the world participate in baseball and softball. The relative risk of serious or fatal injury is very small. Nonetheless, the US Consumer Product Safety Commission reported that be-

tween 1973 and 1980 participation in baseball and softball accounted for the most sport-related deaths in the 5–14-year age group (Rutherford et al., 1981). The majority of these deaths re-sulted from being struck in the chest or head with a thrown or hit ball. Of the 51 deaths 23 occurring during this period were secondary to being struck in the chest by the ball. Commotio cordis, which occurs secondary to forces gener-ated through the chest wall to the myocardium, has been recognized as the most common cause of traumatic death in baseball (Abrunzo, 1991). When struck with a baseball, the relatively thin, compliant chest wall of a child is thought to transmit greater energy to the myocardium than that of the adult, resulting in fatal dys-rhythmias or arrythmia. The next most common category of injury resulting in death involves the head being struck by the ball and conse-quent closed head injury. The greatest risk of being struck in the chest or head is incurred while batting or pitching (Rutherford 1981).

During the period 1983–89, 2655 404 baseball or softball injuries severe enough to result in emergency room visits were recorded in the USA by the National Electronic Injury Surveil-lance System (Janda et al., 1993). This figure does not include visits to physicians and does not represent the full magnitude of injuries. Among injuries in softball approximately 70% have been shown to be consequent to sliding (Janda et al., 1986). The overwhelming majority of sliding injuries occur during deceleration and subsequent contact with a stationary base. The most common types of sliding injuries are ankle fractures and sprains followed by knee trauma including meniscal and collateral liga-ment tears.

Protective equipment

BREAKAWAY BASES

The impact of using breakaway based in base-ball and softball on the reduction of lower extremity injuries, specifically ankle sprains and fractures, is dramatic. In an analysis of injury prevention in recreational softball players

Janda *et al.*, (1990) demonstrated a nearly 300-fold decrease (99:1 reduction) in per game sliding injuries. The medical costs for injuries with stationary bases would be reduced by 98% with the use of breakaway bases. Unfortunately, breakaway bases are nearly twice as expensive as stationary bases; however, the health-care cost saving clearly justifies their use. Breakaway bases have been developed for different age groups, most of which attach via Velcro to a plate that is anchored at ground level. Youth, teen, adult and professional models are available, each of which requires increasingly greater force to dislodge.

Occasionally, changes in sports are not readily accepted by coaches, athletes and governing bodies. Breakaway bases were being developed during the late 1970s and are still not widely used. However, umpires, players and coaches do not report any difficulty in rules interpretation if a base breaks away during the course of a game. If the base dislodges, the attachment plate easily serves as a temporary base to facilitate continuation of play. Every attempt should be made to encourage all governing bodies in baseball and softball to adopt breakaway bases as a standard part of their equipment requirements.

Chest protectors

Chest protectors have been a part of the catchers protective equipment for years. Recently, more attention has been focused on the use of chest protectors for all baseball players in an attempt to prevent commotio cordis. In 1986, the US Consumer Product Safety Commission recommended that baseball players wear chest protectors (King & Viano, 1986). However, the acceptance of chest protectors by batters and defensive players has been poor because of cost and bulkiness.

Recently, manufacturers have begun producing chest protectors for players other than catchers. One model (the athletic safety jacket produced by IPASC is designed with removable sleeve segments to adapt to left- or right-handed

batters and is to be worn sleeveless in the field. Another model is designed to protect the side torso only (the Bat-R-Vest produced by Carroll Industries). Unfortunately, there is serious doubt regarding the efficacy of such devices.

The main purpose of chest protectors is to prevent the occurrence of commotio cordis. A study utilizing an animal model (swine), a child dummy and a 5% Hybrid III female dummy failed to demonstrate a significant advantage from utilization of a variety of chest protectors in reducing impact force (Janda *et al.*, 1992). The conclusions of the authors appear to be primarily related to force impact data. Unfortunately, the velocity of the ball used ($45.3 \, \text{m} \cdot \text{s}^{-1}$) was significantly greater than that experienced in actual play in youth leagues (median = $20 \, \text{m} \cdot \text{s}^{-1}$). Batted balls rarely exceed $26.2 \, \text{m} \cdot \text{s}^{-1}$. (Hale, 1979). Conclusions drawn from the Janda study which tested balls at such a high velocity are suspect regarding the applicability to practice and game situations. While dysrhythmias occurred when utilizing a combination of either closed cell or hard plastic covered chest protectors and softer core baseballs, none were fatal when tested on the chests of swine which suggests the potential for a protective effect from this combination.

The efficacy of chest protectors in general has been questioned since two deaths have been reported in 15-year-old hockey players after being struck in the chest with a hockey puck, in spite of the use of commercially designed and manufactured closed cell chest protectors (Kaplan *et al.*, 1993). The practicality and effectiveness of chest protectors has not been clarified. Until that occurs their use should be considered but not required.

'Soft' balls

Since most catastrophic injuries result from a player being struck in the chest or head by a thrown or hit baseball or softball, attention has been focused on changing the characteristics of the ball. Some manufacturers have introduced baseballs and softballs with reduced hardness characteristics. These balls are manufactured with a polyurethane core rather than the traditional yarn core. The National Operating Committee on Standards for Athletic Equipment (NOCSAE) has developed standards for these lower impact balls (National Operating Committee on Standards for Athletic Equipment, 1989). Laboratory-based testing models that predict the likelihood of head injury based on impact force have been developed. Impact force is based on ball liveliness, hardness and velocity. Little League 12-year-old pitchers are able to throw the ball up to $33.4\,\mathrm{m\cdot s^{-1}}$ (Hale, 1979). Ironically, many baseballs currently in use in Little League are harder than major league balls. Major league ball standards are set at $700\,\mathrm{N\cdot cm^{-2}}$ and some Little League balls at $1050\,\mathrm{N\cdot cm^{-2}}$. Currently, in order for a ball to be labelled 'meets the NOCSAE standard' it must represent no more than a 40% risk of head injury at a velocity of $28.6\,\mathrm{m\cdot s^{-1}}$. Based on this model, balls with a hardness rating of $1050\,\mathrm{N\cdot cm^{-2}}$ (youth leagues) and $700\,\mathrm{N\cdot cm^{-2}}$ (professional leagues) pose a 99% and 80% risk of head injury respectively. These 'soft' baseballs and softballs have recently been introduced to the youth baseball market. In the USA, Worth Sports Co. reports that 10% of

youth league baseballs used during the 1992 season conformed to these new standards. At least one manufacturer produces a series of balls with a range of hardness from a maximum of $300\,\mathrm{N\cdot cm^{-2}}$ to below $175\,\mathrm{N\cdot cm^{-2}}$. According to the NOCSAE model, these balls would be expected to reduce the likelihood of serious injury when the head is struck with a ball at $28.6\,\mathrm{m\cdot s^{-1}}$ to 10% or less, dependent on the hardness (Fig. 15.2).

In a study over an 8-week season conducted by the Youth Sports Institute, comparisons were made between 100 youth baseball teams using soft-core baseballs and 100 teams using the traditional hard-core ball. Minor injury rate caused by impact with the softer balls was 70% lower and no serious injuries occurred. One serious head injury occurred with the hard balls (Seefeldt *et al.*, 1993).

A barrier to the use of new protective equipment can be the manner in which it affects play. Coaches are traditionally reluctant to introduce new products if they perceive that the quality of play will be negatively impacted. The performance standards of the new low impact balls show very little variation from traditional balls. However, there may be as much as 10% variation in distance travelled or angle

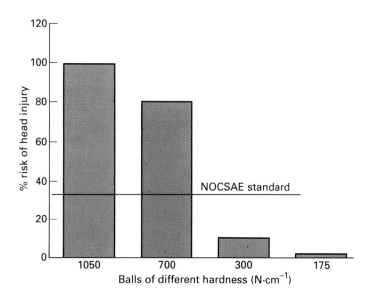

Fig. 15.2 Ball hardness and head injury risk ($28.6\,\mathrm{m\cdot s^{-1}}$ impact). NOCSAE, National Operating Committee on Standards for Athletic Equipment. Redrawn with permission from Worth Sports Co. (1992).

of rebound dependent on the softness of the ball.

Some leagues in the United States are now requiring the use of low impact balls. The American Amateur Baseball Congress now requires the use of soft-core baseballs in its youth division (12 and under) World Series finals (Worth Sports Co., 1992). Based on laboratory analysis and standards developed by NOCSAE as well as preliminary field tests, it appears prudent for physicians to encourage the use of these balls in all sanctioned and recreational baseball and softball activities.

Pitching machines

Pitching machines are not traditionally thought of as protective sports equipment. Their purpose originally was intended to prevent wear and tear on pitchers arms during practice. However, some youth baseball leagues have begun using pitching machines during both practices and competition. One report from an 8–10-year-old youth baseball league revealed a reduction in hitting the batter to zero, a reduction of walks to zero and strike-outs equivalent to when pitchers were used. The ball was hit into play twice as often when a pitching machine was used resulting in more involvement by all players (Dorsey & Benton 1993).

Eye protection

Epidemiology

In 1990, over 37 000 sports-related and recreational eye injuries occurred, of which 68% occurred in those less than 25 years of age, 38% under 15 years of age and 5% under 5 years of age (National Society to Prevent Blindness, 1990).

Baseball and basketball account for the largest number of eye injuries in the 5–24 year age range (Erie, 1991). Baseball has consistently accounted for the greatest occurrence of eye injuries in the 5–14-year-old age range and ranks second among 15–24 year olds (Fig. 15.3). The greatest risk of being hit in the eye is while batting (Jeffers, 1990). The severity of these injuries as well as participation rates for different sports are unavailable precluding the use of relative injury risk data for specific sports. However, in 1985 baseball accounted for nearly 30% of severe sport-related eye injuries (Schein et al., 1988).

Sports can be divided into low, high and very high risk based on occurrence data and inherent risk and rules of individual sports. Boxing, full contact martial arts and wrestling should be considered very high risk because protective eyewear cannot be used in these

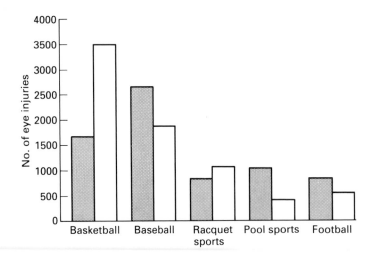

Fig. 15.3 Estimated sports and recreational eye injuries (1990) in 5–14 year olds (□) and 15–24 year olds (□). Redrawn from National Society to Prevent Blindness (1990).

sports. While thumbless boxing gloves have been mandated in some amateur leagues, this regulation is inadequate for eye protection. Examples of high risk sports and recommendations for protective eyewear are shown in Table 15.1. The American Academy of Pediatrics and the American Ophthalmology Association are developing a more definitive sports classification schema and recommendations for use of protective eyewear.

The frequency of sports-related eye injuries makes it essential for athletes, parents, coaches and physicians to be aware of the risks as well as the variety of approved eye protectors. Categories of eye protection devices are described in Table 15.2.

Equipment

The American Society for Testing and Materials, among others in the USA, has been primarily responsible for setting standards for protective eyewear. American Society for Testing Materials standard F803 refers to a basic sports eye protector utilizing polycarbonate lenses for sports involving high speed balls and rackets such as

Table 15.1 Eyewear available in high risk eye injury sports.

Sport	Eye protection
Football	Polycarbonate shield or sports goggles
Ice hockey	Helmet and full face protection
Baseball/softball	Polycarbonate face guard for batting and base running; polycarbonate goggles for fielding
Water polo	Polycarbonate swim goggles
Basketball	Polycarbonate goggles
Badminton/squash/ racquetball/handball	Polycarbonate goggles (lenseless goggles not effective)
Lacrosse	Helmet and full face protection

Table 15.2 Eyewear protection definitions.

Streetwear frames: sturdy daily wear frames with a posterior lip to prevent inward displacement of the lenses

Polycarbonate lenses: designed to fit in streetwear frames or sports goggles. Prescription or non-prescription lenses made of polycarbonate material with a centre thickness of at least 2 mm

Sports goggles: non-hinged protective wear with a moulded frame and temple and prescription or non-prescription polycarbonate lenses with a 3 mm centre thickness

Polycarbonate shield/face guard: molded protective shields or face guards designed to be attached to sports helmets

racquetball, squash, handball and tennis. Open face sport goggles (i.e. frame does not have a full lens) are not acceptable protection for sports involving high speed balls. While standard polycarbonate lenses should be 2 mm in thickness, prescription lenses need to be 3 mm. Occasionally, polycarbonate cannot be used for an especially strong prescription. In this instance, an allyl/resin plastic lens (CR-39) with a 3 mm centre thickness is recommended.

For collision sports such as ice hockey and football an eye/face protector must be securely attached to the helmet. In football, a polycarbonate shield may be attached to the face guard. Although baseball is not considered a collision sport, face as well as eye protection is desirable. Consequently, face guards attached to helmets for batters and base runners should be used by all players. A cage-type face shield (similar to football) or polycarbonate shields are acceptable for this purpose (Fig. 15.4). All helmet devices should be secured with a chin strap. Defensive players should use sport goggles if functionally one-eyed or if they need corrective vision devices to participate.

It is critical that visually impaired athletes use appropriate protective eyewear. In the past, the definition of the functionally one-eyed athlete has been somewhat arbitrary. Most States in the USA will not issue a driver's licence to

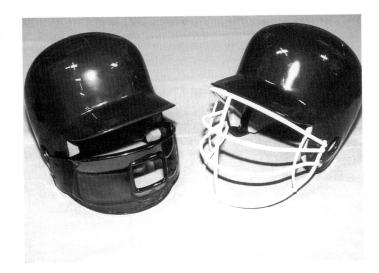

Fig. 15.4 Baseball helmet face guards — polycarbonate and face guard styles.

anyone with a corrected visual acuity that is worse than 20/50 (Federal Highway Administration, 1988). Therefore, anyone with best corrected vision in one eye that is worse than 20/50 should be considered functionally one-eyed.

Ideally, for high risk sports all children would wear protective eyewear. Unfortunately, cost and lack of public awareness make this an unlikely goal. For the functionally one-eyed athlete and those that need glasses for vision correction during sports participation, protective eyewear should be required.

Compliance

Until it becomes socially acceptable and encouraged, voluntary use of protective eyewear by all athletes in high risk sports is unlikely. The appearance of eye protectors on professional athletes (Chris Sabo, baseball; James Worthy and Kareem Abdul Jabar, basketball) will hopefully encourage their use. At the professional level of competition, the 8% reduction in visual field associated with protective eyewear may make the difference between success or failure. However, for most young athletes, this small difference is unlikely to affect the outcome of competition.

Functionally one-eyed athletes or those that require corrective devices for participation in sports can be required or encouraged to use proper eye protection devices during a pre-participation evaluation. It is unusual for athletes involved in community based sport programmes to be required to have a preparticipation evaluation. Therefore, mandated rules through regulatory bodies or sport governance organizations will continue to be necessary. Many national organizations are reluctant to mandate changes at the local area secondary to socioeconomic differences in various geographical locales. Nonetheless, the use of protective eye equipment is very cost-effective relative to injury prevention.

Challenges for future research

• While a great deal of research data regarding injuries. have been developed for secondary and collegiate levels, very little exist for sports involving younger athletes in community-based programmes or clubs. Development of an expanded youth sport injury reporting system should be a priority. In the USA, only catastrophic injuries are reported through emergency room utilization. Development of such a surveillance network would facilitate development of sports protective equipment from a research documented need basis, rather than market forces.

• Currently, manufacturers have the primary responsibility to perform limited testing of new products. Development of a focused surveillance network to evaluate the practical effectiveness of new sports protective equipment is needed. Other information regarding the efficacy of new equipment is available only on an anecdotal basis or limited local studies.

- Sophisticated computer software programs are used in the aerospace industry to predict the consequence of using new equipment or design modifications to a variety of environmental variables. Development of computer-based models that would accurately predict the outcome of utilization of new sports protective equipment prior to field testing is worthwhile.
- There is some indication that soccer players may experience damage to the central nervous system from repeated heading of the ball over a number of years. Documentation of this potential problem and what protective effect, if any, would result from the use of header helmets would be useful before their use becomes widespread due to aggressive marketing techniques.

References

Abrunzo, T. (1991) Commotio cordis. *Am. J. Dis. Child.* **145**, 1279–82.

Dorsey, J. & Benton, R. (1993) Saving young arms and batter's heads. *Pediatrics* **91**, 679–80.

Ellis, T. (1991) Sports protective equipment. *Primary Care* **18**, 889–921.

Erie, J. (1991) Eye injuries: prevention, evaluation, and treatment. *Phys. Sports Med.* **19**, 108–22.

Federal Highway Administration (1988) *Manual on Uniform Traffic Control Devices: Streets and Highways.* Department of Public Transportation, Washington, DC.

Hale, C. (1979) Protective equipment for baseball. *Phys. Sportsmed.* **9**, 46–50.

Janda, D., Hankin, F. & Wojtys, E. (1986) Softball injuries, cost, cause, prevention. *Am. Fam. Phys.* **33**, 143–4.

Janda, D., Maguire, R., Mackesy, D., Hawkins, R., Fowler, P. & Boyd J. (1993) Sliding injuries in college and professional baseball — a prospective study comparing standard and break-away bases. *Clin. J. Sports Med.* **3**, 78–81.

Janda, D., Viano, D., Andrejak, D. & Hensinger, R. (1992) An analysis of preventive methods for baseball induced chest impact injuries. *Clin. J. Sports Med.* **2**, 172–9.

Janda, D., Wojtys, E., Hankin, F., Benedict, M. & Hensinger, R. (1990) A three-phase analysis of the prevention of recreational softball injuries. *Am. J. Sports Med.* **18**, 632–5.

Jeffers, J. (1990) An on going tragedy: pediatric sports-related eye injuries. *Sem. Ophthalmol.* **5**, 216–23.

Kaplan, J., Karofsky, P. & Volturo, G. (1993) Commotio cordis in two amateur ice hockey players despite the use of commercial chest protectors: case reports. *J. Trauma* **34**, 151–3.

King, A. & Viano, D. (1986) *Baseball-Related Chest Impact.* United States Consumer Product Safety Commission, Washington, DC.

Mueller, F. & Shindler, R. (1991) *Annual Survey in Football Injuries Research, 1931–1991,* National Collegiate Athletic Association, Mission, KS.

National Operating Committee on Standards for Athletic Equipment (1989) *Standard Method of Impact Test and Performance Requirements for Baseball/Softball Batters Helmets, Baseballs and Softballs.* NOCSAE, Kansas City, MO.

National Society to Prevent Blindness (1990) *1990 Sports and Recreational Eye Injuries* National Society to Prevent Blindness, Chicago, IL.

Pacelli, L. (1990) Aging helmets to be sidelined. *Phys. Sports Med.* **18**, 15.

Patterson, D. (1987) Legal aspects of athletic injuries to the head and cervical spine. *Clin. Sports Med.* **6**, 197–210.

Roy, M-A., Bernard, D., Roy, B. & Marcotte, G. (1989) Body checking in Pee Wee hockey. *Phys. Sports Med.* **17**, 119–26.

Rutherford, G., Kennedy, J. & McGhee, L. (1981) *Hazard Analysis: Baseball and Softball-Related Injuries to Children 5–14 Years of Age.* US Consumer Product Safety Commission, Washington, DC.

Schein, O., Hibbard, P., Shingleton, B. *et al.* (1988) The spectrum and burden of ocular injury. *Ophthalmology* **95**, 300–5.

Seefeldt, V., Brown, E., Wilson, D. & Walk, S. (1993) *Influence of Low-Compression Versus Traditional Baseballs on Injuries in Youth Baseball.* Institute for the Study of Youth Sport, Michigan State University, East Lansing, MI.

Tator, C. & Edmonds, V. (1984) National survey of spinal injuries in hockey players *Can. Med. Ass. J.* **130**, 875–80.

Tator, C., Edmonds, V., Lapczak, L. & Tator, I. (1991) Spinal injuries in ice hockey programs 1966–1987. *Can. J. Surg.* **34**, 63–9.

Torg, J., Vegso, J. & Sennett, B. (1987) The national football head and neck injury registry: 14-year report on cervical quadriplegia (1971–1984). *Clin. Sports Med.* **6**, 61–72.

Worth Sports Co. (1992) *Worth Safety Report.* (Spring, 1992) *AABC adopts RIF as Official World Series Ball.* Worth Sports Co., Tullahoma, TN.

Chapter 16

Rehabilitation of Children following Sport- and Activity-related Injuries

ANGELA D. SMITH

Importance of rehabilitation

After any injury to the musculoskeletal system, rehabilitation is essential for preventing injury following return to activity — either a recurrent injury or a related injury. A child who has sustained one ankle sprain and does not rehabilitate the injured region fully may sustain a recurrent sprain to the same ankle. An example of a related injury would be patellofemoral pain caused by quadriceps atrophy that occurred while the child was limping from the ankle sprain.

Rehabilitation includes regaining muscle capabilities to the level of full power, strength and endurance. It also includes the return of normal flexibility and neuromuscular coordination. Rehabilitation is important for restoration of full performance. Compliance with a prescribed rehabilitation programme may be difficult even for adults. Older children and adolescents seem to respond best when instructed that the rehabilitation process is aimed at improving their performance. Their parents, guardians and coaches generally respond best when informed that the rehabilitation programme is important for eliminating musculoskeletal 'weak links' that occurred both at the time of injury and during the period of healing. Eliminating these musculoskeletal deficits will help to decrease the possibility of a later, secondary injury.

Some practitioners advocate prehabilitation. Identification of deficits in muscle strength,

flexibility and coordination allows a motivated individual to correct the deficits before beginning a new playing season, or prehabilitate. Available evidence indicates a relationship between flexibility deficits and certain injuries in skeletally immature athletes (Micheli & Ireland, 1987; Smith, 1991). A cross-sectional study of 513 healthy schoolchildren found that the flexibility of the hamstring and posterior hip and trunk muscles begins to decrease after age 6 years, and does not begin to improve again, on average, until 16 years of age (Gurewitsch & O'Neill, 1944). Muscle flexibility can be measured reproducibly by the tests shown in Figs 16.1–16.5. Young male and female non-contact sport participants most likely to sustain overuse injuries have a high degree of ligamentous laxity, poor muscle strength and poor muscle flexibility (Lysens et al., 1989). In contact sports, increased muscle mass and strength seem to reduce the occurrence of certain acute injuries (Cahill & Griffith, 1978). In individual sports such as tennis and swimming, upper body strengthening is thought to reduce injuries to the shoulder (Kibler et al., 1992). The proper balance between the strengths of antagonist muscle groups, such as the quadriceps and hamstrings, may be important in the prevention of injury.

Principles of rehabilitation for children and adolescents

Most of the rehabilitation literature concerning

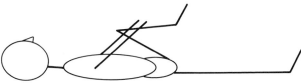
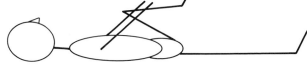

(a) Negative

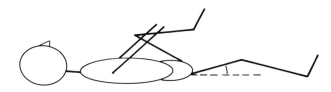

(b) Positive

Fig. 16.1 Thomas test for hip flexor flexibility. Lying supine, the youth grasps one knee up to the chest, flexing the hip until the lumbar spine is flattened against the examining table. In a negative test, the contralateral thigh remains on the table. The Thomas test should be negative. The measurement of a positive test is the angle formed by the table and the femoral shaft.

children relates to individuals with neuromuscular, neurological or congenital musculoskeletal disorders. This author is not aware of controlled studies comparing different methods of rehabilitation of musculoskeletal injuries of children who are otherwise healthy. Therefore, most of the practical information presented in this chapter is based primarily on the author's clinical experience.

Compliance with the programme

Although the exercises that are performed during the rehabilitation process are similar for adults and youth, the methods for ensuring compliance are somewhat different. Children have much shorter attention spans. Therefore, rehabilitation principles must be taught to them in as entertaining and concise a manner as possible. The exercise programme must be organized into brief but highly effective and efficient segments.

Children and adolescents are much less likely than adults to care why rehabilitation programmes should work or why they need to do them. Adolescents do not want to be different from their peers. Teenagers often feel invulnerable. Even though a teenager has just sustained one injury, he or she is unlikely to think that an injury could happen again. Therefore, using the threat of recurrent or related injury as a means to induce compliance is usually ineffective. Concentrating on improving performance is generally a more effective line of reasoning for influencing an adolescent to complete a rehabilitation programme.

Several principles appear to improve compliance with the therapy programme for both children and adolescents. The first principle is to set a defined period of time — generally not longer than 2 months — for meeting the most important goals of the rehabilitation programme. The second principle is that the rehabilitation exercise bouts should be short. Third, a small number of exercises should be prescribed, with emphasis on performing them correctly and regularly. The injured youth must be able to see evidence of progress — such as increasing the amount of weight that can be lifted by 500 g — within short intervals. Programmes should be designed to be as interesting as possible, with built-in incentives, brightly coloured equipment and entertaining explanations to help ensure compliance. Finally, the programme must be integrated into the injured individual's daily and weekly schedules.

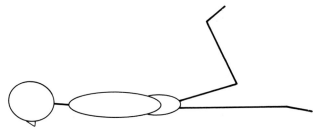

(a) Side view

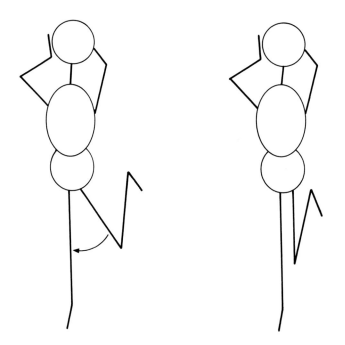

(b) View from above

Fig. 16.2 Modified Ober test for iliotibial band/tensor fasciae latae flexibility. The examiner stabilizes the prone youth's pelvis with one hand and grasps one of the youth's ankles with the other hand. The examiner then abducts the hip, flexes the ipsilateral knee to 90°, and fully extends the hip. Maintaining the hip extension and knee flexion and still grasping the ankle, the examiner then attempts to swing the knee medially until it reaches the midline, for a negative test. A positive test is measured by the angle between the midline and the femoral shaft. The modified test is more reproducible on larger individuals than the original decubitus position (side-lying) test as it is easier to stabilize the pelvis when the patient is prone. Also, the modified test is more sensitive, since gravity is not a factor (D. Gibson, personal communication, 1985).

Defined rehabilitation period

For most injuries of childhood and adolescence, reasonable goals can be met within 1–2 months. The best opportunity for gaining the young person's interest and cooperation is when pain and physical limitations are still present. If the programme is designed to start very slowly, utilizing primarily modalities (treatments administered to the passive patient), and then progressing gradually through weeks of simple isometric exercises that progress too slowly,

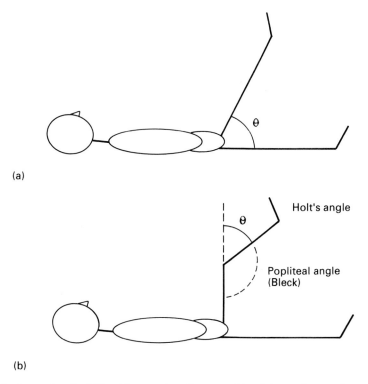

(a)

(b)

Holt's angle

θ

Popliteal angle
(Bleck)

Fig. 16.3 Tests for hamstring flexibility. The examiner flexes one hip of the supine youth to 90°. Maintaining the hip flexion, the examiner then passively extends the ipsilateral knee until resistance is felt. If the youth manages to extend the hip slightly during the test, the examiner will feel the proximal hamstrings slip slightly lateral to the maximum prominence of the ischial tuberosity, and the popliteal angle will appear to improve instantaneously. The popliteal angle is measured between the tibial shaft and the femoral shaft (as described by Bleck in Tachdjian, 1990); by eye, it may be easier to judge the angle between the tibial shaft and a vertical line extended from the femoral shaft, described by Holt (Tachdjian, 1990). (a) For the straight leg raise, the youth is supine and the examiner passively flexes the hip by lifting the foot, with the knee extended, until resistance is felt or the contralateral thigh begins to move upward from the examining table (indicating that the pelvis has rotated). The straight leg raise angle is formed between the extremity and the examining table. (b) The popliteal angle test should measure no greater than 10° (Holt's method), and the straight leg raise should be possible to 85°.

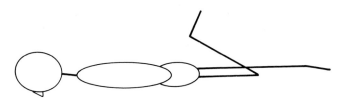

Fig. 16.4 Ely test for rectus femoris flexibility. The child lies prone, with the anterior superior iliac spines touching the table and the knees touching (preventing hip flexion and abduction, respectively). Each knee, tested individually, should flex the same amount as it does with the hip flexed. Children, younger male adolescents, and all young females should be able to touch the heel to the ipsilateral buttock. Mature males may have less knee flexion, even with the hip flexed, due to decreased joint laxity compared with females and children.

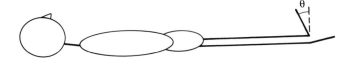

Fig. 16.5 Triceps surae flexibility test. The foot must be supinated slightly to align the tendo Achilles with the shaft of the tibia. Holding it in this position, the examiner passively dorsiflexes the ankle. The examinee keeps the knee extended, and does not attempt active dorsiflexion during the test. Ankle dorsiflexion, with the knee extended, should be at least 10°.

then the window of interest is lost. Optimal therapy includes the most rapid control of pain and swelling possible, in order to begin active therapeutic exercise as soon as possible. For children and adolescents, a therapeutic exercise programme usually begin within the first week following injury or surgery. The therapeutic exercise programme continues throughout the phase of healing and well into the phase of return to activity.

Short rehabilitation exercise bouts

The length of rehabilitation time that seems to encourage compliance among young people is the short period of only $15 \, min \cdot day^{-1}$. However, many health-care professionals design rehabilitation programmes that are all-inclusive and require much more than 15 min to perform. An ideal programme would rehabilitate all abnormal muscle groups related to the problem under treatment. However, few children and adolescents are willing to devote enough time to complete an ideal programme. Therefore, the most critical regions should be treated first. The optimal end-point would be total rehabilitation of all regions affected by the injury. However, given the usually limited period of an injured person's time and interest, it is more important to restore the most severely injured regions to the greatest extent possible than to restore all muscle groups of the injured limb only partially.

Even adults have difficulty completing a very inclusive programme each day. Children, who become bored quickly and who see little value

in the programme, frequently do not perform *any* portion of a programme that takes too long to complete.

Small number of exercises

It is preferable to teach only a very limited number of exercises specific to the particular injury, rather than a large list of related exercises. With a brief, but highly specific, therapeutic programme, the rehabilitating young person can feel accomplishment at having completed the entire group of exercises. This is possible if the entire programme consists of only three or four different exercises that require approximately 15 min to complete correctly. If a more inclusive programme is prescribed, a young person generally chooses to do the easiest exercises first, and then becomes too tired or bored to move on to the more difficult ones, which are usually the most important ones.

In most therapeutic exercise programmes, the easiest exercises to perform tend to be those that are the least useful for improving the condition being treated. The ones that are easiest for the child to perform involve the muscles that are already the strongest, most flexible or best coordinated. Therefore, the practitioner who prefers a more inclusive programme must emphasize the most critical exercises. This can be done by providing written handouts with stars, stickers or underlining to highlight the important exercises. These critical exercises should be performed first in a rehabilitation session. The remaining exercises can be indicated on the written instructions in order of priority, in case the child has sufficient time and motivation after the initial group of exercises are completed.

Visible progress

Like adults, children respond very well to goal-oriented progressions. The more levels on the ladder of goals, the better. Adolescents should take some responsibility for setting the goals, making them as concrete and specific as possible (Danish, 1984; Murphy, 1991). If possible, the injured youth should be able to reach intermediate goals at fairly short intervals. Progress may be indicated by changing colours of elastic bands or tubing, by increasing numbers of repetitions, or by increasing resistance of free weights. In the author's experience, young people are most excited by their progress when they achieve the ability to lift greater amounts of weight, rather than simply increasing numbers of repetitions or strength of elastic bands. For muscle strengthening, a child can frequently increase the resistance by approximately 250 or 500 g after only a very short interval of time, as opposed to a longer interval of time for changing from one strength of elastic band or tubing to the next greater strength.

Interesting and entertaining therapeutic exercise programmes

Practitioners who instruct children and teenagers in therapeutic exercise programmes may need to think of themselves as entertainers as well as teachers. Address the information to be conveyed in brief, interesting ways. For example, use cartoon characters known to a child in order to bring greater interest to the discussion of why and how to perform the programme. For rehabilitating adolescents, parallels with sports stars may be useful. The use of 'gimmicks' is especially appreciated by young people. The most enticing equipment is brightly coloured and appears fun to use. Exercising children and adolescents can be encour-

aged to decorate their therapy equipment with personalized painting or stickers that they like in order to try to increase compliance. Children may record their exercise programme days by sticking stars on a calendar. Adolescents may choose to maintain a personal log of the exercise parameters in a special notebook.

Integration into regular schedule

The exercise professional must help the injured youth to integrate the rehabilitation programme into a daily schedule, 6 days a week. It is unrealistic for most children to perform a long programme more than once a day. In fact, some incentive can be provided by suggesting that the young person perform the programme only 6 days a week, with one day off 'for good behaviour'. Exercises that take only 1–3 min, such as stretching exercises, can be performed any time that the young person is waiting for something. Children frequently wait for rides to and from school, wait for meals or wait for other people. Encourage the injured youth to use these waiting periods for flexibility exercises. More prolonged exercise activities (those that will require 10–15 min) can be integrated into the time periods that children and adolescents have reserved for other activities, such as listening to music or watching television. The coordinator of the rehabilitation programme might suggest that the young person put the exercise equipment in the place where he or she spends the most time with music, television, and so on. Then the child can build some incentive into the programme by planning to do the exercises during the first record or the first television show. The remainder of the individual's agreement is that if the exercise is completed, then the activity (television show, etc.) can be continued at least for an agreed period of time. If the exercise is not completed, then the fun activity terminates. It also helps to have the young person plan some sort of treat on the seventh day (the day off).

Components of the rehabilitation programme

Control of pain and swelling is the first component of the rehabilitation programme. Physical therapy modalities such as ice, compression and elevation — or more expensive, technological modalities such as ultrasound and electrical stimulation — help speed this process. The injured region may need to be supported temporarily with a cast, brace or other device. Exercise of other regions should not be neglected while waiting for the injured region to heal sufficiently to begin the specific rehabilitation for the injury. As soon as possible, range of motion activities are begun, followed by the therapeutic exercise programme. The ultimate goals of the exercise programme include restoration of muscle strength, muscle flexibility and neuromuscular coordination.

Modalities

For children, the best physical therapy modalities include local application of ice, compression and elevation of the injured area. These are useful both for acute and repetitive overuse injuries. These modalities can be provided with simple equipment, including a footstool or chair arm for elevation, an ice bag and an elastic bandage. The modalities can also be provided by the use of sophisticated equipment that provides compression in a pumping manner, compressing the oedema fluid from distal to more proximal regions at the same time that cold is applied locally.

Ultrasound therapy and phonopheresis (the use of ultrasound technology to move anti-inflammatory medication through the superficial tissues) may be useful for children's injuries such as tendonitis and muscle strains. Some evidence suggests a need for caution concerning the use of therapeutic ultrasound in the regions of open growth plates (Gann, 1991). DeForest et al. (1953) produced growth plate injury by repeated direct applications of 5−10 W for 5−10 min to rabbit proximal tibial growth plates; this dosage was substantially higher than dosages generally used today. However, to the author's knowledge, there is no reported series of growth plate injuries resulting from ultrasound used at the currently recommended doses. Therapeutic ultrasound at the energies currently used is probably safe, but consideration should be given to employing other methods for control of pain and swelling of the injured region first, and utilizing ultrasound on skeletally immature individuals only if these prove ineffective. Electrical stimulation may be useful for controlling muscle spasm, particularly paraspinous spasm. It can also be useful for control of pain, especially in the ankle or knee. Some prefer to alternate between the application of heat and ice, using the heat to increase blood flow into the area, but then ending with ice application in order to decrease the inflammatory response.

Therapeutic exercise programme

Therapeutic exercise programmes that are recommended for children and adolescents are similar to those for adults. For a complete programme, all components of the exercising body need to be rehabilitated. This includes not only the injured area, but the muscles and joints that immediately surround the injured area, as well as remote muscles and joints. Anaerobic power must be restored, and aerobic endurance must be either maintained or regained. Realistically, only the most motivated or élite young athletes pursue a rehabilitation programme to this end-point.

FLEXIBILITY AND STRENGTHENING

Special considerations for children involve both flexibility and strengthening. In the growing child, the muscles may be relatively short compared with the bones, which are elongating with growth. In fact, the lack of a normal relationship between bone length and muscle length is frequently an aetiological factor for musculoskeletal injuries in youth. Children have little concept of the appropriate non-ballistic methods for stretching muscles, and these must be taught especially carefully. When explaining the need for warming up the muscles first and stretching them slowly (Strickler *et al.*, 1990), descriptions of caramel candy or pulling toffee can be useful analogies. Many children have experienced the brittleness of cold candy, and they know that the candy stretches better when warm and breaks when cold.

Children should be taught to differentiate the sensation of a stretching muscle (pulling sensation) from a tearing muscle (painful sensation). They should learn to relax into the stretch. Relaxation into a stretch may be enhanced by concentrating on 'letting go' of the muscle during each exhalation while breathing slowly. Contraction of a muscle group, followed by relaxation, may provide greater flexibility gains than static stretching (Etnyre & Abraham, 1986). Each stretch should be held for 20–30 s. Two or three repetitions are probably most time-effective (Taylor *et al.*, 1985).

For strengthening, free weights and elastic tubing have both been used successfully even with young children. Such exercise programmes should be supervised carefully, whether at an exercise facility or at home. If free weights are used, supervision is particularly important. Strength training machines may be used successfully for children. However, if machines are to be utilized, they must be adjusted carefully to fit the child's frame, the child must be instructed appropriately, and the exercise programme should be carefully supervised. Averaging 10 repetitions $\cdot$ set^{-1} has proved safe and effective clinically (Sewall & Micheli, 1986).

RELATIVE REST

In the past, injured children and adolescents were often instructed to stop all play, fitness and sports activities until an injury had healed completely. A young person who suddenly returns to full activity on the day that healing is pronounced to be complete is at risk for recur-

rent injury because of loss of strength, flexibility, coordination and cardiopulmonary endurance. A much safer plan includes determining safe activities that do not risk further injury but allow maintenance of the child's fitness as much as possible. With some injuries, the individual may need to eliminate only a single element from the practice routine. The time that is freed up from normal practice time may be utilized for performing the rehabilitation exercises.

DETERMINE AETIOLOGICAL FACTORS

Another important part of the rehabilitation programme is the elimination of any factors involved in the aetiology of the injury. If the injury was acute, the main causative factor may have involved an unusual accident or an unanticipated collision. However, acute injuries may also be related to training technique, equipment, footwear or playing surface. All of these factors can be examined and changed as needed. Other elements that should be checked are any previous injuries that have not been rehabilitated, and any areas of poor muscle or joint flexibility not directly within the injured region.

The causes of overuse injuries are frequently possible to identify (see Chapter 13). Common causes of overuse injuries include: (i) poor flexibility related to rapid growth; (ii) previous unrehabilitated injuries; (iii) biomechanical problems of the upper or lower extremities, including anatomical malalignment; (iv) problems of training technique; (v) training error; (vi) ill-fitting or inappropriate equipment; (vii) congenital disorders; or (viii) associated diseases. The health-care professional must ask appropriate questions regarding each of these to prevent recurrent or new, unrelated injury.

Medications

Immediately following an acute injury or an operative procedure, children and adolescents may require pain medication. The type and dosage of the medication depend on the severity of the injury. Young children with simple fractures rarely require medication other than a day or so of acetaminophen. Older children and teenagers with more severe injuries accompanied by marked swelling often benefit from non-steroidal anti-inflammatory drugs (NSAIDs) such as ibuprofen, naproxyn or tolmetin sulphate. For the adolescent with a soft tissue injury that is accompanied by marked swelling, such as a sprain, an NSAID may be the medication of choice, due to its possible effect of slightly speeding early ligament healing (Dahners *et al*, 1988). NSAIDs do not affect either oedema or passive muscle strength in the first 24 h following muscle strain injury, according to one study (Almekinders, 1992). Evidence suggests that NSAIDs may actually slow bone healing in fractures (Allen *et al.*, 1980; Elves *et al.*, 1982).

The choice of using medication for the young individual with a significant overuse injury requires more consideration. Those with marked pain and swelling may need anti-inflammatory medication in addition to local treatment (such as ice application) to control symptoms sufficiently to allow rehabilitation. Sometimes it is difficult to convince an adolescent to take a short course of an NSAID in an appropriate dosage that ensures reasonable serum levels throughout the day. Some children and young adolescents report that NSAIDs make them sleepy, so they do not want to take the medication before or during school hours. Many prefer to take medications only at the moment that pain is severe. Explaining the rationale for treatment may help improve compliance with a recommended medication regimen, but even this is only somewhat successful, in this author's experience.

Another group of older children and adolescents who may benefit from NSAID therapy are those with milder overuse injuries, with only slight or no oedema. They should be instructed to use the medication only when in a situation in which there is no risk of further injury to the structure that is being rehabilitated.

For example, a 15-year-old basketball player may take the medication *after* a game or practice, or before performing the therapeutic exercise programme or at bedtime. The rehabilitating athlete should not take the pain-masking medication before an activity that is likely to disrupt the healing process or to cause a different injury because of playing on a weakened limb. Of course, an élite athlete, or an athlete who wishes to play in the final, championship game of a season, may choose to take some risk of further injury and use medication to allow the possibility of competing.

Instructions on athletic activity during rehabilitation

Athletes, coaches and parents may use four simple rules regarding return to activity, as outlined in Table 16.1. The first rule is that the amount of tissue healing that occurs over a 24-h period must exceed the amount of tissue destruction that occurs during that period. An

Table 16.1 Rules for sports participation while injured.

Pain may be present at the end of activity, but must be gone by the next morning, indicating that the amount of tissue injury is probably not exceeding tissue healing

Limping, or favouring the injured limb, means it is too risky to participate in activities where you are not in control of the situation. If you continue in an activity where collision or slipping is likely — and the muscles are not performing in a normal, coordinated manner — then serious, permanent injury could occur

Ability to complete the prescribed exercise programme effectively, 6 days a week, is necessary. If you have so much discomfort following the sport activities that you cannot perform the strengthening exercises properly, then you should either decrease the amount of sport activity or perform the strengthening exercises in the morning

You should not use pain-masking drugs or ice application *before* sport activity, so that you can monitor your body's signals of pain

effective clinical guideline is to allow activity, even if it causes pain, as long as the pain resolves very shortly after the activity is completed. If pain is still present the following morning, then tissue destruction is likely to have exceeded tissue healing, and the athlete must decrease the amount of activity.

The second rule states that activities must be avoided if they cause pain that interferes with the patient's ability to do the therapeutic exercises correctly and efficiently. If athletic activity causes swelling, for example, then the surrounding muscles are inhibited and cannot contract normally. Some adolescents choose to perform the exercise programme early in the morning, when swelling and pain are minimal. If the programme has already been successfully completed for the day, then activities are allowed as long as pain and swelling are again negligible by the next morning.

The third rule is that the athlete cannot compete if the weakened region is likely to lead to further injury. For weight-bearing sports, an individual may continue activity with pain only if he or she is willing to tolerate the pain and has full control of the activity. For example, an athlete may continue to jog on a level surface even if a slight limp is present. However, if an athlete participates in an activity where complete control is not possible, such as a contact sport or a collision sport such as gymnastics or downhill skiing, then activity must stop if the youth feels the least tendency to favour the injured limb, or if any observer notes limping or favouring. If the athlete continues participation under these conditions, with decreased ability to respond to a sudden unexpected application of force, then further injury (possibly severe and permanently disabling) becomes likely.

Finally, an injured youth should not mask pain by the use of medication or physical therapy modalities *before* participating in sport activity. The individual must be able to appreciate any pain that occurs during the activity to guard against further injury.

Psychological aspects of rehabilitation

Most children and teenagers perceive an injury as a temporary interruption that makes them either different and unable to be a part of their usual group (a negative response) or special, with a cast to be signed and a special therapy programme (a positive response). As long as the period of disability is fairly short and the youth believes that full recovery will follow, he or she is likely to comply with a rehabilitation programme with a positive mental attitude. The athlete's parents should be enlisted to assist in the rehabilitation process and the return to activity. 'Parent management' includes allaying the parents' anxieties and helping them to understand the physical injury and the related emotional state of the injured child (Heil, 1993). It also includes teaching them ways to help the child prevent recurrent injury.

Rotella (1988) compares the sequence of emotional responses of an athlete with an injury to those of a person facing death, as described by Kubler-Ross (1969): (i) disbelief, denial and isolation; (ii) anger; (iii) bargaining; (iv) depression; and (v) acceptance and resignation. However, some athletes may perceive an injury as an opportunity to show strength or courage, or as a convenient excuse to end a poor season prematurely. Smith *et al.* (1990) found that the most frequent emotional response of adolescent athletes 1 day following injury were frustration, depression and anger, with anger reported more among adolescents than among adults. The author's experience with young athletes suggests that only the more mature and highly competitive or élite athletes with severe injuries undergo processes that resemble the Kubler-Ross stages. Less emotionally mature adolescents often proceed rapidly to acceptance of the knowledge that a severe injury has precluded the chance to play at the college or professional level; however, they simultaneously deny that it is unsafe to participate in recreational activities that are very likely to increase their disabilities even more.

Some use injury as an excuse to gain relief

from the pressures of sport. Some of these individuals then use recurrent injury or difficulties out of proportion to the usual pain and disability of a given injury, as a reason to stop an activity entirely. Often these children or adolescents have been under severe pressure to succeed from parents or coaches, and injury provides the athlete with the only perceived escape from a sport that is no longer enjoyable. Heil (1993) cautions that if the 'sick role' of prolonged injury recovery persists unexpectedly, then there may be a parent–child relationship problem. The individual's reasoning and coping mechanisms should be identified and dealt with appropriately by the coordinator of the rehabilitation programme and mental health consultants, if needed. The appropriate treatment may include supporting the athlete's desire to decrease the level of participation in the sport — or quit the sport entirely — even though the coach and parents wish the child to continue in the sport at a highly competitive level.

Some young people may confuse the bodily sensations that occur with emotional distress (nausea, muscle tension, chest tightness) with signs of physical illness or injury. According to Heil (1993) such somatization is most common among young athletes, especially when participation is required. The treating physicians and therapists must help the child recognize the differences among these psychophysiological symptoms, the discomforts of an injury that is healing properly, and the discomforts of an injury that is not healing well.

Injured élite athletes may be willing to spend several hours each week on psychological training. Useful psychological mechanisms for coping with an injury include learning to stop self-defeating inner dialogue, replacing it with self-enhancing inner dialogue. Visual imaging of successful scenes of injury recovery and athletic accomplishment and of the body's healing process may be useful (Murphy, 1991). Relaxation techniques are often helpful in self-control of pain. A frequently used technique consists of alternately tightening the muscles of a region for several seconds and then letting go

of all of the tension. Each major muscle group, from trunk to arms to legs, is included sequentially (Rotella, 1988). Mastery rehearsal (imagining successful completion of tasks) and coping rehearsal (actively anticipating potential problems) are other psychological strategies (Rotella, 1988).

Extremely motivated young athletes often spend 6 h daily perfecting their sport skills. For these athletes, injuries are often even more devastating psychologically than they are physically. Rotella has laid out specific programmes for emotional healing that may proceed concomitantly with physical healing. An athlete may follow a system of desensitization hierarchies from simpler through more difficult anxieties that are sport-specific, at a rate that ensures that the athlete will be psychologically ready to return to sport by the time of completion of biological healing and physical rehabilitation. The three processes should be coordinated so that emotions, healing and rehabilitation are all prepared for return to activity at approximately the same time (Rotella, 1988). The athlete proceeds by means of visualization through the desensitization hierarchy, imagining successful completion of each step while remaining in a relaxed state. The desensitization hierarchy for a basketball player could include the following steps: going onto the basketball court for practice, beginning practice with simple sprints, completing more skill-specific drills, shooting over a defensive player in a scrimmage, and so forth, through the most difficult situations that the player can envision (Rotella, 1988).

Simple biofeedback principles may be taught to the recreational athlete. These include relaxation techniques (heart rate is the parameter monitored) and muscle isolation techniques (individual muscle contraction is monitored visually). Muscle isolation techniques are especially useful for strengthening specific muscles. An élite athlete with a serious injury may benefit from sophisticated methods of biofeedback training such as telemetry of heart rate and blood pressure, and electromyography.

Relaxation techniques are useful for pain control and for flexibility training.

Some of the concepts of psychological healing are useful for the average youth who participates in organized sports. Promoting positive thought and stopping negative thoughts encourage progress through a rehabilitation programme. To help maintain a positive self-image, the injured individual should participate in all team activities that are safe, within the parameters of relative rest and the four rules of participation outlined in Table 16.1. Many coaches and teachers allow an injured youth to attend practice or class only if full participation and '100% effort' are allowed, so special communication from a parent and/or physician is often required to set an appropriate programme, based on the above parameters.

Specific examples

It is beyond the scope of this chapter to outline rehabilitation protocols for all types of injuries. However, patellofemoral pain syndrome is discussed to illustrate a rehabilitation programme for one of the most frequently diagnosed overuse injuries of children and adolescents, and ankle sprain illustrates a protocol for rehabilitation of an acute injury frequently occurring in this age group.

Patellofemoral pain syndrome

Patellofemoral pain syndrome is one of the most frequently diagnosed disorders in sports medicine clinics for children and adolescents (see Chapter 12). It may occur as a primary overuse injury, usually in early- to mid-adolescence, or it may result secondary to another injury to the limb that led to muscular imbalance about the knee.

Most young people with patellofemoral pain syndrome present with mild to moderate symptoms. This author's clinical impression is that these individuals respond as well to a loosely supervised home programme as to a closely monitored formal physical therapy programme.

Those with marked inflammation and swelling require a more aggressive initial approach to relieve the inflammation before an independent progressive therapeutic exercise program becomes possible. The more aggressive approach may include NSAID, locally applied therapeutic modalities such as ultrasound or cold compression, McConnell taping (McConnell, 1986), or use of a patella restraining brace with a lateral buttress. The goal of this approach is to allow the injured individual to begin a progressive resistance exercise programme as rapidly as possible, in order to compress the total rehabilitation period as discussed above. In the author's practice, this programme has proved effective in more than 98% of adolescent patients with patellofemoral pain, including patients initially diagnosed with lateral patellar compression syndrome and lower extremity malalignment.

DEFINED REHABILITATION PERIOD

The usual adolescent with mild to moderate symptoms of patellofemoral pain syndrome (either primary or secondary) requires 2 months of therapeutic exercise to decrease the severity of pain by approximately 50%. To resolve the remainder of the symptoms generally requires an additional 1–2 months. However, many adolescents choose to abandon the exercise programme once 90–95% of their pain has resolved.

SMALL NUMBER OF EXERCISES

Most adolescents with patellofemoral pain have both strength deficits and flexibility deficits. A very effective programme that involves a minimal number of exercises is based on straight leg raise progressive resistance exercises (Fig. 16.6), three sets of eight to 12 repetitions done by each leg, alternating right and left sides (even if symptoms are unilateral). The individual increases the amount of exercise, either by adding repetitions or by adding 500 g of weight attached to the ankle, as rapidly as possible. If

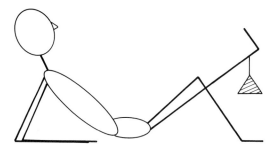

Fig. 16.6 Straight leg raising, to strengthen quadriceps in the treatment of patellofemoral pain. The child leans back on the elbows comfortably. One knee is bent so that the heel of that foot touches the opposite knee. The patient contracts the quadriceps muscles of the straight leg, while observing the position of the patella. Focusing his or her eyes on the vastus medialis muscle, the patient then quickly raises the straight leg until the knees touch lightly. The patella should be pointed up toward the ceiling. This position is held for 5 s, the leg is then lowered slowly for 4 s, and the leg is completely relaxed at its original position on the 10th s. Three sets of eight to 12 repetitions are performed, alternating left and right sides.

the rehabilitating child or adolescent wishes to do another strengthening exercise, then short arc knee extensions from 30 to 0° of flexion, partial squats or cycling are added. Flexibility exercises are included in the programme, depending on the specific deficits noted in the evaluation. For patellofemoral pain, these often include the hamstrings (Fig. 16.7), triceps surae (calf) and quadriceps muscles.

VISIBLE PROGRESS

The exercise prescription for the adolescent with patellofemoral pain includes a frequency of once daily, 6 days a week. Several times each week he or she should be able to increase either the number or repetitions or the weight. Once the individual can complete three sets of 12 repetitions · set^{-1}, then the resistance should be increased by 500 g, and the number of repetitions decreased to eight repetitions · set^{-1}. Repetitions are increased until 12 repetitions are possible at the new resistance, and then another 0·45 kg is added to begin the sequence again. Clinical evidence suggests that a 55-kg adolescent with moderate patellofemoral pain syndrome requires approximately 2 months to be able to straight leg raise 5·5 kg for three sets. At that level, generally half of the pain has resolved. An appropriate end-point for this

55-kg adolescent is three sets of 9 kg. Once this exercise level is achieved, the individual ideally continues lifting this weight for 1 month more, but on a maintenance programme of only three or four times every week. For the next 2 months, the ankle weights should be used once a week, to make certain that the strength gains have been maintained. If possible, the rehabilitated adolescent should then check for maintenance of the strength gains by monthly testing with the 9 kg, for an additional 6 months.

INTERESTING AND ENTERTAINING THERAPEUTIC EXERCISE PROGRAMMES AND INTEGRATION IN THE DAILY SCHEDULE

After the practitioner explains the aetiological factors leading to patellofemoral pain, demonstrating the atrophied or inflexible muscles, the young patient often appears disinterested, and the idea of a boring exercise programme, to be done alone without friends, is distasteful. At this point in the discussion, a question such as 'Do you ever watch TV or talk on the phone?' brings either laughter or smiling nods from parent and patient. Once their interest is regained, the principles of the exercise programme can be disclosed.

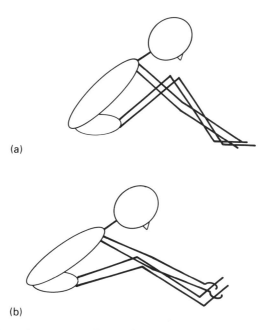

(a)

(b)

Fig. 16.7 Hamstring stretching, for treatment of patellofemoral pain and low back pain. The child sits on a firm, flat surface, with both knees bent, and lightly grasps the lateral sides of the feet (a). Resting the trunk comfortably on the thighs, releasing any tension in the back and shoulders, the patient slowly slides the feet away from the buttocks until a pulling sensation is felt in the hamstrings (b). This position is held for 30 s. Then the trunk is lifted up a few centimetres from the thighs to relax (and the hamstrings may be contracted here, if that technique is desired), the feet are slid distally a bit more, and the trunk is then brought down to the thighs again. This sequence may be repeated several times.

Many centres utilize elastic bands as resistance for quadriceps strengthening. Although the bands are brightly coloured, and although they are among the best equipment for rehabilitation of ankle sprains, they do not allow enough visible progress for the individual with patellofemoral pain. Ankle weights may be purchased, either as a metal weight boot with a bar for adding weight discs, or as a wrap-around device with pockets for inserting sandbag weights. For smaller amounts of weight, socks filled with coins or rocks (weighed on a kitchen scale or at the post office) and wrapped in a figure-of-eight fashion around the foot and ankle, are effective.

The practitioner should help the injured individual develop a programme of incentives for performing the exercises. For example, if a child completes the exercises during the first 15 min of a television show, the reward is to watch the remainder of the show. Similarly, an adolescent who completes the exercises during the first telephone call of the evening may have an agreement to be allowed a second phone call.

Acute ankle sprain, grade II or III

Severe ankle sprains can be treated at home by the patient, but a physical therapist, certified athletic trainer or other health-care professional can help speed the healing and rehabilitation process markedly. The most important difference between a home programme and a formal therapy programme for sprains is the more rapid and more efficient control of pain and swelling in the early phase of professional treatment. In the strengthening phase, the assistance of the practitioner helps the injured individual stay motivated, since the attainment of strength training goals may be difficult for the patient to observe readily. For the final phase of proprioceptive training, a therapy facility generally has better and more interesting equipment than at home.

DEFINED REHABILITATION PERIOD

The healing process of ankle sprains in children and adolescents is dependent on the severity of the injury, the age of the patient and the type of therapy. Utilizing an air-stirrup brace for protected mobilization and an aggressive physical therapy protocol, almost all children and adolescents with severe ankle sprains are able to begin range of motion exercises 1–2 days following the injury, bear full weight by 3–5 days following the injury, and begin strengthening the muscle groups around the ankle within the first 7–10 days. Return to full activity, wearing a protective brace, generally requires 4–8 weeks, depending on the factors noted above.

SMALL NUMBER OF EXERCISES

The formal, supervised, therapy programme that this author recommends for the most rapid effect should be complemented by a home programme, performed on the days that the patient is not seen in the therapy facility. Range of motion exercises are performed several times daily, beginning very early in the rehabilitation process. Simple strengthening exercises for the ankle evertors, invertors, dorsiflexors and plantarflexors require only a few minutes to perform. Stretching of the triceps surae is the final important exercise of the mandatory rehabilitation, but proprioceptive training is highly recommended for regaining full performance capability and for preventing recurrent injury (Tropp et al., 1985).

VISIBLE PROGRESS

Early on, the patient can observe resolution of oedema and ecchymosis. However, later in the rehabilitation process, progress is more subtle, so the assistance of a trained professional is very helpful for interpreting evidence of progress to the patient.

INTERESTING AND ENTERTAINING THERAPEUTIC EXERCISE PROGRAMMES AND INTEGRATION INTO THE DAILY SCHEDULE

Brightly coloured elastic bands or surgical tubing add interest to the strengthening programme. The proprioceptive training and final strengthening phases can be made more entertaining by designing hopping or balancing games that incorporate the exercises. These may be done any time that the patient is waiting for someone or something.

Challenges for future research

• What percentage of overuse injuries are preventable by prehabilitation? No prospective controlled study has adequately investigated a causal relationship between specific flexibility deficits and certain injuries.

• Are home therapy programmes as successful as more closely monitored programmes? Few injured young people have ready access to a physical therapy centre for frequent treatments and monitored exercise. For many simple injuries, the clinical impression is that a simple, brief home programme may produce results similar to those from a formal programme with therapy supervised professionally. For more severe injuries, particularly injuries with prolonged swelling and significant pain, more frequent formal therapy sessions appear to be preferential to home programmes in terms of recovery time and final result.

• Are there differences in the response of injured growing tissues to certain rehabilitation techniques?

• Do modalities such as therapeutic ultrasound and electrical stimulation affect growing bones and soft tissues?

• Is there any effect — deleterious or salutatory — of strength training on growing tissues?

• Although there is no evidence that suggests that strength training (performed appropriately) harms normal growth plates of long bones, is there an effect on the growth plate when the surrounding soft tissues are weakened from injury?

References

Allen, H.L., Wase, A. & Bear, W.T. (1980) Indomethacin and aspirin: effect of nonsteroidal anti-inflammatory agents on the rate of fracture repair in the rat. *Acta Orthop. Scand.* **51**, 595–600.

Almekinders, L.C. (1992) The effects of early anti-inflammatory treatment in muscle strains. *Trans. Orthop. Res. Soc.* **17**, 260.

Cahill, B.R. & Griffith, E.H. (1978) Effect of preseason conditioning on the incidence and severity of high school football knee injuries. *Am. J. Sports Med.* **6**, 180–3.

Dahners, L.E., Gilbert, J.A., Lester, G.E., Taft, T.N. & Paynes, L.Z. (1988) The effect of a nonsteroidal antiinflammatory drug on the healing of ligaments. *Am. J. Sports Med.* **16**, 641–6.

Danish, S. (1984) Psychological aspects in the care and treatment of athletic injuries. In P.E. Vinger & E. Hoerner (eds) *Sports Injuries — The Unthwarted Epidemic*, 2nd edn. PSG Publishing, Littleton, MA.

DeForest, R.E., Herrick, J.F., Janes, J.M. & Kursen, F.H. (1953) Effects of ultrasound on growing bone: an experimental study. *Arch. Phys. Med. Rehab.* **34**, 21–31.

Elves, M.W., Bayley, I. & Roylance, P.J. (1982) The effect of indomethacin upon experimental fractures in the rat. *Acta Orthop. Scand.* **53**, 35–41.

Etnyre, B.R. & Abraham, L.D. (1986) Gains in range of ankle dorsiflexion using three popular stretching techniques. *Am. J. Phys. Med.* **65**, 189–96.

Gann, N. (1991) Ultrasound: current concepts. *Clin. Manage.* **11**, 64–9.

Gurewitsch, A.D. & O'Neill, M.A. (1944) Flexibility of healthy children. *Arch. Phys. Ther.* **25**, 216–21.

Heil, J. (1993) *Psychology of Sport Injury*. Human Kinetics, Champaign, IL.

Kibler, W.B., Chandler, T.J. & Stracener, E.S. (1992) Musculoskeletal adaptations and injuries due to overtraining. *Exerc. Sports Sci. Rev.* **20**, 99–126.

Kubler-Ross, E. (1969) *On Death and Dying*. Macmillan, New York.

Lysens, R.J., Ostyn, M.S., Auweele, Y.V., Lefeevre, J., Vuylsteke, M. & Renson, L. (1989) The accident-prone and overuse-prone profiles of the young athlete. *Am. J. Sports Med.* **17**, 612–19.

McConnell, J. (1986) The management of chondromalacia patellae: a long term solution. *Austral. J. Phys.* **32**, 215–23.

Micheli, L.J. & Ireland, M.L. (1987) Prevention and management of calcaneal apophysitis in children: an overuse syndrome. *J. Pediatr. Orthop.* **7**, 34–8.

Murphy, S. (1991) Behavioral considerations. In R.C. Cantu & L.J. Micheli (eds) *ACSM's Guidelines for the Team Physician*. Lea & Febiger, Philadelphia.

Rotella, R.J. (1988) Psychological care of the injured athlete. In D. Kulund (ed.) *The Injured Athlete*. Lippincott, Philadelphia.

Sewall, L. & Micheli, L.J. (1986) Strength training for children. *J. Pediatr. Orthop.* **6**, 143–6.

Smith, A.D. (1991) A four-year longitudinal study of injuries of élite figure skaters. *Med. Sci. Sports Exerc.* **23**, S151.

Smith, A.D., Stroud, L. & McQueen, C. (1991) Flexibility and anterior knee pain in adolescent élite figure skaters. *J. Pediatr. Orthop.* **11**, 77–82.

Smith, A.M., Scott, S.G., O'Fallon, W.M. & Young, J.L. (1990) Emotional responses of athletes to injury. *Mayo Clin. Proc.* **65**, 38–50.

Strickler, T., Malone, T. & Garrett, W.E. (1990) The effects of passive warming on muscle injury. *Am. J. Sports Med.* **18**, 141–5.

Tachdjian, M.O. (1990) *Pediatric Orthopedics*. W.B. Saunders, Philadelphia.

Taylor, C.C., Seaber, A.B. & Garrett, W.E. Jr (1985) Response of muscle–tendon units to cyclic repetitive stretching. *Trans. Orthop. Res. Soc.* **10**, 84.

Tropp, H., Askling, C. & Gillquist, J. (1985) Prevention of ankle sprains. *Am. J. Sports Med.* **13**, 259–62.

PART 4

NON-ORTHOPAEDIC
HEALTH CONCERNS

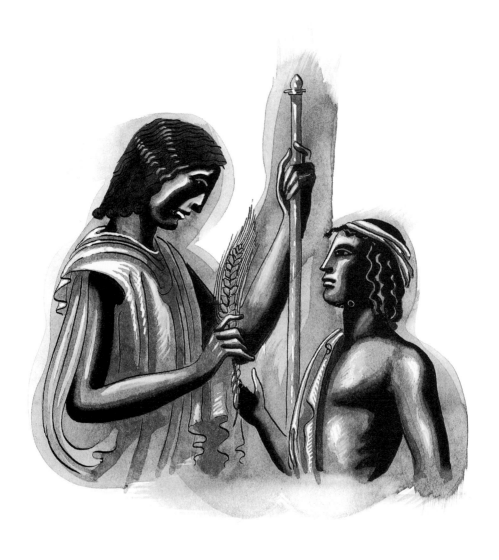

Chapter 17

The Preparticipation Physical Examination

PAUL G. DYMENT

Introduction

There is a substantial risk of injury in most athletic participation, and the purpose of the preparticipation examination is to 'prevent life-threatening or disabling injuries by identifying predisposing factors, recommending preparatory and/or rehabilitative measures, and assisting in matching the participant with an appropriate sport and/or position' (Linder et al., 1981). The preparticipation examination of the young athlete is a time-honoured custom which has only recently come under close scrutiny, with questions about its cost-effectiveness being the subject of several recent commentaries by Linder et al. (1981), Risser et al. (1985), Rowland (1986) and Samples (1986).

The problem is that if a traditional physical examination is performed, i.e. a search for medical abnormalities such as a heart murmur or hernia, only about 1% of athletic teenagers will have an abnormality uncovered; and even these 'abnormalities' usually are such things as an innocent heart murmur, a trace of albuminuria or a transiently elevated blood pressure, none of which will turn out to be of any consequence as far as either athletic participation or eventual health are concerned. Physicians only too often assume from their previous experience examining healthy teenagers that nothing will be detected during a sports examination. The athletes, on their part, are keen to 'pass' the examination, so they volunteer little in the way of an accurate medical history.

This combination of attitudes results in a cursory examination of little value in identifying physical problems which will either affect performance or which may be made worse by participation. In this situation there is little to justify the 'annual sports examination'.

However, the purposes of the preparticipation examination outlined above can be achieved if the examination includes a detailed musculoskeletal evaluation looking for residua of previous sports injuries. Most sports injuries are reinjuries, and if a musculoskeletal assessment is performed as many as 10% of adolescent athletes will be found to have an abnormality requiring advice at least regarding rehabilitation, if not about the wisdom of competition (Thompson et al., 1982). If the physician also has both the time and the privacy to offer personal health maintenance counselling on such issues as sexuality, alcohol and drug abuse, 'safer' sex and coping skills to handle the stresses of adolescence and young adulthood, then the athlete will truly have benefitted from this kind of a visit to the doctor.

Comparison of single and multiple examiners

The most cost-effective and efficient method of examining large numbers of athletes is the stations format, in which a group of health-care professionals (physicians, nurses and athletic trainers) attend, and each member performs part of the examination. Durant et al. (1985)

243

demonstrated that far more abnormalities were detected by such a team than by private physicians performing individual examinations. The obvious disadvantages of this technique are that a complete medical and social history are not obtained, as they would be during a comprehensive physical examination in a physician's office. The only time most high school aged athletes ever see a physician in any one year is for their preparticipation examination, and health maintenance counselling can really only occur during a youth's visit to his or her personal physician's office. Most authorities in adolescent medicine recommend annual health maintenance examinations for teenagers, principally because of the anticipatory guidance offered, and not because of the remote chance of detecting a previously undetected and asymptomatic medical condition.

When youth are being seen for a health maintenance examination, physicians should enquire whether they are planning to participate in competitive athletics, and if so, then the musculoskeletal assessment to be described should be incorporated into that physical examination.

Timing of the examination

The preparticipation examination should occur at least 4 weeks before practice begins in order to allow rehabilitative exercises to become effective in those athletes in whom an incompletely rehabilitated previous injury has been detected during the examination. Sports examinations really need only be performed at entry to high school and again at college entrance. If they are given at these infrequent intervals, however, there must also be a system in place so that an interim medical history (Fig. 17.1) will be obtained prior to each athletic season. If this reveals that there has been a recent injury or serious illness, then the student should undergo another preparticipation physical examination by a physician. The screening of the interim history form could be done by either the school doctor, team physician or school nurse. Without this safeguard in schools that require an annual sports examination, the athlete who undergoes a preparticipation physical examination in August and who sprains an ankle playing football in September, could try-out for the basketball team in November without medical review of the advisability of competing with a recently injured ankle.

Medical history

The Sports Medicine Committee of the American Academy of Pediatrics (AAP) has printed sports preparticipation history and physical forms, and school districts are encouraged to adopt these as standards (Figs 17.1 & 17.2). Note that this medical history form includes both the standard preparticipation history as well as the optional interim history.

Laboratory tests

Neither a haemoglobin/haematocrit nor urinalysis are recommended by the AAP as a necessary part of a preparticipation examination, although they may well be indicated at regular intervals throughout adolescence as part of a health maintenance programme. It is still not clear whether iron deficiency without anaemia affects athletic performance. Even frank iron-deficiency anaemia needs to be fairly significant before there is measurably impaired performance. However, iron deficiency is common amongst female athletes, particularly those engaged in endurance sports (see Chapter 19). A female élite athlete competing in national competition might therefore benefit from a serum ferritin being obtained and supplemental oral ferrous sulphate given if there is evidence that body iron stores are low. This is an expensive test, and some have therefore just recommended giving oral iron supplementation to all endurance athletes throughout their training season.

Sickle cell screening for all athletes in at-risk populations is still controversial (Browne,

1993); it seems that athletes with sickle cell trait present little risk unless they exercise at high altitude or in conditions of high heat and humidity, or other conditions that may induce dehydration, in which case they incur a definite risk of collapse, rhabdomyolysis, hyperkalaemia, renal failure and death (Eichner, 1986). It would therefore be reasonable to screen Black athletes who will be competing under those conditions with a rapid haemoglobin solubility test, following up those positive tests with blood tests for haemoglobin and haemoglobin electrophoresis.

Musculoskeletal assessment

In addition to the usual medical examination, a musculoskeletal examination should be performed — 'the 2-minute orthopaedic examination' (Table 17.1, Figs 17.3–17.14). The AAP physical examination form (Fig. 17.2) was developed to allow a detailed recording of the musculoskeletal assessment. The physician should demonstrate or describe each movement, starting with the neck and working down. Not only should the physician watch for signs of muscular weakness on one side

Table 17.1 The 2-min orthopaedic examination. From the American Academy of Pediatrics (1991) with permission, © 1991.

Figure number	Instructions	Observations
17.3	Stand facing examiner	Acromioclavicular joints, general habitus
17.4	Look at ceiling, floor, over both shoulders; touch ears to shoulders	Cervical spine motion
17.5	Shrug shoulders (examiner resists)	Trapezius strength
17.6	Abduct shoulders 90° (examiner resists at 90°)	Deltoid strength
17.7	Full external rotation of arms	Shoulder motion
17.8	Flex and extend elbows	Elbow motion
17.9	Arms at sides, elbows 90° flexed; pronate and supinate wrists	Elbow and wrist motion
17.10	Spread fingers; make fist	Hand or finger motion and deformities
	Tighten (contract) quadriceps; relax quadriceps	Symmetry and knee effusion; ankle effusion
17.11	'Duck walk' four steps (away from examiner with buttocks on heels)	Hip, knee and ankle motion
17.12	Back to examiner	Shoulder symmetry, scoliosis
17.13	Knees straight, touch toes	Scoliosis, hip motion, hamstring tightness
17.14	Raise up on toes, raise heels	Calf symmetry, leg strength

Sports Participation Health Record. This evaluation is only to determine readiness for sports participation. It should not be used as a substitute for regular health maintenance examinations.

Name _____ Age _____ (yrs) Grade _____ Date _____

Address _____

Sports _____

The Health History (Part A) and Physical Examination (Part C) sections must both be completed, at least every 24 months, before sports participation. The Interim Health History (Part B) needs to be completed at least annually.

Part A — Health History

To be completed by athlete and parent

Yes   No

1. Have you ever had an illness that:
   a. required you to stay in hospital?
   b. lasted longer than a week?
   c. caused you to miss 3 days of practice or a competition?
   d. is related to allergies? (e.g. hives)
   e. required an operation?
   f. is chronic? (e.g. asthma, diabetes)

2. Have you ever had an injury that:
   a. required you to go to an emergency room or see a doctor?
   b. required you to stay in hospital?
   c. required X-rays?
   d. caused you to miss 3 days of practice or a competition?
   e. required an operation?

3. Do you take any medication or pills?

4. Have any members of your family under age 50 had a heart attack, heart problem, or died unexpectedly?

5. Have you ever:
   a. been dizzy or passed out during or after exercise?
   b. been unconscious or had concussion?

Part B — Interim Health History

This form should be used during the interval between prepartication evaluations. Positive responses should prompt a medical evaluation.

1. Over the next 12 months, I wish to participate in the following sports:
   a. _____
   b. _____
   c. _____
   d. _____

Yes   No

2. Have you missed more than 3 consecutive days of participation in usual activities because of an injury this past year?
   a. Site of injury _____
   b. Type of injury _____

3. Have you missed more than 5 consecutive days of participation in usual activities because of an illness, or have you had a medical illness diagnosed that has not been resolved in the past year? If yes, please indicate type of illness _____

4. Have you had a seizure, concussion or been unconscious in the last year?

6. Are you unable to run 1km (2 times around the track) without stopping? ☐ ☐

7. Do you:
   a. wear glasses or contacts? ☐ ☐
   b. wear dental bridges. plates or braces? ☐ ☐

8. Have you ever had a heart murmur, high blood pressure or a heart abnormality? ☐ ☐

9. Do you have any allergies to medicine? ☐ ☐

10. Are you missing a kidney? ☐ ☐

11. When was your last tetanus booster? _____

12. For women
    a. At what age did you experience your first menstrual period? _____
    b. In the last year, what is the longest time you have gone between periods? _____

EXPLAIN ANY "YES" ANSWERS (separate sheet)

I hereby state that to the best of my knowledge, my answers to the above questions are correct.

Signature of athlete _____

Signature of parent _____ Date _____

5. Have you had surgery or been hospitalized in the last year? If yes, please indicate: ☐ ☐
   a. Reason _____
   b. Type of surgery _____

6. List all medications you are presently taking and what condition the medication is for:
   a. _____
   b. _____
   c. _____

   Yes No
7. Are you worried about any problem or condition at this time? ☐ ☐
   If yes, please explain: _____

I hereby state that to the best of my knowledge, my answers to the above questions are correct.

Signature of athlete _____

Signature of parent _____ Date _____

Fig. 17.1 Preparticipation medical history form. Adapted with permission from the American Academy of Pediatrics (1991) © 1991.

Name				Date	Age	Birth date

Name _____ Date _____ Age _____ Birth date _____

Height _____ Vision: R _____/_____ Corrected _____ Uncorrected _____

Weight _____ Vision: L _____/_____ Corrected _____ Uncorrected _____

Pulse _____ Blood pressure _____ Percent body fat _____

	Normal	Abnormal findings	Initials
1. Eyes			
2. Ears, nose and throat			
3. Mouth and teeth			
4. Neck			
5. Cardiovascular			
6. Chest and lungs			
7. Abdomen			
8. Skin			
9. Genitals—hernia (male)			
10. Musculoskeletal: ROM, strength, etc.			
a. neck			
b. spine			
c. shoulders			
d. arms/hands			
e. hips			
f. thighs			
g. knees			
h. ankles			
i. feet			
11. Neuromuscular			
12. Physical maturity (Tanner stage)	1	2 3 4 5	

Comments re abnormal findings _____

_____

Participation recommendations:

1. No participation in _____

2. Limited participation in _____

3. Requires _____

4. Full participation in _____

Physician signature _____

Telephone number _____ Address _____

Fig. 17.2 Physical examination record. Adapted with permission from the American Academy of Pediatrics (1991) © 1991.

Fig. 17.4 (*Opposite*) Look at the ceiling; look at the floor; touch right (left) ear to shoulder; look over right (left) shoulder. The athlete should be able to touch chin to chest, ears to shoulders and look equally over shoulders. Common abnormalities (may indicate previous neck injury): (1) loss of flexion; (2) loss of lateral bending; (3) loss of rotation. Redrawn with permission from Ross Laboratories, Columbus, Ohio.

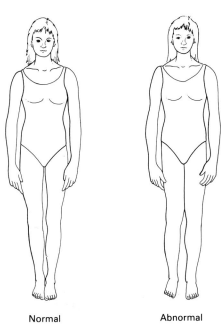

Fig. 17.3 Stand straight with arms at sides. Check for symmetry of upper and lower extremities and trunk. Common abnormalities: (1) enlarged acromioclavicular joint; (2) enlarged sternoclavicular joint; (3) asymmetrical waist (leg length difference or scoliosis); (4) swollen knee; (5) swollen ankle. Redrawn with permission from Ross Laboratories, Columbus, Ohio.

Normal   Abnormal

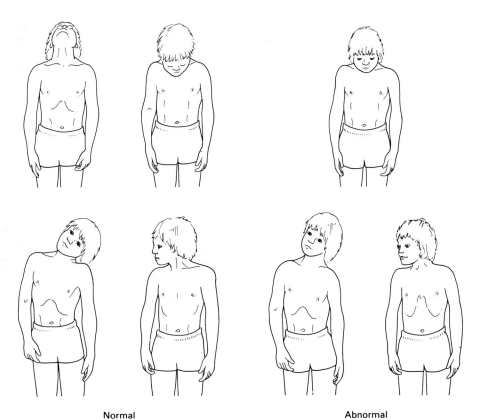

Normal   Abnormal

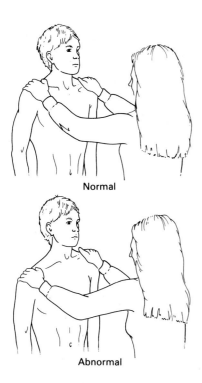

Normal

Abnormal

Fig. 17.5 Shrug shoulders while examiner holds them down. Check that trapezius muscles appear equal; left and right side have equal strength. Common abnormalities (may indicate neck or shoulder problem): (1) loss of strength; (2) loss of muscle bulk. Redrawn with permission from Ross Laboratories, Columbus, Ohio.

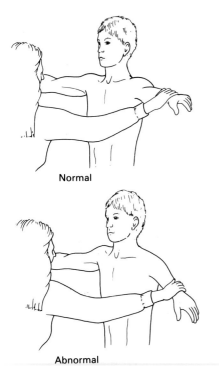

Normal

Abnormal

Fig. 17.6 Hold arms out from sides horizontally and lift while examiner holds them down. Strength should be equal and deltoid muscles should be equal in size. Common abnormalities: (1) loss of strength; (2) wasting of deltoid muscle. Redrawn with permission from Ross Laboratories, Columbus, Ohio.

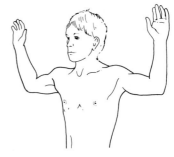

Normal

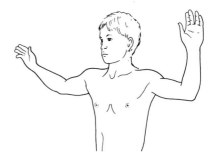

Abnormal

Fig. 17.7 Hold arms out from sides with elbows bent (90°); raise hands back vertically as far as they will go. Check that hands go back equally and at least to upright vertical position. Common abnormality (may indicate shoulder problem or old dislocation) is loss of external rotation. Redrawn with permission from Ross Laboratories, Columbus, Ohio.

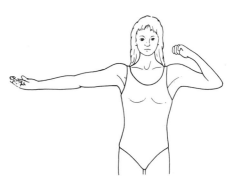

Normal

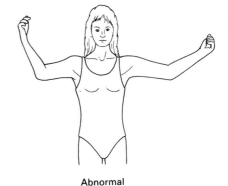

Fig. 17.8 Hold arms out from sides, palms up; straighten elbows completely; bend completely. Check motion is equal left and right sides. Common abnormalities (may indicate old elbow injury, old dislocation, fracture, etc.): (1) loss of extension; (2) loss of flexion. Redrawn with permission from Ross Laboratories, Columbus, Ohio.

Abnormal

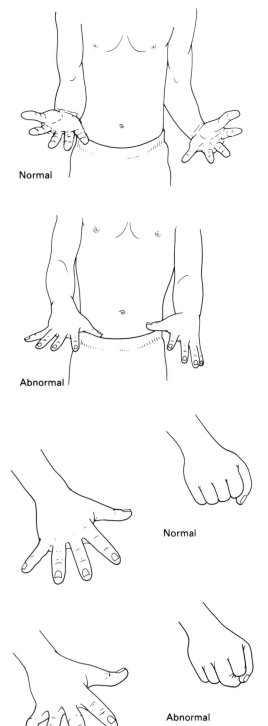

Fig. 17.9 Hold arms down at sides with elbows bent (90°); supinate palms; pronate palms. Palms should go from facing ceiling to facing floor. Common abnormalities (may indicate old forearm, wrist, or elbow injury): (1) lack of full supination; (2) lack of full pronation. Redrawn with permission from Ross Laboratories, Columbus, Ohio.

Fig. 17.10 Make a fist; open hand and spread fingers. First should be tight and fingers straight when spread. Common abnormalities (may indicate old finger fractures or sprains): (1) protruding knuckle from fist; (2) swollen and/or crooked finger. Redrawn with permission from Ross Laboratories, Columbus, Ohio.

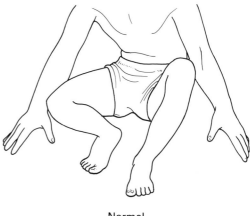

Normal

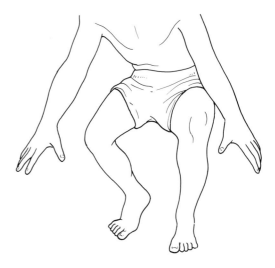

Abnormal

Fig. 17.11 Squat on heels; duck walk four steps and stand up. Check that manoeuvre is painless; heel to buttock distance is equal left and right; knee flexion is equal during walk; rises straight up. Common abnormalities: (1) inability to fully flex one knee; (2) inability to stand up without twisting or bending to one side. Redrawn with permission from Ross Laboratories, Columbus, Ohio.

compared to the other, but the face should also be observed for signs of discomfort during the movements, as pain may not be volunteered because of fear of disqualification.

Although most girls in competitive sports during early adolescence are postpubertal, this is definitely not the case with boys. The size and strength of both boys and girls during childhood is comparable as groups until the onset of puberty. This occurs in girls beginning about 10 years of age with the first appearance of breast buds. Not only do girls begin their sexual maturation about 2 years earlier than

boys, but their entire duration of puberty is quite short, about 2 or 3 years. Conversely, boys generally do not begin puberty until about the age of 12, with the first sign being testicular enlargement, and the entire process can normally last for 4 or 5 years. The time of onset of boys can also occur any time between 10 and 14 years of age and still be normal. This means that any group of 13-year-old boys may well include some who have still not entered puberty, while others may have deep voices, are muscular and are shaving. Ideally, similarly aged boys in early adolescence should be

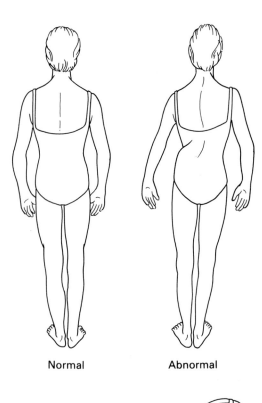

Normal   Abnormal

Fig. 17.12 With back to examiner stand up straight. Check for symmetry of shoulders, waist, thighs and calves. Common abnormalities: (1) high shoulder (scoliosis) or low shoulder (muscle loss); (2) prominent rib cage (scoliosis); (3) high hip or asymmetrical waist (leg length difference or scoliosis); (4) small calf or thigh (weakness from old injury). Redrawn with permission from Ross Laboratories, Columbus, Ohio.

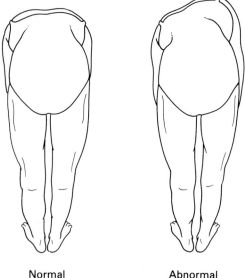

Normal   Abnormal

Fig. 17.13 Bend forward slowly as to touch toes. Check that the patient bends forward straightly and smoothly. Common abnormalities: (1) twists to side (low back pain); (2) back asymmetrical (scoliosis). Redrawn with permission from Ross Laboratories, Columbus, Ohio.

matched for competition by pubertal stage rather than by chronological age. Not only might this reduce the risk of injury to the boy who is physiologically less mature, and there-

fore less muscular, but it also 'evens the playing-field' as athletic ability at this age is more dependent upon boys' degrees of sexual maturity, the development of muscles and bones

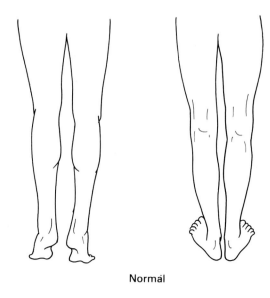

Normal

Abnormal

Fig. 17.14 Stand on heels; stand on toes. Check for equal elevation on right and left sides; symmetry of calf muscles. Common abnormality is wasting of calf muscles (Achilles injury or old ankle injury). Redrawn with permission from Ross Laboratories, Columbus, Ohio.

in response to androgen stimulation, than it is to either innate athletic ability or training. For a detailed discussion of matching of opponents see Chapter 14.

The most widely used assessment of the degree of sexual maturity is the Tanner pubic hair staging system (Figs 17.15 & 17.16). The 'Tanner stage' should be recorded, at least on all adolescent boys, during the preparticipation examination. The early maturing boy, who has

had a size and strength advantage over his classmates for several years, may need to be cautioned by his physician that this success in sports may not continue as the other boys will eventually catch up physically to him, and he may then no longer be as successful in competition as he is now. This advice may prevent disappointment due to unrealized dreams that his early sports success will continue into a professional athletic career. Conversely, the late

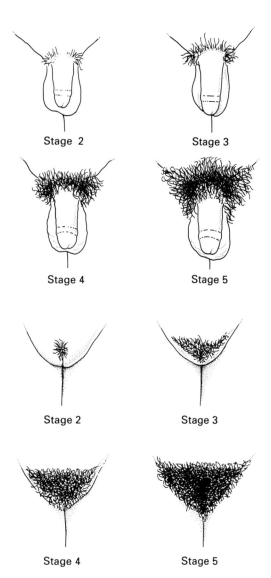

Stage 2

Stage 3

Stage 4

Stage 5

Fig. 17.15 Pubertal development of male pubic hair. Stage 1: prepubertal (not shown). Stage 2: slightly pigmented hair laterally at the base of the penis, usually straight. Stage 3: hair becomes darker, coarser, begins to curl and spreads over the pubes. Stage 4: hair is adult in type but does not extend onto thighs. Stage 5: hair extends onto the thighs and frequently up the linea alba. Adapted with permission from Tanner (1962).

Stage 2

Stage 3

Stage 4

Stage 5

Fig. 17.16 Pubertal development of female pubic hair. Stage 1: prepubertal (not shown). Stage 2: long, slightly pigmented, downy hair along the edges of the labia. Stage 3: darker, coarser, slightly curled hair spread sparsely over the mons pubis. Stage 4: adult type of hair but it does not extend onto thighs. Stage 5: adult distribution including spread along the medial aspects of the thighs. Adapted with permission from Tanner (1962).

developer might well be advised to participate in a non-contact sport such as tennis or swimming. However, if he wants to compete in a contact sport like football, and his parents acknowledge that there is at least a theoretically increased risk of injury during play with bigger and stronger boys and accept this risk, then play would be allowed.

Girls generally have completed puberty before they become active participants in contact sports like football and ice hockey, although this is probably changing. Tanner staging of girls is therefore only rarely, if ever, of significance, but the staging criteria (Fig. 17.16) are included for completeness.

Disqualifying conditions

The AAP has published (1988) a set of recommendations about which medical conditions should preclude participation (Tables 17.2 & 17.3). The American Medical Association (1990)

Table 17.2 Classification of sports. Adapted with permission from the American Academy of Pediatrics (1991) © 1991.

Collision	Limited contact/impact	Non-contact (strenuous)	Non-contact (moderately strenuous)	Non-contact (non-strenuous)
Boxing	Baseball	Aerobic dancing	Badminton	Archery
Field hockey	Basketball	Crew	Curling	Golf
Football	Bicycling	Fencing	Table-tennis	Riflery
Ice hockey	Diving	Field*		
Lacrosse	Equestrian	Running		
Martial arts	Field*	Swimming		
Rodeo	Gymnastics	Tennis		
Soccer	Racquetball	Track		
Wrestling	Skating	Weight-lifting		
	ice			
	roller			
	Skiing:			
	downhill			
	cross country			
	water			
	Softball			
	Squash			
	handball			
	Volleyball			

* Field events: jumping events such as pole-vaulting and high jump are 'limited contact/impact', others are 'non-contact strenuous'.

has accepted it as a replacement for its own much older list of disqualifying conditions which was far more exclusionary and needed revising because of both improvements in safety equipment and increased medical knowledge.

Sudden unexpected death on the playing field is usually due to an unsuspected cardiac abnormality, generally idiopathic hypertrophic cardiomyopathy. Examining physicians should have access to the recommendations for athletic participation for those athletes with a cardiovascular abnormality. These recommendations emanated from a consensus meeting sponsored by the American College of Cardiology (1985) and is more detailed than the AAP list. Other chapters in this volume also discuss the problems of athletic participation of children and adolescents with hypertension (Chapter 31) and cardiac disease (Chapter 22).

Subsequent to the publication of the AAP list of disqualifying conditions a statement concerning allowing athletes infected with the human immunodeficiency virus (HIV) was issued by the AAP (1991). It concluded that, although there was a theoretical risk of HIV transmission during contact sports due to bleeding, this was justification neither for excluding HIV infected athletes from competition nor for routine HIV testing of athletes. Rather it recommended that athletes, coaches and trainers be educated in 'universal precautions', i.e. the use of rubber gloves when stopping a bleeding episode, and the use of bleach solution when cleaning up blood from surfaces such as wrestling mats. The Canadian Academy of Sports Medicine issued a similar statement in 1993. One difference between these two statements is that the Canadian one did not include the AAP's recommendation that 'a physician counseling a known HIV-infected athlete in a sport involving blood

Table 17.3 Recommendations for participation in competitive sports. Adapted with permission from the American Academy of Pediatrics (1991) © 1991.

	Contact/ collision	Limited contact/impact	Non-contact		
			Strenuous	Moderately strenuous	Non-strenuous
Atlantoaxial instability	No	No	Yes[1]	Yes	Yes
Acute illnesses	2	2	2	2	2
Cardiovascular					
Carditis	No	No	No	No	No
Hypertension					
mild	Yes	Yes	Yes	Yes	Yes
moderate	3	3	3	3	3
severe	3	3	3	3	3
Congenital heart disease	4	4	4	4	4
Eyes					
Absence or loss of function of one eye	5	5	5	5	5
Detached retina	6	6	6	6	6
Inguinal hernia	Yes	Yes	Yes	Yes	Yes
Kidney: absence of one	No	Yes	Yes	Yes	Yes
Liver: enlarged	No	No	Yes	Yes	Yes
Musculoskeletal disorders	7	7	7	7	7
Neurological					
History of serious head or spine trauma, repeated concussions, or craniotomy	8	8	Yes	Yes	Yes
Convulsive disorder					
well controlled	Yes	Yes	Yes	Yes	Yes
poorly controlled	No	No	Yes[9]	Yes	Yes[10]
Ovary: absence of one	Yes	Yes	Yes	Yes	Yes
Respiratory					
Pulmonary insufficiency	11	11	11	11	Yes
Asthma	Yes	Yes	Yes	Yes	Yes
Sickle cell trait	Yes	Yes	Yes	Yes	Yes
Skin: boils, herpes, impetigo, scabies	12	12	Yes	Yes	Yes
Spleen: enlarged	No	No	No	Yes	Yes
Testicle: absence or undescended	Yes[13]	Yes[13]	Yes	Yes	Yes

[1] Swimming: no butterfly, breast stroke or diving starts.

[2] Needs individual assessment, e.g. contagiousness to others, risk of worsening illness.

[3] Needs individual assessment.

[4] Patients with mild forms can be allowed a full range of physical activities: patients with moderate or severe forms, or who are postoperative, should be evaluated by a cardiologist before athletic participation.

[5] Availability of American Society for Testing and Materials approved eye guards may allow competitor to participate in most sports, but this must be judged on an individual basis.

[6] Consult ophthalmologist.

[7] Needs individual assessment.

[8] Needs individual assessment.

[9] No swimming or weight lifting.

[10] No archery or riflery.

[11] May be allowed to compete if oxygenation remains satisfactory during a graded stress test.

[12] No gymnastics with mats, martial arts, wrestling or contact sports until not contagious.

[13] Certain sports may require protective cup.

exposure, such as wrestling or football, should inform him of the theoretical risk of contagion to others and strongly encourage him to consider another sport'.

Physicians should be cognizant of what is probably the prevailing bioethical philosophy, at least in the USA, regarding the rights of athletes to compete — that regardless of the severity of the medical condition, if an adult athlete wishes to compete, and fully understands the risks and accepts them, then participation should be allowed. The physician, of course, would be wise to obtain extensive documentation proving the athlete was acting with full knowledge and had signed an informed consent statement. Children and minor adolescents need to be considered differently as both legal theory and law generally preclude parents from subjecting their children to an unwarranted risk. Physicians who approve athletic participation for children who have a medical problem which would disqualify them according to a list compiled by specialists in the field, i.e. the AAP list, need tö know that they are exposing themselves to some considerable medicolegal liability if the child subsequently sustains a related significant injury during competition.

Challenges for future research

Enough research has been done to indicate that the preparticipation examination does have some value in detecting unsuspected medical conditions and residua of previous injuries, both of which could affect athletic performance or health. What is needed now are controlled studies demonstrating the following.

- The cost-effectiveness of annual examinations versus those performed at 2, 3 or 4 years.
- The effectiveness of rehabilitation exercises prescribed for minor previous injuries detected during an examination in preventing reinjuries during the next sport season.
- The effectiveness of the interim medical history at the beginning of each sport season in detecting potential problems.

References

American Academy of Pediatrics (AAP) Committee on Sports Medicine (1988) Recommendations for participation in competitive sports. *Pediatrics* **81**, 737−9.

American Academy of Pediatrics (AAP) Committee on Sports Medicine and Fitness (1991) Human immunodeficiency virus (acquired immunodeficiency syndrome virus) in the athletic setting. *Pediatrics* **88**, 640−1.

American College of Cardiology 16th Bethesda Conference (1985) Cardiovascular abnormalities in the athlete: recommendations regarding eligibility for competition. *J. Am. Coll. Cardiol.* **6**, 1186−90.

American Medical Association Board of Trustees (1990) *Athletic Preparticipation Examination for Adolescents*. AMA, Chicago.

Browne, R.J. & Gillespie, C.A. (1993) Sickle cell trait: a risk factor for life-threatening rhabdomyolysis? *Phys. Sportsmed.* **21**, 80−8.

Canadian Academy of Sport Medicine (1993) HIV as it relates to sport. *Can. J. Sports Med.* **3**, 63−8.

Durant, R.H., Seymore, C., Linder, C.W. & Jay, S. (1985) The preparticipation examination of athletes: comparison of single and multiple examiners. *Am. J. Dis. Child.* **139**, 657−61.

Eichner, E.R. (1986) Sickle cell trait, exercise, and altitude. *Phys. Sportsmed.* **14**. 144−51.

Linder, C.W., Durant, R.H., Seklecki, R.M. & Strong, W.B. (1981) Preparticipation health screening of young athletes: results of 1268 examinations. *Am. J. Sports Med.* **9**, 187−93.

Risser, W.L., Hoffman, H.M., Bellah, G.G. & Green, L.W. (1985) A cost−benefit analysis of preparticipation sports examinations of adolescent athletes. *J. School Health* **55**, 270−3.

Rowland, T.W. (1986) Preparticipation sports examination of the child and adolescent athlete: changing views of an old ritual. *Pediatrician* **13**, 3−9.

Samples, P. (1986) Preparticipation exams: are they worth the time and trouble? *Phys. Sportsmed.* **14**, 180−7.

Tanner, J.M. (1962) *Growth at Adolescence*, 2nd edn. Blackwell Scientific Publications, Oxford.

Thompson, T.R., Andrish, J.T. & Bergfeld, J.A. (1982) A prospective study of preparticipation sports examinations of 2670 young athletes: method and results. *Cleve. Clin. Q.* **49**, 225−33.

Chapter 18

Nutrition for the School-aged Child Athlete

SUZANNE NELSON STEEN

Introduction

Participation in athletics often begins at an early age and has become an important part of growing up for many children. In addition to providing children with opportunities for personal enjoyment, social interaction and skill development, athletic participation can be used to introduce children and their families to sound nutritional practices that may provide an important lifelong health benefit.

Children have the right to enjoy physical activity and to strive for success. This can be compromised if they are misinformed about how much and what foods to eat and drink for activity. The purpose of this chapter is to provide information to help ensure that young athletes are guaranteed appropriate nutrition, compatible with optimal needs for growth an development.

Assessment of nutritional status

The preparticipation physical examination of the child athlete provides an opportunity to initiate a nutritional assessment and integrate sports nutrition into the child's training regimen. The nutritional assessment should include an evaluation of growth dietary intake, and discussion of sports-related practices and issues.

Evaluation of growth

All children should have their weight, height, weight for height, and standard height for age plotted on a growth chart by a qualified health professional (see Figs 18.1–18.4; Hamill *et al.*, 1979).

Routine plotting of these parameters is essential to identify growth patterns that are indicative of acute or chronic malnutrition stunting, failure to thrive) or overnutrition (obesity). Growth retardation, obesity, iron-deficiency anaemia, dental disease and poor academic performance suggest that many children may be at nutritional risk (Meyers, 1989; Splett & Story, 1991).

Because height and weight taken once do not lend themselves to interpretation of growth status, measurements should be recorded at regular intervals in order to accurately reflect the growth patterns of the child (Chumlea, 1993). Usually, normal childhood growth occurs between the 5th and 95th percentile. During the first 2 years of age, some fluctuation in height and weight within the 5th and 95th percentile is expected as both infants and children demonstrate individual spurts in growth. However, children generally maintain their height and weight between the same percentiles (i.e. 50–75th percentile; also referred to as growth channel) during the preschool and early childhood years.

Although individual children differ in their rates of growth they should follow the same

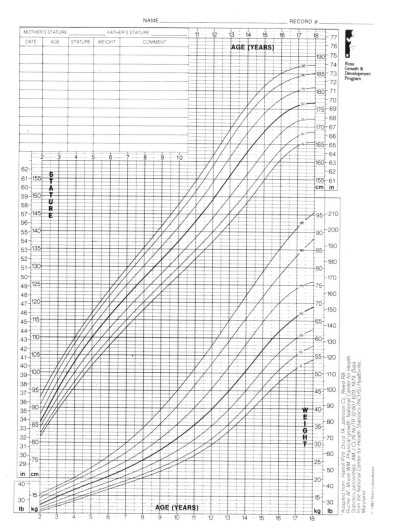

Fig. 18.1 Physical growth NCHS percentiles for boys aged 2–18 years. Reproduced with permission of Ross Products Division, Abbott Laboratories from NCHS Growth Charts, © 1982 Ross Laboratories.

channels. When either height or weight change from the child's usual growth percentiles the aetiology of the change from the child's usual growth percentiles the aetiology of the change should be investigated.

A more precise evaluation of growth is necessary when height and weight fall in markedly different percentiles (i.e. height 25th percentile, weight 75th percentile) since the height and weight of a child should be in proportion to one another. This is assessed by plotting the weight for height. Assessment of weight in relation to height enables assessment of current nutritional status and growth specific to the child's body size. At a single point in time, weight for height is a more sensitive index of appropriate growth than weight for age, as appropriateness of body weight is dependent on total body size not on age.

In contrast to the weight for height assessment, height for age comparison is an index of previous nutritional and growth status. A re-

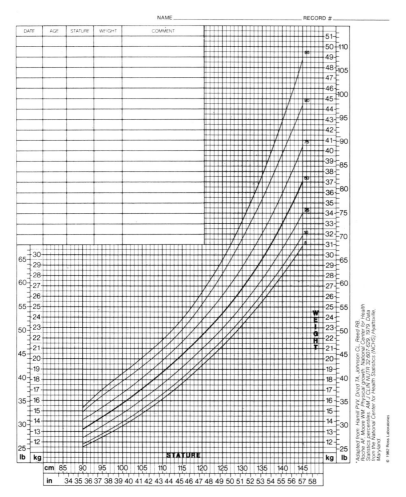

Fig. 18.2 Prepubescent physical growth NCHS percentiles for boys. Reproduced with permission of Ross Products Division, Abbott Laboratories from NCHS Growth Charts, © 1982 Ross Laboratories.

duction in height velocity is slower to develop in the presence of undernutrition than a decrease in weight velocity therefore it is an index of chronic malnutrition.

Age- and sex-specific standards have been developed to separate the genetic contribution of parental stature from other factors that affect a child's linear growth, such as malnutrition or disease. A child's actual height can be adjusted with a factor derived from the average of each parent's height. This method is recommended for evaluating children whose height for age is

less that the 5th percentile (Garm & Rohmann, 1966; Himes et al., 1985).

The actual increments in height and weight during the school-age years are small compared with those of infancy and adolescence. Weight increases an average of 2−3 kg each year until the child is 9 or 10 years old. Then, rate of weight gain increases, which is an initial sign of approaching puberty. Height increments average 5−6 cm·year^{-1} from the age of 2 years until the pubertal acceleration (Chumlea, 1993).

At puberty, children undergo hormonal

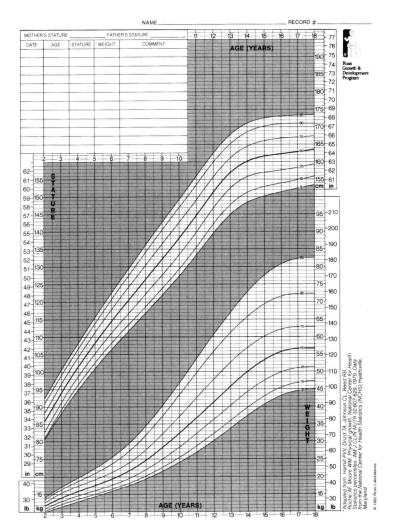

Fig. 18.3 Physical growth NCHS percentiles for girls aged 2–18 years. Reproduced with permission of Ross Products Division, Abbott Laboratories from NCHS Growth Charts, © 1982 Ross Laboratories.

changes that mark the beginning of adolescence and a period of rapid growth which increases nutritional needs. In addition to growth charts, the Tanner stages of sexual development (sexual maturity ratings) can be used to monitor maturing athletes (Tanner, 1962). This numerical system has been established for describing children in terms of how their bodies are changing and developing sexually. By using the Tanner staging syste, the athletic capabilities of children can be estimated so that boys and girls are trained properly and appropriately nourished. Regular monitoring of growth allows trends to be identified early and when necessary appropriate intervention given to ensure that long-term growth is not compromised.

Body composition

As discussed in Chapter 33, the evaluation of body composition in children and youth is complicated by several factors which affect the

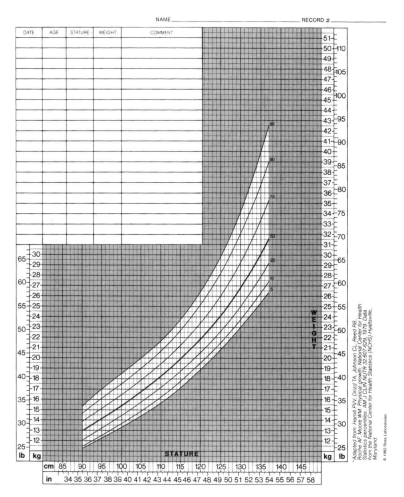

Fig. 18.4 Prepubescent physical growth NCHS percentiles for girls. Reproduced with permission of Ross Products Division, Abbott Laboratories from NCHS Growth Charts, © 1982 Ross Laboratories.

conceptual basis for estimating fat and lean tissue (Boileau *et al.*, 1988; Slaughter *et al.*, 1988; Lohman, 1989). However, when appropriate equations are used, body composition assessment can be an important component in the comprehensive evaluation of health fitness and performance (Boileau *et al.*, 1988). It is well recognized that relative amounts of fat and fat-free mass influence performance. This fact has important implications for physical fitness testing in which performance-based items are used (Boileau & Lohman, 1977; Boileau *et al.*, 1988).

In certain sports, the young athlete may initiate weight loss to meet a certain weight classification (wrestling) or to achieve a low body weight for appearance (gymnasts) (Steen & Brownell 1990; Steen, 1991a). Body composition assessment can be used to identify acceptable variability in body weight based on age and body composition measures to ensure adequate nutrition for normal maturation (Boileau *et al.*, 1988). Whether an optimal amount of body fat for maximal performance exists in young athletes is not clear.

From a practical standpoint, anthropometric measures can be used by a qualified health professional to monitor changes in fatness during training and/or when a prudent weight loss or weight gain regimen is deemed appropriate. These measures should *never* be used in the prepubescent athlete to manipulate body fat in a strict way for sports participation or to set stringent weight requirements. Doing so may adversely affect growth and development. This point needs to be made clear to coaches and parents.

Dietary requirements

School-aged children tend to be repetitious in their food choices, and the foods they include in their diets remain relatively constant from month to month (Thomas-Doberson 1989; Lucas, 1993). In addition to evaluating the caloric and nutrient content of the diet, excess consumption of high calorie low nutrient density foods, unusual foods and consistently omitted food categories should be noted (Thomas-Doberson, 1989; Lucas, 1993).

Methods of dietary assessment

A 24-h recall, food frequency, food record or a combination of these methods can be used to obtain dietary information. Research has shown that most children recall food items fairly reliably, but quantities less accurately (Dwyer *et al*. 1987). The methodology chosen should be adjusted to consider the physical and emotional differences between children and older athletes. Of primary importance is to establish a good rapport with the child to facilitate later recommendations that will be made.

It is also important to interview the parent(s) about their impressions of the child's diet. Ideally, the child and parent(s) should be interviewed separately. Otherwise, children may report what they think the parent wants them to be eating instead of actual intake. Comparing and combining information from both parent and child will provide a complete picture of the child's habits and rationale for consumption of certain foods.

Meal patterns

Meal patterns can be identified by asking children when they typically eat, where they eat and with whom. Does the child eat breakfast? Does the child have lunch at school or at home? What is the frequency of snacking? Are dinners spent with family or eaten alone? What times of day does the child eat meals in relation to practice? Are fluids consumed during/after practice?

Many children skip breakfast (Lucas, 1993). Some studies suggest that children who eat breakfast have a better attitude, school record and problem-solving ability compared to children who do not eat breakfast (Pollitt *et al*., 1981; Simeon & Grantham-McGregor, 1989). In addition, breakfast helps to replenish glycogen stores depleted during an overnight fast, to ensure that the child has adequate energy stores for afternoon training. It is important to encourage children to find foods they like to eat for breakfast. These do not need to be traditional foods. Food composition, not social tradition is the best strategy. Breakfast should provide between a quarter to a third of the nutrients for the day.

The child's lunch may be provided by the school or brought from home. Because food choices are often influenced by the child's friends, it is important to ask the child whom he or she typically eats lunch with and why certain foods are chosen. Studies have shown that the school lunch is usually more nutritious than a lunch brought from home (Ho *et al*., 1991). This is because box lunches typically contain less variety and include only favourite foods (Ho *et al*., 1991). In addition, they are limited to foods that travel well and do not require heating or refrigeration. Even if a nutritious lunch is packed at home, the parent does not necessarily know what portion is eaten, traded or thrown away.

Snacks may significantly contribute to the child's nutrient intake and eating style (Thomas-Doberson, 1989; Lucas 1993). The quality of snacks eaten may determine whether nutrient requirements are being met. Therefore, the frequency of snacking and type of snacks are important considerations. Does the child typically snack during the morning or afternoon? What are the child's favourite snacks? Are they prepared at home or purchased from a vending machine?

Calorie requirements

Calorie requirements should be estimated based on current dietary intake, rate of growth, age and physical activity. Energy needs for the school-aged child are modest compared to the adolescent period of rapid growth and high nutritional demands (Lucas, 1993).

Studies have shown large variability in energy intakes of healthy growing children of the same age and sex (Beal, 1961). For example, a 7-year-old boy and a 10.5-year-old girl approaching puberty have significantly different factors determining their energy needs even though they are in the same recommended dietary allowance (RDA, US standards; National Research Council, 1989) category. The RDA can be used to estimate caloric needs for normal growth and developments per kilograms of body weight as shown in Table 18.1.

If reported energy intake seems low, several factors to consider are whether the child has adequate time to eat, is a finicky eater, trying to lose weight or has an underlying medical problem (Thomas-Doberson, 1989). The nutritionist needs to be cognizant of the significant numbers of children who live in poverty and frequently do not have access to sufficient calories and nutrients (Community Childhood Hunger Identification Project, 1991; Kellogg Children's Nutrition Survey, 1991). Social changes such as unemployment, the increasing number of dual income families, and one-parent families have an impact on the food availability and food selection of children (Kellogg Children's Nutrition Survey, 1991).

In order to estimate how many calories the child may be expending during activity, specific questions should be asked about the training

Table 18.1 Estimated average calories (calculated in $J \cdot kg^{-1}$) and protein needs per kilogram of body weight for children aged 4–14 years. Data from National Research Council (1989). The recommended dietary allowance energy recommendations are derived from longitudinal intake data and represent average energy intake consistent with good health and appropriate growth in healthy individuals. Protein recommendations are determined from the measurement of minimum protein intakes necessary to maintain nitrogen balance in practically all growing, healthy individuals plus a safety factor to account for individual variation.

Age (years)	Calories ($J \cdot kg^{-1}$)	Protein ($g \cdot kg^{-1}$)
4–6	378	1.2
7–10	294	1
11–14 (M)	231	1
11–14 (F)	198	1

F, female; M, male.

schedule. First of all, in what sport(s) is the child involved? Does he or she participate in competitions, and at what level? What have his or her accomplishments been so far? How often do they train, and for how long? Try to estimate the intensity of their sessions by asking them to describe a typical training session.

Caloric expenditures for various activities that are specific for children are presented in Table 18.2. These data can be used as a guide to calculate calories expended per kilogram of body weight. Interestingly, children are more inefficient with their movements and thus potentially require more calories per unit of body weight. For example, compared with adults, children (age 6–8 years old) require 20–30% more oxygen per unit of body weight to run at a particular speed (Åstrand, 1952; Daniels, 1978; Krahenbuhl & Pangrasi, 1983). In older children the difference is less.

Dietary recommendations

What is the most appropriate diet for the child athlete? For the school-aged child, increased caloric needs for training are best met by increasing food intakes across the board, without

Table 18.2 Calorie equivalents of child's activities in kJ per 10 min activity. Adapted from Bar-Or (1983).

Activity	Body weight (kg)									
	20	25	30	35	40	45	50	55	60	65
Basketball	143	181	214	252	286	323	357	395	428	462
Calisthenics	55	71	84	97	109	126	139	151	168	181
Cycling										
$10\,km\cdot h^{-1}$	63	71	84	97	109	122	139	151	164	176
$15\,km\cdot h^{-1}$	92	113	134	151	172	193	210	231	252	273
Figure skating	168	210	252	294	336	378	420	462	504	546
Ice hockey (on-ice time)	218	273	328	382	437	491	546	601	655	706
Running										
$8\,km\cdot h^{-1}$	155	189	218	252	277	302	328	353	378	399
$10\,km\cdot h^{-1}$	202	231	269	307	332	357	386	420	449	475
Soccer (game)	151	189	227	265	302	340	378	416	454	491
Swimming $30\,m\cdot min^{-1}$										
breast	80	101	122	143	160	181	202	223	244	260
front crawl	105	130	155	181	206	235	260	286	311	336
back	71	88	105	126	143	160	176	197	214	231
Tennis	92	118	139	164	185	210	231	256	277	302
Walking										
$4\,km\cdot h^{-1}$	71	80	88	97	109	118	126	134	143	151
$6\,km\cdot h^{-1}$	101	109	118	126	134	143	155	168	181	202

significantly altering the proportions of the micro- or macronutrients of the diet (Smith & Worthington-Roberts, 1989; Steen, 1991b). Planning daily intake around the food pyramid (US Department of Agriculture and US Department of Health and Human Services, 1993) encourages consumption of a variety of foods and serves as a visual guide for planning healthy meals.

As shown in Fig. 18.5, each section of the pyramid represents a food category and gives a range for the number of recommended servings to be consumed daily. Each day, the young athlete should consume at least two to three servings from the milk group, two to three servings from the meat/protein group, four servings from the vegetable group, three servings from the fruit group and nine servings from the bread/grain group. Foods containing the majority of calories from fat or sugars at the top of the pyramid are not eliminated, but should be consumed occasionally as an addition to, and not in place of other nutrient dense foods.

In general, providing servings within these recommended ranges will supply the necessary nutrients and calories (9240 J) that most active children require. However, depending on the frequency, intensity and duration of physical activity the exercising child may need an additional 2100–6300 J each day. Children should be encouraged to distribute calories throughout

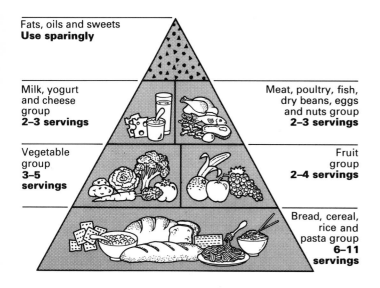

Fig. 18.5 Food guide pyramid — a guide to daily food choices. Developed by the US Department of Agriculture and the Department of Health and Human Services (1993).

the day at regular meal times and snacks. This will ensure the presence of readily available sources of energy to support training activity.

Young athletes can meet their vitamin and mineral needs on diets that include the foods and servings recommended in the food guide pyramid. However, school-aged children often avoid fruits and vegetables which may lead to an inadequate intake of vitamins A, B_6 and C, and folic acid (Science and Education Administration, 1980; Mahan & Rosebrough, 1984). Consumption of calcium- and iron-rich foods may also be suboptimal (Science and Education Administration, 1980; Mahan & Rosebrough, 1984). If the child's intake is low for certain micronutrients, strategies to increase consumption from food should be discussed with the parent (Jennings & Steen, 1993).

In addition to purchasing more healthy foods, favourite foods can be made nutritionally dense or acceptable substitutions made with similar foods. There are many different food choices available that will supply adequate amounts of vitamins and minerals for even the choosiest of eaters. Variety in the family menu will underscore the importance of eating different foods to provide the range of nutrients necessary for growth and development. Ideally, this variety is most easily achieved in regularly scheduled meals at home plus nutritious snacks. In order to be effective in encouraging the child to actually eat the recommended foods, it is important to suggest changes that are compatible with the eating style of the child (Thomas-Doberson, 1989; Steen, 1991b).

Based on the information obtained from the initial questions on dietary patterns and nutritional adequacy, sports nutrition issues that are pertinent for this age group can be considered which include: fluid and electrolyte needs, pre- and postevent meals, weight control practices and food supplements.

Fluid and electrolyte requirements

Children sweat less, have a lower cardiac output, do not tolerate temperature extremes, and acclimatize to heat more slowly than young adults (Haymes *et al.*, 1975; Bar-Or, 1980). All of these factors increase the risk of dehydration. Therefore special emphasis should be placed on ensuring adequate fluid intake in the preadolescent child athlete before, during and after activity.

During activity, fluid consumption may be facilitated by providing children with a personalized bottle and encouraging them to drink 120 ml every 15 min of activity. Supervision of fluid intake is essential, because children do not instinctively drink enough fluid to replace water losses (Bar-Or *et al.*, 1980, 1992). During prolonged exercise, children may not recognize the symptoms of heat strain and push themselves to the point of heat-related illness (Bar-Or, 1980; Bar-Or *et al.*, 1980).

Serial weighing can identify the athlete who is becoming chronically dehydrated during repetitive training. Another practical strategy would be to weigh the athlete during several training sessions and then predict how much fluid the athlete needs for subsequent workouts (O. Bar-Or, personal communication).

Choosing the correct fluids

Plain water is the most economical source of fluid to hydrate the body. Although water is adequate for most children, some children will be more likely to drink sufficient amounts if they are given flavoured fluids. In a recent study, Meyer *et al.* (1994) found that prepubertal and early pubertal girls and boys prefer grape flavour to apple and orange flavours or water. Carbohydrate beverages (6–8% carbohydrate or 15–18 g of carbohydrate per 240 ml) and diluted fruit juice are appropriate choices. Fruit juices should be diluted at least twofold (480 ml of water for every 240 ml of juice). Children should not drink undiluted juice or carbonated soda during activity since they typically contain too much carbohydrate (10–12% carbohydrate) and may cause gastric discomfort. Caffeinated beverages (tea, coffee, cola) should be avoided since they promote diuresis.

Recent research suggests that the optimal electrolyte content in children's fluid replacement drinks may be different from that currently recommended for adults. Meyer *et al.* (1992) have demonstrated that sweat [Na^+] and [Cl^-] tended to increase with maturation while sweat [K^+] was lower in young adults compared with prepubescent females and males. Because children have a lower sweating rate than young adults, total Na^+ and Cl^- losses per kilogram of body weight from sweat were higher in young adults compared with those of the prepubescent and pubescent groups. However, no maturational differences were found in K^+ losses.

The authors speculate that a protective mechanism may exist in children against excessive salt loss, which accompanies their lower sweating rate. Salt tablets should never be given to children as they would potentially contribute to dehydration and irritate the stomach mucosa.

Pre- and postevent meal

The pre-event meal serves two main purposes: (i) to prevent athletes from feeling hungry before or during activity; and (ii) to help supply fuel to the muscles during training and competition. Still, most of the energy needed for any sports event is provided by whatever the child has eaten during the prior week. The most optimal plan is to offer foods 2–3 h before exercise that the child finds pleasing, and that are high in carbohydrate, contain low to moderate amounts of protein, and are low in fat. In addition, at least 240 ml fluid (water or juice) should be encouraged (Jennings & Steen, 1993).

High fat and high protein foods should be avoided because they take longer to digest than carbohydrate foods and, if eaten for the pre-event meal can contribute to indigestion and nausea. Children should also avoid eating simple carbohydrates such as sugar, sweets, honey or soft drinks before exercise. They do not provide 'quick energy', and some athletes are more sensitive than others to changes in blood glucose levels when simple sugars are eaten. Instead, complex carbohydrates which are found in breads, cereals, pasta, rice and other starchy foods should be included in the pre-event meal. These foods are digested relatively quickly, so that the child's stomach is empty and blood sugar level is stable before practice or competition.

Ideally, these guidelines should be considered regarding the pre-event meal for the child. However, some children prefer not to eat because they feel nervous or excited. Under these circumstances, the child should never be pressured to eat; instead, water and juice should be offered.

After exercise, fluids should be offered to promote hydration and complex carbohydrates encouraged to replenish glycogen stores. Some parents may inappropriately use food as a bribe to encourage a winning performance. Parents should be advised that special treats should not be used to reward a child that does well and withheld if not. Whether the child competed successfully or not should have no bearing upon post-exercise intake.

Weight control practices

Sometimes, healthy nutritional practices are disregarded in the pursuit of athletic prowess. The emphasis may be on what will make the child a better athlete, rather than what will make him or her a happy, healthy human being. This may be in part because parents and coaches are not well informed about the child's stage of maturation, nutritional needs, emotions and/or physical ability.

Unfortunately, some parents and coaches have misconceptions about how much the prepubescent child should eat. Some encourage their children to eat excessively, with the erroneous belief that this will build strength and endurance at a faster rate (Smith & Worthington-Roberts, 1989). On the contrary, indiscriminate consumption, in which food intake exceeds the child's caloric requirement, may be the start of a lifelong struggle with obesity.

At the other extreme are parents and coaches who promote a diet restricted in calories and nutrients that may compromise the health of the child (Smith & Worthington-Roberts, 1989). Given the current focus on lowering cholesterol and fat, some parents inappropriately narrow the child's food choices (excluding red meat, dairy products) in an attempt to control weight or to minimize the future risk of heart disease (American Academy of Pediatrics, 1986). Prepubescent children should receive 30% of total calories from fat (American Academy of Pediatrics, 1986), since restriction of fat to lower levels may not adequately support growth and development (American Academy of Pediatrics, 1986). Parents can encourage long-term healthy habits without compromising growth by offering foods with moderate amounts of unsaturated fats and reducing (not eliminating) foods which are high in saturated fats.

Exercise demands by parents or coach to reduce body weight such as running laps, calisthenics or extra practice time can be excessive. Especially during hot temperatures, fatigue, heat-exhaustion and illness can be the result. If the child does need to lose fat weight, a medically supervised weight control plan which focuses on weight monitoring, caloric stabilization and increased activity is recommended (Smith & Worthington-Roberts, 1989; Jennings & Steen, 1993).

The special case of 'making weight'

Scholastic wrestlers must meet a certain weight classification in order to compete. It is a common practice throughout the competitive season for wrestlers to restrict food and fluid intake in order to compete at one to three weight classes below their normal weight (Steen & Brownell, 1990). Wrestlers typically believe that this practice, known as 'making weight', gives them a competitive edge over smaller opponents. Few wrestlers, coaches and parents realize the negative physiological impact this practice may have on their bodies.

Studies have shown that 'making weight' lowers blood and plasma volumes, reduces cardiac function during submaximal work (e.g. higher heart rate, smaller stroke volume and reduced cardiac output), impairs thermoregulation, decreases renal blood flow and renal filtration, and increases electrolyte losses (American Medical Association, 1967; American College of Sports Medicine, 1976). The calorie and micronutrient content of wrestlers' diet during training are typically inadequate (Steen & McKinney, 1986).

From a performance standpoint, 'making weight' can lead to liver and muscle glycogen depletion, dehydration, reduced muscular strength and decreased performance work time (Yarrows, 1988). Since wrestlers rarely regain all of their lost weight after the official weigh-in prior to competition, they may be wrestling under suboptimal conditions.

In an effort to preclude the use of erratic weight loss practices commonly observed among adolescent and collegiate wrestlers, it is imperative to establish healthy weight control guidelines with the prepubescent child. Through nutrition education, coaches, parents and athlete can be informed about the consequences of rapid and extreme weight reduction by fluid and food restriction and healthy alternatives for achieving a suitable competitive weight (Steen & McKinney, 1986).

While the majority of parents are appropriately supportive and considerate of the young child's needs, some are not as well informed about weight control. It is imperative to develop effective strategies to counter a demanding parent who may be exploiting their child for their own satisfaction or personal gain. Nutritional requirements for growth and development must be placed before athletic considerations.

Food supplements

There is no place in the diet of a healthy child for dietary supplements which are often vigorously promoted to athletes of all ages (American Academy of Pediatrics, 1980; American Dietetic Association, 1987; American Medical Association, 1987). Unfortunately, many well-meaning, but misinformed parents and coaches advise children to take supplements in an effort to promote early athletic development, improve performance and as 'health insurance'. However, eventual maturity and athletic prowess does not necessarily depend upon how early a child reaches adolescence, and in any event, the process will not be facilitated by dietary supplements (Smith & Worthington-Roberts, 1989). The adage of 'if some is good then more must be better' does not apply to supplements. On the contrary, if taken in large doses, certain vitamins and minerals can be toxic. Providing children with supplements can

give them a false sense of security and may encourage faulty eating habits. They may assume that their morning dose of supplements provides them with all of the nutrients that they need, so that they can eat sweets and soft drinks instead of cereal and fruit juice.

Another disadvantage of supplement use is that the child athlete may erroneously associate improvements in performance with whatever supplements they are taking. They may be less likely to attribute progress to training, hard work and a balanced diet. This type of false reinforcement may also encourage children to try other types of supplements and substances (including steroids), which can lead to a snowball effect with undesired consequences. Aside from being dangerous, megadose levels of nutrients do not make up for a lack of training or talent or give athletes a competitive advantage.

To move away from this reliance on 'supplement insurance', young athletes need to feel confident about eating 'ordinary foods'. Parents and coaches must emphasize how regular foods promote muscle growth and optimal performance. From a practical standpoint children can be encouraged to keep records of what they eat, when and how hard they train and how their performance improves. These records can be used to illustrate the importance of good dietary and training habits as the cause of improvement rather than leaving the child to erroneously associate athletic accomplishments with a pill or powder (Jennings & Steen, 1993).

The use of megadose levels of vitamin and minerals, protein mixtures, or other special supplements should be denounced as an unhealthy practice (American Academy of Pediatrics, 1980; American Dietetic Association 1987; American Medical Association, 1987). Health professionals need to emphasize that nutrients should come from food, not supplements and provide parents, coaches and children with healthy alternatives for developing strength and stamina. Hopefully, if children understand why these substances are not necessary, they will abstain from using them at an early age and continue to do so during adolescence when peer pressure is amplified.

Conclusion

When working with the prepubescent athlete, the challenge for health professionals is to provide the child, coach and parents with appropriate nutritional information to promote training and performance after meeting needs for growth and development. Meal patterns, and caloric and nutritional adequacy of the diet should be evaluated followed by questions and recommendations about sports-related issues and practices. In addition to promoting a healthy dietary intake, explanation of basic nutritional concepts as they are related to exercise is important to help establish good habits at an early age, and to dispel any misconceptions that the child has already heard of, or will most likely be exposed to as an adolescent.

Challenges for future research

● Currently there is a lack of information regarding sports nutrition recommendations for the school-aged child athlete. As the number of young athletes increases, research is needed to evaluate specific energy, macronutrient and micronutrient requirements for activity in the growing child.

● Body composition assessment and the issue regarding appropriate amount and rate of weight loss are paramount, since extreme measures taken in an attempt to improve performance may compromise normal growth and development.

● Evaluation of hormonal perturbations in the young athlete who chronically restricts intake for appearance (gymnasts, figure skaters, dancers) is also needed to assess the impact on long-term growth.

● Additional research on fluid requirements is needed to further clarify electrolyte losses, the biological implications of the findings, and the practical implications for recommending optimal fluid–electrolyte replacement drinks for children.

● Studies to determine the most effective means of educating child, coach and parent about sports nutrition are key to facilitate the message of the primary importance of growth, with issues of performance being secondary.

References

American Academy of Pediatrics, Committee on Nutrition (1980) Vitamin and mineral supplementation needs in normal children in the United States. *Pediatrics* **66**, 1015.

American Academy of Pediatrics, Committee on Nutrition (1986) Prudent life-style for children, dietary fat and cholesterol. *Pediatrics* **78**, 521.

American College of Sports Medicine (1976) Position stand on weight loss in wrestlers. *Med. Sci. Sports Exerc.* **8**, xi.

American Dietetic Association (1987) Recommendations concerning supplement usage: ADA statement. *J. Am. Diet. Assoc.* **87**, 1342.

American Medical Association (1967) Committee on the Medical Aspects of Sports: wrestling and weight control. *JAMA* **201**, 541.

American Medical Association, Council on Scientific Affairs (1987) Vitamin preparations as dietary supplements and as therapeutic agents. *JAMA* **257**, 1929.

Åstrand, P.O. (1952) *Experimental Studies of Physical Working Capacity in Relation to Sex and Age.* Munksgaard, Copenhagen.

Bar-Or, O. (1980) Climate and the exercising child — a review. *Int. J. Sports Med.* **1**, 53–65.

Bar-Or, O. (1983) *Pediatric Sports Medicine for the Practitioner.* Springer-Verlag, New York.

Bar-Or, O., Blimkie, C.J.R., Hay, J.A., MacDougal, J.D., Ward, D.S. & Wilson, W.M. (1992) Voluntary dehydration and heat intolerance in cystic fibrosis. *Lancet* **339**, 696–9.

Bar-Or, O., Dotan, R., Inbar, O., Rotshtein, A. & Zonder, H. (1980) Voluntary hypohydration in 10–12-year-old boys. *J. Appl. Physiol.* **48**, 104.

Beal, V.A. (1961) Dietary intake of individuals followed through infancy and childhood. *Am. J. Public Health* **51**, 1107.

Boileau, R.A. & Lohman, T.G. (1977) The measurement of human physique and its effect on physical performance. *Orthop. Clin. N. Am.* **8**, 563–81.

Boileau, R.A., Lohman, T.G., Slaughter, M.H., Horswill, C.A. & Stillman, R.J. (1988) Problems associated with determining body composition in maturing youngsters. In E.W. Brown & C.F. Banta (eds) *Competitive Sports for Children and Youth: An*

Overview of Research and Issues, pp. 3–16. Human Kinetics, Champaign, IL.

Chumlea, W.C. (1993) Growth and development. In P.M. Queen & C.E. Land (eds) *Handbook of Pediatric Nutrition*, pp. 3–25. Aspen Publishers, Gaithersburg.

Community Childhood Hunger Identification Project (1991) *A Survey of Childhood Hunger in the United States. Executive Summary*. Food Research Action Center, Washington, DC.

Daniels, J. (1978) Differences and changes in VO_2 among runners 10–18 years of age. *Med. Sci. Sports Exerc.* **10**, 200–12.

Dwyer, J.T., Krall, E.A. & Coleman, K.A. (1987) The problem of memory in nutritional epidemiology research. *J. Am. Diet. Ass.* **87**, 1509–12.

Garn, S.M. & Rohmann, C.G. (1966) Interaction of nutrition and genetics in the timing of growth and development. *Pediatr. Clin. N. Am.* **13**, 353.

Hamill, P.V.V., Drizd, T.A., Johnson, C.L., Reed, R.B., Roche, A.F. & Moore, W.M. (1979) Physical growth: National Center for Health Statistics percentiles. *Am. J. Clin. Nutr.* **32**, 607–629.

Haymes, E.M., McCormick, R.J. & Buskirk, E.R. (1975) Heat tolerance of exercising lean and obese prepubertal boys. *J. Appl. Physiol.* **39**, 457.

Himes, J.H., Roche, A.F., Thissen D. & Moore, W.M. (1985) Parent-specific adjustments for evaluation of recumbent length and stature of children. *Pediatrics* **75**, 304.

Ho, C.S., Gould, R.A. & Jensen, L.N. (1991) Evaluation of the nutrient content of school, sack and vending lunch of junior high school students. *Sch. Food Serv. Res. Rev.* **15**, 85–90.

Jennings, D. & Steen, S.N. (1993) *Sports Nutrition for the Child Athlete*. American Dietetic Association, Chicago.

Kellogg Children's Nutrition Survey (1991) *Executive Summary*. Michigan Kellogg Co., Battle Creek, MI.

Krahenbuhl, G.S. & Pangrasi, R. (1983) Characteristics associated with running performance in young boys. *Med. Sci. Sports Exerc.* **15**, 488.

Lohman, T.G. (1989) Assessment of body composition of children. *Pediatr. Exerc. Sci.* **1**, 19–30.

Lucas, B. (1993) Normal nutrition from infancy through adolescence. In P.M. Queen & C.E. Land (eds) *Handbook of Pediatric Nutrition*, pp. 145–70. Aspen Publishers, Gaithersburg.

Mahan, L.K. & Rosebrough, R.H. (1984) Nutritional requirements and nutritional status assessment in adolescence. In L.K. Mahan & J.M. Rees (eds) *Nutrition and Adolescence*. C.V. Mosby, St Louis.

Meyer, F., Bar-Or, O., MacDougall, D. & Heigenhauser, G.J.F. (1992) Sweat electrolyte loss during exercise in the heat: effects of gender and maturation. *Med. Sci. Sports Exerc.* **24**, 776–81.

Meyer, F., Bar-Or, O., Salsberg, A., Passe, D. (1994) Hypohydration during exercise in children: effect on thirst, drink preferences, and rehydration. *Int. J. Sports Nutr.* **1**, 22–35.

Meyers, A. (1989) Undernutrition, hunger, and learning in children. *Nutr News* **52**, 1.

National Research Council (1989) *Recommended Dietary Allowances*, 10th edn. National Academy Press, Washington DC.

Pollitt, E., Leibel, R.L. & Greenfield, D. (1981) Brief fasting, stress, and cognition in children. *Am. J. Clin. Nutr.* **34**, 1526.

Science and Education Administration (1980) *Nationwide Food Consumption Survey, 1977–78. Preliminary Report No. 2, Food and Nutrient Intakes of Individuals in One Day in the US, Spring, 1977*. US Department of Agriculture, Hyattsville.

Simeon, D.T. & Grantham-McGregor, S. (1989) Effects of missing breakfast on the cognitive functions of school children of differing nutritional status. *Am. J. Clin. Nutr.* **49**, 646.

Slaughter, M.H., Lohman, T.G., Boileau, C.A. *et al.* (1988) Skinfold equations for estimation of body fatness in children and youth. *Hum. Biol.* **60**, 709–23.

Smith, N. & Worthington-Roberts, B. (1989) *Food for Sport*. Bull Publishing, Palo Alto.

Splett, P. & Story, M. (1991) Child nutrition objective for the decade. *J. Am. Diet. Ass.* **91**, 665–8.

Steen, S.N. (1991a) Nutritional considerations for the low body weight athlete. In J.B. Berning & S.N. Steen (eds) *Sports Nutrition for the 1990s: The Health Professional's Handbook*, pp. 153–74. Aspen Publishers, Gaithersburg.

Steen, S.N. (1991b) Nutritional management of the school age child athlete. In J.B. Berning & S.N. Steen (eds) *Sports Nutrition for the 1990s: The Health Professional's Handbook*, pp. 229–54. Aspen Publishers, Gaithersburg.

Steen, S.N. & Brownell, K.D. (1990) Patterns of weight loss and regain in wrestlers: has the tradition changed? *Med. Sci. Sports Exerc.* **22**, 762–8.

Steen, S.N. & McKinney, S. (1986) Nutritional assessment of college wrestlers. *Phys. Sports Med.* **14**, 100–16.

Tanner, J.M. (1962) *Growth at Adolescence*, 2nd edn. Blackwell Scientific Publications, Oxford.

Thomas-Doberson, D. (1989) Dietary assessment and management of the school age child. In M.D. Simko, C. Cowell & M.S. Hreha (eds) *Practical Nutrition: A Quick Reference for the Health Care Practitioner*, pp. 149–60. Aspen Publishers, Gaithersburg.

US Department of Agriculture and US Department of Health and Human Services (1993) *Food Guide Pyramid: A Guide to Daily Food Choices*. USDA/USDHHS, Washington DC.

Yarrows, S.A. (1988) Weight loss through dehydration in amateur wrestling. *J. Am. Diet. Ass.* **88**, 491.

Chapter 19

Iron Deficiency in the Adolescent Athlete

THOMAS W. ROWLAND

Introduction

The iron content of the human body is small — a mere 3.5 g in the mature male — but proper iron nutrition is critical for maintaining good health. Over two-thirds of body iron is incorporated into haemoglobin, where it plays an essential role in haematogenous oxygen transport. A much smaller amount (about 150 mg) fulfils important metabolic functions in iron-containing proteins and enzyme co-factors. These non-haem iron-dependent processes are widespread among the body's systems, a fact reflected by the diverse clinical manifestations observed when iron stores become depleted. Besides anaemia, defective thermoregulation, poor scholastic performance, sensory and behavioural disturbances, alteration of immune function, growth suppression, decreased physical work performance and gastrointestinal derangements have all been related to the iron-deficient state (Oski, 1979; Dallman, 1982).

The negative effect of iron deficiency on physical performance has been recognized since antiquity. Herbert (1965) noted that the ancient Greeks administered iron to their patients complaining of weakness, believing that Mars, the god of war, had given strength to the metal. In more contemporary times, attention to the iron–fitness connection has involved such diverse interests as improving the productivity of undernourished workers in developing nations (Basta et al., 1979), promoting iron-containing tonics to tired housewives, and

maximizing sports performance in competitive athletes (Clement & Sawchuck, 1984). It is upon this latter group that this chapter will focus.

The role of iron in exercise performance and the effect of iron deficiency on young competitive athletes has drawn considerable attention. Research information to date indicates that iron deficiency is common in adolescent females engaged in sports training — affecting nearly 50% in some series — although overt anaemia is unusual. The frequency of non-anaemic iron deficiency is also high in non-athletes, but sports training, particularly distance running, appears to predispose to increased iron losses. Animal studies indicate that non-anaemic iron deficiency impairs endurance exercise capacity, but most studies have failed to support this conclusion in humans.

Given the high frequency of iron deficiency in female athletes and the ease of treatment of this condition with oral iron supplementation, continued investigation into the influence of iron depletion on athletic performance is clearly warranted. In addition, these studies provide the opportunity for gaining insights into the basic physiological mechanisms important for endurance exercise performance.

Iron and exercise performance

Impairment in physical work capacity has traditionally been associated with iron-deficiency anaemia, defined as a haemoglobin concentration of less than $12 \, g \cdot dl^{-1}$ in females and less than $13 \, \mathrm{g} \cdot \mathrm{dl}^{-1}$ in males. Indeed, there is no question that exercise performance is depressed when haemoglobin concentrations fall as a result of depleted iron stores (Woodson, 1984). Adult volunteers who have undergone repeated phlebotomies show a linear relationship between fall in haemoglobin concentration and decline in treadmill endurance time and maximal aerobic power ($\dot{V}o_{2\,max}$) (Ekblom et al., 1972; Woodson et al., 1978). In general, these studies indicate that percentage decrease in haemoglobin approximates the percentage fall in $\dot{V}o_{2\,max}$.

An important report by Gardner et al. (1977) of women working on a tea estate illustrated that diminished work performance can be expected with even small decreases in haemoglobin concentration. In that study, women who had mild iron-deficiency anaemia (haemoglobin concentration between 11 and $11.9 \, \mathrm{g} \cdot \mathrm{dl}^{-1}$) demonstrated a treadmill work time that was 20% less than those with a haemoglobin value over $13 \, \mathrm{g} \cdot \mathrm{dl}^{-1}$. Correction of the anaemia by iron treatment restored normal exercise performance in this and other studies (Dallman, 1982).

While the observation that those with iron-deficiency anaemia have impaired exercise performance is incontrovertible, the mechanism responsible for the decline in physical capacity and maximal aerobic power in these individuals has not been altogether clarified. Certainly the diminished arterial oxygen content in the anaemic subject is at least partially responsible (Woodson et al., 1978). Yet other studies, particularly in animals, indicate an important role of intracellular non-haem iron in energy production critical for normal muscle contractile function. Effects of iron depletion independent of anaemia therefore have the potential for depressing athletic performance.

In contrast to haem iron, which is important in the transport of oxygen to exercising muscle, muscular iron plays key roles in various intracellular functions which are critical for the utilization of energy by contractile proteins. Of body iron 5% is incorporated into myoglobin, which serves as a reservoir for oxygen within the muscle cell. Iron is a component of the cytochromes of the electron transport chain, important in oxidative phosphorylation, and a number of enzymes important in energy metabolism either contain iron or require it is a cofactor, including aconitase, cytochrome oxidase, succinate dehydrogenase and tyrosine hydroxylase (Dallman, 1982; Galan et al., 1984). Thus, although quantitatively much smaller than haem iron, iron within the muscle cell is critical for energy production necessary for normal physical work capacity.

Effect of non-haem iron on performance

Several lines of evidence, mostly in experimental rats, have suggested that deficiency of intramuscular iron can be responsible for decreased work performance in the iron-depleted subject independent of anaemia. Finch et al. (1976) demonstrated that treadmill endurance run time in four groups of non-anaemic rats was related to adequacy of body iron stores. Haemoglobin concentration was maintained constant by intermittent removal and addition of blood through an intravascular catheter. In the 4 weeks prior to testing, rats in group A were fed an iron-deficient diet, group B rats ate a normal diet, and group C animals consumed an iron-deficient diet plus an iron supplement. Group D rats were given an iron-deficient diet but started on iron supplementation at the beginning of the treadmill testing period.

During the exercise testing, rats with a normal or iron-supplemented diet (groups B and C) ran for periods of 16–20 min on serial runs over 4 days, while the iron-deficient animals (group A) could only sustain exercise for 4 min. Group D rats ran for only 4 min at the onset of testing, but while on iron supplementation improved performance to 18 min by the fourth day (Fig. 19.1).

Willis et al. (1990) showed that the improvement in endurance performance in iron-deficient rats treated with iron was remarkably rapid.

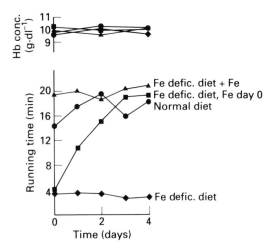

Fig. 19.1 Response of treadmill running time in rates following iron (Fe) treatment (see text). Hb conc., haemoglobin concentration. Redrawn with permission from Finch *et al.* (1976) © by The American Society for Clinical Investigation.

Treadmill endurance time increased over three-fold in severely iron-deficient rats over 15 h after injection of intraperitoneal iron compared to controls, without significant change in haemoglobin concentration.

Several reports in rats indicate that iron-deficient diets cause significant reductions in cytochrome C (Galan *et al.*, 1984), although there appears to be little change in cytochrome oxidase activity. A fall of 20−50% in myoglobin concentration has been reported in rats during the growing period, but this effect of iron depletion has not been duplicated in adult animals (Galan *et al.*, 1984). The greater endurance in the iron-deficient rats after dietary repletion reported by Finch *et al.* (1976) was most closely linked to increased rate of oxidative phosphorylation with α-glycerophosphate as a substrate.

The rapid 15-h improvement in exercise performance in the iron-deficient rats after iron treatment described by Willis *et al.* (1990) occurred without significant change in myoglobin concentration or activity of mitochondrial enzymes. This suggested to the authors that

alterations in exercise performance were likely related to iron's role as an enzyme co-factor.

Several studies in humans have also suggested that changes in work capacity relative to iron nutrition may be independent of haemoglobin concentration. Basta *et al.* (1979) described improved work output in iron-deficient Indonesians which improved after only 1 month of iron supplementation, before any significant rise in haemoglobin. Similarly, Ohira *et al.* (1979) and Ericsson (1970) reported improved exercise performance after treatment of iron-deficient adults, which could not be explained by changes in haemoglobin concentration.

Data regarding iron-dependent metabolic activity within the muscle cell in the depleted state are limited in humans. Celsing *et al.* (1986) reported no change in cytochrome C oxidase activity in biopsy samples of healthy men made iron deficient and anaemic by repeated phlebotomies. In a subsequent study of iron-deficient Indonesian subjects with moderate anaemia (haemoglobin $8 - 10\,g \cdot dl^{-1}$), Celsing *et al.* (1988) could find no differences in iron-dependent enzymes (succinate dehydrogenase, cytochrome C oxidase) and myoglobin concentration compared to non-anaemic controls.

Mechanisms of haem and non-haem iron on work capacity

Studies in animals comparing the effects of deficiency of intramuscular iron (oxygen utilization) to those of iron-deficiency anaemia (oxygen delivery) have provided interesting insights into means by which these two determinants of energy availability might affect different forms of exercise performance. These reports suggest that the ability to utilize oxygen within the cell may be essential for performance of prolonged submaximal exercise (endurance). Conversely, the ability to deliver oxygen, may determine the capacity to achieve peak work such as that performed on a progressive treadmill test (as indicated by $\dot{V}o_{2\,max}$) (Fig. 19.2).

Davies *et al.* (1982) supported this concept

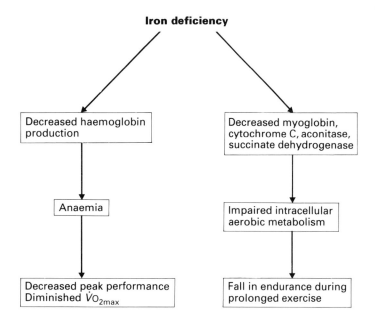

Fig. 19.2 Model of the effects of iron deficiency on sports performance.

with studies of temporal changes in $\dot{V}\text{O}_{2\,\text{max}}$, haemoglobin concentration, and endurance time during iron repletion and transfusions in iron-deficient rats. In the first, young rats were made severely anaemic (haemoglobin $4\,\text{g}\cdot\text{dl}^{-1}$) by feeding an iron-deficient diet. Values for $\dot{V}\text{O}_{2\,\text{max}}$ were 50% of control animals, and treadmill endurance time was 7% of rats with normal haemoglobin levels. These rats had muscle cytochrome oxidase and pyruvate oxidase levels of 44 and 21% of control animals, respectively. During dietary iron repletion, improvements in $\dot{V}\text{O}_{2\,\text{max}}$ paralleled those of haemoglobin concentration during the first 3 days. A significant rise in muscle enzyme concentrations occurred after the fifth day of iron treatment, concomitant with increased treadmill endurance times.

In a second study (Davies *et al.*, 1984), iron-deficient rats with anaemia and decreased skeletal muscle oxidative capacity underwent exercise testing. On a brief treadmill run with progressively increasing workload, $\dot{V}\text{O}_{2\,\text{max}}$ was approximately 50% of normal controls, while time to exhaustion at a constant submaximal intensity was 90% less than controls. Following an exchange transfusion that increased haemoglobin from an average of 3.9 to $9.5\,\text{g}\cdot\text{dl}^{-1}$,

$\dot{V}\text{O}_{2\,\text{max}}$ of the iron-deficient rats increased to within 15% of control animals with no significant improvement in submaximal endurance time.

Current concepts

These data, obtained almost entirely from animal experiments, suggest that iron deficiency can impair exercise performance through decreased oxygen delivery (anaemia) and/or cellular utilization (diminished skeletal muscle oxidative capacity). Iron-deficiency anaemia may principally affect $\dot{V}\text{O}_{2\,\text{max}}$ and peak exercise capacity, while deficiency of intramuscular iron may negatively influence one's ability to sustain prolonged submaximal exercise (endurance).

The extent and means by which anaemia and/or cellular iron deficiency affect exercise performance in humans remains unclarified. Limited information outlined later in this chapter suggests that results from animal experiments cannot necessarily be translated to humans. Still, according to available information, athletes should be concerned about the detection, prevention and treatment of both iron-deficiency anaemia and intramuscular iron depletion. Blood haemoglobin concentration is an easily obtainable marker of the former, but, short of muscle biopsy, there is currently no means of assessing the latter.

Is it possible that depressed skeletal muscle oxidative capacity resulting from iron deficiency can impair athletic performance (particularly endurance) in the absence of anaemia? Lacking a non-invasive marker of muscle oxidative activity, the answer is uncertain. The question bears close scrutiny; however, the following information is clear: (i) while overt anaemia is uncommon, iron deficiency is frequently observed in adolescent females; (ii) the time course of depressed haemoglobin levels and iron-dependent muscle oxidative capacity in the iron-deficient state are not necessarily identical; and (iii) anaemia is a late clinical manifestation of iron depletion.

Assessment of iron deficiency

As noted previously, over two-thirds of body iron is found in haemoglobin, with small but essential amounts involved in intracellular metabolism. The remainder — about 1 g in the adult male and 300 mg in the female — are stored in the liver and reticuloendothelial system, principally as ferritin, an iron−protein complex. Ferritin levels measured in serum directly reflect those in the tissues and therefore are a useful means of estimating stores of body iron.

Initial stages of iron deficiency are marked by a progressive decline is serum ferritin levels. Based on population studies, phlebotomy, bone marrow aspiration and iron absorption measurements, a serum ferritin of less than $12 \, \text{ng} \cdot \text{ml}^{-1}$ is considered consistent with total bone marrow iron depletion (Cook et al., 1976). Some authors have considered levels below $20 \, \text{ng} \cdot \text{ml}^{-1}$ indicative of significant iron deficiency (Newhouse & Clement, 1988).

Iron-deficiency anaemia, with a fall in haemoglobin below $12 \, \text{g} \cdot \text{dl}^{-1}$ in females and $13 \, \text{g} \cdot \text{dl}^{-1}$ in males, is a late development in progressive iron depletion. These levels are typically observed with ferritin levels less than $12 \, \text{ng} \cdot \text{ml}^{-1}$, indicative of less than 100 mg total storage iron.

Frequency of iron deficiency in athletes

Studies of adult athletes have generally indicated lower serum ferritin levels than their non-training peers and a significant frequency of values less than $12 \, \text{ng} \cdot \text{ml}^{-1}$, particularly in distance runners (Rowland, 1989). In these reports the incidence of hypoferritinaemia is consistently greater in female than male athletes. The validity of iron depletion in these athletes is indicated by bone marrow studies demonstrating a total absence of storage iron in a large percentage of these individuals (Wishnitzer et al., 1983).

The concept of 'sports anaemia' has been suggested by the finding of low haemoglobin concentrations in many of these highly trained adult endurance athletes. In most of these reports the mean haemoglobin values of the athletes, although significantly less than those of non-athletes, remain at the lower limit of the normal range (Oscai et al., 1968; Magnusson et al., 1984). It has been argued that this decline in haemoglobin concentration reflects increases in plasma volume that accompanies training, and that the dilution fall in haemoglobin is neither a true anaemia nor detrimental to exercise performance.

Anaemia is unusual in adolescent athletes. In their study of 46 athletes from five varsity college teams, Pate et al. (1979) could find no cases of anaemia. Rowland and Kelleher (1989) reported only one boy with anaemia among 15 male and 15 female high school swimmers. Similarly, in a study of 30 male and 20 female high school cross-country runners, only one boy was found to be anaemic (Rowland et al., 1987).

Brown et al. (1985) investigated the haematological status of 32 adolescent female track athletes. Using a definition of anaemia as haemoglobin concentration of less than

$12.2 \,\mathrm{g} \cdot \mathrm{dl}^{-1}$ in white and less than $11.38 \,\mathrm{g} \cdot \mathrm{dl}^{-1}$ in Black athletes, four of the athletes (12.5%) and one of 31 non-athlete controls (3%) were anaemic. Two of 18 female high school runners (11%) reported by Nickerson and Tripp (1983) were anaemic.

Conversely, the frequency of depressed ferritin levels among teenage athletes, most particularly females, is surprisingly high. As outlined in Table 19.1, studies of high school athletes indicate that approximately one-third to one-half of girls can be expected to have hypoferritinaemia. Iron status in males has not been frequently assessed, but available data indicate a much lower incidence of low ferritin levels (0–17%).

Willows *et al.* (1993) studied 107 athletes (52 male, 55 female) aged between 9 and 18 years to determine if frequency of iron deficiency related to pubertal status. Sports involved were swimming, gymnastics, dancing and running. Mean ferritin levels were higher in the boys, but no significant differences were observed within gender between pre-, mid- and late pubertal athletes (Fig. 19.3).

Serum ferritin levels typically decline in the course of a competitive high school cross-country season. Rowland *et al.* (1987) described a fall in serum ferritin in all nine females and 14

Table 19.1 Frequency of non-anaemic iron deficiency in adolescent athletes.

Subjects	Findings	Reference
Runners (M/F)	45% F, 17% M had ferritin less than $12 \,\mathrm{ng} \cdot \mathrm{ml}^{-1}$ at end of season	Rowland *et al.* (1987)
Runners (F)	67% had ferritin less than $20 \,\mathrm{ng} \cdot \mathrm{ml}^{-1}$	Nickerson & Tripp (1983)
Runners (F)	40% had ferritin less than $20 \,\mathrm{ng} \cdot \mathrm{ml}^{-1}$	Nickerson *et al.* (1985)
Runners (F)	34% had ferritin less than $12 \,\mathrm{ng} \cdot \mathrm{ml}^{-1}$ and transferrin saturation 16%	Nickerson *et al.* (1989)
Runners (F)	44% had ferritin less than $12 \,\mathrm{ng} \cdot \mathrm{ml}^{-1}$ at mid-season	Brown *et al.* (1985)
Swimmers (M/F)	47% F, 0 M had ferritin less than $12 \,\mathrm{ng} \cdot \mathrm{ml}^{-1}$	Rowland & Kelleher (1989)

F, female; M, male.

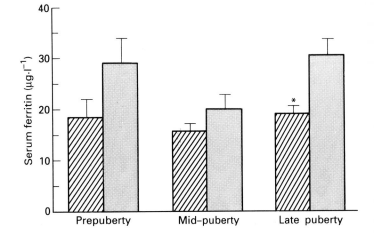

Fig. 19.3 Serum ferritin levels in pre-, mid- and late pubertal male (▥) and female (▨) athletes. Redrawn with permission from Willows *et al.* (1993) © 1993 by Human Kinetics Publishers.

of 17 males during 11 weeks of running training. The average value in the girls fell from $26.6\,ng \cdot ml^{-1}$ at the beginning of the season to $14\,ng \cdot ml^{-1}$ at the end. Respective values for the boys were 29.4 and $23.9\,ng \cdot ml^{-1}$. Similar findings have been reported by others (Frederickson et al., 1983; Rowland et al., 1988; Nickerson et al., 1989), indicating that distance running training predisposes to iron loss. Whether this occurs with other sports is uncertain. Rowland and Kelleher (1989) demonstrated no significant change in average ferritin values in high school swimmers during the course of a season.

While training appears to play some role in diminishing iron stores in high school runners, it is clear that the major factor(s) responsible for hypoferritinaemia in young female athletes is not related to sports participation. The 44% incidence of non-anaemic iron deficiency in high school female track athletes reported by Brown et al. (1985) was not significantly different than the 35% observed in a non-athlete group. Likewise, preseason serum ferritin levels of female adolescent cross-country runners and swimmers reviewed by Rowland et al. (1991) were not significantly different from non-athletes (21.7, 18.9 and $22.5\,ng \cdot ml^{-1}$, respectively, $P > 0.05$). The preseason frequency of hypoferritinaemia (less than $12\,ng \cdot ml^{-1}$) was higher in the athletes (40 and 46.7%) compared to the non-athletes (26.7%), but the differences were not significantly different.

This evidence suggests that the high frequency of non-anaemic iron deficiency in female adolescent athletes largely reflects the common occurrence of hypoferritinaemia in this age group. Still, it appears that sports training, at least distance running, does contribute to a decrease in iron stores during a competitive season.

Aetiologies for iron deficiency

By necessity, iron deficiency must reflect an imbalance between dietary iron intake and losses through haemorrhage, stools, urine and sweat. Normally, iron turnover is small. The daily losses amount to 1.4 and 1 mg in adult females and males, respectively. Only about 10% of dietary iron is absorbed, depending on the form of iron. The recommended daily allowance for iron is often met by males, but the frequency of inadequate dietary iron in females is high.

Foods rich in iron, such as liver, lima beans, shellfish and green vegetables, are not typically relished by adolescents, and the high carbohydrate diet of the endurance athlete who avoids red meat may further diminish dietary iron intake. The average daily iron consumption of the high school female cross-country runners reported by Frederickson et al. (1983) was 14.7 mg. Among the female high school runners described by Nickerson et al. (1985), daily iron intake averaged about 10 mg, with 83% consuming less than 14 mg. Studies in adult endurance athletes have indicated similar results, typically demonstrating that iron intake is less in females than males (Clement & Asmundsen, 1982).

Iron loss through menstrual blood flow is presumably the major factor responsible for the gender-related differences in frequency of hypoferritinaemia in adolescents. Rowland and Kelleher (1989) reported a negative relationship between estimates of menstrual blood loss and serum ferritin levels in high school swimmers. Inadequate dietary iron and menstrual iron loss, therefore, are considered the principal factors responsible for the high incidence of non-anaemic iron deficiency observed in both female athletes and non-athletes in the adolescent age group.

Several mechanisms may be responsible for exaggerated iron losses unique to athletic training. Gastrointestinal bleeding has been frequently observed in highly competitive adult runners, presumably a manifestation of gut ischaemia. This may occur in high school athletes as well. Of the 20 female high school cross-country runners reported by Nickerson et al. (1989) seven of nine with iron deficiency had at least one stool containing a level of haemoglobin greater than $4\,mg\cdot g^{-1}$ using haem-compound testing. Only two of 11 without iron deficiency had similar findings.

Red blood cell haemolysis resulting from athletic training has long been suspected of increasing iron losses (Miller, 1990). Mechanical disruption of erythrocytes from trauma to capillaries of the feet as well as contracting muscles could accelerate red cell breakdown during sports training and competition. Haemolysis will only lead to iron loss in the urine when red cell fragmentation is brisk, however, since released iron from haemolysis can be re-used by the body to form new erythrocytes.

Some studies have demonstrated haemolysis in adult athletes by decreased serum haptoglobin levels or increased plasma-free haemoglobin (Miller, 1990). However, Nickerson et al. (1989) reported no significant differences in urine or serum haemoglobin or myoglobin in iron-deficient compared to iron-sufficient high school runners.

Rowland and Kelleher (1989) found no changes in serum haptoglobin levels in high school swimmers during training. The scant information in adolescent athletes, then, does not support haemolysis as a significant factor in iron losses from sport training in this age group.

Excessive sweating, haematuria and myoglobin losses from rhabdomyolysis have also been suggested as possible avenues of iron loss in athletes. In high school cross-country runners, Nickerson et al. (1989) observed no significant contributions to iron deficiency from any of these processes.

Non-anaemic iron deficiency and athletic performance

Available research information indicates that iron-deficiency anaemia does not pose a frequent threat to adolescent athletes. Conversely, non-anaemic iron deficiency, can be expected in up to one-half of female high school athletes, an incidence which can be anticipated to increase in runners during a training season. It is obviously important, therefore, to determine if this substantial number of young athletes is at risk for impaired sports performance.

In accord with current concepts of the role of iron in physical work performance, researchers can translate this concern into a key question: can low ferritin levels in the absence of anaemia reflect an impairment of iron-dependent cellular metabolic processes within skeletal muscle? The question is not easily addressed, as there is no means of assessing such intracellular functions short of muscle biopsy. As an alternative approach, then, investigators have approached this issue by examining performance outcomes of athletes with known non-anaemic iron deficiency.

According to the model based on current animal research data outlined earlier in this review, it would be expected that non-anaemic iron deficiency should (i) not affect $\dot{V}o_{2\,max}$; (ii) not influence exercise time on brief progressive treadmill tests to exhaustion; (iii) shorten endurance time on treadmill tests conducted at a particular submaximal work load; and (iv) negatively influence performance in endurance athletic events.

Several studies have addressed these issues, either by examining the effects of an induced iron-deficient state or by evaluating responses to iron treatment in deficient athletes. Most have involved adult subjects and have measured performance in the laboratory setting.

Maximal oxygen uptake

Non-anaemic iron deficiency does not affect maximal oxygen uptake in humans. All eight studies addressing this question have demonstrated no differences in $\dot{V}o_{2\,max}$ between subjects in the iron-replete and iron-deficient state (Schoene et al., 1983; Celsing et al., 1986; Matter et al., 1987; Rowland et al., 1988; Newhouse et al., 1989; Yoshida et al., 1990; Fogelholm et al., 1992; Klingshirn et al., 1992). This includes the two reports described below indicating diminished performance in those who were iron deficient (Rowland *et al.*, 1988; Yoshida *et al.*, 1990).

Progressive maximal exercise tests

Newhouse *et al.* (1989) studied the effects of iron supplementation (320 mg ferrous sulphate daily) on 40 female endurance runners ages 18–40 years with initial serum ferritin of less than $12 \text{ ng} \cdot \text{ml}^{-1}$ and blood haemoglobin of more than $12 \text{ g} \cdot \text{dl}^{-1}$. Results of maximal treadmill run time, Wingate anaerobic test, muscle biopsy for citrate synthetase and α-glycerophosphate dehydrogenase activity were unchanged compared to those of matched placebo-treated subjects after 8 weeks of iron treatment.

Matter *et al.* (1987) evaluated 11 adult female marathon runners with serum ferritin levels of less than $40 \text{ ng} \cdot \text{ml}^{-1}$ and normal haemoglobin values. Following treatment with iron, no significant changes were observed in maximal treadmill run time, maximal aerobic power, peak lactate levels or anaerobic threshold, despite a rise in ferritin concentrations. The mean pretreatment ferritin level of $30 \text{ ng} \cdot \text{ml}^{-1}$ was, however, greater than that usually considered indicative or iron depletion.

In a double-blind study, Rowland *et al.* (1988) studied the effects of iron treatment of seven female high school cross-country runners with initial ferritin levels of less than $20 \text{ ng} \cdot \text{ml}^{-1}$ and normal haemoglobin levels. Mean serum ferritin level rose from 8.7 to $26.6 \text{ ng} \cdot \text{ml}^{-1}$ on 4 weeks treatment with 975 mg daily of ferrous sulphate. Six of seven subjects improved treadmill endurance time (range 0.03–1.92 min on a progressive protocol), while times of non-anaemic iron-deficient placebo-treated controls declined.

Schoene *et al.* (1983) examined the effects of 2 weeks of iron treatment on cycle exercise performance in nine young adult female athletes with hypoferritinaemia and borderline haemoglobin levels (mean $12.2 \text{ g} \cdot \text{dl}^{-1}$). Treatment caused ferritin and haemoglobin to rise, but maximal cycle time and $\dot{V}\text{O}_{2\,\text{max}}$ were unchanged.

Maximal lactate levels, however, were significantly decreased.

Submaximal treadmill endurance tests

According to animal studies, effects of non-anaemic iron deficiency on cellular aerobic function would be expected to be most prominently manifest as depressed performance on prolonged submaximal endurance tests. Both studies in humans using this type of exercise protocol have failed to show such an effect.

Celsing *et al.* (1986) could not demonstrate any effect of non-anaemic iron deficiency on submaximal treadmill endurance time or maximal oxygen uptake in male adults using an artificially induced iron-deficiency state. The subjects were initially made iron-deficient anaemic by repeated phlebotomies over a 9-week period, which resulted in the expected decline in endurance run time. Testing was then repeated after transfusion corrected the anaemia but left the subjects with low ferritin levels. In this non-anaemic iron-deficient condition the running endurance performance and $\dot{V}\text{O}_{2\,\text{max}}$ returned to normal.

Klingshirn *et al.* (1992) studied the responses of iron supplementation on 18 iron-deficient non-anaemic female endurance runners aged 22–39 years. All had ferritin levels of less than $20 \text{ ng} \cdot \text{ml}^{-1}$ and haemoglobin of more than $12 \text{ g} \cdot \text{dl}^{-1}$. Treadmill testing was performed before and after 8 weeks of iron therapy (320 mg ferrous sulphate daily), which increased the mean ferritin level from 11.6 to $23.4 \text{ ng} \cdot \text{ml}^{-1}$. Endurance run time at approximately 80% $\dot{V}\text{O}_{2\,\text{max}}$ increased significantly after iron treatment (from 66.47 to 83.23 min). This 25% improvement was not, however, different from that observed in placebo-treated subjects.

Endurance athletic events

Assessment of alterations in physical capacity of athletes resulting from iron deficiency should optimally be conducted in terms of actual competitive performance. Such investigations are rendered difficult by the influence of multiple variables which can affect athletic performance, including weather, diet, terrain, emotional factors and team morale.

Yoshida *et al.* (1990) treated six female college-aged runners who had non-anaemic iron deficiency (ferritin of less than $20 \, ng \cdot ml^{-1}$) with 200 mg ferrous citrate and vitamins three times daily for 8 weeks. During this period, in which runners ran $32-48 \, km \cdot day^{-1}$, mean serum ferritin level rose from 13.7 to $21.2 \, ng \cdot ml^{-1}$ with respective haemoglobin levels of 13 and $13.2 \, g \cdot dl^{-1}$. Following treatment a significant improvement in 3000-m run performance was observed (from approximately 281 to $291 \, m \cdot min^{-1}$) compared to placebo-treated subjects who showed no change.

Conclusion

While it is difficult to form definite conclusions on the basis of these studies, there is sufficient information to doubt whether non-anaemic iron deficiency commonly affects endurance performance in humans. As a corollary, these data also suggest that most individuals who have low ferritin and normal haemoglobin values do not have impaired intracellular iron-dependent energy metabolism. It is of interest to those concerned with high school athletes, however, that the two studies reviewed above which involve the youngest subjects both showed an influence of hypoferritinaemia on performance (Rowland *et al.*, 1988; Yoshida *et al.*, 1990). Clearly, this question deserves additional research attention.

There is reason to suspect that some individuals with depressed ferritin levels and borderline low haemoglobin values (i.e. about $12 \, g \cdot dl^{-1}$ in females) may in fact be impaired in performance by true mild anaemia. Lamanca and Haymes (1989) demonstrated this in a study of 8 weeks of iron supplementation in 20 active women aged 19–35 years with a ferritin concentration of less than $20 \, ng \cdot ml^{-1}$. After treatment, the cycle submaximal endurance time

increased 38% (from 37.3 to 51.4 min), while endurance time in hypoferritinaemic untreated controls showed little change (from 46.3 to 45.9 min). However, the mean haemoglobin levels increased significantly in both groups (from 12.7 to $13.5 \, g \cdot dl^{-1}$), making it impossible to tell if change in endurance time in the iron-treated group was due to correction of mild anaemia or increase in serum ferritin. These findings do suggest, however, the possibility that some individuals with low ferritin levels and haemoglobin values in the expected normal range can be at risk for impaired performance on the basis of a true mild anaemia.

Management guidelines

Maintenance of appropriate levels of body iron is important for endurance athletes to assure maximal performance. It is difficult, however, to formulate definitive guidelines for assuring proper iron nutrition based on current research information. Still, certain recommendations can be made:

1 It is intuitively obvious that promoting a diet rich in iron would be expected to help protect athletes from significant iron depletion. However, this approach by itself is not likely to provide an adequate solution. Even a well-rounded diet contains an average of $5-6 \, mg$ of iron per 4200 J, hardly enough to significantly raise iron stores in an athlete with overt iron deficiency or ongoing iron losses (Clement & Sawchuck, 1984). Still, it would appear prudent to encourage intake of iron-rich foods which should be acceptable to adolescent athletes such as lean red meat, poultry, iron-enriched breakfast cereals and green vegetables.

2 The current experimental data do not support the practice of routine 'blind' oral iron supplementation (i.e. without the benefit of ferritin or haemoglobin determinations) for athletes. Overt iron-deficiency anaemia is unusual, and the evidence that non-anaemic hypoferritinaemia is detrimental to sports performance is not substantial.

3 Routine screening of athletes with serum

ferritin and/or haemoglobin determinations is unwarranted. Testing for serum ferritin is expensive and would require at least two ferritin determinations (at the beginning and middle) of the competitive season. The rarity of iron-deficiency anaemia precludes the wisdom of routine haemoglobin determinations.

4 There is sufficient experimental information, however, to recommend that serum ferritin and haemoglobin determinations are important in any athlete whose performance levels are not meeting expectations or whose competitive performance is declining. In those with documented iron deficiency, a short-term trial of oral iron therapy is appropriate and carries little risk (see below). Therapeutic doses of oral iron (180 mg elemental iron daily divided into three doses) will usually raise serum ferritin levels to above $20 \, ng \cdot ml^{-1}$ after 4–6 weeks. If iron prophylaxis is indicated, the dose should be approximately $105 \, mg$ elemental iron $\cdot day^{-1}$. Nickerson *et al.* (1989) found that this dose prevented fall in serum ferritin in female high school cross-country runners during training. In a separate study, 60 mg daily did not prevent a decrease in serum ferritin levels (Nickerson *et al.*, 1985).

5 Whether athletes with known non-anaemic iron deficiency (serum ferritin of less than $12 \, ng \cdot ml^{-1}$) but with appropriate sports performance should be treated with oral iron supplementation is not clear. The author suggests that such treatment during the competitive season can be justified, since (i) these athletes may be predisposed to overt iron-deficiency anaemia; (ii) some athletes with low ferritin levels but 'normal' haemoglobin values may actually have subtle anaemia, as indicated by a rise in haemoglobin concentration with iron treatment; and (iii) iron deficiency may have a broad influence on the health of adolescents, including altered cognitive function, susceptibility to infection and gastrointestinal disease.

Are there risks to oral iron supplementation? Gastrointestinal effects of short-term iron treatment (constipation, diarrhoea, gastric distress) are infrequent and usually minor. During iron treatment stools typically turn black and this may invalidate some tests for detection of occult stool blood (Herbert, 1965). Gastrointestinal zinc absorption may be disturbed in individuals on oral iron supplementation (Solomons *et al.*, 1983), but whether this occurs in athletes taking iron — and whether this has peformance or health implications — is unknown.

If all athletes were treated with oral supplementation 'blindly', one in 400 receiving iron would have haemochromatosis, a genetic disorder characterized by excessive absorption and storage of iron (Smith, 1990). Clinical manifestations of abnormal iron accumulation (cirrhosis, cardiomyopathy diabetes) generally do not appear until the fifth or sixth decade of life, and are unusual in women (who constitute only about 10% of cases). The risk of short-term iron therapy to normally menstruating female adolescents with this disease would seem to be small.

Challenges for future research

The issues regarding iron deficiency in adolescent athletes raised by the current pool of information should serve as priorities for future research efforts.

● How significant is the effect of intramuscular iron deficiency on exercise performance independent of anaemia?

● Can this effect occur in the absence of low haemoglobin concentrations?

● If lack of intracellular iron is important to performance independent of anaemia, how can it be detected clinically?

● How should non-anaemic iron deficiency be interpreted by the training athlete?

● Is there a threshold of serum ferritin level which is indicative of performance-threatening iron deficiency?

● Are there young athletes who are at particular risk for iron deficiency anaemia?

It is also important to know whether or not iron deficiency has particular significance to growing athletes. The unique needs for iron during the pubertal growth spurt may create a high risk period for iron deficiency.

References

Basta, S.S., Soekirman, S. & Karyadi, D. (1979) Iron deficiency anemia and the productivity of adult males in Indonesia. *Am. J. Clin. Nutr.* **32**, 916–25.

Brown, R.T., McIntosh, S.M., Seabolt, V.R. Daniel, W.A. (1985) Iron status of adolescent female athletes. *J. Adolesc. Health Care* **6**, 349–51.

Celsing, F., Blomstrand, E., Werner, B., Pihlstedt, P. & Ekblom, B. (1986) Effects of iron deficiency on endurance and muscle enzyme activity in man. *Med. Sci. Sports Exerc.* **18**, 156–61.

Celsing, F., Ekblom, B., Sylven, C., Everett, J. & Åstrand, P.O. (1988) Effect of chronic iron deficiency anaemia on myoglobin content, enzyme activity, and capillary density in the human skeletal muscle. *Acta Med. Scand.* **223**, 451–7.

Clement, D.B. & Asmundsen, R.C. (1982) Nutritional intake and hematological parameters in endurance runners. *Phys. Sportsmed.* **10**, 37–43.

Clement, D.B. & Sawchuck, L.L. (1984) Iron status and sports performance. *Sports Med.* **1**, 65–74.

Cook, J.D., Finch, C.A. & Smith, N.J. (1976) Evaluation of the iron status of a population. *Blood* **48**, 449–55.

Dallman, P.R. (1982) Manifestations of iron deficiency. *Sem. Hematol.* **19**, 19–30.

Davies, K.J.A., Donovan, C.M., Refino, C.J., Brooks, G.A., Packer, L. & Dallman, P.R. (1984) Distinguishing effects of anemia and muscle iron deficiency on exercise bioenergetics in the rat. *Am. J. Physiol.* **246**, E535–43.

Davies, K.J.A., Maguire, J.J., Brooks, G.A., Dallman, P.R. & Packer, L. (1982) Muscle mitochondrial bioenergetics, oxygen supply, and work capacity during dietary iron deficiency and repletion. *Am. J. Physiol.* **242**, E418–27.

Ekblom, B., Goldbarg, A.N. & Gullbring, B. (1972) Response to exercise after blood loss and reinfusion. *J. Appl. Physiol.* **33**, 175–80.

Ericsson, P. (1970) The effect of iron supplementation on the physical work capacity in the elderly. *Acta Med. Scand.* **188**, 361–74.

Finch, C.A., Miller, L.R., Inamidar, A.R., Person, R., Seiler, K. & Mackler, B. (1976) Iron deficiency in the rat. Physiological and biochemical studies of muscle dysfunction. *J. Clin. Invest.* **58**, 447–53.

Fogelholm, M., Jaakkola, L. & Lampisjarvi, T. (1992) Effects of iron supplementation in female athletes with low serum ferritin concentrations. *Int. J. Sports Med.* **13**, 158–62.

Frederickson, L.A., Puhl, J.L. & Runyan, W.S. (1993) Effect of training on indices of iron status of young cross country runners. *Med. Sci. Sports Exerc.* **15**, 271–6.

Galan, P., Hercberg, S. & Touitou, Y. (1984) The activity of tissue enzymes in iron-deficient rat and man: an overview. *J. Biochem. Physiol.* **77B**, 647–53.

Gardner, G.W., Edgerton, V.R. & Senewiratne, B. (1977) Physical work capacity and metabolic stress in subjects with iron deficiency anemia. *Am. J. Clin. Nutr.* **30**, 910–17.

Herbert, V. (1965) Drugs effective in iron deficiency and other hypochromic anemias. In L.S. Goodman & S. Gillman (eds) *The Pharmacologic Basic of Therapeutics*, 3rd edn, pp. 1394. Macmillan; New York.

Klingshirn, L.A., Pate, R.R., Bourque, S.P., Davis, J.M. & Sargent, R.G. (1992) Effect of iron supplementation on endurance capacity in iron-depleted female runners. *Med. Sci. Sports Exerc.* **24**, 819–24.

Lamanca, J. & Haymes, E. (1989) Effects of dietary iron supplementation on endurance. *Med. Sci. Sports Exerc.* **21** (Suppl.), S77 (abstract).

Magnusson, B., Hallberg, I., Rossander, I. & Swolin, B. (1984) Iron metabolism and 'sports anemia'. II. A hematological comparison of élite runners and control subjects. *Acta Med. Scand.* **216**, 157–64.

Matter, M., Stittfal, T., Graves, J. *et al.* (1987) The effect of iron and folate therapy on maximal exercise performance in female marathon runners with iron and folate deficiency. *Clin. Sci.* **72**, 415–22.

Miller, B.J. (1990) Haematological effects of running. *Sports Med.* **9**, 1–6.

Newhouse, I.J. & Clement, D.B. (1988) Iron status in athletes: an update. *Sports Med.* **5**, 337–52.

Newhouse, I.J., Clement, D.B., Taunton, J.E. & McKenzie, D.C. (1989) The effects of prelatent/latent iron deficiency on physical work capacity. *Med. Sci. Sports Exerc.* **21**, 263–8.

Nickerson, H.J., Holubets, M., Tripp, A.D. & Pierce. W.G. (1985) Decreased iron stores in high school runners. *Am. J. Dis. Child.* **139**, 1115–19.

Nickerson, H.J., Holubets, M.C., Weiler, B.R., Haas, R.G., Schwartz, S. & Ellefson, M.E. (1989) Causes of iron deficiency in adolescent athletes. *J. Pediatr.* **114**, 657–63.

Nickerson, H.J. & Tripp, A.D. (1983) Iron deficiency in adolescent cross country runners. *Phys. Sportsmed.* **11**, 60–6.

Ohira, Y., Edgerton, V.R., Gardner, G.W., Senewiratne, B., Barnard, R.J. & Simpson, D.R. (1979) Work capacity, heart rate, and blood lactate responses to iron treatment. *Br. J. Haematol.* **41**, 365–72.

Oscai, L.B., Williams, B.T. & Hertig, B.A. (1968) Effect of exercise on blood volume. *J. Appl. Physiol.* **24**, 622–4.

Oski, F.A. (1979) The nonhematologic manifestations of iron deficiency. *Am J. Dis. Child.* **133**, 315–22.

Pate, R.R., Maguire, M. & Van Wyke, J. (1979) Dietary iron supplementation in women athletes. *Phys. Sportsmed.* **7**, 81–9.

Rowland, T.W. (1989) Iron deficiency and supplementation in the young endurance athlete. In O. Bar-Or (ed.) *Advances in Pediatric Sport Sciences*, Vol. II. Biological Issues, pp. 169–90. Human Kinetics, Champaign, IL.

Rowland, T.W., Black, S.A. & Kelleher, J.F. (1987) Iron deficiency in adolescent endurance athletes. *J. Adolesc. Health Care* **8**, 322–6.

Rowland, T.W., Deisroth, M.B., Green, G.M. & Kelleher, J.F. (1988). The effect of iron therapy on the exercise capacity of non-anemic iron-deficient adolescent runners. *Am. J. Dis. Child.* **142**, 165–9.

Rowland, T.W. & Kelleher, J.F. (1989) Iron deficiency in athletes. Insights from high school swimmers. *Am. J. Dis. Child.* **143**, 197–200.

Rowland, T.W., Stagg, L. & Kelleher J.F. (1991) Iron deficiency in adolescent girls. Are athletes at increased risk? *J. Adolesc. Health Care* **12**, 22–5.

Schoene, R.B., Escourrou, P., Robertson, H.T., Nilson, K.L., Parsons, J.R. & Smith, N.J. (1983) Iron repletion decreases maximal exercise lactate concentrations in female athletes with minimal iron-deficiency

anemia. *J. Lab. Clin. Med.* **102**, 306–12.

Smith, L.H. (1990) Overview of hemochromatosis. *West. J. Med.* **153**, 296–308.

Solomons, N.W., Pineda, O., Viteri, F. & Sandstead, H.H. (1983) Studies on the bioavailability of zinc in humans: mechanism of the intestinal interaction of nonheme iron and zinc. *J. Nutr.* **113**, 337–49.

Willis, W.T., Gohil, K., Brooks, G.A. & Dallman, P.R. (1990) Iron deficiency: improved exercise performance within 15 hours of iron treatment in rats. *J. Nutr.* **120**, 909–16.

Willows, N.D., Grimston, S.K., Roberts, D., Smith, D.J. & Hanley, D.A. (1993) Iron and hematologic status in young athletes relative to puberty: a cross-sectional study. *Pediatr. Exerc. Sci.* **5**, 367–76.

Wishnitzer, R., Vorst, E. & Berrebi, A. (1983) Bone marrow depression in competitive distance runners. *Int. J. Sports Med.* **4**, 27–30.

Woodson, R.D. (1984) Hemoglobin concentration and exercise capacity. *Ann. Rev. Respir. Dis.* **129** (Suppl.), S72–5.

Woodson, R.D., Wills, R.E. & Lenfant, C. (1978) Effect of acute and established anemia on O_2 transport at rest, submaximal, and maximal work. *J. Appl. Physiol.* **44**, 36–43.

Yoshida, T., Udo, M., Chida, M., Ichioka, M. & Makiguchi, K. (1990) Dietary iron supplement during severe physical training in competitive female distance runners. *Sports Training Med. Rehab.* **1**, 279–85.

Chapter 20

Eating Disorders in the Young Athlete

JACK H. WILMORE

Introduction

Eating and weight disorders have become a major focus of clinical medicine since the 1980s and 1990s. Of the two primary eating and weight disorders, anorexia nervosa has been considered a clinical syndrome since the late nineteenth century, at which time the term was coined and described (Strober, 1986). Bulimia nervosa, as a syndrome, was first introduced in 1976, although the authors used the term bulimarexia to differentiate between binge eating, i.e. bulimia, and the binge−purge syndrome (Boskind-White & White, 1986). The term bulimia is now the accepted term to describe the binge−purge syndrome. While appropriately referred to as eating and weight disorders, throughout the remainder of this chapter these two disorders will simply be referred to as eating disorders.

Why has there been such an increased focus on and concern for these two eating disorders over the past 10−15 years? First, it is important to understand that eating disorders are found predominantly in late adolescent and early adult females. Males probably represent less than 10% of all cases (American Psychiatric Association, 1987; Anderson, 1992). Rodin and Larson (1992) have made a strong case implicating sociocultural influences as major forces leading to what appears to be an increasing prevalence in disordered eating. Physical attractiveness and appearance are major concerns among late adolescents and young adults. With

an increasing emphasis on 'thinness' or 'leanness', females are hormonally at a distinct disadvantage. At the onset of puberty, oestrogen levels increase leading to, among other alterations, an increased deposition of body fat. The adolescent female is thus faced with a paradox, a hormonally induced increase in body fat and a socioculturally driven desire to be thin.

In the arena of athletics, the potential for eating and weight disorders in certain subpopulations of female athletes, and male athletes to a lesser extent, is slowly being acknowledged, although recognition of this potential has occurred only during the past 10 years. Added to the same sociocultural factors impacting on the non-athlete are demands to be thin for optimizing performance. This demand to be thin can come from:

1 The appearance sports such as gymnastics, figure skating and diving where the athlete is scored on the basis of appearance during the performance.

2 The endurance sports where low body weight is equated with a more efficient performance, and thus a faster time for a given distance.

3 Weight-class sports, such as boxing, weight- or power-lifting and wrestling, where goal weight must be met before competition is allowed. Jockeys also fall into this category.

The vulnerability of athletes for eating disorders is compounded by the psychological make-up of the élite athlete who is generally goal-oriented, perfectionistic and under the tight control of a strong parent or coach. It is also possible that individuals who are more prone to eating disorders are drawn to sports competition.

Definitions and criteria

For a better understanding of eating disorders and their aetiology, it is first necessary to provide a precise definition as to what constitutes a frank eating disorder. Many individuals, particularly athletes, have unusual eating patterns, so it is important to understand that a clinical eating disorder must meet established diagnostic criteria. These diagnostic criteria are published periodically in the American Psychiatric Association's *Diagnostic and Statistical Manual (DSM) of Mental Disorders*, the most recent being the third edition, revised (DSM-III-R), published in 1987 (American Psychiatric Association, 1987). According to the DSM-III-R, eating disorders are characterized by gross disturbances in eating behaviour, and include anorexia nervosa, bulimia nervosa, pica (craving for unnatural types of food) and rumination disorder (regurgitation of food) of infancy. This discussion will focus on anorexia nervosa and bulimia nervosa, since the other two disorders are not problems in the athletic domain.

Anorexia nervosa is a disorder characterized by:

1 A refusal to maintain body weight over a minimal level considered normal for age and height.

2 A distorted body image.

3 An intense fear of fatness or gaining weight while, in fact, remaining underweight.

4 Amenorrhoea (American Psychiatric Association, 1987).

Table 20.1 lists the diagnostic criteria for anorexia nervosa. Patients with anorexia 'feel fat' whilst remaining underweight. The author has viewed a videotape of a patient with anorexia being interviewed by her physician, an eating disorders specialist. The patient was bedridden due to the fact that she had become so emaciated that she was unable to sit or stand. During the interview, the physician

Table 20.1 Diagnostic criteria for anorexia nervosa (DSM-IV). From American Psychiatric Association (1994).

- Refusal to maintain body weight over a minimally normal weight for age and height (e.g. weight loss leading to maintenance of body weight 15% below that expected), or failure to make expected weight gain during period of growth, leading to body weight below 15% of that expected
- Intense fear of gaining weight or becoming fat, even though underweight
- Disturbance in the way in which one's body weight or shape is experienced, undue influence of body shape and weight on self-evaluation, or denial of the seriousness of current low body weight
- In postmenarchal females, amenorrhoea, i.e. the absence of at least three consecutive menstrual cycles (a woman is considered to have amenorrhoea if her periods occur only following hormone, e.g. oestrogen, administration)
- *Restricting type*: during the episode of anorexia nervosa, the person does not regularly engage in binge eating or purging behaviour (i.e. self-induced vomiting or the misuse of laxatives or diuretics)
- *Binge eating/purging type*: during the episode of anorexia nervosa, the person regularly engages in binge eating or purging behaviour (i.e. self-induced vomiting or the misuse of laxatives or diuretics)

demonstrated the severity of this disorder by totally encircling the patient's mid-thigh with his thumb and middle finger, the tips of his finger and thumb touching. Even in this severely depleted state, the patient was remarking to the physician how fat she was, and how she needed to continue to lose additional weight. The patient with anorexia restricts eating to lose weight, and is typically obsessed with exercise. Purging through self-induced vomiting, and/or the use of laxatives and diuretics, can also be a part of this syndrome, which may indicate the coexistence of bulimia nervosa.

Anorexia nervosa occurs predominantly in females (approximately 95%) and its onset is usually during adolescence, but can occur up to the early thirties (American Psychiatric Association, 1987). Mortality rates vary between 5 and 18% (American Psychiatric Association, 1987). There appears to be a familial pattern to the disorder, and its onset is often associated with a stressful life situation. Perfectionistic or 'model children' and those who are slightly over-weight, are considered high risk populations.

The DMS-III-R diagnostic criteria for bulimia nervosa are presented in Table 20.2. Bulimics are characterized by the following:

1 Recurrent episodes of rapid consumption of a large amount of food in a discrete period of time (binge eating).

2 A feeling of lack of control over eating during these feeding binges.

3 Purging behaviour including self-induced vomiting and/or the use of laxatives or diuretics.

4 Strict dieting or fasting, or vigorous exercise to prevent weight gain.

Table 20.2 Diagnostic criteria for bulimia nervosa (DSM-IV). From American Psychiatric Association (1994).

- Recurrent episodes of binge eating. An episode of binge eating is characterized by both of the following:
    (a) eating, in a discrete period of time (e.g. within any 2-h period), an amount of food that is definitely larger than most people would eat in a similar period of time in similar circumstances; and,
    (b) a sense of lack of control over eating during the episode (e.g. a feeling that one cannot stop eating or control what or how much one is eating)
- Recurrent inappropriate compensatory behaviour in order to prevent weight gain, such as self-induced vomiting, misuse of laxatives, diuretics or other medications, fasting, or excessive exercise
- The binge eating and inappropriate compensatory behaviours both occur, on average, at least twice a week for 3 months
- Self-evaluation is unduly influenced by body shape and weight
- The disturbance does not occur exclusively during episodes of anorexia nervosa
- *Purging type*: the person regularly engages in self-induced vomiting or the misuse of laxatives or diuretics
- *Non-purging type*: the person uses other inappropriate compensatory behaviours, such as fasting or excessive exercise, but does not regularly engage in self-induced vomiting or the misuse of laxatives or diuretics

5 Persistent overconcern with body shape and weight (American Psychiatric Association, 1987).

The eating binge typically includes high caloric density foods (sweets), usually eaten inconspicuously or secretly. By using vomiting to relieve abdominal discomfort, the individual can continue the binge. As with anorexia nervosa, bulimia nervosa begins in adolescence or in early adulthood (American Psychiatric Association, 1987). Parents of bulimics are frequently obese, and bulimics have often been obese during adolescence.

Vomiting itself can become a pleasurable and addictive behaviour. Bulimics have referred to their vomiting episodes as 'a rush' or 'a real high'. Vomiting can occur as frequently as 20 or more episodes a day, and it is not unusual for bulimics to have excessive disruption of tooth enamel from the acid in the vomitus, requiring extensive dental repair (Pomeroy & Mitchell, 1992). Bulimia seldom results in death, however, severe electrolyte disturbances from purging behaviours, particularly hypokalaemia, can lead to lethal cardiac arrythmias (Pomeroy & Mitchell, 1992).

The National Collegiate Athletic Association has recently taken a strong interest in eating disorders in collegiate athletes. They have released (1990) a three-part videotape series on eating disorders with accompanying written materials, articles and posters, which are intended to be distributed to athletic administrators, coaches, trainers and athletes. Among these materials is a list of warning signs designed specifically for athletes. This list is presented in Table 20.3. It is important to realize, however, that a qualified health professional, trained in diagnosing and treating eating disorders, must make the actual diagnosis of an eating disorder.

Prevalence

Obtaining information regarding the prevalence of eating disorders has become of major concern in order to document what some have

Table 20.3 Warning signs for anorexia nervosa and bulimia nervosa, from the National Collegiate Athletic Association, Kansas City, Missouri, 1990.

Warning signs for anorexia nervosa
- Dramatic loss in weight
- A preoccupation with food, calories, and weight
- Wearing baggy or layered clothing
- Relentless, excessive exercise
- Mood swings
- Avoiding food-related social activities

Warning signs for bulimia nervosa
- A noticeable weight loss or gain
- Excessive concern about weight
- Bathroom visits after meals
- Depressive moods
- Strict dieting followed by eating binges
- Increasing criticism of one's body

Note: the presence of one or two of these signs does not necessarily indicate an eating disorder. Absolute diagnosis should be made by appropriate health professionals.

considered to be a major epidemic during the past 5–10 years. Prevalence data are generally lacking, but what data are available for the USA as a whole, and for female and male athletic populations will be presented.

In the US population

In the general population of the USA, the prevalence of anorexia nervosa is estimated to be from as low as one in 800 to as high as one in 100 females between 12 and 18 years of age (American Psychiatric Association, 1987). For bulimia nervosa, early studies of college students estimated the prevalence at between 8 and 19% of college women and up to 5% of college men (Drewnowski *et al.*, 1988). More recent studies have provided estimates which are substantially lower. Schotte and Stunkard (1987), in their study of University of Pennsylvania undergraduate and graduate students, estimated a rate of only 1.3% for women and 0.1% for men using the strict DSM-III-R diagnostic criteria for bulimia nervosa. Drewnowski *et al.* (1988), using a telephone

survey of a national probability sample of 1007 college students to determine prevalence rates, reported values of 1% for women and 0.2% for men. Kurtzman *et al.* (1989) assessed the prevalence of eating disorders among 716 females from selected student populations at a major West Coast university. Overall prevalence across the total sample was 2.1% at the time of the survey, and 4.8% at any time during the student's life. The difference between these three recent studies with relatively low prevalence rates and the earlier studies with relatively high prevalence rates is more than likely due to the lack of application of strict criteria for determination of anorexia nervosa or bulimia nervosa, i.e. the DSM-III-R criteria. A number of individuals who have bulimic-type behaviour do not meet the stringent criteria of a minimum average of two binge episodes a week for at least 3 months.

Female athletes

Prevalence figures in athletic populations are limited. First, very few studies have addressed the issue of eating disorder prevalence in athletes. Second, of those studies that have attempted to address this issue, most have had very small and restricted sample sizes. Finally, most of these studies have failed to use the strict DSM-III-R criteria. This final point is an important one, for there may be many athletes who demonstrate bulimic behaviour, yet who do not meet the DSM criteria for bulimia nervosa.

Most of these studies have used surveys or inventories to establish prevalence data in athletic populations. The two measures used most frequently are the eating attitudes test (EAT) (Garner & Garfinkel, 1979) and the eating disorders inventory (EDI) (Garnet *et al.*, 1983). The most recent version of EAT contains 26 items, where the person responds to a series of statements, e.g. 'I am terrified about being overweight', 'I vomit after I have eaten', and 'I give too much time and thought to food'. Each item is rated on a six-point scale with descriptors ranging from 'always' to 'never'. The EDI is a 64-item questionnaire with eight subscales addressing the following areas:

1 Drive for thinness.
2 Bulimia.
3 Body dissatisfaction.
4 Ineffectiveness.
5 Perfectionism.
6 Interpersonal distrust.
7 Interceptive awareness.
8 Maturity fears.

A summary of those studies that have been conducted on female athletes to date is presented in Table 20.4. These studies have been grouped by sport where possible. It is impressive to note the very high prevalence of suspected or confirmed eating disorders in these athletic populations. Even with the limitations noted earlier in this section, it seems obvious that certain segments of the athletic population are at high risk for disordered eating. The actual prevalence may, in fact, be considerably higher than that noted in Table 20.4. This will be illustrated in the following two examples by data collected in the Department of Kinesiology and Health Education at the University of Texas at Austin.

In the first study (J.H. Wilmore, K.D. Brownell and J. Rodin, unpublished data, 1987), a large questionnaire on training history, menstrual history and eating disorders, which contained EAT, was administered to a group of 110 élite female athletes representing seven different sports. The questionnaires were administered by a physician and graduate student, and each athlete was encouraged to complete the questionnaire and return it to our laboratory. Total anonymity was assured. Completed questionnaires were returned by 87 of the athletes (79.1% return). Not a single athlete scored in the disordered eating range of the EAT and there were few indications of serious disorders in other parts of the questionnaire. During the subsequent 2-year period, 18 of these athletes had received either in-patient or out-patient treatment for eating disorders. It could be argued that these 18 athletes with documented

eating disorders were among the 23 athletes who did not return their questionnaires. Since the questionnaire was completed anonymously we had no way of determining if this did, in fact, occur. However, this is a moot point, since the results of the survey indicated that eating disorders were not a serious problem in this group of athletes, yet 16.4% exhibited clinically disordered eating.

In a second study (Wilmore et al., 1992), 14 nationally ranked women distance runners were administered the EDI. Of the total, nine runners were amenorrhoeic and five were eumenorrhoeic. The EDI identified three of these athletes as having 'possible' problems, but not clear eating disorders. Of the nine amenorrhoeic runners, seven were subsequently diagnosed as having an eating disorder that required either or both in-patient and out-patient treatment: four were subsequently diagnosed as having anorexia nervosa, two as having bulimia nervosa and one as having both. None of the eumenorrhoeic group were subsequently diagnosed as having an eating disorder. Two of the three identified by the EDI as 'possible' later received treatment for an eating disorder.

These examples illustrate that at least for populations of female athletes, the use of questionnaires, inventories, surveys or self-reports may not be valid. Considering the very nature of eating disorders, it is not surprising that a certain subset of those with disordered eating would attempt to hide or mask their problem. Further, even though anonymity was assured, many of these athletes may have feared that their coaches would somehow be able to discern individual responses, even though the coaches were not allowed to look at the resulting questionnaires.

Thus, it is reasonable to state that female athletes are at higher risk than the normal population for eating disorders. Further, the prevalence data obtained to date may be underestimating the actual risk. Finally, athletes in sports where additional body weight may hinder optimal performance, and athletes in

Table 20.4 A summary of studies surveying the prevalence of eating disorders in female athletes. In those studies in which both males and females were studied, the results for both are reported. Adapted from Brownell and Rodin (1992).

	Subjects	Measure of eating disorder	Outcome of the study	Reference
Dancers	55 female ballet dancers in regional and national companies	EAT, self-report	33% self-reported anorexia or bulimia	Brooks-Gunn *et al.* (1987)
	21 female university dancers	EAT	33% of the dancers and 13.8% of the controls scored in the range symptomatic for anorexia	Evers (1987)
	Female ballet dancers, 10 with stress fractures, 10 without and 10 controls	EAT, structured interview using DSM-III-R criteria for eating disorders	Trend (NS) for stress fractured dancers to have higher EAT scores; greater incidence of eating disorders in stress fracture group	Frusztajer *et al.* (1990)
	35 female ballet students, age 11–14 years, followed for 2–4 years	EDI	At follow-up, 16% of subjects had anorexia nervosa and 14% had bulimia nervosa or a 'partial syndrome'	Garner *et al.* (1987)
	55 white and 11 Black female dancers in national and regional companies	EAT, self-report	15% of white dancers reported anorexia nervosa and 19% reported bulimia nervosa, while no Black dancers reported either	Hamilton *et al.* (1985)
	49 female ballet dancers, 19 from highly select and 13 from lower select American companies, and 17 Chinese highly select	EAT, self-report	11% of highly selected and 46% of less selected American dancers, and 24% of Chinese highly selected dancers experienced anorexia, bulimia and purging behaviour	Hamilton *et al.* (1988)
Figure skaters	17 male and 23 female figure skaters	EAT	48% of the females and none of the men had EAT scores in the range of anorexia nervosa (> 30)	Rucinski (1989)
Gymnasts	42 female college gymnasts, 17–22 years of age	Michigan State University Weight Control Survey	62% were using at least one pathogenic form of weight control (self-induced vomiting: 25%; diet pills: 24%; fasting: 24%; diuretics: 12%; laxatives: 7%	Rosen *et al.* (1986)

Runners	1908 female and 2634 male runners responding to a survey in *Runner's World*	EAT questions on eating and diet concerns	38% of females and 23% of males indicated they ate excessively and out of control at least once a month, while 6% of females and 3% of males did this at least three times · week^{-1}. 26% of females and 4% of males have purged at least once, and 4% of the females and 0.7% of the males purged at least three times · week^{-1}	Brownell *et al.* (1988)
	93 élite female runners, 75 eumenorrhoeic and 18 amenorrhoeic	Nutrition and Menstrual Patterns Questionnaire	13% reported a history of anorexia; 25% reported undesired binge eating; and 9% stated that they binged and purged. A total of 34% reported atypical eating behaviours	Clark *et al.* (1988)
	13 amenorrhoeic and 19 eumenorrhoeic runners	Interview by a psychiatrist to establish DSM-III-R criteria	62% of the amenorrhoeic runners and none of the eumenorrhoeic runners and none of the eumenorrhoeic runners reported eating disorders	Gadpaille *et al.* (1987)
	125 female distance runners, white and Black (% distribution not indicated)	EAT, EDI	14% (18 runners) were symptomatic for anorexia nervosa, no mention was made of percentage symptomatic for bulimia	Weight & Noakes (1987)
Swimmers	487 girls and 468 boys, 9–18 years of age	Michigan State University Weight Control Survey	15.4% of the girls and 3.6% of the boys used pathogenic weight loss techniques. In a subgroup trying to lose weight, 12.7% of the girls and 2.7% of the boys used vomiting; 10.7 and 6.8% respectively used diet pills; 2.5 and 4.1% respectively used laxatives; and 1.5 and 2.8% respectively used diuretics	Dummer *et al.* (1987)

Continued

Table 20.4 *Continued*

	Subjects	Measure of eating disorder	Outcome of the study	Reference
Mixed sports	695 college athletes, 55% women from eight sports and 45% men from seven sports	Questionnaire developed using DSM-III-R criteria	21.4% of the males and 25.1% of the females were eating $<2520\,kJ \cdot day^{-1}$. 8.6 and 14.7% respectively used fasting; 7.3 and 13.4% respectively used fad diets; 3.5 and 7.3% respectively used self-induced vomiting; 2.9 and 4.5% respectively used laxatives; 1.9 and 4.2% respectively used diuretics; and 1.9 and 1% respectively used enemas	Black & Burckes-Miller (1988)
	518 Norwegian female élite athletes in various sports	EDI, self-report	47% were dieting, 25% used pathogenic weight control techniques and 12% reported having eating disorders	Borgen (1990)
	Females: 35 athletes in sports stressing leanness, 32 in sports not stressing leanness, and 101 non-athletes	EDI	8.6% of athletes in sports stressing leanness and 3 non-athletes demonstrated a tendency toward eating disorders, and 11.4 and 3%, respectively, showed preoccupation with weight. Athletes in sports not stressing leanness had no problems	Borgen & Corbin (1987)
	12 female gymnasts on the Swiss national team; 18 highly trained female swimmers; 34 non-athletic schoolgirls	EDI	Preoccupation with weight: swimmers (11%), gymnasts (1%); controls (6%); body dissatisfaction: swimmers (NS); body dissatisfaction: swimmers (38%), gymnasts (1%); controls (9%) ($P<0.01$); more swimmers scored high on three EDI subscales compared to the other two groups ($P<0.05$)	Benson *et al.* (1990)
	Females: 64 college athletes in 'thin' build sports, 62 athletes in 'normal' build sports and 64 college student controls	EDI	Athletes in 'thin' build sports had greater weight concerns, more body dissatisfactions and more dieting than normal build athletes and controls, even though body weights were lower. Overall EDI scores were not different between groups	Davis & Cowles (1989)

Sample	Measures	Results	Source
224 college female athletes in six sports	EAT	18.5% of the female athletes surveyed exhibited behaviour characteristic of an eating disorder	Gustafson (1989)
126 athletes from unspecified sports	EDI, eating disorder attitudes and behaviours using DSM-III-R diagnostic criteria	Athletes had lower scores on all eating disorders measures than other groups surveyed	Kurtzman et al. (1989)
Junior and senior high school female students: 87 athletes from track, swimming, gymnastics and ballet; 41 with eating disorders; and 120 controls	Self-reports of dieting, vomiting, or eating disorders	Frequent dieting, vomiting and claimed anorexia nervosa was more common in athletes than normal controls, but less common than eating disordered subjects	Mallick et al. (1987)
15 males and 15 females in each of three groups: obligatory runners, obligatory weight-lifters, sedentary controls	Three subscales of EDI	Runners and weight-lifters had greater eating disturbances than controls; females had greater pathology than males	Pasman & Thompson (1988)
182 female college athletes in nine sports from two major midwestern universities	Questionnaire on dieting and weight control practices	32% practiced at least one pathogenic weight control behaviour, including self-induced vomiting: 14%; laxatives: 16%; diet pills: 25%; and diuretics 5%	Rosen et al. (1986)
103 female weight-lifters and body builders (12 competitive, 89 non-competitive and two unknown) and 92 female controls	EDI	Weight-lifters and body builders scored significantly higher on the drive for thinness subscale of the EDI; were more preoccupied with weight; were more terrified of becoming fat; were more obsessed with food; and had a higher use of laxatives. Of the competitive weight-lifters, 42% used to be anorexic, 67% were terrified of becoming fat and 50% experienced uncontrollable urges to eat	Walberg & Johnston (1991)

EAT, eating attitudes test; EDI, eating disorders inventory; DSM-III-R, *Diagnostic and Statistical Manual*, 3rd edn (revised); NS, not significant.

Table 20.5 A summary of studies surveying the prevalence of eating disorders in male athletes. In those studies in which both males and females were studied, the results for both are reported. Adapted from Brownell and Rodin (1992).

	Subjects	Measure of eating disorder	Outcome of the study	Reference
Figure skaters	17 male and 23 female figure skaters	EAT	48% of the females and none of the men had EAT scores in the range of anorexia nervosa (> 30)	Rucinski (1989)
Runners	1908 female and 2634 male runners responding to a survey in *Runner's World*	EAT questions on eating and diet concerns	38% of females and 23% of males indicated they ate excessively and out of control at least once a month, while 6% of females and 3% of males did this at least three times · week^{-1}. 26% of females and 4% of males have purged at least once, and 4% of the females and 0.7% of the males purged at least three times · week^{-1}	Brownell *et al.* (1988)
Swimmers	487 girls and 468 boys, 9–18 years of age	Michigan State University Weight Control Survey	15.4% of the girls and 3.6% of the boys used pathogenic weight loss techniques. In a subgroup trying to lose weight, 12.7% of the girls and 2.7% of the boys used vomiting; 10.7 and 6.8% respectively used diet pills; 2.5 and 4.1 respectively used laxatives; and 1.5 and 2.8 respectively used diuretics	Dummer *et al.* (1987)
Wrestlers	42 wrestlers from two college teams	Open-ended interview	In addition to using food deprivation (21%), sauna (51%), fluid restriction (58%), and rubber or plastic suits (42%), wrestlers on one team used laxatives (5%), diuretics (5%) and vomiting (11%) to lose weight	Steen & Brownell (1986)
	63 college and 368 high school wrestlers	Questionnaire was developed to assess weight control and nutrition practices	Fasting at least once a week: 44% of high school and 63% of college wrestlers; vomiting at least once a week: 5% of high school and 2% of college students; laxatives at least	Steen & Brownell (1990)

	Sample	Assessment	Results	Reference
			once a week: 5% of high school and 3% of college students; diuretics at least once a week: 4% of high school and 3% of college students	
	125 high school wrestlers	32-item wrestler survey (many items taken from Michigan State University Weight Control Survey)	Wrestlers had tried or regularly used the following: fasting (51%), exercise in rubber suit (34%), diet pills (14%), diuretics (10%), laxatives (8%) and vomiting (15%)	Weissinger et al. (1991)
	49 high school wrestlers and a group of non-wrestlers	Questionnaire to determine weight control techniques	The wrestlers used dieting (73%), binging (27%), vomiting (8%), sweating (64%), fluid restriction (17%), fasting (10%) and exercise (76%) as methods of weight control	Woods et al. (1998)
Mixed sports	695 college athletes, 55% women from eight sports and 45% men from seven sports	Questionnaire developed using DSM-III-R criteria	21.4% of the males and 25.1% of the females were eating $< 2520 \mathrm{kJ} \cdot \mathrm{day}^{-1}$; 8.6 and 14.7% respectively used fasting; 7.3 and 13.4% respectively used fad diets; 3.5 and 7.3% respectively used self-induced vomiting; 2.9 and 4.5% respectively used laxatives; 1.9 and 4.2% respectively used diuretics; and 1.9 and 1.0% respectively used enemas	Black & Burckes-Miller (1988)
	26 male wrestlers, 21 male swimmers and cross-country skiers	EAT, Restraint Questionnaire, Body Image Assessment	Higher EAT scores in wrestlers due to higher scores on weight fluctuation and dieting. No overall differences in estimates of body size	Enns et al. (1987)
	10 male jockeys	EAT	The majority reported food avoidance, saunas and laxative abuse. Diuretics and appetite suppressants were used. Binging was common, but vomiting was unusual	King & Mezey (1987)
	15 males and 15 females in each of three groups: obligatory runners, obligatory weight-lifters, sedentary controls	Three subscales of EDI	Runners and weight-lifters had greater eating disturbances than controls; females had greater pathology than males	Pasman & Thompson (1988)

EAT, eating attitudes test; EDI, eating disorders inventory; DSM-III-R, *Diagnostic and Statistical Manual*, 3rd edn (revised).

those sports where athletic performance is judged, at least in part, by the appearance of the athlete, comprise a subset of the female athletic population that would have to be considered at high risk for disordered eating.

Male athletes

Since males account for less than 5% of all diagnosed anorexia and less than 10% of all diagnosed bulimia, it would be predicted that male athletes would also represent a small percentage of eating disordered athletes. While the data for women are few and incomplete, there are far less data available for male athletes. The few studies that have been published are summarized in Table 20.5. As suspected, while there are symptoms of pathogenic eating behaviours in some of these athletes, the percentages are low compared to female athletes. The sport of wrestling appears to be the one sports for males that has the highest potential for disordered eating.

Related disorders — the triad

In the example given on p. 291 (Wilmore et al., 1992), it was noted that of 14 élite female distance runners, seven were later diagnosed with eating disorders. These seven athletes represented seven of the nine athletes who were amenorrhoeic. Again, none of the eumenorrhoeic athletes have yet been treated for disordered eating. Gadpaille et al. (1987), using the DSM-III criteria, conducted psychiatric interviews of 13 amenorrhoeic and 19 eumenorrhoeic distance runners. Within the amenorrhoeic group, 11 of the 13 reported major affective disorders in themselves or in first- and second-degree relatives, and eight of the 13 reported eating disorders in themselves. No eating disorders or major affective disorders were noted in the eumenorrhoeic runners, and only one from this group had first-degree relatives with major affective disorders. They also reported that 12 of the 13 amenorrhoeic runners

were vegetarians, compared with only three vegetarians among the 19 eumenorrhoeic runners.

Brooks-Gunn et al. (1987) reported similar results in a group of 55 female ballet dancers from national and regional classical ballet companies. Using EAT and self-report of anorexia nervosa or bulimia nervosa, one-third of the dancers reported having had an eating problem. Analysis of the eating disorders by menstrual status revealed that 50% of those who were amenorrhoeic had self-reported eating disorders, compared to only 13% for the eumenorrhoeic and 13% for the oligomenorrhoeic groups. Rippon et al. (1988) studied the relationship between elevated scores for the EAT and EDI, and menstrual dysfunction in 88 predominantly lean female marathon runners, ballet dancers and fashion models. Menstrual dysfunction was equally common in all groups, as was the incidence of elevated EAT and EDI scores. Menstrual dysfunction was most closely associated with elevated EAT test scores.

Weight and Noakes (1987), however, were not able to substantiate this link between disordered eating and menstrual status. In their study of 125 women runners, only 18 (14%) of the runners were reported to have anorexia nervosa on the basis of both the EDI and EAT measures. Of these 18 runners, only five also had a low body mass and a past history of amenorrhoea. The issue of bulimia was not addressed in this study.

Brownell et al. (1987) made an important observation in their review of the literature on athletic amenorrhoea. In three separate studies, amenorrhoeic runners consumed substantially fewer total calories a day than equally trained eumenorrhoeic runners. These differences generally ranged from 1260 to 2100 $J \cdot day^{-1}$, and the differences were independent of either total or fat-free body weight. Additional studies have been published since the publication of this study, and all of these studies are summarized in Table 20.6. It is clear, with the exception of the Wilmore et al. (1992) study,

Table 20.6 Caloric intake in distance runners and controls by menstrual status. Values expressed in absolute terms and relative to weight and fat-free mass (FFM).

Units	Amenorrhoeic or oligomenorrhoeic runners	Eumenorrhoeic runners	Eumenorrhoeic controls	Reference
$kJ \cdot day^{-1}$	5342	7203	—	Marcus *et al.* (1985)
	6817	8253	—	Drinkwater *et al.* (1984)
	7266	9450	—	Nelson *et al.* (1986)
	6644	10458	7090	Kaiserauer *et al.* (1989)
	9034	10454		Deuster *et al.* (1986)
	7266	8123	7459	Myerson *et al.* (1991)
	7480	7098	7404	Wilmore *et al.* (1992)
$kJ \cdot kg\ weight^{-1} \cdot day^{-1}$	108	134	—	Marcus *et al.* (1985)
	125	142	—	Drinkwater *et al.* (1984)
	126	171	—	Nelson *et al.* (1986)
	135	193	115	Kaiserauer *et al.* (1989)
	183	200	—	Deuster *et al.* (1986)
	142	159	123	Myerson *et al.* (1991)
	147	137	123	Wilmore *et al.* (1992)
$kJ \cdot kg\ FFM^{-1} \cdot day^{-1}$	120	151	—	Marcus *et al.* (1985)
	150	172	—	Drinkwater *et al.* (1984)
	161	213	—	Nelson *et al.* (1986)
	151	219	150	Kaiserauer *et al.* (1989)
	206	228	—	Deuster *et al.* (1986)
	166	189	164	Myerson *et al.* (1991)
	164	152	162	Wilmore *et al.* (1992)

that the amenorrhoeic runners either eat less than eumenorrhoeic runners, or they under-report what they eat.

It is tempting to conclude from the above that amenorrhoea secondary to exercise training is linked to disordered eating and malnutrition. However, just as eating disorder surveys are suspect in a population with a high prevalence of eating disordered athletes, nutritional surveys must be equally suspect. The linkage is certainly sufficiently strong to suggest that this would be an important area for further study. For a more detailed discussion of the possible relationship between amenorrhoea and athletic activity, see Chapter 21.

The third member of this triad is bone mineral disturbances. Cann *et al.* (1984) and Drinkwater *et al.* (1984) were the first to report the disturbing finding that while exercise generally improves bone health, those athletes who are training and are amenorrhoeic have a reduction in bone density and bone mineral content. In the Drinkwater *et al.* (1984) study, female amenorrhoeic runners with a chronological age of 24.9 years had an average bone mineral density equivalent to that of women 51.2 years of age. In a follow-up study, Drinkwater *et al.* (1986) reported that bone mineral density increased with the resumption of menses. However, more recently, further follow-up of these women indicated that bone mineral density remained well below the average for their age group 4 years after resumption of normal menses (Drinkwater *et al.*, 1990).

Two related points need to be addressed. First, Prior *et al.* (1990) measured the density of spinal bone on two occasions 1 year apart in ovulatory female runners with regular menstrual cycles. These women were training intensely and they were compared to women with regular cycles who were sedentary. Bone loss over this 1-year period was strongly associated with ovulatory disturbances (anovulatory cycles and cycles with short luteal phases), but was unrelated to level of physical activity. Thus, it appears that menstrual dysfunction, not intense endurance training, is primarily responsible for the bone loss observed in amenorrhoeic athletes with training.

Second, athletes must be aware of the potential for fracture when they become amenorrhoeic. Warren *et al.* (1986) reported a strong relationship between both the age at menarche and the presence of secondary amenorrhoea with fractures. Of the observed fractures 69% were stress fractures, mostly in the metatarsals. Myburgh *et al.* (1990) have also reported an increased risk of stress fracture in athletes with low bone density, and the presence of amenorrhoea was identified as a major contributing factor. For a more detailed discussion of the relationship between bone metabolism and athletic activity, see Chapter 9.

Thus, there is increasing evidence that disordered eating, menstrual dysfunction and bone mineral disorders form a triad of disorders. It could well be that disordered eating, including malnutrition, is the initiating factor or triggering mechanism. Certainly, additional research is essential to determine more clearly the interrelationships between these three variables.

Conclusion

In summary, athletes are at an increased risk for eating disorders, particularly female athletes in endurance sports or appearance sports. Disordered eating can lead to menstrual dysfunction and disorders of bone. It is important to do everything possible to prevent the onset of serious eating disorders. Realistic weight limits must be established for athletes, and athletes must be encouraged to eat balanced diets, not limiting protein, fat, carbohydrate, micronutrients and total calories to the point where normal physiological function is compromised.

Challenges for future research

Future research in the area of disordered eating and athletics should concentrate on the following areas:

● Identify the actual prevalence of disordered eating in athletes in all high risk sports. Too often, coaches and administrators are unwilling to discuss issues related to disordered eating as they do not perceive that there is a problem. Actual prevalence data would provide a starting point for these discussions.

● Development of a means by which athletes at risk for disordered eating can be identified early prior to the actual onset of disordered eating so that preventive measures can be introduced.

● Development of effective preventive measures to reduce the onset of disordered eating.

● Determine the detrimental effects of disordered eating on performance. Since a potential trigger point for disordered eating is the athlete's desire to lose weight to perform better, it is important to be able to demonstrate that dropping weight too low can have the opposite effect.

● Better define the interrelationships of those factors involved in the female athlete triad to determine cause and effect. It is possible that the disruption of normal menstrual function might be the single most important sign of impending deterioration in health and performance.

Acknowledgements

This chapter was reproduced, in part, from Wilmore (1991) with permission.

References

American Psychiatric Association (1987) *Diagnostic and Statistical Manual of Mental Disorders*, 3rd edn (revised), pp. 65–9 APA, Washington, DC.

American Psychiatric Association (1994) *Diagnostic and Statistical Manual of Mental Disorders*, 4th edn. APA, Washington, DC.

Anderson, A. (1992) Eating disorders in males: a special case? In K.D. Brownell, J. Rodin & J.H. Wilmore (eds) *Eating, Body Weight and Performance in Athletes: Disorders of Modern Society*. Lea & Febiger, Philadelphia.

Benson, J.E., Allemann, Y., Theintz, G.E. & Howald, H. (1990) Eating problems and calorie intake levels in Swiss adolescent athletes. *Int. J. Sports. Med.* **11**, 249–52.

Black, D.R. & Burckes-Miller, M.E. (1988) Male and female college athletes: use of anorexia nervosa and bulimia nervosa weight loss methods. *Res. Q. Exerc. Sport* **59**, 252–6.

Borgen, J.S. (1990) Pathogenic weight control behavior and self-reported eating disorders among Norwegian female élite athletes. *Pediatr. Exerc. Sci.* **2**, 174 (abstract).

Borgen, J.S. & Corbin, C.B. (1987) Eating disorders among female athletes. *Phys. Sportsmed.* **15**(2), 89–95.

Boskind-White, M. & White, W.C. (1986) Bulimarexia: historical-sociocultural perspective. In K.D. Brownell & J.P. Foreyt (eds) *Handbook of Eating Disorders: Physiology, Psychology, and Treatment of Obesity, Anorexia, and Bulimia*, pp. 353–66. Basic Books, New York.

Brooks-Gunn, J., Warren, M.P. & Hamilton, L.H. (1987) The relation of eating problems and amenorrhea in ballet dancers. *Med. Sci. Sports Exerc.* **19**, 41–4.

Brownell, K.D. & Rodin, J. (1992) Prevalence of eating disorders in athletes. In K.D. Brownell, J. Rodin & J.H. Wilmore (eds) *Eating, Body Weight and Performance in Athletes: Disorders of Modern Society*, pp. 128–45. Lea & Febiger, Philadelphia.

Brownell, K.D., Rodin, J. & Wilmore, J.H. (1988) Eat, drink, and be worried? *Runner's World* 28 August.

Brownell, K.D., Rodin, J. & Wilmore, J.H. (eds) (1992) *Eating, Body Weight and Performance in Athletes: Disorders of Modern Society*. Lea & Febiger, Philadelphia.

Brownell, K.D., Steen, S.N. & Wilmore, J.H. (1987) Weight regulation practices in athletes: analysis of metabolic and health effects. *Med. Sci. Sports Exerc.* **19**, 546–56.

Cann, C.E., Martin, M.C., Genant, H.K. & Jaffe, R.B. (1984) Decreased spinal mineral content in amenorrheic women. *JAMA* **251**, 626–9.

Clark, N., Nelson, M. & Evans, W. (1988) Nutrition education for élite female runners. *Phys. Sportsmed.* **16**(2), 124–36.

Davis, C. & Cowles, M. (1989) A comparison of weight and diet concerns and personality factors among female athletes and non-athletes. *J. Psychosom. Res.* **33**, 527–36.

Deuster, P.A., Kyle, S.B., Moser, P.B., Vigersky, R.A., Singh, A. & Schoomaker, E.B. (1986) Nutritional intakes and status of highly trained amenorrheic and eumenorrheic women runners. *Fertil. Steril.* **46**, 636–43.

Drewnowski, A., Hopkins, S.A. & Kessler, R.C. (1988) The prevalence of bulimia nervosa in the US college student population. *Am. J. Publ. Health* **78**, 1322–5.

Drinkwater, B.L., Bruemner, B. & Chesnut III, C.H. (1990) Menstrual history as a determinant of current bone density in young athletes. *JAMA* **263**, 545–8.

Drinkwater, B.L., Nilson, K., Chestnut, C.H. III, Bremner, W.J., Shainholtz, S. & Southworth, M.B. (1984) Bone mineral content of amenorrheic and eumenorrheic athletes. *New Engl. J. Med.* **311**, 277–81.

Drinkwater, B.L., Nilson, K., Ott, S. & Chesnut, C.H. III (1986) Bone mineral density after resumption of menses in amenorrheic athletes. *JAMA* **256**, 380–2.

Dummer, G.M., Rosen, L.W., Heusner, W.W., Roberts P.J. & Counsilman, J.E. (1987) Pathogenic weight-control behaviors of young competitive swimmers. *Phys. Sportsmed.* **15**(5), 75–86.

Enns, M.P., Drewnowski, A. & Grinker, J.A. (1987) Body composition, body size estimation, and attitudes toward eating in male college athletes. *Psychosom. Med.* **49**, 56–64.

Evers, C.L. (1987) Dietary intake and symptoms of anorexia nervosa in female university dancers. *J. Am. Diet. Ass.* **87**, 66–8.

Frusztajer, N.T., Dhuper, S., Warren, M.P., Brooks-Gunn, J. & Fox, R.P. (1990) Nutrition and the incidence of stress fractures in ballet dancers. *Am. J. Clin. Nutr.* **51**, 779–83.

Gadpaille, W.J., Sanborn, C.F. & Wagner, W.W. (1987) Athletic amenorrhea, major affective disorders, and eating disorders. *Am. J. Psychiatr.* **144**, 939–42.

Garner, D.M. & Garfinkel, P.E. (1979) The eating attitudes test: an index of the symptoms of anorexia. *Psychol. Med.* **9**, 273–9.

Garner, D.M., Garfinkel, P.E., Rockert, W. & Olmsted,

M.P. (1987) A prospective study of eating disturbances in the ballet. *Psychother. Psychosom.* **48**, 170.

Garner, D.M., Olmsted, M.P. & Polivy, J. (1983) The
eating disorder inventory: a measure of cognitive–
behavioral dimensions of anorexia nervosa and
bulimia. In *Anorexia Nervosa: Recent Developments
in Research*, pp. 173–84. Alan R. Liss, New York.

Gustafson, D. (1989) Eating behaviors of women
college athletes. *Melpomene J.* **8**, 11–12.

Hamilton, L.H., Brooks-Gunn, J. & Warren, M.P.
(1985) Sociocultural influences on eating disorders
in professional female ballet dancers. *Int. J. Eat.
Dis.* **4**, 465–77.

Hamilton, L.H., Brooks-Gunn, J., Warren, M.P. &
Hamilton, W.G. (1988) The role of selectivity in the
pathogenesis of eating problem in ballet dancers.
Med. Sci. Sports Exerc. **20**, 560–5.

Kaiserauer, S., Snyder, A.C., Sleeper, M. & Zierath, J.
(1989) Nutritional, physiological, and menstrual
status of distance runners. *Med. Sci. Sports Exerc.*
21, 120–5.

King, M.B. & Mezey, G. (1987) Eating behaviour of
male racing jockeys. *Psychol. Med.* **17**, 249–53.

Kurtzman, F.D., Yager, J., Landsverk, J., Wiesmeier,
E. & Bodurka, D.C. (1989) Eating disorders among
selected female student populations at UCLA. *J.
Am. Diet. Ass.* **89**, 45–53.

Leon, G.R. (1991) Eating disorders in female athletes.
Sports Med. **12**, 219–27.

Mallick, M.J., Whipple, T.W. & Huerta, E. (1987)
Behavioral and psychological traits of weight-
conscious teenagers: a comparison of eating-
disordered patients and high- and low-risk groups.
Adolescence **22**, 157–67.

Marcus, R., Cann, C., Madvig, P. *et al.* (1985) Menstrual function and bone mass in élite women
distance runners. *Ann. Int. Med.* **102**, 158–63.

Myburgh, K.H., Hutchins, J., Fataar, A.B., Hough,
S.F. & Noakes, T.D. (1990) Low bone density is an
etiologic factor for stress fractures in athletes. *Ann.
Int. Med.* **113**, 754–9.

Myerson, M., Gutin, B., Warren, M.P. *et al.* (1991)
Resting metabolic rate and energy balance in
amenorrheic and eumenorrheic runners. *Med. Sci.
Sports Exerc.* **23**, 15–22.

Nelson, M.E., Fisher, E.C., Catsos, P.D. *et al.* (1986)
Diet and bone status in amenorrheic runners. *Am.
J. Clin. Nutr.* **43**, 910–16.

Pasman, L. & Thompson, J.K. (1988) Body image and
eating disturbance in obligatory runners, obligatory weightlifters, and sedentary individuals. *Int. J.
Eat. Dis.* **7**, 759–69.

Pomeroy, C. & Mitchell, J.E. (1992) Medical issues in
the eating disorders. In K.D. Brownell, J. Rodin &
J.H. Wilmore (eds) *Eating, Body Weight and Per-*

formance in Athletes: Disorders of Modern Society.
Lea & Febiger, Philadelphia.

Prior, J.C., Vigna, Y.M., Schechter, M.T. & Burgess,
A.E. (1990) Spinal bone loss and ovulatory disturbances. *New Engl. J. Med.* **323**, 1221–7.

Rippon, C., Nash, J., Myburgh, K.H. & Noakes, T.D.
(1988) Abnormal eating attitude test scores predict
menstrual dysfunction in lean females. *Int. J. Eat.
Dis.* **7**, 617–24.

Rodin, J. & Larson, L. (1992) Social factors and the
ideal body shape. In K.D. Brownell, J. Rodin & J.H.
Wilmore (eds) *Eating, Body Weight and Performance
in Athletes: Disorders of Modern Society.* Lea &
Febiger, Philadelphia.

Rosen, L.W., McKeag, D.B., Hough, D.O. & Curley,
V. (1986) Pathogenic weight-control behavior in
female athletes. *Phys. Sportsmed.* **14**(1), 79–86.

Rucinski, A. (1989) Relationship of body image and
dietary intake of competitive ice skaters. *J. Am.
Diet. Ass.* **89**, 98.

Schotte, D.E. & Stunkard, A.J. (1987) Bulimia versus
bulimic behaviors on a college campus. *JAMA* **258**,
1213–15.

Smith, N.J. (1980) Excessive weight loss and food
aversion in athletes simulating anorexia nervosa.
Pediatrics **66**, 139–42.

Steen, S.N. & Brownell, K.D. (1986) Nutrition assessment of college wrestlers. *Phys. Sportsmed.* **14**,
100–16.

Steen, S.N. & Brownell, K.D. (1990) Patterns of weight
loss and regain in wrestlers: has the tradition
changed? *Med. Sci. Sports Exerc.* **22**, 762–8.

Strober, M. (1986) Anorexia nervosa: history and
psychological concepts. In K.D. Brownell & J.P.
Foreyt (eds) *Handbook of Eating Disorders: Physiology,
Psychology, and Treatment of Obesity, Anorexia, and
Bulimia*, pp. 232–46. Basic Books, New York.

Walberg, J.L. & Johnston, C.S. (1991) Menstrual function
and eating behavior in female recreational weight
lifters and competitive body builders. *Med. Sci. Sports
Exerc.* **23**, 30–6.

Warren, M.P., Brooks-Gunn, J., Hamilton, L.H., Warren,
L.F. & Hamilton, W.G. (1986) Scoliosis and fractures
in young ballet dancers: relation to delayed menarche
and secondary amenorrhea. *New Engl. J. Med.* **314**,
1348–53.

Weight, L.M. & Noakes, T.D. (1987) Is running an
analog of anorexia? A survey of the incidence of
eating disorders in female distance runners. *Med.
Sci. Sports Exerc.* **19**, 213–17.

Weissinger, E., Housh, T.J., Johnson, G.O. & Evans,
S.A. (1991) Weight loss behavior in high school
wrestling: wrestler and parent perceptions. *Pediatr.
Exerc. Sci.* **3**, 64–73.

Wilmore, J.H. (1991) Eating and weight disorders in

the female athlete. *Int. J. Sport Nutr.* **1**, 104–17.

Wilmore, J.H., Wambsgans, K.C., Brenner, M. *et al.* (1992) Is there energy conservation in amenorrheic compared with eumenorrheic distance runners? *J.* *Appl. Physiol.* **72**, 15–22.

Woods, E.R., Wilson, C.D. & Masland, R.P. (1988) Weight control methods in high school wrestlers. *J. Adolesc. Health Care* **9**, 394–7.

Chapter 21

Delayed Puberty in Girls and Primary and Secondary Amenorrhoea

ALAN D. ROGOL

Introduction

The purpose of this chapter is to describe the pubertal process in girls, its variation in timing and the effects of pathophysiological processes on its onset, progression and completion. Since the emphasis of this volume is on the athlete, the effects of athletic training are considered in greater depth than other causes of delayed puberty and primary or secondary amenorrhoea.

Normal pubertal development

Growth and sexual maturation in both boys and girls is a complex process involving the dynamic interplay of genetic constitution, nutrition and a number of hormones. Ultimate height, the biological timing of pubertal development, and the tempo and degree of that development are encoded in the genetic constitution. However, the process of pubertal development can be significantly modified by alterations in nutritional intake, psychological state and hormonal activity.

Female adolescent development has been extensively reviewed by Tanner and colleagues (Marshall & Tanner, 1969). They have developed a staging system that defines the normal progression of adolescent sexual development as well as defining some of the variations (particularly in onset) that are considered to represent the range of normal. Their method simply relies on a careful physical examination of the child or adolescent and does not require any

endocrine laboratory or radiological studies. Female sexual maturation is characterized by pubic hair development (see Chapter 39) as well as by changes in breast size and contour.

Although puberty progresses in an orderly process, there is much variability in its onset and completion. Once entrained, however, the variability between stages (tempo), although present, is much less. Given this basic premise, one can describe how adolescent females mature and have a firm basis for accurately pinpointing alterations and aberrations of this developmental process. Pubic hair and breast development are divided into five stages of maturation, which are shown in Tables 21.1 and 21.2. The greatest variation is in the age of onset of pubertal development; that is usually heralded by breast budding; although in 10–20% of girls pubic hair development will precede breast enlargement (Tables 21.1–21.3). These two events, however, may be considerably disparate; for example, among girls in breast stage III, all stages of pubic hair development may be noted as 25% may have none (Tanner stage I) and 10% will have reached full adult status (Tanner stage V) (Tanner, 1990). For details about the methods for assessing the Tanner stages, see Chapter 39.

The uterus begins to enlarge early in puberty attaining a threefold increase by breast stage III and virtually a fivefold increase at full maturity. The ovaries may begin to increase in size well before external signs of puberty become apparent as many small primordial follicles mature

Table 21.1 Pubic hair development in the female.

Stage	Characteristics	Age (years) and mean (95% confidence limits)
I	Prepubertal, no sexual hair	
II	Sparse growth of long, slightly pigmented hair over mons veneris or labia majora	11.7 (9.2–14.1)
III	Further darkening and coarsening of hair with spread over the symphysis pubis	12.4 (10.2–14.6)
IV	Hair is adult in character but not in distribution, has not spread to medial surface of the thighs	13 (10.8–15.1)
V	Hair is adult with extension to the medial thighs	14.4 (12.2–16.7)

Table 21.2 Breast development.

Stage	Characteristics	Age (years) and mean (95% confidence limits)
I	Prepubertal	
II	Breast budding, widening of areola with elevation of the breast and papilla as a small mound	11.1 (9.0–13.3)
III	Continued enlargement of both breast and areola but without separation of their contours	12.2 (10.0–14.3)
IV	Formation of the areola and papilla as a secondary mound projecting above the contour of the breast	13.1 (10.8–15.3)
V	Adult, project of the papilla only with the areola recessed to the contour of the breast. Not all girls pass through stage V; others may maintain stage IV development	15.3 (11.9–18.8)

to a stage in which follicle-stimulating hormone (FSH) bound to its receptor induces the aromatase enzyme system and the production of oestrogen.

Most girls will experience menarche between 2 and 2.5 years later. In the USA the average age at menarche is 12.8 ± 1.2 (SD) years. The sequence of these events is shown in Fig. 21.1.

Table 21.3 Typical age ranges for normal female pubertal development.

Characteristics	Age (years) and mean (95% confidence limits)
Breast budding	11.2 (9.0–13.3)
Pubic and axillary hair (adrenarche)	11.7 (9.3–14.1)
Menarche	12.8 (10.8–14.8)

At menarche there is a considerable range of breast development. Most girls are in breast stage IV (projection of the nipple and areola above the level of the rest of the breast, see Table 21.2). However, some 25% are in breast stage III, with a small percentage in stage II. Similarly, most girls at menarche are in pubic hair stages III or IV, but some are in stage V, and a very few have yet to have pubarche (stage I).

Menarche does not necessarily mark the end of sexual development or mean that the adolescent has attained full reproductive capacity, since ovulation does not occur with each cycle. Young women have great variability in their menstrual cycles (Vollman, 1977) and appear particularly susceptible to stressors (e.g. psychological and athletic) that may alter the function of the brain–hypothalamic–pituitary–ovarian axis (see below).

Growth at adolescence occurs relatively early in girls — in some, peak height velocity is reached soon after breast buds appear. When menarche occurs, the height velocity is declining. On average girls will continue to grow 6 cm after menarche (95% confidence limits, 0–12 cm) (Tanner, 1990). The adolescent growth spurt is also accompanied by alterations in body shape and size. In fact the greatest alterations in the sexually dimorphic characteristics occur during adolescent development. Nearly all skeletal and muscular dimensions (lengths, breadths and girths) are altered during pubertal maturation, although not necessarily in a proportional manner. The greatest sexual dimorphism occurs at the shoulders and hips. Girls have a very large adolescent increase in bi-iliac diameter, but a much smaller one (compared to boys) in the bi-acromial diameter. Other skeletal changes at puberty include widening of the pelvic inlet.

The tempo of the pubertal growth spurt refers to the rate at which the child passes through these developmental stages. Although the timing of the onset of puberty may be quite variable, this biological parameter (rather than a 'chronological' one) demonstrates considerably less dispersion. For example, the variation (95% confidence interval) for the age at menarche is 11–15 years in terms of chronological age, but only 12–14 years in terms of

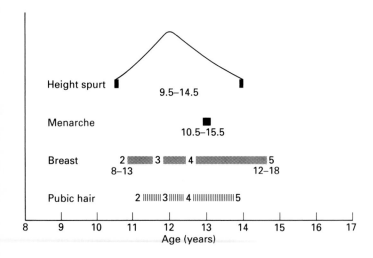

Fig. 21.1 Diagram of sequence of events at puberty. An average girl is represented in relation to the scale of ages: the range of ages within which some of the changes occur is indicated by the figures below them. Redrawn with permission from Marshall and Tanner (1969).

skeletal (bone) age (Tanner, 1990). In part, the tempo of pubertal development is determined genetically as is the final height and body habitus, although all may be affected by undernutrition or hormonal deficiencies.

Body composition and the relative proportions of fat and fat-free mass (and its subdivisions into water, bone and muscle) also change predictably during puberty. Fat-free mass, bone mass and per cent body fat are nearly equal in prepubertal boys and girls; by full maturity women have almost twice the body fat, but only two-thirds the fat-free body mass and skeletal mass of men. Children are chemically as well as biologically immature when compared to adults (who have a diminished amount of total body water compared to less mature individuals). Excess subcutaneous fat can be stored at several sites. The health implications can be (and increasing evidence shows that they are) vastly different (Bouchard et al. 1993). Traditional measures of anthropometry have been expanded to take into account these concepts of regional distribution of fat, since there is growing evidence that abdominal fat and upper body truncal fat are more closely related to health risk than any other fat depots (Bouchard et al., 1993).

Considerable recent evidence suggests that body fat content and its regional distribution, especially to the abdominal area, are related to increased oestrogen levels and lower androgen : oestrogen ratios in plasma (de Ridder et al., 1990). The earlier maturing girl has an abdominal accumulation of fat (Frisancho & Flegel, 1982). Whether the tempo of puberty contributes to body composition and fat patterning has not been adequately studied.

Hormonal control of puberty in the female

Growth hormone (GH)

Gonadal steroid hormones are important for the growth process since they are responsible in large part for the augmented GH secretion characteristic of the adolescent growth spurt of maturing girls (Rose et al., 1991). The increase in mean GH level is most evident at night and occurs, as it does in boys (Mauras et al., 1987; Martha et al., 1989), by an increase in the amplitude of the GH pulse rather than in the frequency of release. In both girls and boys the amount of GH released is inversely correlated to the body mass index [BMI = body mass (kg) · length^{-2} (m)] (Rose et al., 1991; Martha et al., 1992).

Gonadotrophins

Pulsatile release of luteinizing hormone (LH) is found at all stages of pubertal development, especially since the newer, third generation LH assays that faithfully track biologically active hormone have been used. With these assays truly pulsatile LH (and FSH) release can be detected in prepubertal (stage I) as well as early pubertal children. Such secretion could be distinguished from that in children with permanent hypogonadotrophic hypogonadism (Haavisto et al., 1990). From early puberty onward the data are consistent (although not quantitatively) with those from many previous studies using less sensitive assays. They show augmented, pulsatile release of LH — at first, only at night — followed by a period of unbalanced secretion with the great majority at night, and finally to the adult pattern of intermittent pulsatile release with a frequency of one pulse approximately every 90 min in the early follicular phase of the menstrual cycle. The ovary is stimulated to produce increasing quantities of oestradiol by the increasing concentrations of biologically active gonadotrophins.

Primary amenorrhoea without sexual development

Constitutional (normal) variations of growth and adolescent development

The normal ranges for growth (and sexual development) are often defined as the 95%

confidence intervals for children at a specific chronological age. Individuals outside of this statistically defined range may be uncommon, but not necessarily abnormal; they may represent constitutional (i.e. physiological) variants. Final height depends also on the adult heights of the parents. On average the adult height of a girl will be the average of her mother's height and that of her father minus 13 cm:

$$\text{Final height} = \frac{\text{maternal height} + (\text{paternal height} - 13\,\text{cm})}{2}.$$

The 13 cm difference is to put the father on the same height percentile on the chart for females that he has on the chart for males. Children with constitutionally delayed growth and adolescent development usually have normal birth weight and length. The growth rate is normal for the first 6–12 months, but then decreases significantly over the next 1–2 years until the child has a steady, although low normal growth velocity at approximately 2.5–3 years. This slow, but steady rate continues for the major portion of the next decade. However, the normal early pubertal deceleration (pre-adolescent 'dip') in growth velocity is often prolonged and accentuated in magnitude.

These constitutional variants are often characterized by a familial occurrence and a normal relationship between the timing of the onset of puberty and skeletal maturation. However, constitutional delayed growth and adolescence may be diagnosed only following careful evaluation that excludes other causes of delay and longitudinal follow-up that shows normal sexual development. The further below the 3rd percentile (approximately −2SD) the young girl finds herself, the less likely that constitutional explanations are correct.

MANAGEMENT

Most girls will require only reassurance. If therapy is needed, it is usually with gonadal steroid hormones, often 0.3–0.6 mg daily conjugated equine oestrogens or ethinyl oestradiol, 5–20 μg daily for several months. If prolonged therapy is necessary, the addition of medroxy-progesterone acetate 10 mg daily for 10–14 days of each month to induce menstrual periods is prudent. The latter is rarely necessary for girls with constitutional delay, but is required for those with hypogonadotrophic hypogonadism (see below).

Pathological variations in growth and adolescent development

HYPOGONADOTROPHIC HYPOGONADISM

Hypogonadotrophic hypogonadism defines the status of absent gonadotrophin secretion; but, it is not in and of itself a pathological diagnosis. There are both familial and sporadic causes and the differential diagnosis is broad (Table 21.4). Isolated gonadotrophin deficiency as noted in a number of sporadic conditions or familial clustering is usually hypothalamic in origin; that is, it is one of a number of disorders of the gonadotrophin-releasing hormone (GnRH) pulse generator rather than a failure of the pituitary to produce gonadotrophins. After a period of priming of the gonadotropes with GnRH, they can begin to secrete gon-

Table 21.4 Differential diagnoses of hypogonadotrophic hypogonadism

Isolated gonadotrophin deficiency
Syndromes (among others)
Kallmann
Prader–Labhardt–Willi
Laurence–Moon–Bardet–Biedl
Multiple pituitary hormone deficiencies
Hypothalamic–pituitary tumours
Functional gonadotrophin deficiency
severe systemic and chronic disorders
hypothyroidism
Cushing's disease
hyperprolactinaemia
severe exogenous obesity
malnutrition (including anorexia nervosa)
exercise-induced conditions
psychogenic
radiation therapy

adotrophins in synchrony with the rhythmic (pulsatile) administration of exogenous GnRH. This form of treatment can produce normal puberty in permanently hypogonadotrophic individuals and induce normal, fertile menstrual cycles.

The various syndromes noted have GnRH deficiency in common, but differ in their other characteristics. Kallmann's syndrome is accompanied by anosmia, due to defective development of the olfactory bulbs; the Prader–Labhardt–Willi syndrome by obesity, short stature, hypogonadism, small hands and feet (acromicria), mental retardation and infantile hypotonia; the Laurence–Moon–Bardet–Biedl syndrome by retinitis pigmentosa, postaxial polydactyly, obesity and hypogonadism.

Multiple pituitary hormone deficiencies may be congenital (usually hypothalamic in origin) and either part of an inherited constellation of findings or sporadic. If GH or thyroid-stimulating hormone (TSH) concentrations are also subnormal, growth as well as adolescent development will be delayed. These, of course, should permit an earlier diagnosis than if gonadotrophin deficiency is isolated. Gonadotrophin deficiency (along with other deficiencies) may occur in association with midline cranial defects, such as septo-optic dysplasia (underdevelopment of the optic discs or nerves and usually an absent septum pellucidum; Hanna et al., 1989).

A long list of tumours of the hypothalamic and pituitary regions may cause a hypogonadotrophic state. These are relatively uncommon in children, except for craniopharyngioma. This tumour is usually suprasellar and may be asymptomatic well into the second decade when it may present as headache, visual disturbances, short stature and/or growth failure, delayed puberty or diabetes insipidus. Visual field deficits (including bilateral temporal hemianopsia), optic atrophy or papilloedema may be noted on physical examination. Laboratory evaluation often confirms the deficits in pituitary hormone release; however, the circulating concentration of prolactin may be increased due to the interruption of hypothalamic dopamine inhibition of prolactin release. Radiographically, the tumour may be solid or cystic with evidence of calcification. Other central nervous system (CNS) disorders that may lead to delayed puberty include infiltrative diseases such as Langerhan's cell histiocytosis; particularly the type formerly known as Hand–Schueller–Christian disease. Diabetes insipidus is the most common endocrinopathy (due to infiltration of the supraoptic hypothalamic nucleus), although growth failure (GH deficiency) and delayed puberty (gonadotrophin deficiency) are relatively common. The pathogenesis is apparently infiltration of the hypothalamic neurones producing the specific releasing hormones.

Radiation therapy to the CNS for leukaemia or for other tumours may result in hypothalamic dysfunction. Although GH deficiency is most common, a small minority of patients will have partial or complete gonadotrophin (releasing hormone) deficiency (Richards et al., 1976; Rappoport & Brauner, 1989) or even precocious puberty.

Severe, chronic systemic disorders, often with attendant malnutrition, may cause slow growth and delayed adolescent development. Weight loss of virtually any cause to less than 80–85% of ideal body weight will often produce hypothalamic GnRH deficiency. When the weight is regained, puberty can commence or continue. If adequate nutrition and body weight are maintained in conditions such as Crohn's disease or in chronic pulmonary or renal disease, sufficient gonadotrophin release usually occurs to initiate and maintain pubertal development. Anorexia nervosa is a special condition (see below) in which weight loss and significant psychological dysfunction occur simultaneously. Weight gain is often enough to permit these mainly young women to obtain pubertal development; however, severe psychological distress may in and of itself continue the hypogonadotrophic state.

Hyperprolactinaemia due to a pituitary tumour is very uncommon in adolescent girls.

However, if present it may inhibit the hypothalamic control of gonadotrophin release. A
common cause of mild hyperprolactinaemia is
therapy with antidopaminergic agents such as
chlorpromazine. In most cases, however, these
adolescents will show some pubertal development, although they may not attain menarche
or may have secondary amenorrhoea. Both
Cushing's disease and hypothyroidism are
listed as causes of delayed adolescence without
sexual development. More often they merely
delay sexual development or prolong the time
before menarche.

HYPERGONADOTROPHIC HYPOGONADISM
(GONADAL FAILURE)

The list of definable causes of hypergonadotrophic hypogonadism without sexual development is small. The overwhelming majority of
these females have Turner's syndrome 45,X
gonadal dysgenesis) or one of its many variants.
Girls with this condition grow slowly beginning
in the second or third year of life; they may
have many of the associated stigmata: lymph-
oedema at birth, webbed neck, multiple pigmented naevi, disorders of the heart (left-sided)
and kidneys (horseshoe) and great vessels (e.g.
coarctation of the aorta) and small hyperconvex
fingernails. As they get older there is significant short stature, growth failure and absence
of adolescent development, often in the presence of either pubic or axillary hair. The latter
is due to an appropriate adrenarche with failure
of gonadarche. Although less severe, short
stature and even some adolescent development
may occur with chromosomal mosaicism; the
dictum that any short, poorly growing, sexually
infantile girl has Turner's syndrome until
proven otherwise, is useful since this condition
is so prevalent (approximately one in 2500
newborn phenotypic females).

The term pure gonadal dysgenesis refers
to 46,XX phenotypic females who have streak
ovaries; this condition may be inherited as an
autosomal recessive trait. Affected girls are of
average height, have none of the stigmata of

Turner's syndrome, but have elevated (to the
menopausal range) circulating levels of gonadotrophins, especially FSH, since the streak ovary
produces neither steroid hormones nor inhibin.

The availability of recombinant human GH
has made mandatory early diagnosis of Turner's
syndrome (i.e. much earlier than the subsequent delayed puberty), since treatment with
GH is not only efficacious in increasing the
growth rate, but most probably will add 8–10 cm
to the average adult height of approximately
146 cm for untreated females with Turner's
syndrome. Low dose replacement therapy with
0.15–0.3 mg of conjugated oestrogens should
be delayed as long as possible since even small
doses of oestrogen may rapidly accelerate
skeletal development. After 6–12 months
medroxyprogesterone acetate (5–10 mg) is
added on days 12–25 of the month to induce
menstrual cycles. Subsequently, the oestrogen
dose is increased to 0.6–1.25 mg on days 1–25
of the month.

For completeness, galactosaemia is mentioned. Pre- or postnatal ovarian failure is
caused, perhaps, by an abnormal metabolite of
galactose, and is later manifested by delayed
puberty. This condition should be detected at
birth by the mandated screening procedure or
by symptoms in the perinatal period. Gonadal
steroid hormone treatment is the same as noted
for young women with Turner's syndrome.

Primary amenorrhoea with sexual development

The disorders described here assume some
form of ovarian function — at least enough to
permit the ovary to produce enough oestrogen
to feminize the adolescent, but not necessarily
enough to induce menarche. This is a hetero-
geneous group of disorders, consisting mainly
of anomalies of the distal reproductive tract.

Disorders of the outflow tract and uterus

Often the anomalies of the vagina or uterus are
part of a syndrome of malformations including

abnormalities of the skeletal and renal systems — the Rokitansky–Küster–Hauser syndrome is the most common (Pinsky, 1974; Griffin et al., 1976).

The simplest single disorder is that of the imperforate hymen, which does not permit the outward passage of uterine mucous and endometrial blood. These accumulate in the vagina (hydrocolpos) or uterus (hydrometrocolpos) and produce a bulging hymen; and/or one may elicit a vague history of abdominal pain that may have monthly exacerbations.

Müllerian agenesis or hypoplasia leads to disorders of the upper portion of the vagina and uterus. These disorders produce a very short vagina ending in a blind pouch and primary amenorrhoea; however, the differential diagnoses include imperforate hymen, other disorders of the vagina and the androgen insensitivity syndromes (see below).

Disorders of the ovary

The common disorders of the ovary, Turner's syndrome and XX 'pure' gonadal dysgenesis usually present as primary amenorrhoea without sexual development and are discussed above. A small percentage of girls with Turner's syndrome — especially those with mosaic variants — may have sexual development including menarche. Those with the more advanced stages of development are often not as short as the typical young woman with, classic 45,X gonadal dysgenesis (approximately 146 cm).

Premature menopause may occur at any age or stage of sexual development. Although this presents mainly as secondary amenorrhoea (see below), occasionally primary amenorrhoea may be the presenting complaint. The pathogenesis may include circulating antiovarian antibodies, either as a rare singular entity or more commonly as part of an expanded syndrome of antiendocrine tissue autoimmune syndrome (e.g. Addison's disease).

Radiation therapy or chemotherapy for Hodgkin's disease or other haematopoietic malignancies can cause premature ovarian failure. The nitroso compounds 1,3-bis(2-chloroethyl)-1-nitrosourea (BCNU) and 1-(-2-chloroethyl)-3-cyclohexyl-1-nitrosourea (CCNU) or procarbazine used for the chemotherapy of other malignancies can produce ovarian failure, but amenorrhoea is usually secondary.

Androgen insensitivity syndromes and other disorders of androgen action

COMPLETE ANDROGEN INSENSITIVITY (TESTICULAR FEMINIZATION)

This syndrome (with some incomplete varieties) is the most common form of male pseudohermaphroditism. There is no genital ambiguity, and these 46,XY individuals have the external appearance of normal females. At puberty they have a growth spurt and feminize completely, except that they have no pubic or axillary hair. The circulating levels of androgens are high, and significant quantities of oestrogen are produced by the aromatization process. The oestrogen receptors are intact, permitting development along female lines, but there is a defect in the androgen receptor that does not permit the production of androgen-dependent proteins. Since the chromosomal complement is XY, there are no internal female genital structures that derive from the Müllerian ducts, uterus and fallopian tubes. The vagina is short and ends in a blind pouch, since the upper portion is derived from the Müllerian duct system. Incomplete forms of androgen insensitivity occur, but they often present with ambiguous genitalia and partial male differentiation.

DISORDERS OF ANDROGEN ACTION

This group also includes the syndromes associated with deficiency of 5α-reductase, the enzyme that reduces testosterone to dihydrotestosterone. A series of reports concerning patients in the Dominican Republic have described families with a 46,XY chromosomal complement raised as females, who underwent a striking degree of virilization at puberty. The genitalia had a female appearance at birth and throughout childhood with a single perineal opening and a short vaginal pouch. As expected there are no Müllerian derivatives.

Secondary amenorrhoea

In adolescents the most common single cause of secondary amenorrhoea is pregnancy. Hypergonadotrophic amenorrhoea is most often due to variants of Turner's syndrome (mosaicism) and less commonly to the other causes noted above, including surgical removal of the ovaries and uterus. Chronic anovulation of central (hypothalamic and suprahypothalamic) origin is, however, very common in the adolescent and includes partial forms of isolated gonadotrophin deficiency described earlier. This syndrome represents a large array of conditions whose final pathway usually includes disruption of the GnRH signal to the pituitary gonadotropes (see Table 21.4). These conditions are represented schematically in Fig. 21.2. This diagram shows the interrelationships among the various purported factors that often lead to secondary amenorrhoea.

Weight loss: related conditions

Simple weight loss is a very common cause of secondary amenorrhoea especially when social pressure in the West is placed on adolescents to be thin. These adolescent women do not fulfil the strict psychiatric criteria for anorexia nervosa, although this latter condition is a well-described antecedent to secondary amenorrhoea (see Chapter 20). A useful differential point for diagnosis is that amenorrhoea uniformly follows weight loss in the former condition, but often precedes weight loss in young women with anorexia nervosa. Its extreme form is noted in the desert-dwelling hunter-gatherers of the Kalahari desert (!Kung San). Poor nutrition during the months of drought with increased energy expenditure to gather food and wood leads to low body weight and suppression of ovulation. During the rainy season, when food is more abundant and the work to gather food and fuel is less intense, the women regain cyclic ovulatory function and exhibit a peak time of giving birth exactly 9 months after attainment of maximal weight (van der Walt *et al.*, 1978).

The important clinical features of anorexia are listed in Table 21.5. Malnutrition is often extreme and may far outstrip that of simple

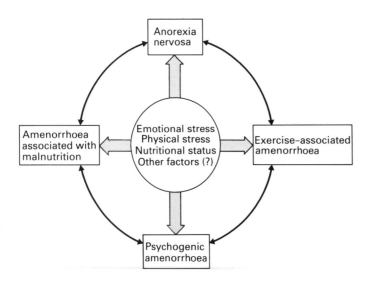

Fig. 21.2 Schematic representation of postulated associations among various forms of hypothalamic chronic anovulation and commonly linked factors. These disorders appear to be closely interrelated. From Rebar (1983) with permission.

Table 21.5 Clinical features of anorexia nervosa. From Yen (1986).

Marked predominance of females
Relentless dieting in an obsessive pursuit of thinness
Emaciation
Cold intolerance
Morbid fear of losing control over dietary intake and
    body weight
Desire to maintain or to regress to prepubertal body
    habitus
Amenorrhoea
    Primary or secondary
    Preceding, during or following weight loss
Hyperactive, intense, commonly obsessive−
    compulsive personality
Lack of self-perception and of ability to discriminate
    body image
Family environment with domineering and/or
    insensitive parent

---

weight loss. The psychoneuroendocrine aspects may be secondary to the central inhibition of the GnRH pulse generator due to metabolic signals from the inadequately nourished peripheral organs and/or may be due to primary psychogenic causes. In either case there is inadequate GnRH stimulation to the gonadotropes; this certainly may be considered a protective mechanism to prevent the caloric drain of the menstrual cycle and pregnancy. Other neuroendocrine correlates include disorders of the circadian pattern of cortisol release indicative of significant activation ('stress'), but with suppression of adrenal androgen release. In a similar manner the hypothalamic−pituitary−thyroid axis is affected with a proportionately more profound decrease in triiodothyronine (T_3) than in thyroxine (T_4) − (and an increase in reverse T_3 (rT_3). Teleologically, this pattern may serve as a protective mechanism to decrease the caloric expenditure (fuel savings), as manifest by significant and often severe abnormalities of thermoregulation.

Hyperprolactinaemia

Hyperprolactinaemia is a common cause of secondary amenorrhoea in women of repro-

ductive age; however, it is relatively uncommon in adolescents. Microadenomas and therapy with dopamine-antagonist drugs are the more common aetiologies of hyperprolactinaemia. Therapy of the former with dopamine agonists (e.g. bromocriptine) both restores cyclic ovulation and reduces the size of the tumour.

Psychogenic hypothalamic amenorrhoea

Secondary amenorrhoea may occur in women with depressive illness and in those with a history of other significant psychological stresses. These stressors usually lead to hypogonadotrophism based on inadequate suprahypothalamic stimulation of the hypothalamic GnRH pulse generator (Lachelen & Yen, 1978). The mechanism may be related to inadequate positive feedback by oestrogen or prolonged oestrogen negative feedback (Santen et al., 1978).

Exercise-associated conditions

Delayed menarche, luteal phase dysfunction and secondary amenorrhoea have been associated with chronic endurance training such as long-distance running and ballet dancing (Cumming & Rebar, 1983; Keizer & Rogol, 1990). Although reproductive system alterations are relatively common in chronically exercising women, no single aetiology has been found. This is not surprising given the multiplicity of factors involved: dietary changes, the hormonal effects of acute bouts of exercise performed chronically, probable alterations in steroid hormone metabolism and of altered body composition and the psychological and physical stress of the exercise itself (Fig. 21.3) (Rebar, 1984).

Interpretation of the available epidemiological and cross-sectional data does not provide a clear depiction of the pathogenetic mechanism(s) responsible for the reported alterations. A wide range for the prevalence of 'athletic amenorrhoea' has been reported: 1−43% compared to 2.5% in the general popu-

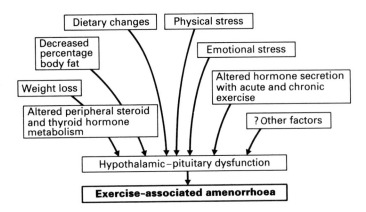

Fig. 21.3 Some factors apparently involved in the pathophysiology of exercise-associated amenorrhoea. From Rebar (1984) with permission.

lation (for reviews see Bonen & Keizer 1984; Loucks & Horvath, 1985; Keizer & Rogol, 1990). This range is due, to a large degree, to methodological limitations, including the definition of amenorrhoea which varies from 4 to 12 months, and wide variations which are included in the reports regarding chronological age, gynaecological age, prior menstrual status, co-incident health problems, and training duration and intensities. Younger competitive athletes appear to have a much higher incidence than older recreational joggers.

Collectively, available cross-sectional studies indicate that the incidence of amenorrhoea is considerably higher in young, intensively training competitive athletes than in the general population. However, it must be recognized that alterations in cycle length may occur that do not produce amenorrhoea. For example, three aberrations — the short luteal phase, luteal phase insufficiency and anovulation — can easily be missed when only menstrual data are obtained. The highest incidence (5–7%) of anovulatory cycles is found in the early postmenarcheal years (Vollman, 1977). The shortened luteal phase (Strott *et al.*, 1970) may be regarded as a sequel to aberrant folliculogenesis (Sherman & Korenman, 1974; DiZerega *et al.*, 1981). However, a luteal phase of less than 10 days is also characteristic of the early postmenarcheal years with a reported incidence of approximately 55% at less than 5 years of gynaecological age (Vollman, 1977). The avail-

able data indicate that strict standardization of gynaecological age, type of training and training volume and intensity according to the subject's capabilities (standardized on lactate threshold or maximal oxygen uptake) is needed to compare data that might link exercise and athletic menstrual disorders.

Cross-sectional studies in intensively training adolescents have revealed that menstrual cycle lengths are not different from controls, whereas luteal phase insufficiency, short luteal phase and anovulation are much more common in young athletes. There is an indication (Marx *et al.*, 1986) that different types of activity evoke different hormonal responses, although selection criteria cannot be excluded. Oestradiol, progesterone and FSH levels have been consistently lower in intensively training adolescents or young women, whereas LH levels are either not different or higher than in controls. In more mature women who began to train at a later gynaecological age, the prevalence of secondary amenorrhoea is much lower than in younger individuals. There are very few longitudinal studies available in which the length of the phases of the menstrual cycle were determined before and after training. Most involve few subjects, few hormone determinations or a relatively short training period. Bullen *et al.* (1984) showed that modest training at 70% of $\dot{V}O_{2\,max}$ caused subtle changes in urinary hormone excretion. This study and that of Bonen and Keizer might be biased by the relatively short training period and the more moderate exercise intensity. The follow-up study by Bullen et al. (1985) carefully showed marked alterations in reproductive system function, e.g. lack of midcycle LH surge despite few indications of menstrual cycle disorders. However, the very marked vigorous training schedule over 2 months may have confounded the results since some of the women may have been overreached or overtrained (Keizer & Rogol, 1990). Thus, a sudden increase in training volume and/or intensity may alter reproductive system function. Boyden et al. (1984) investigated 19 eumenorrhoeic (mean age 29.3 years) moderately trained women preparing for a marathon during 14–15 months of training ($48–80\,km \cdot week^{-1}$). Although menstrual cyclicity remained unaltered, subtle reproductive changes occurred including decreased LH and oestradiol (single samples) and a decreased GnRH responsivity (in contrast to highly trained competitive runners; Veldhuis et al., 1985).

Although many possible mechanisms of altered brain–hypothalamic–pituitary–gonadal function in endurance training women (Keizer & Rogol, 1990) have been proposed, none has been unequivocally proven. The mechanism of stress-altered GnRH and gonadotrophin release in runners has been suggested to include mediation by corticotrophin-releasing hormone (CRH) and central endorphin pathways (Loucks & Horvath, 1985; Villaneuva et al., 1986; Ding et al., 1988; Loucks et al., 1989). These mechanisms may be involved in many forms of hypothalamic (central) amenorrhoea (Biller et al., 1990). Thus in both eumenorrhoeic and amenorrhoeic runners, these mechanisms along with others may conspire to alter reproductive function. Although there are relatively direct effects of the endorphins and CRH on the adrenocorticotrophic hormone (ACTH) rhythm and on the brain–GnRH–gonadotrophin–gonadal axis, there are a host of other indirect actions at multiple hierarchical levels. Exercise activates the hypothalamic–pituitary–adrenal axis acutely to varying degrees depending upon the intensity and duration of exercise (Farrell et

al., 1983) and probably diminishes the firing rate of the GnRH pulse generator by increasing local levels of pro-opiomelanocortin-related peptides.

Others have suggested an interaction between the brain–hypothalamic–pituitary–adrenal and gonadal axes. Loucks et al. (1989) reported a blunted ACTH response to CRH and very mild hypercortisolism despite normal ACTH levels. Gambacciani et al. (1986) speculate from data in rats that a loss of negative feedback of cortisol at the level of the hippocampus may lead to increased CRH levels in the hypothalamus, which subsequently inhibits GnRH release. Taken together these data point to a central (brain or hypothalamic) mediation of altered gonadotrophin release with a major input of the brain–hypothalamic portion of the adrenal axis. Similar results (? due to 'stress') have been reported in non-exercising women with hypothalamic amenorrhoea (Biller et al., 1990). In addition to a certain poorly defined predisposition of certain women to menstrual cycle disorders, there is apparently a relationship between physical training and reproductive system alterations in endurance training women. However, evidence suggests that training must exceed a certain duration and/or intensity to inhibit pulsatile GnRH release. One may hypothesize that 'overreaching' or 'overtraining' (see Kuipers & Keizer, 1988, for definitions) may play an important role in altering the reproductive system. According to this thesis, a certain amount of training and/or a sudden increase in the amount or intensity of training is required to become 'overreached'. In this case, inappropriate or incomplete adaptation has occurred (Selye, 1939).

Our own prospective studies in older, previously sedentary women (average age 31.4 ± 1.4 years, 17.8 ± 0.9 years beyond menarche) produced remarkably little alteration in clinical reproductive status (e.g. menstrual cyclicity) in eumenorrhoeic, previously non-training women, despite running almost 1300 km in the first year (Rogol et al., 1992). Minimal changes were noted in the pulsatile release of LH indicating little, if any alteration in the hypo-thalamic GnRH pulse generator. We conclude that a progressive exercise programme of moderate distance and intensity does not significantly alter the robust reproductive system of gynaecologically mature eumenorrhoeic women. Thus, the so-called 'athletic amenorrhoea' reported in cross-sectional studies may result from associated, or prior, non-exercise dependent variables (especially younger gynaecological age and diminished body weight) that alone or in the aggregate affect the activity of the hypothalamic−pituitary−ovarian axis.

Challenges for future research

- To determine the genetic, nutritional and hormonal (especially gonadotropin, gonadal and growth hormone axis) mechanisms that subserve alterations in body composition and the regional distribution of fat in girls at adolescence. This is to determine (i) influence on menarche itself; and (ii) the mechanisms by which endurance exercise alters these relationships.
- To determine the nutritional, stress and hormonal mechanisms for secondary amenorrhoea in athletes and their non-exercising cohort.
- To determine the influence of the CRH−pituitary−adrenal axis on the GnRH−pituitary−gonadal axis and its modulation by exercise.

References

Biller, B., Federoff, H. & Koenig, J. (1990) Abnormal cortisol secretion and responses to corticotropin-releasing hormone in women with hypothalamic amenorrhea. *J. Clin. Endocrinol. Metab.* **70**, 311−17.

Bonen, A. & Keizer, H. (1984) Athletic menstrual cycle irregularity: endocrine response to exercise and training. *Phys. Sports Med.* **12**, 78−94.

Bouchard, C., Després, J-P. & Mauriège, P. (1993) Genetic and nongenetic determinants of regional fat distribution. *Endocr. Rev.* **14**, 72−93.

Boyden, T.W., Pamenter, R.W., Stanforth, P., Rotkis, T. & Wilmore, J. (1984) Impaired gonadotropin responses to gonadotropin-releasing hormone stimulation in 20 endurance-trained women. *Fertil. Steril.* **41**, 359−63.

Bullen, B., Skrinar, G., Beitins, I. *et al.* (1984) Endurance training effects on plasma hormonal responsiveness and sex hormone excretion. *J. Appl. Physiol. Respir. Environ. Exerc. Physiol.* **56**, 1453−63.

Bullen, B., Skrinar, G., Beitins, I., VonMering G., Twinbull, B. & McArthur, J. (1985) Induction of menstrual cycle disorders by strenuous exercise in untrained women. *New Engl. J. Med.* **312**, 1349−53.

Cumming, D. & Rebar, R. (1983) Exercise and reproductive function in women: a review. *Am. J. Indust. Med.* **4**, 113−25.

de Ridder, C., Bruning, P., Zonderland, M. *et al.* (1990) Body fat mass, body fat distribution and plasma hormones in early puberty in females. *J. Clin. Endocrinol. Metab.* **70**, 888−93.

Ding, J-H., Sheckter, C., Drinkwater, B., Soules, M. & Bremner, W. (1988) High serum cortisol levels in exercise associated amenorrhea. *Ann. Int. Med.* **108**, 530−4.

DiZerega, G., Turner, C., Stouffer, R., Anderson, L., Channing, C. & Hodgen, G. (1981) Suppression of follicle-stimulating hormone-dependent folliculo-genesis during the primate ovarian cycle. *J. Clin. Endocrinol. Metab.* **52**, 451−6.

Farrell, P., Garthwaite, T. & Gustafson, A. (1983) Plasma adrenocorticotropin and cortisol responses to submaximal and exhaustive exercise. *J. Appl. Physiol. Respir. Environ. Exerc. Physiol.* **55**, 1441−4.

Frisancho, A. & Flegel, P. (1982) Advanced maturation with centripetal fat pattern. *Hum. Biol.* **54**, 717−27.

Gambacciani, M., Yen, S. & Rasmussen, D. (1986) GnRH release from the mediobasal hypothalamus: *in vitro* inhibition by corticotropin-releasing factor. *Neuroendocrinology*, **43**, 533−6.

Griffin, J., Edwards, C. & Madden, J. (1976) Congenital absence of the vagina. *Ann. Int. Med.* **85**, 224.

Haavisto, A-M., Dunkel, L., Petterson, K. & Huhtaniemi, I. (1990) LH measurements by *in vitro* bioassay and a highly sensitive immunofluoro-metric assay improve the distinction between boys with constitutional delay of puberty and hypogon-adotropic hypogonadism. *Pediatr. Res.* **27**, 211−14.

Hanna, C., Mandel, S. & LaFranche, S. (1989) Puberty in the syndrome of septo-optic dysplasia. *Am. J. Dis. Child.* **143**, 186−9.

Keizer, H. & Rogol, A. (1990) Physical exercise and menstrual cycle alterations: what are the mechanisms? *Sports Med.* **10**, 218−35.

Kuipers, H. & Keizer, H. (1988) Overtraining in élite athletes. *Sports Med.* **6**, 79−92.

Lachelin, G. & Yen, S. (1978) Hypothalamic chronic anovulation. *Am. J. Obstet. Gynecol.* **130**, 825−31.

Loucks, A. & Horvath, S. (1985) Athletic amenorrhea: a review. *Med. Sci. Sports Exerc.* **17**, 56−72.

Loucks, A., Mortola, J., Girton, L. & Yen, S. (1989) Alterations in the hypothalamic−pituitary−

ovarian, and the hypothalamic–pituitary–adrenal axes in athletic women. *J. Clin. Endocrinol. Metab.* **68**, 402–11.

Marshall, W.A. & Tanner, J. (1969) Variations in pattern of pubertal changes in girls. *Arch. Dis. Child.* **44**, 291–303.

Martha Jr, P., Gorman, K., Blizzard, R., Rogol, A. & Veldhuis, J. (1992) Endogenous growth hormone secretion and clearance rates in normal boys as determined by deconvolution analysis: relationship to age, pubertal status and body mass index. *J. Clin. Endocrinol. Metab.* **74**, 336–44.

Martha Jr, P., Rogol, A., Veldhuis, J., Kerrigan, J., Goodman, D. & Blizzard, R. (1989) Alterations in the pulsatile properties of circulating growth hormone concentrations during puberty in boys. *J. Clin. Endocrinol. Metab.* **69**, 563–70.

Marx, K., Kische, B., Lenz, H. & Hoffmann, P. (1986) Die Gonadotropin and Sexualsteroide während des Menstruationszyklus bei jungen sporttreibenden Frauen. *Med. Sport* **26**, 51–4.

Mauras, N., Blizzard, R., Link, K., Johnson, M., Rogol, A. & Veldhuis, J. (1987) Augmentation of growth hormone secretion during puberty: evidence for a pulse amplitude-modulated phenomenon. *J. Clin. Endocrinol. Metab.* **64**, 596–601.

Pinsky, L. (1974) A community of human malformation syndromes involving the Müllerian ducts, distal extremities, urinary tract and ears. *Teratology* **9**, 65–79.

Rappoport, R. & Brauner, R. (1989) Growth and endocrine disorders secondary to cranial irradiation. *Pediatr. Res.* **25**, 561–7.

Rebar, R.W. (1983) The reproductive age: chronic anovulation. In G.B. Serra (ed.) *The Ovary*, pp. 217–40. Raven Press, New York.

Rebar, R.W. (1984) Effect of exercise on reproductive function in females. In J.R. Givens (ed.) *The Hypothalamus in Health and Disease*, p. 245. Year Book, Chicago.

Richards, G., Wara, W., Grumbach, M., Kaplan, S., Sheline, G. & Conte, F. (1976) Delayed onset of hypopituitarism: sequelae of therapeutic irradiation of central nervous system, eye and middle ear tumors. *J. Pediatr.* **89**, 533–9.

Rogol, A., Weltman, A., Weltman, J. *et al.* (1992)

Durability of the reproductive axis in eumenorrheic women during 1 year of endurance training. *J. Appl. Physiol.* **72**, 1571–80.

Rose, S., Municchi, G., Barnes, K. *et al.* (1991) Spontaneous growth hormone secretion increases during puberty in normal girls and boys. *J. Clin. Endocrinol. Metab.* **73**, 428–35.

Santen, R., Friend, J., Trejanowski, D., Davis, B., Samojlike, E. & Barden, C. (1978) Prolonged negative feedback suppression after estradiol administration: proposed mechanism of eugonadal secondary amenorrhea. *J. Clin. Endocrinol. Metab.* **47**, 1220–9.

Selye, H. (1939) The effect of adaptations to various damaging agents on the female sex organs in the rat. *Endocrinology*, **25**, 615–24.

Sherman, B. & Korenman, S. (1974) Measurement of plasma LH FSH, estradiol and progesterone in disorders of the human menstrual cycle: the short luteal phase. *J. Clin. Endocrinol. Metab.* **38**, 89–93.

Strott, C., Cargille, C., Ross, G. & Lipsett, M. (1970) The short luteal phase. *J. Clin. Endocrinol. Metab.* **30**, 246–51.

Tanner, J. (1990) *Foetus into Man: Physical Growth from Conception to Maturity*, pp. 1–103. Harvard University Press, Cambridge.

van der Walt, L., Wilmsen, E. & Jenkins, T. (1978) Unusual sex hormone patterns among desert-dwelling hunter-gatherers. *J. Clin. Endocrinol. Metab.* **46**, 658–63.

Veldhuis, J., Evans, W., Demers, L., Thorner, M., Wakat, D. & Rogol, A. (1985) Altered neuroendocrine regulation of gonadotropin secretion in women distance runners. *J. Clin. Endocrinol. Metab.* **61**, 557–63.

Villaneuva, A., Schlosser, C., Hopper, B., Liu, J., Hoffmah, D. & Rebar, R. (1986) Increased cortisol production in women runners. *J. Clin. Endocrinol. Metab.* **63**, 133–6.

Vollman, R. (1977) *The Menstrual Cycle*. W.B. Saunders, Philadelphia.

Yen, S.S.C. (1986) Chronic anovulation due to CNS–hypothalamic–pituitary dysfunction. In S.S.C. Yen & R.B. Jaffe (eds) *Reproductive Endocrinology*, 2nd edn, pp. 500–45. W.B. Saunders, Philadelphia.

Chapter 22

Cardiological Concerns in the Young Athlete

REGINALD L. WASHINGTON

Introduction

Congenital heart diseases (present at birth) comprise a number of specific conditions and occur at a rate of eight per 1000 births (Labarthe *et al.*, 1990). It is important to establish the safety of physical activity in this population and encourage continuation of physical activity according to their individual limits. Acquired heart disease (occurring after birth) may be encountered in children interested in participating in physical activities. The majority of these individuals may participate in all physical activities without limitations; however, there are exceptions. Just as the child with congenital heart disease, these children should be individually evaluated and their limitations personally set.

Perhaps the largest category of children who have a cardiovascular concern are individuals in whom the cardiovascular system is normal but who are perceived to have cardiovascular disease. The child with the functional heart murmur is the most common example of this. These children are often restricted in their physical activities by their parents or by their health-care providers.

Murmurs

Murmurs are commonly heard in children, and it is estimated that up to 85% of young athletes have heart murmurs (Shaffer, 1974). The majority of these murmurs are of the functional or innocent variety (synonymous terms) (Table 22.1). Often, these murmurs are appreciated for the first time during a preparticipation physical examination (see Chapter 17). Once the murmur is heard, several questions are raised:

1 Is the murmur functional or organic?

2 If the murmur is organic, should participation in physical activity be limited?

3 What type of evaluation should be completed before participation in physical activity is allowed?

The most common murmur heard in childhood is the Still's murmur (Cantwell & Murray, 1990). This murmur is characterized by a medium to high pitched slightly vibratory or moaning quality. It is best heard along the lower left sternal border but radiates widely from the apex to the upper left sternal border. It is best appreciated when the individual is supine and decreases dramatically in intensity when the patient is upright or standing. The murmur is confined to systole and is never heard in diastole. This murmur is characteristically intermittent and is most pronounced

Table 22.1 Functional murmurs.

Systolic
   vibratory Still's murmur
   pulmonary flow murmur
   peripheral pulmonary branch stenosis murmur
   mammary souffle murmur
Continuous
   venous hum
   continuous mammary souffle

318

with activities that increase cardiac output including anxiety, fever or exercise.

Another common functional murmur is the venous hum. This murmur is characterized as a continuous rather blowing murmur best heard in the right or left supra- and infraclavicular areas. This murmur is best appreciated when the individual is sitting and generally is inaudible when the individual is supine or becomes inaudible with various manipulations that obstruct the return of venous blood from the neck to the heart (gentle external jugular compression). This murmur also becomes inaudible when the individual moves his or her head from side to side or up and down. If the murmur persists throughout all of these manoeuvres and continues to be heard when the individual is supine, the differential diagnoses must include patent ductus arteriosus.

Organic murmurs are generally characterized by their harshness rather than their intensity (a functional murmur may in fact be grade III−VI). Organic murmurs are generally not vibratory in nature and are not drastically affected by body position. Organic murmurs may represent very mild cardiovascular defects (atrial septal defect, ventricular septal defect) or may be part of a more complex cardiovascular problem (stenotic valves, cyanotic heart disease). The experienced clinician may have little difficulty discriminating between functional murmurs and organic murmurs. If there is any question, the individual should be referred to an experienced clinician or perhaps a paediatric cardiologist.

If further evaluation is necessary, this assessment should begin with a thorough history of the individual as well as his or her immediate family. Adverse response to exercise should be included in this interrogation. A thorough physical examination, looking for signs of cardiovascular disease, should also be completed. Various laboratory examinations may be appropriate, for example electrocardiogram (ECG), chest X-ray, echocardiogram, and so on.

The presence of an organic murmur alone is not grounds for prohibiting physical murmurs.

There are over 300 different types of organic murmurs. Many individuals with organic murmurs (from congenital or acquired defects) do not have haemodynamic impairment and are capable of full active involvement in physical activities (Gutgesell et al., 1986). The decision to allow an individual to participate in physical activities should be left to the primary healthcare provider and each case must be considered individually. Useful guidelines for the practising physician who needs to advise patients about sports participation were laid down at the Sixteenth Bethesda Conference on Cardiovascular Abnormalities in the Athlete (McNamara et al., 1985). This report focuses on the principle that different activities vary considerably in their emotional and physical demands, and, therefore, an individual's eligibility for a given activity must be considered in relation to the physiological demands of that sport.

Dysrhythmias

When a child is suspected of having a dysrhythmia, a thorough history should be obtained. Questions should be asked regarding the frequency, intensity and number of episodes, as well as the time of day that the episodes occur. Often dysrhythmias are associated with exercise, medications, caffeine intake or drug use and/or abuse. Associated symptoms include headache, nausea, vomiting, loss of vision, syncope or near syncope.

A variety of modalities are used in the diagnosis and characterization of dysrhythmias. In addition to the history outlined above, an ECG is often very helpful in characterizing a particular dysrhythmia. On occasion, however, long-term recording devices (24-h Holter monitor or 15−30-s patient activated monitor) are useful.

Children who have been evaluated and diagnosed with a dysrhythmia may require treatment before physical activity is allowed (Zipes et al., 1985). Some dysrhythmias require special pacemakers that are designed to suppress the irregular rhythm and to readjust the heart rate back to a normal rhythm. Other individuals require medication to suppress dysrhythmias.

Not all dysrhythmias in children are pathological. A wandering atrial pacemaker is a clinical situation in which two separate foci in the atria are 'competing with each other'. During this circumstance, the heart rhythm may appear to be irregular. A similar situation is a sinus dysrhythmia during which a single focus in the atrium is initiating an irregular but adequate impulse. The above two conditions are benign and no exercise restrictions are required. Some dysrhythmias are more complex and need further evaluation (Table 22.2).

A more complex dysrhythmia results from premature ventricular contraction (PVC). In this situation, a focus in the ventricle initiates a premature contraction by the ventricle. On auscultation, the rhythm is irregular and is followed by a 'compensatory pause'. The beat following the compensatory pause is often more forceful and is perceived by the individual as a skipped beat. An ECG should be obtained when this diagnosis is suspected. If the PVCs appear to be uniform (and therefore unifocal), do not appear in couplets and disappear when the heart rate reaches approximately $140-150$ beats $\cdot$ min^{-1}, then there are no exercise restrictions. If, on the other hand, the PVCs are not uniform (and thereby multifocal), appear in couplets or runs or do not disappear with exercise, then further evaluation is warranted before athletic participation is allowed.

Another dysrhythmia is the premature atrial contraction. This dysrhythmia is very common and results from a separate focus in the atrium initiating a premature atrial beat or contraction.

Table 22.2 Common dysrhythmias needing evaluation.

Premature ventricular contraction
Premature supraventricular contraction
Atrial flutter
Supraventricular tachycardia
Heart block

This dysrhythmia is easily discernible on ECG, is benign and requires no further evaluation or activity restriction.

Supraventricular tachycardia is also known as paroxysmal atrial tachycardia. This dysrhythmia results from an abnormally rapid conduction of an atrial impulse into the ventricle. Supraventricular tachycardia is typically episodic and occurs in paroxysms. The supraventricular tachycardic heart rate is usually very fast (greater than $180-200$ beats $\cdot$ min^{-1}). This dysrhythmia requires further evaluation and perhaps medical treatment before athletic participation is allowed.

In individuals with complete congenital heart block, there is no transmission of electrical impulses from the atria to the ventricles. If the ventricular heart rate is sufficient for adequate cardiac output ($50-60$ beats $\cdot$ min^{-1} at rest) then these individuals usually have no symptoms. People with complete congenital heart block, however, rarely attain a heart rate of greater than $90-100$ beats $\cdot$ min^{-1} during vigorous exercise. Often an exercise test is required to establish the limits of their physical activity. A rate responsive pacemaker is very helpful in allowing these individuals to participate in vigorous physical activity. They should be under the care of a physician before being allowed to participate.

Individuals who experience more complex dysrhythmias, including atrial flutter and fibrillation, junctional tachycardia, ventricular tachycardia or multifocal ventricular dysrhythmias, should be referred to a cardiologist for evaluation, and possible treatment, before athletic participation is allowed.

Dysrhythmias may be associated with structural congenital heart defects. These individuals should be under the care of a cardiologist before physical activity is allowed.

Syncope

Near syncope has vasovagal signs and symptoms. These individuals often complain of not feeling well and may be dizzy. They are often cold, clammy and sweaty with a thready pulse and a low blood pressure but do not lose consciousness. In syncope, the above presyncopal symptoms are followed by loss of muscle tone and consciousness. There are many causes of syncope including vasodepressor syncope (the common faint), primary and secondary cardiovascular syncope, vascular syncope and non-cardiovascular syncope (O'Laughlin & McNamara, 1990) (Table 22.3).

The vasodepressor syncope or fainting is commonly characterized by a sudden fall in blood pressure associated with dizziness, light headedness or loss of consciousness and is accompanied by prominent symptoms of autonomic activity (pallor, perspiration, nausea, hyperventilation and tachycardia) (O'Laughlin & McNamara, 1990). This event may be initiated by environmental stimuli such as anxiety or the sight of blood. The typical faint is preceded by a prodrome; therefore, the individual usually has some warning and avoids physical injury. The syncopal episode lasts less than 1 min. If the environmental stimulus is identified (crowds, hunger, heat, dehydration, pain or emotion) and eliminated, full athletic participation may be allowed.

Cardiovascular syncope may be the result of congenital heart disease (cyanotic heart disease, low cardiac output or myocardial infarction) or may be secondary to cardiovascular disease (dysrhythmia). In these individuals, the syncopal episode will be accompanied by historical facts and physical findings that will suggest the cardiovascular aetiology. These individuals require careful evaluation and diagnosis before being allowed to participate in physical activity.

Vascular syncope is also known as vasodepressor syncope or orthostatic syncope (Thilenius *et al.*, 1991). The mechanism for this reaction begins with reduced left ventricular filling secondary to pooling of blood in the lower parts of the body during standing. This reduction in left ventricular volume results in the stimulation of the special receptors that are located in the left ventricle that cause a reflex slowing of the heart rate and vasodilation of the blood vessels (especially in the brain). This is a paradoxical response and is seen in individuals who are prone to vasodepressor syncope. When these individuals are closely observed (as during a tilt test), there is a normal rise in heart rate by 20 or so beats $\cdot$ min^{-1} in response to upright tilting. This level of tachycardia is maintained for several minutes but is quickly followed by a precipitous fall in blood pressure and heart rate with the complete cessation of sinus activity and profound nodal bradycardia. Often severe vasovagal symptoms are evident. These individuals often require pharmacological intervention before being allowed to participate in physical activities.

Non-cardiac causes of syncope include, but are not limited to, hypoxia, hypoglycaemia, hyperventilation, seizures, vertigo, hysteria and severe migraine headaches (O'Laughlin & McNamara, 1990). In evaluating an individual who has experienced presyncope or syncope, a thorough history is required followed by a physical examination. The results of the history and physical examination should help dictate which laboratory evaluations are in order (ECG, tilt test, exercise test, glucose determinations). Referral to a neurologist may be necessary.

The amount of activity restrictions imposed should be determined individually and is dependent upon the aetiology of the syncopal event. The practitioner should be confident that the proper diagnosis has been made before allowing the individual to participate in physical activity.

Table 22.3 Major causes of syncope.

Cardiac
  dysrhythmia (e.g. heart block)
  obstructive lesion (e.g. aortic stenosis)
  low cardiac output
Non-cardiac
  vasovagal
  micturition, defaecation
  orthostatic
  seizure
  hypoglycaemia, hypovolaemia
  psychogenic

Chest pain

It is not uncommon for the preadolescent or adolescent athlete to complain of chest pain that may or may not be associated with physical activity (Table 22.4). When chest pain occurs, it is common for the child, parent, coach or physician to assume that the aetiology of this chest pain is related to the cardiovascular system and that it may signal serious or even life-threatening cardiovascular disease (Pantell & Goodman, 1983). An extensive review of chest pain and its management was recently published and will be highlighted here (Duster, 1990). The physician is obliged to rule out cardiovascular disease as a primary cause of chest pain and this is usually reassuring. However, it is also the responsibility of the physician to determine, if possible, the cause of the chest pain. In order to make this determination, five features of the pain must be evaluated: (i) duration; (ii) quality; (iii) factors that provoke the pain; (iv) factors that relieve the pain; and (v) location of the pain (Duster, 1990).

Pain that is secondary to musculoskeletal problems is often brief in nature and occurs with specific stimuli. Visceral pain on the other hand may last for hours although the level of intensity may change throughout the duration of the pain. Pain as the result of myocardial ischaemia is short in duration and often described as pressure or a dull aching sensation.

Identifying associated factors will often help determine the cause of the pain. For example,

pain that occurs immediately after the ingestion of food or liquids might suggest oesophageal origin; pain that is provoked by a particular movement or position is often musculoskeletal in origin; myocardial ischaemia and resultant pain is usually provoked by exercise and relieved by rest.

The list of non-cardiac causes of chest pain is quite extensive and may include any obvious aetiology such as trauma, costochondritis, the slipping rib syndrome, muscle strain, spasm or fatigue.

Perhaps the most common cause of chest pain in children is the precordial catch syndrome (Duster, 1990). These sharp pains are felt in the anterior chest, at or near the cardiac apex. This pain lasts from 30 s to 3 min and is often aggravated by deep breathing and relieved by shallow respirations. It is a benign condition.

Pulmonary causes of chest pain include inflammation of the pleura, asthma and the presence of pleural effusions.

The gastrointestinal tract may be the cause of referred chest pain. Disorders of the stomach, duodenum, biliary and less commonly colonic, pancreatic, hepatic and peritoneal disease may be the cause of upper abdominal or chest area pain (Duster, 1990).

The most unusual cause of chest pain is the circulatory system. Chest pain that is the result of the cardiovascular system often is accompanied by a history of syncope or presyncope, palpitations, previous cardiac surgery or perhaps a positive family history of early sudden unexpected death (Duster, 1990). If chest pain occurs acutely in an individual with Marfan's syndrome or Turner's syndrome, acute dissection of the aorta should be suspected. Dissection of the aorta is a true medical emergency and this individual should be transported immediately to the nearest diagnostic facility. Diseases of the pericardium include post-traumatic pericardial effusion which is another cause of chest pain in children. Diseases of the coronary artery may also result in chest pain. Anomalies of the origin of a coronary artery

Table 22.4 Chest pain.

Non-cardiac
    chest wall (e.g. costochondritis)
    lungs
    gastrointestinal
    psychogenic
Cardiac
    pericarditis
    coronary artery
    valve disease
    conduction defects

or entrapment of a coronary artery are two common varieties that result in chest pain.

Another important cardiovascular cause of chest pain is unrecognized hypertrophic cardiomyopathy with its resultant ischaemia and coronary insufficiency. These individuals often require the help of a cardiologist to make the proper diagnosis. Aortic stenosis (sub-valvular, valvular and supravalvular) also may cause chest pain, with or without exertion. Appropriate murmurs are often present.

The evaluation of an individual with chest pain begins with a careful and thorough history. Appropriate laboratory studies may include, but are not limited to, a chest radiograph, ECG, echocardiogram and perhaps exercise testing.

The majority of children who undergo such an evaluation are diagnosed with musculo-skeletal chest pain (Duster, 1990). Precordial catch syndrome is also a frequent cause of chest pain in children who have been evaluated. True cardiovascular origin of chest pain in children is rare.

The child with known congenital heart disease

It is impractical to define the same limits for all patients with congenital heart disease. In addition, some individuals with a particular defect have undergone surgery while others have not. Those who are unoperated may have minor defects that are inconsequential. Others are not operated on because the defect is too complex and is not amenable to surgery. Furthermore, individuals who have undergone corrective or palliative surgery may not have had a successful result. In summary, the spectrum of congenital cardiovascular disease is too broad to list specific recommendations.

The Sixteenth Bethesda Conference on Cardiovascular Abnormalities in the Athlete have published their recommendations regarding eligibility for competition (McNamara et al., 1985) which lists 20 rather common conditions based on anatomy as well as severity. In order to make proper recommendations regarding participation in activities, certain baseline data will be required including a thorough history and physical examination. In some instances, an ECG and chest radiogram are useful. Often, an exercise tolerance test, 24 h ECG and cardiac catheterization, with or without angiography, is required before proper recommendations are made. The reader is referred to this paper before making recommendations for participation in individuals with congenital heart disease.

The child with acquired heart disease

Rheumatic fever is a defuse inflammatory disease of the connective tissue involving chiefly the heart, joints, brain, blood vessels and subcutaneous tissues (Stollerman, 1975). The syndrome is a delayed sequela of an upper respiratory tract infection that is the result of group A β-haemolytic streptococcal infection. In the acute stages, rheumatic fever presents with a combination of arthritis, carditis, chorea, subcutaneous nodules and a distinctive rash. The only permanent sequela from rheumatic fever is cardiac involvement, which occurs in 40–50% of individuals (Stollerman, 1975). The prognosis is excellent for subjects to escape carditis during an initial attack of rheumatic fever. The prognosis worsens with increasing severity of the initial carditis and its sequelae. Individuals who have recovered from the acute phase of rheumatic fever and do not have carditis, may participate in all athletic activities. At no time is rheumatic fever contagious. Individuals who have cardiovascular sequelae (usually mitral or aortic valve disease) should be under the care of a cardiologist and their activity limitations must be tailored individually.

Kawasaki's disease is an acute febrile syndrome of unknown aetiology that usually is observed in children under the age of 4 years. The most serious sequelae of Kawasaki's disease are the cardiovascular complications including arteritis and aneurysms of the coronary arteries. These children should be under the care of a cardiologist. If they have no aneurysms demonstrated in their coronary arteries, their exercise is unrestricted. Because the long-term prognosis of individuals with Kawasaki's disease is unknown, and coronary artery aneurysms have been discovered as late as 7–10 years after the initial illness; sequential follow-up with a cardiologist is recommended.

Mitral valve prolapse occurs in between 1 and 8% of children (Washington, 1993). Most paediatric patients with mitral valve prolapse should not be restricted from any type of physical activity or competition. Patients who have had a history of syncope, family history of sudden death related to mitral valve prolapse, chest pain that is intensified by exercise, dysrhythmias or mitral regurgitation should be cleared by a cardiologist before being allowed to participate in vigorous physical activities.

Sudden unexpected death

Most athletes who die suddenly are not known to have a cardiac abnormality (Garson, 1985). Most young individuals with cardiac disease who die suddenly and unexpectedly do not do so during exercise. Sudden death has been demonstrated to be related to exercise or physical activity in only 10% of the cases of sudden unexpected death in children who were known to have heart disease (Garson, 1985). Those individuals who experience sudden cardiac death have cardiac abnormalities that are inapparent prior to death. These abnormalities are rarely identified, despite a thorough preparticipation physical examination. Disorders such has hypertrophic cardiomyopathy or abnormalities of the coronary arteries are two of the more common cardiac causes of sudden unexpected death.

Indications for exercise testing

Exercise testing is useful in evaluating the cardiopulmonary system during vigorous physical activity. Recent advances in technology now allow for the direct and indirect measurement of oxygen uptake, cardiac output, determination of cardiac reserve and the evaluation of various abnormal cardiovascular events during exercise. The addition of pulmonary function evaluation during exercise testing is of value in evaluating individuals with chronic lung disease such as cystic fibrosis. These exercise studies should be conducted by individuals experienced in exercise testing of children and adolescents. Table 22.5 lists the most common indications for exercise testing in this age group.

Conclusion

When the preparticipation physical examination is performed, a thorough history should also be obtained. This history should contain questions regarding cardiac symptoms (near syncope, syncope, chest pain, palpitations, etc.) as well as questions regarding immediate family members who may have experienced sudden death or dysrhythmias during exercise. Since the majority of individuals who die suddenly during exercise do not have clinically apparent cardiac disease, nothing more than a general thorough preparticipation physical examination is warranted.

The majority of children with cardiovascular disorders may participate in most, if not all, physical activities. It is important to emphasize that decisions regarding sports participation in children who have cardiovascular disease must be made individually. It is the primary responsibility of their health-care providers to evaluate their individual cardiovascular problems and to set individual limits of physical activity.

Table 22.5 Indications for paediatric exercise testing.

Evaluate specific symptoms and signs which may be related to exercise

Identify abnormal adaptive responses occurring in children with cardiac and other disorders

To assess the effectiveness of specific medical and surgical treatment

To estimate level of functional or capacity during exercise

Challenges for future research

• Physical activity and physical fitness are important for health. In adults, higher levels of physical activity have been associated with a reduced incidence of coronary artery disease, hypertension, non-insulin dependent diabetes mellitus, depression, cancer and total mortality (Baranowski *et al.*, 1992). These hypokinetic diseases generally manifest themselves among adults and not children. To evaluate the efficacy of physical activity and physical fitness on the health of children, end-points other than manifest disease must be used. Further research is needed to establish what these end-points should be.

• The assessment of physical activity among children in field research continues to be impeded by major limitations in the available methods and the absence of 'gold standards'. Youth-oriented laboratory 'gold standards' and field measures must be developed by future research.

• The validity and reliability of common field tests used to measure physical fitness are not well documented. Valid measures of health-related fitness in children and youth need to be identified and documented.

• Limited data are available on the cardiovascular and metabolic responses among children to exercise. This is true not only in the child with cardiovascular disease but also in the healthy child. Further research is needed to document the benefit of exercise in children.

• As cardiovascular science progresses, increasing numbers of children with heart disease are reaching adolescence and young adulthood. These individuals need to remain physically active. Further research is needed to evaluate the safety and efficacy of this physical activity.

References

Baranowski, T., Bouchard, C., Bar-Or, O. *et al.* (1992) Assessment, prevalence, and cardiovascular benefits of physical activity and fitness in youth. *Med. Sci. Sports Exerc.* **24**, S237−47.

Cantwell, J. & Murray, P. (1990) Evaluation and management of the athlete with a heart murmur. *Your Patient Fitness* **2**, 3−7.

Duster, M. (1990) Chest pain. In A. Garson, J. Bricker & D. McNamara (eds) *The Science and Practice of Pediatric Cardiology*, 1st edn, pp. 1947−50. Lea & Febiger, Philadelphia.

Garson, A. (1985) Sudden death in a pediatric cardiology population, 1958−1983: relation to prior arrhythmias. *J. Am. Coll. Cardiol.* **5**, 138B−41.

Gutgesell, H., Gessner, I., Vetter, B., Yabek, S. & Norton, J. (1986) Recreational and occupational recommendations for young patients with heart disease. A statement for physicians by the Committee on Congenital Cardiac Defects of the Council on Cardiovascular Disease of the Young, American Heart Association. *Circulation* **74**, 1195A−8.

Labarthe, D., Kosinetz, C. & Jones, T. (1990) Epidemiology. In A. Garson, J. Bricker & D. McNamara (eds) *The Science and Practice of Pediatric Cardiology*, 1st edn, pp. 135−51. Lea & Febiger, Philadelphia.

McNamara, D., Bricker, J., Galioto, F., Graham, T., James, F. & Rosenthal, A. (1985) Task force I congenital heart disease. *J. Am. Coll. Cardiol.* **6**, 1200−8.

O'Laughlin, M. & McNamara, D. (1990) Syncope. In A. Garson, J. Bricker & D. McNamara (eds) *The Science and Practice of Pediatric Cardiology*, 1st edn, pp. 1929−46. Lea & Febiger, Philadelphia.

Pantell, R. & Goodman, B. (1983) Adolescent chest pain: a prospective study. *Pediatrics* **71**, 881.

Shaffer, T. (1974) Cardiac evaluation for participation in school sports. *JAMA* **228**, 398.

Stollerman, G. (1975) *Rheumatic Fever and Streptococcal Infection*. Grune & Stratton, New York.

Thilenius, O., Quinones, J., Husayni, T. & Novak, J. (1991) Tilt test for diagnosis of unexplained syncope in pediatric patients. *Pediatrics* **87**, 334−8.

Washington, R. (1993) Mitral valve prolapse and active youth. *Phys. Sports Med.* **21**, 136−44.

Zipes, D., Cobb, L., Garson, A., Gillette, P., James, G., Lazzara, R. & Rink, L. (1985) Task force VI: arrhythmias. *J. Am. Coll. Cardiol.* **6**, 1225−32.

Chapter 23

Physiological and Health Aspects of Exercise in Hot and Cold Climates

BAREKET FALK

Introduction

Body temperature may be regulated by behavioural and physiological means. Behavioural means of temperature regulation involve the conscious selection of a suitable microenvironment. Physiological temperature regulation involves the control of metabolic heat production, blood flow from the core to the periphery and sweating.

During exercise, metabolic heat produced by the working muscles may be as high as 15–20 times that produced during rest. The heat is convected from the body core to the periphery and is subsequently dissipated through evaporation, convection, conduction or radiation from the body to the environment. Thermoregulation may be affected by the environmental conditions, and the physical and physiological state of the body. The environmental conditions that affect thermoregulation are ambient temperature, air humidity and wind velocity. Physical factors affecting thermoregulation include body size, composition and body surface area to mass ratio. For any given environmental conditions and physical characteristics, the physiological response to exercise in the heat may be affected by factors such as the individual's state of acclimatization, aerobic fitness or hydration. It is not clear how these factors affect the thermoregulatory response to cold exposure.

This chapter outlines the differences in thermoregulation between children and adults

and the possible changes which occur during adolescence in the physiological response to exercise in the heat and in the cold. The early signs and symptoms of various heat and cold disorders are described to facilitate their early identification. Finally, the adverse effects of hyperthermia and hypothermia and their prevention are discussed.

Thermoregulation: children, adolescents and adults

The effectiveness of thermoregulation is reflected by heat and cold tolerance, and by the stability of body temperatures and heart rate while performing various tasks in the heat and cold. Numerous studies have investigated the response of children and adolescents to exercise in the heat. In comparison, there are few studies which have examined the effects of cold exposure on children or adolescents (Tables 23.1 & 23.2). This section outlines the differences in heat and cold tolerance between children and adults and the possible physical and physiological reasons for these differences.

Heat tolerance

In a thermoneutral environment, exercise tolerance and thermoregulation seem to be similar among children and adults (Drinkwater *et al.*, 1977; Davies, 1981; Delmarche *et al.*, 1990), and children are capable of reaching thermal balance (Gullestad, 1975), with 'no subjective

Table 23.1 Studies comparing the thermoregulatory response to exercise in the heat and cold between children or adolescent and adults.

Subjects	Environment	Exercise task	Children versus adults: findings	Reference
Heat				
8 boys, 5 girls, 8 men (athletes)	$T_{db} = 21°C$ $T_{wb} = 17°C$	68% $\dot{V}O_{2\,max}$ 60-min treadmill	Same final T_{re} $\downarrow$ Evaporative loss $\uparrow T_{sk}$ Greater proportion of heat dissipated through radiation and convection	Davies (1981)
11 boys (versus men)	20°C, 20% RH	60% $\dot{V}O_{2\,max}$	Same final T_{re} $\downarrow$ Evaporative loss $\uparrow$ Radiative and convective heat loss	Delmarche *et al.* (1990) (versus Bittel & Henane, 1975)
5 girls, 5 women	28°C, 45% RH	30% $\dot{V}O_{2\,max}$, 2 × 50-min treadmill	Similar tolerance $\downarrow$ Evaporative loss $\uparrow$ Dry heat loss $\uparrow$ Final T_{re} $\downarrow$ Cardiac output $\downarrow$ Stroke index	Drinkwater *et al.* (1977)
	35°C, 65% RH and 48°C, 10% RH	30% $\dot{V}O_{2\,max}$, 2 × 50-min treadmill	$\downarrow$ Tolerance $\uparrow$ Final T_{re} $\downarrow$ Cardiac output $\downarrow$ Stroke index Similar proportion of dry and evaporative heat loss	
7 lean, 5 obese girls (versus lean and obese women)	$T_{eff} = 21.1$ $T_{eff} = 26.7$ $T_{eff} = 29.4$ $T_{eff} = 32.2$	$4.8\,km \cdot h^{-1}$, 5% grade, 3 × 20-min treadmill	$\downarrow$ Tolerance $\uparrow$ Dry heat loss per kg $\uparrow$ Evaporative loss per kg (but $\uparrow$ metabolic load per kg)	Haymes *et al.* (1974) (versus Bar-Or *et al.*, 1969)
7 lean and 5 obese boys (versus lean and obese men)	$T_{eff} = 21.1$ $T_{eff} = 26.7$ $T_{eff} = 29.4$ $T_{eff} = 32.2$	$4.8\,km \cdot h^{-1}$, 5% grade, 3 × 20-min treadmill	$\uparrow T_{re}, T_{sk},$ HR $\downarrow$ Sweating rate $\uparrow$ Heat storage per kg	Haymes *et al.* (1975) (versus McCormick & Buskirk, 1974)
15 boys, 16 men	43°C, 20% RH	50% $\dot{V}O_{2\,max}$, 3 × 20-min cycle	$\downarrow$ Sweating rate $\downarrow$ Sweating sensitivity $\uparrow$ Gland population density	Inbar (1978)
17 girls, 8 women, 18 boys, 8 men	42°C, 20% RH	50% $\dot{V}O_{2\,max}$, 2 × 20-min cycle	$\downarrow$ Sweating rate $\downarrow$ Na^+ and Cl^- loss in sweat	Meyer *et al.* (1992)
7 children, 2 men	30°C, 55% RH	7 km march	$\uparrow$ Rise in body temperature $\downarrow$ Sweating rate	Sohar & Shapira (1965)
5 boys, 5 men	$T_{db} = 49°C$ $T_{wb} = 26.6°C$	$5.6\,km \cdot h^{-1}$ treadmill	$\downarrow$ Tolerance $\uparrow T_{sk}$ $\downarrow$ Evaporative loss	Wagner *et al.* (1972)
Cold				
8 boys, 11 men	5°C	30% $\dot{V}O_{2\,max}$, 40-min cycle	$\uparrow T_{re}$ $\uparrow \dot{V}O_2$ $\downarrow T_{sk}$	Smolander *et al.* (1992)

$\uparrow$, Higher in children; $\downarrow$, lower in children; HR, heart rate; RH, relative humidity; T_{db}, dry bulb temperature; T_{eff}, effective temperature; T_{re}, rectal temperature; T_{sk}, skin temperature; T_{wb}, wet bulb temperature.

Table 23.2 Studies in which the thermoregulatory response to exercise in the heat and cold was studied in children and adolescents.

Subjects	Environment	Exercise task	Findings	Reference
Heat				
10–12-year-old boys	39°C, 45% RH	45% $\dot{V}O_{2\,max}$, 3.5-h inter-mittent cycle	Voluntary dehydration accompanied by rise in T_{re}	Bar-Or *et al.* (1980)
9–14-year-old boys and girls, healthy versus cystic fibrosis	32°C, 45% RH	45% $\dot{V}O_{2\,max}$, 20-min bouts cycle	Voluntary dehydration greater among cystic fibrosis patients than among healthy children	Bar-Or *et al.* (1992)
8–10-year-old boys	<24.5°C, <90% RH	60% $\dot{V}O_{2\,max}$, 30 min	No effect of T_a on tolerance	Blanchard (1987)
10–13-year-old boys	30°C, 80% RH	6 km·h⁻¹, 60-min treadmill	T_{re} reached plateau after 30 min. Endomorphy related to decreased thermoregulatory effectiveness	Docherty *et al.* (1986)
36 boys (varying pubertal stages)	42°C, 20% RH	50% $\dot{V}O_{2\,max}$, 3 × 20-min cycle	Increase in sweating rate with increase in pubertal stage. Increase rate of sweat gland lactate excretion with increase in pubertal stage	Falk *et al.* (1991b)
36 boys (varying pubertal stages)	42°C, 20% RH	50% $\dot{V}O_{2\,max}$, 3 × 20-min cycle	Similar plasma aldosterone after exercise-heat stress, regardless of pubertal stage. Increase in plasma prolactin after exercise-heat stress, with increase in pubertal stage	Falk *et al.* (1991a)
36 boys (varying pubertal stages)	42°C, 20% RH	50% $\dot{V}O_{2\,max}$, 3 × 20-min cycle	Similar rate of heat production and heat loss, regardless of pubertal stage	Falk *et al.* (1992a)
31 boys (varying pubertal stages, followed longitudinally)	42°C, 20% RH	50% $\dot{V}O_{2\,max}$, 3 × 20-min cycle	Increase in sweating rate with physical maturity. No change in the rate of rise of T_{re}	Falk *et al.* (1992b)
11-year-old boys	22°C, 35–55% RH	31–39, 45–56, 61–69% $\dot{V}O_{2\,max}$, cycle	Thermal balance reached in all exercise intensities	Gullestad (1975)
8–10-year-old boys	T_{db} = 43°C T_{wb} = 24°C	40 W, 3 × 20-min cycle	Acclimatization can be achieved by exercise in the heat or by training in thermoneutral conditions	Inbar *et al.* (1981)
8–14-year-old girls	30°C, 50% RH	50% $\dot{V}O_{2\,max}$, cycle	Subjective intolerance	Mackie (1982)
Boys and girls	Tropical climate	60% $\dot{V}O_{2\,max}$, 4 × 20-min cycle	Voluntary dehydration in the sun and in the shade	Rodriguez *et al.* (1990)

Continued

Table 23.2 *Continued*

Subjects	Environment	Exercise task	Findings	Reference
Cold				
8–18-year-old boys and girls	$T_{water} = 20.3°C$	$30\,m \cdot min^{-1}$ swim	Direct relationship between rate of cooling and adiposity and body surface area to mass ratio	Sloan & Keatinge (1973)
11-year-old boys and girls	5°C versus 22°C	Ventilatory threshold 30-min cycle	Higher $\dot{V}O_2$, $\dot{V}E$, HR, lactate and RPE in the cold	

RPE, rate of perceived exertion; T_a, ambient temperature; T_{water}, water temperature. For other abbreviations, see footnote to Table 23.1.

handicap' (Mackova *et al.*, 1984). As ambient temperature rises above 40°C, tolerance in children seems to be lower (Drinkwater *et al.*, 1977; Haymes *et al.*, 1974 versus Bar-Or *et al.*, 1969; Wagner *et al.*, 1972); whereas mean body temperature (Sohar & Shapira, 1965; Wagner *et al.*, 1972; Leppaluoto, 1988) or heat storage per kilogram of body mass (Haymes *et al.*, 1974; Drinkwater *et al.*, 1977) are higher compared to adults. The reduced tolerance and deficient thermoregulation often seen in children compared to adults are associated with lower sweating rates among children (Sohar & Shapira, 1965; Wagner *et al.*, 1972; Haymes *et al.*, 1974; Meyer *et al.*, 1992), and thus lower evaporative cooling.

A lower heat tolerance exhibited by girls compared to women (Drinkwater *et al.*, 1977) was characterized by complaints such as dizziness and nausea. Similar findings were noted by Orenstein *et al.* (1983) among two young subjects (15-year-old cystic fibrosis patient and 16-year-old healthy control) but not in adults exercising in the heat. Jokinen *et al.* (1990) reported a decrease in blood pressure following, although not during, exposure to extreme heat among children but not among adults. This was accompanied by vasovagal collapses in two cases. In a recent study comparing pre-, mid- and late-pubertal boys exercising at 50% $\dot{V}O_{2\,max}$ in the heat (42°C, 20% relative humidity), there were no differences in premature

cessation of testing among the three groups (Falk *et al.*, 1992a). However, the reasons for early cessation differed. A greater proportion of prepubertal boys ended the session early due to headache and subjective exhaustion, while among the late-pubertal boys, early cessation was accompanied by an elevated rectal temperature without subjective distress. It is suggested that the lower heat tolerance observed among children compared to adults is due, at least in part, to inadequate cardiovascular adjustment.

In a warm environment, when ambient temperature is similar to, or slightly higher than, skin temperature, children seem to tolerate at least 1 h of exercise at a moderate intensity (Haymes *et al.*, 1974, 1975; Drinkwater *et al.*, 1977; Docherty *et al.*, 1986; Piekarski *et al.*, 1986; Delmarche *et al.*, 1990), although not in all cases (Mackie, 1982). When compared to adults, however, children's body temperature and heat storage are sometimes higher (Sohar & Shapira, 1965; Haymes *et al.*, 1975; Drinkwater *et al.*, 1977). Thus, possible differences between children and adults in warm, yet not extreme, environments may become apparent only after a prolonged exposure.

Cold tolerance

There is only one reported study in which cold stress was severe enough to result in a decrease in body temperature among exercising children and adolescents (Sloan & Keatinge, 1973). Subjects within the age range of 8–18 years, swam at a speed of $30 \, \text{m} \cdot \text{min}^{-1}$, where water temperature was 20.3°C. The younger children were able to stay in the water for a shorter period and had a greater drop in oral temperature compared to the more mature swimmers. The authors reported a direct correlation between the rate of cooling and the surface area to body mass ratio. Additionally, there was an inverse relationship between the rate of cooling and the extent of subcutaneous adiposity. These results demonstrate the importance of body dimensions and composition to thermoregulation in the cold.

Smolander *et al.* (1992) reported that in spite of obvious differences in body dimensions, pre- and early-pubescent boys were able to maintain their body temperature as effectively as adults while exercising (30% $V_{O_{2\,max}}$) in the cold (5°C). The children's strategy was to increase their metabolic rate and vasoconstrict peripheral vessels to a greater degree than the adults. The age-related difference in strategy was also apparent among two boys and two adults of similar body dimensions, which suggests that these different 'strategies' were related to maturation and not merely body size. Similar differences in the thermoregulatory strategy between children and adults were reported during rest in cool conditions (16–20°C) (Wagner *et al.*, 1974; Araki *et al.*, 1980).

Bar-Or (1989) suggested that some of the inconsistencies in the literature, regarding the effectiveness of thermoregulation among children compared to adults, may be explained by the varying environmental conditions. Figure 23.1 demonstrates the hypothesis that the effectiveness of thermoregulation among children is comparable to that of adults in moderate conditions but may be deficient in extreme environmental conditions, when the skin to air temperature gradient is large.

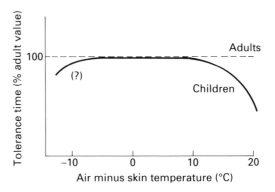

Fig. 23.1 Schematic representation of heat and cold tolerance among children (———) compared to adults (– – –) in relation to the skin to air temperature gradient. Redrawn from Bar-Or (1989).

Physical and physiological characteristics related to thermoregulation

The apparent difference in thermoregulatory effectiveness between children and adults may be attributed to several physical and physiological differences which diminish with pubertal growth and maturation (Table 23.3).

BODY DIMENSIONS

The higher surface area to mass ratio among children allows them to rely on convective and radiative heat loss and to depend less on evaporative cooling in a thermoneutral or warm environment (Gullestad, 1975; Davies, 1981; Delmarche *et al.*, 1990). However, in more extreme hot or cold environmental conditions, the high surface area to mass ratio becomes a liability. In the heat, the body absorbs heat from the environment and evaporative cooling may not be sufficient for adequate thermoregulation. In the cold, the body dissipates body heat to the environment and cannot always compensate by increasing metabolic heat production.

METABOLIC AND CIRCULATORY CHARACTERISTICS

The oxygen cost of locomotion per unit mass is

Table 23.3 Changes occurring during puberty which might influence thermoregulation.

Change	Effect on thermoregulation
Decrease in body surface area to mass ratio	Decrease in heat gain in a hot environment Decrease in heat loss in a cold environment
Increase in body density among boys*	Increase in the specific heat of the body
Decrease in body density among girls	Decrease in the specific heat of the body
Decrease in oxygen cost of walking or running	Decrease in metabolic heat production per kg body mass
Increase in maximal cardiac output	Enhancement of peripheral perfusion and therefore, convective heat loss
Increase in blood volume per body surface area	Decrease in the proportion of blood volume necessary for adequate peripheral perfusion and therefore, enhance perfusion of muscles
Increase in sweat gland size	Increase in sweat gland output
Increase in sweat gland sensitivity	Decrease in sweat threshold and time to sweat onset Increase in sweating rate
Increase in sweat gland anaerobic metabolism	Increase in sweating rate
Change in hormonal status	Change in sweat electrolyte composition

* Not consistent in all studies.

higher among children compared to adults (Robinson, 1938; Åstrand, 1952; MacDougall et al., 1983), resulting in a higher metabolic heat production. This places an added strain on the thermoregulatory system during exercise in the heat. In the cold, the elevated metabolic heat production may be advantageous. However, Smolander et al. (1992) argue that the higher increase in metabolic rate among chil-

dren relative to adults exercising in the cold may leave them with smaller reserves for prolonged exercise.

Children have a smaller blood volume, especially when expressed relative to surface area or to body mass (Åstrand, 1952). Thus, they require a larger proportion of their blood volume for adequate peripheral perfusion, particularly when the heat-dissipating system is stressed (Drinkwater et al., 1977). This, coupled with the greater reduction in stroke volume during heat stress (Jokinen et al., 1990) and with the lower cardiac output at high exercise intensities in children (Bar-Or et al., 1971), limits the potential of heat convection from the body core to the periphery and subsequently to the environment. It is suggested that the larger proportion of total blood volume necessary to maintain adequate cooling by peripheral flow among children, may result in inadequate perfusion of muscles and the central nervous system, and contribute to the previously reported lower heat tolerance.

The circulatory response to cold stress among children is not well documented. Several studies reported a lower skin temperature among children compared to adults during rest (Wagner et al., 1974; Araki et al., 1980; Smolander et al., 1992) and during exercise (Smolander et al., 1992) in the cold. The lower skin temperature reflects a decrease in skin blood flow and hence, reduced heat loss to the periphery. Heart rate has been reported to be elevated (Marsh et al., 1992) as well as depressed (Mackova et al., 1984), among children exercising in the cold (5°C), compared to comfortable conditions (22°C). Unfortunately, neither of the latter two studies compared the children's response to that of adults.

SWEATING RESPONSE

For any given environmental and metabolic load, the sweating rate in children is much lower compared to adults (see Bar-Or, 1980, 1989 for reviews). Children exhibit lower sweating rates whether expressed per body surface area (Kawahata, 1960; Wagner *et al.*, 1972; Drinkwater *et al.*, 1977; Inbar, 1978; Araki *et al.*, 1979; Davies, 1981; Meyer *et al.*, 1992), or per gland (Kawahata, 1960; Huebner *et al.*, 1966; Lobeck & McSherry, 1967; Foster *et al.*, 1969). Nevertheless, the maximal sweating rates of children and adults remains unknown, as is whether or not these are limiting factors in thermoregulation. Furthermore, when sweating rate, as reported in previous studies, was related to the metabolic load (standardized for body mass and $\dot{V}_{O_2\,max}$) there was no clear age-related difference (B. Falk & R. Dotan, unpublished observations). Thus, it is possible that children are able to take advantage of their large surface area and dissipate sufficient heat via convection, conduction and radiation, without relying on sweat evaporation. This possibility needs to be clarified.

A recent study extended the previously reported differences in sweating rate between children and adults by comparing pre-, mid- and late-pubertal boys who exercised at 50% $\dot{V}_{O_2\,max}$ in 42°C, 20% relative humidity (Falk *et al.*, 1992b). Sweating rate per body surface area and per gland increased with physical maturity (Fig. 23.2). Furthermore, regular follow-up of these boys over a period of 18 months revealed a longitudinal increase in sweating rate (Falk *et al.*, 1992c). However, the results did not clearly demonstrate whether sweating rate increases progressively through puberty or, coinciding with the growth spurt and hormonal changes, there is also a sudden enhancement of the sweating mechanism.

The changes which occur in the sweating response from childhood to adulthood may be explained by changes in sweat gland size and by modifications in sweat gland function.

Sweat gland size and population density

During childhood, sweat gland size is directly related to age ($r = 0.77$) and to height ($r = 0.81$) (Landing *et al.*, 1968). Sato and Sato (1983) also reported that large glands (biopsied from adults) exhibited an enhanced sweating rate

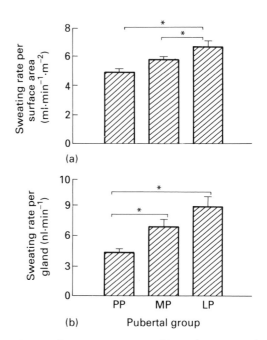

Fig. 23.2 Sweating rate (a) per skin surface area, and (b) per gland among pre-, mid- and late-pubertal boys (PP, MP, LP, respectively) exercising in the heat (50% $\dot{V}_{O_2\,max}$; 42°C, 20% relative humidity). Adapted with permission from Falk *et al.* (1992a,b).

compared with small glands. In view of the relationship between sweat gland function and size, it is tempting to speculate that the difference in glandular size of children compared to adults (Cawley *et al.*, 1963; Lobeck & McSherry, 1967; Landing *et al.*, 1968; Wolfe *et al.*, 1970) may be partly responsible for the difference in the sweating response.

The total number of sweat glands is believed to be determined by the age of 2–3 years (Kuno, 1956) and does not change thereafter. Therefore, as the body surface area increases with age, the population density (number per unit area) of sweat glands decreases (Szabo, 1962; Huebner *et al.*, 1966; Lobeck & McSherry, 1967; Foster *et al.*, 1969; Bar-Or, 1980, 1989; Falk *et al.*, 1992b). The proportion of sweat gland counts on the extremities and central body region may change during the pubertal growth period. The effect that such a change in proportion may have on evaporative cooling is unknown.

When the heat-activated sweat glands response to exercise in the heat was compared among pre-, mid- and late-pubertal boys (Falk *et al.*, 1992b), the distribution of sweat over the skin differed with increasing physical maturity. The younger boys had numerous small sweat beads per unit of skin area, while the more physically mature boys had fewer but larger sweat beads per unit of skin area. However, the percentage of skin area covered by all drops did not differ among groups and therefore, might have resulted in similar evaporative cooling (Fig. 23.3). If this is indeed the case, then, in view of the lower whole body sweating rate among the younger boys, their pattern of sweat distribution may facilitate more efficient cooling. This possibility needs to be examined experimentally.

Sweating sensitivity and sweat gland metabolism

Several studies reported a greater increase in skin temperature among children compared to adults at a given heat load (Wagner *et al.*, 1972; Drinkwater *et al.*, 1977; Araki *et al.*, 1979; Delmarche *et al.*, 1990). This may be explained by a delay in the onset of sweating among children. Indeed, Araki *et al.* (1979; as illustrated by Bar-Or, 1989) demonstrated that during exercise in the heat, sweating began after a 0.2°C rise in rectal temperature in men, compared to a 0.7°C rise in boys. Thus, the sweat gland sensitivity to an increase in body temperature may be lower among children compared to adults. Some evidence suggests that during puberty, along with the growth of the sweat glands, there is also an increase in sensitivity to cholinergic (Sato & Sato, 1983) and adrenergic (Wada, 1950) stimuli, contributing to an elevated sweating rate.

The differences in sweating rate observed among children and adults (Kawahata, 1960; Wagner *et al.*, 1972; Drinkwater *et al.*, 1977; Inbar, 1978; Araki *et al.*, 1979; Davies, 1981; Meyer *et al.*, 1992), and the increase in sweating

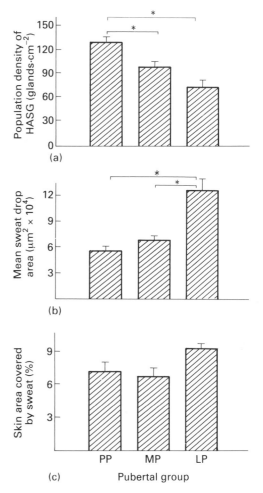

Fig. 23.3 (a) Population density of heat-activated sweat glands (HASG), (b) sweat bead area, and (c) the percentage of skin area covered by sweat among pre-, mid- and late-pubertal boys (PP, MP, LP, respectively) exercising in the heat (50% $\dot{V}o_{2\,max}$; 42°C, 20% relative humidity). Adapted with permission from Falk *et al.* (1992b).

rate observed through puberty (Falk *et al.*, 1992c) may also be explained by the increase in the metabolic capacity of the sweat glands during puberty. Lactate is a product of anaerobic glycolysis at the sweat gland and the rate of lactate excretion is used as an index of sweat gland metabolism (Wolfe *et al.*, 1970; Fellmann *et al.*, 1985; Falk *et al.*, 1991b). It was recently demonstrated that among pubertal boys, sweat-

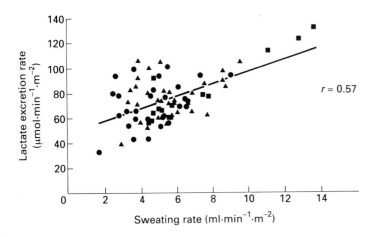

Fig. 23.4 The relationship between lactate excretion rate per gland and sweating rate per gland among pre- (●), mid- (▲) and late-pubertal (■) boys exercising in the heat (50% $\dot{V}_{O_2\,max}$; 42°C, 20% relative humidity). $P < 0.01$. Adapted from Falk *et al.* (1991b).

ing rate is directly related to lactate excretion rate per gland (Fig. 23.4) and that the latter increases with physical maturity among boys (Falk *et al.*, 1991b). This increase in glandular anaerobic metabolism may be analogous to the increase in glycolytic enzymes in muscle (Eriksson & Saltin, 1974), and the increase in anaerobic muscle power (Falk & Bar-Or, 1993) observed during puberty. Thus, it is possible that the increase in sweating rate seen from childhood to adulthood is partly due to an increase during puberty in the capacity of the anaerobic energy pathway in sweat glands.

HORMONAL STATUS

Of the hormones which are associated with pubertal changes, two have been implicated in thermoregulation: (i) testosterone (Kawahata, 1960); and (ii) prolactin (Brisson *et al.*, 1986; Boisvert *et al.*, 1988). A sudorific effect of testosterone was demonstrated by Kawahata (1960) in 70–81-year-old men, but Rees and Shuster (1981) failed to show a similar effect among 20–35-year-old men and women. The authors suggested that changes in sweating rate may be initiated by androgens at puberty but their effect does not appear to be maintained in later years.

Prolactin has been shown to increase in response to thermal stress (Brisson *et al.*, 1986; Kaufman *et al.*, 1988; Kukkonen-Harjula *et al.*,

1988; Laatikainen *et al.*, 1988; Melin *et al.*, 1989) among adults, as well as among children (Falk *et al.*, 1991a; Jokinen *et al.*, 1991). It has also been implicated in affecting electrolyte composition in adults (Robertson *et al.*, 1986; Kaufman *et al.*, 1988; Kulczycki & Robertson, 1988; Robertson, 1989) and in adolescents (Falk *et al.*, 1991a). However, its exact role is sweat gland function is unclear.

The endocrine response to exercise in the heat has been studied extensively in adults, mainly in relation to hormones associated with fluid and electrolyte balance (see Francesconi, 1988 and Francesconi *et al.*, 1989 for reviews), but has scarcely been studied in children. Increases in aldosterone and other stress-related hormones similar to those observed in adults were recently reported among children (Jokinen *et al.*, 1991) and adolescents (Falk *et al.*, 1991a) during rest and exercise in the heat, respectively. Nevertheless, it is still unclear how particular hormones may modify the thermoregulatory response during growth and maturation.

The endocrine response to cold stress has been studied in adults (e.g. Leduc, 1961; Suzuki *et al.*, 1967; Goldstein-Golaire *et al.*, 1970) but not in children. It is therefore unknown if this response is different among children or if, indeed, differences in the thermoregulatory response to cold can be explained by hormonal differences between children and adults.

Heat disorders: identification

Athletes exercising in the heat can experience various heat-related disorders ranging in intensity and severity from hypotension and headache to a potentially fatal heat stroke. Often the victims of hyperthermia are young, healthy and highly motivated individuals who are unaware of the early symptoms of heat illness. In fact, since hyperthermia is not associated with any painful sensation, motivated athletes may even increase exercise intensity during the last stages of competition, when hyperthermia is likely to occur.

Heat disorders have frequently been divided into three syndromes: (i) heat cramps; (ii) heat exhaustion; and (iii) heat stroke. However, the three syndromes are not always distinct and an overlap exists in the signs and symptoms of each condition (Table 23.4). In fact, some argue that the various heat-related illnesses may be a continuum rather than separate, distinct patho-

Table 23.4 Symptoms and signs of heat disorders from Bar-Or (1983), Callaham (1979), Hubbard and Armstrong (1988), Shapiro and Seidman (1990), Shibolet et al. (1962, 1967, 1970) and Knochel (1974).

Symptom or sign	Heat cramps	Heat exhaustion (SD)	Heat exhaustion (WD)	Heat stroke
Pain	+	+*		
Headache	+*			
Nausea	+*	+	+	
Vomiting		+*		
Diarrhoea				+*
Thirst			+	
Fatigue, weakness		+	+	+
Loss of skin turgor		+	+	+
Dry skin				+*
Apathy		+	+	
Coma				+
Confusion, agitation, seizures, convulsions				+
Hypotension				+
Tachycardia		+	+	+
Flattened or inverted T waves				+*
High rectal temperature		+ (< 41°C)	+ (< 41°C)	+ (> 41°C)
Pupillary changes				+*
Hyperventilation				+
Oliguria and anuria				+*
Hypernatraemia			+	
Hyponatraemia	+	+		
Hypochloraemia	+			
Low urine sodium	+	+		
High urine nitrogen, CPK, creatinine, inorganic phosphate	+*			
Acute renal failure				+*
Clotting dysfunction				+*

* Sometimes.
SD, salt depletion; WD, water deprivation.

physiological entities (Shibolet *et al.*, 1967; Costrini *et al.*, 1979; Hubbard & Armstrong, 1988).

Heat cramps are painful, involuntary spasms of skeletal muscle (often the hamstring and gastrocnemius), and are associated with electrolyte imbalance and inadequate circulation to active muscle tissue (Hubbard, 1990). The localized contractions affect a few muscle bundles and, as one bundle relaxes, an adjacent bundle contracts (Hubbard & Armstrong, 1988).

Heat exhaustion, whether due to salt depletion or water deprivation, is characterized by profuse sweating and cutaneous flushing accompanied by headache, dizziness, nausea or vomiting. Rectal temperature is elevated (around 40°C in severe cases) and haemoconcentration may be present. Heat exhaustion may occur among athletes as well as spectators in seemingly harmless environmental conditions (e.g. a warm day with a moderate breeze) (Bar-Or, 1983), or it may develop over several days (Hubbard & Armstrong, 1988). Squire (1990) reports that a national junior Olympic track-and-field meet held during the last 3 days of July 1983 in southeastern USA, cumulative fluid losses resulted in an increased incidence of heat disorders. Most distance events were held on the first day of competition and the remainder took place on the second day. However, the greatest incidence of heat illness was observed on the third day of the meet (nine cases per 100 competitors, compared with two and five cases during the first and second day, respectively).

Heat stroke differs from heat exhaustion in that it involves a higher rectal temperature (over 41°C) and central nervous system dysfunctions such as disorientation, confusion or coma. In the later stages, it may also be accompanied by a lack of sweating and pale, dry skin (Shibolet *et al.*, 1967; Shapiro & Seidman, 1990). Heat stroke is a life-threatening medical emergency and, along with complications in the central nervous system, it is associated with adverse effects on the cardiovascular, pulmonary and gastrointestinal systems, with acute renal failure and electrolyte imbalance (see Shapiro & Seidman, 1990 for review). Since differentiation between heat exhaustion and heat stroke may sometimes be difficult, it is therefore recommended that all heat exhaustion cases be treated as potential heat stroke cases.

Treatment of all heat disorders should focus on reduction of body temperature and rehydration. A lower body temperature may be achieved by simply stopping activity, or moving to a shaded area, or more drastically, by cool (Shapiro & Seidman, 1990) or ice-cold (Costrini, 1990) water immersion, depending on the severity of the symptoms. Rehydration may be achieved by oral ingestion or, in more severe cases, by administration of fluids intravenously (for detailed treatment procedures see Costrini, 1990; Shapiro & Seidman, 1990).

Prevention of heat disorders

All heat disorders are *preventable*. With adequate precompetition and preseason preparation, which involve sound hydration practices, proper conditioning and acclimatization, and identification of athletes at risk, all heat disorders may be averted.

Hydration

During exercise, especially in the heat, sweating rate is elevated. If not accompanied by sufficient drinking, it will result in a net fluid loss and a state of hypohydration. When water is available *ad libitum*, children (Bar-Or *et al.*, 1980, 1992) and adults (Pugh *et al.*, 1967; White & Ford, 1983) do not drink sufficiently to replenish fluid loss. Recent studies suggest that when the available beverage is flavoured, involuntary dehydration may be prevented, particularly among children (Wilk *et al.*, 1994).

Hypohydration results in a reduction of plasma volume, stroke volume and cardiac output, and an elevation in heart rate during submaximal exercise. This strain on the cardiovascular system compromises thermoregulation in that both skin blood flow (Fortney *et al.*, 1984; Kenney *et al.*, 1990) and sweating rate (Ekbolm *et al.*, 1970; Greenleaf & Castle, 1971; Fortney *et al.*, 1984; Sawka *et al.*, 1985, 1989) may be reduced. This has been demonstrated in adults but has not been confirmed in children (Bar-Or *et al.*, 1980). Nevertheless, in view of the lower sweating rate among children and the added reliance on radiative and convective heat loss, and therefore on skin blood flow, it is likely that hypohydration is more detrimental in children than in adults. In fact, Bar-Or *et al.* (1980) demonstrated that for each 1% weight loss, there was a higher increase in rectal temperature among children exercising in the heat, compared to adults (Fig. 23.5).

Many athletes, such as wrestlers, boxers, body builders or judoka, commonly lose 3–5% of their body weight before competition in order to 'make weight' (Tcheng & Tipton, 1976; Serfass *et al.*, 1984; Caterisano *et al.*, 1988; Yarrows, 1988). In fact, some wrestlers, mostly those in the light weight categories, lose 10% or more of their body weight before competition (Tipton & Tcheng, 1970). This is in spite of the

widely reported decrements in physical performance, including reduced muscle strength (Bosco *et al.*, 1968; Torranin *et al.*, 1979; Webster *et al.*, 1990), anaerobic capacity (Saltin, 1964; Torranin *et al.*, 1979; Webster *et al.*, 1990), and aerobic power (Webster *et al.*, 1990) as a result of dehydration.

Dehydration is often accompanied by a disruption of electrolyte balance and by electrolyte loss through sweat and urine. Therefore, physiological function may be impaired. Controversy exists over the necessity of replacing electrolytes lost during exercise and the advantages or disadvantages of consuming electrolytes- or carbohydrate-containing beverages (White & Ford, 1983; Murray, 1987; Johnson *et al.*, 1988). Nevertheless, the major advantage of the many commercially available 'athletic' beverages is their enhancement of water absorption and prevention of hypohydration (Johnson *et al.*, 1988).

Once hypohydration sets in, it is very difficult to correct it during exercise. Therefore, adequate hydration level must be ascertained before participation in any physical activity. This can be achieved with 7–8 ml of fluids per kilogram of body weight (e.g. 300–400 ml for 42–45 kg child), 20–30 min before warm-up. Although a large fluid volume empties faster from the stomach (Costill & Saltin, 1974), it is uncomfortable for the athlete. Therefore during activity it is recommended to drink small volumes (2–3 ml per kilogram of body weight, or 90–135 ml for a 45 kg child) at short intervals (every 15 min) (Bar-Or, 1983). The current American College of Sports Medicine (1987) position statement on the prevention of thermal injuries during distance running recommends that drinking stations be situated every 2–3 km during an organized road race. This would probably be sufficient for children participating in such races, provided they drink at every station. In sports such as soccer, rugby or field hockey, if environmental conditions are stressful (Table 23.5), it suggested that the game be divided into quarters rather than halves in order to provide an additional short break for

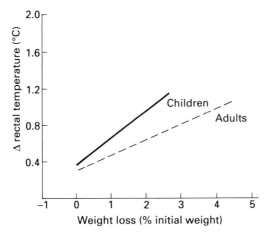

Fig. 23.5 Comparison of the relationship between the level of hypohydration, expressed as percentage change in initial body weight, and the rise in rectal temperature among children (———) and adults (———). Adapted from Bar-Or *et al.* (1980); redrawn with permission from Bar-Or (1983).

Table 23.5 Modification in athletic activity using the wet bulb globe temperature (WBGT)* index. Adapted from American College of Sports Medicine (1987), Bar-Or (1983) and Squire (1990).

WBGT °C	Risk of thermal disorders	Modification of activity
> 28	Very high	Stop all athletic activities
23–28	High	Stop activities of individuals at risk, such as the unacclimated, unfit, obese, and those with a history of heat disorders Increase rest periods of all other participants Reduce exercise intensity Increase fluid intake
18–23	Moderate	Increase rest periods and fluid intake Be alert for signs and/or symptoms of heat disorders
10–18	Low	All activities are allowed
< 10	Low	All activities are allowed but beware of signs of hypothermia

* WBGT = $0.7\,T_{wb} + 0.2\,T_g + 0.1\,T_{db}$, where T_{wb} = wet bulb temperature, T_g = black globe temperature, and T_{db} = dry bulb temperature.

rehydration (Squire, 1990). The fluid selected should stimulate further drinking and athletes should be encouraged to drink beyond thirst quenching. Electrolyte- and carbohydrate-containing beverages may stimulate thirst and encourage further fluid consumption, especially when grape- or orange-flavoured (Meyer et al., 1994). In view of the lower sodium and chloride loss among children compared to adults (Gibson & Di Sant' Agnes, 1963; Dill et al., 1966; Araki et al., 1979; Hjelm et al., 1986; Kirk & Westwood, 1989; Falk et al., 1991a; Meyer et al., 1992), children may require more dilute beverages compared to adults. This, however, has not been proven experimentally. In addition, cold water is more palatable than lukewarm water and empties faster from the stomach (Costill & Saltin, 1974).

Acclimatization and acclimation

Heat acclimatization and acclimation are the processes by which the body adapts to heat stress — naturally or via repeated exposures, respectively. The physiological adaptations include (i) an enhanced sweating rate at any given rectal temperature (Wyndham, 1967; Henane & Valatx, 1973; Nadel et al., 1974; Shvartz et al., 1979; Libert et al., 1983); (ii) an enhanced skin blood flow at any given rectal temperature (Roberts et al., 1977; Robert & Wenger, 1979); and (iii) an increase in plasma volume (Senay et al., 1976; Shapiro et al., 1981; Armstrong et al., 1987). In addition, there may be a redistribution of sweat (Shvartz et al., 1979), and a marked reduction in sweat and urine salt concentration, resulting in diminished salt loss (Armstrong et al., 1987). Finally, glycogen utilization rate during exercise may also be reduced (Kirwan et al., 1987). These adaptations lead to improved thermoregulation, enhanced physical performance in the heat and greater thermal comfort.

Children and adolescents are able to acclimate to heat similar to adults. The main difference is in the rate of acclimation, as demonstrated by Inbar (1978) during a 2-week acclimation programme (Fig. 23.6) (Bar-Or, 1983). Wagner *et al.* (1972) demonstrated a lower level of acclimation among adolescent boys compared to men following an 8-day protocol. Additionally, Inbar *et al.* (1981) reported no increase in sweating rate but an increase in the population density of heat-activated sweat glands after acclimation in 8–10-year-old boys. The latter may reflect a better distribution of sweat, as suggested by Shvartz *et al.* (1979).

Conversely, the subjective difficulty at a given physiological strain was shown to decrease at a faster rate among boys compared to men during acclimation (Bar-Or & Inbar, 1977). Although this may appear advantageous, it is also potentially dangerous because children may be reluctant to stop activity during exercise in the heat.

Proper acclimation is particularly important early in the athlete's competitive season, during the transitory and unpredictable spring season, and for those athletes who travel to warmer geographical regions. There are several reports of heat stroke among high school football players during the first practices of the season (Fox *et al.*, 1966; Redfearn & Murphy, 1969; Barcenas *et al.*, 1976), which may have been prevented with proper acclimation. In adults, reasonable acclimation may be attained following four to seven exposures to exercise (>50% $\dot{V}O_{2\,max}$) and heat, and eight to 14 exposures may be sufficient for maximal acclimation (Armstrong & Maresh, 1991). Children and adolescents may require a longer exposure programme. Conversely, less stringent protocols, which involve exercise in a thermoneutral environment or rest in the heat, rather than exercise in the heat, are apparently sufficient for acclimation among children (Inbar *et al.*, 1981). It is also important to remember that since acclimation increases sweating rate, it also increases fluid loss. Therefore, sound hydration practices, as described above, should be emphasized.

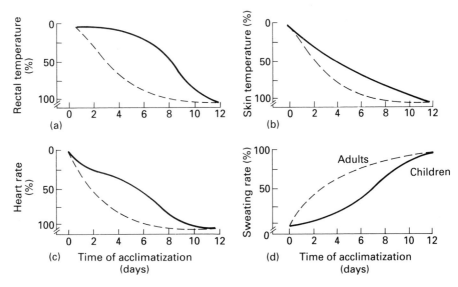

Fig. 23.6 Physiological adaptations during the course of heat acclimation among 8–10-year-old boys (———) and 20–33-year-old men (— — —). Adaptations in (a) rectal temperature, (b) skin temperature, (c) heart rate, and (d) sweating rate are expressed as per cent of final acclimation value, where baseline values are 0%. Schematic representation from Bar-Or (1980); redrawn with permission from Bar-Or (1983).

Loss of acclimation is fairly rapid. Williams *et al.* (1967) demonstrated that, among adults, over 50% of the acclimation effect on the rise in rectal temperature was lost within 3 weeks of no heat exposure. Moreover, over 50% of the adaptation in sweating rate disappeared within 1 week. It is unknown whether the rate of loss of acclimation is similar among children and adolescents but the advantages of acclimation should not be taken for granted beyond a few days (Armstrong & Maresh, 1991).

Conditioning

It is widely accepted that physical training in a thermoneutral environment improves the physiological responses to heat stress (see Armstrong & Pandolf, 1988 for review). A high $\dot{V}o_{2\,max}$ *per se* may not be as important in influencing exercise-heat tolerance as the physiological adaptations which result from physical training (e.g. increased blood volume, enhanced cardiovascular function).

Delmarche *et al.* (1990) did not observe any relationship between $\dot{V}o_{2\,max}$ (range 43–65 ml · min^{-1} · kg^{-1}) and the thermoregulatory response to rest in the heat among prepubertal boys. Likewise, Araki *et al.* (1980) reported no difference in body temperature in response to a passive heat load among prepubertal boys before and after training. Conversely, the same authors (Matsushita & Araki, 1980) observed a higher sweating rate at any given rectal temperature among trained boys compared to untrained boys. Similarly, Inbar *et al.* (1981) reported that among 8–10-year-old boys, heat acclimation can be achieved either by rest in the heat or by mere physical conditioning (training at 65% $\dot{V}o_{2\,max}$) in thermoneutral conditions. Thus, it appears that physical training can enhance thermoregulation among children, although the mechanism may be different than that in adults. Nevertheless, the fit child and adolescent will tolerate better an exercise-plus-heat stress.

Environmental conditions

At high ambient temperatures radiative and convective heat loss is diminished, or even reversed, and reliance is placed upon evaporative cooling. High humidity further stresses the thermoregulatory system in that sweat evaporation and thus, evaporative cooling, is reduced. Heat disorders can occur even in a relatively mild ambient temperature when humidity is high (Pugh *et al.*, 1967; Murphy, 1979; Assia *et al.*, 1985). In fact, fatal heat stroke in a high school football player was reported in 24°C but 97% relative humidity (Murphy, 1979). Conversely, windy conditions can improve heat dissipation by enhancing evaporation.

In contrast, windy conditions present an added risk for cold injuries when air temperature is low. Additionally, an aqueous environment or wet clothes also increase the risk for hypothermia.

The most commonly applied heat stress index is the wet bulb globe temperature (WBGT) (American College of Sports Medicine, 1987), which takes into account temperature, humidity and solar radiation. Portable heat stress monitors which measure these three variables and compute WBGT are commercially available (Hughson *et al.*, 1983) and are recommended for all organizers of outdoor athletic events. Modification for outdoor activities, according to the WBGT index are outlined in Table 23.6. In addition, it is recommended that in summer, activities be planned for the early morning or evening hours. The worst situation is on a hot day with a high relative humidity, high solar radiation and little wind, especially in the spring, when participants are not yet heat acclimatized.

Clothing should also be suitable for the environmental conditions. Loose, lightweight or net-like material is appropriate for hot humid days, and provided solar radiation is not excessive, skin should be exposed to allow for sweat evaporation. It should be noted that most sunscreen lotions are lipid-based and may, therefore, hinder sweat evaporation. Foot-

Table 23.6 Drugs which may affect thermo-regulation.

Drug	Effect on thermoregulation
Thyroid hormone	Increases metabolic rate and thus, heat production
Amphetamines, LSD	Increase metabolic rate and thus, heat production
Diuretics	Predispose to hypohydration. Alter electrolyte balance
Anticholinergics	Decrease sweating and thus, decrease evaporative cooling
Vasodilators	Increase skin blood flow and thus, increase heat gain in a hot environment and increase heat loss in cold environment
β-blockers	Increase sweating and may lead to dehydration
Antihistamines	Decrease sweating and thus, decrease evaporative cooling

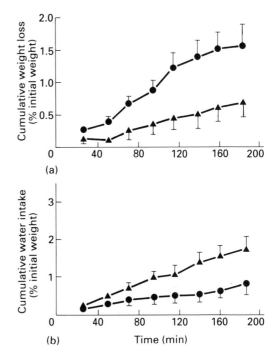

Fig. 23.7 (a) Cumulative weight loss, and (b) cumulative water intake among 9–14-year-old children with cystic fibrosis (●) and healthy children (▲) during exercise (45% $\dot{V}o_{2\,max}$) in the heat (31–33°C, 43–47% relative humidity). Adapted with permission from Bar-Or et al. (1992) © 1992 by The Lancet Ltd.

ball helmets and equipment, long-sleeved heavy rugby jerseys and fashionable track body suits will impede heat loss and impair thermoregulation.

Paediatric populations at high risk for heat disorders

Identifying individuals at high risk for heat dysfunction is fundamental in preventing heat-related disorders. Several diseases which involve the sweating mechanism (e.g. cystic fibrosis, sweating insufficiency syndromes, diabetes mellitus) or the cardiovascular system (e.g. congenital heart disease, diabetes mellitus) may impair the effectiveness of thermoregulation. For example, Bar-Or et al. (1992) demonstrated that children with cystic fibrosis underestimate their fluid requirements and, compared to healthy children, have a greater weight loss during a 3-h exposure to exercise-heat stress (Fig. 23.7). Thus, these children are more prone to hypohydration and to the detrimental effects associated with hypohydration. The reader is referred to Bar-Or

(1983) for further discussion of clinical conditions in which thermoregulation may be affected.

Drug abuse, although not common among children, is becoming problematic among adolescents (Hindmarsh & Opheim, 1990; Oetting & Beauvais, 1990). Drug abuse may alter thermoregulatory function due to physiological or behavioural effects. Drugs such as amphetamines and other stimulants may increase heat production and body temperature (Clark, 1987), diuretics will predispose the individual to hypohydration and electrolyte imbalance, while β-blockers and atropine can adversely affect the cardiovascular system and sweating (Gordon et al., 1984; Simpson et al., 1986; Kolka et al., 1987). It is unknown how anabolic steroids may affect the thermoregulatory response to exercise in the heat. Drugs which have been suggested to affect thermoregulation are listed in Table 23.6.

Among otherwise healthy children, two cases deserve special attention: obesity and prior heat-illness.

OBESITY

Obese individuals have a lower heat tolerance than lean individuals. This has been demonstrated among men (McCormick & Buskirk, 1974), women (Bar-Or et al., 1969) and prepubertal boys (Haymes et al., 1975) (Fig. 23.8) but has not been confirmed among prepubertal girls (Haymes et al., 1974).

There are several factors which limit the ability of obese individuals to tolerate heat. The insulation provided by subcutaneous fat

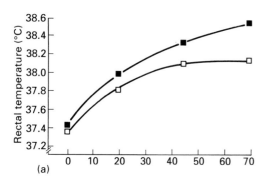

(a)

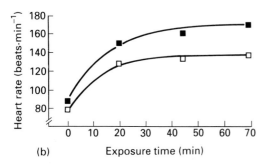

(b) Exposure time (min)

Fig. 23.8 Comparison of the rise in (a) rectal temperature and (b) heart rate among lean (□) and obese (■) boys exercising in the heat (4.8 km · h⁻¹, 5% grade; 40–42°C, 25% relative humidity). Data from Haymes et al. (1975); redrawn with permission from Bar-Or (1983).

in a cold environment is associated with a lower heat conductance and thus, compromised heat dissipation in a hot environment. In addition, the lower specific heat of fat ($1.68\,kJ \cdot g^{-1} \cdot {}^{\circ}C^{-1}$), means that a given heat load will induce a greater rise in body temperature among children with increased body fat. Therefore, a given exercise-heat stress will result in a higher rise in body temperature and lower heat tolerance among obese compared to lean individuals. In fact, Docherty et al. (1986) reported that, among prepubertal boys exercising in the heat, endomorphy was correlated with hyperthermia.

Obese individuals also have a lower percentage of total body water per kilogram compared to lean individuals and are thus more susceptible to the adverse effects of hypohydration (Bar-Or et al., 1976).

Finally, obese children are often characterized by a low physical activity level accompanied by low physical fitness. Since the rise in body temperature is proportional to the relative exercise intensity, obese children are at a disadvantage when participating in a given activity with their peers.

PRIOR HEAT-ILLNESS

Several investigators have suggested that individuals who have previously suffered from heat stroke are predisposed to suffer subsequent heat disorders (Robinson et al., 1976; Epstein et al., 1983; Kenney, 1985), even in conditions which would not precipitate heat disorders among other individuals. It is unknown whether this is due to an inherent susceptibility to heat stroke, or to an irreversible damage incurred during the first episode (Keren et al., 1981; Epstein et al., 1983). However, as noted by Epstein (1990), in those heat stroke victims where dehydration was the underlying cause, a normal response to a standard exercise-heat test is observed after 6 weeks. Whatever the reason for the initial episode of any heat disorder, the individual with such a history should be more cautious about exercising in the heat.

Cold injuries: identification and prevention

Cold injuries may be superficial (frostbite) or systemic (hypothermia). Early signs and symptoms of frostbite include local pain and red skin which may become white with an increase in severity.

To the author's knowledge, there are no reports of hypothermia (rectal temperature < 35°C) among children during exercise in the cold. This is due to the fact that the elevated metabolic rate, which characterizes most athletic activities, compensates for the body heat lost to the periphery. Smolander *et al.* (1992) reported that children were able to exercise in the cold (5°C) and maintain their core temperature similar to adults (Fig. 23.9). In order to do so, they 'needed' to increase their metabolic heat production to a greater extent than the adults. Thus, the authors argue that in physical activity of longer duration, children may experience earlier exhaustion.

During exercise in the cold outdoors, one must consider the windchill factor. When air temperature is 0°C, for example, a $24 \, \text{km} \cdot \text{h}^{-1}$ air velocity will result in a perceived air tempera-

ture equivalent to −10.5°C; a $40 \, \text{km} \cdot \text{h}^{-1}$ air velocity will bring perceived air temperature down to −16°C. The windchill factor is important not only in winter sports but may also be significant during running or cycling, where the relative air velocity may result in cold injury to exposed skin. This applies similarly to children and adults.

Heat conduction in the water can be 25 times greater than in air. Additionally, with increased body movements, there is an increase in heat convection. Thus, exercise in the water can result in a much greater rate of heat loss, compared to exercise on land. The greater body surface area to mass ratio of children, compared to adults, presents a disadvantage during swimming and results in a greater heat loss (Sloan & Keatinge, 1973). Obese children can partly compensate for this liability due to the insulative effect of subcutaneous fat. Similarly, prepubertal girls are characterized by lower subcutaneous fat compared to women and may therefore be more susceptible to hypothermia (Sloan & Keatinge, 1973).

In contrast to heat acclimation, there appears to be only limited adaptation to cold (Young, 1988), which is mainly characterized by an elevated skin blood flow to frequently exposed extremities (Krog *et al.*, 1960). This adaptation, which may help to prevent frostbite, has been demonstrated in adults but has not been studied in children. Elevated physical fitness reduces the risk of heat injuries but does not appear to prevent cold injuries (Adams & Heberling, 1958). Indeed, well-trained individuals are usually characterized by a thin layer of subcutaneous fat and may therefore be more susceptible to cold injuries.

Finally, prevention of hypothermia is dependent on proper clothing. Clothing material should allow for some insulation, yet permit sweat evaporation. In especially cold conditions, hat and gloves are recommended, since a large portion of body heat is lost from the head and hands. During exercise in cool water (< 23°C), it is recommended to allow children to exit and warm up every 10−15 min.

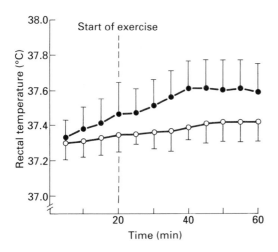

Fig. 23.9 Rectal temperature (mean ± SE) in boys (●) and in men (○) during rest and exercise (30% $\dot{V}_{O_2 \, max}$) in 5°C. Redrawn with permission from Smolander *et al.* (1992).

Paediatric populations at high risk

Two paediatric subpopulations are at an especially high risk for cold-related disorders during exercise: (i) underweight children; and (ii) children suffering from exercise-induced bronchoconstriction. Those children who are underweight, whether as a result of mal-nourishment or anorexia nervosa, are characterized by a thin layer of subcutaneous fat. Thus, their low insulation results in a greater heat loss to the environment and a greater risk of hypothermia.

One of the mechanisms which explain exercise-induced bronchoconstriction involves respiratory heat loss and airway cooling. When the inspired air is cold, there is an increase in its prevalence among children and adults (Strauss et al., 1977). Thus, it is recommended when possible to breathe through the nose during exercise in the cold. Shturman-Ellstein et al. (1978) demonstrated that children were able to breathe through the nose while exercising at 50–70% $\dot{V}o_{2\,max}$. At higher exercise intensities, nasal breathing may become impossible.

Challenges for future research

The physiological effects and health-related aspects of exercise in the heat or in the cold have been extensively investigated in adults but scarcely in children. There is a particular lack of information with regard to cold exposure. The following list presents some topics which merit further research.

• It is well established that the sweating rate in children relative to their body surface area or per gland, is lower compared to adults. However, it is unclear whether the sweating rate in children relative to the metabolic load, which is dependent on body mass and physical fitness, is also lower than that of adults. It is yet unknown whether sweating rate increases during adolescence due simply to an increase in body dimensions and sweat gland size, or due to hormonal and metabolic changes which are part of the maturation process. For example, it is unclear: (i) how particular hormones and neurotransmitters affect sweat gland function and sweat composition; (ii) whether sweat distribution is affected by growth — in particular, whether or not children can utilize evaporative cooling more efficiently than adults by activating more glands, yet producing less sweat per unit area; and (iii) whether children produce less sweat because they are limited by a maximal sweating rate or because they dissipate sufficient heat via convection and radiation.

• Involuntary hypohydration has been documented in children and in adults. The effects of hypohydration on thermoregulation and on exercise performance may be more detrimental in children, compared to adults. These effects have not been properly investigated, possibly due to ethical considerations. In addition, the possible effects of maturation on thirst perception, affecting fluid replacement, also need to be given further attention.

• Children respond to cold exposure with a greater increase in metabolic rate compared to adults. There is also indirect evidence that suggests enhanced vasoconstriction among children. Further study is needed to clarify the circulatory and hormonal response to cold exposure among children, and how this response may be affected by maturation.

• No information is available on the possible acclimation or adaptation process to cold among children and adolescents and how enhanced or reduced physical fitness may affect the response to cold during childhood and adolescence.

• Most studies investigate the response to heat or cold among young or adolescent boys. By comparison, there is relatively little information on girls and on possible gender-related differences in thermoregulation and in heat and cold tolerance.

• Theoretically, children are more susceptible to heat- or cold-induced disorders. There are some experimental data to support this statement. However, there are no epidemiological data on the relative risk in children to various heat- or cold-related injuries. This information is particularly important in view of the increasing participation of children in outdoor sports.

• Finally, the use of drugs and ergogenic aids is becoming popular among adult as well as adolescent athletes. There is very little information on how these drugs or supplements may affect thermoregulation and the susceptibility to heat- or cold-related disorders.

Acknowledgements

The author wishes to acknowledge Raffy Dotan for the helpful comments and critical review of this manuscript.

References

Adams, T. & Heberling, E.J. (1958) Human physiological responses to a standardized cold stress as modified by physical fitness. *J. Appl. Physiol.* **13**, 226.

American College of Sports Medicine (1987) Position statement on the prevention of thermal injuries during distance running. *Med. Sci. Sports Exerc.* **19**, 529–33.

Araki, T., Toda, Y., Matsushita, K. & Tsujino, A. (1979) Age differences in sweating during muscular exercise. *Jap. J. Fitness Sports Med.* **28**, 239–48.

Araki, T., Tsujita, J., Matsushita, K. & Hori, S. (1980) Thermoregulatory responses of prepubertal boys to heat and cold in relation to physical training. *J. Hum. Ergonom.* **9**, 69–80.

Armstrong, L.E., Costill, D.L. & Fink, W.J. (1987) Changes in body water and electrolytes during heat acclimation: effects of dietary sodium. *Aviation, Space Environ. Med.* **58**, 143–8.

Armstrong, L.E. & Maresh, C.M. (1991) The induction and decay of heat acclimatization in trained athletes. *Sports Med.* **12**, 302–12.

Armstrong, L.E. & Pandolf, K.B. (1988) Physical training, cardiorespiratory physical fitness and exercise-heat tolerance. In K.B. Pandolf, M.N. Sawka & R.R. Gonzalez (eds) *Human Performance Physiology and Environmental Medicine at Terrestrial Extremes*, pp. 199–226. Benchmark Press, Indianapolis.

Assia, E., Epstein, Y. & Shapiro, Y. (1985) Fatal heat stroke after a short march at night: a case report. *Aviation, Space Environ. Med.* **56**, 441–2.

Åstrand, P.O. (1952) *Experimental Studies of Physical Work Capacity in Relation to Sex and Age.* Munksgaard, Copenhagen.

Barcenas, C., Hoeffler, H.P. & Lie, J.T. (1976) Obesity, football, dog days and siriasis: a deadly combination. *Am. Heart. J.* **92**, 237–44.

Bar-Or, O. (1980) Climate and the exercising child — a review. *Int. J. Sports Med.* **1**, 53–65.

Bar-Or, O. (1983) *Pediatric Sports Medicine for the Practitioner*, pp. 259–99. Springer-Verlag, New York.

Bar-Or, O. (1989) Temperature regulation during exercise in children and adolescents. In C.V. Gisolfi & D.R. Lamb (eds) *Perspectives in Exercise Science and Sports Medicine*, Vol. II. *Youth Exercise and Sports*, pp. 335–62. Benchmark Press, Indianapolis.

Bar-Or, O., Blimkie, C.J.R., Hay, J.A., MacDougall, J.D., Ward, D.S. & Wilson, W.M. (1992) Voluntary dehydration and heat intolerance in cystic fibrosis. *Lancet* **339**, 696–9.

Bar-Or, O., Dotan, R., Inbar, O., Rotshtein, A. & Zonder, H. (1980) Voluntary hypohydration in 10–12-year-old boys. *J. Appl. Physiol.* **48**, 104–8.

Bar-Or, O., Harris, D., Bergstein, V. & Buskirk, E.R. (1976) Progressive hypohydration in subjects who vary in adiposity. *Israel J. Med. Sci.* **12**, 800–3.

Bar-Or, O. & Inbar, O. (1977) Relationship between perceptual and physiological changes during heat acclimatization in 8–10-year-old boys. In H. Lavalee & R.J. Shephard (eds) *Frontiers of Activity and Child Health*, pp. 205–14. Pelican, Quebec.

Bar-Or, O., Lundergren, H.M. & Buskirk, E.R. (1969) Distribution of heat-activated sweat glands in obese and lean men and women. *J. Appl. Physiol.* **26**, 403–9.

Bar-Or, O., Shephard, R.J. & Allen, C.L. (1971) Cardiac output of 10–13-year-old boys and girls during submaximal exercise. *J. Appl. Physiol.* **30**, 219–23.

Bittel, J. & Henane, R. (1975) Comparison of neutral exchanges in men and women under neutral and hot conditions. *J. Physiol.* (London) **250**, 475–89.

Blanchard, S. (1987) *Effects of ambient temperature and relative humidity on 8- and 10-year-old children involved in endurance activities working at 60% of maximal oxygen consumption.* PhD dissertation, University of Maryland.

Boisvert, P., Brisson, G.R., Peronnet, F., Fortier, M. & Senecal, L. (1988) Inhibiting action of selective face cooling and of bromocriptine mesylate on blood prolactin response induced by exercise. *Can. J. Sports Sci.* **13**, 6P.

Bosco, J.S., Greenleaf, J.E. & Terjung, R.L. (1968) Effects of progressive hypohydration on maximal isometric muscular strength. *J. Sports Med.* **8**, 81–6.

Brisson, G.R., Audet, A., Ledoux, M., Matton, P., Pellerin-Massicotte, J. & Perronet, F. (1986) Exercise-induced blood prolactin variations in trained adult males: a thermic stress more than an osmotic stress. *Horm. Res.* **23**, 200–6.

Callaham, M.L. (1979) *Emergency Management of Heat*

Illness, pp. 1–23. Emergency Physician Series. Abott Laboratories, North Chicago.

Caterisano, A., Camaione, D.N., Murphy, R.T. & Gonino, V.J. (1988) The effect of differential training on isokinetic muscular endurance during acute thermally induced hypohydration. *Am. J. Sports Med.* **16**, 269–73.

Cawley, E.P., Weary, P.E. & Hsu, Y.T. (1963) Cystic fibrosis and eccrine sweat gland size. *Arch. Dermatol.* **88**, 97–102.

Clark, W.G. (1987) Changes in body temperature after administration of antipyretics, LSD, delta 9-·THC and related agents: II. *Neurosci. Biobehav. Rev.* **11**, 35–96.

Costill, D.L. & Saltin, B. (1974) Factors limiting gastric emptying during rest and exercise. *J. Appl. Physiol.* **37**, 679–83.

Costrini, A. (1990) Emergency treatment of exertional heatstroke and comparison of whole body cooling techniques. *Med. Sci. Sports Exerc.* **22**, 15–18.

Costrini, A.M., Pitt, H.A., Gustafson, A.B. & Uddin, E.E. (1979) Cardiovascular and metabolic manifestations of heatstroke and severe heat exhaustion. *Am. J. Med.* **66**, 296–302.

Davies, C.T.M. (1981) Thermal responses to exercise in children. *Ergonomics* **24**, 55–61.

Delmarche, P., Bittel, J., Lacour, J.R. & Flandrois, R. (1990) Thermoregulation at rest and during exercise in prepubertal boys. *Eur. J. Appl. Physiol.* **60**, 436–40.

Dill, D.B., Hall, F.G. & van Beaumont, W. (1966) Sweat chloride concentration: sweat rate, metabolic rate, skin temperature and age. *J. Appl. Physiol.* **21**, 99–106.

Docherty, D., Eckerson, J.D. & Hayward, J.S. (1986) Physique and thermoregulation in prepubertal males during exercise in a warm, humid environment. *Am. J. Physiol. Anthropol.* **70**, 19–23.

Dotan, R. & Bar-Or, O. (1980) Climatic heat stress and performance in the Wingate anaerobic test. *Eur J. Appl. Physiol.* **44**, 237–43.

Drinkwater, B.L., Kupprat, I.C., Denton, J.E., Christ, J.L. & Horvath, S.M. (1977) Response of prepubertal girls and college women to work in the heat. *J. Appl. Physiol.* **43**, 1046–53.

Ekblom, B., Greenleaf, C.J., Greenleaf, J.E. & Hemansen, L. (1970) Temperature regulation during exercise dehydration in man. *Acta Physiol. Scand.* **79**, 475–83.

Epstein, Y. (1990) Heat intolerance: predisposing factor or residual injury? *Med. Sci. Sports Exerc.* **22**, 29–35.

Epstein, Y., Shapiro, Y. & Brill, S. (1983) Role of surface-to-mass ratio and work efficiency in heat intolerance. *J. Appl. Physiol.* **54**, 831–6.

Eriksson, B.O. & Saltin, B. (1974) Muscle metabolism during exercise in boys aged 11 to 16 years com-

pared to adults. *Acta Paediatr. Belg.* **28** (Suppl.), 257–65.

Falk, B. & Bar-Or, O. (1993) Longitudinal changes in peak aerobic and anaerobic mechanical power of circumpubertal boys. *Pediatr. Exerc. Med.* **5**, 318–31.

Falk, B., Bar-Or, O. & MacDougall, J.D. (1991a) Aldosterone and prolactin response to exercise in the heat among circumpubertal boys. *J. Appl. Physiol.* **71**, 1741–5.

Falk, B., Bar-Or, O. & MacDougall, J.D. (1992a) The thermoregulatory response of pre-, mid- and late-pubertal boys to exercise in dry heat. *Med. Sci. Sports Exerc.* **24**, 688–94.

Falk, B., Bar-Or, O., MacDougall, J.D. & Calvert, R. (1992b) Sweat gland response to exercise in the heat among pre-, mid- and late-pubertal boys. *Med. Sci. Sports Exerc.* **24**, 313–19.

Falk, B., Bar-Or, O., MacDougall, J.D., Goldsmith, C. & McGillis, L. (1992c) A longitudinal analysis of the sweating response of pre-, mid- and late-pubertal boys during exercise in the heat. *Am. J. Hum. Biol.* **4**, 527–35.

Falk, B., Bar-Or, O., MacDougall, J.D., McGillis, L., Calvert, R. & Meyer, F. (1991b) Sweat lactate in exercising children and adolescents of varying physical maturity. *J. Appl. Physiol.* **71**, 1735–40.

Fellmann, N., Labbe, Gachon, A-M. & Coudert, J. (1985) Thermal sweat lacate in cystic fibrosis and in normal children. *Eur. J. Appl. Physiol.* **54**, 511–16.

Fortney, S.M., Wenger, C.G., Bove, J.R. & Nadel, E.R. (1984) Effect of hyperosmolality on control of blood flow and sweating. *J. Appl. Physiol.* **57**, 1688–95.

Foster, K.G., Hey, E.N. & Katz, G. (1969) The response of the sweat glands of the newborn baby to thermal stimuli and intradermal acetylcholine. *J. Physiol.* **203**, 13–29.

Fox, E.L., Mathews, D.K. & Kaufman, W.S. (1966) Effects of football equipment on thermal balance and energy cost during exercise. *Res. Q. Am. Ass. Health Phys. Educ. Recr.* **37**, 332–9.

Francesconi, R.P. (1988) Endocrinological responses to exercise in stressful environments. *Exerc. Sports Sci. Rev.* **16**, 255–84.

Francesconi, R.P., Sawka, M.N., Hubbard, R.W. & Pandolf, K.B. (1989) Hormonal regulation of fluid and electrolytes: effects of heat exposure and exercise in the heat. In J.R. Claybaugh & C.E. Wade (eds) *Hormonal Regulation of Fluid and Electrolytes*, pp. 45–85. Plenum Press, London.

Gibson, L.E. & Di Sant' Agnes, PA. (1963) Studies of salt excretion in sweat. *J. Pediatr.* **61**, 855–67.

Goldstein-Golaire, J., Vanhaelst, L., Bruno, O.D., Lecirco, R. & Copinjschi, G. (1970) Acute effects of cold on blood levels of growth hormone, cortisol, and thyrotropin in man. *J. Appl. Physiol.* **29**, 622–6.

Gordon, N.F., Kruger, P.E., van Rensburg, J.P., van

der Linde, A., Kielblock, A.J. & Cilliers, J.F (1984) Effect of beta-adrenoreceptor blockade on thermoregulation during prolonged exercise in the heat. *Med. Sci. Sports Exerc.* **16**, 138 (abstract).

Greenleaf, J.E. & Castle, B.L. (1971) Exercise temperature regulation in man during hypohydration and hyperhydration. *J. Appl. Physiol.* **30**, 847–53.

Gullestad, R. (1975) Temperature regulation in children during exercise. *Acta Paediatr. Scand.* **64**, 257–63.

Haymes, E.M., McCormick, R.J. & Buskirk, E.R. (1974) Heat tolerance of exercising lean and heavy prepubertal girls. *J. Appl. Physiol.* **36**, 566–671.

Haymes, E.M., McCormick, R.J. & Buskirk, E.R. (1975) Heat tolerance of exercise lean and obese prepubertal boys. *J. Appl. Physiol.* **39**, 457–61.

Henane, R. & Valatx, J.L. (1973) Thermoregulatory changes induced during heat acclimatization by controlled hyperthermia in man. *J. Physiol.* **230**, 255–71.

Hindmarsh, K.W. & Opheim, E.E. (1990) Drug abuse prevalence in western Canada and the north west territories: a survey of students in grades 6–12. *Int. J. Addict.* **25**, 301–5.

Hjelm, M., Brown, P. & Bridden, A. (1986) Sweat sodium related to amount of sweat after sweat test in children with and without cystic fibrosis. *Acta Paediatr. Scand.* **75**, 652–6.

Hubbard, R.W. (1990) Heatstroke pathophysiology: the energy depletion model. *Med. Sci. Sports Exerc.* **22**, 19–28.

Hubbard, R.W. & Armstrong, L.E. (1988) The heat illnesses: biochemical, ultrastructural and fluid–electrolyte considerations. In K.B. Pandolf, M.N. Sawka & R.R. Gonzales (eds) *Human Performance Physiology and Environmental Medicine at Terrestrial Extremes*, pp. 305–60. Benchmark Press, Indianapolis.

Huebner, D.E., Lobeck, C.C. & McSherry, N.R. (1966) Density and secretory activity of eccrine sweat glands in patients with cystic fibrosis and healthy controls. *Pediatrics* **38**, 613–18.

Hughson, R.L., Standl, L.A. & Mackie, J.M. (1983) Monitoring road racing in the heat. *Phys. Sports Med.* **11**, 94–105.

Inbar, O. (1978) *Acclimatization to dry and hot environment in young adults and children 8–10 years old.* EdD dissertation, Columbia University.

Inbar, O., Bar-Or, O., Dotan, R. & Gutin, B. (1981) Conditioning vs. exercise in heat as methods for acclimatizing 8–10 year old boys to dry heat. *J. Appl. Physiol.* **50**, 406–11.

Johnson, H.L., Nelson, R.A. & Consolazio, C.F. (1988) Effects of electrolyte and nutrient solutions on performance and metabolic balance. *Med. Sci. Sports Exerc.* **20**, 26–33.

Jokinen, E., Valimaki, I., Antila, K., Seppanen, A. & Tuominen, J. (1990) Children in sauna: cardiovascular adjustment. *Pediatrics* **86**, 282–8.

Jokinen, E., Valimaki, I., Marniemi, J., Seppanen, A., Irjala, K. & Simkell, O. (1991) Children in sauna: hormonal adjustments to intensive short thermal stress. *Acta Physiol. Scand.* **80**, 370–4.

Kaufman, F.L., Mills, D.E., Hughson, R.L. & Peake, G.T. (1988) Effects of bromocriptine on sweat gland function during heat acclimatization. *Horm. Res.* **29**, 31–8.

Kawahata, A. (1960) Sex differences in sweating. In H. Yoshimura, K. Ogata & S. Itoh (eds) *Essential Problems in Climatic Physiology.* Nankodo, Kyoto.

Kenney, W.L. (1985) Physiological correlates of heat intolerance. *Sports Med.* **2**, 279–86.

Kenney, W.L., Tankersley, C.G., Newswanger, D.L., Hyde, D.E., Puhl, S.M. & Turner, N.L. (1990) Age and hypohydration independently influence the peripheral response to heat stress. *J. Appl. Physiol.* **68**, 1902–8.

Keren, G., Epstein, Y. & Magazanik, A. (1981) Temporary heat intolerance in a heatstroked patient. *Aviation, Space Environ. Med.* **52**, 116–17.

Kirk, J.M. & Westwood, A. (1989) Interpretation of sweat sodium results — the effect of patient age. *Ann. Clin. Biochem.* **26**, 38–43.

Kirwan, J.P., Costill, D.L., Kuipers, H. *et al.* (1987) Substrate utilization in leg muscle of men after heat acclimation. *J. Appl. Physiol.* **63**, 31–5.

Knochel, J.P. (1974) Environmental heat illness. An eclectic review. *Arch. Int. Med.* **133**, 841–64.

Kolka, M.A., Stephenson, L.A., Bruttig, S.P., Cadarette, B.S. & Gonzalez, R.R. (1987) Human thermoregulation after atropine and/or pralidoxime administration. *Aviation Space Environ. Med.* **58**, 545–9.

Krog, J., Folkow, B., Fox, R.H. *et al.* (1960) Hand circulation in the cold of Lapps and North Norwegian fisherman. *J. Appl. Physiol.* **15**, 651.

Kukkonen-Harjula, K., Oja, P., Laustiola, K. *et al.* (1989) Haemodynamic and hormonal responses to heat exposure in a Finnish sauna bath. *Eur. J. Appl. Physiol.* **58**, 543–50.

Kulzycki, L.L. & Robertson, M.T. (1988) The sweat chloride concentration and prolactin activity in cystic fibrosis. *Scand. J. Gastroenterol.* **223** (Suppl. 143), 28–30.

Kuno, Y. (1956) *Human Perspiration.* C.C. Thomas, Springfield, IL.

Laatikainen, T., Salminen, K., Kohvakka, A. & Pettersson, J. (1988). Response of plasma endorphins, prolactin and catecholamines in women to intense heat in a sauna. *Eur. J. Appl. Physiol.* **57**, 98–102.

Landing, B.H., Wells, T.R. & Williamson, M.L. (1968) Studies on growth of eccrine sweat glands. In D.B. Cheek (ed.) *Human Growth: Body Composition, Cell*

Growth, Energy and Intelligence. pp. 382–94. Lea & Febiger, Philadelphia.

Leduc, J. (1961) Catecholamine production and release in exposure and acclimatization to cold. *Acta Physiol. Scand.* **183** (Suppl.), 1–101.

Leppaluoto, J. (1988) Human thermoregulation in sauna. *Ann. Clin. Res.* **20**, 240–3.

Libert, J.P., Candas, V. & Vogt, J.J. (1983) Modifications of sweating responses to thermal transients following heat acclimation. *Eur. J. Physiol.* **50**, 235–46.

Lobeck, C.C. & McSherry, N.R. (1967) The ionic composition of pilocarpine induced sweat in relation to gland output during aging and cystic fibrosis. *Mod. Prob. Pediatr.* **10**, 41–57.

McCormick, R.J. & Buskirk, E.R. (1974) Heat tolerance of exercising lean and obese middle-aged men. *Fed. Proc.* **33**, 441 (abstract).

MacDougall, J.D., Roche, P.D., Bar-Or, O. & Moroz, J.R. (1983) Maximal aerobic capacity of Canadian school children: prediction based on age-related oxygen cost of running. *Int. J. Sports Med.* **4**, 194–8.

Mackie, J.M. (1982) *Physiological responses of twin children to exercise under conditions of heat stress.* MSc thesis, University of Waterloo.

Mackova, J., Sturmova, M. & Macek, M. (1984) Prolonged exercise in prepubertal boys in warm and cold environments. In J. Illmarinen & I. Valimaki (eds) *Children and Sports*, pp. 135–41. Springer-Verlag, Heidelberg.

Marsh, M.L., Mahon, A.D. & Naftzger, L.A. (1992) Children's physiological responses to exercise in a cold and neutral temperature. *Proceedings of the North American Society of Pediatric Exercise Medicine Meeting.* Miami, Florida.

Matsushita, K. & Araki, T. (1980) The effect of physical training on thermoregulatory responses of preadolescent boys to heat and cold. *Jap. J. Phys. Fitness* **29**, 69–74.

Melin, B., Cure, M., Pequignot, J.M. & Bittel, J. (1989) Body temperature and plasma prolactin and nor-epinephrine relationships during exercise in a warm environment: effect of dehydration. *Eur. J. Appl. Physiol.* **58**, 146–51.

Meyer, F., Bar-Or, O., MacDougall, D. & Heigenhauser, G.H. (1992) Sweat electrolyte loss during exercise in the heat: effects of gender and maturation. *Med. Sci. Sports Exerc.* **24**, 776–81.

Meyer, F., Bar-Or, O., Salsberg, A. & Passe, R. (1994) Hypohydration during exercise in children: effect on thirst, drink preferences, and rehydration. *Int. J. Sports Nutr.* **4**, 22–35.

Murphy, R.J. (1979) Heat illness and athletics. In R.H. Strauss (ed.) *Sports Medicine and Physiology*, pp. 320–7. W.B. Saunders, Philadelphia.

Murray, R. (1987) The effects of consuming carbohydrate–electrolyte beverages on gastric emptying

and fluid absorption during and following exercise. *Sports Med* **4**, 322–51.

Nadel, E.R., Pandolf, K.B., Roberts, M.F. & Stolwijk, J.A.J. (1974) Mechanisms of thermal acclimation to exercise and heat. *J. Appl. Physiol.* **37**, 515–20.

Oetting, E.R. & Beauvais, F. (1990) Adolescent drug use: findings of national and local surveys. *J. Consult. Clin. Psychol.* **58**, 385–94.

Orenstein, D.M., Henke, K.G., Costill, D.L., Doershuk, C.F., Lemon, P.J. & Stern, R.C. (1983) Exercise and heat stress in cystic fibrosis patients. *Pediatr. Res.* **17**, 267–9.

Pierkarski, C., Morfeld, P., Kampmann, B., Ilmarinen, R. & Wenzel, H.G. (1986) Heat-stress reactions of the growing child. In J. Rutenfranz, R. Mocellin & F. Lkint (eds) *Children and Exercise XII*, pp. 403–12. Human Kinetics, Champaign, IL.

Pugh, L.G.C., Crobett, J.L. & Johnson, R.H. (1967) Rectal temperatures, weight losses and sweat rates in marathon running. *J. Appl. Physiol.* **23**, 347–52.

Redfearn, J.A. Jr & Murphy R.J. (1969) Letter: history of heat-stroke in a football trainee. *JAMA* **208**, 699–700.

Rees, J. & Shuster, S. (1981) Pubertal induction of sweat gland activity. *Clin. Sci.* **60**, 689–92.

Roberts, M.F. & Wenger, C.B. (1979) Control of skin circulation during exercise and heat stress. *Med. Sci. Sports* **11**, 36–41.

Roberts, M.F., Wenger, C.B., Stotwijk, J.A.J. & Nadel, G.R. (1977) Skin blood flow and sweating changes following exercise training and heat acclimation. *J. Appl. Physiol.* **43**, 133–7.

Robertson, M.T. (1989) Prolactin, human nutrition and evolution, and the relation to cystic fibrosis. *Med. Hypoth.* **29**, 87–99.

Robertson, M.T., Boyajian, M.J., Patterson, K. & Robertson, W.V.B. (1986) Modulation of the chloride concentration of human sweat by prolactin. *Endocrinology* **119**, 2439–44.

Robinson, S. (1938) Experimental studies of physical fitness in relation to age. *Int. Z. Angew. Physiol. Einschl. Arbeitsphysiol.* **10**, 251–323.

Robinson, S., Wiley, S.L., Myhre, L.G., Bondurant, S. & Mamlin, J.J. (1976) Temperature regulation of men following heat-stroke. *Israel J. Med. Sci.* **12**, 786–95.

Rodriguez, J.R., Rivera, M.A., Rivera, A., Bar-Or, O., Mayol, P. & Frontera, W.R. (1990) Body fluid balance during exercise in chronically heat acclimatized children: a field study. *Med. Sci. Sports Exerc.* **22**, S89 (abstract).

Saltin, B. (1964) Aerobic and anaerobic work capacity after dehydration. *J. Appl. Physiol.* **19**, 1114–18.

Sato, K. & Sato, F. (1983) Individual variations in structure and function of human eccrine sweat glands. *Am. J. Physiol.* **245**, R203–8.

Sawka, M.N., Tatzka, W.A. & Pandolf, K.B. (1989)

Temperature regulation during upper body exercise: able-bodied and spinal cord injured. *Med. Sci. Sports Exerc.* **21**, S132–40.

Sawka, M.N., Young, A.J., Francesconi, R.B., Muza, S.R. & Pandolf, K.B. (1985) Thermoregulation and blood responses during exercise at graded hypohydration levels. *J. Appl. Physiol.* **59**, 1394.

Senay, L.C., Mitchell, D. & Wyndham, C.H. (1976) Acclimation in a hot, humid environment: body fluid adjustments. *J. Appl. Physiol.* **40**, 786–96.

Serfass, R.D., Stull, G.A. & Alexander, J.F. (1984) The effects of rapid weight loss and attempted rehydration and endurance of the handgripping muscles in college wrestlers. *Res. Q.* **55**, 46–52.

Shapiro, Y., Hubbard, R.W., Kimbrough, C.M. & Pandolf, K.B. (1981) Physiological and hematological responses to summer and winter dry-heat acclimation. *J. Appl. Physiol.* **50**, 792–8.

Shapiro, Y. & Seidman, D.S. (1990) Field and clinical observations of exertional heat stroke patients. *Med. Sci. Sports Exerc.* **22**, 6–14.

Shibolet, S., Coll, R., Gilat, T. & Sohar, E. (1967) Heatstroke: its clinical picture and mechanism in 36 cases. *Q. J. Med.* **36**, 525–47.

Shibolet, S., Fisher, S., Gilat, T., Bank, H. & Heller, H. (1962) Fibrinolysis and hemorrhages in fatal heat stroke. *N. Engl. J. Med.* **266**, 169–73.

Shibolet, S., Lancaster, M.C. & Danon, Y. (1970) Heat stroke: a review. *Aviat. Space Environ. Med.* **47**, 280–301.

Shturman-Ellstein, R., Zeballos, R.J., Buckey, J.M. *et al.* (1978) The beneficial effect of nasal breathing on exercise-induced bronchoconstriction. *Am. Rev. Respir. Dis.* **118**, 65.

Shvartz, E., Bhattacharya, A., Sperinde, S.J., Brock, P.J., Sciaraffa, D. & van Beaumont, W. (1979) Sweating responses during heat acclimation and moderate conditioning. *J. Appl. Physiol.* **46**, 675–80.

Simpson, K.H., Green, J.H. & Ellis, F.R. (1986) Effect of glycopyrrolate and atropine on thermoregulation after exercise. *Br. J. Clin. Pharmacol.* **22**, 579–86.

Sloan, R.E. & Keatinge, W.R. (1973) Cooling rates of young people swimming in cold water. *J. Appl. Physiol.* **35**, 371.

Smolander, J., Bar-Or, O., Korhonen, O. & Ilmarinen, J. (1992) Thermoregulation during rest and exercise in the cold in pre- and early pubescent boys and in young men. *J. Appl. Physiol.* **72**, 1589.

Sohar, E. & Shapira, Y. (1965) The physiological reactions of women and children marching during heat. *Proc. Israel Physiol. Pharmacol. Soc.* **1**, 50.

Squire, D.L. (1990) Heat illness: fluid and electrolyte issues for pediatric and adolescent athletes. *Pediatr. Clin. N. Am.* **37**, 1085–109.

Strauss, R.H., McFadden, E.R., Ingram, R.H. & Jaeger, J.J. (1977) Enhancement of exercise-induced asthma by cold air. *New Engl. J. Med.* **297**, 743.

Suzuki, M., Tonoue, T., Matsuzaki, S. & Yamamoto, K. (1967) Initial response of human thyroid, adrenal cortex, and adrenal medulla to acute cold exposure. *Can. J. Physiol. Pharmacol.* **45**, 423–32.

Szabo, G. (1962) The number of eccrine sweat glands in human skin. *Adv. Biol. Skin* **3**, 1–5.

Tcheng, T. & Tipton, C. (1976) Iowa wrestling study: anthropometric measurements and the prediction of a 'minimal' body weight for high school wrestlers. *Med. Sci. Sports* **8**, 101–4.

Tipton, C. & Tcheng, T. (1970) Iowa wrestling study: weight loss in high school students. *JAMA* **214**, 1269–74.

Torranin, C., Smith, D.P. & Byrd, R.D. (1979) The effects of acute thermal dehydration on isometric and isotonic endurance. *J. Sports Med.* **19**, 1–9.

Wada, M. (1950) Sudorific action of adrenalin on the human sweat glands and determination of their excitability. *Science* **111**, 376–7.

Wagner, J.A., Robinson, S. & Marino, R.P. (1974) Age and temperature regulation of humans in neutral and cold environments. *J. Appl. Physiol.* **37**, 562.

Wagner, J.A., Robinson, S., Tzankoff, S.W. & Marino, R.P. (1972) Heat tolerance and acclimatization to work in the heat in relation to age. *J. Appl. Physiol.* **33**, 616–22.

Webster, S., Rutt, R. & Weltman, A. (1990) Physiological effects of a weight loss regimen practised by college wrestlers. *Med. Sci. Sports Exerc.* **22**, 229–34.

White, J. & Ford, M.A. (1983) The hydration and electrolyte maintenance properties of an experimental sports drink. *Br. J. Sports Med.* **17**, 51–8.

Wilk, B., Meyer, F. & Bar-Or, O. (1994) Effect of electrolytes and carbohydrate drink content on voluntary drinking and fluid balance in children. *Med. Sci. Sports Exerc.* **26**, S205.

Williams, C.G., Wyndham, C.H. & Morrison, J.F. (1967) Rate of loss of acclimatization in summer and winter. *J. Appl. Physiol.* **22**, 21–6.

Wolfe, S., Cage, G., Epstein, M., Tice, L., Miller, H. & Gordon, R.S. Jr (1970) Metabolic studies on isolated human eccrine sweat glands. *J. Clin. Invest.* **49**, 1880–4.

Wyndham, C.H. (1967) Effect of acclimatization on the sweat rate/rectal temperature relationship. *J. Appl. Physiol.* **22**, 27–30.

Yarrows, S.A. (1988) Weight loss through dehydration in amateur wrestling. *J. Am. Diet. Ass.* **88**, 491–3.

Young, A. (1988) Human adaptation to cold. In K.B. Pandolf, M.N. Sawka & R.R. Gonzalez (eds) *Human Performance Physiology and Environmental Medicine at Terrestrial Extremes*, pp. 401–34. Benchmark Press, Indianapolis.

PART 5

PSYCHOSOCIAL ISSUES

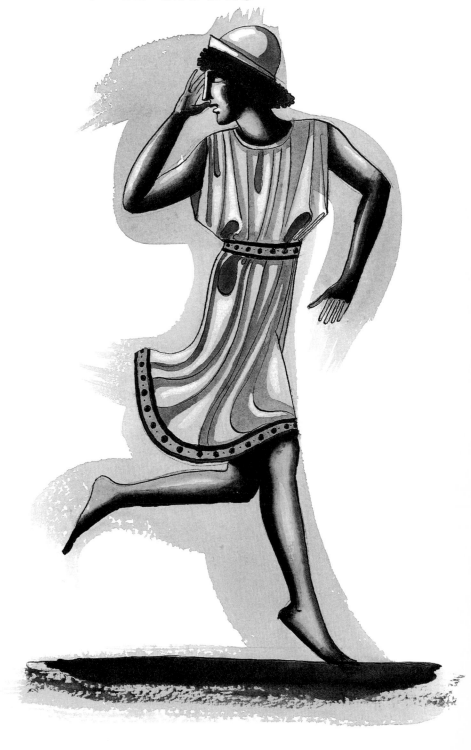

Chapter 24

Socialization through Sports

JAY COAKLEY

Introduction

Does sport participation have an impact on social development? Does it involve special learning experiences? Does it promote learning that carries over into other spheres of life? Does it build character? Most people connected with sport would answer affirmatively to these questions. They may qualify their answers, but they generally believe that sport participation teaches people, especially young people, useful lessons applicable to social life.

Such a set of beliefs is not new. In fact, during the mid-nineteenth century British public schools incorporated competitive sports into their curricula because administrators were convinced that rule-governed physical games produced loyal, disciplined, moral and patriotic young men fit for leadership in civil and military life. Others have since believed that organized sports were especially useful in re-shaping the cultural orientations of colonized peoples and immigrants, and directing the working classes in industrial societies to embrace a commitment to production norms. The 'muscular Christian' groups in Europe and North America during the mid- to late-nineteenth century tied physical exercise and sport participation to the expression of moral character. More recently, organized sports have been widely perceived as wholesome activities consisting of special character building experiences.

During the first half of this century debates about socialization through sport were rare; it was widely assumed that participation in organized competitive sports automatically produced discipline, commitment to following rules, and a desire to achieve socially accepted goals. These assumptions about socialization through sport were not systematically questioned and investigated until the late 1950s. Since then numerous studies have been done, mostly designed to test the validity of beliefs about the perceived character building consequences of sport participation. A review of this research is useful in assessing what we know about sport and the social development of individuals.

Research on socialization

Research on socialization through sport generally assumes that socialization is a combined process of social interaction and social development — that socialization occurs through social relationships, and that through socialization people learn about their connections to the social world and about how their social worlds are organized, maintained and changed.

However, most research done prior to the 1980s ignored the dynamic social interaction processes involved in socialization and simply attempted to identify hypothesized developmental outcomes (or products) associated with sport participation. This research was based on what has been called an internalization model of socialization (Wentworth, 1980) and it involved correlational analyses of quantitative survey data collected from subjects identified either as sport participants or non-participants. Since the early 1980s there has been a shift away from using the overly deterministic internalization model toward using an interactionist model that emphasizes the dynamic quality of the social relationships through which socialization occurs. Research based on an interactionist model generally involves interpretive analyses of qualitative data collected through case studies, in-depth interviews or observations and field studies.

Research based on an internalization model of socialization

Until recently, most studies of socialization through sport focused on identifying the impact of sport participation on the lives of those who participated in some type of organized sport programme; research subjects were usually white males in US high schools, although a handful of studies included 10−14 year olds in their samples. The assumption underlying these studies was that socialization involved a process of internalization through which people, especially young people, were 'moulded' and 'shaped' by sport experiences. Sport participants were assumed to be passive learners who internalized the norms and orientations believed to be a part of organized, competitive sports. These norms and orientations were assumed to be transmitted to participants through significant others such as coaches, parents and siblings, and occasionally, peers. Various measures of conformity, deviance, achievement and social success were used as the primary indicators of socialization.

CROSS-SECTIONAL SURVEYS

The methodology used in most studies based on the internalization model involved correlational analyses of cross-sectional survey data. Data were generally collected in connection with larger studies of the characteristics of American high school students, and analysis consisted of statistical comparisons of the measured characteristics of students who were identified as members of varsity sport teams in the schools and students who were so-called 'non-athletes' (at least within the context of the schools). Pretest and post-test research designs were seldom used in these studies so it was impossible to distinguish between the actual socialization effects of sport participation and the selection effects associated with high school varsity sports. In other words, researchers could not say whether any differences they found between so-called 'athletes' and 'non-athletes' could be attributed to participation itself, or whether the differences simply existed prior to trying out, being selected for and actually playing on sport teams. This was a problem because US high school varsity sport programmes, due to their élitist emphasis, have long encouraged self-selection and involved the use of selection criteria designated by coaches and other adults in authority positions.

In addition to these research design problems, cross-sectional studies on socialization through sport also had problems because researchers tended to assume that all forms of participation in organized, competitive sports involved a unique and consistent set of character shaping experiences, that all participants equally shared those experiences, and that the experiences were not generally available to those who did not participate in organized sport (McCormack & Chalip, 1988). The combination of these assumptions and the simplistic research designs used in these studies led to confusing and contradictory findings about socialization through sport. Researchers could say little about whether sport participation actually contributed to the development of positive character traits, whether it turned young people into better students and occupationally successful adults, whether it promoted conformity, reduced delinquency rates, inculcated conservative social and political attitudes, or inspired strong achievement orientations and moral development (McPherson & Brown, 1988; Coakley, 1993).

It should be noted that few of these studies

focused on preadolescent children. Part of the reason for this was that researchers emphasized quantitative methods that were difficult to use when gathering data from and about children. Widely used scales and questionnaires were not always valid or reliable when administered to young children. And even when they were, it was difficult for researchers to assume that sport participation in the lives of young children was so separate from other socialization experiences that they ought to try to isolate its developmental consequences.

LONGITUDINAL RESEARCH

Studies using longitudinal research designs in which survey data are collected at different points in time from the same respondents through repeated measures have eliminated some of the problems of cross-sectional studies. Although longitudinal studies have also tended to use samples drawn from students in American high schools, they have enhanced our understanding of socialization through sport. The results of these studies show that participation in interscholastic sport programmes is not random and that the consequences of participation are negligible when viewed in the light of the normal developmental changes occurring during adolescence (Hauser & Lueptow, 1978; Melnick *et al.*, 1988; Rees *et al.*, 1990; Spreitzer, 1992).

One of the most informative longitudinal studies was performed by Spreitzer (1992). He analysed data from a national probability sample of some 12 000 males and females at about 1100 public and private secondary schools in the USA. Data were collected from high school sophomores and seniors in 1980 with follow-up surveys of the same respondents in 1982, 1984 and 1986. Spreitzer found that when compared with other students the young people participating in varsity sports were disproportionately from economically privileged backgrounds and initially had above average cognitive abilities, self-esteem and records of academic performance. This apparent 'selection' pattern was common to participation in

nearly all organized, school sanctioned extracurricular activities, not just varsity sports. Self-selection, encouragement from others and externally imposed informal and formal selection criteria all combined to form a differential recruitment process that made young people in these programmes different from those who did not participate. But differences were *not* attributable to sport participation in itself. Spreitzer (1992) also noted that this differential recruitment was especially prominent in organized, competitive sports since the selection and filtering processes in competitive sports often begin years earlier in youth programmes in which participation criteria may be strict and uniformly used by adults who control player selection processes.

Spreitzer (1992) also found that dropping out of varsity sports was not random. Students who discontinued varsity sport participation between their sophomore and senior years were disproportionately from less advantaged backgrounds and had lower levels of cognitive abilities, lower self-esteem, lower grade averages and were less likely to be in a college preparatory curriculum. Furthermore, he found that young women were twice as likely as young men to drop out during this period. Each of these findings suggests that in addition to a 'selection' process there is a 'filtering' process that occurs in connection with certain organized sports. Spreitzer also noted that separating the effects of sport participation from the socialization effects of participating in other experiences was especially difficult because varsity athletes were more likely than other students to become involved in additional extracurricular activities while in school. Therefore, they may have had access to social experiences with peers and relationships with supportive adults that were not enjoyed by their peers who participated in neither varsity sports nor other formally organized extracurricular activities.

In the remainder of his analysis Spreitzer (1992) found 'no clear association between athletic participation as a high school senior and psychological well-being six years later',

nor did he find significant relationships between sport participation and patterns of
alcohol use, level of self-esteem, age of marriage
or birth of first child. There was a modest
positive association between participation and
educational attainment, but varsity sport participation was a much weaker predictor than
other factors, and it was relevant only for white
males as opposed to all females and Black males.

Spreitzer concluded his analysis with a
warning and some advice. He warned that conclusions about socialization through sport
based on comparisons between so-called 'athletes' and 'non-athletes' should take note of
'antecedent social background characteristics'
(1992, p. 12). And he advised that arguments
supporting organized sport programmes
should emphasize the intrinsic rewards associated with participation rather than unsubstan-
tiated beliefs about sport as a character builder.
Other research (cf. Coakley, 1993) seems to
support his advice.

Research based on interactionist models of socialization

Fortunately, what we know about socialization
through sport does not stop with the findings
of correlational analyses inspired by an internalization model. Recent research is more often
based on interactionist models of socialization.
These models call for the use of data collection
techniques that capture the dynamic nature of
the interaction through which socialization
occurs. They are based on the assumption that
socialization is a two-way process and that
human beings are agents who actively participate in the social construction of their own
social worlds and in the socialization processes
that occur in those worlds. This assumption
leads researchers to recognize that people who
participate in sport do not simply internalize
moral lessons imparted by external sources of
influence such as parents and coaches. It also
leads them to more carefully attend to processes
of negotiation, resistance, struggle and transformation that are a part of socialization itself.

Instead of focusing on social learning and individual responses to the social environment, as
is the case when an internalization model is
used, researchers using interactionist models
generally focus on processes of social relations
associated with sport, identity formation
among sport participants, and the social transformation of sport itself.

The best way to illustrate the findings of
research based on interactionist models is to
provide overviews of actual studies. The following six examples of studies have been selected because they use a variety of data collection
procedures, focus on various types of sport
participants, and call attention to different
dimensions of socialization processes. (These
six examples are adapted from Coakley, 1993.)
Again, studies of young children are rare, partly
due to the privacy and informed consent issues
associated with using qualitative methods
which demand long periods of access to a wide
range of situations in the children's lives.

Sport participation and the moral socialization of children: a study of Little Leaguers

Fine (1987) used an interactionist model of
socialization to guide his study of the participants on 10 Little League teams in five different
leagues. Data were collected over 3 years
through participant observations and informal
conversations and interviews. In his observations and analysis Fine gave detailed attention to the specific situations in which children
are exposed to moral guidelines for behaviour.
He found that moral socialization through sport
involved a complex process through which
young people redefined and transformed the
idealized rules and moral lessons offered by
adults into concerns that fit their own immediate needs, primarily needs for acceptance
among peers. Social acceptance among fellow
Little Leaguers was achieved through efforts to
'be a man' in a traditional moral sense. This led
these preadolescent boys to choose behaviours
that expressed autonomy and established distance between themselves and anyone defined

as weak and submissive, i.e. girls and younger children. Since being identified with girls or younger children interfered with being defined as 'men', the boys on youth teams tended to mimic stereotypical models of traditional masculinity. This tendency was seldom discouraged by coaches; in fact, it was sometimes used by coaches to motivate the boys to play in aggressive ways. This process led to the reproduction of a masculinity grounded in displays of toughness and dominance, and to expressions of disdain for females and any boys seen as unable to fend for themselves or unwilling to engage in daring or bold behaviours.

Fine also found that boys seldom accepted at face value the moral messages stressed by coaches and parents. But coaches and parents seldom detected this resistance to and transformation of moral messages because the boys quickly learned to present themselves in ways that expressed and reaffirmed the 'moral truths' proclaimed by adults; the boys also learned that to avoid sanctions when caught violating rules, they had to use particular expressions of 'moral rhetoric' that appeased adults. These preadolescent boys did not simply ignore the moral talk offered by adults or see it as useless, but they did transform it to fit their own definitions of the situation. Furthermore, the boys evaluated the rhetoric used by adults by comparing it to actual adult behaviour. When there were contradictions between rhetoric and behaviour the boys raised questions about the credibility of the adults and the moral messages they proclaimed. The boys did not overtly reject the values promoted by parents and coaches, but they did question them and creatively adapt them to fit their own lives.

Fine's study shows that socialization through sport is a problematic process. It does not happen according to some prescribed recipe. Instead, it emerges out of a combination of the concerns of those who control sport structures and the participants themselves, even when the participants are children. Participants may lack formal power relative to those who organize control sport programmes,

but that does not men they simply internalize the values promoted by the organizers and controllers; instead, they interpret and transform those values in the light of tasks and issues important in their lives and in the peer or subcultural groups in which they seek acceptance.

Sport participation and the development of identity: a study of male intercollegiate athletes

Adler and Adler (1991) also used an interactionist model to guide their decade-long study of the identities of men on a high profile college basketball team. Through a combination of observation, participant observation, and both formal and informal in-depth interviews with athletes, coaches and others associated with the basketball programme, data were collected on how the self-conceptions of college student athletes changed in connection with their sport participation. Their major finding was that young men on high profile intercollegiate teams usually became so engulfed in their athlete roles that they made adjustments and compromises in their academic lives. This 'role engulfment' involved increasing commitments to identities based exclusively on sport participation. These commitments were consistently and clearly reinforced by coaches, students, fans, community members and teammates. Thus, being an athlete became a 'master status' for these young men, and the athletic subculture became the context in which they set goals, evaluated themselves and defined their identities.

Although Adler and Adler suspected that intercollegiate athletes learned something about the importance of focusing their attention on specific tasks and delaying gratification while specific goals were pursued, they found nothing to suggest that these lessons might be carried over by the athletes to other spheres of their lives. This conclusion is tied to the fact that role engulfment often involves a heightened salience of a situation-specific identity that is unique and unrelated to other identities and contexts. However, the process of role engulfment is itself problematic. For example, research inspired by Adler and Adler's study found that unlike male athletes, female intercollegiate athletes did not make exclusive commitments to athletic identities or make revisions in academic standards and goals (Meyer, 1990). This suggests that gender and gender relations mediates the meanings attached to sport experiences and the integration of sport into a person's life.

Accepting pain and injury as a normal part of sport participation: a study of the sport career of an amateur wrestler

Curry's (1992) study of the sport career of an amateur wrestler focused on the socialization that occurs as an athlete deals with pain and injuries often associated with sport participation. Curry's case study used biographical data collected through three 2-h interviews over a 2-month period. These interviews followed several years of observing the wrestling team on which this young man (in his early twenties) participated. Curry's analysis clearly outlines the socialization process through which many athletes come to define pain and injury as normal parts of their sport experiences.

The young wrestler studied by Curry initially learned to define pain and injury as a routine part of sport participation simply by observing other wrestlers and interacting with people connected to the sport. As he progressed to higher levels of competition he became increasingly aware of how the endurance of pain and injury were commonplace among fellow athletes and former athletes who were now coaches. Over time this young man learned the following in connection with his wrestling career.

1 To 'shake off' minor injuries.

2 To see special treatment for minor injuries as a form of coddling.

3 To express desire and motivation by playing while injured or in pain.

4 To avoid using injury or pain as excuses for not practising or competing.

5 To use physicians and trainers as experts whose roles were to keep him competing when not healthy.

6 To see pain-killing anti-inflammatory drugs as necessary performance-enhancing aids.

7 To commit himself to the idea that all athletes must pay a price as they strive for excellence.

8 To define any athlete (including himself) unwilling to pay the price or to strive for excellence as morally deficient.

Finally, through a combination of injuries to his spine and knees, and repeated injuries that disfigured his ears ('cauliflower ear' is common among long-time wrestlers), he become a role model for younger wrestlers.

The socialization experiences associated with this young man's wrestling career clearly illustrate what has been described as the 'sport ethic' (Hughes & Coakley, 1991). By adopting the sport ethic athletes learn to define sacrifice, risk, pain and injury as the price one must pay to be accepted as an athlete in competitive sports. In many sport groups the sport ethic provides the criteria to evaluate oneself and others as athletes and to gain status among peers. When these criteria are accepted uncritically, athletes often overconform to them to the point that they jeopardize the health and physical well-being of themselves and others. And they do this in the name of duty, honour, loyalty and self-respect. Use of the sport ethic to evaluate self and others has been noted in other research on socialization through sport (Ewald & Jiobu, 1985; Sabo & Panepinto, 1990; Nixon, 1991).

Sport rituals and community socialization processes: a study of sport in the culture of a small town

Foley (1990) studied the connection between sport events and community socialization processes in a small Texas town by using field methods (observation, participant observation, and informal and formal interviews) over a 2-year period. His analysis was guided by popular culture theory and an interactionist model of socialization. His goal was to view the socialization process from a broad, holistic perspective. In particular, Foley wanted to examine the extent to which sport served as a site for cultural practices through which community members might resist and transform the capitalist, racial and patriarchal order that defined social life in their town. He found that sport in general and high school football in particular were important community rituals that partially constituted a general socialization process in the social life of the town.

Although Foley set out to examine sport as a site for progressive practices challenging the dominance of a small élite group who controlled capital resources in the town, he found few examples. Resistance and counterhegemonic cultural practices did occur, but they produced few effects beyond specific individuals and immediate situations. This led Foley to conclude that high school sports in small towns are quite likely to reproduce and reaffirm the status quo even when the status quo works to the disadvantage of many, especially women, minorities and low income people.

Foley's work indicates that socialization through sport occurs in connection with the economic, political and cultural systems that make up the everyday culture of a community. Although sports can serve as sites for social practices that might actually change the culture of a community in some way, or the ways in which young people see themselves and their connections to the community at large, Foley found that high school sports are social rituals that reproduce the forms of social inequality in race, class and gender relations that characterize life in many communities. Ethnographic research done by Eder and Parker (1987) in a racially mixed high school in a medium-sized, American mid-western community supports Foley's findings: highly visible extracurricular activities such as varsity sports and cheerleading reproduce gender inequities in the peer culture of the school. Other research indicates that this process has occurred throughout history (O'Hanlon, 1980) and across cultural settings (Carrington et al., 1987).

Sport participation and the social construction of masculinity: a study of socialization among male athletes

Messner (1992) combined feminist theory with an interactionist model of socialization to study the ways in which masculinities (i.e. different ideas about masculinity) were socially constructed in connection with men's athletic careers. Open-ended in-depth interviews were conducted with 30 former athletes from different racial and social class backgrounds to discover how gender identities developed and changed as men interacted with the socially constructed world of sports. Messner notes that the men in his study began their first sport experiences with already gendered identities; in fact, their emerging identities during childhood were associated with their initial attraction to sport. The men had not entered sports as 'blank slates' ready to be 'filled in' with culturally approved masculine orientations and behaviours. Instead, as their athletic careers progressed, these men constructed orientations, relationships and experiences 'consistent with the dominant values and power relations of the larger gender order'. Overall, their masculinity was based on (i) limited definitions of public success; (ii) relationships with men in which bonds were shaped by homophobia (i.e. a generalized fear of and objection to all homosexuality and homosexuals) and misogyny (a general disdain for women); and (iii) a willingness to use their bodies as tools of domination regardless of consequences for health or general well-being. This socially constructed masculinity influenced how these men presented themselves in public as well as their relationships with women, and it engendered a continuing sense of insecurity about issues related to their 'manhood'.

Messner also found that socialization through sports is a complex process that does not always simply and unambiguously reproduce a gender order in which all men have power and privilege. For example:

1 Sport participation brought many of the men in his study temporary public recognition, but

discouraged formation of needed intimate relationships with other men and with women.

2 It enabled the men to develop physical competence, but frequently led to chronic health problems.

3 It offered career opportunities, but opportunities varied depending on the sexual preferences and the racial and class backgrounds of the men.

4 It provided guidelines on how to be a man, but the involvement and success of women in sport raised serious questions for those who had learned that becoming a man necessarily involved detaching themselves from all things female.

Messner's research indicates that sport participation is a process through which men enhance their public status, create non-intimate bonds of loyalty with each other, perpetuate patriarchal relationships with women, and construct masculinity in a way that privileges some men over others. This process is sometimes challenged by participants, but transformations of sport and sport experiences are difficult to initiate because sport itself has been constructed in ways that perpetuate the notion that male privilege is grounded in nature and biological destiny. Messner's work calls attention to the fact that gender is a social construction and that sport offers a fruitful site for exploring the formation of gender identities as part of the overall process of socialization through sport. This has also been noted in Palzkill's (1990) research on women in élite, amateur sports.

Changing sport to create alternative socialization experiences: a study of women softball players

Birrell and Richter (1987) used feminist theory informed by interactionist and cultural studies approaches to study the way in which sport was socially constructed by selected women involved in recreational slow-pitch softball leagues in two communities. Intensive interviews and observations over 4 years focused on the ways feminist consciousness might inform and structure women's sport experiences, the interpretation of those experiences, and the integration of the experiences into women's lives. Birrell and Richter reported that the women in their study were concerned with developing and expressing skills, playing hard and challenging opponents, but that they wanted to do these things without adopting orientations characterized by (i) an overemphasis on winning; (ii) power relationships between players and coaches; (iii) social exclusion and skill-based élitism; (iv) an ethic of risk and endangerment; and (v) the derogation of opponents. In other words, the women attempted to create alternative sport experiences that were 'process oriented, collective, supportive, inclusive, and infused with an ethic of care'.

Birrell and Richter found that creating an alternative to sport forms that promoted male interests could not be done without extended struggle. Transformations in the way teams were organized and the way games were played came slowly over the 4-year research period, but they did come. This provided the women with a sense of satisfaction, enjoyable sport experiences, and reaffirmation of their collective feminist consciousness and feelings of political empowerment.

Birrell and Richter's research illustrates that sport is not so much a product as it is a process of invention. This invention process is grounded in the consciousness and collective reflection of the participants themselves, and it is shaped by their conversations about experiences, feelings, decisions, behaviours, accounts of and responses to incidents, and a combination of individual and collective conclusions about the connection between sport and the lives of the participants. In other words, not only is sport a social construction, but so too are the consequences of participation. This is crucial to remember when socialization through sport is being discussed.

Summary

These six examples of research illustrate current approaches to socialization through sport. Each study highlights some dimension of socialization as it occurs in connection with sport participation and shows that participation itself is a social process with emergent qualities tied to the interests of those involved and the context in which it occurs. This means that it makes much more sense to frame discussions of socialization through sport in terms of human agency, cultural practices, struggle, power relations and social construction than it does to frame them in terms of specific measurable character traits of athletes and former athletes as they might compare to the character traits of 'non-athletes'.

Conclusion

This discussion of socialization through sport highlights major changes in the conceptual and methodological approaches used in research, and major research findings. Until the late 1970s an internalization model was used to guide research. According to this model human beings were assumed to be passive learners who internalized the norms and orientations associated with being an athlete. These norms and orientations were assumed to be transmitted through important social relationships. This gave the impression that athletes were naive, powerless actors simply responding to and internalizing the world around them. Research findings based on this conceptualization of socialization have been confusing, although longitudinal studies suggest that participation in organized, competitive sports does not so much change people as much as it provides a context in which important social relationships might be established, nurtured and maintained; these relationships then become the foundation of socialization experiences.

Researchers have more recently realized that sport and sport experiences are social construc-tions and that interactionist research models are needed to capture the dynamics of socialization through sport. Use of interactionist models has been encouraged by a growing awareness among social science researchers that sports and sport participation are parts of larger processes of social relations encompassing gender, class, race, ethnicity and sexual orientations. Since sports are themselves parts of social and cultural formations, socialization through sport cannot be separated from the economic and political practices that often constrain people's choices and activities, nor can it be separated from human agency and processes of resistance and transformation. This means that socialization through sport cannot be approached in terms of unreflexive responses to specific events, relationships and external forces. Socialization research has begun to take into account the fact that sport participation is a socially constructed process mediated by power relations and the consciousness and collective reflection of participants. Research based on interactionist models has begun to uncover the dynamics of differing social realities in sport, and to contextualize those realities so we can better understand how sport practices are connected to larger social and cultural formations.

Challenges for future research

In the light of recent conceptual and methodological developments, future research on socialization through sport faces the following challenges:

• Developing research methodologies that can be effectively and ethically used to understand the role of physical activities and sport in the lives of young children, and the way children see themselves, their connections to others, and their abilities to control and alter the social worlds in which they live their lives.

• Discovering the ways in which social relationships among participants in sport serve to mediate, extend or subvert the moral messages and lessons that coaches, parents, and other adults often try to associate with sport participation.

• Outlining the range of different meanings associated with being an athlete among people at different stages in their lives, and how those meanings change over time.

• Explaining the ways in which the sport experiences of individuals and groups are combined with experiences related to gender, race, ethnicity/nationality, class and sexual orientation, and then integrated into the social construction of identities.

• Discovering the ways in which identities associated with sport participation inform decisions about what people do in sport and in other spheres of life as they move from childhood to and through adulthood.

• Clearly specifying when sport and sport participation lead to the reproduction *or* the transformation of dominant forms of social relations in groups, organizations, communities and societies.

• Identifying the processes through which alternative forms of sport may be developed to meet the collective concerns of groups seeking experiences that do not reproduce inequities related to gender, race and ethnicity, and social class.

These topics do not deal with the question of whether sport builds character. Instead, they are based on the recognition that sport experiences are diversified, given different meanings over time and from one person to the next, and integrated into people's lives in different ways. The question of whether sport builds character has been misleading and has, until recently, inhibited research on the process of sport participation itself. Research on the role of sports in the lives of children in particular is often difficult to conduct due to the privacy and informed consent issues; these issues are especially difficult to deal with when conducting qualitative research that involves long-term access to the life experiences of children. And it is qualitative research that is needed as we attempt to discover more about socialization through sport.

References

Adler, P.A. & Adler, P. (1991) *Backboards and Blackboards: College Athletes and Role Engulfment.* Columbia University Press, New York.

Birrell, S. & Richter, D.M. (1987) Is a diamond forever? Feminist transformations of sport. *Women's Studies Int. Forum* **10**, 395–409.

Carrington, B., Chivers, T. & Williams, T. (1987) Gender, leisure and sport: a case-study of young people of South Asian descent. *Leisure Studies* **6**, 265–79.

Coakley, J. (1993) Sport and socialization. *Exerc. Sport Sci. Rev.* **21**, 169–200.

Curry, T. (1992) A little pain never hurt anyone: athletic career socialization and the normalization of sports injury. *Symbolic Interact.* **16**, 273–90.

Eder, D. & Parker, S. (1987) The cultural production and reproduction of gender: the effect of extracurricular activities on peer-group culture. *Sociol. Educ.* **60**, 200–13.

Ewald, K. & Jiobu, R.M. (1985) Explaining positive deviance: Becker's model and the case of runners and bodybuilders. *Sociol. Sport J.* **2**, 144–56.

Fine, G.A. (1987) *With the Boys: Little League Baseball and Preadolescent Culture.* University of Chicago Press, Chicago.

Foley, D.E. (1990) The great American football ritual: reproducing race, class, and gender inequality. *Sociol. Sport J.* **7**, 111–35.

Hauser, W.J. & Lueptow, L.B. (1978) Participation in athletics and academic achievement: a replication and extension. *Sociol. Q.* **19**, 309–9.

Hughes, R.H. & Coakley, J. (1991) Positive deviance among athletes: the implications of overconformity to the sport ethic. *Sociol. Sport J.* **8**, 307–25.

McCormack, J.B. & Chalip, L. (1988) Sport as socialization: a critique of methodological premises. *Social Sci. J.* **25**, 83–92.

McPherson, B.D. & Brown, B. (1988) The structure, processes, and consequences of sport for children. In F.L. Smoll, R.A. Magill & M.J. Ash (eds) *Children in Sport*, pp. 265–86. Human Kinetics, Champaign, IL.

Melnick, M.J., Vanfossen, B.E. & Sabo, D.E. (1988) Developmental effects of athletic participation among high school girls. *Sociol. Sport J.* **5**, 22–36.

Messner, M.A. (1992) *Power at Play: Sports and the Problem of Masculinity.* Beacon Press, Boston.

Meyer, B.B. (1990) From idealism to actualization: the academic performance of female collegiate athletes. *Sociol. Sport J.* **7**, 44–57.

Nixon, H.L. (1991) *Accepting the risks and pain of sports injuries: understanding the nature of 'consent' to play.* Paper presented at the North American Society for the Sociology of Sport Conference, Milwaukee, November.

O'Hanlon, T. (1980) Interscholastic athletics, 1900–1940: shaping citizens for unequal roles in modern industrial states. *Educ. Theory* **30**, 89–103.

Palzkill, B. (1990) Between gymshoes and high-heels — the development of a lesbian identity and existence in top class sport. *Int. Rev. Sociol. Sport* **25**, 221–33.

Rees, C.R., Howell, F.M. & Miracle, A.W. (1990) Do high school sports build character? A quasi-experiment on a national sample. *Social Sci. J.* **27**, 303–15.

Sabo, D.F. & Panepinto, J. (1990) Football ritual and the social reproduction of masculinity. In M.A. Messner & D.F. Sabo (eds) *Sport, Men, and the Gender Order*, pp. 115–26. Human Kinetics, Champaign, IL.

Spreitzer, E. (1992) *Does participation in interscholastic athletics affect adult development? A longitudinal analysis of an 18–24 age cohort.* Paper presented at the American Sociological Association Conference, Pittsburgh, August.

Wentworth, W.M. (1980) *Context and Understanding: An Inquiry into Socialization Theory.* Elsevier, New York.

Chapter 25

Self-esteem and Perceptions of Competence in Youth Sports: Theory, Research and Enhancement Strategies

MAUREEN R. WEISS AND VICKI EBBECK

Introduction

Christine, a 10-year-old soccer player in a local YMCA league, often shows apathy during practices and competitions, which is characterized by a cursory show of effort, an unhappy demeanour and low performance levels. Hannah portrays a stark contrast to her teammate: she readily looks forward to participation, puts forth a high level of intensity during play, performs up to her potential and exhibits pride and pleasure in her accomplishments. Why do these two individuals think, feel and behave so differently? One possible answer is their self-perceptions in the domain of sport. Christine perceives a low sense of physical capabilities, while Hannah possesses a high level of competence perceptions. These differing self-perceptions, in turn, result in variations in motivation, performance and emotional reactions to sport participation.

This chapter will focus on the important individual characteristic of self-perceptions, generally defined as thoughts and feelings by individuals about themselves as persons, in general, or their abilities in a particular achievement domain such as sports, academics or social activities. We will specifically focus on the self-perceptions of: (i) general self-esteem (i.e. self-appraisal of oneself as a person); and (ii) perceptions of competence (i.e. evaluation of one's capabilities to perform in a specific domain or situation). This topic is important because self-perceptions have been found to

explain differences in levels of performance, achievement behaviours (e.g. effort, persistence) and positive and negative emotional reactions among young participants in sport. More specifically, an understanding of self-esteem and perceptions of physical competence may provide a window for explaining the varying behaviours and motivation of the many Christines and Hannahs (and Charlies and Harolds) as they pursue their sporting experiences.

Our objective is to illuminate an understanding of how self-perceptions are formed and how they influence behaviour in the physical domain. To do this, theories of self-perceptions and associated empirical research are reviewed in order to explain the mechanisms underlying self-esteem and perceived competence. Then, strategies for enhancing physical perceptions of competence and general self-esteem will follow, and challenges for future research will conclude this chapter.

Self-esteem

Terminology

The study of self-perceptions has produced a plethora of terms that are akin to a foreign language. A certain degree of interpretation is necessary, therefore, in order to differentiate key terms, although specific definitions are not provided in this chapter and may not even be desirable (Hattie, 1992). What is most essential is to identify the unique characteristics that are associated with self-esteem in order to highlight the importance of this construct.

Undoubtedly, most discussion regarding terminology has revolved around the two terms *self-concept* and *self-esteem*. The meaning of the two terms and how they are related continues to be the focus of considerable debate (Berger & McInman, 1993). Traditionally, self-concept has been aligned with self-description, while self-esteem has been identified with the process of self-evaluation (Weiss, 1987; Fox, 1988). This distinction, however, is arguably too simplistic for the following reasons: (i) self-description and self-evaluation are not readily distinguishable (Shavelson *et al.*, 1976); (ii) self-concept has been construed to include an evaluative component (Shavelson *et al.*, 1976; Wylie, 1979); and (iii) self-evaluation is not exclusively associated with self-esteem but also terms such as self-acceptance (Waite *et al.*, 1990). A more appropriate approach to conceptualizing self-concept and self-esteem is to consider self-esteem as part of an individual's self-concept (Fleming & Courtney, 1984). Self-conceptions logically encompass self-esteem given that self-conceptions have been broadly defined by Markus and Wurf (1987) so as to include 'self-representations that can be the subject of conscious reflection' (p. 305). Thus, self-esteem is one of a myriad of self-conceptions that in combination comprise the self-concept.

Early notions of the self-concept as a stagnant and unitary entity have been replaced by the contention that the self-concept represents both a dynamic and multidimensional self-system (Markus & Wurf, 1987; Oosterwegel & Oppenheimer, 1993). According to Markus and colleagues (Markus & Kunda, 1986; Markus & Wurf, 1987), a subset of self-conceptions will be accessible or working at any one time that is comprised of core self-conceptions as well as surrounding tentative self-conceptions. The core self-conceptions are central to defining the self and tend to be always accessible, unlike the tentative self-conceptions whose accessibility is dependent upon the immediate social situation. Being a good athlete could represent a core self-conception for an individual who also tentatively views himself or herself as insensitive after laughing at an injured teammate. Examples of the different self-conceptions include real (how people actually perceive themselves) and ideal (how people would like to be) selves that can be perceived from the individual's own perspective or from the perspective of others (Oosterwegel & Oppenheimer, 1993). Most attention in the literature has been paid to how people perceive their ability or adequacy across a variety of domains that represent academic, social, physical and personal development (Harter, 1986; Marsh & Peart, 1988). With regard to physical development, four specific self-conceptions have been identified including (i) sport competence; (ii) physical strength; (iii) physical conditioning; and (iv) body attractiveness (Fox & Corbin, 1989; Whitehead, 1991).

Recognizing the many and varied self-conceptions that exist within this self-system raises the question as to what exactly is unique about self-esteem. Therefore, it is necessary to identify the discerning features of self-esteem that in combination make self-esteem unlike any other self-conception. Most importantly, self-esteem involves an individual's assessment of his or her own worth (Coopersmith, 1981; Harter, 1986; Rosenberg, 1986). High self-esteem individuals view themselves favourably and are satisfied with themselves, whereas low self-esteem individuals tend to lack self-respect and feel inadequate. Second, self-esteem is context-free and subsequently viewed as a more global construct than domain-specific self-conceptions (Wylie, 1979; Harter, 1986). Furthermore, self-esteem is not merely an aggregate of domain-specific self-conceptions but an independent construct (Harter, 1987). Third, self-esteem development is a function of particular influencing factors that help define what does and does not constitute self-esteem. For example, the formation of self-esteem is contingent upon domain-specific self-conceptions while another global, positive self-regard construct such as self-acceptance is unconditional and not influenced by perceptions of competence or adequacy (Waite *et al.*, 1990). Knowing the factors that influence self-esteem development provides a greater understanding about the nature of self-esteem. Consequently, the factors that influence self-esteem are identified and discussed in the following conceptual framework that delineates the determinants and consequences of self-esteem development.

Conceptual framework

A conceptual model that can identify the constructs affected by self-esteem as well as the constructs that impact self-esteem development is clearly beneficial. The consequences of self-esteem explain why it is desirable for people to have high self-esteem, while the determinants of self-esteem suggest how self-esteem might be enhanced. Harter (1987) has proposed such a model that illustrates the interconnectedness of self-esteem and related constructs. The model was grounded in existing conceptual frameworks and theories, and has been empirically tested with children. An adapted version of Harter's original model is shown in Fig. 25.1.

The two consequences of self-esteem depicted in Harter's model include affect and motivation. Self-esteem influences motivation both directly and indirectly via affect, although the indirect relationship is stronger than the direct relationship. Consequently, an individual's personal evaluation of worth will result in certain emotions that, in turn, will determine an individual's motivation or choice of activities, effort and persistence. High self-esteem is likely to produce feelings of happiness, pride and satisfaction which are in contrast to the feelings of sadness, depression and anxiety that may result from low self-esteem. It is then expected that positive affect will encourage behaviours such as seeking optimal challenges, exerting maximum effort and persisting over time, and that negative affect will lead to avoidance of challenging tasks, minimal effort and withdrawal. These very different emotions and behaviours of high and low self-esteem individuals certainly highlight the need to examine the factors and underlying mechanisms that determine an individual's level of self-esteem.

One determinant of self-esteem discussed by Harter is domain-specific self-conceptions. Specifically, self-esteem is thought to be influenced by perceptions of competence or adequacy in achievement domains that are perceived to be important. This notion is derived from the work of James (1890) and suggests that an individual who perceives he or she is competent in a particular domain will experience increased self-esteem, if the individual values competence in that particular domain. Thus the athlete who thinks he or she

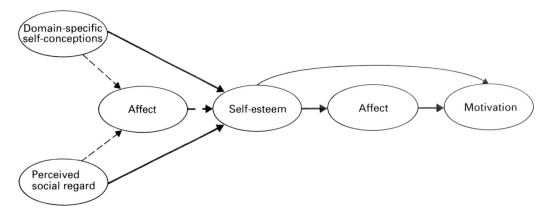

Fig. 25.1 Antecedents–consequences model of self-esteem. Adapted from Harter (1987).

is talented in sport and believes that being good at sports is important will likely benefit from increased feelings of worthiness. Moreover, an individual with low perceptions of competence in a domain that is valued will experience decreased self-esteem. Supposedly, it is only in those domains considered unimportant to the individual that perceptions of competence will not affect self-esteem development. To date, the literature has supported a positive relationship between domain-specific self-conceptions and self-esteem, but research results suggest that only a small amount of the variance in self-esteem is accounted for by the perceived importance of being competent in a particular domain (Marsh, 1986). The interplay among self-esteem, self-conceptions and perceived importance further pertains to the process of discounting (Harter, 1986). According to this phenomenon, individuals protect their self-esteem by discounting the importance of those domains in which self-conceptions are low and endorsing the importance of those domains associated with positive self-conceptions. Therefore, low self-esteem can result not only from low perceptions of competence in domains that are perceived to be important, but also from the inability to discount the importance of domains associated with negative self-conceptions.

Another determinant of self-esteem in Harter's model is perceived social regard or how individuals perceive they are regarded by others. If individuals think that they are positively regarded by significant others, then self-esteem will increase; self-esteem will decrease if individuals perceive that they are viewed unfavourably by others. Consequently, self-esteem is a social construction susceptible to how individuals appraise the views of others about the self. This idea stems from Cooley (1902) who coined the phrase 'looking-glass self' suggesting that individuals come to see themselves through others. Conceivably, self-esteem could be protected by an individual surrounding himself or herself with select people who appear to view the individual favourably, so that one's personal evaluation of worth would reflect the perceived positive evaluation of others. Perceived social regard, then, serves to accentuate the role played by social interactions in the development of self-esteem.

A final determinant of self-esteem is affect. Harter's model did not identify affect as an antecedent of self-esteem (hence the use of broken lines in Fig. 25.1), but there is sufficient support in the literature to suggest that self-conceptions and perceived social regard influence affect which subsequently influences self-esteem. First, affect is thought to be a consequence of the subset of self-conceptions that are active at any one time (Salovey & Rodin, cited in Markus & Wurf, 1987). Ebbeck and Weiss (1992), for example, found an indirect relationship in which affect experienced in sport mediated the physical self-conception/ self-esteem relationship was stronger than a direct relationship between self-conception of physical ability and self-esteem. Second, the notion of perceived social approval where people imagine how they are seen and judged by others is going to include an affective element where individuals feel, for example, proud or mortified (Hattie, 1992). Third, the relationship between affect and self-esteem is considered bidirectional so that an emotion such as anxiety can impact or be impacted by self-esteem (Coopersmith, 1981; Rosenberg, 1989). Future research may reveal that the predominant emotions influencing self-esteem are different emotions to those generated by self-esteem, but for now the main concern is to include affect as a viable determinant of self-esteem development. Therefore, in combination, the determinants of self-esteem demonstrate that cognitions, social interactions and affect are all central to how an individual evaluates his or her worth.

Empirical research

The self-esteem construct has received considerable attention in the empirical literature.

Studies conducted in the physical activity setting with children and adolescents often include a self-report measure of self-esteem. Self-esteem has been examined in relation to the acquisition of motor skills, fitness levels and different physical education instructional techniques (see Gruber, 1986). A particularly fertile area, however, for investigating self-esteem has been organized youth sports. Sport is a valued achievement domain in many societies that is characterized by overt displays of ability and inability, and represents a microcosm of complex social interactions. The sport context has stimulated a variety of research questions that have incorporated self-esteem and resulted in the examination of self-esteem across studies utilizing diverse investigative approaches. A brief review of these studies provides an idea about the current status of self-esteem research in youth sports.

A common research design involves the assessment of self-esteem in order to explore group differences. In such cases, the average self-esteem score for each group is statistically compared with other group means on the same variable. For example, fourth and fifth grade participants in organized sport reported significantly higher levels of self-esteem than non-participants (Roberts et al., 1981). With a sample of 10–15-year-old male soccer players, Passer (1983) found that high competitive-trait-anxious individuals had significantly lower self-esteem scores than low competitive-trait-anxious individuals, although the magnitude of the difference was small. In a study that replicated and extended Passer's work with male and female youth baseball and softball players, Brustad and Weiss (1987) also found that high competitive-trait-anxious males had significantly lower self-esteem scores than low competitive-trait-anxious males, but the findings for the girls indicated a non-significant relationship between levels of competitive trait anxiety and self-esteem. Furthermore, Richman and Rehberg (1986) investigated karate students and discovered that the novice group was significantly lower in self-esteem than the three

groups with higher skill levels. These descriptive studies provide an account of the similarities and differences in self-esteem across categories of individuals.

Self-esteem has also been explored in field-based studies that entail an experimental intervention. The purpose of these studies is to determine whether individuals exposed to a particular treatment experience levels of self-esteem that are significantly greater than the self-esteem levels of individuals not exposed to the treatment. Smith et al. (1979), for example, randomly assigned 31 Little League baseball coaches to either a training or control group at the start of the season. Trained coaches were instructed in the use of positive coaching behaviours such as providing encouragement and instruction. After controlling for player self-esteem scores that were obtained a year earlier, postseason measures of self-esteem suggested that individuals who played for the trained coaches felt significantly better about themselves than individuals who played for the control coaches. Smoll et al. (1993) similarly compared the self-esteem scores of Little League baseball players who were coached by either trained or control coaches. After controlling for preseason levels of self-esteem, postseason self-esteem scores were not significantly different for individuals who played for the trained and control coaches. Low self-esteem children who played for the trained coaches, however, experienced significantly higher levels of self-esteem at the end of the season than low self-esteem individuals who played for the control coaches. This finding suggests that interventions may not be equally beneficial for all individuals and that the examination of subgroup differences across low, medium and high self-esteem individuals should also be considered in research designs.

A final collection of studies that incorporate self-esteem have examined predictors of self-esteem or the influence of self-esteem on other variables. Hines and Groves (1989) assessed which of several factors associated with basketball competition predicted self-esteem development. The findings revealed that positive subjective ratings by the coach of each player's ability as well as participating for fun and skill development reasons were the factors that resulted in higher levels of self-esteem. Ebbeck and Stuart (1993), in a study involving youth football players, found that perceived football competence, the perceived importance to the individual of being a good football player and the perceived importance to the team of being a good football player collectively predicted self-esteem and accounted for 47% of the variance in self-esteem. Both perceived football competence and individual importance significantly contributed to explaining self-esteem, although perceived football competence was the strongest predictor. The outcomes, as opposed to predictors, of self-esteem were investigated by Brustad (1988) in a study that examined the influence of self-esteem, along with other intrapersonal and socialization factors, on affect experienced in sport. Results pertaining to self-esteem were consistent for boys and girls participating in a youth basketball league and revealed that self-esteem significantly and negatively predicted competitive trait anxiety; however, self-esteem was not predictive of levels of enjoyment. Therefore, the findings from these studies provide some support for the conceptual model that has been proposed regarding the antecedents and consequences of self-esteem.

An alternative model of self-esteem development conceived specifically for the physical domain has been proposed by Sonstroem and Morgan (1989). This model is characterized by a continuum of self-perceptions that increase in generality. Improvement in physical ability produces positive self-efficacy (task-specific self-confidence) which subsequently increases perceived physical competence which, in turn, enhances self-esteem. Self-esteem might also be enhanced as a function of greater physical acceptance (feeling good about one's physical appearance) which results from increased perceived competence. Initial support for this model has recently been documented with male

adolescent swimmers (Sonstroem et al., 1993). Continued model testing with child and adolescent samples will undoubtedly be the focus of future studies.

The empirical interest in self-esteem that has been demonstrated to date in the literature is encouraging. Obviously the study of self-esteem development in the youth sport setting has proven to be both feasible and relevant. Despite the progress that has been made, however, there are several concerns regarding the current trends in self-esteem research that need to be addressed if a comprehensive understanding of self-esteem is to be achieved in the future. A relatively limited number of self-esteem studies have been conducted, which is surprising given the extensive history associated with the topic and the importance so frequently attached to the study of self-esteem. Certainly most studies have not employed a conceptual or theoretical guiding framework which would help decipher not only if group differences exist or if an intervention is effective but also why self-esteem is significantly higher for some people and in some situations. Finally, the measures used to assess self-esteem in some instances could be challenged because the one-dimensional view of self-esteem upon which certain measures are based is inconsistent with the current multidimensional approach to the self-system (Harter, 1986). Therefore, opportunities exist for re-evaluating and subsequently improving the process by which self-esteem is studied in youth sports so that research in this area continues to be profitable.

Perceptions of physical competence

While self-esteem was defined as an individual's global evaluation of worth as a person, perceptions of competence refer to one's description and evaluation of, as well as affect toward, their abilities in a *particular domain* (e.g. academics, sport, social relationships) or *subdomain* (e.g. mathematics, swimming, peer acceptance). Thus, in line with terminology presented in the previous section, perceptions of competence can be equated with domain-specific self-conceptions. When considering the child's self-perceptions in the physical domain, we are interested in how perceptions of physical competence are developed and, subsequently, how these self-appraisals influence future motivated behaviour such as adherence to an activity programme, persistence at difficult skills and the intrinsic desire to continue participation.

Several theories highlight the role of competence perceptions in predicting motivation, emotions and performance (Bandura, 1977; Harter, 1978, 1981; Nicholls, 1984; Deci & Ryan, 1985; Eccles & Harold, 1991). For example, central constructs in Harter's competence motivation theory include perceptions of competence and locus of control, influence from significant others and emotional reactions to performance. Specifically, mastery attempts on the part of youngsters which result in perceptions of success, positive reinforcement by significant others, enhanced perceptions of competence and control, and positive affective reactions are likely to be continued and be characterized by effort, persistence and intensity. Thus, major theories of motivation, although different in their central foci, all identify self-perceptions of competence as a crucial personal characteristic driving participation choice, effort and persistence.

The empirical research to date has examined self-perceptions in the physical domain in two primary ways. One set of studies has focused on understanding antecedents, or sources of developing self-perceptions, such as mastery experiences, social influences and emotional investment in and effort exerted toward activity. The other set of studies has primarily examined the consequences of perceived ability such as affective reactions, motivation and sport performance. The major findings from both these approaches are presented in turn.

Sources of competence perceptions in the physical domain

In the sport setting, countless opportunities exist to form judgements about self-competencies. Communication from significant others such as parents, coaches, teammates and spectators; the comparison of ability to same-age peers; indices of how quickly skills are learned and improved and the achievement of specific skill goals are all common information sources. Other salient information includes (i) performance statistics; (ii) amount of playing time or player status; (iii) game outcome and win/loss record; (iv) the degree of attraction toward or enjoyment of the activity and, conversely, the level of nervousness experienced prior to competitions. These sources are used by youngsters to form expectations and evaluations of their competence.

AGE-RELATED DIFFERENCES

A series of studies by Horn and colleagues demonstrates age-related preferences in children's use of information to form judgements of physical competence (Horn & Hasbrook, 1986; Horn & Weiss, 1991; Horn et al., 1993). Specifically, children under the age of 10 years indicated they rely more heavily upon (i) adult feedback such as parents, teachers/coaches and spectators; (ii) game outcome; and (iii) attraction toward or enjoyment of sport than do children 10–14 years of age. Older youth, in contrast, prefer peer comparison and evaluation as a primary means to judge competence. This reliance upon the peer group begins to decline in the later adolescent years (16–18 years), and greater emphasis is placed on self-referenced information such as degree of exerted effort, skill improvement over time, self-motivation and personal goal achievement. From middle childhood through late adolescence, then, there is a shift from adult feedback and peer comparison/evaluation to internal cues and personal comparison as salient information sources by which to determine levels of physical competence.

In addition to age-related preferences for sources of information, research indicates that young children are inaccurate in their competence ratings when compared to objective performance evaluations (Stipek & Mac Iver, 1989; Horn & Weiss, 1991). In fact, little or no correlation between actual and perceived competence exists for children under the age of 10 years. As children mature through the elementary and middle school years, they become increasingly capable of accurately estimating their physical competence. Horn and Weiss found that increases in accuracy of self-perceived competence could be attributed, at least in part, to the shift in sources of information relied upon by younger and older children. As children shifted in emphasis from adult feedback to peer comparison and evaluation, accuracy in estimating personal competence increased. However, these researchers also showed that children who underestimated their competencies in relation to actual competence almost exclusively relied upon the use of peer comparison and evaluation. Therefore, children need to be encouraged to use a wide range of information sources, both internal and external, in order to make accurate and positive judgments of their competence. Table 25.1 depicts the sources of competence information that are used most frequently by and distinguish age groups.

GENDER PREFERENCES FOR INFORMATION SOURCES

Research across middle and late childhood has revealed no gender differences on preferences for information (Horn & Hasbrook, 1986, 1987; Horn & Weiss, 1991). However, differences show up starting in early adolescence and extend through young adulthood (Ebbeck, 1990; Horn et al., 1993). Specifically, Horn et al. found that adolescent female athletes placed greater importance on the use of self-comparison information and feedback from peers, coaches and spectators than male athletes, who identified competitive outcomes (e.g. game statistics, win/loss record) and speed/ease of learning skills as primary forms of judging personal competence.

PERSONALITY CHARACTERISTICS AND COMPETENCE SOURCES

Two studies suggest that preferences for competence information sources are related to psychological characteristics such as perceived ability, locus of control, self-esteem and dispositional anxiety (Horn & Hasbrook, 1987; Weiss et al., 1992). Horn and Hasbrook found that children of 10–14 years of age who were higher in perceived physical competence placed emphasis upon peer comparison and evaluation, coach feedback, self-referenced information (e.g. skill improvement) and attraction for sport involvement — a wide variety of informational sources — for judging personal competence. Children higher in external locus of control were associated with higher scores on game outcome as a source of information. Weiss et al. (1992) simultaneously examined trait anxiety, perceived physical competence and self-esteem with sources of competence information among 8–13-year-old youth. Younger children who were relatively high in trait anxiety and low in perceived competence indicated primary use of information in the form of worry and nervousness before games, little reliance upon peer comparison and evaluation, as well as self-referenced information such as effort exerted and skill improvement. In contrast, older children with the same pattern of psychological characteristics used social comparison and evaluation as their information source of choice,

Table 25.1 Age-related differences in sources of information used to judge physical competence.

Age (years)	Sources*
8–9	Game outcome
	Adult feedback (parents, coaches)
10–13	Peer comparison and evaluation
14–15	Peer evaluation
16–18	Self-comparison/internal information
	Goal achievement
	Sport attraction/enjoyment

* All age groups use a variety of information sources to judge personal competence. The sources in this list represent those that have been shown to distinguish these age groups.

and assigned low importance to self-referenced information and parental feedback.

Taken together, these findings indicate that sources of information children and adolescents rely upon to form judgements of physical competence vary by age, gender and personality characteristics. Specific research studies have further explored the influence of significant others on self-perceptions of competence in the physical domain. The degree of positive and negative influence from the social environment surrounding sport has received considerable interest and attention in the public eye. Only recently have studies systematically examined the potential effects that parents, peers and coaches have on self-perceptions of competence developed in the sporting domain.

PARENTS

Eccles and Harold (1991) recently tested aspects of their expectancy-value model of activity choice with approximately 875 third to sixth grade male and female children. They found that boys scored significantly higher than girls on perceptions of sport competence, usefulness of sport learning, enjoyment of sport activities and importance of doing well in sport. To examine the possible origins of these differences, skill aptitude tests, ratings of parental beliefs and perceptions of gender-role stereotypes were obtained. Results indicated that motor skill tests favoured boys but the variance explained by gender was very low (2%). Strong differences were found on the other two variables: (i) both boys and girls indicated that it was more important for boys than for girls to have ability in sport; and (ii) boys indicated that it was more important to their parents that they do well and participate in sport than did girls. Finally, the more girls saw sport as appropriate for girls (and boys as appropriate for boys), the higher their evaluation of sport-related abilities, and the extent that children thought that their parents placed importance on being involved and excelling in sport, the higher their perceived competencies in sport.

The important role of parents in developing

self-perceptions was also reported by Felson (1989) in a study of fourth to eighth grade boys and girls. Children's reflected appraisals (beliefs about parents' perceptions of their sporting ability) were predictive of their own appraisals of ability. That is, children who perceived that their parents regarded their abilities highly also appraised their competencies highly, and the contrary for children who perceived low parental perceptions. Similarly, Dempsey et al. (1993) found a moderate correlation ($r = 0.41$) between children's perceived competence in moderate to vigorous physical activity and parents' perception of their child's physical competence. Finally, Brustad (1993) examined the influence of parental attitudes (enjoyment of and value toward physical activity) and encouragement on fourth-grade children's perceived physical competence, importance attached to being physically active and attraction to physical activity. A path analysis indicated that parental enjoyment of activity was predictive of their encouragement which, in turn, influenced children's perceived competence and importance attached to physical activity. This relationship was linked to gender, with boys perceiving higher competence in, assigning more importance to and perceiving greater encouragement to participate in sport from parents than girls.

PEERS

The child's peer group, including close friends, teammates and classmates, is a salient source of competence information from late childhood through the adolescent years (Horn & Hasbrook, 1986; Horn & Weiss, 1991; Horn et al., 1993). Despite this consistent finding, few studies have delved into the degree to which peers provide this important function. One finding, however, is that physical competence is strongly related to peer acceptance and social status, for boys and girls (Eitzen, 1975; Feltz, 1978; Evans & Roberts, 1987; Chase & Dummer, 1992; Weiss & Duncan, 1992). For example, Weiss and Duncan found that children (ages 8–13 years) who rated themselves as physically competent and who were rated by teachers as competent in sport were also those children who felt accepted by their peers and who were identified by teachers as competent in peer relationships.

COACHES

The coach has been singled out in youth sport publications as a salient source of development of positive self-perceptions, affect and motivation (e.g. Gould, 1988; Martens, 1990). Only a handful of studies, however, have been conducted to verify empirically these claims. Horn (1985) comprehensively examined the influence of coaching behaviours on physical self-perceptions among junior high school-aged female softball players. Results indicated that, above and beyond actual skill improvement over the season, observed measures of positive reinforcement decreased and criticism increased levels of perceived competence in young athletes. Although these results were opposite to hypothesized relationships, Horn attributed these findings to the degree of appropriateness of the reinforcement provided for performances of the athletes. The use of criticism by the coach was not simply a negative remark made in response to errors; instead, this behaviour was characterized as a verbal criticism of performance followed by information on how to improve in subsequent attempts. Many of the positive statements, however, were non-contingent to performance, often characterized by remarks of 'good job', 'way to go', and the like, and which may have decreased self-perceptions because the lack of information feedback may have conveyed the message that higher levels of performance were not attainable.

Black and Weiss (1992) replicated and extended Horn's (1985) study by examining perceptions of contingent coaching behaviour on young athletes' perceptions of competence, enjoyment and intrinsic motivation. Male and female age-group swimmers ranging in age from 10 to 18 years completed measures of their coaches' use of praise, information, encourage-

ment and criticism in response to desirable and undesirable performances, as well as self-perceptions, affect and motivational variables such as perceived effort, challenge and choice. Results supported Horn's findings in that contingent praise and information following good performances, and contingent encouragement and encouragement combined with information following skill errors, were associated with higher levels of perceived competence, success, enjoyment, challenge and effort. The combination of findings from these two studies point to the importance of the quality of coaching feedback and reinforcement on competence perceptions.

In summary, research on antecedents or sources of competence perceptions in the physical domain support contemporary motivational theories and underscore the crucial influences exerted by parents, friends and coaches. The research, though sparse, consistently points to the salience of a network of social support in attempts to enhance young athletes' perceived competence, enjoyment and motivation to continue participation in the physical domain.

Consequences or correlates of physical competence perception

Perceived competence has been implicated as a central construct in nearly every theory of motivation, and empirical research in the sport setting strongly supports this high ranking. Variations in self-ability perceptions have been found to relate to positive and negative affective responses to performance, achievement cognitions and motivated behaviour such as causal attributions for performance, locus of control and preference for challenge, and actual sport performance. Obviously, the influence of self-perceptions of competence on these variables maximizes the probability of positive experiences and continued participation in the physical domain.

PERCEIVED COMPETENCE AND AFFECTIVE RESPONSES

Several studies have demonstrated that children's perceptions of their physical competence are related to or directly influence positive (e.g. enjoyment, pride, happiness) and negative (e.g. boredom, anxiety, anger) affect in the physical domain. Scanlan and Lewthwaite (1986) found that 9–14-year-old wrestlers who perceived themselves to be high in physical ability experienced more enjoyment during the season than their low perceived ability peers. In a retrospective study of former élite figure skaters (Scanlan et al., 1989), perceived competence was the major source of enjoyment in competitive experiences. Perceived competence was operationally defined as mastery of skills, competitive and performance achievement, and demonstration of athletic ability. Interestingly, Scanlan et al. (1993), in a study of ethnically diverse children and youth 10–15 years of age, did not find perceived competence to be a significant predictor of sport enjoyment.

In Brustad's (1993) study reported earlier, parental influences on attraction to or liking of physical activity was mediated by the child's perceived competence in sport, which was the strongest contributor explaining the variance in attraction toward sport. Ebbeck and Weiss (1992) found that levels of perceived sport competence directly influenced experiences of positive and negative affect which, in turn, significantly influenced ratings of self-esteem. That is, children who reported higher levels of self-perceptions of sport ability experienced high levels of positive (pride, satisfaction, happy, excited) and low levels of negative (unhappy, guilty, angry) affect in sport.

PERCEIVED COMPETENCE AND ACHIEVEMENT COGNITIONS

In addition to affective consequences, achievement-related cognitions such as locus of control and causal attributions are related to varying levels of perceived physical competence. Locus or perceptions of control refer to the individual's determination of whether internal (e.g. ability, effort) or external (e.g. significant others, task difficulty, luck) factors are responsible for performance outcomes. Weiss et al. (1986) found that children higher in perceived physical competence were associated with higher scores on internal locus of control and lower external control perceptions. Perceptions of competence were, in turn, strongly predictive of performance and motivation. Specifically, perceived competence was associated with a preference to perform hard, challenging skills and the development of using internal criteria to determine performance levels. Weiss and Horn (1990) investigated the accuracy of children's estimates of physical competence and found that children who underestimated their competence reported higher levels of external and unknown loci of control than their accurate and overestimating peers. That is, these children whose perceptions were considerably lower than teacher's ratings of actual competence indicated that powerful others were responsible for their performance successes and failures, or that they did not know what or who controlled their behaviour.

Similar to perceptions of performance control, causal attributions deal with the explanations children give for perceived performance outcomes. According to Weiner's (1985) theory of achievement motivation, attributions for performance influence future motivated behaviour and performance through the mediation of affective responses and future expectations of success. Thus, attributions following success which can be classified as internal, stable and controllable (e.g. ability) are associated with positive affect, expectations and motivation. Following unsuccessful outcomes, unstable and controllable attributions are seen as positive influences on future motivated behaviour such as reasons related to poor decision-making, incorrect strategy or insufficient practice. However, stable and uncontrollable factors (e.g. inherent ability) would likely attenuate one's desire to try again.

Given this conceptualization, Weiss *et al.* (1990) examined the relationship between perceived physical competence and attributions for sport performance among 8–13-year-old children. They found support for theoretical predictions in that children who were higher in perceived competence made attributions for perceived success that were more internal, stable and personally controllable than did low perceived competence children. Moreover, children in the upper quartile of perceived competence scores could be discriminated from their lower quartile peers on the basis of perceived success, future success expectations and stability attributions.

PERCEIVED COMPETENCE, MOTIVATION AND SPORT PERFORMANCE

Studies examining the relation between perceived competence and indices of motivation have supported the powerful influence of self-perceptions. Early studies found that sport participants and non-participants (and drop-outs) could be distinguished based on levels of perceived physical competence (Roberts *et al.*, 1981; Feltz & Petlichkoff, 1983). However, Klint (1985) found that gymnasts who discontinued their participation in a competitive club actually scored higher in perceived physical and social competence than those who persisted. Further, Ulrich (1987) did not find a significant difference between sport participants and non-participants on perceived physical competence in 5–10-year-old children. Klint and Weiss (1987) followed these results with a study that examined the link between perceptions of competence and particular motives for participating. Indeed, children higher in perceived physical competence were associated with higher scores on reasons related to skill development, while those who scored higher in perceived social competence or peer acceptance cited friendships and team atmosphere as primary reasons for involvement. This study supported theoretical notions that children are motivated to demonstrate competence in those achievement domains in which they perceive themselves to have higher ability.

In studies reported earlier, quantity and quality of perceived physical competence were also associated with intrinsic motivation measures, notably preference for challenge, independent mastery and curiosity, as well as actual performance (Weiss *et al.*, 1986, 1989; Weiss & Horn, 1990). Weiss *et al.* (1986) found that youngsters higher in perceived competence positively and directly influenced levels of intrinsic motivation and sports performance. Similarly, Weiss *et al.* (1989) found that gymnasts' self-efficacy with regard to competitive performance was highly predictive of subsequent scores on five out of six events. Finally, Weiss and Horn found that underestimating children reported lower challenge motivation than children with accurate or overestimated competence perceptions.

In sum, the studies reported here demonstrate a strong relationship between competence perceptions in the physical domain and affective responses, perceptions of performance control and attributions for performance outcomes, and intrinsic motivation. Children with positive self-appraisals of ability experience higher levels of positive and lower levels of negative affect, an internal locus of control or self-determination and higher preferences for challenge and independent mastery in sport. Given that educators strive to maximize enjoyable experiences, intrinsic desire, and independence of mastery in students, strategies that focus on enhancing self-perceptions of competence and general self-esteem are critical.

Strategies for enhancing self-esteem and perceived competence

Information from theory and research in the physical domain concerning the development of self-esteem and perceived competence indicate recommendations for enhancement strategies that can be implemented by parents, teachers and coaches. These strategies can be categorized as mastery experiences, social support, maximizing positive affect and self-regulated learning or individual control strategies (Weiss, 1991).

Mastery experiences

Information pertaining to mastery of sport skills was found to be a salient source by which children judged their physical competence. This included self-referenced or personal comparison criteria such as ease in learning new skills, degree of effort exerted, achievement of skill goals and amount of skill improvement. It also included more norm-referenced or outcome information as game statistics, winning or losing, and comparison to and evaluation from same-age peers. Because norm-referenced sources tend to be overemphasized in the sport environment, it is strongly recommended that mastery experiences be defined as *optimal challenges* for each child, which are difficult, but attainable, goals that are customized to the individual's current skill capabilities and opportunities for improvement. In this way, children are motivated to achieve individualized and realistic personal standards of success.

TASK ANALYSIS OF DEVELOPMENTAL PROGRESSIONS

One way in which to provide optimal challenges, and thus ensure enhanced self-perceptions, is for teachers and coaches to outline a task analysis of the sport skills and strategies to be learned, which serve as short-term goals for children to strive for. In this way, the activity is matched to the child, and not the child to the activity as is the case with norm-referenced standards adopted in many classrooms and sport teams. For example, the American Red Cross has carefully considered the developmental progressions to be taught with each swimming stroke, and USA wrestling has adopted the 'seven basic skills' of proper skill execution and technique in which each skill is dependent upon successful mastery of the one preceding it.

GAME MODIFICATIONS

Equipment, facilities and rules can be changed in order to provide youth with more opportunities for practice, feedback and reinforcement for desirable performances and skill errors, and thus optimal learning and mastery of skills. Changes in equipment might include shorter baskets in basketball to encourage proper shooting technique, narrower goals in soccer to emphasize passing and shooting skills, and softer volleyballs and baseballs to reduce the fear of pain and injury and, thus, focus efforts on learning skills. With regard to facilities, boundaries could be made narrower to encourage accuracy and teamwork, as well as increase opportunities for practising certain skills such as inbounds passing and receiving. Rule changes that emphasize a mastery approach include smaller numbers per side (e.g. soccer, volleyball), elimination of complex rules (e.g. off-sides in soccer, infield fly rule and balk in baseball), and modifications that emphasize maximal participation and learning. These may include batting through the order in softball, an established amount of playing time (e.g. two quarters in basketball), and stopping the game to allow coaches and officials to explain the nature of rule violations (e.g. interrupt a basketball game to explain a moving screen).

Social support strategies

MODELLING

Modelling refers to the cognitive, affective and behavioural changes that occur as a result of observing adults and peers (Schunk, 1989). A review of the modelling research with youth indicates that certain strategies or types of models can maximize the development of positive self-perceptions and, ultimately, skill performance (Weiss *et al.*, 1993). For example, similar models, who are matched to observer characteristics such as age, gender and ability level, serve to enhance attention and motivation through observer perceptions that, 'If she (he) can do it, so can I!' Therefore, educators are encouraged to use multiple demonstrators in the sport setting so that child observers can identify with at least one of these models and feel confident about trying and performing the target skills or strategies.

Many complex sport skills pose an element of danger or fear in child observers, such as diving, gymnastics tricks, taking a charge in basketball, sliding in baseball and a take-down in wrestling. Some children, especially with low perceived competence and high anxiety, will not have an opportunity to master skills because they will not even try. In this case, coping models may provide a salient and successful means of enhancing self-perceptions and approach behaviours. A coping model is one that initially verbalizes and demonstrates the same fears and low self-confidence experienced by observers, but who gradually overcomes uncertainties and performs the skill successfully. Coping models influence self-confidence through information provided about what strategies to use in overcoming avoidance, as well as motivating observers through perceived similarity and bonding.

FEEDBACK AND REINFORCEMENT

The literature on parental and coach feedback strongly suggests that the quality, rather than the quantity, of verbal and non-verbal communication is a stronger influence on self-esteem and perceptions of competence. Contingent (i.e. based on performance) and appropriate (i.e. based on level of mastery) feedback and reinforcement were identified as the key ingredients for enhancing self-perceptions. This means that, in response to desirable performances, parents and coaches should respond with praise followed by information on how to improve on the next attempt or trial. The praise should not be overly excessive nor should mediocre performance (based on the child's potential) be reinforced. An attitude that skill errors are a part of the learning process and signify a temporary, rather than permanent, setback is critical for the development of positive self-perceptions. That is, adults and peers should encourage young athletes following an inappropriate skill response and provide appropriate information for adjusting subsequent performance.

The sport setting is one that naturally emphasizes the competitive aspects of participation, and thus encourages comparison to and evaluation from peers about levels of physical competence. However, the research indicates that peer comparison and evaluation is not always the most appropriate or accurate source of information with which youth should estimate their abilities. Children and youth differ in numerous ways such as physical size, biological maturity, importance attached to success in certain achievement domains, and years of experience in and knowledge base about a specific sport. Therefore, peer comparison and evaluation should be just one of the many sources of information children use to determine their physical competence. Feedback and reinforcement on the part of parents and coaches should emphasize the use of internal criteria or personal comparison information such as achievement of self-set goals, degree of effort exerted, attraction toward or enjoyment of sport and improvement relative to previous levels of performance. These standards of comparison enhance children's self-perceptions of competence and control, and serve to enhance their intrinsic desire and continued sport participation.

MASTERY MOTIVATIONAL CLIMATE

A mastery motivational climate refers to structuring the environment so that emphasis is placed on defining success in terms of learning and improving skills, rather than performance in comparison to others or event outcome (Ames, 1992). To do this, individualistic rather than competitive rewards are emphasized, where learners are recognized for achieving self-set goals independently, rather than beating a teammate or attaining the best time or score. An emphasis is heavily placed on individual effort as a means of mastering skills and attributing performance outcomes, so that increased effort and persistence will result in successful accomplishments. This contrasts an emphasis on ability attributions for performance outcome, where performance failures are seen as inadequate ability and may result in negative self-perceptions, affect and attenuated motivation.

Specific strategies for fostering a mastery motivational climate and, subsequently, positive self-perceptions, could include modelling and reinforcement of form or technique, and ignoring performance outcome, in the learning phase of sport skills. This would ensure that attention and motivation are directed toward the process, rather than the product, of skill performance. Emphasis on the use of self-comparison sources of information (e.g. personal improvement, effort expenditure) would help compromise the tendency for young performers to solely compare their abilities to same-age peers. Recognition to performers for desirable but often neglected efforts such as 'sportsperson of the week', 'unsung hero award', 'team player of the game' and 'most inspirational player' also reinforces a mastery orientation. Reinforcement of effort and persistence, improvement from past performance and positive attitude toward the sport learning process needs to be emphasized to balance out the salience placed on competitive and peer-oriented goals and rewards inherent in sport.

Maximizing positive affect

Theory and research on self-esteem and competence perceptions in the physical domain identified affect as an antecedent and consequent variable. Therefore, another approach to maximize the development of positive self-conceptions is to enhance positive affect such as enjoyment, pride, satisfaction, happiness and excitement. For example, adults can make sport a positive emotional experience by keeping practices and competitions fun as well as achievement-oriented, and by matching the difficulty of sport skills and goals to the developmental capabilities of the participants. Leadership styles and communication that focus on improving skills, allowing shared decision making, showing care and empathy toward athletes, and providing contingent positive feedback also maximize the probability of positive emotional experiences in the sport environment. While these strategies are enhancing positive affective reactions, research has shown that they also reduce the possible onset of negative affective responses such as anxiety, shame and disappointment.

Self-regulated learning strategies

Structuring the sport setting to foster mastery experiences and the careful use of social support strategies might be labelled as environmental-based influences of self-perceptions. In addition to strategies which originate in the social environment, researchers are increasingly alluding to the need for children and youth to take control of their own learning and performance through the use of self-regulated learning or individual control strategies (Schunk, 1989; Weiss, 1995). Self-regulated learning refers to the child as an active agent in his or her choice, control and achievement of self-set goals, and children who are effective with using self-regulated strategies are characterized as high in self-perceptions, internal locus of control and intrinsic motivation to continue participation in achievement-related activities.

Self-regulated learning is comprised of three processes: (i) self-observation; (ii) self-judgement or evaluation; and (iii) self-reinforcement (Bandura, 1986). Self-observation entails monitoring of one's behaviours through the use of self-recording and other strategies. Self-judgement is a process whereby learners compare present performance level with desired goals; and, self-reinforcement refers to the positive or negative self-evaluations concerning progress toward goal attainment.

The successful learning of all three of these phases characterizes the self-regulated learner. The strategies that have been identified for developing self-regulated learning skills include several of those already discussed: modelling, attributional feedback, social comparison and reward contingencies. Additional acquisition strategies include goal setting, self-monitoring progress through logs or other recording devices, and strategy training (e.g. self-instructional talk, attribution retraining and anxiety management). Parents, teachers and coaches can systematically provide opportunities for children and youth to become self-regulated learners through a variety of these strategies. The reader is referred to Weiss (1995) for a more detailed discussion of self-regulated learning and its associated strategies. A summary of enhancement strategies for self-esteem and perceived competence can be found in Table 25.2.

Challenges for future research

The strategies outlined above provide guidelines for practitioners, but guidelines must also be established for researchers who will continue to explore self-esteem and perceived competence in future studies. Several suggestions regarding research directions as well as improved methodologies have already been discussed in the literature (Sonstroem, 1984; Weiss, 1993).

Table 25.2 Strategies for enhancing self-esteem and perceived competence.

Mastery experiences
   developmental progressions
   game modifications
Social support
   modelling
   feedback and reinforcement
   mastery motivational climate
Positive affect
Self-regulated learning
   self-observation
   self-evaluation
   self-reinforcement

The intent here, therefore, is merely to identify several of the more prominent challenges awaiting researchers interested in studying self-esteem and perceived competence in the youth sport setting.

• Recognize the need for ongoing research. A systematic line of research is necessary that examines self-esteem and perceived competence in youth sport. Self-esteem and perceived competence play an important role in understanding human behaviour and deserve increased attention in the literature. Pre-existing ideas of nebulous constructs that are difficult to investigate scientifically must be replaced by the conviction that self-esteem and perceived competence offer exciting possibilities for future research.

• Couch research questions within a theoretical or conceptual framework. A guiding framework is extremely useful because it offers an explanation as to why groups are significantly different or an intervention is successful. Most of the conceptualizing about self-esteem and perceived competence has originated in psychology. Therefore, the applicability to sport of established theories and models needs to be tested and any modifications incorporated that provide a better representation of the youth sport experience. Ideally, future research conducted in the physical domain will foster original hypotheses regarding the self-system that will contribute to the existing knowledge base.

• Adopt a multidimensional approach. Part of the intrigue associated with the self-system as it is currently conceptualized is that it is multifaceted and, consequently, inadequately studied by way of a single variable. It is not enough to individually examine self-esteem or perceived competence because a true understanding of the complexity of self-perceptions can only result from investigating multiple variables in any given study. The context-free variable of self-esteem should be investigated along with domain-specific self-conceptions. Cognitive components are best examined in relation to affective, social and behavioural components. The sophistication of future studies needs to be increased in order to match the sophistication of the self-system.

- Explore subgroup differences across various levels of self-perceptions. Too frequently research designs average scores for an entire sample and fail to document the interesting findings for individuals categorized as high, medium or low on a self-perception variable such as self-esteem or perceived competence. Clearly such a strategy as exploring subgroup differences requires additional planning in terms of the choice of sample (so as to ensure that each subgroup is adequately represented) and the number of subjects involved. Nevertheless, certain research questions definitely lend themselves to this design which should be employed more often in future research studies.

- Use valid and reliable measures. The relatively recent changes in how the self-system is conceptualized have dated earlier measures that were developed to align with earlier notions. Arguments have been made for the limited value of measures that assess the self-concept as if it were a one-dimensional construct (Harter, 1986). The use of single-item measures to operationalize constructs has also been challenged (Schutz & Gessaroli, 1993), and certainly single items have been employed to measure variables such as perceived competence. Therefore, future research studies that investigate self-esteem and perceived competence need to utilize sound assessment tools that will most likely reflect the true nature of self-perceptions.

References

Ames, C.A. (1992) Achievement goals, motivational climate, and motivational processes. In G. Roberts (ed.) *Motivation in Sport and Exercise*, pp. 161–76. Human Kinetics, Champaign, IL.

Bandura, A. (1977) Self-efficacy: toward a unifying theory of behavioral change. *Psychol. Rev.* **84**, 191–215.

Bandura, A. (1986) *Social Foundations of Thought and Action: A Social Cognitive Theory*. Prentice-Hall, Englewood Cliffs, NJ.

Berger, B.G. & McInman, A. (1993) Exercise and the quality of life. In R.N. Singer, M. Murphy &

L.K. Tennant (eds) *Handbook of Research on Sport Psychology*. Macmillan, New York.

Black, S.J. & Weiss, M.R. (1992) The relationship among perceived coaching behaviors, perceptions of ability, and motivation in competitive age-group swimmers. *J. Sport Exerc. Psychol.* **14**, 309–25.

Brustad, R.J. (1988) Affective outcomes in competitive youth sport: the influence of intrapersonal and socialization factors. *J. Sport Exerc. Psychol.* **10**, 307–21.

Brustad, R.J. (1993) Who will go out and play? Parental and psychological influences on children's attraction to physical activity. *Pediatr. Exerc. Sci.* **5**, 210–23.

Brustad, R.J. & Weiss, M.R. (1987) Competence perceptions and sources of worry in high, medium, and low competitive trait anxious young athletes. *J. Sport Psychol.* **9**, 97–105.

Chase, M. & Dummer, G. (1992) The role of sport as a social status determinant for children. *Res. Q. Exerc. Sport* **63**, 418–24.

Cooley, C.H. (1902) *Human Nature and the Social Order*. Scribner, New York.

Coopersmith, S. (1981) *The Antecedents of Self-esteem*. Consulting Psychologists Press, Palo Alto, CA.

Deci, E.L. & Ryan, R.M. (1985) *Intrinsic Motivation and Self-determination in Human Behavior*. Plenum Press, New York.

Dempsey, J.M., Kimiecik, J.C. & Horn, T.S. (1993) Parental influence on children's moderate to vigorous physical activity participation: an expectancy-value approach. *Pediatr. Exerc. Sci.* **5**, 151–67.

Ebbeck, V. (1990) Sources of performance information in the exercise setting. *J. Sport Exerc. Psychol.* **12**, 56–65.

Ebbeck, V. & Stuart, M.E. (1993) Who determines what's important? Perceived competence, individual importance, and group importance as predictors of self-esteem in youth football players. *Pediatr. Exerc. Sci.* **5**, 253–62.

Ebbeck, V. & Weiss, M.R. (1992) *Antecedents of children's self-esteem: an examination of perceived competence and affect in sport*. Paper presented at the annual meeting of the Association for the Advancement of Applied Sport Psychology, Colorado Springs, CO, October.

Eccles, J.S. & Harold, R.D. (1991) Gender differences in sport involvement: applying the Eccle's expectancy-value model. *J. Appl. Sport Psychol.* **3**, 7–35.

Eitzen, D.S. (1975) Athletics in the status system of male adolescents: a replication of Coleman's *The Adolescent Society*. *Adolescence* **10**, 167–276.

Evans, J.R. & Roberts, G.C. (1987) Physical competence and the development of children's peer relations. *Quest* **39**, 23–35.

Felson, R.B. (1989) Parents and the reflected appraisal process: a longitudinal analysis. *J. Personal. Soc. Psychol.* **56**, 965–71.

Feltz, D.L. (1978) Athletics in the status system of female adolescents. *Rev. Sport Leisure* **3**, 98–108.

Feltz, D.L. & Petlichkoff, L.M. (1983) Perceived competence among interscholastic sport participants and dropouts. *Can. J. Appl. Sport Sci.* **8**, 321–35.

Fleming, J.S. & Courtney, B.E. (1984) The dimensionality of self-esteem: II. Hierarchical facet model for revised measurement scales. *J. Personal. Soc. Psychol.* **46**, 404–21.

Fox, K.R. (1988) The self-esteem complex and youth fitness. *Quest* **40**, 230–46.

Fox, K.R. & Corbin, C.B. (1989) The physical self-perception profile: development and preliminary validation. *J. Sport Exerc. Psychol.* **11**, 408–30.

Gould, D. (1988) Your role as a coach. In V. Seefeldt (ed.) *Handbook for Youth Sports Coaches*, pp. 19–32. American Association for Health, Physical Education, Recreation and Dance (AAHPERD), Reston, VA.

Gruber, J. (1986) Physical activity and self-esteem development in children. A meta-analysis. In H. Echert (ed.) *Effects of Physical Activity on Children and Growth: The Academy Papers*, pp. 30–48. Human Kinetics, Champaign, IL.

Harter, S. (1978) Effectance motivation reconsidered. *Hum. Dev.* **21**, 34–64.

Harter, S. (1981) A model of intrinsic mastery motivation in children: individual differences and developmental change. In W.A. Collins (ed.) *Minnesota Symposium on Child Psychology* Vol. 14, pp. 215–55. Lawrence Erlbaum, Hillsdale, NJ.

Harter, S. (1986) Processes underlying the construction, maintenance, and enhancement of the self-concept in children. In J. Suls & A. Greenwald (eds) *Psychological Perspectives on the Self*, Vol. 3, pp. 137–81. Lawrence Erlbaum, Hillsdale, NJ.

Harter, S. (1987) The determinants and mediational role of global self-worth in children. In N. Eisenberg (ed.) *Contemporary Topics in Developmental Psychology*, pp. 219–42. Wiley, New York.

Hattie, J. (1992) *Self-concept.* Lawrence Erlbaum, Hillsdale, NJ.

Hines, S. & Groves, D.L. (1989) Sports competition and its influence on self-esteem development. *Adolescence* **24**, 861–9.

Horn, T.S. (1985) Coaches' feedback and changes in children's perceptions of their physical competence. *J. Educ. Psychol.* **77**, 174–86.

Horn, T.S., Glenn, S.D. & Wentzell, A.B. (1993) Sources of information underlying personal ability judgments in high school athletes. *Pediatr. Exerc. Sci.* **5**, 263–74.

Horn, T.S. & Hasbrook, C.A. (1986) Informational components influencing children's perceptions of their physical competence. In M.R. Weiss & D. Gould (eds) *Sport for Children and Youths*, pp. 81–8. Human Kinetics, Champaign, IL.

Horn, T.S. & Hasbrook, C.A. (1987) Psychological characteristics and the criteria children use for self-evaluation. *J. Sport Psychol.* **9**, 208–21.

Horn, T.S. & Weiss, M.R. (1991) A developmental analysis of children's self-ability judgments in the physical domain. *Pediatr. Exerc. Sci.* **3**, 310–26.

James, W. (1890) *The Principles of Psychology*, Vol. 1. Henry Holt, New York.

Klint, K.A. (1985) *Participation motives and self-perceptions of current and former athletes in youth gymnastics.* Unpublished master's thesis, University of Oregon.

Klint, K.A. & Weiss, M.R. (1987) Perceived competence and motives for participating in youth sports: a test of Harter's competence motivation theory. *J. Sport Psychol.* **9**, 55–65.

Markus, H. & Kunda, Z. (1986) Stability and malleability of the self-concept. *J. Personal. Soc. Psychol.* **51**, 858–66.

Markus, H. & Wurf, E. (1987) The dynamic self-concept: a social psychological perspective. *Ann. Rev. Psychol.* **38**, 299–337.

Marsh, H.W. (1986) Global self-esteem: its relation to specific facets of self-concept and their importance. *J. Personal. Soc. Psychol.* **51**, 1224–36.

Marsh, H.W. & Peart, N.D. (1988) Competitive and cooperative physical fitness training programs for girls: effects on physical fitness and multidimensional self-concepts. *J. Sport Exerc. Psychol.* **10**, 390–407.

Martens, R. (1990) *Successful Coaching.* Human Kinetics, Champaign, IL.

Nicholls, J.G. (1984) Achievement motivation: conceptions of ability, subjective experience, task choice, and performance. *Psychol. Rev.* **91**, 328–46.

Oosterwegel, A. & Oppenheimer, L. (1993) *The Self-System: Developmental Changes between and Within Self-concepts.* Lawrence Erlbaum, Hillsdale, NJ.

Passer, M.W. (1983) Fear of failure, perceived competence, and self-esteem in competitive-trait-anxious children. *J. Sport Psychol.* **5**, 172–88.

Richman, C.L. & Rehberg, H. (1986) The development of self-esteem through the martial arts. *Int. J. Sport Psychol.* **17**, 234–9.

Roberts, G.C., Kleiber, D.A. & Duda, J.L. (1981) An analysis of motivation in children's sport: the role of perceived competence in participation. *J. Sport Psychol.* **3**, 206–16.

Rosenberg, M. (1986) *Conceiving the Self.* Robert E. Krieger, Malabar, FL.

Rosenberg, M. (1989) *Society and the Adolescent Self-image.* Wesleyan University Press, Middletown, CO.

Scanlan, T.K., Carpenter, P.J., Lobel, M. & Simons,

J.P. (1993) Sources of enjoyment for youth sport athletes. *Pediatr. Exerc. Sci.* **5**, 275–85.

Scanlan, T.K. & Lewthwaite, R. (1986) Social psychological aspects of competition for male youth sport participants: IV. Predictors of enjoyment. *J. Sport Psychol.* **8**, 25–35.

Scanlan, T.K., Stein, G.L. & Ravizza, K. (1989) An in-depth study of former élite figure skaters: II. Sources of enjoyment. *J. Sport Exerc. Psychol.* **11**, 65–83.

Schunk, D.H. (1989) Social cognitive theory and self-regulated learning. In B.J. Zimmerman & D.H. Schunk (eds) *Self-Regulated Learning and Academic Performance*, pp. 83–110. Springer-Verlag, New York.

Schutz, R.W. & Gessaroli, M.E. (1993) Use, misuse, and disuse of psychometrics in sport psychology research. In R.N. Singer, M. Murphey & L.K. Tennant (eds) *Handbook of Research in Sport Psychology* pp. 901–17. Macmillan, New York.

Shavelson, R.J., Hubner, J.J. & Stanton, G.C. (1976) Self-concept: validation of construct interpretations. *Rev. Educ. Res.* **46**, 407–41.

Smith, R.E., Smoll, F.L. & Curtis, B. (1979) Coach effectiveness training: a cognitive–behavioral approach to enhancing relationship skills in youth sport coaches. *J. Sport Psychol.* **1**, 59–75.

Smoll, F.L., Smith, R.E., Barnett, N.P. & Everett, J.J. (1993) Enhancement of children's self-esteem through social support training for youth sport coaches. *J. Appl. Psychol.* **78**, 602–10.

Sonstroem, R.J. (1984) Exercise and self-esteem. In R. Terjung (ed.) *Exercise and Sport Sciences Reviews*, Vol. 12, pp. 123–55. Franklin Institute, Philadelphia.

Sonstroem, R.J., Harlow, L.L. & Salisbury, K.S. (1993) Path analysis of a self-esteem model across a competitive swim season. *Res. Q. Exerc. Sport* **64**, 335–42.

Sonstroem, R.J. & Morgan, W.P. (1989) Exercise and self-esteem: rationale and model. *Med. Sci. Sports Exerc.* **21**, 329–37.

Stipek, D. & Mac Iver, D. (1989) Developmental change in children's assessment of intellectual competence. *Child Dev.* **60**, 521–38.

Ulrich, B.D. (1987) Perceptions of physical competence, motor competence, and participation in organized sport: their interrelationships in young children. *Res. Q. Exerc. Sport* **58**, 57–67.

Waite, B.T., Gansneder, B. & Rotella, R.J. (1990) A sport-specific measure of self-acceptance. *J. Sport Exerc. Psychol.* **12**, 264–79.

Weiner, B. (1985) An attributional theory of motivation and emotion. *Psychol. Rev.* **92**, 548–73.

Weiss, M.R. (1987) Self-esteem and achievement in children's sport and physical activity. In D. Gould & M.R. Weiss (eds) *Advances in Pediatric Sport Sciences*, Vol. 2. *Behavioral Issues*, pp. 87–119. Human Kinetics, Champaign, IL.

Weiss, M.R. (1991) Psychological skill development in children and adolescents. *The Sport Psychol.* **5**, 335–54.

Weiss, M.R. (1993) Psychological effects of intensive sports participation on children and youth: self-esteem and motivation. In B.R. Cahill & A.J. Pearl (eds) *Intensive Participation in Children's Sports*, pp. 39–69. Human Kinetics, Champaign, IL.

Weiss, M.R. (1995) Children in sport: an educational model. In S. Murphy (ed.) *Sport Psychology Interventions*, pp. 39–69. Human Kinetics, Champaign, IL.

Weiss, M.R., Bredemeier, B.J. & Shewchuk, R.M. (1986) The dynamics of perceived competence, perceived control, and motivational orientation in youth sports. In M.R. Weiss & D. Gould (eds) *Sport for Children and Youths*, pp. 89–101. Human Kinetics, Champaign, IL.

Weiss, M.R. & Duncan, S.C. (1992) The relation between physical competence an peer acceptance in the context of children's sport participation. *J. Sport Exerc. Psychol.* **14**, 177–91.

Weiss, M.R., Ebbeck, V. & Horn, T.S. (1992) *Children's psychological characteristics and preferences for information sources regarding physical competence.* Paper presented at the annual meeting of the North American Society for the Psychology of Sport and Physical Activity, Pittsburgh, PA, June.

Weiss, M.R., Ebbeck, V. & Wiese-Bjornstal, D.M. (1993) Developmental and psychological factors related to children's observational learning of physical skills. *Pediatr. Exerc. Sci.* **5**, 301–17.

Weiss, M.R. & Horn, T.S. (1990) The relation between children's accuracy estimates of their physical competence and achievement-related characteristics. *Res. Q. Exerc. Sport* **61**, 250–8.

Weiss, M.R., McAuley, E., Ebbeck, V. & Wiese, D.M. (1990) Self-esteem and causal attributions for children's physical and social competence in sport. *J. Sport Exerc. Psychol.* **12**, 21–36.

Weiss, M.R., Wiese, D.M. & Klint, K.A. (1989) Head over heels with success: the relationship between self-efficacy and performance in competitive youth gymnastics. *J. Sport Exerc. Psychol.* **11**, 444–51.

Whitehead, J.R. (1991) *Preliminary validation of the physical self-perception profile questionnaire for seventh and eighth grade students.* Paper presented at the annual meeting of the North American Society for the Psychology of Sport and Physical Activity, Pacific Grove, CA.

Wylie, R.C. (1979) *The Self-Concept*, Vol. 2. *Theory and Research on Selected Topics*. University of Nebraska Press, Lincoln, NE.

Chapter 26

Emotional Stress and Anxiety in the Child and Adolescent Athlete

DANIEL GOULD AND ROBERT C. EKLUND

Introduction

Highly organized sport for young athletes exists throughout the world (Weiss & Gould, 1986). These activities have been widely supported by adults based on the belief that there are a broad variety of positive outcomes associated with participation. Clearly there are potential motoric benefits as a consequence of the child or adolescent learning to utilize his or her body in the skilful ways demanded by the sport activity. Also, a variety of positive outcomes are anticipated in the cognitive and effective domains. For example, it is assumed that the young athlete will have fun in this setting. Furthermore, there is a belief that the social interactions inherent in sport will provide opportunities for lessons about competition, values and social skills (Estrada *et al.*, 1988).

However, despite the fact that youth sport has flourished during this century, there have been critics suggesting that the special learning opportunity sport provides may not be as safe and idyllic as frequently depicted. Competitive stress, in particular, has been a point of central concern throughout the history of youth sport (Berryman, 1988). Contemporary literature, for example, have discussed this topic using phrases such as 'psychological trauma' (Smilkstein, 1980) and 'child abuse' (Tutko & Burns, 1978).

In recent years, sport psychology researchers interested in youth sport have begun systematic research programmes examining the effects of competitive sports participation on young athletes. These efforts have begun to pay dividends for understanding psychosocial stress and hence have provided information to guide professional practice in the youth sport setting. This chapter examines emotional stress and anxiety in the child and adolescent athlete by summarizing this research literature.

For the purposes of this chapter, participation in competitive sport is defined as athletic involvement where the child attends scheduled competitions and organized practices under the supervision of an adult leader. Unfortunately, paediatric sport psychology researchers have not characterized young athletes with the same precision as paediatric exercise physiology researchers with regard to the maturational categories such as prepubescent, pubescent and postpubescent. Hence, this line of research can only be discussed relative to the chronological age of young athletes.

Stress as a process

There have been a number of problems confounding common understandings of competitive stress including the notion that stress is inherently good or bad. Youth sport critics have suggested that stress is always unsatisfactory and potentially harmful to young athletes. Conversely, advocates have regarded competitive stress as one of the favourable aspects of the youth sport setting, providing a valuable learning opportunity for the young athlete.

However, these value-laden perspectives are both inappropriate because stress researchers have shown that stress can have both positive and negative effects (Selye, 1974).

Adding further confusion to common understandings of competitive stress is that the term 'stress' is informally used in at least two different ways. The first usage invokes stress as a situational variable, something in the environment, that may challenge the response resources of an individual (e.g. the stress of a championship game will test Sally's metal). The second usage refers to stress as psychological reaction to environmental events (e.g. Billy experienced a great deal of stress playing in the championship game). The meaning of 'stress' in each of these instances is *not* synonymous (Smith & Smoll, 1982). For example, one young athlete may perceive a championship game as very stressful emotionally while another may not perceive the same game as stressful at all. Hence it is important to make a distinction between potential stressors in the environment and the young athlete's perception of psychological stress.

Many researchers investigating this area have adopted a process definition of stress to manage the previously identified problems. The process conceptualization emphasizes that stress involves a dynamic interaction between environmental and personal factors (Lazarus & Folkman,

1984). According to this view, the competitive situation is not itself stress inducing nor are stable personality factors strong predictors of stress. Rather, a particular environment may or may not provoke a stress response depending on the individual's cognitive appraisal of the situation and his or her available coping resources. Furthermore, viewing stress as a process allows us to understand that consequences associated with the process may be positive, negative or neutral.

Smith and Smoll have posited one model of the stress process that has received considerable attention in youth sport literature (Smith, 1986a). As can be observed in Fig. 26.1, this conceptual model is composed of situational, cognitive, physiological, and coping and task behaviour components. Hypothesized relationships between these components are also illustrated. Finally, this model illustrates that personality and motivational variables affect and interact with the model components.

Situational component

In examining stress as a process, neither the particular objective competitive situation that a young athlete encounters (e.g. participating in a championship game, playing in front of one's parents) nor the personal or environmental resources available (e.g. the child's sport skill

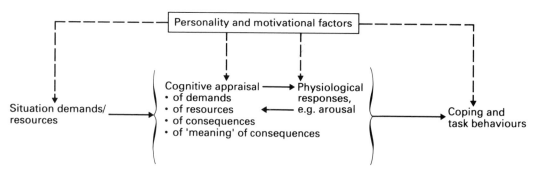

Fig. 26.1 A conceptual model of stress showing hypothesized relationships among situational, cognitive, physiological and behavioural components. Motivational and personality variables are assumed to affect and interact with each of the components. Redrawn with permission from Smith (1986a) © 1986 by Human Kinetics.

level and social support network) are as import-ant as the interaction between these two sets of factors (Smith & Smoll, 1982). Whenever demands are encountered in the competitive environment, resources are mobilized to meet these demands and stress is experienced as a consequence of the relative balance or im-balance between demands and resources. Further, the relative balance between demands and resources determines whether the stress experience is positive, negative or neutral.

More specifically, stress will likely be in-significant or unlikely to be perceived at all when there is little imbalance between re-sources and demands (e.g. two evenly matched wrestlers in a practice match). A young athlete will probably view a situation as challenging if demands slightly exceed resources (e.g. a highly skilled swimmer participating in the city finals). However, a situation featuring a substantial imbalance between demands and resources will likely be regarded as stressful. In the case of a substantial imbalance favouring demands (e.g a back-up hockey goalkeeper facing league-leading scorers in a championship game), stress will likely have the effective consequence of high levels of nervousness or anxiety states. By contrast, stress in the form of boredom and stagnation is a likely consequence of a substan-tial imbalance favouring resources (e.g. an inter-nationally ranked tennis player confined to local high school competition).

Although stress may result from excessive external demands (e.g. opponent superiority), Smith and Smoll (1982) emphasize that situ-ational demands may also emanate from within the individual. Personal or motivational factors such as desired goals, personal performance standards or even unconscious motives or con-flicts contribute to the perception of the com-petitive situation and influence the salience of the array of environmental demands. For example, a young athlete obsessed with per-fectionism may experience a great deal of stress, without any reference to an opponent, purely as a consequence of his or her expectations of self. Also, memories of past performance as

well as anticipation of future consequences may interact with the current situation to in-fluence the young athlete's perception of the setting.

Cognitive component

The situational component of Smith and Smoll's (1982) model emphasizes that the stress is a consequence of an interaction between de-mands and resources. The second component of this model focuses upon the individual's cognitive appraisal of a situation. The emotional intensity with which individuals respond to situations does not depend upon the actual balance between situational demands and re-sources but rather upon what the child believes to be true about the situation. For example, a child's belief that he or she is out-classed by an opponent is a psychological reality of much greater importance in the stress process than an objective assessment suggesting that the child is more than capable of mastering the competitive demands. Clearly, the child's appraisal of the demands of the situation and the available resources may or may not be objectively accurate and, again, personality and motivational factors such as individual differ-ences in self-esteem, confidence and trait anxiety can influence the amount of stress experienced.

Additionally, Smith and Smoll (1982) have indicated that cognitive evaluation of a situation also extends beyond an assessment of demands and resources. People also appraise the possible consequences of failure to master the demands as well as the implications or meaning of such a failure. A situation is more likely to be appraised as stressful if a perceived imbalance threatens harm (e.g. injury or embarrassment) or loss of desired goals (e.g. a league championship) than if the outcome is of no consequence (a loss in practice). There is certainly the possibility of distortion, both exaggeration or underesti-mation, in evaluating the likelihood of a variety of consequences as well as in the meaning of these consequences. For example, a very skilled young athlete may experience a great deal of self-imposed stress over an unfounded concern about parental rejection over the unlikely possibility of losing to a particular inexperienced opponent. Hence, it is not the objective probability of any particular consequence or its actual importance influencing the stress process but rather what the individual *holds* to be true.

Physiological component

As can be seen in Fig. 26.1, the physiological component of the model is reciprocally related to the cognitive appraisal component of the model. Although the primacy of affect versus cognition is debatable (Lazarus, 1984; Zajonc, 1984), the model that Smith and Smoll (1982) have specified assumes cognitive mediation between the situational component and physiological responses. More specifically, it is assumed that cognitive appraisal of threat results in physiological arousal as a part of the mobilization of resources to deal with the situation. However, the reciprocal relationship between these two components indicates that resulting physiological arousal serves as feedback concerning the intensity of the emotion being experienced which in turn influences the appraisal of the situation. Hence, there is an ongoing cycle of appraisal and reappraisal by physiological arousal levels. For example, a young wrestler may have worries about being able to compete with a particular opponent leading to physiological symptoms of anxiety (e.g. racing heart, increased perspiration, etc.). Recognition of and concern about the physiological symptoms may in turn lead to the wrestler having additional concerns about his ability perform adequately and so on.

Behavioural component

The final component of Smith and Smoll's (1982) stress process model consists of task-oriented, social and coping behaviours that occur in response to the situation (as appraised through cognitive processes and physiological responses). The behaviours — both social and sport performance — that an individual emits in the setting can be influenced by his or her perception of the situation. Performance may suffer or be enhanced as a consequence just as behaviour may become more pro- or anti-social when individuals experience competitive stress. Further, the athlete may engage in coping behaviours to manage competitive stress. The adequacy of these coping behaviours affects the balance between demands and resources as well as the ongoing appraisal process. Successful coping may allow the young athlete to appraise the balance between situational demands and available resources favourably. However, coping behaviours are not always effective in redressing a perceived imbalance between resources and demands (Compas, 1987). Regardless, the young athlete who perceives his or her responses (sport performance, social and/or coping) as lacking is more likely to experience negative affect. For example, the realization by a young tennis player that his or her passing shots are simply not precise enough to be effective against a particular opponent can have the affective consequence of additional competitive anxiety.

State and trait anxiety

In addition to defining stress itself, terms frequently associated with stress — state and trait anxiety — must be defined before the stress process and its ramifications can be fully understood. State anxiety is a possible byproduct of the stress process and the one which negative connotations of stress are most often associated. Specifically, state anxiety is defined as 'an existing or current emotional state characterized by feelings of apprehension and tension and associated with activation of the organism' (Martens, 1977). In essence, state anxiety is a negative feeling experienced at a particular moment in time. It is a feeling everyone at some time in their life has noticed, from butterflies experienced a few minutes before an athletic competition to that queasy feeling in one's stomach before giving a public speech for the first time.

Trait anxiety is closely associated with state anxiety. However, unlike state anxiety, trait anxiety is considered to be an enduring attribute or a part of one's personality. Trait anxiety is defined as 'a predisposition to perceive certain environmental stimuli as threatening or nonthreatening and to respond to these stimuli with varying levels of state anxiety' (Martens, 1977). A young athlete's trait anxiety would be conceptualized within the personal and motivational factors part of Smith and Smoll's (1982) stress model and hence could influence all four components of the model. Trait anxiety is important because it has been consistently shown to influence one's level of state anxiety. For example, a high trait anxious child will tend to perceive evaluative environments, like competition, as very threatening and, as a consequence, experience increases in state anxiety. In contrast, when a low trait anxious child is placed in the same competitive environment, he or she is less likely to perceive the environment to be as threatening and therefore is less likely to experience marked increases in state anxiety. Thus, the level of state anxiety a child experiences in evaluative environments is directly related to his or her level of trait anxiety.

Stress research in youth sport

A number of investigators have begun to examine stress in children's sport. There have been a number of questions of central interest to youth sport researchers and progress has been made toward understanding the stress process in these areas. These questions include:
1 Do youth sport participants experience too much stress?
2 What are the consequences of athletic stress?
3 What are the factors related to state and trait anxiety in young athletes?
4 Do children and adults differ in their perception and responses to stress?
These questions are addressed below.

Too much stress

A fundamental question at issue surrounding youth sport has regarded the desirability of levels of state anxiety experienced by young athletes as a consequence of competitive stress. Critics of youth sport have suggested that competitive stress generates excessive levels of state anxiety that can negatively affect the mental health of the child athlete (Martens, 1978). Conversely, youth sport proponents have argued that the very beauty of youth sport is that young athletes *do* experience stress but not at excessive levels and in a 'safe' environment that allows children to learn how to cope with stress successfully.

A great deal of energy has been devoted to examining the levels of state anxiety experienced by young athletes to address the question of whether or not competitive stress is excessive in youth sport. Studies examining levels of state anxiety can be classified into three major types.
1 Psychophysiological assessments of state anxiety experienced before, during and immediately after athletic competitions.
2 Survey assessments of state anxiety and anxiety-related symptoms associated with athletic competition.
3 Assessments of state anxiety occurring before, during and immediately after athletic competition using validated self-report state anxiety inventories.
Each of these areas are summarized below.

Several investigators (Skubic, 1955; Hanson, 1967; Lowe & McGrath, 1971) have examined levels of state anxiety experienced by young athletes using physiological indices of stress such as heart rate or galvanic skin response. For example, Skubic (1955), in the earliest study of this issue, assessed physiological stress in 9–15-year-old boys participating in Little League baseball and physical education class softball competitions via galvanic skin response. Few differences were found between the groups and it was concluded that the state anxiety experienced during competitive youth baseball was not greater than that experienced in a physical education class competition.

In a youth baseball study, Lowe and McGrath (1971) examined respiration and heart rates prior to batting under conditions of varying game importance (e.g. based on league standings, won−loss records) and situation criticality (e.g. score, number of outs, position of runners on base). It was found that physiological state anxiety was positively related to game importance and increased situation criticality. Unfortunately, assessments in non-evaluative or other forms of competition were not made.

These two investigations of physiological indices of state anxiety associated with youth sports competition illustrate typical findings in the area. Specifically, these studies suggest that overall either few differences in state anxiety exist between youth sport and other competitive environments (physical education class competitions) or that high but short-lived elevations in state anxiety occur during events. However, such results must be interpreted with some caution because Dishman (1989) has recently cited evidence suggesting that elevated physiological state anxiety as assessed by heart rate during youth sport competition does not appear to differ from that occurring during recreational play or bicycle ergometer tests. Hence, these physiological changes associated with athletic competition may not result from the competitive setting *per se*, but rather from the physical activity itself. Notwithstanding this caution, it is important to take note of evidence of a relationship between heightened state anxiety during events and game importance and situation criticality.

Taking a different approach, a number of investigators (Skubic, 1955; Hale, 1961; McPherson *et al.* 1980; Purdy *et al.* 1981; Ralio, 1982; Gould *et al.* 1983a; Feltz & Albrecht, 1986; Tierney, 1988) have asked either the young athlete or their parents to rate the degree of anxiety-related symptoms associated with or as a consequence of athletic competition. In most cases one or two questions pertaining to this issue were posed as part of a larger youth sport survey project and hence the findings are somewhat superficial and difficult to interpret. However, the results of these studies do provide clues as to levels of state anxiety experienced by youth sport participants.

Among findings emerging in survey investigations, Skubic (1955) found that approximately one-third of the Little League baseball players interviewed reported contest-related sleeping difficulties. Thirty-three per cent of the male and 56% of the female youth swimmers surveyed by McPherson *et al.* (1977) reported experiencing some emotional stress. Feltz and Albrect (1986) reported that 41% of their sample of élite young distance runners reported becoming nervous and worried in races but half of these young athletes indicated that this nervousness *helped* their performance. Interestingly, Hale (1961) reported that 97% of the fathers of Little League baseball participants he surveyed indicated that their sons were not affected by participation.

Despite problems with non-validated instruments and superficiality, these results suggest that some, but clearly not the majority of young athletes engaged in competition experience high levels of competitive state anxiety and associated symptoms.

Finally, a number of investigators (Scanlan & Passer, 1978, 1979; Simon & Martens, 1979; Bump *et al.* 1985) have used validated self-report state anxiety instruments to assess levels of state anxiety experienced before, during and after competitive youth sport events.

For example, Simon and Martens (1979) conducted the most extensive investigation of state anxiety experienced in competitive and non-competitive sport settings. State anxiety levels of 749 boys (9−14 years of age) were assessed in practice settings and just prior to required school activities (e.g. classroom tests and physical education class competitions), non-required non-sport competitive activities (band solos and band group competition) and non-school sports (baseball, basketball, tackle football, gymnastics, ice hockey, swimming and wrestling) using the competitive state anxiety inventory for children (CSAIC) (Martens, 1977). Differences between practice and competitive state anxiety levels were examined as well as comparisons among the various competitive activities.

Not surprisingly precompetitive state anxiety was found to be elevated over practice levels, although the overall change was not excessive. For example, the mean precompetitive state anxiety score for the entire sample was 16.87 (possible scores on the CSAIC range from 10 to 30). Of particular interest in the study by Simon and Martens (1979) was the comparison of state anxiety levels of boys participating in sport to boys participating in other competitive activities not typically the focus of parental concern (band solos, band group competition, etc.). Band solo participation elicited the greatest state anxiety ($M = 21.48$) followed by individual sport participation (for wrestling $M = 19.52$; for gymnastics $M = 18.52$) while physical education competition elicited the lowest levels of anxiety ($M = 14.47$). However, it was noted that substantial individual differences existed. Relatively few of the boys experienced what could be considered extremely high levels of competitive state anxiety (scoring in the upper quartile of possible CSAIC scores or above 25 out of 30) while the vast majority of boys (82%) reported scores between 10 and 20 or the lower half of the scale.

Bump *et al.* (1985) also examined state anxiety levels of young athletes by administering the CSAIC to 13 and 14-year-old boys prior to competitive tournament wrestling matches. Among the 112 participants, similar to the findings of Simon and Martens (1979) for wrestlers, prematch state anxiety levels averaged 18.9 (out of a possible 30). Again, relatively few of the boys reported experiencing extremely high levels of state anxiety with only 9% scoring in the upper quartile of possible CSAIC scores (> 25). These results are consistent with other studies (Scanlan & Passer, 1978, 1979) conducted in this area and reveal that the majority of children participating in competitive youth sports are not experiencing excessive levels of

state anxiety as a result of their competitive experience.

Summarizing across approaches to studying levels of state anxiety and associated symptoms in young athletes, then, the results have shown that the vast majority of children involved in competitive sport are not experiencing high levels of stress. Hence, critics of organized competitive sport programmes for children may be incorrect in their claims relative to the excessive levels of stress placed on young athletes and therefore concerns about excessive stress should not prevent parents from encouraging their children from becoming involved in sport.

Notwithstanding this conclusion, the evidence also shows that a small, but significant, minority of young athletes experience high levels of stress which may be manifested in such symptoms as insomnia and a loss of appetite. If, for example, only 5–10% of the estimated 1 million children in Australia (Robertson, 1986), 18 million children in Brazil (Ferreira, 1986), 2.5 million children in Canada (Valeriote & Hansen, 1986), 25 million children in the USA (Martens, 1988) and 23 million children in the former USSR (Jefferies, 1986) involved in organized sport experience excessive stress, this alone would involve about 3.5–7 million youngsters. Efforts need to be made to identify young athletes who are susceptible to heightened state anxiety and the youth sport situations related to heightened anxiety states in young athletes.

Consequences of athletic stress on the child

Excessive competitive stress has been associated with a variety of undesirable outcomes. It has been linked, for example, to sport withdrawal among young athletes (Gould & Petlichkoff, 1988), sport burnout (Smith, 1986b; Coakley, 1992; Gould, 1993), reduced performance (Scanlan *et al.* 1984; Gould *et al.* 1991) and reduced fun and satisfaction (Scanlan & Passer, 1978, 1979; Scanlan & Lewthwaite, 1984). Further, Orlick and Botterill (1975) suggested, in studying a sample of 8- and 9-year-old sport non-participants, that anticipation of competitive stress may be a barrier to sport entry for some children. Also identified have been associations with potential health-threatening effects such as a loss of sleep (Skubic, 1955; State of Michigan, 1978) and appetite (Skubic, 1955). Although tentative links have been established in these areas, few conclusions can be reached with any degree of certainty at this time because of the limited number of studies.

A further area of recent concern with regard to health-related effects has been a potential association between high levels of stress and the incidence or severity of injury in sport competition. For example, Smith *et al.* (1990) examined 451 male and female high school athletes participating in basketball, wrestling and gymnastic competition on the variables of life events, social support, coping skills and sport participation time lost to injury. While no significant direct relationship between positive or negative life change scores and injury-related time loss was observed, when social support and coping variables were considered in conjunction with negative major life changes, significant associations were observed. Specifically, high school athletes with low levels of social support and low coping skills who experienced negative stress from major life changes tended to exhibit greater subsequent injury-related time loss. Subsequently, Smith *et al.* (1992) have found evidence to suggest that the relationship between major negative sport-specific life events and ensuing injury-related time loss may be most profound for adolescents who have a lower tolerance for arousal than their high sensation seeking counterparts.

Although there is some evidence to suggest that reduced performance is a consequence of high state anxiety (Scanlan *et al.*, 1984; Gould *et al.*, 1991), the assumption that increased state anxiety always negatively influences the performance of the young athlete requires additional examination. Research with adult athletes (see Gould & Krane, 1992 for a review) has shown that increased state anxiety does not always lead to inferior performance and may,

at times, enhance performance. This notion is reinforced by findings in youth sport survey literature indicating that significant percentages of junior élite runners (39%) and wrestlers (50%), ranging in age from 9 to 19 years, identify anxiety and nervousness as facilitating performance (Gould *et al.*, 1983a; Feltz & Albrecht, 1986).

Critics of youth sport have suggested that young athletes may develop an aversion to challenge through the experience of excessive levels of stress during sport participation. Hence, there has been the question of whether or not the stress of sport participation negatively influences a child's competitive trait anxiety or enduring predisposition to perceive competition as threatening. Unfortunately, there is a paucity of research examining this important question. In one of the few studies conducted with children, Magill and Ash (1979) found no competitive trait anxiety differences between fourth grade youth sport participants and non-participants. Non-participant fifth graders, however, were higher in trait anxiety than were fifth grade participants. By contrast, Feltz and Albrecht (1986), in studying 28 élite 10–15-year-old youth distance runners, found competitive trait anxiety levels which were slightly higher than norms for comparable age and gender groups. Finally, Raviv (1981) detected no competitive trait anxiety differences in a 1-year longitudinal study of 37 matched pairs of Israeli sport club and non-participant children.

The equivocal and limited nature of the research linking trait anxiety with sports participation precludes definitive conclusions regarding the effects of competitive youth sport participation on the trait anxiety of young athletes. Half of the studies revealed no evident differences and the remaining studies suggest that participants, at most, have only slightly elevated levels of trait anxiety compared to non-participants. Before definitive conclusions can be derived more studies of a longitudinal nature are needed and potential moderator variables (e.g. extent of involvement, success level) mediating the relationship between partici-pation status and competitive trait anxiety must be assessed.

In contrast, Martens (1978) has suggested that there are potential long-term positive con-sequences of exposure to competitive stress. Specifically, Martens has hypothesized that stress in the sport setting may act as a sort of stress vaccination which stimulates the devel-opment of general coping strategies, as a vaccine stimulates protection against disease. This notion, as yet unexamined, implies that ex-posure to appropriate levels of stress may help the young athlete to learn stress coping skills transferable to other life settings. Investigations examining the veracity of Martens' (1978) vaccine stress consequence hypothesis (and re-lated questions such as what might constitute an optimal dosage of stress) are certainly of interest but have yet to be conducted.

Further comprehensive investigations into the consequences of competitive stress are clearly required. Although appropriate levels of competitive stress are thought to have posi-tive affective, psychological and behavioural consequences, there is no clear evidence for this. However, it can be concluded that excess-ive competitive stress can have negative physi-cal and behavioural consequences on the young athlete. Further, the long-term ramifications of competitive stress are unknown both in terms of the number of children afflicted with nega-tive consequences or the nature of potential benefits. Lines of systematic research are needed, particularly longitudinal investi-gations, that examine long-term effects of com-petitive athletic stress on children.

Factors related to state and trait anxiety

It is imperative that personal and situational factors associated with competitive state and trait anxiety are identified. The reasons for this include the following two factors. First, a sub-stantial minority of youth sport participants are at risk of experiencing negative conse-quences associated with excessive anxiety and knowledge of such factors provides the basis for intervention efforts. Second, the identifi-cation of these factors is important to ensure that ill-advised efforts do not put additional young participants at risk. Fortunately, over the last decade youth sport researchers have conducted relatively extensive research upon factors related to competitive state anxiety (Scanlan & Passer, 1978, 1979; Gould et al., 1991, 1983b; Scanlan & Lethwaite, 1984; Feltz & Albrecht, 1986) and trait anxiety (Passer, 1983; Brustad & Weiss, 1987; Brustad, 1988; Newton & Duda, 1992) in young athletes that enable practitioners to better identify children who are susceptible to heightened levels of competi-tive stress and for helping then ensure that youth sport settings are not excessively stressful.

The typical approach to identifying factors associated with state anxiety in young athletes consists of assessing state anxiety levels in children immediately prior to and following a competition. Information about various per-sonality factors (e.g. self-esteem) and demo-graphics (e.g. years of experience in sport) collected at a previous non-stressful time (e.g. practice) are used to predict levels of pre- and postcompetitive state anxiety. Scanlan (1986) has summarized this research and identified a number of personal and situational factors as-sociated with competitive state anxiety. These include:

1 Competitive trait anxiety
2 Self-esteem.
3 Fun.
4 Satisfaction.
5 Personal performance expectancies.
6 Worries about failure and adult evaluation.

Trait anxiety, as previously defined, is a part of a young athlete's personal make-up or per-sonality that predisposes the young athlete to perceive evaluative and competitive environ-ments as threatening or non-threatening. High trait-anxious youth sport participants tend to respond to potentially stressful situations, like competition, with nervousness or high state anxiety levels. By contrast, low trait-anxious participants do not tend to respond to competitive situations with the same levels of state anxiety. Self-esteem also has been associated with state anxiety. Specifically, the lower the young athlete's self-esteem, the higher the state anxiety level experienced in stressful situations.

It has been found that fun is related to state anxiety. When winning and losing are controlled, youth sport participants perceiving more fun in their experience of the competition experience less state anxiety. Conversely, when young athletes experience less fun, it is likely that they experience more state anxiety. Similarly, when winning and losing are factored out, state anxiety after the game has been found to be related to the amount of satisfaction young athletes perceive in their performance. Specifically, young athletes tend to experience less state anxiety when they perceive more satisfaction from participating in a game and vice versa.

Personal and team performance expectancies are also related to state anxiety. The lower the young athlete's expectancy relative to his or her personal ability to perform, the greater the state anxiety experienced. Also, the lower the young athlete's confidence relative to his or her team's ability to perform well, the more state anxiety that is experienced.

Finally, worries about failure and adult expectations and social evaluation are associated with elevations in state anxiety. An interesting finding from an investigation conducted by Scanlan and Lewthwaite (1984) and replicated by Gould et al. (1991) suggests that increased parental pressure to participate is associated with increased levels of state anxiety among youth sport participants. It was found that young wrestlers perceiving that it was important to their parents to have them participate in the sport experienced more state anxiety than athletes who did not perceive parental pressure to participate.

There are two readily apparent situational factors that have been associated with heightened state anxiety in youth sport participants. The first is victory versus defeat. Young athletes who win games experience less state

anxiety than young athletes who lose (Scanlan & Passer, 1979). Second, as the Lowe and McGrath's (1971) youth baseball data illustrates, the greater importance placed on a particular event, the more stressful it is for the individual.

Some research exists specifically examining sources of stress for the junior élite athlete (secondary school-aged athletes competing in national level competition). The typical paradigm for this type of research involves having these athletes rate the importance and frequency of the specific stress sources they experience on a seven-point Likert scales (1, don't experience very much; 7, experience a great deal). A typical question that might be asked of the young athlete is: 'do you worry about participating in championship meets?' Through this research, a number of stress sources for the junior élite athlete have emerged.

For example, Gould et al. (1983b) examined sources of stress in 400 junior élite wrestlers (13–19 years of age) at a national tournament. The highest rated stress sources for these junior élite competitors were 'performing up to their levels of ability', 'improving on their last performance', 'participating in championship meets', 'not performing well', 'losing', 'not making weight' (which is probably sport-specific) and 'being able to get mentally ready to wrestle'. In all these cases, at least 41% of the individuals sampled rated these items as very important in terms of stress sources for them.

A similar study using the same instrument was conducted by Feltz and Albrecht (1986) examining sources of stress in élite secondary school-aged distance runners. They found that 'performing up to their ability', 'improving on their last performance', 'participating in championship meets', 'not performing well', and 'not being able to get mentally ready' were all major stress sources for these young runners. Again, these sources were all rated as very important by at least 41% and as high as 54% of the sample.

These results reveal that élite junior competitors (age 9–19 years) are primarily concerned about fear of failure and concerns over performance evaluations. Closely associated with worries are feelings of inadequacy such as concerns about an inability to mentally prepare themselves to perform well. Hence, two major stress sources to be recognized when dealing with élite junior level athletes are fear about failure/performance evaluation and feelings of inadequacy.

In summary then, the research on state anxiety before and after games and associated factors has helped provide a useful profile of personal and situational factors that are associated with heightened state anxiety in organized youth sport settings. Knowledge of these factors can help physicians, parents and adult leaders identify young athletes who experience high levels of state anxiety in sport, and in turn, take steps toward reducing this stress. Further, such information can be useful in helping to ensure that additional young athletes are not put at risk.

Several investigators (Passer, 1983; Brustad & Weiss, 1987; Brustad, 1988; Newton & Duda, 1992) have also begun to examine factors associated with high competitive-trait-anxiety in young athletes. This is an important area of study because the personality disposition of high competitive-trait-anxiety has been one of the factors most consistently related to elevated levels of high state anxiety in young athletes. A better understanding of the high trait-anxious young athlete and factors related to his or her high trait anxiety should assist youth sport leaders in helping 'at risk' young athletes cope with stress of athletic competition (Gould, 1993).

Passer (1983) was the first investigator to study the high competitive-trait-anxious youth sport participant. In particular, he compared 163 high and low competitive-trait-anxious youth soccer players (aged 10–15 years) on self-esteem, performance expectation, criticism for failure expectations, perceived competence, and performance- and evaluation-related worries. Results revealed that the high as compared to low anxious players worried more frequently about losing, not playing well, and

coach parent and teammate evaluations. It was concluded that high competitive-trait-anxious young athletes perceived fear of evaluation and failure as major sources of threat.

In a similar investigation, Brustad and Weiss (1987) studied 55 male baseball players and 55 female softball players (aged 9–13 years). Results revealed that high as compared to low competitive-trait-anxious boys reported lower levels of self-esteem and more performance worries but, interestingly, no significant differences were found for the girls. In a follow-up investigation, Brustad (1988) studied 207 youth basketball players. Results again revealed that high competitive-trait-anxious boys demonstrated lower levels of self-esteem but this time, a similar pattern of results were found for the girls. Higher competitive trait anxious athletes also demonstrated more frequent evaluation and performance-related worries.

Recently, Newton and Duda (1992) have found evidence to suggest that there is a link between achievement goal orientations and multi-dimensional trait anxiety in young athletes. In the current effort towards examining sport achievement motivation, two primary goal perspectives (a task orientation and an ego orientation) underlying perceptions of success have come under considerable scrutiny. Task-oriented conceptions of success are self-referenced and associated with the belief that hard work, improving and meeting the demands of the task are the primary goals of the activity. By contrast, ego-oriented conceptions of success are associated with the belief that superiority over others in the contest (winning) is the primary goal.

In examining the association between multi-dimensional trait anxiety and goal orientations among 124 male and female tennis players ($M = 12.71$ years, $SD = 2.10$ years), Newton and Duda (1992) found that the ego orientation was related to increased multidimensional trait anxiety and particularly for those young tennis players who held a very strong ego orientation combined with a moderate task orientation. Hence, young athletes who use victory as a primary gauge of personal success in their sporting efforts while only placing minimal or moderate emphasis upon improvement and effort tend to see sport competition as much more threatening than young athletes who place greater emphasis upon improvement and effort.

Taken together, these results show that the high trait anxious youth athlete is likely to perceive failure and/or negative evaluation from significant others as emotionally very aversive. Hence there is a need to reduce evaluation potential for these young athletes, to enhance their low self-esteem and ensure success. Further, evidence from recent goal-orientation research suggests that efforts to help these young athletes learn to interpret success and failure may be important. Specifically, high trait anxious young athletes, in particular, need to learn to evaluate their performance from a task-orientation conception of success (hard work, improving and meeting and demands of the task) while keeping ego-oriented conceptions of success (superiority over others) in perspective.

Paediatric–adult differences in perception and response to competitive stress in sport

O. Bar-Or (personal communication, 20 August 1992) identified several important questions for paediatric sport psychologists interested in anxiety and stress. In particular, he asks if children differ from adolescents and adults in their emotional responses to stressors. If so, what are the characteristic sport-related responses of the child as compared to the adolescent and/or the adult and, furthermore, are certain stressors unique to children's sports?

Unfortunately, few studies have been conducted to address these issues and, to the authors' knowledge, no investigations have been conducted that directly examine whether children, adolescents and adults differ in their perceptions of and responses to competitive stress in sport. Some investigators (Scanlan et al. 1991; Gould et al. 1992) have examined sources of stress in studies of élite (mostly adult) athletic populations and compared their

findings to previously discussed studies of stress sources and predictors of state anxiety in young athletes. The conclusions of these comparisons are best summarized by Scanlan et al. (1991, p. 118):

> The results show that élite and youth sport athletes have similar competition-related stressors: namely, worrying about failure, performing poorly, and losing. The extant stress literature's exclusive focus on competition leaves future research to determine whether the élite athlete's stressors outside of competition (e.g. interpersonal conflict, time and financial demands or costs, perfectionism) generalize to youth sport athletes.

A common area across child, adolescent and adult sport participants has been that trait anxiety has been shown to be a consistent predictor of state anxiety (Martens et al. 1990). That is, high trait-anxious adult, adolescent and child athletes consistently experience higher levels of state anxiety in competition than their low trait-anxious counterparts.

However, in one of the few areas where children and adults have been directly compared, equivocal findings have resulted when levels of trait anxiety are examined (Martens et al., 1990). Specifically, some studies have found younger athletes to exhibit lower levels of trait anxiety than older athletes while other investigations have identified no such differences among age classifications. Martens et al. (1990) contend, however, that to understand these equivocal findings, the interrelationship between age, situational factors and trait anxiety must be considered. For instance, in studies where younger athletes exhibit lower levels of trait anxiety than older athletes, observed differences may result from the fact that younger children have not yet learned to view competition as evaluative threats to their self-esteem. The question remains then, whether age-related trait anxiety differences would exist when the intensity of the competitive situation was controlled.

In summary, the few studies that have been

conducted to compare children and adults in their perceptions of and response to anxiety and stress show that children and adults are more similar than different. Extreme caution must be made in drawing these conclusions, however, because so few developmentally based studies have been conducted that simultaneously compare athletes of different ages and control for potential moderator variables such as the intensity of the competitive situation. This is certainly an area ripe for future research.

Conclusion

In this chapter, the literature on competitive stress accompanying competitive sport participation for the young athlete has been examined. The following elements have been identified:

1 The stress process.
2 The levels of state anxiety experienced by young athletes.
3 The consequences of athletic stress.
4 Factors associated with state and trait anxiety.
5 Comparisons of child and adult perceptions of and responses to anxiety and stress.

Our understanding of the stress process in the youth sport is certainly far from complete but nonetheless there are a number of recommendations for guiding practice and future research directions that can be forwarded directions.

Stress, youth sport and recommendations for practice

1 Competitive stress in young athletes results from the complex interplay between situational factors and personal characteristics inherent in the child. Therefore, efforts must be made to consider both types of factors in the youth sport setting rather than simply attributing stress solely to the child or the situation.

2 Personal characteristics of children most likely to experience high levels of state anxiety include high levels of competitive-trait-anxiety, low self-esteem, and low personal and team performance expectancies. Also, these children experience less fun and satisfaction in the youth sport setting and worry about failure and adult evaluation. Special attention is warranted with children exhibiting these characteristics (Gould, 1993).

3 Environments where the young athlete is uncertain about the expectations of others and his or her ability to perform as well as being laden with social evaluation and importance placed upon competitive performance and contest outcome are most likely to provoke a stress response. Efforts to engineer the environment to reduce uncertainty, evaluative components and importance placed upon contest outcome can help moderate the situational effects in the stress process.

4 Children should not be discouraged from participating in competitive sport because of concerns about competitive stress because the vast majority of youth sport participants are *not* experiencing excessive levels of state anxiety nor do they appear to differ from their non-athletic counterparts in trait anxiety.

5 A significant minority of participants *do* suffer from high levels of competitive stress. Efforts must be made to identify and assist these children so that their youth sport experience represents a positive developmental opportunity rather than an onerous aversive struggle.

6 Although contest outcome is a salient and important aspect of the sport setting, young athletes, particularly high trait-anxious young athletes, need to learn to evaluate their performances on the basis of hard work, improvement and meeting the demands of the task while keeping winning and losing in perspective. Efforts must be made to assist young athletes to interpret their sporting experience not only in terms of outcome but also through improvement, effort and attainment of performance goals.

Challenges for future research

• Studies examining heightened state and trait anxiety in young athletes involved in 'intensive competition' such as league, regional, national and or world championships are needed (Gould *et al.*, 1992). To date, most of the research has *not* been conducted on young athletes who have been involved in these types of intense training regimens.

• Comparisons of state and trait anxiety, as well as sources of athletic stress in samples of children, adolescents and adults are badly needed. In particular, research on the question of whether children differ from adolescents and adults in their emotional responses to stressors is needed (O. Bar-Or, personal communication, August 1992). And, if so, what the sport-related typical responses are of children versus adolescents versus adult athletes.

• Paediatric exercise physiologists have found it very useful to examine specific characteristics of young athletes developmentally or maturationally classified as prepubescent, pubescent and postpubescent rather than strictly according to chronological age. Paediatric sport psychology researchers, however, have generally pooled all data into a young athlete category or simply related findings to chronological age categories. Future research is needed to determine if the same growth- and maturation-related evolution identified in many exercise physiology variables holds true regarding emotional stress and anxiety. Moreover, it has been suggested that children are characterized by separate physical, social–emotional and intellectual developmental patterns (Martens, 1978). Investigation linking anxiety and stress responses to these varying patterns are badly needed.

• Longitudinal investigations that examine long-term effects of competitive athletic stress on children are warranted.

• An assessment is needed of the potential positive consequences associated with experiencing stress in sport competition. For example, is Martens' (1978) stress vaccine hypothesis tenable? Does exposure to small doses of stress in youth sport prepare or vaccinate a young athlete for handling more severe stress levels later in life? And, if so, what is the optimal dosage of stress needed for such a vaccine effect to occur?

• Considerable attention has been paid to identifying stress sources surrounding athletic competition for children. However, it is unclear whether or not newly identified noncompetitive stressors which affect élite adult athletes (e.g. financial costs of participating, time demands) apply to youth sport athletes (Scanlan *et al.*, 1991).

• Qualitative research methodologies (e.g. indepth interviews) should be used to examine stress and anxiety responses in young athletes. Qualitative approaches are needed because virtually all the youth sport stress and anxiety investigations have employed a quantitative paradigm. However, recent stress and anxiety research conducted on élite athletes (Scanlan *et al.*, 1991; Gould *et al.*, 1992) has found qualitative approaches to be especially useful in identifying important new variables of interest and previously unexamined relationships. This type of approach would be especially useful in examining previously unexplored areas such as the potential positive consequences of experiencing stress in sports competitions.

References

Berryman, J.W. (1988) The rise of highly organized sports for preadolescent boys. In F.L. Smoll, R.A. Magill & M.J. Ash (eds) *Children in Sport*, 3rd edn, pp. 3–16. Human Kinetics, Champaign, IL.

Brustad, R.J. (1988) Affective outcomes in competitive youth sport: the influence of intrapersonal and socialization factors. *J. Sport Exerc. Psychol.* **10**, 307–21.

Brustad, R.J. & Weiss, M.R. (1987) Competence perceptions and sources of worry in high, medium, and low competitive trait-anxious young athletes. *J. Sport Psychol.* **9**, 97–105.

Bump, L., Gould, D., Petlichkoff, L., Peterson, K. & Levin, R. (1985) *The relationship between achievement orientations and state anxiety in youth wrestlers*. Paper presented at the North American Society for the Psychology of Sport and Physical Activity Conference, Gulfpark, MS. May.

Coakley, J. (1992) Burnout among adolescent athletes: a personal failure or a social problem. *Sociol. Sport J.* **9**, 271–85.

Compas, B.E. (1987) Coping with stress during childhood and adolescence. *Psychol. Bull.* **101**, 393–403.

Dishman, R.K. (1989) Exercise and sport psychology in youth 6 to 18 years of age. In C.V. Gisolfi & D.R. Lamb (eds) *Perspectives in Exercise and Sports Medicine*, Vol. 2. *Youth, Exercise and Sport*, pp. 47–97. Benchmark Press, Indianapolis, IN.

Estrada, A.M., Gelfand, D.M. & Hartmann, D.P. (1988) Children's sport and the development of social behaviors. In F.L. Smoll, R.A. Magill & M.J. Ash (eds) *Children in Sport*, 3rd edn, pp. 251–62. Human Kinetics. Champaign, IL.

Feltz, D.L. & Albrecht, R.R. (1986) Psychological implications of competitive running. In R.M. Weiss & D. Gould (eds) *Sports for Children and Youth*, pp. 225–30. Human Kinetics, Champaign, IL.

Ferreira, M.B.R. (1986) Youth sport in Brazil. In M.R. Weiss & D. Gould (eds) *Sports for Children and Youth*, pp. 11–15. Human Kinetics, Champaign, IL.

Gould, D. (1993) Intensive sports participation and the prepubescent athlete: competitive stress and burnout effects. In B. Cahill & A.J. Pearl (eds) *Intensive Training and Participation in Youth Sports*, pp. 19–38. Human Kinetics, Campaign, IL.

Gould, D., Eklund, R.C., Petlichkoff, L., Peterson, K. & Bump, L. (1991) Psychological predictors of state anxiety, and performance in age-group wrestlers. *Pediatr Exerc. Sci* **3**, 198–208.

Gould, D., Horn, T. & Spreemann, J. (1983a) Competitive anxiety in junior élite wrestlers. *J. Sport Psychol.* **5**, 58–71.

Gould, D., Horn, T. & Spreemann, J. (1983b) Sources of stress in junior élite wrestlers. *J. Sport Psychol.* **5**, 159–71.

Gould, D., Jackson, S.A. & Finch, L. (1992) *Sources of stress experienced by national champion figure skaters*. US Olympic Committee Sports Science Grant Final Report.

Gould, D. & Krane, V.I. (1992) The arousal–athletic performance relationship: current status and future directions. In T. Horn (ed.) *Advances in Sport Psychology*, pp. 119–42. Human Kinetics, Champaign, IL.

Gould, D. & Petlichkoff, L. (1988) Participation motivation and attrition in young athletes. In F.L. Smoll, R.A. Magill & M.J. Ash (eds) *Children in Sport*, 3rd (edn), pp. 161–78. Human Kinetics, Champaign, IL.

Hale, C.J. (1961) Injuries among 771,810 Little League baseball players. *J. Sports Med. Phys. Fitness*, 3–7.

Hanson, D.L. (1967) Cardiac response to participation in Little League baseball competition as determined by telemetry. *Res. Q.* **38**, 384–8.

Jefferies, S.C. (1986) Youth sport in the USSR. In M.R. Weiss & D. Gould (eds) *Sports for Children and Youth*, pp. 21–6. Human Kinetics, Champaign, IL.

Lazarus, R.S. (1984) On the primacy of cognition. *Am. Psychol.* **39**, 124–9.

Lazarus, R.S. & Folkman, S. (1984) *Stress, Appraisal and Coping*. Springer-Verlag, New York.

Lowe, R. & McGrath, J.E. (1971) *Stress, arousal and performance: some findings calling for a new theory*. Report No. AF1161–67. Air Force Office of Strategic Research, Washington DC.

McPherson, B., Martinuk, R., Tihanyi, J. & Clark, W. (1980) The social system of age group swimmers, parents and coaches. *Can. J. Appl. Sport Sci.* **4**, 142–5.

Magill, R.A. & Ash, M.J. (1979) Academic, psychosocial and motor characteristics of participants and nonparticipants in children's sports. *Res. Q.* **50**, 230–40.

Martens, R. (1977) *Sports Competition Anxiety Test*. Human Kinetics, Champaign, IL.

Martens, R. (1978) *Joy and Sadness in Children's Sports*. Human Kinetics, Champaign, IL.

Martens, R. (1988) Youth sport in the USA. In F.L. Smoll, R.A. Magill & M.J. Ash (eds) *Children in Sport*, 3rd edn, pp. 17–23. Human Kinetics, Champaign, IL.

Martens, R., Vealey, R.S. & Burton, D. (eds) (1990) *Competitive Anxiety in Sport*. Human Kinetics, Champaign IL.

Newton, M.L. & Duda, J.L. (1992) *The relationship of goal perspectives to multidimensional trait anxiety in adolescent tennis players*. Paper presented at the North American Society for the Psychology of Sport and Physical Activity Conference, Pittsburgh, PA. June.

Orlick, T. & Botterill, C. (1975) *Every Kid Can Win*. Nelson-Hall, Chicago IL.

Passer, M.W. (1983) Fear of failure, fear of evaluation, perceived competence and self-esteem in competitive-trait anxious children. *J. Sport Psychol.* **5**, 172–88.

Purdy, D.A., Haufler, S.E. & Eitzen, D.S. (1981) Stress among child athletes: perceptions by parents, coaches and athletes. *J. Sport Behav.* **4**, 32–44.

Ralio, W.S. (1982) The relationship of sport in childhood and adolescence to mental and social health. *Scand. J. Sports Med.* **29** (Suppl.), 135–45.

Raviv, S. (1981) Reactions to frustration, level of anxiety and loss of control of children participating in competitive sports. In E. Geron, A. Mashiach, N. Dunkelman, S. Raviv, Z. Levin & E. Nakash (eds) *Children In Sport: Psychosociological Characteristics*, pp. 72–94. Wingate Institute, Netanya, Israel.

Robertson, I. (1986) Youth sport in Australia. In M.R. Weiss & D. Gould (eds) *Sports for Children and Youth*, pp. 5–10. Human Kinetics, Champaign, IL.

Scanlan, T.K. (1986) Competitive stress in children. In M.R. Weiss & D. Gould (eds) *Sport for Children and Youth*, pp. 113–18. Human Kinetics, Champaign, IL.

Scanlan, T.K. & Lewthwaite, R. (1984) Social psychological aspects of competition for male youth sport participants: I. Predictors of competitive stress. *J. Sport Psychol.* **6**, 208–27.

Scanlan, T.K., Lewthwaite, R. & Jackson, B.L. (1984) Social psychological aspects of competition for male youth sport participants: II. Predictors of performance outcomes. *J. Sport Psychol.* **6**, 422–9.

Scanlan, T.K. & Passer, M. (1978) Factors related to competitive stress among male youth sports participants. *Med. Sci. Sports* **10**, 103–8.

Scanlan, T.K. & Passer, M. (1979) Sources of competitive stress in young female athletes. *J. Sport Psychol.* **1**, 151–9.

Scanlan, T.K., Stein, G.L. & Ravizza, K. (1991) An indepth study of former élite figure skaters. III. Sources of stress. *J. Sport Exerc. Psychol.* **13**, 103–20.

Selye, H. (1974) *Stress without Distress.* New York: New American Library.

Simon, J. & Martens, R. (1979) Children's anxiety in sport and nonsport evaluative activities. *J. Sport Psychol.* **1**, 160–9.

Skubic, E. (1955) Emotional responses of boys to Little League and Middle League competitive baseball. *Res. Q.* **26**, 342–52.

Smilkstein, G. (1980) Psychological trauma in children and youth in competitive sport. *J. Fam. Prac.* **10**, 737–9.

Smith, R.E. (1986a) A component analysis of athletic stress. In M.R. Weiss & D. Gould (eds) *Sport for Children and Youth*, pp. 107–11. Human Kinetics, Champaign, IL.

Smith, R.E. (1986b) Toward a cognitive-affective model of athletic burnout. *J. Sport Psychol.* **8**, 36–50.

Smith, R.E., Ptacek, J.T. & Smoll, F.L. (1992) Sensation seeking, stress, and adolescent injuries: a test of stress-buffering, risk-taking, and coping skills hypotheses. *J. Personal. Soc. Psychol.* **62**, 1016–24.

Smith, R.E. & Smoll, F.L. (1982) Psychological stress: a conceptual model and some intervention strategies in youth sports. In R.A. Magill, M.J. Ash & F.L. Smoll (eds) *Children in Sport*, 2nd edn, pp. 178–95 Human Kinetics, Champaign, IL.

Smith, R.E., Smoll, F.L. & Ptacek, J.T. (1990) Conjunctive moderator vulnerability and resiliency: life stress, social support and coping skills, and adolescent sport injuries. *J. Pers. Soc. Psychol.* **58**, 360–70.

Smoll, F.L. & Smith, R.E. (1989) Competitive stress and young athletes. In C.C. Teitz (ed) *Scientific Foundations of Sports Medicine*, pp. 375–90. B.C. Decker, Philadelphia, PA.

State of Michigan (1978) *Joint Legislative Study on Youth Sports Programs: Phase II. Agency Sponsored Sports.* State of Michigan, East Lansing, MI.

Tierney, J. (1988) Stress in age-group swimmers. *Swimming Tech.* **24**, 9–14.

Tutko, T. & Burns, W. (1978) The child superstar: a curse or a blessing. *Tennis USA* March, 40–48, 56.

Valeriote, T. & Hansen, L. (1986) Youth sport in Canada. In M.R. Weiss & D. Gould (eds) *Sports for Children and Youth*, pp. 17–20. Human Kinetics, Champaign, IL.

Weiss, M.R. & Gould, D. (1986) (eds) *Sport for Children and Youth.* Human Kinetics, Champaign, IL.

Zajonc, R.B. (1984) On the primacy of affect. *Am. Psychol.* **39**, 117–23.

Chapter 27

Intelligence of Child and Adolescent Participants in Sports

EMA GERON

Introduction

The importance of intelligence in sports activity is often emphasized in the literature of sport psychology and physical education. In addition to the physical strain, participation in sport also demands intellectual effort. To learn to use motor skills appropriately, the athlete needs to understand their structure and the situations in which they have to be utilized, to analyse and evaluate the movement execution and to adapt it to the requirements of the situation. Participation in competition requires the athlete to refine problem-solving and quick decision-making techniques as well as to develop an understanding of his or her own behaviour and feelings.

Despite the recognition of its role in sport, intelligence is the least studied aspect in the field of sport psychology as well as in the specific area of child and youth sport psychology. In his review of psychological studies on child and youth sports, Gould (1982) did not report even one publication devoted to intelligence.

Publications to date on intelligence in sport represent mainly theoretical speculations, hypotheses and general ideas. The few empirical studies on this topic were mostly concentrated on the relationship between intelligence and motor performance, the academic achievements of athletes and, recently, the role of separate intellectual and cognitive processes in sport.

Intelligence of children and adolescents

Although intelligence is a relatively stable personality characteristic, defined to a large extent by heredity, it changes and develops with age. Its role in child and youth sports may be understood by taking into account the rules of intelligence development and its specific characteristics in childhood. In describing the intellectual development of children, Piaget (1953) stressed that the child's intelligence differs profoundly from that of the adult. It develops through fixed developmental sequences which are qualitatively different from one another, each subsequent stage always being of a higher degree.

According to Piaget, the cognitive activity of infants during the sensorimotor stage (from birth to 18 months), includes perceptions which appear during and together with the children's motor activity, and are expressed by the child's motor behaviour. The stage of preoperational thinking (from 18 months to 7 years) includes acquisition of symbolic functions based on the development of language. At this stage children's thinking differs by egocentricity, unilateral centralization, immobility, realism, irreversibility and transductive conclusions. The stage of concrete operations (7–12 years) is distinguished by mobile intellectual activity and reversible transformations. But intellectual operations during this stage are still related to concrete objects, situations and activities.

The stage of formal operations (from 12 years onwards) characterizes the intellectual activity of adolescents. This activity becomes independent of the situational environment and is manifested by conclusions based on hypothetical assumptions. Children begin to think in abstract terms. They move from concrete and egocentric explanations to more abstract and formal comprehension. Their ability to analyse and evaluate themselves also increases.

Criticism of Piaget's view during the past two decades denies that a child's thoughts differ profoundly from adult thinking, and claims that concepts in children appear much earlier, i.e. before the age of 7 years (Waxman, 1991). Some studies also established that stages in the intellectual development are not defined by age alone. Individual differences in intellectual ability, as well as the influence of environment and learning, may change age boundaries in the developmental stages (Goebel & Harris, 1980).

Comprehensive studies on the intellectual development of the child and adolescent participants in sport are almost lacking. Various authors have occasionally described children's intellectual capabilities facilitating participation in movement activity and competitive sports.

According to these descriptions children become intellectually ready to participate in sport at the age of 7 years. At this age they are able to concentrate, categorize, select, organize their perceptions, make decisions and solve problems (Singer, 1984). According to Cratty (1984), children from the age of 4 to 7 years, in which impulsivity begins to decrease, may develop abilities in planning and analysing movement activity. After the age of 8 years in girls, and somewhat later in boys, cognitive strategies may be adopted. At age 7–11 years, which Corlitt (1973) called 'the skill hungry age', children become more creative and independent in using movement. They differentiate and combine movements, make efforts in spatial orientation and use movement images as models. Their movement learning abilities develop and the use of learning strategies expands. However, before the age of 12 years, children often have problems in concentration. To overcome these, Cratty (1984) proposed to teach the children to verbalize their thoughts, and to use the 'self-talk' method (inner speech determining how to behave) which is already possible in 10–11-year-old children. Sugden and Connell (1982) pointed out that until the age of 12 years children have difficulties in information processing. Children 4–6 years old do not use any strategies in information processing. They cannot rehearse and cannot organize information processing alone. This becomes possible at about the age of 9 years. Children's thoughts begin to be focused on social relations at age 7–11 years (Corlitt, 1973; Cratty, 1984) and this enables the development of their moral thinking. Jantz (1975), studying children aged 7–12 years, found that moral thinking matures after the age of 9 years.

Adolescence (age 12–16 years) is the developmental period in which participation in sport is the most fruitful, and the age at which changes in intelligence are the most crucial. The most outstanding psychological characteristic of this period is the move from dependence to independence. This move concerns not only behaviour and attitudes but also thinking, creativity, problem-solving, decision-making and cognitive style.

According to Cratty (1984), the development of abstract thinking in adolescents facilitates the appreciation of shapes, forms and rhythms of movements. Sensitivity to movement exertion increases and thus control and fluency in movement improves. Adolescents may experience changes in movement flow, evaluate aesthetic aspects and quantitative parameters of movements. Unlike small children, adolescents understand the purposes of movement and therefore they may differentiate among types of movement: whether actions, expressions or play (Corlitt, 1973). Comparing adolescents with children aged 5–7 and 9–10 years, Goebel and Harris (1980) found that adolescents show a greater ability to formulate hypotheses and solve problems. Their limitations are that they still base choices on actual and not on expected probability, that they select and process information slowly and that they have difficulties in acquisition strategies for attentional allocation.

Relationships between intelligence and motor ability in children and adolescents

The idea that intelligence and motor performance are related is based on Rousseau's concept of integrated development and Sherrington's view of body−mind unity. This idea stimulated elaboration of hypotheses about the role of motor activity in improving intellectual development and studies examining the relationships between intellectual and motor abilities.

Influenced by the idea of Piaget (1953), that movement experience precedes cognitive development and is a necessary basis for it, physical educators, psychologists and clinicians of the 1950s and 1960s developed various physical education programmes for intellectual development. The construction of these programmes were based on two different principles. Some authors, assuming inherent links between intelligence and motor activity, expected that movement exercises stimulating the functions of the central nervous system may improve intellectual achievement. This supposition directed the elaboration of motor programmes for helping children with intellectual or learning problems and also for enhancing the academic achievements of normal children (Getman, 1952; Kephart, 1964; Corder, 1966; Delacato, 1966; Ismail, 1967; Kiphard & Huppertz, 1968).

The most striking promoter of the second conception, used in the construction of movement programmes for intellectual improvement, was Cratty (1972). He did not accept the view that improvement of intelligence may be a direct result of motor exercises, and explained the positive effect of movement education on the mental activity through the introduction of cognitive demands during motor performance. He suggested that movement exercises may improve intellectual activity if they require the children to think, select, plan and solve problems. Such movement programmes were presented by Cratty and Martin Sister (1969), Frostig (1970) Humphrey and Sullivan (1970), Mosston (1966), Sharpe (1979) and some recent authors (Pauwels & Mols, 1981; Geron & Reches, 1984; Kohen-Raz et al., 1984; Laporte, 1984; Sherrill, 1986; Gorman et al., 1990).

Studies undertaken to tackle directly the nature of the relationship between intelligence and motor abilities were begun in the second half of the 1960s. Ismail and Gruber (1967) studied 10−13-year-old boys and girls divided into three groups according to their level of academic achievements. The children were tested for intelligence, measured by the IQ of OTIS (unpublished test of A.S. Otis) and the Stanford academic achievement test, as well as for various motor aptitudes and physical abilities. Simple and multiple correlations, among 42 items, were computed for the total group of subjects, as well as separately for boys and girls, and for high, medium and low achievers in school. Regression equations were adopted to test the predictive power of different motor variables for intelligence. This study was replicated by Kirkendall and Ismail (1970) adding discriminant and factor analysis. Another replication of the study with children of the same age was carried out by Ismail et al. (1969) in the UK. Investigations on this topic with socially deprived adolescents (14−17 years old) were conducted by Kirkendall and Gruber (1970), using canonical correlation.

The results of all these investigations were reviewed by Ismail (1972) and Gruber (1975). They reported that only some specific physical and motor variables correlated with intelligence. Physical growth was not found to relate with intelligence. Speed, strength, power and accuracy showed a positive relationship with academic achievement, but not with level of intelligence (IQ). Positive relations were found between intelligence and academic achievement and the motor abilities of coordination, balance and kinaesthetic sense. These relations were more pronounced in girls than in boys. Factor analysis in all groups extracted a factor composed of the motor variables coordination and balance (which had the highest loadings), IQ and the Stanford academic achievement score. This factor was called 'academic development'. According to the regression analysis, the motor items, coordination and balance, were found to have the highest predictive power for intellectual achievement.

Other studies on the intelligence–motor abilities relationship further confirmed the main findings of the Ismail group and emphasized the specificity of these relationships, regarding defined motor and intelligence items. Schewe (1977) and Singer (1968), testing elementary level schoolchildren, found that fine coordination is the motor ability which correlates best with a child's intelligence. Gaskin (1971) and Jeffries (1978), testing male participants in school-level sports, found that non-verbal intelligence is related more highly with the student's play abilities than verbal intelligence.

Studies suggested that the intelligence–motor abilities relationship changes according to the level of intelligence. Nettlebeck and Kirby (1983) found high correlations between intelligence and reaction time when studying together mentally retarded, normals and children with above average IQ. However, when the children with extreme levels of IQ were excluded from the analysis, the correlation between intelligence and reaction time dropped. Campbell and Noldy-Cullum (1985) found low correlations between motor and intellectual performance when studying only normal children and high correlations for retarded children. The intelligence–motor abilities relationship depends also on the characteristics of the tested motor activity. Hayashi and Yamaoka (1965), who studied children during physical education classes, and Kashiwabara et al. (1966), who tested child athletes, found that the correlation

between motor and intellectual achievements change curvilinearly according to the duration of the motor performance.

Many authors stressed the role of age in the intelligence–motor abilities relationship. A common inference is that this relationship is stronger in younger than in older children. However, it does not decrease gradually and uniformly with age. Dibner and Korn (1969) found that performance of motor tasks may be a predictor of academic achievement in kindergarten children, but not so well in first graders. It is not a predictor in second graders but becomes a moderate predictor in grades 3 and 4. Chissom (1971) found higher relations between three motor variables and academic achievement in first graders and lower in third graders. However, coordination in particular was found to relate higher with academic achievement in third grade and lower in first grade. Using ball placement tasks, Thomas and Chissom (1972) found that coordination also appears as the best predictor of intelligence for pre-schoolars and for first and second graders.

The intelligence–motor abilities relationship was also studied by comparing motor activity of subjects with different levels of intelligence and intelligence of children with different levels of motor achievement. A popular approach is the comparison of the motor activity of normal and mentally retarded children. Mentally retarded children often suffer from disturbances in exertion of motor acts. That is why disturbed movement exertion in early childhood may predict future intellectual delay. Silva et al. (1982) reported that children with motor disturbances at age 3 and 5 years, demonstrate at age 7 low levels of intelligence and low reading abilities. However, according to Rarick (1980) motor disturbance in children with low intelligence does not always indicate a low level of motor abilities. Mentally retarded children often have normal possibilities in the performance of movements, but limitations in intelligence do not allow them to know how to perform.

Comparisons between children with different

levels of physical fitness did not show that they differ intellectually. Railo (1969) found that physical fitness and school achievement did not correspond. However, children with a low IQ, unlike those with a high IQ, dropped in physical fitness with age.

As for participation in sport, there is a lot of evidence confirming its positive relationship with intelligence. Ruffer (1965) compared personality and academic achievements of 50 physically active and 50 non-active boys and found that the active group had higher academic averages and higher levels of intelligence than the non-active. Boulton (1966) tested the level of intelligence in 330 14−15-year-old boys who were both participants and non-participants in sport. He divided them into five groups according to their level of intelligence. Of the group with the lowest intelligence 75% did not participate in sport and only 4% of them participated in more than two sports. In contrast among the children with the highest intelligence only 34% did not participate in any sport and 41% participated in more than two sports.

A general conclusion of the studies about the intelligence − motor abilities relationship is that it does exist. However, it is neither always direct nor global, and it involves only special intellectual and motor variables and depends on additional factors. The main direction of this relationship is that motor capabilities predict and facilitate intellectual development. Defined motor abilities, such as coordination and balance were found as predicting intellectual achievement. Specially organized motor activities or physical education programmes facilitate the children's intellectual development.

Conversely, intelligence, although not a predictor of motor achievements stimulates participation in motor activity and sport. Highly intelligent children are more active motorically than those with low intelligence. Particularly, non-verbal intelligence was found to facilitate performance in motor activity.

The intelligence−motor abilities relationship itself was found to change according to level of intelligence. This relationship is stronger in children with extreme levels of intelligence than in normals. Factors affecting this relationship also include age and gender.

Academic achievements of child athletes

The broad popularity of youth sports and the increasing number of children and adolescents involved in it raises the question whether participation of children in sport, and especially in competitive sport, is beneficial or harmful to their socialization and mental development. As sport becomes an important part of children's lives, the nature of its influence is obviously crucial. Participants in youth sports range from 7 to 18 years of age. This parallels the age at which they receive their basic academic preparation. Therefore, the relationship between school and sport, and the coordination of their demands, are central issues in children's sport today.

A common belief exists that athletes are inferior students and that participation in sports limits their chances of academic success. Studies testing this viewpoint have found it to be incorrect. Child athletes have normal and often above normal levels of academic achievement. McIntosh (1966) studied 14 000 students at London comprehensive schools and found that the higher the academic attainments, the greater was the chance of participation in school sports teams. Start (1967) presented four studies, each carried out with a large number of students from different secondary schools, and repeatedly found that students at the low 25% in academic achievement did not attain success and status in school sport. The hypothesis that students with low academic achievement attempt to retrieve status through participation in sport was also not confirmed. Children low in academic achievements and with high achievements in sport appear to be exceptional. Kaminski and Ruoff (1979) reported an investigation on 100 10−14-year-old child participants in competitive sport.

Their lifestyle and academic achievements were compared with those of non-participants in sport matched according to age, sex, intelligence, social status, members of family and type of school. Despite their very intensive involvement in sporting activities and long time spent in sport preparation, the student athletes did not differ from the other children in school achievements. Dunkelman (1981) compared 11−12-year-old students of so-called 'sport classes' with their counterparts who attended ordinary classes at the same school, matched according to sex, socioeconomic status and intelligence. The groups were compared in grade average, mathematics and comprehension. The students of the 'sport classes' showed better scores in mathematics than the ordinary students and the scores of comprehension and grade average were equal for both groups. After a year's follow-up at a new school level, academic achievement of the non-athletes decreased, while that of the athletes did not change.

Differences were found in the academic achievement of boy and girl participants in competitive sports. Buhrmann (1972) reported that boy athletes are usually higher in academic achievement than girl athletes. Dunkelman (1981) who compared groups of participants and non-participants in sport, found that non-participant girls are higher in academic achievement than boys, while among the student athletes boys have higher academic achievement than girls. She related this finding with the fact that boys participate in sports more actively than girls.

The relatively high academic achievement of child athletes raises questions about the factors which may determine this phenomenon. Many authors attribute it to the influence of sport on the general lifestyle, behaviour and some personality characteristics of child athletes. Schurr and Brookover (1970) tested and confirmed the hypothesis that high academic achievements in student athletes is due to their high self-confidence. Kaminski and Ruoff (1979) explained it by the habits acquired in sport

regarding how to organize time, concentrate and persist in goal seeking, as well as by the self-confidence that sport develops in athletes. Singer (1984) also stressed the role of time organization in the lifestyle of the child athletes. Some authors stress the role of social factors. Chambers (1991) stated that academic awareness is cultivated in young athletes, by combining athletic participation with school service and leadership activities. Schafer and Armer (1964) attributed the high academic achievement of student athletes to a combination of several factors: (i) high achievement motivation; (ii) influence of movement activity; (iii) efficient use of time; (iv) help of teachers, coaches and peers; (v) being graded leniently; (vi) drive for high grades (to be eligible for sport); (vii) high self-concept; and (viii) external and internal pressures.

An ecological approach, presuming the role of the environmental and situational conditions, has been introduced to explain the effect of sport on children's academic achievement (Rarick, 1973; Seefeldt et al., 1978; Smith & Smoll, 1978). Geron et al. (1981) compared the effect of sport organized by sport clubs out of school and the effect of school's 'sport classes' on the academic achievement of 11−12-year-old children. Academic achievement was found to be higher when the student athletes performed sports in a school setting. Similar findings have been reported by Williams (1988). Using a self-completion questionnaire, he studied 14−15-year-old students from six different schools and found that those with the highest academic attainments were participants in school sport teams, whereas the participants in physical activity outside school were lower in academic achievement.

The conclusion is that sport does not hamper the academic attainments of children. On the contrary, it may stimulate children's academic activities. Such an effect is mediated by the behavioural characteristics that sport cultivates in athletes and by the lifestyle that it established for them. The influence of sport on academic achievement depends also on the environmental conditions in which sport is practiced. A natural milieu which may facilitate the positive effect of sport on the academic achievements is the school environment.

Intelligence of child and adolescent participants in competitive sport

Intelligence and motor learning

The belief exists that success in learning motor skills depends on the level of intelligence. Indeed, motor learning needs some intellectual processes such as understanding the movement structure, planning and modelling the forthcoming execution, comparing the execution with the movement image, and evaluating the performance. It is known also that intelligent people use some learning procedures more successfully. Examples are mental practice (mental rehearsal of the motor act), whole practice (learning a skill by the execution of the motor act as a whole rather than part by part) and transfer (the influence of a skill learned before on the acquisition of a new one). However, studies reveal that success in motor learning does not relate directly to level of intelligence (Start, 1964; Geron, 1976).

Success in motor learning also does not relate to level of intellectual development according to age. Singer (1984) states that the difficulties in learning motor skills are the same in children and adults and they depend on the motor experience, but not on the level of intelligence. Children and adults do not differ in level of success in learning but in the manner by which they learn. Yando *et al.* (1978) found that children of different ages (4, 7, 10 and 14 years) use different learning models adapted to their cognitive and physical capabilities. Weiss (1983) studied children aged 4−5 and 7−8 years, when they learned a motor task. She found that the older group, who had higher attentional and verbal abilities may use equally verbal and non-verbal models during motor learning, while the 4−5 year olds learn only after observation of the model. Differences between children with different levels of intellectual development appear only when they learn difficult motor tasks or learn in complex situations.

Sugden (1984) indicates that children of different ages (8, 12 and 15 years) differ in the learning of a dual task. However, after 5 days intensive practice during which the task difficulty decreased, these differences disappeared. He found also that children of different age groups (7 and 12 years) and different levels of intelligence (with IQ of 50−70 and normals) did not differ in learning team handball, during a standard learning situation. When the situation was changed and became more complicated the learning success of the younger and mentally retarded children became significantly lower than that of the older and intellectually normal children. According to Sugden this difference is due to the children's insufficiences in information processing, the demands to which increase in complex situations and during learning of difficult tasks.

Being unaffected by the level of general intelligence motor learning may be facilitated by the availability of intellectual abilities important in the specific motor activity. Geron (1976) using, over a 3-month period, a planned observation on 9−11-year-old girls learning gymnastics, found that the number of repetitions needed for successful execution of the motor tasks did not correlate with level of intelligence, but correlated significantly ($r = 0.45$ and 0.53; $P < 0.01$) with two cognitive abilities: (i) concrete creativity (the ability to construct concrete images); and (ii) abstract formal creativity (the ability to construct abstract geometrical forms); both of these obviously have important roles in learning gymnastic skills.

A conclusion follows that the acquisition of motor skills is not related to the level of general intelligence. Limitations in the children's motor learning process appear only during difficult learning situations: during learning of complex tasks, during high attentional demands or during variations in the learning situation. Such conditions require high levels of information processing which children up to 12 years of age cannot realize alone without external help. Thus, an adaptation of the learning process to the children's motor and cognitive capabilities is necessary.

The acquisition of motor skills is facilitated by intellectual abilities appropriate to the learned motor tasks.

Sport-specific intelligence

The idea that athletes use a specific kind of intellectual activity is relatively old. There are special terms which denote this activity as 'motor (or movement) intelligence', 'perceptual intelligence' and 'non-verbal intelligence'. Attempting to describe the characteristics of sport-specific intelligence Rieder (1984) states that it appears in sport tactics and strategies, and in the planning and organization of competitive behaviour. Carroll (1972) and Yates (1975) claim that non-verbal communication, the capacity to contact with others by bodily movements and to decode the movement activity of others, are characteristics of sport-specific intelligence. Fleury et al. (1982) and Geron (1975) found that the intellectual activity of athletes is distinguished by speed, anticipation and automatism. Some authors define sport-specific intelligence as a specific form of information processing (Fleury et al., 1982; Isaacs & Finch, 1983). Fisher (1984) presented a comprehensive description of sport-specific intelligence as a form of perceptual intelligence. Its main role, according to Fisher, is to answer the environmental demands using perceptions, memory, attention, verbalization and visualization. Sport-specific intelligence appears in the search, detection and selection of the cues relevant to the sport's tasks. It appears in adaptation of the attentional focus and the cognitive style to the needs of the sport activity. Fisher also stressed the role of sport-specific intelligence in the regulation of the athlete's inner state. Sport-specific intelligence includes a special trend to the use of past knowledge and thus helps the athletes to make decisions using a very limited amount of new information.

Fisher's paper is the only one devoted specifically to sport intelligence. It is, however, based on observations and not on empirical studies.

Empirical studies on sport-specific intelligence are oriented merely to detect separate intellectual manifestations in specific kinds of sport. Early studies used comparisons between athletes and non-athletes. Recent studies introduce comparisons between experts and novices in sport. The differences found between these groups led to the conclusion that sport-specific intelligence is a consequence of experience in sport. However, some findings hinted that sport-specific intelligence is also related to particular personality characteristics. Eysenck et al. (1982) in a series of studies revealed that athletes according to their personality are predominantly extroverts. Robinson (1985) found that extroverts in contrast to introverts are more successful in solving non-verbal than verbal intelligence tests. Kirkcaldy and Siefen (1991) explained non-verbal intelligence with the domination of motor associative functions in the brain, distinguishing extroverts from introverts, in whom sensory associations dominate. These findings led to the hypothesis that sport-specific intelligence, being predominantly non-verbal intelligence, is a manifestation of an extrovert personality and of the domination of motor associative functions in the brain. Such a hypothesis is expected to be tested in young athletes in whom intellectual behaviour is not already moderated by learning and experience. Until now, however, studies on sport intelligence in children have been very scanty, and have almost never used comparisons according to experience, age and personality together.

Fourcade (1975) carried out a series of investigations on decision-making in child athletes and non-athletes. The findings indicated that decision-making of non-athletes is less dynamic and with low speed. Geron (1975) tested decision-making in adolescent girls (15−18 years old) who were either experts or novices in basketball. They had to observe play situations and then decide on how the player holding the ball should act, and to react accordingly.

Experts outperformed the novices in speed and correctness of decisions. When in addition the girls were asked to make the decisions aloud, the thought processes of the experts were found reduced and several parts of them were not expressed verbally. This finding suggests that sport expertise has provoked automation of thought processes which transform them into non-verbal acts.

Stevens (1977) studied tactical thoughts in children (7–12 years old) who were either, basketball players or non-athletes. After observing a basketball game, they were required to draw and describe it. The results indicated that tactical thoughts developed gradually in children according to age and experience. Five types of players' interactions were outlined. Specific to the child athletes was that they subordinated the players in groups and that the actions which they described concerned the typical structure of the sports activity.

The above studies ascertained that the intellectual activity of child athletes is distinguished by speed, correctness, automation and fitness to the sport situations. However, these studies did not create opportunities for differentiation between the effects of age, expertise and personality.

Attempts to compare children of different ages and sport experience in their capacity of anticipation in ball sports were undertaken by Abernethy (1988) and Tenenbaum et al. (1992). Anticipation of ball movement introduces two intellectual processes: (i) selection of the input information; and (ii) allocation of attention. These functions develop in children slowly and relatively late. However, Wickens (1974) found that the ability to select information and organize it depends also on task-specific practice.

The purpose of Abernethy's study was to define at what age sport experience may affect anticipation. He studied four groups of experts and four groups of novices in badminton, aged 10–13, 14–16, 17–19 and over 20 years. All subjects were tested by a film occlusion task, presenting eight different badminton strokes. Subjects were asked to predict the landing positions of the strokes. The findings showed that children's anticipation is affected by three factors: (i) environmental conditions (the level of occlusion); (ii) age; and (iii) experience, which interacted with each other. Increase of the occlusion led to more incorrect anticipation in all subjects. However, the anticipation levels of experts was always higher than that of novices in each level of occlusion. Age did not improve the anticipation of novices, but child experts improved it at each subsequent age level. Sport experience influenced attentional allocation also. While novices anticipated using cues of the racquet position only, expert athletes may use several different cues.

The study, carried out by Tenenbaum et al. (1992) included three groups of tennis players: (i) adults with about 12 years sport experience; (ii) children 12–13 years old with 4 years experience; and (iii) child novices 10–11 years old with only 1 year experience. They were tested by a film occlusion task demonstrating six ball strokes. Analysis concerned the amount and direction of errors in anticipation of the ball location and also the subject's confidence in his or her own anticipation. The findings almost repeated those by Abernethy. They stress the role of the input information and of sport experience for correct anticipation. In addition, Tenenbaum et al. found that experience does not reduce all errors in anticipation and that anticipation during some strokes is influenced mainly by age and not by experience. (No differences were found between the two child groups.) Self-confidence did not influence correctness of anticipation. Self-confidence itself increases with the increase in the amount of input information, but only in expert players. These findings show that the athlete's capacity of anticipation is not related to self-confidence but that expertise in sport improving anticipation increase self-confidence.

The studies on 'sport intelligence' presented initial information which showed that manifestation of intellectual activity specific for sport may appear even in childhood. However, there exist differences in 'sport intelligence' of children and adults. Several intellectual capabilities specific for athletes develop later and relatively slower in children, e.g. attentional allocation which develops with maturity. Other intelligence capabilities are affected mainly by sport experience. Studies on anticipation, however, revealed that this intellectual capability improved in athletes as a result of interaction between situational factors (the input information), age and experience.

Intelligence profiles in child athletes

The specific intelligence of athletes is presumed to appear not only in separate intellectual capabilities but also in the athlete's intelligence profile (Cratty, 1972). Intelligence profiles express the relationships among the fundamental components of intelligence. These components are independent of one another and are not directly subordinate to general intelligence. That is why intelligence is defined as multidimensional (Cratty, 1972) and its dimensions as components of a complex, which may relate among them in different ways.

The dimensions (the fundamental components) of intelligence are intellectual activities often manifested as abilities. Such are the functions of analysis, abstraction, concretization, analogy, categorization, creativity and others. Some of them are further classified as concrete or formal (abstract) and as verbal or non-verbal.

Intelligence profiles are studied using intelligence test batteries which include a series of subtests, each measuring a separate intelligence dimension. The profiles are constructed using the quantitative determination of the developmental level of each dimension.

Intelligence profiles of athletes are rarely studied. Geron (1979) and Levin (1981, 1984) attempted to construct intelligence profiles of child athletes using the Meili's intelligence test – the Analytischer Intelligenztest (1971). This test was developed as an instrument for vocational selection. It includes six subtests, five of which are non-verbal. The evaluation

procedure uses profiles, constructed graphically on the bases of six rays arranged radially and expressing quantitatively six intelligence dimensions: (i) abstract analysis; (ii) concrete analysis; (iii) analogy; (iv) concrete thinking; (v) abstract (formal) non-verbal creativity; and (vi) concrete verbal creativity.

A study on the intelligence profiles of child novices in gymnastics (Geron, 1979) was done in order to clarify whether the specific intelligence profile, which was established in gymnasts experts during a previous study (Geron, 1975), is due to sport experience or is an inherent individual characteristic which appears in childhood before the child's involvement in sport and which may facilitate the engagement in sport. Average intelligence profiles were constructed and analysed separately for boys and girls aged 8–10 years old, who were accepted into a gymnastic training programme after a year of thorough selection. The Meili test was administered before the selection procedure to all candidates for the training programme (360 children). The scores of the 109 children accepted to this programme were later compared with the scores of two control groups: (i) a group of 169 children non-participants in sport of the same age, same district and schools; and (ii) a group of 17 children of the same age, accepted in a training course for children talented in tennis.

Using the Meili's intelligence test, Levin (1981) constructed intelligence profiles of children involved in track-and-field activity. The test was administered to 145 children 11–12 years old, candidates for sport classes specializing in track-and-field events. Comparison was carried out between the intelligence profiles of the 75 children involved in these classes, and 1 year successfully participated in them and the 70 children who appeared as not able enough to get on with track-and-field events. In another study Levin (1984) investigated differences in the intelligence profiles of child athletes of various sports and ages. The Meili test was administered to child athletes 10–12 and 13–15 years old, active participants in two individual sports (swimming and gymnastics) and in two team sports (soccer and basketball). In the individual sports boys and girls were tested separately while in team sports only boys were tested. For each gender and age about 30 subjects were involved in the study. The intelligence profiles of the child athletes were compared with the norms of the Meili test for the country, elaborated for the same age and sex on the bases of 2000 Israeli children.

The scores in the three studies were analysed using graphic constructions of the intelligence profiles, discriminant analysis and intercorrelations between the six tested intelligence dimensions.

The results showed that child athletes are distinguished by specific intelligence profiles, which vary according to the sport (Fig. 27.1). In the intelligence profiles of child gymnasts the dimension of abstract formal non-verbal creativity dominates. They are also classified

higher in concrete thinking but significantly lower than non-athletes in concrete verbal creativity. In the intelligence profiles of children succeeding in track-and-field events, analytical thinking (abstract and concrete) and analogy dominate significantly. Swimmers outperform the norms in abstract analysis, analogy and concrete thinking. Soccer players are distinguished from the norms by being better only in concrete creativity, while basketball players excel in concrete creativity, concrete thinking and abstract analysis. The profiles of the children tennis players excel in comparison with the children non-participants in sport and participants in other sports at a higher level of all intelligence dimensions. Concrete verbal creativity dominated in their profiles also.

A general finding is that in the intelligence profiles of the child participants in ball sports (tennis, basketball and soccer) the dimension of the concrete verbal creativity dominates. In

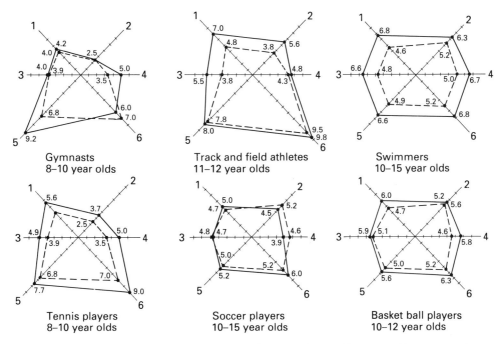

Fig. 27.1 Intelligence profiles in different sports: boy athletes (———) and boy non-athletes (– – – –). Intelligence dimensions: (1) abstract analysis; (2) concrete analysis; (3) analogy; (4) concrete thinking; (5) abstact (formal) creativity; and (6) concrete creativity. Based on Geron (1979), Levin (1981, 1984) and unpublished data.

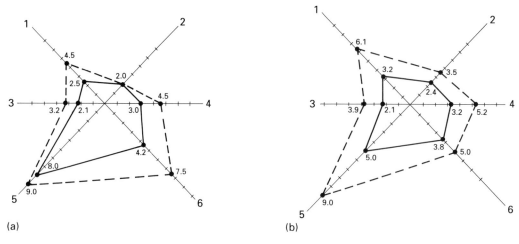

Fig. 27.2 Intelligence profiles of child gymnasts according to sex and age: (a) girls, and (b) boys; 8–9 years old; (———), and 9–10 years old (– – – –). Intelligence dimensions, see Fig. 27.1. Based on Geron (1979).

contrast, in the profile of the gymnasts the non-verbal formal creativity prevails. In the profiles of track-and-field athletes and swimmers, the dimensions of analysis and analogy are the most developed. Most of the tested athletes achieved relatively higher scores than non-athletes in concrete thinking.

The intelligence profiles of the child gymnasts and of the participants in the track-and-field events were determined according to the scores obtained before the child's involvement in sports. Their typical structures were clearly manifested in 8–9-year-old children before they began to practice gymnastics and in 11–12-year-old novices in track-and-field events. These findings support the supposition that intelligence profiles are not a product of sport experience. This is further confirmed by the fact that intelligence profiles of young children are more typically structured than profiles of older children.

The formation of the intelligence profiles of child athletes differs according to gender. The specific profile of gymnasts was manifested in girls at the age of 8 years and in boys at the age of 9 years (Fig. 27.2). The profiles of the participants in track-and-field events were more typically structured in boys than girls. Such age and gender differences were not found in the

intelligence profiles of child non-athletes (Fig. 27.3).

The multivariate correlation analysis between the intelligence dimensions of the child gymnasts established lower correlations (between 0.14 an 0.38) than in non-athletes (between 0.29 and 0.50). Differences were also found in the intercorrelations between the intelligence dimensions of children accepted and not accepted in the track-and-field sport classes. The correlations between the intelligence dimensions of the child gymnasts and their motor abilities, showed lack of uniformity. Namely, the intelligence dimensions which dominated in the child's profiles did not correlate with the child's motor abilities. This finding may be interpreted as supporting the idea that the formation of the typical intellectual structure in athletes are independent of their motor development.

The specific structure of the intelligence profiles of athletes is displayed in the inequality of the developmental level of the intelligence dimensions. One may suppose that the domination of some dimensions in the intelligence structure is what facilitates the performance of sport activities, which need the respective cognitive functions. Thus, the examination of the intelligence profiles of athletes, as well as

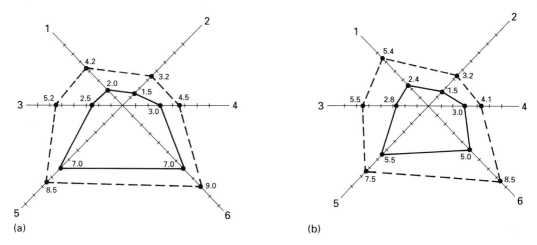

Fig. 27.3 Intelligence profiles of child non-athletes according to sex and age: (a) girls, and (b) boys; 8–9 years old (———), and 9–10 years old (– – – –). Intelligence dimensions, see Fig. 27.1. Based on Geron (1979).

the examination of the level of their various intelligence dimensions, may be fruitful in understanding some of the sources of success of children in specific sports. The findings suggested that the specific organization of the intelligence profiles of athletes is not due to sport experience. It appears before beginning the active sport activity and in relatively early childhood. Sport experience as well as maturation conceal the structure of the profile by newly developed cognitive capabilities.

Although very limited, the data on the intelligence profiles of child athletes suggested that their determination may help the selection of children who are talented in sports and the orientation of the children to these kinds of sport in which, from the cognitive aspect, they have higher prospects of succeeding.

Conclusion

Intelligence is a personality characteristic promoting success in each human performance. Practice and research also revealed its significant role in sport activity. This role is due mainly to two factors: (i) the existing mutual relationship between intelligence and motor performance; and (ii) the need of self-regulation

during sport activity (and especially during competition).

The intelligence–motor abilities relationship is manifested in that:

1 Intelligence in its elementary form is born during the infant's motor activity and later during the child's development it transforms into a necessary component of this activity. This is why quality of motor performance in early childhood may predict future intellectual development, and organized motor activity in childhood may stimulate intellectual development.

2 Intelligence facilitates motor performance. Intelligent children participate more actively and more successfully in sport than those with a lower intelligence. Successful development of defined intelligence dimensions and intellectual abilities as well as specific intelligence profiles support success in sport learning and performance.

3 Research reveals that the mutual relation between intelligence and motor performance is not general but specific. Specific motor characteristics predict intellectual development. Specific intelligence abilities, dimensions and profiles may facilitate learning and performance of motor and sport activities. Experience in defined types of sporting activity stimulates the development of specific intellectual capabilities.

4 The intelligence–motor abilities relationship is more clearly manifested in early developmental stages. In later stages of the child's development the influence of maturation, learning and environmental effects obscure this relationship.

The practical value of the studies on the intelligence–motor abilities relationship is that they open the possibility of predicting intellectual and motor achievements, to select motor activities, which may stimulate intellectual development and to select children for appropriate sports.

The second factor which defines the role of intelligence in sport is the requirements of sport for adequate self-regulation of behaviour. During competitions, athletes should process in a very short time complex and varied information and have to make adequate decisions in continually arising problem-solving situations. The experience in answering these requirements stimulates the development of relevant intellectual capabilities, which may develop in child athletes earlier than in children who do not participate in sport. These intellectual capabilities form the so-called 'sport-specific intelligence'. Speculation exists that this is based on certain characteristics of the personality and specific brain functions. However, research findings reveal the primary role of sport experience in the development of 'sport-specific intelligence'. But one may suppose that individual characteristics may serve as dispositions for successful expertise effect on the development of 'sport-specific intelligence'.

These generalizations on the role of intelligence in children's sports are obviously very general and almost completely hypothetical. This is due to the nature and quality of the studies that have been carried out on this topic, most of which are comparatively out of date, sporadic, fragmentary and incomplete. They suffer also from some methodological shortcomings. The developmental approach, recommended for the psychology of children's

sport (Weiss & Bredemeier, 1983) and particularly important for intelligence studies, has been rarely used. Analyses of data are often insufficient and use obsolete techniques. Some of the research findings need additional verifications and further detail.

Challenges for future research

Studies concerning the intelligence of child athletes have been very restricted in number. This makes the identification of topics for future research on this issue an arduous task so only the main trends are outlined here.

There are two main directions which should be adopted in future studies: the first concerns the methodological specification of any possible studies, and the second concerns the definition of the objects of research.

Methodological specifications

- Existing studies are directed at investigating the mutual effects between intelligence and motor and sport activity among children. Findings show that these effects vary according to additional factors such as individual characteristics of the children (age, gender, level of experience and others) and environmental conditions in which sport occurs. This fact reveals the necessity to modify the questions of the study: not to enquire about the existence of effects but about the conditions in which they may be realized. Such a modification of the study questions will direct the investigations to searching the modes of regulating the effect of sport on the child's intellectual development and to utilizing the child's intellectual capacities in reaching success in sport.

- Future investigators of the intelligence of child athletes will be faced with the necessity of solving problems related to the means for testing the athlete's intelligence. Recently, sport psychologists developed specific psychological tools (tests, inventories, questionnaires) for testing the psychological characteristics and states of participants in sport. Should intelligence of athletes be tested also by specific sport-intelligence tests? This depends on the object of the study. General intelligence development of child athletes obviously should be tested by general intelligence tests, which permit comparisons between athletes and non-athletes. However, the effect of specific sport situations as well as the expertise effect of sport on the intelligence capabilities of the children need to be studied by specific measurement tools adapted to sport. Until now such tools have not been available. An attractive challenge to future studies will be to investigate the opportunities of the existing intelligence tests for studying child athletes, to adapt some of them to the specific needs of sport, and eventually to develop new sport intelligence tests. One of the difficulties in this endeavour is the great diversity in the intellectual characteristics of athletes in varying types of sports. A selection of common elements among them may enable the creation of more general intelligence tests and overcome the extreme specialization of the objects of testing. The next step will be the adaptation of the tests to the children's ages.

● An important methodological requirement for future studies on intelligence of child athletes is the introduction of longitudinal measurements. Such measurements have not been carried out until now, although they are necessary in studies on the intellectual development and on the effects of sport experience.

The objects of future research

● Studies on important topics, whose findings are not comprehensive and convincing enough, need to be replicated. Such replications will be useful in the completion and verification of the findings about the effect of sport on the academic achievements of child athletes; the age affect on the intelligence−motor abilities relationship; the age and gender differences in the intelligence profiles of child athletes; the adaptation of the motor learning strategies on the child's cognitive capabilities and so on.

● New studies are necessary in two main areas:

(i) on the intellectual development of child athletes; and (ii) on the specific intellectual characteristics of young athletes, taking into consideration 'sport-specific intelligence' and intelligence profiles.

● Studies on child athletes in various scientific areas have included as an important object of their research the follow-up of the normal development of the child athlete. Although intellectual development of children has always been regarded as a vital issue, there have been no serious studies devoted to the intellectual development of children participants in sport. Many questions related to this issue are still open. Does participation in sport change the normal course of the child's intellectual development, its stages and their age boundaries? Is intellectual development of child athletes different from that of child non-athletes? Is intellectual development different in child participants in various sports?

● In connection with these general questions, additional questions arise, one of which concerns the intelligence−motor abilities relationship. Does it appear in the same form in child athletes and non-athletes? It was expected that participation in sport would reinforce this relationship. However, some studies (Geron, 1976, 1979) pointed out that in child gymnasts the relationship between intellectual and motor capabilities is weaker than in non-participants in sport. Thus, new questions arise. Is this fact valid for children participants in other sports? Does the intelligence−motor abilities relationship change according to sport experience? What is the reason for the reduction of the intelligence−motor abilities relationship in child gymnasts?

● Today, special institutions are being established for the preparation of young athletes in many countries: sport schools, classes, hostels, training camps, and so on. Do these institutions contribute to a more favourable effect of sport on the intellectual development of the youth involved? Are they beneficial to the athlete's academic achievement, to the enlargement of the child's intellectual interests and to the stimulation of their congitive activity? Future research is to be confronted with these questions.

• Learning in sport in some specific way is also related to intellectual development. Being independent of level of intelligence (Start, 1964; Geron, 1976; Singer, 1984; Sugden, 1984) it needs to be adapted to the cognitive capabilities of the child participants in sport (Yando *et al.*, 1978; Weiss, 1983). Learning strategies used in surmounting difficulties during learning in sport are based on cognitive activities (imagination, inner speech, attentional allocation and others) which develop in children with age. That is why each learning strategy may be used by children of different age in different ways. Determining what learning strategies and how and when they should be used by child athlete of different ages are questions which await investigation.

• Until now, studies on the specific intellectual characteristics of child athletes have been very limited, and needs to be extended. Two kinds of specific intellectual characteristics for athletes may be defined: (i) the characteristics subsumed to the so-called 'sport-specific intelligence'; and (ii) the intelligence profiles. 'Sport-specific intelligence' was found to be a result of experience in sport, while sport profiles are supposed to be inherited.

The main method which the studies on 'sport-specific intelligence' characteristics use, is a comparison between athletic experts and novices. For studies testing children, it is also advisable to introduce comparisons between child and adult athletes, as well as comparisons among child athletes of different age groups. As the 'sport-specific intelligence' characteristics develop during sport practice, they are, most probably, also influenced by the requirements of the specific sports. This is why research on these characteristics should also use comparisons between children participating in different sports.

There are general 'sport-specific intelligence' characteristics which distinguish participants in many and perhaps in all sports. Their study would prove to be especially useful. Such characteristics, for example, are the ability to decode movements, the ability to communicate non-verbally, speed of thinking, automation of thinking and others. A relatively general 'sport-specific intelligence' characteristic is tactical thinking, which until now has been investigated in adult athletes. Its exploration in child athletes may be very helpful for coaches of children. Coaches need to know to what extent children may self-determine their own tactical behaviour, and what part of the tactic should be elaborated by the coach's intervention. Research is also necessary on two other general intelligence characteristics contributing to tactical thinking: (i) the automation of thinking; and (ii) the speed of thinking. Is the automation of thinking available and recommended in childhood? Can speed of thinking be stimulated and developed in children? Are the strategies used suitable for children?

An intriguing question not usually studied is the question concerning the influence of personality on the development of sport-intelligence characteristics. Do some personality characteristics (extroversion, field dependence, self-confidence and others) support the development of 'sport-specific intelligence'? Is 'sport-specific intelligence' always related to non-verbal thinking? Studies on 'sport-specific intelligence' characteristics of child athletes will be considerably helped if one can use a taxonomy on the intelligence characteristics which distinguish athletes. Such a document may guide the research for determining which of the intellectual characteristics are already developed in child athletes and at what age this occurs.

• Studies on the intelligence profiles of child athletes are only in their early stages and are expected to be extended in different sports and age levels. It will be beneficial to build constructions of intelligence profiles using various intelligence tests and including more intelligence dimensions. Studies will be necessary for determining the predictability of the intelligence profiles for children's involvement in sport activities, success in sport learning and achievement in sports.

References

Abernethy, B. (1988) The effect of age and expertise upon perceptual skill development in racquet sport. *Res. Q. Exerc. Sport* **59**, 210–21.

Boulton, S.M. (1966) Relationships between mental ability, physique and various competitive game activities of adolescent boys in comprehensive school. *Res. Papers Phys. Educ.* **3**, 3–13.

Buhrmann, H.G. (1972) Scholarship and athletics in junior high school. *Int. Rev. Sport Sociol.* **7**, 119–28.

Campbell, K.B. & Noldy-Cullum, N. (1985) Mental chronometry. II. Individual differences. In B.D. Kirckaldy (ed.) *Individual Differences in Movement*, pp. 147–68. MIP Press, Lancaster.

Carroll, J. (1972) Deception in games playing. In H.T.A. Whiting (ed.) *Readings in Sports Psychology*, pp. 238–46. Henry Kimpton, London.

Chambers, S.T. (1991) Factors affecting elementary school students participation in sport. *Element. School J.* **91**, 413–19.

Chissom, B.S. (1971) A factor analytical study of the relationship of motor factors to academic criteria for first and third grade boys. *Child Dev.* **42**, 1133–43.

Corder, W.O. (1966) Effect of physical education on intellectual, physical and social development of educable mentally retarded boys. *Except. Child.* **32**, 357–64.

Corlitt, H. (1973) Development of movement concepts in the child. In J.D. Brooke & H.I. Whiting (eds) *Human Movement: A Field of Study*, pp. 277–94. Henry Kimpton, London.

Cratty, B.J. (1972) *Physical Expressions of Intelligence*. Prentice Hall, Englewood Cliffs, NJ.

Cratty, B.J. (1984) *Psychological Preparation and Athletic Excellence*. Movement Publications, New York.

Cratty, B.J. & Martin Sister, M.M. (1969) *Perceptual-motor Efficiency in Children*. Lea & Febiger, Philadelphia.

Delacato, C.H. (1966) *Neurological Organization on Reading*. C.C. Thomas, Springfield, IL.

Dibner, A.S. & Korn, E.J. (1969) Group administration of the Bender gestalt test to predict early school performance. *J. Clin. Psychol.* **25**, 263–8.

Dunkelman, N. (1981) Level of academic achievement of child-participants in sport. In E. Geron, A. Mashiach, N. Dunkelman, S. Raviv, Z. Levin & E. Nakash (eds) *Children in Sport: Psychosociological Characteristics*, pp. 56–63. Wingate Monograph Series No. 11. Wingate Institute, Israel.

Eysenck, H.J., Nias, D.K.B. & Cox, D.B. (1982) Sport and personality. *Adv. Behav. Res. Ther.* **4**, 1–56.

Fisher, A.C. (1984) Sport intelligence. In W.F. Straub & J.M. Williams (eds) *Cognitive Sport Psychology*, pp. 42–50. Sport Science Associates, Lansing, NY.

Fleury, M., Bard, C. & Carriere, L. (1982) Effects of reduction of processing time and level of expertise in a multiple-choice decision task. *Percept. Motor Skills* **55**, 1279–88.

Fourcade, J. (1975) Approche quantitative de l'influence de la personalite sur l'activite decisionnelle (Quantitative approach to the influence of the personality on decision-making). In *Travaux Scientifiques du CRSSA de Lyon*, pp. 127–130. Centre de Reserches du Service de Sante des Armee, Lyon.

Frostig, M. (1970) *Movement Education: Theory and Practice*. Follet Educational, Chicago.

Gaskin, P.R. (1971) Mental ability and success in a test of motor ability. *Br. J. Phys. Educ.* **2**, 20–3.

Geron, E. (1975) *Methoden und Mitteln zur Psychischen Vorbereitung des Sportlers* (Methods and Means of Psychological Preparation of Athletes). Verlag Karl Hofmann, Schorndorf.

Geron, E. (1976) Intelligence and motor learning ability in gymnastics. In U. Simri (ed.) *Motor Learning in Physical Education and Sport*, pp. 90–8. Proceedings of an International Seminar. Wingate Institute, Israel.

Geron, E. (1979) Sport giftedness (in gymnastics) and intelligence in children. *Int. J. Sport Psychol.* **10**, 18–30.

Geron, E., Mashiach, A., Dunkelman, N., Raviv, S., Levin, Z. & Nakash, E. (1981) A research project on the psycho-sociological characteristics of participants in sport classes in school. In E. Geron, A. Mashiach, N. Dunkelman, S. Raviv, Z. Levin & E. Nakash (eds) *Children in Sport: Psycho-Sociological Characteristics*, pp. 7–43. Wingate Monograph Series No. 11. Wingate Institute, Israel.

Geron, E. & Reches, I. (1984) The effect of a self-assessment approach during physical education on the perceptual-motor development of 7–8 year old children. In U. Simri, D. Eldar & S. Lieberman (eds) *Pre-school and Elementary School Children and Physical Activity*, pp. 54–63. Proceedings of the 26th ICHPER Congress. Em. Gill Publishing House, Israel.

Getman, G.N. (1952) *How to Develop your Child's Intelligence. A Research Publication*. G.N. Getman, Luverne, MI.

Goebel, B.L. & Harris, E.L. (1980) Cognitive strategy and personality across age levels. *Percept. Motor Skills* **50**, 803–11.

Gorman, D.R., Zody, J.M., Rrown, B.S., Debrezze, R. & Edwards W.H. (1990) Multivariate relationships of IQ with motor performance in children referred to a diagnostic motor development clinic. *Clin. Kinesiol.* **44**, 107–10.

Gould, D. (1982) Sport psychology in the 1980s: status, direction and challenge in youth sports research. *J. Sport Psychol.* **4**, 203–18.

Gruber, J.J. (1975) Exercise and mental performance. *Int. J. Sport Psychol.* **6**, 28–40.

Hayashi, T. & Yamaoka, S. (1965) Research of the influence of physical activity on intellectual work. *Res. J. Phys. Educ.* (Japan) **10**, 15–18.

Humphrey, J.H. & Sullivan, D.D. (1970) *Teaching Slow Learners Through Active Games.* C.C. Thomas, Springfield, IL.

Isaacs, L.D. & Finch, A.E. (1983) Anticipatory timing of beginning and intermediate tennis players. *Percept. Motor Skills* **57**, 451–4.

Ismail, A.H. (1967) The effect of a well organized physical education programme on intellectual performance. *Res. Phys. Educ.* **1**, 31–8.

Ismail, A.H. (1972) Integrated development. In J.E. Kane (ed.) *Psychological Aspects of Physical Education and Sport*, pp. 1–37. Routledge & Kegan Paul, London.

Ismail, A.H. & Gruber, J. (1967) *Integrated Developments: Motor Aptitudes and Intellectual Performance.* Charles E. Merrill, New York.

Ismail, A.H., Kane J. & Kirkendall, D.R. (1969) Relationships among intellectual and nonintellectual variables. *Res. Q.* **40**, 83–92.

Jantz, R.K. (1975) Moral thinking in male elementary pupils as reflected by perception by basketball rules. *Res. Q.* **46**, 414–21.

Jefferies, M.S. (1978) Relationship of football with academic ability and nonverbal intelligence. *Br. J. Phys. Educ.* **9**, 15–16.

Kaminski, G. & Ruoff, B.A. (1979) Kinder in Hochleistungssport (Children in high achievement sport). In H. Gabler, H. Eberspacher, E. Hahn, J. Kern & G. Schilling (eds) *Praxis der Psychology in Leistungssport*, pp. 200–24. Verlag Bartels & Wernitz, Berlin.

Kashiwabara, K., Kobayashi, T. & Kondo, M. (1966) The influence of physical activity on the mental work. *Res. J. Phys. Educ.* (Japan) **11**, 16–22.

Kephart, N.C. (1964) Perceptual-motor aspects of learning disabilities. *Except. Child.* **31**, 201–6.

Kiphard, E.J. & Huppertz, H. (1968) *Erziehung durch Bewegung* (Movement Education). Durr, Bad Godesberg.

Kirkcaldy, B.D. & Seifen, G. (1991) Personality correlates of intelligence in a clinical group. *Psychol. Rep.* **69**, 947–52.

Kirkendall, D.R. & Gruber, J.J. (1970) Canonical relationships between the motor and intellectual achievement domains in culturally deprived high school pupils. *Res. Q.* **41**, 498–502.

Kirkendall, D.R. & Ismail, A.H. (1970) The discriminating power of nonintellectual variables among three discrete intellectual groups. In J. Kenyon (ed.) *Contemporary Psychology of Sport*, pp. 481–7. Athletic Institute, Chicago.

Kohen-Raz, R., Hecht, O. & Ayalon, T. (1984) Possible effects of structured physical education on scholastic progress of culturally disadvantaged first graders. In U. Simri, D. Eldar & S. Lieberman (eds) *Preschool and Elementary School Children and Physical Activity*, pp. 64–8. Proceedings of the 26th ICHPER Congress. Em. Gill Publishing House, Israel.

Laporte, W. (1984) The impact of the integrated movement education on motor and intellectual behavior of children in the first year of the primary school. In U. Zimri, D. Eldar & S. Lieberman (eds) *Preschool and Elementary School Children and Physical Activity*, pp. 69–78. Proceedings of the 26th ICHPER Congress. Em. Gill Publishing House, Israel.

Levin, Z. (1981) Intelligence in children participating in sports. In E. Geron, A. Mashiach, N. Dunkelman, S. Raviv, Z. Levin & E. Nakash (eds) *Children in Sport: Psychosociological Characteristics*, pp. 64–71. Wingate Monograph Series No. 11. Wingate Institute, Israel.

Levin, Z. (1984) Intelligence structure of elementary school age athletes. In U. Simri, D. Eldar & S. Lieberman (eds) *Preschool and Elementary School Children and Physical Activity*, pp. 79–88. Proceedings of the 26th ICHPER Congress. Em. Gill, Israel.

McIntosh, P.C. (1966) Mental ability and success in school sport. *Res. Phys. Educ.* **1**, 1–3.

Meili, R. (1971) *Analytischer Intelligenztest* (Analytical Test of Intelligence). Verlag Hans Huber, Bern.

Mosston, M. (1966) *Teaching Physical Education.* Charles E. Merrill, Columbus, OH.

Nettlebeck, T. & Kirby, N.H. (1983) Measures of timed performance and intelligence. *Intelligence* **7**, 39–52.

Pauwels, J.M. & Mols, H. (1981) Ball games: the body and the mind. Relationship between intelligence and a number of motor abilities and skills in 12 year old boys and girls. In J.C. DePotter (ed.) *Adapted Physical Activities*, pp. 149–58. Proceeding of an international Symposium, Edition de l'Universitée de Bruxelles, Bruxelles.

Piaget, J. (1953) *The Origins of Intelligence in the Child.* Routledge & Kegan Paul, London.

Railo, W.S. (1969) Physical fitness and intellectual achievement. *Scand. J. Educ. Res.* **2**, 103–20.

Rarick, G.L. (1973) Competitive sports in childhood and early adolescence. In G.L. Rarick (ed.) *Physical Activity: Human Growth and Development*, pp. 364–86. Academic Press, New York.

Rarick, G.L. (1980) Cognitive-motor relationships in the growing years. *Res. Q. Exerc. Sport* **51**, 174–92.

Rieder, H. (1984) Kognitive Fahigkeiten als Training-saufgabe im Leistungssport (Cognitive capacities as a purpose of coaching in achievement sport). In H. Rieder (ed.) *Sport Psychology-International*, pp. 43–62. CPS Verlag, Koln.

Robinson, D.R. (1985) How personality relates to intelligence tests performance: implications for a theory of intelligence, aging research and personality assessment. *Personal. Ind. Diff.* **6**, 203–16.

Ruffer, W.A. (1965) A study of extreme physical activity groups of young men. *Res. Q.* **36**, 183–96.

Schafer, W. & Armer, J.J. (1964) Athletes are not inferior students. *Trans-Action* **6**, 21.

Schewe, H. (1977) Evaluation of relationship between intellectual and motor ability in children. *Fed. Int. d'Educ. Phys. Bull.* **47**, 35–40.

Schurr, T. & Brookover, W. (1970) Athletes, academic self-concept and achievement. *Med. Sci. Sports* **2**, 96–9.

Seefeldt, V.D., Gilliam, T., Blievernich, D. & Russel, B. (1978) Scope of youth sport programs in the state of Michigan. In F.L. Smoll & R.E. Smith (eds) *Psychological Perspectives in Youth Sports*, pp. 17–67. Hemisphere, Washington DC.

Sharpe, P.J. (1979) Contribution of aspects of movement education to the cognitive development of infant school children. *J. Hum. Move. Stud.* **5**, 125–40.

Sherrill, C. (1986) Fostering creativity in handicapped children. *Adap. Phys. Activ. Q.* **3**, 236–49.

Silva, P.A., McGee, R. & Williams, S. (1982) Prospective study of the association between delayed motor development at ages three and five and low intelligence and reading difficulties at age seven: a report from the Dunedin multidisciplinary child development study. *J. Hum. Move. Stud.* **8**, 187–93.

Singer, R.N. (1968) Interrelationships of physical, perceptual-motor and academic variables in elementary school children. *Percept. Motor Skills* **27**, 1323–32.

Singer, R.N. (1984) What do children want in youth sport? In H. Rieder (ed.) *Sport Psychology International*, pp. 115–26. B.P.S. Verlag, Koln.

Smith, R.E. & Smoll, F.L. (1978) Sport and the child, conceptual and research perspectives. In F.L. Smoll & R.E. Smith (eds) *Psychological Perspectives in Youth Sport*, pp. 3–13. Hemisphere, Washington DC.

Start, K.B. (1964) Intelligence and the improvement in a gross motor skill after mental practice. *Br. J. Educ. Psychol.* **34**, 85–8.

Start, K.B. (1967) Sporting and intellectual success among English secondary school children. *Int. Rev. Sport Sociol.* **2**, 47–54.

Stevens, T.R. (1977) Cognitive structure in sport tactics: a preliminary investigation. In P. Stevens (ed.) *Studies in the Anthropology of Play*, Part 4, pp. 175–84. Leisure Press, New York.

Sugden, D.A. (1984) The learning of motor skills by children of different intellectual abilities. In U. Simri, D. Eldar & S. Lieberman (eds) *Preschool and Elementary School Children and Physical Activity*, pp. 149–53. Proceedings of the 26th ICHPER Congress. Em. Gill, Israel.

Sugden, D.A. & Connell, R.A. (1982) Information processing in children's motor skills. *Phys. Educ. Rev.* **2**, 123–41.

Tenenbaum, G., Kolker, N., Sade, S. & Liebermann, D. (1992) Anticipation and confidence of decisions related to skilled performance. Report presented at the Ribstein Center for Research and Sport Medicine Sciences, Wingate Institute, Israel.

Thomas, J.R. & Chissom, B.S. (1972) Relationships as assessed by canonical correlation between perceptual motor and intellectual abilities for pre-school and early elementary age children. *J. Motor Behav.* **4**, 23–9.

Waxman, S.R. (1991) Contemporary approaches to concept development. *Cog. Dev.* **6**, 105–18.

Weiss, M.R. (1983) Modeling and motor performance: a developmental perspective. *Res. Q. Exerc. Sport* **54**, 190–7.

Weiss, M.R. & Bredemeier, B.J. (1983) Developmental sport psychology: a theoretical perspective for studying children in sport. *J. Sports Psychol.* **5**, 216–30.

Wickens, C.D. (1974) Temporal limits of human information processing: a developmental study. *Psychol. Bull.* **81**, 739–55.

Williams, A. (1988) Physical activity patterns among adolescents — some curriculum implications. *Phys. Educ. Rev.* **11**, 28–39.

Yando, R., Seitz, V. & Zigler, E. (1978) *Imitation: A Developmental Perspective*. Wiley, New York.

Yates, J.B. (1975) Physical education as symbolic interaction: an interpretation of the hidden messages of the physical education curriculum. *Bull. Phys. Educ.* **11**, 13–18.

Chapter 28

The Drop-out Dilemma in Youth Sports

LINDA M. PETLICHKOFF

Introduction

For more than two decades, youth sport researchers have studied the drop-out dilemma in organized sport (for reviews see Gould & Horn, 1984; Gould & Petlichkoff, 1988; Weiss & Petlichkoff, 1989). Current estimates indicate that, on average, 35% of the children and adolescents involved in youth sports withdraw from organized sport each year (Gould, 1987). Furthermore, research conducted in the USA reveals that participation in youth sports declines dramatically between the ages of 11 and 13 years (State of Michigan, 1976, 1978a,b; Athletic Footwear Association, 1990).

Early efforts to explain the drop-out phenomenon left some youth sport researchers questioning the structure of organized sport (Orlick, 1973, 1974; Orlick & Botterill, 1975). Orlick (1974), for example, interviewed 60 athletic drop-outs ranging in age from 7 to 18 years who had participated in one of four sports the previous year. The results revealed that 67% of the sample discontinued their involvement because of the overemphasis placed on winning. In an earlier investigation, Orlick (1973) found that 75% of the 8- and 9-year-old non-participants sampled did not become involved in sport because they thought they were 'not good enough' to make the team or play on a regular basis. Orlick concluded that, at times, an overemphasis placed on winning and a fear of failure greatly influenced some children's decisions to withdraw from sport.

Other studies (Robertson, 1981; Sefton & Fry, 1981; Athletic Footwear Association, 1990) lend support to the notion that programme emphases such as too much time, emphasis placed on winning and too much pressure, as well as dislike for the coach contribute significantly to the decline in sport participation. Robertson (1981) assessed reasons for dropping out of sport with a sample of 12-year-old former Australian athletes (353 females and 405 males) and determined that approximately 40% of the sample cited reasons such as 'too boring', 'not having fun' and 'lack of playing time' for discontinuing their involvement. Sefton and Fry (1981) assessed reasons for discontinuing swimming with 86 former swimmers ranging in age from 6 to 22 years. The two primary reasons for dropping out of swimming were (i) too time-consuming (31%); and (ii) a degree of dissatisfaction with practice (27%). Another reason cited for discontinuing involvement in age-group swimming focused on the coach's behaviour suggesting that he or she either played favourites or was overdemanding. Once again, these results prompted some youth sport researchers to criticize the structure and emphasis of programmes and cited these factors as primary contributors to sport withdrawal.

Contributing also to the decline in sport participation, however, is the fact that children develop interests in both other sports and non-sport activities. In fact, when all studies are considered together, 'conflicts of interests' or 'other things to do' appear to be the most often cited reasons for dropping out of sport (Gould & Horn, 1984). Sapp and Haubenstricker (1978) found that older athletes ($n = 404$), ranging in age from 11 to 18 years, who indicated they did not plan to participate next year, cited other activities (64%) and working (44%) as important reasons for dropping out of sport. Gould *et al.* (1982) found that 49% of the former swimmers ($n = 50$) between the ages of 10 and 18 dropped out of swimming because they had 'other things to do'. Similar results were reported also in several of the studies cited earlier in this chapter (Athletic Footwear Association, 1980; Robertson, 1981; Sefton & Fry, 1981). Drop-outs sampled in the Athletic Footwear Association (1990) investigation indicated they wanted to try non-sport activities and/or they needed more study time, as reasons for their withdrawal from sport.

More recent evidence suggests that dropping out of sport may reflect a normal trial-and-error sampling children do in search of an enjoyable activity and/or an achievement domain in which they can demonstrate competence (Burton & Martens, 1986; Burton, 1988; Weiss & Petlichkoff, 1989; Petlichkoff, 1993a). That is, a number of activities exist in and outside school that children can become involved in while they are growing up. As their days become filled with these activities, decisions are made as to whether they can maintain the quality of their sport involvement along with all the other activities (Weiss & Petlichkoff, 1989). Withdrawing from sport in these instances represents more of a developmental process rather than a departure predicated upon negative outcomes, poor coaching or an overemphasis placed on winning — not that these do not exist.

Given these plausible explanations for youth sport withdrawal, researchers have realized that simply identifying reasons for sport withdrawal may no longer be appropriate. Rather, a better understanding of the factors influencing a child's decision to drop out of sport should be the primary focus of youth sport withdrawal research. This chapter is structured to examine youth sport withdrawal from a process-oriented approach focusing on factors that may contribute to the child's withdrawal from sport.

The first section provides a clarification of current terms used to describe drop-outs from youth sports. Such clarification is necessary because the term drop-out fails to capture the essence of the phenomenon. This traditional term represents the end-product — the child no longer being involved in sport — and carries with it a negative connotation. The second section synthesizes the research conducted to date through the model of youth sport withdrawal forwarded by Gould (1987). Special emphasis in this section is placed on the child's decision-making process of weighing the costs against the benefits (i.e. the rewards and costs) of being involved in sport, as well as whether the child has any control over the decision to withdraw from sport. The third section focuses on the major issues facing youth sport researchers and identifies challenges for future research on youth sport withdrawal.

Defining the process

One of the major barriers paediatric sport scientists have encountered in an effort to explain the drop-out dilemma in youth sports focuses on definitional hurdles. Most of the early research classifies children and adolescents into one of the following categories.

1 Participant: an athlete who is currently participating in a specific sport programme.

2 Drop-out: an individual who is no longer involved in that particular programme.

3 Non-participant: an individual who has never been involved in that particular programme (Weiss & Petlichkoff, 1989).

Typically, these classifications were made after the fact and assessed the individual's current status of sport involvement or non-involvement. These definitions infer an all-or-nothing meaning to sport participation or withdrawal.

What these terms fail to capture is the rather complex process that contributes to the child's withdrawal from sport. Researchers utilizing these more traditional definitions cannot evaluate, for example, whether or not:

1 The individual develops an interest in another sport or an activity outside of sport.

2 The child's withdrawal is permanent or temporary.

3 The child actually has a choice in the decision to withdraw from sport.

4 The end-result (sport withdrawal) is detrimental to the child's psychological well-being. The process that leads to sport withdrawal, then, may completely alter how researchers define the phenomenon.

Evidence suggests (Klint & Weiss, 1986; Weiss & Petlichkoff, 1989) that drop-outs fit into various categories based on the process that leads to their withdrawal from organized sport. Klint and Weiss, for example, identified three types of drop-outs:

1 The volunteer drop-out: an individual who was not necessarily unhappy in his or her present situation but wanted to sample other sports or activities.

2 The resistant drop-out: a child or adolescent who still valued sport participation but was unhappy in the present situation.

3 The reluctant drop-out: an individual forced out because of injury or the cost of the programme.

It is obvious from these definitions that the resistant and reluctant drop-outs present more cause for alarm than does the volunteer drop-out. That is, resistant or reluctant drop-outs may have experienced more negative affect associated with their departure from sport and these feelings may influence whether or not they return to sports or other activities in the future. In contrast, voluntary drop-outs may be sampling various achievement domains in an effort to find an activity that they are reasonably good at, given their present ability or interest level. Hence, this reaffirms the notion that differences may exist among drop-outs based on factors influencing their decision to withdraw.

Lindner et al. (1991) have taken an interesting approach to delineate voluntary withdrawal from competitive sport. These authors also identified three types of potential drop-outs: (i) the sampler drop-out; (ii) the participant drop-out; and (iii) the transfer drop-out. These definitions are based on the individual's level of participation and commitment prior to dropping out of sport. The sampler drop-out was identified as an individual who was briefly involved in a sport with the specific purpose of 'trying it out' (Burton & Martens, 1986; Lindner et al., 1991). This individual had not made a commitment to the sport and may have been a once only participant (e.g. season) in one or more sports (i.e. trial-and-error sampling). An individual who fits into this classification may approach sport involvement as a way of being with friends or as something to do after school or during summer recess.

The participant drop-out was an individual who had committed his or her time to one or more sports for a number of years and may have competed at various levels of competition (i.e. recreational, competitive or national). For this individual, dropping out may have occurred when the sport no longer met his or her needs. Or, this athlete may have been experiencing a classic case of 'burn-out' — a phenomenon differentiated from voluntary withdraw (Smith, 1986).* The participant drop-out may, at times, return to another sport, return to the same sport at another level, or drop out completely from sport (Klint & Weiss, 1986; Lindner et al., 1991).

The third type of drop-out identified was the transfer drop-out who, based on traditional definitions, drops out because he or she is no longer involved in a particular programme. However, this individual may have re-entered sport at another level or may be currently participating in another sport.

---

* Smith (1986) differentiates between the sport burn-out and sport drop-out based on cognitive-affective issues resulting from competitive stress. Specifically, Smith defines burn-out as the psychological, emotional and physical withdrawal from sport resulting from chronic stress. Drop-out, on the other hand, results from a change of interests and/or value reorientation and is the focus of this chapter.

Inherent in all of these definitions is the notion that different factors contributed to the individual's withdrawal or transfer from sport. Moreover, the majority of these definitions do not infer negative connotations associated with the more traditional definitions of drop-out that embrace an all-or-nothing meaning of sport participation or withdrawal. Such a conclusion does not suggest that dropping out of sport is always positive (e.g. resistant drop-out); rather, it calls for a better understanding of the process involved in youth sport withdrawal.

Hence, a need exists to classify drop-outs according to factors (i.e. sport- or milieu-related) that influence an individual to withdraw from sport (Lindner et al., 1991), as well as to assess the current status of his or her involvement or non-involvement in sport and non-sport activities. By redirecting the focus from reasons for dropping out, as in the early research, to factors that interact to influence the decision to withdraw from sport, sport scientists and practitioners may intervene more appropriately in the process to provide a positive sport experience for children and adolescents. Furthermore, once researchers understand the process, dropping out of sport may not carry with it the negative connotation that it has endured in the past (Orlick, 1973; Orlick & Botterill, 1975; Lee & Owen, 1984).

A model of youth sport withdrawal

In an effort to describe and explain the drop-out phenomenon as a process, Gould (1987) generated a model of youth sport withdrawal (Fig. 28.1).* The majority of attrition research has focused on component 4 of the model, motivation for youth sport withdrawal. Specifically, descriptive studies cited earlier in this

chapter indicate that children and adolescents withdraw from sport for a variety of reasons and that these reasons are typically associated with personal (i.e. lack of ability, skills do not improve, lack of success) and situational (i.e. lack of playing time, lack of social support, programme emphasis) factors. More recently, youth sport researchers have utilized several theoretical frameworks that are thought to underlie surface level reasons for sport withdrawal (Maehr & Nicholls, 1980; Harter, 1981; Smith, 1986) to better explain the phenomenon (see component 4b). It appears that children and adolescents who withdraw from youth sport differ on their achievement orientations, as well as their perception of ability, from those individuals who remain involved in sport (i.e. drop-outs tend to have a lower perception of ability than those individuals who remain involved in sport). Although much has been gained through the assessment of reasons and underlying theoretical constructs, a need exists for youth sport researchers to examine systematically the remaining three components.

The first component, sport withdrawal, is defined on a continuum ranging from activity-specific to domain-general. Activity- or sport-specific withdrawal refers to the individual who drops out of one sport to enter another sport or activity, whereas domain- or sport-general withdrawal suggests that the individual leaves sport completely and never participates again. These two terms more appropriately capture the essence of sport withdrawal and the definitions put forward by Klint and Weiss (1986) and Lindner et al. (1991).

Permanent drop out from sport

Several investigations lend support to the notion that sport withdrawal may best be represented on such a continuum. Gould et al. (1982), for example, reported that 80% of the drop-outs sampled from a group of 10–18 year olds on a swimming programme re-entered sport at the same or different level during the following season. Moreover, 68% of those

---

* The discussion related to this model is limited to the first three components. The reader is referred to Gould (1987), Gould and Petlichkoff (1988) and Petlichkoff (1994) for an explanation of the underlying theories thought to influence sport participation and withdrawal.

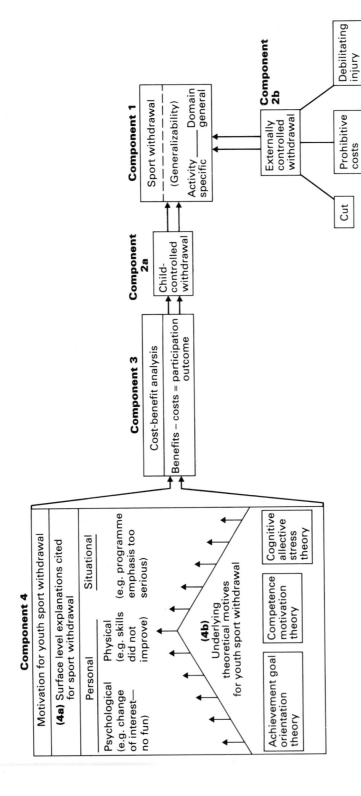

Fig. 28.1 A model of youth sport withdrawal. Redrawn with permission from Gould (1987).

sampled were actively involved in other sport programmes. Similarly, Klint and Weiss (1986) indicated that 95% of the gymnasts sampled changed levels rather than totally withdrew from the sport of gymnastics. Such evidence strongly supports the concept that sport withdrawal (i.e. sport-specific factors) is not always permanent. However, Petlichkoff (1982) found that 59% of the junior and high school athletes interviewed (aged 13–18 years) stated they had not participated in organized sport since discontinuing, nor did they have plans for future involvement (i.e. domain-general factors).

Petlichkoff *et al.* (unpublished data, 1991) surveyed a number of interscholastic athletes, ranging in age from 15 to 18, identified by their coaches as drop-outs from the previous year and found that many of these drop-outs fell into the sport-specific classification of sport withdrawal. That is, several athletes looked for other sports (e.g. cross-country, track and field) where participation was not limited by the number of athletes allowed to play on the team. Results also suggest that some high school athletes found it difficult to be involved in more than one sport and often 'dropped out' (usually from the sport in which they received little playing time) to devote more time to another sport or activity. In fact, a number of athletes who withdrew completely from sport indicated they were involved in activities outside sport (e.g. music, rodeo, school clubs, etc.) at the time of the interview. It appears, then, that lack of playing time greatly influences whether athletes 'stick it out', transfer to another sport or activity, or withdraw completely from sport.

Hodge and Zaharopoulos (1991) found that sport-specific and sport (domain)-general withdrawal also exists in New Zealand. Specifically, Hodge and Zaharopoulos surveyed a random sample of drop-outs from the sports of rugby and netball to determine reasons for dropping out, as well as current involvement in sport. Out of the 150 drop-outs identified, who ranged in age from 12 to 19 years, 38.7% were classified as sport-specific drop-outs, while 61.3% were classified as sport-general drop-

outs. These results suggest that the majority of athletes who withdrew from the sports of rugby and netball did not transfer to another sport activity; rather, they dropped out of sport completely.

These findings prompted Hodge and Zaharopoulos (1991) to enquire whether these two former groups of participants differed significantly on measures of self-concept. Results revealed that sport-specific drop-outs scored higher on their physical ability self-concept and general/global self-concept than sport-general drop-outs. Hence, it appears that individuals who withdraw completely from sport tend to have a lower perception of both their physical ability and general self-concept than those who transfer to different sports. It is difficult to ascertain, however, whether the lower ratings resulted from dropping out of sport or whether these lower ratings of self-concept (general and physical ability) contributed to their decision to withdraw completely from sport.

In summary, research (Klint & Weiss, 1986; Gould, 1987; Hodge & Zaharopoulos, 1991; Lindner *et al.*, 1991; Petlichkoff *et al.*, unpublished data, 1991) supports the notion that sport withdrawal should be defined on a continuum that assesses current status of involvement or non-involvement in sport, as well as the factors that contribute to the decision to withdraw from sport. More importantly, preliminary data (Hodge & Zaharopoulos, 1991; Petlichkoff *et al.*, unpublished data, 1991) indicate that drop-outs (sport-specific versus domain-general) differ on their self-concept and the type of sport they transfer to once they have dropped out of a sport. It appears that most children and adolescents who transfer sports become involved in sports that are participation-based (e.g. cross-country, track and field) rather than sports limited in the number of participants (e.g. basketball, volleyball) where most slots are reserved for the better players. It may be concluded that factors such as lack of ability or type of sport may be major contributors to sport withdrawal and, at times, may not be under the child's control.

Control over the decision to withdraw

An overriding assumption in most of the research conducted to date is that withdrawing from sport is voluntary (Gould, 1987; Lindner *et al.*, 1991). That is, the child made the decision to drop out, transfer sports or change levels of competition. This is not always the case, however. Gould (1987) indicates that child-controlled withdrawal occurs when the child makes the decision to withdraw from sport, whereas externally controlled withdrawal occurs when the child is cut from the team, the programme costs make it prohibitive to participate, or the child suffers a season-ending or career-ending injury (see Fig. 28.1, components 2a and 2b). Although little, if any, research exists that distinguishes between these two types of withdrawal, most studies infer that withdrawal from sport is under the child's control (i.e. voluntary).

CHILD-CONTROLLED WITHDRAWAL

Implicit in child-controlled withdrawal is the notion that the child weighs the costs and benefits of their present situation to determine whether to remain involved in or withdraw from sport (see Fig. 28.1, component 3). For the most part, children become involved in situations to maximize the rewards and minimize the costs (Thibaut & Kelly, 1959). It has been proposed that individuals consider the perceived benefits of a situation minus the costs relative to their own standards of satisfaction. When a change occurs (i.e. sport no longer meets their needs), it forces them to re-evaluate the participation outcome against other opportunities seen as more or less satisfying than the present situation. If the perceived costs outweigh the perceived benefits of being involved in sport, and other activities are evaluated as more attractive, then some children may choose to withdraw from sport (Gould, 1987). Conversely, if no alternative is perceived as more satisfying than the present situation, a child may remain involved in the present situation.

Coakley and White (1992), for example, illus-

trate how the decision to withdraw does not result from unpleasant feelings toward sport. After interviewing 34 men and 26 women (aged 13–23 years) in England about their sport experience, it was determined that adolescents considered such factors as competence, past experiences, personal preferences, as well as external factors such as money, parents and friends before making the decision to withdraw from sport.* Some of these individuals decided to change activities or levels, and experienced feelings of positive affect as they became involved in other sports or activities.

Petlichkoff (1993b), however, found that individuals who remained involved in high school sports and received little playing time (i.e. survivors) had lower ratings of perceived ability than those individuals who voluntarily dropped out of sport. This trend in the data suggests that drop-outs may realize they have little possibility of playing and maintain their higher perception of ability by dropping out of sport (Roberts, 1984). Hence, drop-outs may look for alternative activities that may be more satisfying than their present situation so they can leave sport (Burton & Martens, 1986). Conversely, survivors may turn to the social aspects of being involved in interscholastic sport. Results from Petlichkoff's investigation indicate that survivors were more social approval-oriented than drop-outs. These results may infer that survivors more easily adapt to their lack of playing time by measuring their success as 'sticking it out' or 'being part of the team' and decide to remain involved in sport.

If the decision to drop out is truly the child's decision, then, there may be little cause for alarm. That is, as children sample different achievement domains, researchers and practitioners should anticipate a certain degree of dropping out (Burton & Martens, 1986; Weiss & Petlichkoff, 1989). These 'drop-outs' may still enjoy the sport; however, as they grow older they realize their physical size, skill or time

---

* In the Coakley and White (1992) investigation, only three individuals were older than 18 years of age.

commitment may limit their future success. As long as the child maintains a certain degree of self-worth and does not view his or her withdrawal as negative, this departure from sport may be in his or her best interest.

In contrast, if the decision to withdraw resulted from negative feelings toward sport, then sport scientists should be concerned with an early departure from sport. Sport withdrawal attributed to factors such as (i) programme emphasis; (ii) an overdemanding coach; and (iii) lack of playing time that influences the athlete's perception of ability or self-esteem (i.e. resistant drop-out) should be the primary target of our concern (Klint & Weiss, 1986; Weiss & Petlichkoff, 1989). In these instances, sport-related factors contributed to the decision to withdraw and may influence whether the child returns to sport in the future.

EXTERNALLY CONTROLLED WITHDRAWAL

In externally controlled withdrawal, the child has virtually no control over the decision to withdraw from sport. Moreover, it is anticipated that this type of withdrawal may be more closely associated with negative affect. Gould (1987) identified such factors as being 'cut' from the programme, prohibitive costs and a debilitating injury as potential contributors to an early departure from sport and indicated that these factors are rarely, if at all, assessed (see Fig. 28.1, component 2b).

Structure of sport. The organizational structure of sport programmes, at times, contributes to children and adolescents being eliminated or cut from programmes. As children become involved in organized sport at the novice levels, most programmes adopt a philosophy that guarantees participation for all. That is, administrators of youth sport programmes structure the situation so that any child who wants to play is placed on a team. As children and adolescents move up through the organizational structure, fewer slots become available and team selection is often based on some kind of try-out. This process results in some children

and adolescents being eliminated from programmes (overtly or covertly) because they are not good enough or because they cannot adhere to the rigours of the programme. Although few studies have examined the ramifications of this type of withdrawal, Petlichkoff (1993b) indicated that 'cuttees' (i.e. individuals who were involuntarily cut from the team) rated their perceived ability and level of satisfaction lower than individuals who remained involved in or voluntarily withdrew from sport.

Prohibitive cost. A small percentage of children and adolescents are eliminated from participating in sport because of the prohibitive costs of a programme. Some coaches make it mandatory to attend off-season training sessions or sport camps that require a substantial registration fee that some children (or parents) cannot afford to pay. Soon, these athlete's skills lag behind those actively involved and, eventually, these individuals are eliminated from future participation.

Sports such as tennis, gymnastics, competitive soccer and golf inadvertently limit continued involvement to more advanced developmental and competitive levels because of the costs associated with specialized training, coaching and facilities. Females, for example, who become involved in a gymnastics programme that teaches movement activities and tumbling skills soon find themselves by the age of 10 or 11 determining their future success. At times, if a child shows potential in the sport of gymnastics, in America it may cost $US80−300 per month to join a club team (Y.S. Sandmire, personal communication, December 1993). Although some clubs may offer scholarships to athletes who show potential, the majority of these athletes and their parents will have made a substantial financial commitment before scholarships become available. Children and adolescents, as well as their parents, often have to assess whether the monetary commitment will be minimized by the potential achievement of the child. For some of these children, the decision will be to drop out of a sport they still enjoy (i.e. reluctant drop-out).

Although little attention has been paid to prohibitive costs as a factor that may restrict participation, future research should assess its potential, especially at points of transition in sport participation. That is, when children move from organized youth sport programmes to school-sponsored programmes or to developmental and/or national sport programmes, some children may be eliminated because of the costs of uniforms and equipment, travel expenses and training. More importantly, as children and adolescents grow older, fewer inexpensive community-based programmes exist in which to participate.

Injury. For some athletes, a season-ending or career-ending injury may contribute to an untimely departure from sport. Although some researchers (Ogilvie & Howe, 1982; Ogilvie & Taylor, 1993) indicate that this type of withdrawal can have devastating psychological ramifications, some evidence suggests that this type of departure may be viewed as a socially acceptable method of withdrawing from a negative situation. Klint and Weiss (1986), for example, found that two gymnasts actually caused their own injuries so they would have an acceptable reason to leave their sport. Petlichkoff (1982) found, after further probing, that several athletes who cited injury as their primary reason for withdrawing from sport used that as an excuse to drop out of a negative situation where they received little playing time or the coach played favourites. These individuals indicated that many peers and significant others empathized with their injury-induced withdrawal allowing the majority of these children to feel positive about their departure. Unfortunately, these are the only two studies that followed up survey results to assess the status of injured athletes who had withdrawn from sport.

It may be concluded, then, that externally controlled withdrawal may be more detrimental to the child's overall well-being than child-controlled withdrawal because the child has little, if any, input into the decision. At times,

sport organizers, coaches and parents create an élitist system in organized sport where only the better players continue to participate. One by one, children are left with fewer programmes to participate in because they may not be good enough. Hence, it should not be surprising that 80% of the children and adolescents who participate in organized sport drop out by the time they reach the age of 17 years (State of Michigan, 1978a). Does participation decline or are there just fewer places for children and adolescents to play? Until children and adolescents are followed through participation phases, researchers can only speculate as to whether some of these external factors contribute to the attrition process or whether the child just makes a decision to leave sport.

Taken together, Gould's (1987) model of youth sport withdrawal has provided an excellent framework to synthesize the existing literature on attrition in youth sport. It establishes also the need to view attrition as a complex process affected by a wide range of interacting factors and introduces the concepts of child- and externally controlled withdrawal. These terms best describe the actual events that are taking place within the realm of youth sports. That is, some children and adolescents are actively involved in the decision-making process of sport withdrawal and seek out opportunities (sport or non-sport) that they are relatively good at, whereas other children are eliminated with virtually little input into the withdrawal process.

Major issues in sport withdrawal research

The research conducted to date on the topic of attrition in youth sport has provided paediatric sport scientists with a better understanding of the phenomenon; however, several issues still remain. Weiss and Petlichkoff (1989) identified a number of missing links associated with the drop-out dilemma in youth sports that researchers and practitioners should consider while they actively seek solutions for sport withdrawal. Although several of these issues have been alluded to throughout this chapter (i.e. definitional hurdles, temporary versus permanent withdrawal, type of sport, lack of playing time), it is important to identify and briefly discuss several of the other issues. Specifically, it is necessary for researchers and practitioners to: (i) follow children through participation phases; (ii) examine developmental differences; and (iii) determine how the social structure of sport influences the withdrawal process.

Following children through participation phases

The majority of investigations on attrition in youth sport have obtained data after the child has withdrawn from sport. This one point in time assessment may not accurately depict the ongoing process that led to the child's departure from sport (Petlichkoff, 1993b). As indicated earlier, this type of assessment cannot determine whether the child's perception of ability was lower because of dropping out of sport or whether that child had a lower perception of ability before he or she became involved in sport. A longitudinal approach that incorporates survey and interview techniques may also allow researchers to determine whether motives change with age or whether contextual factors such as playing time, coaching behaviours and competitive emphasis of the programme influence the child's decision-making process (Weiss & Petlichkoff, 1989). Until children are followed through different levels of sport involvement, researchers can only infer that dropping out of sport is detrimental to the child's well-being.

Barnett et al. (1992), for example, examined whether players trained by coaches who participated in a coaching effectiveness training (CET) workshop returned to sport at a higher rate the following year than athletes who had played for untrained coaches. The results indicated that 95% of the players of the CET-trained coaches returned to sport the following

year while only 74% of the players of the untrained coaches played the next year. The players of trained coaches cited 'conflict of interest' as the reason for not returning, whereas players of untrained coaches cited more negative reasons such as not having fun, too much pressure, lack of ability or the coach playing favourites as reasons for not returning to sport. These more negative reasons, however, do not necessarily identify the factors that contributed to 'not having fun' or 'too much pressure'. Hence, these results suggest that participation patterns (i.e. returning to sport the next year) may be influenced by the coach–athlete interactions the previous year.

Developmental differences

Little attention has been paid to developmental issues in youth sport withdrawal; however, the few investigations that have examined age-related issues have found differences between younger and older athletes who drop out of sport. Orlick (1974) and Orlick and Botterill (1975), for example, found that all elementary school-aged children cited an overemphasis on winning (40% because they did not play and 60% because they were not successful), whereas the majority of high school-aged drop-outs withdrew because of conflicts of interest. Similar differences are reported in Sapp and Haubenstricker (1978).

One factor that may contribute to the child's withdrawal is that the sport programme may lack developmentally appropriate activities. That is, if children find themselves in programmes that fail to modify games or rules, emphasize winning rather than skill improvement, then some individuals may experience a lack of success and eventually drop out of sport or look for alternative situations. Hence, to maximize the youth sport experience, it is essential for paediatric sport scientists to examine developmental differences (Weiss & Petlichkoff, 1989).

Social structure of sport

Weiss and Petlichkoff (1989) have challenged the youth sport researcher to examine the interaction of the social context and the initial motivation of children to determine how this influences sport persistence and withdrawal. Researchers cannot continue to assess only the child's perceptions; rather, assessments are needed that determine whether a league's philosophy either matches or conflicts with the child's motivation for being involved in sport. Some evidence suggests that the motivational climate (i.e. goals of the programme, mastery-oriented versus ability-oriented goals) may influence the child's perception of ability and eventually may determine whether the child adapts to the situation or withdraws (Roberts, 1992).

Conclusion and recommendations

This chapter was structured to examine youth sport withdrawal from a process-oriented approach. Specifically, Gould's (1987) model of youth sport withdrawal was used to argue that:
1 There is a need for better definitions that truly depict the process of sport withdrawal.
2 Dropping out of sport may represent trial-and-error sampling which is normal within the process of growing up.
3 Sport withdrawal does not represent an all-or-nothing level of participation (i.e. sport withdrawal is not always permanent).
4 Children are, at times, actively involved in the decision-making process to withdraw from sport.

Although youth sport researchers and practitioners have a better understanding of the process of youth sport withdrawal and the factors that influence the decision to withdraw from sport, there certainly is more that can be done to advance our knowledge on such an important topic.

Challenges for future research

• As suggested throughout this chapter, youth must be followed up throughout their participation phases. This would allow youth sport researchers and administrators to determine if the participation decline is due to past experience and success or whether children develop interests in other sport or non-sport activities. Longitudinal studies are severely lacking in this area of study.
• Youth sports organizations should work with paediatric sport scientists to establish a pre- and postparticipation assessment to determine why children become involved in organized youth sport; and, once involved, what motivates some of these individuals to continue in or withdraw from sport.
• Paediatric sport scientists need to assess whether differences exist among various groups of youth sport drop-outs. That is, do gender-, age- and maturation-related differences exist in the process of sport withdrawal? Unfortunately, few investigations have been designed with the purpose of examining gender- and age-related differences.
• Likewise, a need exists to determine whether socioeconomic as well as ethnic background influence the sport participation and withdrawal process. Most studies conducted to date assess predominantly white children involved in sport (Weiss & Petlichkoff, 1989).
• There has been no research conducted to date to determine whether different 'drop-out stories' exist for individuals who drop out of team sports versus individual sports. Evidence (Petlichkoff et al., unpublished data, 1991) suggests, however, that some high school athletes dropped out of team sports to become involved in individual sports. This change in sport may indicate that individual sports focus more on skill improvement and measuring success against personal standards of excellence rather than winning or losing. It may be important to determine whether team sports have a higher rate of attrition than individual sports.
• Qualitative research methodologies are

needed to examine factors not accounted for in survey research that has relied so heavily on quantitative assessments. Follow-up informal interviews have enhanced traditional data collection and has tapped into the interactive power of some context variables that tend to influence the decision-making process of children involved in organized youth sports.

• A need exists to determine if sport withdrawal is detrimental to the child's psychological well-being. Given the current research findings, this type of conclusion may only be inferred. More importantly, it was such a conclusion that became the catalyst for this line of research.

Acknowledgements

Portions of this chapter are based on previously published work by the author (Gould & Petlichkoff, 1988; Weiss & Petlichkoff, 1989; Petlichkoff, 1992, 1993a, 1994). The author would like to thank Steven Dorigan and Anne Schorzman for their helpful comments on an earlier draft of this manuscript.

References

Athletic Footwear Association (1990) *American Youth Sports Participation*. Athletic Footwear Association, North Palm Beach.

Barnett, N.P., Smoll, F.L. & Smith, R.E. (1992) Effects of enhancing coach–athlete relationships on youth sport attrition. *Sport Psychol.* **6**, 111–27.

Burton, D. (1988) The dropout dilemma in youth sport: documenting the problem and identifying solutions. In R.M. Malina (ed.) *Young Athletes: Biological, Psychological, and Educational Perspectives*, pp. 245–66. Human Kinetics, Champaign, IL.

Burton, D. & Martens, R. (1986) Pinned by their goals: an exploratory investigation into why kids drop out of wrestling. *J. Sport Psychol.* **8**, 183–97.

Coakley, J. & White, A. (1992) Making decisions: gender and sport participation among British adolescents. *Sociol. Sport J.* **9**, 20–35.

Gould, D. (1987) Understanding attrition in children's sport. In D. Gould & M.R. Weiss (eds) *Advances in Pediatric Sport Sciences*, Vol. 2. *Behavioral Issues*, pp. 61–85. Human Kinetics, Champaign, IL.

Gould, D., Feltz, D., Horn, T. & Weiss, M.R. (1982)

Reasons for discontinuing involvement in competitive youth swimming. *J. Sport Behav.* **5**, 155–65.

Gould, D. & Horn, T. (1984) Participation motivation in young athletes. In J.M. Silva & R.S. Weinberg (eds) *Psychological Foundations of Sport*, pp. 359–70. Human Kinetics, Champaign, IL.

Gould, D. & Petlichkoff, L. (1988) Participation motivation and attrition in young athletes. In F. Smoll, R. Magill & M. Ash (eds) *Children in Sport*, 3rd edn, pp. 161–78. Human Kinetics, Champaign, IL.

Harter, S. (1981) The development of competence motivation in the mastery of cognitive and physical skills: is there a place for joy? In G.C. Roberts & D.M. Landers (eds) *Psychology of Motor Behavior and Sport — 1980*, pp. 3–29. Human Kinetics, Champaign, IL.

Hodge, K. & Zaharopoulos, E. (1991) *Participation motivation and dropouts in high school sport*. Executive Summary Report. School of Physical Education, Dunedin.

Klint, K. & Weiss, M.R. (1986) Dropping in and dropping out: participation motives of current and former youth gymnasts. *Can. J. Appl. Sport Sci.* **11**, 106–14.

Lee, C. & Owen, N. (1984) Preventing dropout: a psychological viewpoint. *Sports Coach* **8**, 20–3.

Lindner, K.J., Johns, D.P. & Butcher, J. (1991) Factors in withdrawal from youth sport: a proposed model. *J. Sport Behav.* **14**, 3–18.

Maehr, M. & Nicholls, J. (1980) Culture and achievement motivation: a second look. In N. Warren (ed.) *Studies in Cross-Cultural Psychology*, Vol. 3, pp. 221–67. Academic Press, New York.

Ogilvie, B.C. & Howe, M.A. (1982) Career crisis in sport. In T. Orlick, J.T. Partington & J.H. Salmela (eds) *Mental Training for Coaches and Athletes*, pp. 176–83. Coaching Association of Canada, Ottawa.

Ogilvie, B.C. & Taylor, J. (1993) Career termination in sports: When the dream dies. In J.M. Williams (ed.) *Applied Sport Psychology: Personal Growth to Peak Performance*, 2nd edn, pp. 356–65. Mayfield, Palo Alto, CA.

Orlick, T.D. (1973) Children's sport — a revolution is coming. *Can. Ass. Health, Phys. Educ. Recr. J.* Jan/Feb, 12–14.

Orlick, T.D. (1974) The athletic dropout — a high price of inefficiency. *Can. Ass. Health, Phys. Educ. Recr. J.* Nov/Dec, 21–7.

Orlick, T.D. & Botterill, C. (1975) *Every Kid Can Win*. Nelson-Hall, Chicago.

Petlichkoff, L.M. (1982) *Motives interscholastic athletes have for participation and reasons for discontinued involvement in school sponsored sports*. Unpublished master's thesis, Michigan State University, East Lansing.

Petlichkoff, L.M. (1992) Youth sport participation and withdrawal: is it simply a matter of *fun*? *Pediatr. Exerc. Sci.* **4**, 105–10.

Petlichkoff, L.M. (1993a) Coaching children: understanding the motivational process. *Sport Sci. Rev.* **2**, 48–61.

Petlichkoff, L.M. (1993b) Relationship of player status and time of season to achievement goals and perceived ability in interscholastic athletes. *Pediatr. Exerc. Sci.* **5**, 242–52.

Petlichkoff, L.M. (1994) Dropping out of sport: speculation versus reality. In D. Hackfort (ed.) *Psycho-Social Issues and Interventions in Elite Sports*, pp. 60–87. Sport Sciences International, Vol. 1. Peter Lang, Frankfurt.

Roberts, G.C. (1984) Toward a new theory of motivation in sport: the role of perceived ability. In J.M. Silva & R.S. Weinberg (eds) *Psychological Foundations of Sport*, pp. 214–28. Human Kinetics, Champaign, IL.

Roberts, G.C. (1992) Motivation in sport and exercise: conceptual constraints and convergence. In G. Roberts (ed.) *Motivation in Sport and Exercise*, pp. 3–29. Human Kinetics, Champaign, IL.

Robertson, I. (1981) *Children's perceived satisfactions and stresses in sport*. Paper presented at the Australian Conference on Health, Physical Education and Recreation Biennial Conference, Melbourne.

Sapp, M. & Haubenstricker, J. (1978) *Motivation for joining and reasons for not continuing in youth sport programs in Michigan*. Paper presented at the AAHPERD National Convention, Kansas City.

Sefton, J.M.M. & Fry, D.A.P. (1981) *A Report on Participation in Competitive Swimming*. Canadian Amateaur Swimming Association, Saskatoon.

Smith, R.E. (1986) Toward a cognitive-affective model of athletic burnout. *J. Sport Psychol.* **8**, 36–50.

State of Michigan (1976) *Joint Legislative Study on Youth Sports Programs – Phase I*. Michigan State University, Youth Sport Institute, East Lansing.

State of Michigan (1978a) *Joint Legislative Study on Youth Sports Programs – Phase II*. Michigan State University, Youth Sport Institute, East Lansing.

State of Michigan (1978b) *Joint Legislative Study on Youth Sports Programs – Phase III*. Michigan State University, Youth Sport Institute, East Lansing.

Thibaut, J.W. & Kelley, H.H. (1959) *The Social Psychology of Groups*. Wiley & Sons, New York.

Weiss, M.R. & Petlichkoff, L.M. (1989) Children's motivation for participation in and withdrawal from sport: identifying the missing links. *Pediatr. Exerc. Sci.* **1**, 195–211.

PART 6

DISEASE AND
THE YOUNG ATHLETE

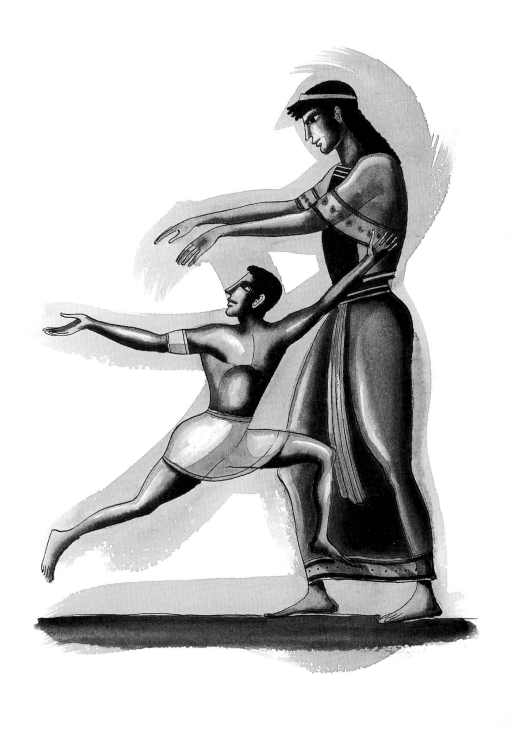

Chapter 29

Asthma and Sports

DAVID M. ORENSTEIN

Background and historical aspects

Highlights of the historical aspects of asthma are discussed in several sources (McFadden & Ingram, 1980; Sakula, 1988; Phelan *et al.*, 1990). Asthma has been referred to at least since Hippocrates (McFadden & Ingram, 1980) but in the early centuries the term was a synonym for breathlessness (McFadden & Ingram, 1980). In the second century AD, Galen wrote about asthma, attributing most respiratory symptoms to thick secretions that dripped into the lung from the brain (McFadden & Ingram, 1980) Thomas Willis (1621–1675) separated asthma from other respiratory disorders, and established the notion that patients with asthma are subject to variable symptoms, triggered by various stimuli:

> An asthma is a most terrible disease, for there is scarce anything more sharp and terrible than the fits thereof. But as to the evident causes, there are many, and also of diverse sorts. Asthmatical persons can endure nothing violent, or unaccustomed; from excess of cold or heat, from any vehement motion of the body or mind, by any grave change of the air, or of the year, or of the slightest errors about things not natural, yea, from a thousand other occasions, they fall into fits of difficult breathing.   (Willis, 1684)

Sir John Floyer wrote an entire book devoted to asthma in 1698. His major contribution may have been the recognition of the importance of bronchial smooth muscle:

> ...in the Asthmatic fit, the Muscular Fibres of the Bronchi...of the Lungs are contracted and that produces the Wheezing Noise, which is most observable in the Expiration...   (Sakula, 1984)

The relationship between exercise and asthma was recognized at least as far back as the second century AD, when Arateus the Cappadocian observed: 'If from gymnastics or other exercise the breathing become labored, it is called asthma' (Ghory, 1975). Floyer also recognized exercise-induced asthma (EIA), and differentiated among types of exercise more and less likely to produce it (McFadden & Ingram, 1980). The list of activities producing asthma had been modified somewhat by three centuries later (Fitch, 1975) but our understanding of the mechanisms underlying EIA had not progressed much and would not do so until the early 1970s, when the role of water and heat loss from the airways began to be elucidated. These factors will be discussed below.

One other point of historical note is the role of the emotions in asthma, particularly EIA. At several stages in the history of medicine, asthma has been viewed as a psychiatric illness. How better to explain the phenomenon of an apparently healthy individual, engaging in vigorous activity, who stops exercising and then suddenly acts as though breathing were nearly impossible, and who then within a matter of minutes, without any intervention, becomes perfectly comfortable again? Fortunately, our current understanding of the complex chemical and mechanical interactions within the bronchial tree of patients with asthma has freed us from these notions, and freed patients with reactive airways from the stigma of a psychiatric disorder.

Epidemiology

Asthma is the most common chronic illness in childhood, currently affecting between 5 and 15% of children (Gergen et al., 1988) for a total of some 2.7 million children in the USA (Taylor & Newacheck, 1992). It is increasing in prevalence (Taylor & Newacheck, 1992). Differences in prevalence rates from different studies may be explained by different ways of collecting data (parent questionnaire, bronchial challenge in a school population, physician diagnosis) and different definitions of asthma. Definitions of asthma are difficult to find, and one prominent pulmonologist has said, 'It's like love — we all know what it is, but who would trust anybody else's definition?' (S. Permutt quoted in Gross, 1980). More recently, the Expert Panel of the National Heart, Lung, and Blood Institute National Asthma Program (1991) have stated:

> the generally agreed-on definition of asthma recognizes that asthma is a lung disease with the following characteristics: (1) airway obstruction that is reversible (but not completely so in some patients) either spontaneously or with treatment; (2) airway inflammation and (3) increased airway responsiveness to a variety of stimuli.

Asthma accounts for some 7.3 million days restricted to bed and 10.1 million days missed from school each year (Taylor & Newacheck, 1992). Finally, 30% of children with asthma have some limitation of activity, compared with 5% of non-asthmatic children (Taylor & Newacheck, 1992).

Just as there has been some question about the prevalence of asthma in the general population, so too has there been some question

about the incidence of EIA in patients known to have asthma, with rates varying from 50 to 80% (Lemanske & Henke, 1989). Currently, most experts agree that the incidence is closer to 100%, given the appropriate exercise challenge (McFadden, 1987).

EIA is not restricted to patients with recognized asthma, as it has also been reported to occur in children with a history of croup (Loughlin & Taussig, 1979), allergic rhinitis (Pierson et al., 1972), cystic fibrosis (Silverman et al., 1978) or bronchopulmonary dysplasia (Badger et al., 1987). Perhaps most importantly, EIA has been found to occur in children and adolescents without any other recognized abnormalities, including as many as 10−15% of high school (Rupp et al., 1992) and college (Rice et al., 1985) athletes.

Exercise-induced asthma

Clinical course

EIA consists of cough, wheeze, chest tightness, chest pain, difficulty breathing or any combination of these symptoms during exercise, or, much more characteristically, shortly following exercise, usually with resolution within 30−90 min. Symptoms may or may not reappear 4−8 h later. The symptoms are accompanied by pulmonary function abnormalities consistent with narrowing of intrathoracic airways. Typically, during the exercise session itself, there is little or no difficulty; in fact, expiratory airflows during exercise are actually increased above baseline in most people with asthma (Jones, 1966) (Fig. 29.1).

Some authors have used the term exercise-induced bronchospasm (EIB) for this phenomenon. I have employed the term EIA throughout this chapter for two reasons. First, an informal survey of 51 recent articles from the medical literature on the topic revealed 37 that referred to EIA and only 14 that referred to EIB. Second, a more compelling reason is that the term 'bronchospasm' may imply that the sole mechanism of airway narrowing is bronchial smooth muscle contraction, while the possible roles of

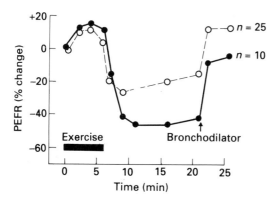

Fig. 29.1 Typical course of exercise-induced asthma in children (○) and adults (●), assessed by measurements of peak expiratory flow rate (PEFR). Each point is the mean for the numbers of subjects indicated. Redrawn from Godfrey (1974).

airway inflammation and oedema in addition to the smooth muscle contributions are more explicitly included in 'asthma'.

The exercise most likely to elicit the symptoms of EIA is typically short and intense: bouts 6–10 min long, at an intensity sufficient to raise the subject's heart rate to 80% of its maximum, are the most asthmagenic (Fitch, 1975; Godfrey et al., 1975). Shorter sessions are less potent stimuli for EIA (Fitch, 1975; Godfrey et al., 1975), and lower intensity exercise will not be as reliable in calling forth the asthmatic response (Fitch, 1975, Godfrey et al., 1975). Longer sessions will not worsen EIA, and may even lessen it — the 'run-through' phenomenon (Fitch, 1975; Godfrey et al., 1975). Extremely strenuous (supramaximal), brief, exercise bouts may provide an even more potent stimulus for the production of EIA (Inbar et al., 1981).

Ambient conditions before, during and after the exercise session influence the magnitude of the response. It has long been observed that cold air is more asthmagenic than warm air. Haas et al. (1986) cite Salter (1864) as having speculated in 1864 that EIA was caused by 'the rapid passage of fresh and cold air over the bronchial mucous membrane'. Within the past few decades, experimental evidence has supported the role of cold inspired air as a cause of EIA (Wells et al., 1960; Strauss et al., 1977; Sakula, 1984) (Fig. 29.2). It also appears that dry

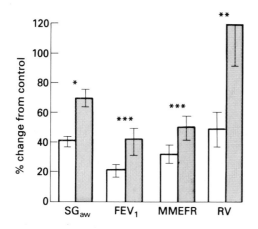

Fig. 29.2 Relative effects of exercise while subjects were breathing air at ambient (□, 24.5 ± 1.1°C) and cold (▨, −13.5 ± 2.6°C) temperatures. The data are expressed as a percentage change from control values. The heights of the bars are mean values, and the vertical lines represent 1 SE of the mean. SG$_{aw}$, specific airway conductance; FEV$_1$, forced expiratory volume in 1 s; MMEFR, maximal mid-expiratory flow rate; RV, residual volume. *, $P < 0.001$; **, $P < 0.01$; ***, $P < 0.05$. Redrawn from Strauss et al. (1977).

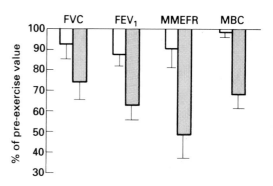

Fig. 29.3 Air humidity and EIA. Pulmonary functions of 10 6–14-year-old girls and boys measured 10 min after each of two treadmill walks. The children were free-breathing in a climatic chamber with air temperature of 25–26°C and humidity 25% ('dry') (▨) or 90% ('humid') (□) relative humidity. FVC, forced vital capacity; FEV$_1$, forced expiratory volume in 1 s; MMEFR, maximal mid-expiratory flow rate; MBC, maximal breathing capacity. Vertical lines denote 1 SE of the mean. Redrawn from Bar-Or (1983); data originally from Bar-Or et al. (1977).

air is more asthmagenic than humidified air (Bar-Or *et al.*, 1977) (Fig. 29.3).

Not surprisingly, polluted air also worsens EIA: in seven subjects with asthma studied by Sheppard *et al.* (1981) 5 min of cycle exercise did not result in a decrease in airway conductance if the patients breathed room air, but did result in significant decreases in airway conductance if they breathed 1 p.p.m. of sulphur dioxide (SO_2) during exercise. Resting airway calibre also influences the response to exercise (Anderson, 1983): Linna *et al.* (1990) studied 84 Finnish children with asthma, and found that the lower the maximal mid-expiratory flow rate (MMEFR, a sensitive measure of small airway patency), the greater the fall in expiratory airflow after an exercise challenge (Fig. 29.4).

The form of exercise seems to influence the amount of airway obstruction that follows it. Several studies in the 1970s suggested that the asthmagenicity of running was greater than cycling, which in turn was greater than arm exercise, and all of these greater than swimming, in inducing an asthmatic response (Fitch, 1975). More recent studies indicate that if the volume, temperature and humidity of the inspired air are held constant among the land-based challenges, the asthmatic response will be equal (Kilham *et al.*, 1979). However, several studies have shown that swimming is less asthmagenic than treadmill running, even if minute ventilation and the temperature and humidity of the inspired air are controlled (Inbar *et al.*, 1980), indicating that there must be factors other than airway heat and water flux that differentiate swimming from other forms of exercise in regard to initiating EIA (Fig. 29.5).

An interesting and important feature of EIA is referred to as the refractory period: a second bout of exercise performed within 1–2 h after the first exercise challenge causes much less airflow obstruction than the initial challenge (Edmunds *et al.*, 1978) (Fig. 29.6). This phenomenon will be discussed at greater length in the next section.

Pathophysiology

Centuries after the initial recognition of EIA, there are still many unanswered questions about the pathophysiology of this phenomenon.

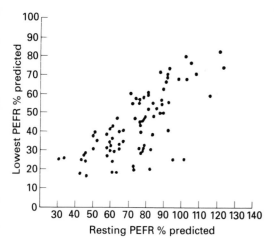

Fig. 29.4 Influence of resting pulmonary function on EIA. Individual values for the per cent fall in peak expiratory flow rate (PEFR) for 80 patients following an exercise challenge, in relation to the pre-exercise value of PEFR, are expressed as a percentage of the predicted value. Redrawn from Anderson (1983).

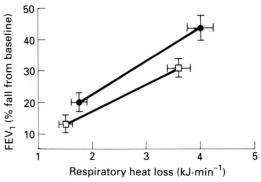

Fig. 29.5 The protective nature of swimming as a function of respiratory heat loss. Thirteen 9–17-year-old patients with asthma ran (●) and swam (□) while inhaling either dry (8% relative humidity) or humid (98–100% relative humidity) air. Air temperature was 24.5°C and water temperature 31.6°C. Oxygen consumption and minute ventilation were equated in both activities. FEV_1 fall, postexercise decrease as a percentage of pre-exercise forced expiratory volume in 1 s. Error bars represent SE of the mean. Redrawn from Bar-Or (1983); data from Bar-Yishay (1982).

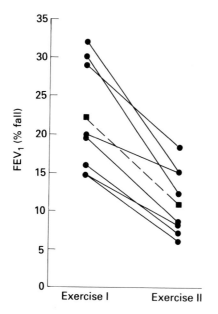

Fig. 29.6 Refractory period in EIA showing a smaller decrease in forced expiratory volume in 1 s (FEV$_1$) after a second exercise challenge performed 60 min after the first challenge. Redrawn from Hamielec *et al.* (1988).

However, recent work has helped to elucidate underlying mechanisms, and we now understand much more than we did just a decade ago.

HEAT AND WATER EXCHANGE

As noted above, it has long been observed that EIA is more likely and more severe in cold air. In the late 1970s and early 1980s, a number of investigators provided experimental evidence to support these observations, and to suggest that airway heat exchange plays a central role in the production of EIA, even when the exercise is not in cold environments. Before reviewing these experiments, it is worth considering the mechanisms employed by the airways to condition inspired air (McFadden & Ingram, 1979). Air that is cooler than body temperature and less than fully saturated with water vapour is warmed and humidified by transfer of heat and water from the airway mucosa. This heat transfer occurs partly by convection, and once

the air is warmed, its capacity to hold water increases, allowing for further heat transfer by evaporation from the airway mucosa (McFadden & Ingram, 1979). Evaporation occurs even at 37°C, if the inspired air is less than fully saturated with water vapour. This process is usually completed in the upper airway, but with large minute ventilation, as is required for vigorous exercise, the heat transfer capacity of the upper airways may be surpassed (particularly if the inspired air is cold and dry), and the heat transfer responsibilities are shared by the intrathoracic airways, perhaps as deep as the tenth generation of airways (McFadden, 1987). The corollary of the exchange of heat to the inspired air is the loss of heat from the airways, and the resulting lower than normal temperatures deep within the lung. A temperature probe directly within the anterior segment of the right lower lobe in subjects breathing cold air (−9°C) during exercise has documented temperatures as low as 31°C, compared to 34.6°C at rest (Gilbert *et al.*, 1988).

There is now considerable evidence that this phenomenon of airway cooling associated with transfer of heat and water to large volumes of inspired air accounts for an important part of EIA. Chen and Horton (1977) showed that asthmatic subjects who exercised breathing warm, humidified air had much less EIA than they did when they performed the same exercise breathing dry room air. Deal *et al.* (1979b) duplicated those findings. They then had the patients at rest breathe volumes of cold air equal to those they breathed during exercise, and showed a degree of airway obstruction following the hyperpnoea equal to that which followed the exercise (Deal *et al.*, 1979a). Again this response was abolished if the inspired air was warmed and humidified (Deal *et al.*, 1979a). These investigators illustrated a close correlation between total respiratory heat exchange and degree of airway obstruction (Fig. 29.7).

Heat exchange within the airways is important in the pathogenesis of EIA, but it is not clear how. In what ways are asthmatic airways different from normal airways in the response to heat flux? Aitken and Morini (1985) reported

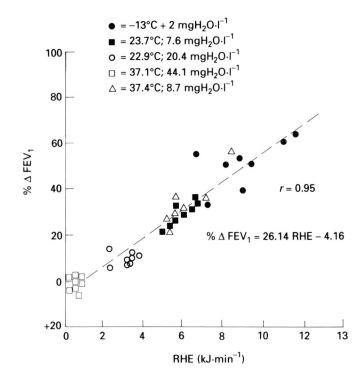

● = −13°C + 2 mgH$_2$O·l^{-1}
■ = 23.7°C; 7.6 mgH$_2$O·l^{-1}
○ = 22.9°C; 20.4 mgH$_2$O·l^{-1}
□ = 37.1°C; 44.1 mgH$_2$O·l^{-1}
△ = 37.4°C; 8.7 mgH$_2$O·l^{-1}

$r = 0.95$

$\% \Delta FEV_1 = 26.14\ RHE - 4.16$

% Δ FEV$_1$

RHE (kJ·min^{-1})

Fig. 29.7 Relationship between respiratory heat exchange (RHE) during exercise and postexertional percentage change in 1-s forced expiratory volume (%ΔFEV$_1$). Redrawn from Deal *et al.* (1979a).

that both normal and asthmatic subjects experience a fall in airways conductance (which would be expected to cause a fall in expiratory airflow) when their airways extract heat from inspired air, but that the response of the asthmatic subjects 5–10 min afterwards is much greater than that in the normal subject. Furthermore, when heat is added to the airways (via inspiration of large volumes of hot air), the normal subjects increase airway conductance, while the asthmatic subjects show dramatic falls in conductance (Aitken & Morini, 1985). As these authors point out, the response in normal airways is consistent with *in vitro* responses of airway smooth muscle strips, which relax (and have diminished constrictor responses to histamine) when warmed (Souhrada & Souhrada, 1981). The different response in asthmatic airways is consistent with McFadden's study that showed postexercise bronchoconstriction to be related more to the speed and degree of airway rewarming than to the amount of heat loss during exercise (McFadden *et al.*, 1986).

Lemanske and Henke (1989) have speculated that this phenomenon may be an airway analogue of the reactive hyperaemia seen in skin that is cooled and rapidly rewarmed: 'if parallel events occurred in the bronchial vascular bed, engorgement and edema formation in the mucosa and submucosa would result...[and] compromise airflow'.

It has been suggested that the water content of inspired air is more important than its temperature: 'it is the osmotic and not the cooling effects induced by the vaporization of water that is the more important factor determining EIA' (Hahn *et al.*, 1984a). The fact that some, but not all, diuretics, when inhaled as an aerosol, block EIA has suggested that electrolyte transport in the airways may somehow be involved in EIA, but the mechanisms are not yet clear (Bianco *et al.*, 1988; O'Donnell *et al.*, 1992).

MEDIATORS OF INFLAMMATION

One of the explanations for the route by which

airway cooling or other exercise-related factors actually cause bronchoconstriction, airway oedema or both, is the elucidation of mediators of inflammation, such as histamine, neutrophil chemotactic factor (NCF) and various leukotrienes (Lee *et al.*, 1983a, 1984; Manning *et al.*, 1990). One of the earliest pieces of evidence that mediators — especially those of mast cell origin — might be important in the pathogenesis of EIA was that sodium cromolyn (a mast-cell stabilizer) prevents EIA in a large proportion of asthmatic patients (Godfrey & Konig, 1976). Several studies have shown that atopic patients who exercise while they breathe cold dry air experience EIA and have elevated circulating levels of histamine, NCF or both (Anderson *et al.*, 1981; Barnes & Brown, 1981;

Nagakura *et al.*, 1983; Lee *et al.*, 1984). Of interest, these studies have also shown the absence of these mediators in the circulation following isocapnic hyperventilation, despite equal degrees of airways obstruction (Barnes & Brown, 1981; Lee *et al.*, 1983a; Nagakura *et al.*, 1983) (Fig. 29.8). This suggests a possible role for these mediators in EIA, but not in hyperventilation-induced asthma, and also suggests that heat loss alone is not sufficient to release these mediators from mast cells.

Further evidence that mediators of inflammation are important in causing EIA (as opposed to being mere epiphenomena of EIA) comes from two studies showing inhibition of EIA by MK-571 (Manning *et al.*, 1990) or ICI 204,219 (Finnerty *et al.*, 1992), both potent antagonists of the receptor for leukotriene D_4 (Fig. 29.9).

Another leukotriene blocker, A-64077, has been shown to block the development of bronchoconstriction induced by hyperventi-

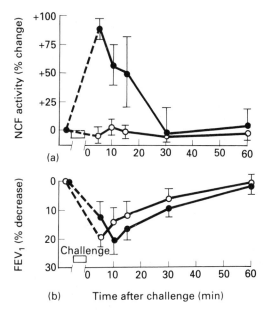

(a)

(b)   Time after challenge (min)

Fig. 29.8 Neutrophil chemotactic factor (NCF) activity (a) and forced expiratory volume in 1 s (FEV_1) (b) after exercise (●) and isocapnic hyperventilation (ISH) (○) in six atopic patients with asthma. The mean NCF activity (neutrophils per high-power field) for exercise and ISH were 115 and 110, respectively. There were significant increases in NCF 5 and 10 min after exercise, but no significant change after ISH. Open bar; period of challenge. Redrawn from Nagakura *et al.* (1983).

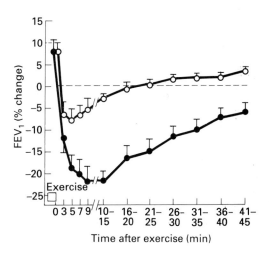

Time after exercise (min)

Fig. 29.9 Inhibition of EIA by MK-571, a potent antagonist of the receptor for leukotriene D_4. Mean (± SEM) change in forced expiratory volume in 1 s over time after exercise, after treatment with MK-571 (○) or placebo (●). Measurements were made immediately after exercise and every 2 min thereafter until the FEV_1 began to improve. Treatment with MK-571 significantly reduced the maximal fall in FEV_1 after exercise and shortened the recovery time. Redrawn from Manning *et al.* (1990).

lation of cold dry air in patients with asthma (Israel *et al.*, 1990). This lends further support for the role of mediators of inflammation in the genesis of airway obstruction after exercise or hyperventilation, but makes less clear the distinctions between the two methods of producing airway blockage.

LESSONS FROM THE REFRACTORY PERIOD

As already discussed, many patients with EIA develop less intense EIA after a second bout of exercise that follows the initial exercise challenge by 2 h or less. It is not yet known why this occurs. The initial challenge need not be severe enough to have caused EIA itself in order to afford protection from the second challenge (Reiff *et al.*, 1989; Wilson *et al.*, 1990). Furthermore, although either exercise or resting hyperventilation of cool dry air produces a refractory period to a similar challenge (Rosenthal *et al.*, 1990), it is not clear that this similarity can be attributed to airway heat loss. Exercise with warm humid air does not cause EIA, but does induce refractoriness to a subsequent exercise challenge (Ben-Dov *et al.*, 1982), while resting hyperventilation of warm humid air causes neither asthma nor refractoriness to a subsequent challenge of cold dry air hyperventilation (Bar-Yishay *et al.*, 1983). This suggests that something specific about exercise itself is inducing refractoriness.

The possibility that the airway smooth muscle is unable to contract during the refractory period has been disproved, since patients who are refractory to exercise challenge are able to have brisk bronchoconstrictor responses to inhaled histamine (Hahn *et al.*, 1984b) or allergen (Weiler-Ravell & Godfrey, 1981). It has been suggested that various mediators, including histamine, may help explain the refractory period: with this theory, mediators are released, especially from mast cells, with the initial challenge, and the mediator stores within the mast cells take up to 2 h to be replenished (Edmunds *et al.*, 1978; Ben-Dov *et al.*, 1982).

THE LATE ASTHMATIC RESPONSE

It has been reported by some investigators that some patients with asthma will suffer not just an immediate but also a late reduction in expiratory airflow, 4–10 h later, associated with chest tightness, wheezing or both (Lee *et al.*, 1983b; Speelberg *et al.*, 1991) (Fig. 29.10). Patients who experience these late responses have been shown to have increased circulating levels of NCF, while those patients who have only the immediate response have only an initial rise in NCF.

Other investigators (Rubinstein *et al.*, 1987; Speelberg *et al.*, 1991; Boner *et al.*, 1992) have been unable to reproduce these results, and point out that a biphasic fall in expiratory flow rates may be characteristic of the diurnal variation seen in some patients, irrespective of prior exercise challenge. These differing findings may possibly be explained by a recent Italian study in which bronchoscopy and bronchial biopsies were performed 3 h after exercise on 2 separate days (Crimi *et al.*, 1992). This study suggested that 'exercise may enhance mast cell degranulation and eosinophilic inflammation of the airways, and...a delayed bronchoconstriction after exercise is not specific to EIA but is more likely the result of fluctuations in lung function associated with airway inflammation' (Crimi *et al.*, 1992).

Diagnosis

In most cases of children or adolescents with recognized asthma, diagnosing EIA is not challenging: the report by the youngster of exercise-associated cough, chest pain or dyspnoea can be assumed to be caused by the underlying problem, and to be EIA (Nixon & Orenstein, 1988). The most appropriate test in these cases is a therapeutic trial of a regimen designed to block EIA (see below). Only if the symptoms are inordinately severe or worrying to the patient, family or physician, or if they are not prevented by appropriate treatment, should more testing be carried out. A major exception

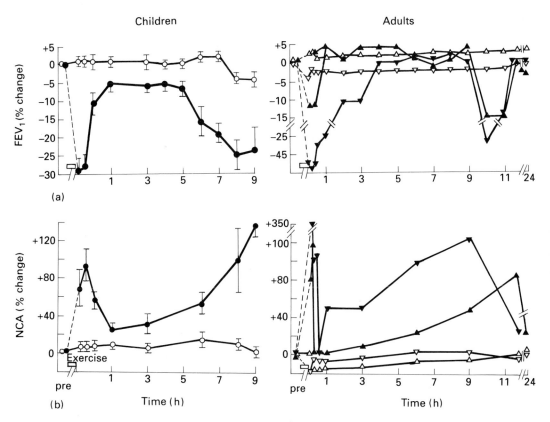

Fig. 29.10 Percentage changes from baseline forced expiratory volume in 1 s (FEV_1) (a) and neutrophil chemotactic activity (NCA) (b) during the control day (open symbols) and after exercise (solid symbols) in 13 children and two adults who had the late asthmatic responses to exercise. The value in the children are means ± SEM; individual values are given for the adults. NCA was measured in 11 of the children. The increases in NCA in these subjects were statistically significant at 5, 15 and 30 min, and at 3, 6, 8 and 9 h. The horizontal bars on the abscissa represent the exercise period. Redrawn from Lee *et al.* (1983b).

to this generalization must always be kept in mind: if the sole exercise-related complaint is dyspnoea, the culprit may be deconditioning; the young asthmatic patient may be out of breath because of poor conditioning, only indirectly (or not at all) related to his or her asthma. The area of fitness is more fully discussed below.

In evaluating the otherwise healthy youngster with atypical presentation of asthma, such as exercise-associated chest pain (Wiens *et al.*, 1992), cough or dyspnoea in the absence of other evidence of asthma, an exercise challenge test may be helpful.

EXERCISE TEST

Challenge tests for diagnosing EIA should take into account some important features of its pathophysiology and clinical course: EIA is most likely following 6–10 min of exercise intense enough to raise the heart rate to 80% of its maximum (about 170 beats · min^{-1} for most paediatric tests) (Fitch, 1975; Godfrey *et al.*, 1975). Cold dry air heightens and warm humid air diminishes EIA (Deal *et al.*, 1979b), therefore testing should be carried out in a setting with relatively stable ambient conditions, ideally with dry air (most hospital and clinical settings ordinarily have dry air). The mode of exercise should also be considered. As discussed above, given the appropriate intensity, the form of dry-land exercise (cycle ergometer, treadmill, 'free-range' running) probably does not matter, but swimming is not an appropriate challenge (except in the very special case of a youngster with symptoms which are difficult to understand during or after swimming), since it seems to be less asthmagenic than other forms of exercise (Inbar et al., 1980; Yishay et al., 1982; Bar-Or & Inbar, 1992).

EIA responses peak between 3 and 20 min after exercise (Cropp, 1975). Therefore, it makes sense to measure pulmonary function before the exercise challenge, for a baseline value, and again at roughly 3-min intervals, beginning immediately afterwards, until about 20 min after exercise. Different investigators have used different pulmonary function parameters as their preferred measurement and different degrees of change in those parameters for diagnosing EIA. Table 29.1 shows Cropp's criteria for diagnosing mild, moderate and severe EIA, based on values expressed as a percentage of pre-exercise values (Cropp, 1979). In our laboratory, we prefer to see forced vital capacity (FVC) relatively unchanged after exercise, since that reassures us that a decreased

forced expiratory flow (FEF) between 25 and 75% of vital capacity, for example, is not simply a reflection of fatigue, or a poorer effort after a tiring session on the exercise cycle or treadmill.

Some investigators suggest comparing the lowest postexercise pulmonary function values with the best values — either during exercise (Silverman & Anderson, 1972) or after bronchodilator inhalation (Jones, 1966) — rather than just with the pre-exercise baseline. We routinely administer bronchodilator (salbutamol, by metered-dose inhaler) after the 20-min postexercise pulmonary function measurement, and compare the lowest postexercise value with the highest value, which is usually the immediate postbronchodilator value. Whatever test is chosen and whatever parameters are used, false negative tests are not at all uncommon (Nixon & Orenstein, 1988), and some investigators suggest repeat testing within a week (Godfrey, 1974) if the first test is negative. Even on repeat testing the tests are not as sensitive as some of the literature would suggest, and false negative tests, or tests with smaller decrements in expiratory flow rates than in Table 29.1, even in children with known EIA, are reasonably common (Orenstein, 1993). One cannot interpret these tests in a clinical vacuum; rather, the whole history, and, in many cases, the patient's

Table 29.1 Criteria for the diagnosis of mild, moderate and severe exercise-induced asthma (EIA). Adapted from Cropp (1979).

Test	Postexercise measurement		
	Mild EIA (%)	Moderate EIA (%)	Severe EIA (%)
SG_{aw}	51−70	30−50	< 30
PEFR	61−75	40−60	< 40
FEF_{25-75}	61−75	40−60	< 40
FEV_1	66−80	50−65	< 50
FVC	81−90	70−80	< 70

SG_{aw}, specific airway conductance; PEFR, peak expiratory flow rate; FEF_{25-75}, forced expiratory flow between 25 and 27% of vital capacity, also referred to as maximal mid-expiratory flow rate; FEV_1, forced expiratory volume in 1 s; FVC, forced vital capacity.
FEF_{25-75} is thought to reflect the status of the small bronchi, while the other measurements are more related to the large airways.

response to a trial of pre-exercise β_2-agonist, cromolyn or nedocromil (see under prevention below) help confirm the diagnosis.

COLD AIR CHALLENGE

Some laboratories have begun to substitute a cold air challenge for the more traditional exercise challenge in their attempts to diagnose EIA (Zach *et al.*, 1984). In these tests, patients at rest breathe cold (typically $< 3°C$) dry air for 3–7 min at a minute ventilation comparable to that which they would have used during exercise — approximately 20 times the forced expiratory volume (FEV) in 1 s (Strauss *et al.*, 1977), or two-thirds of the predicted maximum voluntary ventilation (Deal *et al.*, 1980). Pulmonary function measurements are made before and at 3-min intervals after the challenge, just as with the standard EIA tests (McLaughlin & Dozor, 1983). During these tests, end-tidal carbon dioxide tensions must be monitored, and carbon dioxide occasionally added to the inspired air, in order to prevent the bronchoconstriction caused by hypocapnia (McFadden *et al.*, 1977). Another approach sometimes employed is to have the patient breathe cold dry air during an exercise challenge (Orenstein, 1993).

Fitness

FITNESS LEVELS

Most (Cropp & Tanakawa, 1977; Clark & Cochrane, 1988; Strunk *et al.*, 1988; Garfinkel *et al.*, 1992), but not all (Ingemann-Hansen *et al.*, 1980), studies have shown that patients with asthma have lower aerobic fitness than their non-asthmatic peers. This is not very surprising, since exercise can induce an asthma attack, and because airway obstruction would be expected to limit exercise tolerance. However, the fascinating and important fact emerging from recent studies is that the limited fitness in patients with asthma seems not to be related

very closely to their degree of airway obstruction (Strunk *et al.*, 1988; Garfinkel *et al.*, 1992), but to be much more closely related to their levels of habitual activity (Fig. 29.11) (Garfinkel *et al.*, 1992). Nevertheless, between half and two-thirds of the patients in one study reported that they did not exercise more because they 'get short of breath/wheeze' when they exercise, a finding not corroborated by objective testing in the laboratory after the inhalation of a single dose of a β_2-agonist (Garfinkel *et al.*, 1992; Schwartzenstein, 1992).

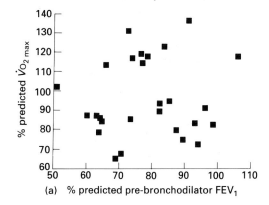

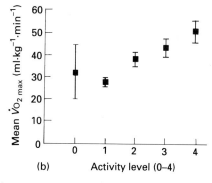

Fig. 29.11 Relationships between fitness and resting pulmonary function (a) and habitual activity level (b) in a group of patients with asthma. There is no relationship between fitness (expressed as per cent predicted maximum oxygen consumption — $\dot{V}_{O_2\,max}$) and degree of pulmonary dysfunction, whereas there is a relationship between fitness and habitual activity. Redrawn from Garfinkel *et al.* (1992).

EXERCISE CONDITIONING

The beneficial effects of exercise conditioning programmes in young patients with asthma have been noted for some time (Petersen & McElhenney, 1965; Geubelle *et al.*, 1971; Fitch *et al.*, 1976; Graff-Lonnevig *et al.*, 1980; Nickerson *et al.*, 1983; Bar-Or, 1985; Bundgaard *et al.*, 1984; Orenstein *et al.*, 1985; Varray *et al.*, 1991; Bar-Or & Inbar, 1992; Schwartzenstein, 1992). These benefits have ranged from the very subjective including (i) improved ability to participate in activities, including school and church programmes and sports; (ii) acceptance by peers; (iii) decrease in emotional upset, and recognition that sickness need not be a way of life (Bar-Or, 1983); and (iv) decrease in the intensity of wheezing attacks (Varray *et al.*, 1991); to the objective. The latter includes (i) increased running performance (Nickerson *et al.*, 1983); and (ii) increased peak oxygen consumption (Orenstein *et al.*, 1985; Varray *et al.*, 1991), indicating increased aerobic fitness, and increased oxygen pulse (Orenstein *et al.*, 1985) suggesting increased cardiac stroke volume which is also consistent with improved aerobic fitness, and increased ventilatory threshold (the point at which minute ventilation abruptly increases out of proportion to changes in oxygen consumption) (Varray *et al.*, 1991) (see Chapter 4) (Fig. 29.12). The types

of training have varied, and have included swimming (Varray *et al.*, 1991) and jogging (Nickerson *et al.*, 1983; Orenstein *et al.*, 1985). Not all studies have included the use of inhalers (see prevention below) prior to conditioning sessions, but some have (Orenstein *et al.*, 1985), and it seems prudent to do so (Schwartzenstein, 1992). The now well-known experience of the 1984 US Olympic team highlights the potential for patients with asthma to respond to exercise conditioning programmes, and the possibility of engaging in an active lifestyle, including competitive sports: 67 of 597 athletes on the team had EIA, and these 67 athletes won 41 medals (15 gold, 21 silver, five bronze), in sports as diverse as wrestling, track and field, basketball and field hockey, as well as the less-surprising water polo and swimming (Monahan, 1986).

EFFECT OF CONDITIONING

Although early reports suggested that exercise programmes diminish airway obstruction in the patient in response to exercise (Oseid & Haaland, 1978), these early reports failed to control for changes in minute ventilation. That is, patients were challenged with a workload after their conditioning programme equal to the preconditioning challenge, and most often were found to have a smaller EIA response.

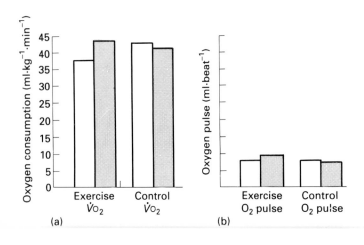

(a)   (b)

Fig. 29.12 Increased peak oxygen consumption ($\dot{V}O_2$) (a) and oxygen pulse (oxygen consumption per heart beat) (b) for 13 children with asthma (exercise) before (□) and after (▨) a 4-month jogging programme and 13 similar patients (control) who did not exercise. Note significantly increased oxygen consumption and oxygen pulse for the exercise group and no change for the control patients. Data from Orenstein *et al.* (1985).

However, if the patients became more aerobically fit, it is expected that their ventilatory threshold will have increased, and therefore a vigorous work rate which might have been above the ventilatory threshold prior to conditioning might well be below the ventilatory threshold after conditioning. By definition of the ventilatory threshold, this means that the patient will have a lower minute ventilation at this same work rate after having become more fit with the conditioning programme. Breathing a smaller volume of air puts less stress on the air conditioning capacity of the airways, and thus provides a smaller stimulus for EIA (see above). Most studies that have taken this principle into consideration (Nickerson et al., 1983; Fitch et al., 1986) have concluded that exercise conditioning does not diminish EIA. There is one very carefully performed study (Haas et al., 1986) that does suggest that the EIA response may be smaller after training. No studies suggest worsened EIA after conditioning.

Prevention

PHARMACOTHERAPY

Pharmacotherapy for EIA has been reviewed recently (Morton & Fitch, 1992). The main classes of drugs that may have some use in preventing EIA are cromolyn sodium (and its analogues), β-adrenergic agonists, methyl xanthines, corticosteroids, anticholinergic agents and calcium channel blockers.

Cromolyn sodium (Intal). Cromolyn is a disodium salt, developed in the 1960s. It is useful in chronic asthma, particularly in those patients with an allergic component to their asthma. In the chronic asthmatic, cromolyn may take weeks before its effects are seen. Therefore, it is perhaps surprising that it is also very effective acutely in blocking EIA, if administered 15–20 min prior to exercise (Fig. 29.13).

It may block EIA completely in 40% of subjects, and partly in more than 70% of subjects (Godfrey & Konig, 1976). Its effects are

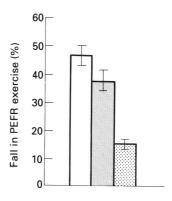

Fig. 29.13 Mean percentage change from pre-exercise peak expiratory flow rate (PEFR) after pre-exercise treatment with no drug (□), placebo (▨) or cromolyn (▨), $n = 31$. Adapted from Godfrey (1974).

dose related (Morton & Fitch, 1992). Cromolyn is unique, or nearly so, among therapeutic agents for its lack of side-effects. Its mode of action is not completely clear, but most clinicians credit its effect to its apparent ability to stabilize mast cell membranes (Morton & Fitch, 1992), and thus inhibit the release of chemical mediators (Cox & Altounyan, 1970). It may also act by inhibiting phosphodiesterase activity, inhibiting reflex mechanisms or modifying calcium flux across cell membranes (Lemanske & Henke, 1989). Cromolyn's protective effect lasts about 2 h, but in combination with terbutaline, protection lasts twice as long (Woolley et al., 1990). Cromolyn sodium is available in three forms: a powder contained within a capsule ($20\,mg \cdot capsule^{-1}$), inhaled via a Spinhaler®, a metered-dose inhaler ($1\,mg \cdot puff^{-1}$) and a nebulizer solution ($20\,mg \cdot amp^{-1}$). Nedocromil sodium is a compound related to cromolyn sodium, with comparable potency and efficacy, and comparable freedom from toxicity (Morton & Fitch, 1992).

β-adrenergic agonists. Among cell membrane receptors, the β-adrenergic receptors are important in the control of intestinal motility, the rate and intensity of cardiac contractions, relaxation or contraction of bronchial smooth muscle and arterial smooth muscle. Stimulation of the β_1-receptors increases cardiac rate and contractility and influences intestinal motility, while stimulation of β_2-receptors dilates bronchial smooth muscle. Recent years have seen the development of relatively selective β_2-agonists, that have potent bronchial smooth muscle relaxant effect, with little cardiac stimulation. These agents, including albuterol (USA) or salbutamol (rest of the world), metaproterenol, terbutaline, bitolterol, fenoterol and salmeterol, are the mainstay in the treatment of the bronchospastic component of asthma, be it chronic or acute, including EIA. These were the first-line drugs for both prevention and treatment of asthma, until recently, when the primary role of airways inflammation in the pathogenesis of asthma became appreciated, and when concern has been raised about the possible dangers of these agents when used as maintenance therapy for chronic asthma (Sears et al., 1990; Spitzer et al., 1992). The β_2-agonists are still accepted as very safe and effective for symptomatic relief of asthma and prevention of EIA. When inhaled 10–20 min prior to exercise, these agents block EIA in virtually all subjects. Their protective effect ranges between 1 (metaproterenol), 2 (terbutaline) and 4 h (salbutamol) (Lemanske & Henke, 1989). As already mentioned, the combination of cromolyn and terbutaline increases the length of time of protection from EIA from 2 h for each agent alone to 4 h (Woolley et al., 1990). Most of these drugs are available in oral or inhaled form (metered-dose inhaler or nebulizer solution), the inhaled route being preferable because of speed of action and lack of side-effects. Currently, a β_2-agonist delivered by metered-dose inhaler 15 min prior to exercise is probably the most potent and reliable means of preventing EIA in the largest number of subjects (Morton & Fitch, 1992).

Methyl xanthines. Theophylline was for many years the preferred drug for treatment of chronic asthma in the USA. More recently, though, the availability of agents with better anti-inflammatory action (cromolyn and cortico-steroids) and better bronchodilator effect (β_2-agonists) has relegated theophylline to the third tier in the classification of helpful drugs for asthma. Theophylline is effective in preventing EIA in about 80% of subjects (Ellis, 1984), but its rather narrow therapeutic window, considerable toxicity and slow onset of action have made it a poor choice for young athletes with EIA (Lemanske & Henke, 1989).

Corticosteroids. These are extremely effective in preventing and treating airways inflammation and oedema in chronic asthma, and the inhaled steroids, with very little systemic absorption, have recently moved into the forefront as the first-line maintenance drug in adult asthma (Barnes, 1989). Inhaled steroids may have some ability to block EIA in children who have been taking the medication for 1–3 weeks (Lemanske & Henke, 1989), probably by attenuating bronchial reactivity (Fig. 29.14). However, their importance lies more in their role in controlling baseline airway inflammation. When these agents are taken regularly, they can help maintain optimal airway patency, thereby reducing the effect of any subsequent narrowing following exercise (or allergen challenge), and can also increase the effectiveness of a low dose pre-exercise β_2-agonist aerosol in preventing EIA in children (Henriksen & Dahl, 1983).

Anticholinergic agents. Since vagal input increases resting bronchomotor tone, anticholinergic agents like atropine may cause bronchodilatation in some people. Ipratropium bromide (Atrovent) is a quarternary ammonium derivative of atropine, and when taken by metered-dose inhaler, is absorbed only poorly, thus reducing atropine-like side-effects (dry mouth, visual problems, etc.). Ipratropium bromide has become a useful agent for some patients, but has only moderate effectiveness in preventing EIA (Lemanske & Henke, 1989).

Calcium channel blockers. These new agents are finding use in many different medical settings. As Lemanske (Lemanske & Henke, 1989) and

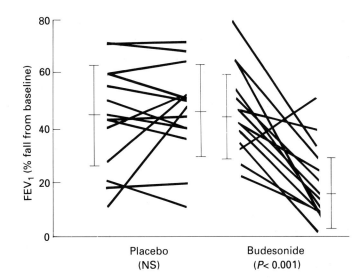

Fig. 29.14 Individual percentage falls in forced expiratory volume in 1 s (FEV$_1$) induced by exercise before and after 3 weeks of treatment with budesonide aerosol and its placebo. Means and SD are shown. Redrawn from Henriksen and Dahl (1983).

Middleton (Middleton, 1984) point out, the pathological processes in the airways of patients with asthma are calcium-dependent: 'excitation–contraction coupling in smooth muscle, stimulus–secretion coupling in mast cells and mucous glands ... and the movement and activation of inflammatory cells'. The calcium channel blockers nifedipine and verapamil have been shown to be effective in blocking EIA, while diltiazem has not (Lemanske & Henke, 1989).

Fig. 29.15 and Table 29.2 show the comparative effects of some of the drugs most commonly used for EIA.

LEGAL AND BANNED ASTHMA DRUGS IN COMPETITIVE SPORT

The list of allowed and disallowed medications is different for each school, and therefore I will not attempt to categorize these drugs for young athletes. For intercollegiate competition in the USA and competition under the aegis of the International Olympic Committee, there is a standard list of legal and banned drugs. Table 29.2 lists most of the drugs relevant to asthma, and is adapted from Morton and Fitch (1992).

Additionally, certain medications used for allergic conditions, such as antihistamines, are

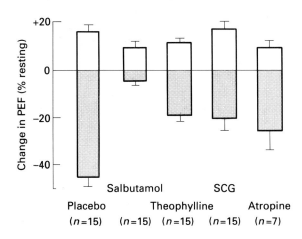

Fig. 29.15 Bronchodilatation during exercise (□) and bronchoconstriction after exercise (▨) expressed as a per cent change from the resting value immediately before exercise but after receiving the drugs indicated. The bars show ± SEM. PEF, peak expiratory flow rate; SCG, sodium cromoglycate. Redrawn from Godfrey and Konig (1976).

Table 29.2 Drugs commonly used for exercise-induced asthma (EIA), their route of administration, effectiveness, whether they are legal or banned for intercollegiate and international competition, and whether they are used prophylactically, for treatment or both.

Medication	Route of administration	Effectiveness in EIA	Legal or banned	Prophylaxis (P); therapeutic (T)
Cromolyn sodium	Aerosol	Good	Legal	P
Nedocromil sodium	Aerosol	Good	Legal	P
β_2-agonists				
Salbutamol	Aerosol	Excellent	Legal	P, T
	Oral	Good	Banned	P, T
Terbutaline	Aerosol	Excellent	Legal	P, T
	Oral	Good	Banned	P, T
Orciprenaline	Aerosol	Excellent	Legal	P, T
Salmeterol	Aerosol	Excellent	Legal	P, T
Clenbuterol	Aerosol	Excellent	Banned	P, T
Theophylline	Oral	Good	Legal	P, T
Ipratropium bromide	Aerosol	Fair	Legal	T
Steroids				
Beclomethasone	Aerosol	?	Legal	P, T
Budesonide	Aerosol	Fair	Legal	P, T
Prednisone	Oral	?	Banned	T
Prednisolone	Oral	?	Banned	T

approved, while others such as ephedrine, pseudoephedrine, phenylephrine and phenyl-propanolamine are banned (Lemanske & Henke, 1989).

Ergogenic properties of anti-asthma drugs. Some of the agents used in treating and preventing asthma have properties that might theoretically give a boost to muscular performance: amino-phylline has been shown to increase the contractility of the diaphragm (Aubier *et al.*, 1981), and of cardiac muscle (Matthay & Mahler, 1986), while certain selective β_2-agonists have been associated with increases in muscle mass in farm animals (Baker *et al.*, 1984). Yet, the preponderance of evidence seems to indicate that neither theophylline (Morton *et al.*, 1989), nor salbutamol (Meeuwisse *et al.*, 1992; Morton *et al.*, 1992; Signorile *et al.*, 1992) influences power output or athletic performance in non-asthmatic athletes or non-athletes. It seems that the main effect of these drugs is to relieve the abnormal narrowing of the asthmatic athlete's bronchi, thus allowing him or her to compete on an equal footing (equal breathing) with the athlete not burdened with an abnormal bronchial tree. Other β-agonists, including clenbuterol, may indeed have ergogenic properties, and are appropriately banned.

NON-PHARMACOLOGICAL MEANS

It is possible to take advantage of our understanding of the pathophysiology of EIA to employ non-pharmacological means that can be successful in preventing, or attenuating EIA.

Warm inspired air. As simple a procedure as wrapping a scarf around the face, or using a simple mask over the nose and mouth, can increase the temperature and humidity of the inspired air by mixing inspired air with exhaled air. This reduces the stimulus to EIA and the likelihood of an attack (Brenner *et al.*, 1980; Schachter *et al.*, 1981) (Fig. 29.16).

Warm-up exercise. It is possible to take advantage of the refractory period by exercising in

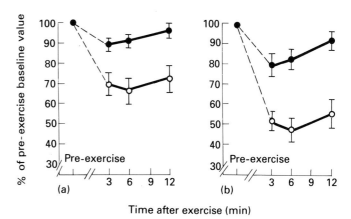

Fig. 29.16 Average pulmonary function indices, (a) FEV$_1$ and (b) maximal mid-expiratory flow rate, while breathing room air (○) and with mask (●) at 3, 6 and 12 min after exercise, expressed as a per cent of baseline value (mean ± SE for 10 subjects). Redrawn from Brenner *et al.* (1980).

the 30–90 min prior to competition. The first ('warm-up') session need not be vigorous enough to induce EIA itself in order to block EIA (Reiff *et al.*, 1989). It is not clear whether short sprints or longer, less intense, warm-ups are better. The best warm-up for preventing EIA and not interfering with performance is best determined by the individual based on experience, and will likely vary from athlete to athlete, and perhaps from sport to sport.

Select the appropriate sport. Since the stimulus that is most likely to cause EIA is non-swimming exercise vigorous enough to raise the heart rate to 170 beats · min^{-1} or so for 6–10 min, especially in cold air, this knowledge can in some cases help direct the aspiring asthmatic athlete towards a sport or event of relatively low asthmagenicity, such as swimming, or events that are shorter or longer in duration, like sprints or distance running or cycling. Stop-and-go sports may also be included and be of low asthmagenicity. Lifting, throwing or jumping events are not likely to provoke much difficulty. Of course, the physician, coach or parent does not always have the luxury of being able to steer the young athlete towards an 'appropriate' sport; instead the young runner may have trouble during her or his event, and wants help with that event. The miler will not appreciate being advised to take up the shot put.

Miscellaneous. Hypnosis has been shown to help block EIA in some subjects (Ben-Zvi *et al.*, 1982), perhaps through influencing resting bronchomotor tone via vagal routes, or perhaps by altering ventilation.

Practical approach to the young athlete with asthma

In most cases, diagnosing a youngster with EIA will be straightforward. If a child or adolescent already carries the diagnosis of asthma, then exercise-related symptoms of chest pain, shortness of breath, cough or wheeze can generally be assumed to be related to the underlying reactive airways, and as part of the evaluation, can be treated as such. Lack of a quick response to appropriate EIA prevention should prompt further investigation. Exercise testing to determine the youngster's level of fitness should be carried out, as many people with asthma will have restricted their own activity, or had it restricted by physicians, parents, teachers or coaches, to the point of substantial deconditioning. The poorly fit individual might well suffer shortness of breath with an aerobic or anaerobic challenge beyond his or her capabilities. In these cases, more exercise, in a rational conditioning programme is indicated.

It is important that asthmatic athletes have excellent care for and control of their asthma, with special attention being paid to the underlying airways inflammation. Only when the asthma and the airway inflammation is well-controlled will the exercise-related component be readily prevented. Then, non-pharmacological approaches, such as wearing a face mask or scarf while exercising in cold weather, may help. If this proves ineffective, pretreatment with a β_2-agonist inhaler should be tried. If inadequate, the dose can be doubled. The next step should be the addition of inhaled cromolyn sodium. If these are not completely successful, the cromolyn dose can be doubled. A final pharmacological addition can be ipratropium bromide. Finally, if these are all unsuccessful, it is important to review again the state of control of the underlying airways inflammation, and perhaps to conduct exercise tests in the laboratory setting with the various medications. Figure 29.17 gives a schematic approach to the child athlete with asthma.

It is fortunate that the vast majority of youngsters with asthma are able to engage in a normal active life, including competitive athletics. Caring for these young athletes is truly one of the most satisfying activities a physician can engage in.

Challenges for future research

Much has been learned about asthma and sports over the past several hundred years, especially the past two decades. Yet, there are still some unknown areas, particularly concerning pathogenesis:
- What precisely is the role of water and heat loss in causing EIA?
- What is it about exercise itself beyond the respiratory heat exchange that leads the susceptible airway to become narrower?

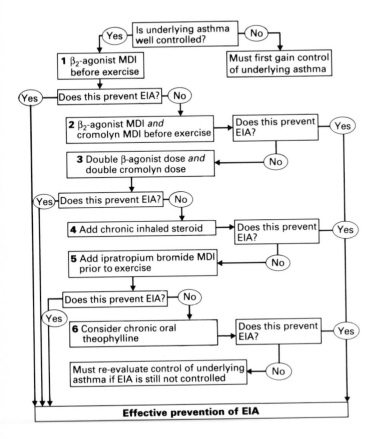

Fig. 29.17 Flow chart for selecting drugs to prevent exercise-induced asthma (EIA). MDI, metered dose inhaler. Adapted from Morton and Fitch (1992).

- Where do the various mediators of inflammation fit in?
- What is the role of NCF, and is this particular factor the same as interleukin 8?
- How can the fact that swimming is less asthmagenic than other forms of exercise be explained: is it body position, water immersion or another as yet undefined factor?
- Finally, what of treatment? Do the β-agonists have ergogenic properties, or are there important differences among them that would make one member of the class 'fair' and another unfair?

References

Aitken, M. & Morini, J. (1985) Effect of heat delivery and extraction on airway conductance in normal and in asthmatic subjects. *Am. Rev. Resp. Dis.* **131**, 357–61.

Anderson, S. (1983) Current concepts of exercise-induced asthma. *Allergy* **38**, 289–302.

Anderson, S., Bye, P., Schoeffel, R., Seale, J., Taylor, K. & Ferris, L. (1981) Arterial plasma histamine levels at rest and during and after exercise in patients with asthma: effects of terbutaline aerosol. *Thorax* **36**, 259–67.

Aubier, M., Troyer, A., Sampson, M., Macklem, P. & Roussos, C. (1981) Aminophylline improves diaphragmatic contractility. *New Engl. J. Med.* **305**, 249–52.

Badger, D., Ramos, A., Lew, C., Platzker, A., Stabile, M. & Keens, T. (1987) Childhood sequelae of infant lung disease: exercise and pulmonary function abnormalities after bronchopulmonary dysplasia. *J. Pediatr.* **110**, 693–9.

Baker, P., Dalrymple, R., Ingle, D. & Ricks, C. (1984) Use of an adrenergic agent to alter muscle and fat deposition in lambs. *J. Anim. Sci.* **59**, 1256–61.

Bar-Or, O. (1983) Pediatric sports medicine for the practitioner. In *Physiologic Principles to Clinical Applications*, pp. 88–109. Springer-Verlag, New York.

Bar-Or, O. (1985) Physical conditioning in children with cardiorespiratory disease. *Exerc. Sport Sci. Rev.* **13**, 305–34.

Bar-Or, O. & Inbar, O. (1982) Swimming and asthma. Benefits and deleterious effects. *Sports Med.* **14**, 397–405.

Bar-Or, O., Neuman, I. & Dotan, R. (1977) Effects of dry and humid climates on exercise-induced asthma in children and preadolescents. *J. Allergy Clin. Immunol.* **60**, 163–8.

Bar-Yishay, E., Ben-Dov, I. & Godfrey, S. (1983) Refractory period after hyperventilation-induced asthma. *Am. Rev. Resp. Dis.* **127**, 572–4.

Bar-Yishay, E., Gur, I., Inbar, O. *et al.* (1982) Differences between swimming and running as stimuli for exercise-induced asthma. *Eur. J. Appl. Physiol.* **48**, 387–97.

Barnes, P. (1989) A new approach to the treatment of asthma. *New Engl. J. Med.* **321**, 1517–27.

Barnes, P. & Brown, M. (1981) Venous plasma histamine in exercise and hyperventilation-induced asthma in man. *Clin. Sci.* **61**, 159–62.

Ben-Dov, I., Bar-Yishay, E. & Godfrey, S. (1982) Refractory period after exercise-induced asthma unexplained by respiratory heat loss. *Am. Rev. Resp. Dis.* **125**, 530–4.

Ben-Zvi, Z, Spohn, W., Young S. & Kattan, M. (1982) Hypnosis for exercise-induced asthma. *Am. Rev. Resp. Dis.* **125**, 392–5.

Bianco, S., Vaghi, A. Rouschi, M. & Pasargiklian, M. (1988) Prevention of exercise-induced bronchoconstriction by inhaled frusemide. *Lancet* **ii**, 252–5.

Boner, A., Vallone, G., Chiesa, M., Spezia, E., Fambri, L. & Sette, L. (1992) Reproducibility of late phase pulmonary responses to exercise and its relationship to bronchial hyperreactivity in children with chronic asthma. *Pediatr. Pulmonol.* **14**, 156–9.

Brenner, A., Weiser, P., Krogh, K. & Loren, M. (1980) Effectiveness of a portable face mask in attenuating exercise-induced asthma. *JAMA* **244**, 2196–8.

Bundgaard, A., Ingemann, H.T. & Halkjaer, K.J. (1984) Physical training in bronchial asthma. *Int. Rehab. Med.* **6**, 179–82.

Chen, W. & Horton, D. (1977) Heat and water loss from the airways and exercise-induced asthma. *Respiration* **34**, 305–13.

Clark, C. & Cochrane, L. (1988) Assessment of work performance in asthma for determination of cardiorespiratory fitness and training capacity. *Thorax* **43**, 745–9.

Cox, J. & Altounyan, R. (1970) Nature and modes of action of disodium cromoglycate (Lomudal). *Respiration* **27**, (Suppl.), 292–309.

Crimi, E., Balbo, A., Milanese, M., Miadonna, A., Rossi, G. & Brusasco, V. (1992) Airway inflammation and occurrence of delayed bronchoconstriction in exercise-induced asthma. *Am. Rev. Respir. Dis.* **46**, 507–12.

Cropp, G. (1975) Grading, time course, and incidence of exercise-induced airway obstruction and hyperinflation in asthmatic children. *Pediatrics* **56** (Suppl.), 868–79.

Cropp, G. (1979) The exercise bronchoprovocation test: standardization of procedures and evaluation of response. *J. Allergy Clin. Immunol.* **64**, 627–33.

Cropp, G. & Tanakawa, N. (1977) Cardiorespiratory adaptations of normal and asthmatic children to exercise. In J. Dempsey & C. Reed (eds) *Muscular Exercise and the Lung*, pp. 265–78. University of Wisconsin Press, Madison, WI.

Deal, E. Jr, McFadden, E. Jr & Ingram, R. Jr (1979a) Hyperpnea and heat flux: initial reaction sequence in exercise-induced asthma. *J. Appl. Physiol. Respir. Environ. Exerc. Physiol.* **46**, 476–83.

Deal, E. Jr, McFadden, E. Jr, Ingram, R. Jr, Breslin, F. & Jaeger, J. (1980) Airway responsiveness to cold air and hyperpnea in normal subjects and in those with hay fever and asthma. *Am. Rev. Resp. Dis.* **121**, 621–8.

Deal, E., McFadden, E., Ingram, R. Jr, Strauss, R. & Jaeger, J. (1979b) Role of respiratory heat exchange in production of exercise-induced asthma. *J. Appl. Physiol.* **46**, 467–75.

Edmunds, A., Tooley, M. & Godfrey, S. (1978) The refractory period after exercise-induced asthma: its duration and relation to the severity of exercise. *Am. Rev. Respir. Dis.* **117**, 247–54.

Ellis, E. (1984) Inhibition of exercise-induced asthma by theophylline. *J. Allergy Clin. Immunol.* **73**, 690–2.

Expert Panel of the National Heart, Lung and Blood Institute (1991) National Asthma Program. Guidelines for the diagnosis and management of asthma. *J. Allergy Clin. Immunol.* **88**, 425–34.

Finnerty, J. Wood-Baker, R., Thomson, H. & Holgate, S. (1992) Role of leukotrienes in exercise-induced asthma. Inhibitory effect of ICI 204219, a potent leukotriene D$_4$ receptor antagonist. *Am. Rev. Respir. Dis.* **145**, 746–9.

Fitch, K. (1975) Comparative aspects of available exercise systems. *Pediatrics* 56 (Suppl.), 904–7.

Fitch, K., Blitvich, J. & Morton, A. (1986) The effect of running training on exercise-induced asthma. *Ann. Allergy* 57, 90–4.

Fitch, K., Morton, A. & Blanksby, B.A. (1976) Effects of swimming training on children with asthma. *Arch. Dis. Child.* **51**, 190–4.

Garfinkel, S., Kesten, S., Chapman, K. & Rebuck, A. (1992) Physiologic and nonphysiologic determinants of aerobic fitness in mild to moderate asthma. *Am. Rev. Respir. Dis.* **145**, 741–5.

Gergen, P., Mullaly, D. & Evans, R. (1988) National survey of prevalence of asthma among children in the United States, 1977–80. *Pediatrics* **81**, 1–7.

Geubelle, F., Ernould, C. & Jovanovich, M. (1971) Working capacity and physical training in asthmatic children, at 1800 m altitude. *Acta Paediatr. Scand.* (Suppl. 217), 93–8.

Ghory, J. (1975) Exercise and asthma: overview and clinical impact. *Pediatrics* 56 (Suppl.), 844–6.

Gilbert, I., Fouke, J. & McFadden, E. Jr (1988) Intra-airway thermodynamics during exercise and hyperventilation in asthmatics. *J. Appl. Physiol.* **64**, 2167–74.

Godfrey, S. (1974) *Exercise Testing in Children*. W.B. Saunders, Philadelphia.

Godfrey, S. & Konig, P. (1976). Inhibition of exercise-induced asthma by different pharmacological pathways. *Thorax* **31**, 137–43.

Godfrey, S., Silverman, M. & Anderson, S. (1975) The use of the treadmill for assessing exercise-induced asthma and the effect of varying the severity and duration of exercise. *Pediatrics* 56 (Suppl.), 893–8.

Graff-Lonnevig, G., Bevegard, S., Eriksson, B. *et al.* (1980) Two years' follow-up of asthmatic boys participating in a physical activity program. *Acta Paediatr. Scand.* **69**, 347–52.

Gross, N.J. (1980) What is this thing called love? — Or, defining asthma. *Am Rev. Respir. Dis.* **121**, 203–4.

Haas, F., Levin, N., Pasierski, S., Bishop, M. & Axen, K. (1986) Reduced hyperpnea-induced bronchospasm following repeated cold air challenge. *J. Appl. Physiol.* **61**, 210–14.

Hahn, A., Anderson, S., Morton, A., Black, J. & Fitch, K. (1984a) A reinterpretation of the effect of temperature and water content of the inspired air in exercise-induced asthma. *Am. Rev. Respir. Dis.* **130**, 575–9.

Hahn, A., Nogrady, S., Tumilty, D., Lawrence, S. & Morton, A. (1984b) Histamine reactivity during the refractory period after exercise-induced asthma. *Thorax* **39**, 919–23.

Hamielec, C.M., Manning, P.J. & O'Byrne, P.M. (1988) Exercise refractoriness after histamine inhalation in asthmatic subjects. *Am. Rev. Resp. Dis.* **138**, 794–8.

Henriksen, J. & Dahl, R. (1983) Effects of inhaled budesonide alone and in combination with low-dose terbutaline in children with exercise-induced asthma. *Am. Rev. Respir. Dis.* **128**, 993–7.

Inbar, O., Alvarez, D. & Lyons, H. (1981) Exercise-induced asthma — a comparison between two modes of exercise stress. *Eur. J. Respir. Dis.* **62**, 160–7.

Inbar, O., Dotan, R., Dlin, R., Neuman, I. & Bar-Or, O. (1980) Breathing dry or humid air and exercise-induced asthma during swimming. *Eur. J. Appl. Physiol. Occup. Physiol.* **44**, 43–50.

Ingemann-Hansen, T., Bundgaard, A., Halkjaer-Kristensen, J., Siggaard-Andersen, J. & Weeke, B. (1980) Maximal oxygen consumption rate in patients with bronchial asthma: the effect of β$_2$-adrenoreceptor stimulation. *Scand. J. Clin. Lab. Invest.* **40**, 99–104.

Israel, E., Dermarkarian, R., Rosenberg, M. *et al.* (1990) The effects of a 5-lipoxygenase inhibitor on asthma induced by cold, dry air. *New Engl. J. Med.* **323**, 1740–4.

Jones, R. (1966) Assessment of respiratory function in the asthmatic child. *Br. Med. J.* **2**, 297–5.

Kilham, H., Tooley, M. & Silverman, M. (1979) Running, walking, and hyperventilation causing asthma in children. *Thorax* **34**, 582–6.

Lee, T., Assoufi, B. & Kay, A. (1983a) The link between exercise, respiratory heat exchange, and the mast cell in bronchial asthma. *Lancet* i, 520–2.

Lee, T., Nagakura, T., Papageorgiou, N., Cromwell, O., Iikura, Y. & Kay, A. (1984) Mediators in exercise-induced asthma. *J. Allergy Clin. Immunol* **73**, 634–9.

Lee, T., Nagakura, T., Papageorgiou, N., Ikura, Y. & Kay, A. (1983b) Exercise-induced late asthmatic reactions with neutrophil chemotactic activity. *New Engl. J. Med.* **308**, 1502–5.

Lemanske, R. Jr & Henke K. (1989) Exercise-induced asthma. In C. Gisolfi & D. Lamb (eds) *Youth, Exercise, and Sport*, pp. 465–511. *Perspectives in Exercise Science and Sports Medicine*. Benchmark Press, Indianapolis, IN.

Linna, O. (1990) Influence of baseline lung function on exercise-induced response in childhood asthma. *Acta Paediatr. Scand.* **79**, 664–9.

Loughlin, G. & Taussig, L. (1979) Pulmonary function in children with a history of laryngotracheobronchitis. *J. Pediatr.* **94**, 365–9.

McFadden, E. (1987) Exercise-induced asthma. Assessment of current etiologic concepts. *Chest* **91**, 151S–7.

McFadden, E. & Ingram, R. Jr (1979) Exercise-induced asthma. Observations on the initiating stimulus. *New Engl. J. Med.* **301**, 763–9.

McFadden, E. & Ingram, R.J. (1980) Asthma: perspectives, definition, and classification. In A. Fishman (ed.) *Pulmonary Diseases and Disorders*, 1st edn, pp. 562–6. McGraw-Hill, New York.

McFadden, E.J., Lenner, A. & Strohl, K. (1986) Post-exertional airway rewarming and thermally induced asthma. New insights into pathophysiology and possible pathogenesis. *J. Clin. Invest.* **78**, 18–25.

McFadden, E. Jr, Stearns, D., Ingram, R. Jr & Leith, D. (1977) Relative contributions of hypocarbia and hyperpnea as mechanisms in post-exercise asthma. *J. Appl. Physiol.* **42**, 22–7.

McLaughlin, F. & Dozor, A. (1983) Cold air inhalation challenge in the diagnosis of asthma in children. *Pediatrics* **72**, 503–9.

Manning, P., Watson, R., Margolskee, D., Williams, V., Schwartz, J. & O'Byrne, P. (1990) Inhibition of exercise-induced bronchoconstriction by MK-571, a potent leukotriene D_4-receptor antagonist. *New Engl. J. Med.* **323**, 1736–9.

Matthay, R. & Mahler, D. (1986) Theophylline im-proves global cardiac function and reduces dyspnea in chronic obstructive lung disease. *J. Allergy Clin. Immunol.* **78**, 793–9.

Meeuwisse, W., McKenzie, D., Hopkins, S. & Road, J. (1992) The effect of salbutamol on performance in élite nonasthmatic athletes. *Med. Sci. Sports Exerc.* **24**, 1161–6.

Middleton, E. Jr (1984) Airway smooth muscle, asthma, and calcium ions. *J. Allergy Clin. Immunol.* **73**, 643–50.

Monahan, T. (1986) Sidelined asthmatics get back in the game. *Phys. Sports Med.* **14**, 61–6.

Morton, A. & Fitch, K. (1992) Asthmatic drugs and competitive sport. An update. *Sports Medicine* **14**,l 228–42.

Morton, A., Papalia, S. & Fitch, K. (1992) Is salbutamol ergogenic? The effects of salbutamol on physical performance in high-performance nonasthmatic athletes. *Clin. J. Sports Med.* **2**, 93–7.

Morton, A., Scott, C. & Fitch, K. (1989) The effects of theophylline on the physical performance and work capacity of well-trained athletes. *J. Allergy Clin. Immunol.* **83**, 55–60.

Nagakura, T., Lee, T., Assoufi, B., Newman-Taylor, A., Denison, D. & Kay, A. (1983) Neutrophil chemotactic factor in exercise- and hyperventilation-induced asthma. *Am. Rev. Resp. Dis.* **128**, 294–6.

Nickerson, B., Bautista, D., Namey, M., Richard, W. & Keens, T. (1983) Distance running improves fitness in asthmatic children without pulmonary complications or changes in exercise-induced bronchospasm. *Pediatrics* **71**, 147–52.

Nixon, P. & Orenstein, D. (1988) Exercise testing in children. *Pediatr. Pulmonol.* **5**, 107–22.

O'Donnell, W., Rosenberg, M., Niven, R., Drazen, J. & Israel, E. (1992) Acetazolamide and furosemide attenuate asthma induced by hyperventilation of cold, dry air. *Am. Rev. Respir. Dis.* **146**, 1518–23.

Orenstein, D. (1993) Assessment of exercise pulmon-ary function. In T. Rowland (ed.) *Pediatric Lab-oratory Exercise Testing: Clinical Guidelines*, pp. 141–63. Human Kinetics, Champaign, IL.

Orenstein, D., Reed, M., Grogan, F. & Crawford, L. (1985) Exercise conditioning in children with asthma. *J. Pediatr.* **106**, 556–60.

Oseid, S. & Haaland, K. (1978) Exercise studies on asthmatic children before and after regular physical training. In B. Eriksson & B. Furberg (eds) *Swimming Medicine IV*, pp. 32–41. University Park Press, Baltimore.

Petersen, K. & McElhenney, T. (1965) Effects of a physical fitness program upon asthmatic boys. *Pediatrics* **35**, 295–9.

Phelan, P., Landau, L. & Olinsky, A. (1990) *Respiratory Illness in Children*, 3rd edn. Blackwell Scientific Publications, Oxford.

Pierson, W., Bierman, W., Kawabori, I. & Van Arsdel, P. (1972) The incidence of exercise-induced bronchospams in 'normal' and 'atopic' children. *J. Allergy Clin. Immunol.* **49**, 129A–30.

Reiff, D., Choudry, N., Pride, N. & Ind, P. (1989) The effect of prolonged submaximal warm-up exercise on exercise-induced asthma. *Am. Rev. Respir. Dis.* **139**, 479–84.

Rice, S., Bierman, C., Shapiro, G., Furukawa, C. & Pierson, W. (1985) Identification of exercise-induced asthma among intercollegiate athletes. *Ann. Allergy* **55**, 790–3.

Rosenthal, R., Laube, B., Hood, D. & Norman, P. (1990) Analysis of refractory period after exercise and eucapnic voluntary hyperventilation challenge. *Am. Rev. Respir. Dis.* **141**, 368–72.

Rubinstein, I., Levison, H., Slutsky, A., Hak, H., Wells, J., Zamel, N. & Rebuck, A. (1987) Immediate and delayed bronchoconstriction after exercise in patients with asthma. *New Engl. J. Med.* **317**, 482–5.

Rupp, N., Guill, M. & Brudno, D. (1992) Unrecognized exercise-induced bronchospam in adolescent athletes. *Am. J. Dis. Child.* **146**, 941–4.

Sakula, A. (1984) Sir John Floyer's *A Treatise of the Asthma* (1698). *Thorax* **39**, 248–54.

Sakula, A. (1988) A history of asthma. The FitzPatrick Lecture 1987. *J. Roy. Coll. Phys. Lond.* **22**, 36–43.

Salter, H. (1864) *On Asthma: Its Pathology and Treatment.* Blanchard & Lea, Philadelphia.

Schachter, E., Lach, E. & Lee, M. (1981) The protective effect of a cold weather mask on exercise-induced asthma. *Ann. Allergy* **46**, 12–16.

Schwartzenstein, R. (1992) Asthma: to run or not to run? (editorial). *Am. Rev. Respir. Dis.* **145**, 739–40.

Sears, M., Taylor, D., Print, C. *et al.* (1990) Regular inhaled beta-agonist treatment in bronchial asthma. *Lancet* **336**, 1391–6.

Sheppard, D., Saisho, A., Nadel, J. & Boushey, H. (1981) Exercise increases sulfur dioxide-induced bronchoconstriction in asthmatic subjects. *Am. Rev. Respir. Dis.* **123**, 486–591.

Signorile, J., Kaplan, T., Applegate, B. & Perry, A. (1992) Effects of acute inhalation of the bronchodilator, albuterol, on power output. *Med. Sci. Sports Exerc.* **24**, 638–42.

Silverman, M. & Anderson, S. (1972) Standardization of exercise tests in asthmatic children. *Arch Dis. Child.* **47**, 882–9.

Silverman, M., Hobbs, F., Gordon, I. & Carswell, F. (1978) Cystic fibrosis, atopy and airways lability. *Arch. Dis. Child.* **53**, 873–7.

Souhrada, M. & Souhrada, J. (1981) The direct effect of temperature on airway smooth muscle. *Respir. Physiol.* **44**, 311–23.

Speelberg, B., Panis, E., Bijl, D., van Herwaarden, C. & Bruynzeel, P. (1991) Late asthmatic responses after exercise challenge are reproducible. *J. Allergy Clin. Immunol.* **87**, 1128–37.

Spitzer, W., Saissa, S., Ernst, P. *et al.* (1992) The use of β-agonists and the risk of death and near death from asthma. *New Engl. J. Med.* **326**, 501–6.

Strauss, R., McFadden, E., Ingram, R., Jr & Jaeger, J. (1977) Enhancement of exercise-induced asthma by cold air. *New Engl. J. Med.* **297**, 743–7.

Strunk, R., Rubin, D., Kelly, L. & Sherman, B. (1988) Determination of fitness in children with asthma. *Am. J. Dis. Child.* **142**, 940–4.

Taylor, W. & Newacheck, P. (1992) Impact of childhood asthma on health. *Pediatrics* **90**, 657–62.

Varray, A., Mercier, J., Terral, C. & Prefaut, C. (1991) Individualized aerobic and high intensity training for asthmatic children in an exercise readaptation program. Is training always helpful for better adaptation to exercise? *Chest* **99**, 579–86.

Weiler-Ravell, D. & Godfrey, S. (1981) Do exercise and antigen-induced asthma utilize the same pathways? *J. Allergy Clin. Immunol.* **67**, 391–7.

Wells, R.J., Walker, J. & Hickler, R. (1960) Effects of cold air on respiratory airflow resistance in patients with respiratory-tract disease. *New Engl. J. Med.* **263**, 268–73.

Wiens, L., Sabath, R., Ewing, L., Gowdamarajan, R., Portnoy, J. & Scagliotti, D. (1992) Chest pain in otherwise healthy children and adolescents is frequently caused by exercise-induced asthma. *Pediatrics* **90**, 350–3.

Willis, T. (1684) *Practice of Physick. Pharmaceutice Rationalis or the Operation of Medicines in Humane Bodies.* Thomas Dring, London.

Wilson, B., Bar-Or, O. & Seed, L. (1990) Effects of humid air breathing during arm or treadmill exercise on exercise-induced bronchoconstriction and refractoriness. *Am. Rev. Respir. Dis.* **142**, 349–52.

Woolley, M., Anderson, S. & Quigley, B. (1990) Duration of protective effect of terbutaline sulfate and cromolyn sodium alone and in combination on exercise-induced asthma. *Chest* **97**, 39–45.

Zach, M., Polgar, G., Kump, H. & Kroisel, P. (1984) Cold air challenge of airway hyper-reactivity in children: practical application and theoretical aspects. *Pediatr. Res.* **18**, 469–78.

Chapter 30

Juvenile Diabetes and Sports

HARRY DORCHY AND JACQUES R. POORTMANS

Type I diabetes in children and adolescents

For general references, the reader is referred to a recent general textbook edited by Alberti *et al.* (1992) and for paediatric references to specific textbooks by Bougnères *et al.* (1990), Brink (1987), Czernichow and Dorchy (1989), Travis *et al.* (1987) and Kelnar (1995).

Aetiology and epidemiology

DEFINITION

Diabetes mellitus is not a disease, but a syndrome with a number of different causes. Clinically, it is characterized by hyperglycaemia and glycosuria. If untreated, it may progress to acidosis and ketosis, dehydration, coma and death. Diabetes of juvenile onset is usually due to a deficiency in the endogenous supply of insulin by the pancreatic β-cells and should therefore be treated by the administration of insulin. Insulin-dependent diabetes mellitus (IDDM) is now called type I diabetes. Total exhaustion of the β-cells, however, may take several years.

PATHOGENESIS AND NATURAL HISTORY

The destruction of the pancreatic β-cells is autoimmune in nature. However, the aetiology and pathogenesis of type I diabetes are not totally understood. Both heredity and precipi-

tating factors are involved. The prevalence of IDDM in first-degree relatives is between 5 and 15%. The associations between IDDM and the HLA antigens located in the human major histocompatibility complex (MHC) on the short arm of chromosome 6, suggests that the genes which encode these antigens determine disease susceptibility. More than 95% of Caucasian diabetics have either HLA-DR3 or HLA-DR4. However these two antigens are found in 50% of healthy controls. Subsequent studies using DNA technology have shown that putative diabetes susceptibility or protection genes map close to, or are part of, the HLA DQ locus. The DQA1*0301-DQB1*0302/DQA1*0501-DQB1*0201 heterozygous genotype occurs in about 30% of type I patients but not more than 1% of controls, thereby conferring a relative risk of over 30% (Dorchy *et al.*, 1993).

The concordance for diabetes in identical twins is less than 50%, suggesting that genetic markers alone do not explain the appearance of IDDM which needs one or more environmental factors playing an important role in the induction of β-cell destruction. Evidence has accumulated incriminating viruses such as Coxsackie viruses (particularly B4), cytomegaloviruses, congenital rubella, and so on. Toxic agents (nitrosamine) and nutritional factors — mainly bovine milk serum albumin — are also involved (Karjalainen *et al.*, 1992).

Clinical onset of the disease results from the near complete destruction of the β-cells. The pathological process that precedes clinical onset

455

extends for months or years: this period is called 'prediabetes'.

The diagnosis, signs and symptoms of overt type I diabetes are rather uniform: polyuria, polydipsia, fatigue and weight loss appear in a few days or weeks. Once treatment has been started, many children experience a period of remission in the course of the first months of the disease, the so-called 'honeymoon', during which the need for insulin is reduced or even disappears completely; the remission may last for several weeks or months but is never permanent (Fig. 30.1).

EPIDEMIOLOGY

In Europe, the incidence of IDDM follows a north–south gradient, being very high in Scandinavia. Before the age of 15 years, the risk of IDDM for a Finnish child is sevenfold higher than for a French child, incidence being 29 and four per 100 000 per year respectively. The reasons are unknown. In the USA, the incidence of IDDM, in the age range 0–20 years, is 15.4 per 100 000 per year in Caucasians, and 10.6 in Black people. Japan is the country with the lowest known incidence: 1.7 per 100 000 per year. In European countries, epidemiological studies show evidence of increasing incidence of IDDM. Incidence peaks during puberty with an earlier peak (1 or 2 years) in girls than in boys. After 40 years of age, the risk for IDDM is low.

Reliable studies on prevalence of IDDM (number of cases per 1000 subjects of the same ages) are rare. Under 15 years, prevalence of IDDM is 0.24 in France, 1.1 in England, 1.3 in USA and 1.9 in Finland.

Treatment

AIMS

Treatment should permit the diabetic child or adolescent to lead a life free from side-effects such as hypoglycaemia, hyperglycaemia and ketosis, growth delay and psychological difficulties. The ultimate aim is to prevent the vascular, renal and neurological complications. Ideally, therefore, blood glucose should be maintained at normal levels throughout the day and night; however, this is almost impossible in the diabetic child, except during the remission period. The determination of glycosylated or glycated haemoglobin levels (total glycated haemoglobin HbA_1 or the fraction HbA_{1c}) may provide a good criterion of overall metabolic control. It should be measured

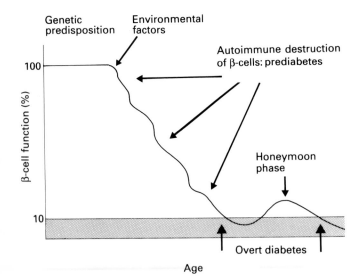

Fig. 30.1 Natural history of type I diabetes.

regularly (every 2 months) because it provides an index of glucose control over the preceding 8 weeks. Figure 30.2 shows the mean annual HbA_{1c} that can be achieved in unselected young diabetic patients during the first 2 years of diabetes — while a residual insulin secretion determined by the C-peptide level is possible — and in young patients with a diabetes duration longer than 2 years and without residual endogenous insulin secretion (Dorchy, 1994).

INSULIN

Commercially available 'human' insulins are grouped into three classes according to their duration of action:
1 Type 1: rapid-acting (<8 h).
2 Type 2: intermediate-acting ($12-24$ h).
3 Type 3: long-acting (>24 h).

Until adolescence, it is often possible to achieve good metabolic control with two injections per day of a mixture of type 1 and type 2 insulins, before breakfast and before dinner, at a total dose between 0.5 and $1.5 \, U \cdot kg^{-1}$ (after the transitory remission period that may appear during the first months following the clinical onset of the disease). The actions of these four insulins in two injections are mainly assessed from the results of self-monitoring of blood glucose (SMBG) with strips read by a meter or, eventually, from the results of urine glucose

measurements which represent an average of blood glucose levels over the time that the urine is collected. Figure 30.3 shows that the midday analysis before lunch reflects the action of type 1 insulin injected in the morning. The evening analysis before dinner reflects the action of type 2 insulin injected in the morning. The bedtime analysis reflects the action of type 1 insulin injected in the evening. Morning analysis reflects the action of type 2 insulin injected in the day before towards the end of the afternoon. From the age of 10 years onwards a child should be able to adjust his or her own insulin dosage. The two injections per day insulin therapy is easy because no injection is needed during school hours. However, it is necessary to have a balanced died divided into six meals, according to the action profile of the insulins used and to physical exercise, at more or less fixed hours (Fig. 30.3).

If a young diabetic patient wants to benefit from a greater freedom with respect to daily life and dietary habits, he or she needs to shift to the basal-prandial or basal-bolus insulin therapy. Figure 30.4 shows an example of such a treatment: a type 3 insulin (long-acting or basal insulin) is administered at bedtime, and three bolus of type 1 insulin are injected before each meal. The use of pen injectors has made this system more convenient. Basal insulin may also be given as a type 2 insulin at bed-

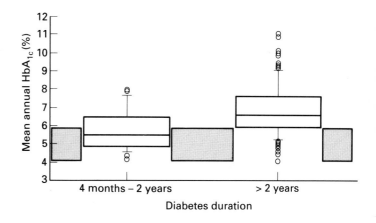

Fig. 30.2 Comparison of mean annual HbA_{1c} levels (shown by the 10, 25, 50, 75 and 90th percentiles) in 23 children with a diabetes duration between 4 months and 2 years (i.e. with a possible residual insulin secretion), and in 129 young patients with a diabetes duration from 2 to 27 years (and without any residual endogenous insulin secretion). HbA_{1c} was determined by high performance liquid chromatography (normal range: 4.4–6.0%). ☐, normal values of HbA_{1c}. Adapted from Dorchy (1994).

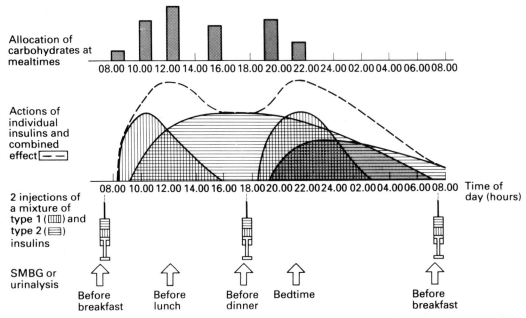

Fig. 30.3 Insulin activities and allocation of carbohydrates in a child giving himself two daily injections of a mixture of rapid-acting and intermediate-acting insulins, and performing blood or urine glucose measurements four times a day. SMBG, self-monitoring of blood glucose. Adapted from Czernichow and Dorchy (1989).

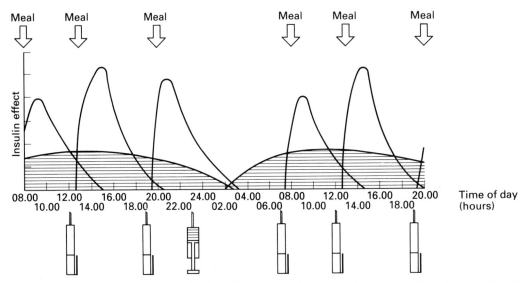

Fig. 30.4 Basal-bolus insulin therapy. Basal insulin (▤) is administered at bedtime, and three boluses of rapid-acting insulin are injected 30 min before each meal. Adapted from Czernichow and Dorchy (1989).

time and in a small morning dose. However, to obtain good metabolic control, it is often necessary to intensify SMBG because dose alteration of type 1 insulin may not be only guided by preprandial blood glucose measurements, but also by postprandial blood glucose targets (Dorchy, 1994). Overall, for adolescents and adults, if they intend to engage in sport and competition, it is the method of choice.

With the introduction of insulin pens, the indications of insulin pump therapy are quite limited in children and young adults.

Insulin therapy cannot fully restore physiological changes in insulin levels as seen in normal children. Moreover, the important exercise-induced changes in insulin secretion cannot be reproduced when insulin is injected subcutaneously. Consequently various states of insulin excess or insulin lack may occur (Kemmer & Berger, 1992).

DIET

Diabetic children should have normal energy intake for their age with an optimal dietary balance as follows: (i) 55% of the energy as carbohydrate (modest amount of sucrose and other refined sugars; preference for unrefined sugars with fibre); (ii) 30% as fat (saturated fats: < 10%; cholesterol: < 300 mg · day^{-1}; mono-unsaturated fats: 10%; saturated fats: 10%); and (iii) 15% as protein (in adults: 0.8 g · kg^{-1}; in children: 1–1.5 g · kg^{-1}). Energy intake may fluctuate from day to day according to physical exercise. To impose a fixed, weighed and measured diet is not required for optimal glycaemic control and is undesirable for psychological reasons. A diet that simply restricts the carbohydrate intake automatically results in an excessive intake of fat which is harmful to the blood vessels. Overall energy restriction prevents normal growth (Dorchy et al., 1979). It is necessary for the athlete to have a well-balanced diet, adapted daily to both insulin activity and physical exercise.

The use of alternative sweeteners is acceptable. Sodium intake should be less than 3 g · day^{-1}. Needs for minerals and vitamins are not influenced by diabetes.

Complications

HYPERGLYCAEMIA AND KETOACIDOSIS

Diabetic ketoacidosis (DKA) is the metabolic consequence of a severe insulin deficiency. All stages of DKA, from the earliest increases in blood glucose through to increasing generation of ketone bodies, ketonaemia and acidaemia, may be steps in the process leading to coma and death if appropriate intervention does not occur. DKA takes from several hours to several days to develop. Most cases of incipient DKA can be recognized very early by well-educated younger patients. In recent years, the severity of DKA at clinical onset of diabetes is decreasing.

HYPOGLYCAEMIA

Hypoglycaemia (blood glucose concentration lower than 60 mg · dl^{-1} or 3.3 mmol · l^{-1}) is the commonest metabolic complication of diabetes. The major causes of hypoglycaemia are insulin excess, delayed or inappropriate food intake and unpredicted physical exercise. Figure 30.5 summarizes the main features of hypoglycaemia according to blood glucose level. Symptoms result from neuroglycopaenia and from activation of adrenergic or cholinergic defence mechanisms. Some patients are unable to recognize the symptoms, which may lead to severe hypoglycaemia and coma. The reasons for hypoglycaemia unawareness are complex and poorly understood but include loss of epinephrine response and autonomic neuropathy. Patients who attempt to achieve normal blood glucose levels are at higher risk and they have to monitor their glycaemia more frequently.

In practice, for treatment of mild hypoglycaemia, we advise the child to eat 5–20 g of some rapidly metabolized sugar (glucose tablets, soft drinks, and so on) and few a grams of some 'slowly absorbed' carbohydrate such

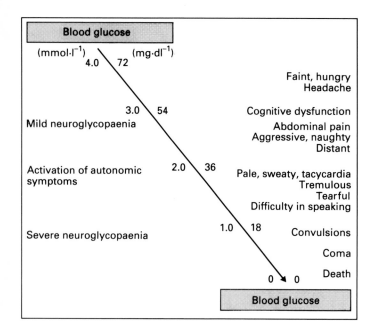

Fig. 30.5 Features of hypoglycaemia according to the blood glucose level. Adapted from Greene (1992).

as bread, in order to prevent recurrent blood glucose fall. The peak glycaemic response occurs after about 30 min. If the child is unable to swallow sugar, a member of the family or school staff should inject glucagon i.m. or s.c. (<10 years of age: 0.5 mg; >10 years of age: 1 mg = full dose). Consciousness returns within 5–10 min but glucagon may provoke headache and nausea. A new device is being produced for nasal administration of glucagon. If glucagon is ineffective, hypertonic glucose solution must be given i.v.

MICROANGIOPATHY, NEUROPATHY
AND NEPHROPATHY

With improvements in treatment, life expectancy has been extended and the principal aim of long-term treatment today is to avoid or at least delay the development of degenerative complications. It appears that chronic hyperglycaemia is an important causal factor, even in those which are partially genetically determined. Before engaging in regular physical activities, type I diabetic adolescents and adults need to be examined carefully for the presence of retinal, neurological or renal complications which can be present after puberty. In recent years, it has become increasingly apparent that functional and reversible abnormalities precede the structural and irreversible lesions that characterize diabetic complications (Dorchy, 1994).

Compared with simple ophthalmoscopy, fluorescein angiography is twice as effective in diagnosing early retinopathy. The first sign seems to be leaks of fluorescein that may precede the appearance of microaneurysms. Incipient retinopathy is not found before 12 years of age and 3 years of diabetes duration. The mean duration of diabetes before occurrence of the first abnormalities is 8–9 years, and the mean age at which they occur is 16–17 years (Verougstraete et al., 1991).

Neurophysiological studies may reveal abnormalities of the central and peripheral nervous systems even in the absence of clinical signs, i.e. depression of tendon reflexes, diminution of vibration perception and paraesthesia, that are only rarely found in adolescents. Reduction of sensory and motor nerve conduction velocities is related to the degree of metabolic control, even at the onset of diabetes. Slowing of motor conduction velocity in the peroneal nerve is found in 30% of diabetic adolescents and young adults after a mean duration of diabetes of 13 years. Neuropathy of the autonomic nervous system is rare in adolescents. The factors that most positively relate to pathological electrocerebral activity detected via electroencephalogram (EEG) are frequent and severe hypoglycaemic attacks, comas and/or convulsions. Minor hypoglycaemic episodes seem to be unrelated to EEG changes.

Renal complications are less common than retinopathy and neuropathy. Diabetic nephropathy develops in 30% of type I diabetics after 20 years of disease duration. At diagnosis of diabetes, renal blood flow and glomerular filtration rate (GFR) are elevated. During the first decade hyperfiltration persists in 30% of patients, after which GFR returns to normal although microalbuminuria is detectable. This abnormal albumin excretion, between 20 and 200 $\mu g \cdot min^{-1}$ or 30−300 $mg \cdot day^{-1}$, cannot be measured by routine strips such as Albustix. This stage does not appear before puberty and 5 years of diabetes duration. Increased microalbuminuria is highly predictive for progression to clinical nephropathy during the third decade after diabetes onset, characterized by macroproteinuria ($>300\,mg \cdot day^{-1}$). Macroproteinuria signals the progression to renal insufficiency and no interventionary measures have been shown to be effective. However, at the stage of microalbuminuria, tight glycaemic control and treatment of the frequently associated increased blood pressure, may slow or stop the development to renal insufficiency.

Lipoprotein abnormalities are common in type I diabetes, even in children and adolescents, and are partially responsible for premature atherosclerosis. Increased levels of triglycerides, total cholesterol, low-density lipoprotein (LDL) cholesterol and apolipoprotein B are correlated to the levels of glycated haemoglobin (Willems & Dorchy, 1990).

Education and the paediatric diabetes medical team

MULTIDISCIPLINARY TEAM

Children and adolescents with IDDM should be routinely referred to a paediatric diabetes centre having a multidisciplinary team (paediatric diabetologist, dietician, specialized nurses, social worker, psychologist, and so on) experienced and conversant with young patients. Children should learn to accept their disease and, from the age of 10 years onwards, they should be able to carry out their own treatment without the need for continuous recourse to parents or doctors. In our experience, the education of the child and the family takes approximately 2 weeks in the hospital. The child is then followed up 6−12 out-patient visits yearly. Patients may benefit from a holiday camp where they will learn to treat themselves and come to realize that they are not rare or isolated cases (Dorchy & Ernould, 1990). For diabetic children and adolescents who want to exercise, sports camps offer teaching programmes for self-management of their metabolic control. A nurse visitor trained in paediatric diabetology should make regular visits, at home or at school, to assist children and adolescents with their daily psychological as well as social and medical problems.

PSYCHOLOGICAL PROBLEMS

The intelligence of diabetic children is normal. Most are anxious about their disease and fairly amenable to adult authority. Psychological tests reveal a tendency towards inhibition and introversion, even though the child's behaviour may be extrovert. Many are very attached to their mothers because of their dependency on daily treatment. Dietary problems preoccupy their thoughts.

At adolescence, all these phenomena are accentuated, and behavioural problems may be seen. Refusal of treatment is frequently the first indication of trouble. The difficulty in psychological treatment arises from the contradiction between the need for close supervision and the need for instilling increasing levels of independence. The high occurrence of 'cheating' should prompt doctors and health visitors to be particularly alert in order to reduce the incidence of episodes of poor metabolic control which in turn increase the risk of degenerative complications.

Metabolic adaptation during physical exercise in the diabetic child

Isolated exercise

MOBILIZATION OF SUBSTRATES

The sequential utilization of energy substrates is governed by the same mechanisms in the diabetic subject correctly dosed with insulin as in the normal adult (Wahren et al., 1978). Although there is no documented information on diabetic children and adolescents, it is believed that anaerobic alactic reactions are the same as those of healthy subjects.

Even though the hepatic production of glucose is quantitatively the same in diabetics and non-diabetics alike, it appears that diabetics have a gluconeogenic capacity three times that of non-diabetics (Sestoft et al., 1977). Among other anomalies, because of a reduced activity of mitochondrial pyruvate dehydrogenase in diabetics (Hagg et al., 1976), a lesser proportion of glucose taken up by the muscle is oxidized (Wahren et al., 1975). The lesser overall oxidative capacity of the diabetic is compensated for by an increased utilization of fatty acids. In diabetics, the uptake of fatty acids by working muscle may reach 33% compared with 27% in healthy subjects (Wahren et al., 1975). The postexercise ketonaemia observed in the normal population is also seen in diabetics, except that the ketone bodies do not constitute an appreciable source of energy during exercise for diabetics.

In conclusion, it can be said that the diabetic subject relies more on lipid metabolism during long-term exercise than the normal subject.

Conversely, the participation of the diabetic in a physical activity programme increases the oxidative capacity of skeletal muscle enzymes, thus increasing the aerobic capacity, as is the case in the normal subject (Saltin et al., 1979).

IMPORTANCE OF INSULIN IN THE PERIPHERAL UPTAKE OF GLUCOSE

Degree of metabolic control

In the diabetic adult during insulin deficiency, and therefore in a poor degree of metabolic control, i.e. hyperglycaemic and ketotic, Berger et al. (1977) observed that exercise accentuates hyperglycaemia and ketosis, leading to extreme fatigue.

In the case of the diabetic adolescent, we were able to demonstrate that the beneficial effect of physical activity on glucose disappearance rate depended on the insulin dose of the subjects. In a series of four clinical studies, we measured the effect of an exercise work rate equal to 50% $\dot{V}_{O_2 \, max}$ on the coefficient of assimilation (K) of intravenously injected glucose as a function of insulin dose. The results presented in Fig. 30.6 show the following findings.

1 In diabetics receiving insulin intravenously in amounts greater than was necessary to saturate the insulin receptors at rest, exercise increased K by 36% (Dorchy et al., 1976).

2 In diabetics injected intramuscularly with their usual dose of insulin, the K value increased by 160% during exercise (Dorchy et al., 1977b).

3 In diabetics injected intramuscularly with their usual dose of insulin, the K value 30 min after exercise was 73% of the exercise K value and 146% of the resting K value of experiment b (Dorchy et al., 1980).

4 In insulin-deprived diabetics, K did not change during exercise (Dorchy et al., 1977a) (Fig. 30.7).

In diabetic children deprived of insulin, K does not increase: the presence of insulin is thus necessary for the beneficial effects of exercise on the assimilation of glucose, playing at least a permissive role (Dorchy et al., 1977a).

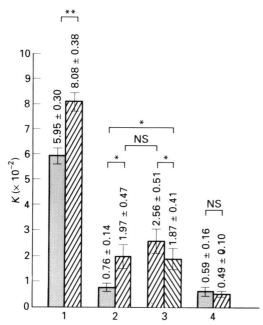

Fig. 30.6 The influence of physical activity equivalent to 50% $\dot{V}o_{2\,max}$ on the coefficient of glucose disappearance rate (K) in diabetic adolescents: 1, receiving $300\,mU \cdot kg^{-1}$ of insulin intravenously (Dorchy *et al.*, 1976); 2, following usual dose intramuscularly, during exercise (Dorchy *et al.*, 1977b); 3, with their usual dose of insulin, 30 min after exercise (Dorchy *et al.*, 1980); 4, insulin-deprived (Dorchy *et al.*, 1977a). $* = P < 0.05$; $** = P < 0.01$; NS, not significant; ▢, rest; ▨, effort; ◩, recovery.

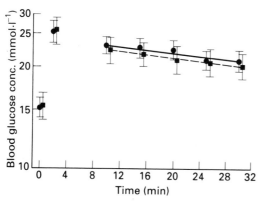

Fig. 30.7 In diabetics deprived of insulin for 24 h, physical activity (■) does not increase the coefficient of glucose disappearance rate K, over rest (●) during a bout of hyperglycaemia by intravenous injection (at time o). K at rest $= 0.59 \times 10^{-2}$; K during effort $= 0.49 \times 10^{-2}$. Adapted from Dorchy *et al.* (1977a).

Insulin deficiency facilitates an enhanced liver glucose output during exercise although it does not permit an uptake of glucose into the working muscles (Zinman *et al.*, 1977). At higher insulin concentrations, other factors than insulin itself were implicated in the increased glucose tolerance during physical activity:

1 Haemodynamic changes (Garratt *et al.*, 1972; Hespel *et al.*, 1995).

2 Activity of humoral factors other than insulin such as insulin-like growth factor-1 (IGF-1) (Couturier *et al.*, 1971).

3 Involvement of kinins and prostaglandins (Dietze, 1982).

4 Modifications of the sensitivity and number of insulin receptors (Soman *et al.*, 1979; Pedersen *et al.*, 1980; Bonen *et al.*, 1985).

5 Activation of skeletal muscle glucose transporters (GLUT 4) (Bonadonna *et al.*, 1993).

6 Glucose arterialized venous blood-deep venous blood difference which seems to be a major determinant of body sensibility to insulin (Ebeling *et al.*, 1995).

The prolongation of muscular avidity for glucose after cessation of muscular effort could result from the exercise-increased affinity and number of available muscle insulin receptors, which favours muscle glycogen repletion. The repletion of hepatic glycogen stores also plays a role. Insulin is also indispensable in this phase of recuperation (Maehlum, 1979). Thus, adequate insulin therapy is required to allow the full benefit of muscular activity on glucose assimilation. It is only under these conditions that metabolic adaptation to exercise in diabetics is of the same order as that seen in non-diabetics. Krentowski *et al.* (1981) have shown that prolonged physical exercise in diabetics under correct insulin therapy follows the same metabolic progression as in normal subjects.

If the insulin dosage is too high, the increase in muscular assimilation combined with the shut-down of liver glucose production may result in a severe hypoglycaemia. Figure 30.8 shows glucose homeostasis during exercise in the cases of insulin lack and excess.

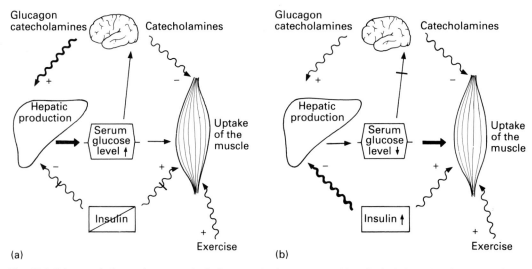

Fig. 30.8 Schema of glucose homeostasis during exercise in presence of insulin lack (a) or insulin excess (b). Straight arrows indicate fuel fluxes; wavy arrows indicate stimulatory and inhibitory effects. Adapted from Kemmer and Berger (1992).

In brief, sport and physical activity can be recommended to child and adolescent diabetics under the express condition that metabolic equilibrium is maintained at all times. Physical activity does not replace insulin. If insulin therapy is optimal, increased glucose disappearance rate during exercise continues after muscle activity has ceased, and could manifest itself in a postexercise hypoglycaemia.

Intrasubject blood glucose responses to prolonged moderate-intensity exercise are reliable and repeatable when pre-exercise, exercise and insulin regimens are kept constant (McNiven Temple *et al.*, 1995).

Recently, Johansson *et al.* (1992) have shown that C-peptide may be of biological importance with regard to glucose uptake by exercising muscles. This finding could be of clinical interest because the equimolar secretion of C-peptide and insulin by the β-cells disappears in most IDDM patients 2 years after the clinical onset of the disease (Dorchy *et al.*, 1982).

Injection site, depth of injection, temperature

Koivisto and Felig (1978) have shown that bicycle pedalling increases the rate of insulin resorption from an injection in the thigh more than from an injection in the arm or abdomen. The conclusion drawn from this was that in order to avoid hypoglycaemia, it is better not to inject the insulin in an active muscle. Kemmer *et al.* (1979) concurred after having shown that hypoglycaemia may occur even when the injection site is not an active muscle group, and advised a large decrease in insulin dose when the peak action of injected insulin occurs during a period of physical exercise. Intramuscular compared with subcutaneous thigh injection of insulin followed by bicycle exercise induces a marked increase in insulin absorption and a substantial fall in plasma glucose (Frid *et al.*, 1990). Warm ambient temperatures (30°C) are associated with three- to fivefold higher insulin absorption and significantly lower blood glucose concentration than cool temperature (10°C) regardless of exercise (Rönnemaa & Koivisto, 1988; Rönnemaa *et al.*, 1991).

Glucose transporters

Over the past 10 years, several laboratories have shown that glucose transport by facilitated diffusion is mediated by a family of tissue-specific membrane glycoproteins (Mueckler, 1990). The adipocyte–muscle transporter (GLUT 4) is expressed exclusively in tissues that are insulin sensitive with respect to glucose uptake. It is believed that the insulin-stimulated glucose disposal mainly takes place through activation of GLUT 4 (Bonadonna *et al.*, 1993), whereas somatostatin-induced acute hypo-insulinaemia does not seem to affect trans-membrane transport or uptake of glucose. However, recently, Handberg *et al.* (1992) showed that the total content of skeletal muscle GLUT 4 is a poor predictor for *in vivo* response to near physiological insulin concentrations in healthy human subjects. Additionally, in type I diabetics, GLUT 4 levels are unaltered in skeletal muscle and do not correlate with important physiological factors. So, in human diabetes, there is tissue-specific regulation of glucose transporters and changes in transporter expression do not explain *in vivo* insulin-resistant glucose uptake (Kahn, 1992). There are no data on GLUT 4 in diabetic children and adolescents.

COUNTERREGULATORY HORMONES

Wasserman *et al.* (1992) observed in dogs that marked insulinopaenia contributes directly, i.e. independently of metabolic and hormonal environment, to the exacerbation of gluco-regulation during exercise in the diabetic state by both limiting the rises in glucose uptake and metabolism, and by enhancing hepatic glucose production. Moreover, in diabetics under conditions of hypoinsulinism, physical activity stimulates an abnormal increase in glucagon, cortisol, growth hormone and catecholamines (Berger *et al.*, 1977; Kemmer & Berger 1983), which aggravates the hyper-glycaemia, lipolysis and ketosis. Kemmer and Berger (1983) have proposed that intense physical exercise should not be engaged in when glycaemia is greater than $300 \, mg \cdot dl^{-1}$ and as long as marked acetonuria is detectable. Conversely, in the case of well-controlled diabetes, the counterregulatory hormones behave

in the same manner during exercise in diabetics as in control subjects.

Under adequate insulin therapy, the risk of hypoglycaemia during physical activity is due to the absence of a decrease in circulating insulin, which occurs in the non-diabetic. Moreover, hyperinsulinaemia may result from insulin liberated from subcutaneous stores. Blockage of glucose production eventually leads to hypoglycaemia. There is a greater risk of severe hypoglycaemia in patients with a poor glucagon and adrenaline response to lowered blood glucose (Kleinbaum & Shamoon, 1983). Furthermore, the lack of adrenaline response hinders these diabetics in anticipating hypoglycaemic episodes; so much so that it becomes aggravated before the subject even thinks of taking sugar (Heller *et al.*, 1987). Bolli *et al.* (1984) proposed a test to single out those patients at risk of hypoglycaemia by inadequate response of counterregulatory hormones.

EFFECTS ON RENAL FUNCTION

Intense physical activity considerably alters various aspects of renal function including reducing GFR and renal blood flow, and increasing reabsorption of water and electrolytes (Poortmans, 1984, 1990). The postexercise proteinuria which becomes evident within 30 min after activity is a function more of the intensity of the exercise than of its duration (Poortmans & Labilloy, 1988), and usually disappears within hours of the exercise (Poortmans *et al.*, 1983). Kidney function during exercise in healthy and diabetic subjects has been recently reviewed (Poortmans & Vanderstraeten, 1994).

It is well established that renal function is disturbed in the young diabetic which is characterized by increased GFR, increased glomerular permeability to plasma proteins, and thickening of the basal membrane of the glomerulus. Mogensen and Vittinghus (1975) introduced a technique to discriminate abnormal glomerular function in diabetics. A light workload (100 W) on a cycle ergometer is sufficient to elicit marked albuminuria in diabetic subjects, whereas the healthy subject shows no significant variation in urinary albumin excretion for this same exercise intensity. This seems to be the case for moderate submaximal exercise, but not for maximal exercise. We have shown that exercise to exhaustion induces, in the adolescent diabetic, albuminuria that is not different from that found in healthy subjects under the same conditions (Poortmans *et al.*, 1976, 1982) (Fig. 30.9). We have concluded that an exercise test leading to exhaustion does not give any additional information other than the basal excretion of proteins. The cause of this postexercise proteinuria is an increase in glomerular permeability and saturation of the tubular reabsorption of filtered protein (Poortmans *et al.*, 1988a). The transitory nature of these disturbances leads to the conclusion that exercise, even intense exercise, does not permanently compromise the function of the kidney. However, Johansson *et al.* (1987) suggested that the sympathoadrenergic effects on heart rate, renal haemodynamics and renal water homeostasis during exercise are blunted in diabetic children and adolescents. Also, Chase *et al.* (1992) reported that early renal damage is related to further elevations in resting and exercise blood pressure in diabetic adolescents.

Physical training

INCREASED INSULIN SENSITIVITY

Physical activity increases insulin sensitivity. Those who have experienced sports camps of several weeks duration for young diabetics have found that insulin requirement decreases during, and for 2 or 3 days following, physical activity. It has been shown in humans, using the hyperinsulinaemic euglycaemic clamp, that glucose utilization under insulin stimulation is still increased 24 h after a single prolonged burst of exercise only in previously active muscles (Annuzzi *et al.*, 1991). Burstein *et al.* (1985) showed that only 60 h after cessation of physical training did the affinity and number of erythrocytic insulin receptors return to the level of untrained, control subjects. Unfortunately, there is no study on the effect of endurance training on the muscle insulin receptors of adolescent diabetics. It has been proposed that increased insulin sensitivity in peripheral receptors after training could be due to the increased activity of certain mitochondrial enzymes (Wallberg-Henriksson *et al.*, 1982). Moreover, insulin sensitivity is directly associated with muscle mass, and inversely related to adipose tissue mass (Yki-Jarvinen & Koivisto, 1983). Costill *et al.* (1979) studied

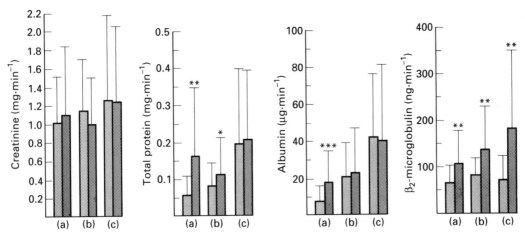

Fig. 30.9 Urinary output of creatinine, total protein, albumin and β₂-microglobulin in 21 young diabetic subjects (■) and 21 control subjects (□): (a) at rest; (b) during maximal exercise; and (c) during recovery. * = $P < 0.05$; ** = $P < 0.01$; *** = $P < 0.001$. Adapted from Poortmans *et al.* (1982).

training adaptations in the skeletal muscle of juvenile diabetics. They reported that muscle tissue of young diabetics who are in moderate insulin balance adapt to endurance training in a similar way to that of non-diabetic men, showing an increase in skeletal muscle enzymes such as lipoprotein lipase, carnitine palmityl-transferase, succinate dehydrogenase and hexokinase. Additionally, the diabetics showed a 41% greater improvement in the measurement of muscle lipid oxidation after training than did the non-diabetic group.

In exercise-trained rats, it has been reported that exercise training increases GLUT 4 proteins in rat skeletal muscle homogenates (Ploug et al., 1990; Goodyear et al., 1992). This increase in GLUT 4 may be the primary factor in explaining the phenomena of increased basal and insulin-stimulated glucose uptake in the skeletal muscle of exercise-trained animals. No such studies exist in diabetic patients.

RELATIONSHIP TO DEGREE OF CONTROL

The favourable role of regular physical training in metabolic control, measured by glycosylated haemoglobin, is still controversial in the paediatric literature. Thus, while Dahl-Jorgensen et al. (1980), Campaigne et al. (1984) and Huttunen et al. (1989) have demonstrated decreases of glycosylated haemoglobin after an exercise programme of several weeks, other authors have noted no change (Baevre et al., 1985; Landt et al., 1985; Rowland et al., 1985; Stratton et al., 1987). Arslanian et al. (1990) have demonstrated that insulin-mediated glucose disposal was positively related to the state of physical fitness as assessed by $\dot{V}o_{2\,max}$ and negatively related to HbA$_1$. It is nonetheless important to note that the physical work capacity of trained diabetics is clearly increased (Campaigne et al., 1984; Baevre et al., 1985; Landt et al., 1985; Stratton et al., 1987).

MODIFICATIONS IN LIPID PROFILE

It is well known that hyperlipidaemia is an important risk factor for cardiovascular disease

which can begin in childhood (Inkeles & Eisenberg, 1981), and is often associated with diabetes (Goldberg, 1981). Anomalies of lipid metabolism seem partially linked to metabolic control of diabetic children and adolescents (Richard et al., 1983; Jos et al., 1985; Strobl et al., 1985; Willems & Dorchy, 1990). Regular physical activity can improve the lipid profile in diabetic adults, notably by the elevation of the high-density lipoprotein (HDL) cholesterol fraction (Moore et al., 1983; Wallberg-Henriksson et al., 1983; Cook et al., 1986). A single episode of high volume resistance exercise is also capable of modifying plasma lipid lipoprotein concentration in a direction (increased HDL-cholesterol, HDL-c) and magnitude comparable to an acute bout of endurance exercise (Wallace et al., 1991). Conversely, other authors have noted no favourable effect of physical training on plasma lipoprotein profile. The discrepancies may be a function of the intensity of the exercise performed (Hughes et al., 1990). In diabetic adolescents, Austin et al. (1993) have demonstrated that the state of physical fitness is an important correlate of lipid levels: the higher the physical fitness level, the lower the plasma total cholesterol LDL-c and Lp(a). This could be an important aspect of physical fitness in alleviating the risk of cardiovascular disease. $\dot{V}o_{2\,max}$ did not correlate with HDL or very low-density lipoprotein (VLDL).

EFFECT ON KIDNEY FUNCTION

Physical training induces a reduction in post-exercise proteinuria in adult and adolescent diabetics, relative to sedentary control subjects, as long as the activity remains submaximal (Poortmans, 1984). When the exercise is of maximal intensity, there are no differences in renal response between trained and untrained subjects (Poortmans, 1984). We have examined the effects of regular physical training (6 h · day^{-1} for 2 weeks) on a mixed group of diabetic boys and girls, aged between 11 and 18 years (Poortmans et al., 1988b). A physical capacity test was undertaken before and after training. The results clearly demonstrate a 50% reduction in the postexercise urinary excretion of albumin and of β_2-microglobulin following training (Table 30.1). Thus, it seems that regular physical training has a beneficial effect on the renal transfer of plasma proteins.

TREATMENT OF OBESITY

Exercise induces negative energy balance either directly or by enhancing meal thermogenesis, increasing resting metabolic rate, and/or decreasing food intake. However, energy cost of exercise *per se* is minimal, and thermic effect of food is negligible. Exercise training may be advantageous in conjunction with a low calorie diet because it helps to maintain resting metabolic rate and fat-free mass (Calles-Escandon & Horton, 1992). Moreover, as obesity is associated with an insulin resistance and as physical training has a beneficial effect on insulin sensitivity, physical training programmes have to be recommended. The prescription of a low calorie diet is facilitated by the use of basal-bolus insulin therapy.

There are two situations in the diabetic when obesity may be the result of management: (i) the overcontrolled patient who is forced to consume extra calories often as a result of too much insulin (Somogyi's syndrome); and (ii) the patient who attempts to normalize blood glucose by insulin administration alone.

Physical work capacity

CONFLICTING STUDIES

Interest in the effects of muscular exercise in diabetic children dates from the first work of Larsson *et al.* (1962), who studied physical work capacity and the influence of training in diabetic adolescents. Following this initial study, conflicting papers have been published. Sterky (1963) and Jakober *et al.* (1983) confirmed the work of Larsson in demonstrating that the physical work capacity of young diabetics is inferior to that of a healthy control population. Conversely, Rutenfranz *et al.* (1968) was only

able to show this in the adolescent group, whereas the younger children were able to perform normally. Elo *et al.* (1965), Hebbelinck *et al.* (1974) and Hagan *et al.* (1979) found that the work capacity of diabetic adolescents did not differ from their healthy counterparts.

Most of these studies are based on the physical work capacity (PWC_{170}, heart rate of 170 beats·min^{-1}) test, on a cycle ergometer, as an indirect measurement of aerobic work capacity. The little information which exists on the maximal oxygen consumption of young diabetics is not consistent. According to the work of Larsson *et al.* (1964) and Persson and Thoren (1980), the $\dot{V}O_{2\ max}$ in diabetic boys is reduced, but within healthy limits, as measured by Hagan *et al.* (1979).

We have studied, in a preliminary project, the PWC and oxygen consumption of a group of 33 IDDM young patients aged from 10 to 17 years (Baran & Dorchy, 1982). The relative mechanical power, maximal oxygen consumption and maximal ventilation were less than those of a normal age-matched reference population.

DEGREE OF METABOLIC CONTROL

The conflicting results in the literature are possibly due to:
1 The arbitrary choice of the reference population whose anthropometric characteristics are not paired with the diabetic group.
2 The degree of metabolic control which was not objectively evaluated.

We have carried out a study (Poortmans *et al.*, 1986), the aims of which were:
1 To investigate the PWC of normal and diabetic adolescents matched by anthropomorphic data.
2 To determine if there is a relationship between PWC and the degree of metabolic control as evaluated by glycosylated haemoglobin.

The study included 17 diabetic adolescents and 17 normal subjects matched for age (16.2 ± 0.7 versus 16.6 ± 1.0 years), weight (57.6 ± 2.9 versus 56.8 ± 3.1 kg), height (165.2 ± 3.2 versus 165.7 ± 3.1 cm) and habitual physical activity.

Table 30.1 Urinary protein excretion before and after training in 21 young diabetic subjects (±SEM). Adapted from Poortmans et al. (1988b).

Urinary output	Before training			After training		
	Rest	Postexercise 15*	Postexercise 45†	Rest	Postexercise 15*	Postexercise 45†
Creatinine (mg·min^{-1})	0.79 ± 0.08	0.84 ± 0.07	0.79 ± 0.08	0.91 ± 0.10	1.62 ± 0.15‡§	1.54 ± 0.15‡§
Total protein (µg·min^{-1})	63 ± 9	221 ± 49‡	190 ± 43‡	74 ± 17	300 ± 57‡	162 ± 35‡
Albumin (µg·min^{-1})	26.8 ± 3.4	58 ± 13.1‡	20.5 ± 4.2	16.5 ± 4.7	24.3 ± 10.2§	20.5 ± 5.8
β$_2$-microglobulin (ng·min^{-1})	100 ± 19	1300 ± 475‡	203 ± 55	84 ± 13.4	462 ± 90‡§	224 ± 55

* Postexercise 15th minute.
† Postexercise 45th minute.
‡ $P < 0.05$ between rest and postexercise for the same session.
§ $P < 0.05$ between post- and pretraining sessions.

The length of time since diagnosis of diabetes was 7.8 ± 1.4 years, and the total glycosylated haemoglobin (HbA$_1$) was $9.2 \pm 0.7\%$. All subjects were tested on a cycle ergometer using a progressive protocol wherein the power was increased by 30 W every 3 min until exhaustion. Respiratory measures were taken using the open circuit technique.

The results of the primary cardiorespiratory measures for all subjects are presented in Table 30.2. The diabetic group was further subdivided according to the level of HbA$_1$, where good metabolic control corresponds to a level of HbA$_1$ less than 8.5%, and insufficient control is taken as HbA$_1$ greater than 8.5%. At rest, there was no significant difference between the three groups for heart rate, oxygen uptake and respiratory quotient. Meanwhile, the control group had a slightly higher pulmonary ventilation. During physical activity, the maximal workload supported by the control group was significantly higher than that of the two diabetic groups. There was a negative correlation between the maximal workload and the level of HbA$_1$ ($r = -0.63$; $P < 0.01$). The heart rate of the insufficiently controlled diabetics was less than that of the control group. Furthermore, $\dot{V}_{O_2 \, max}$ was significantly higher with healthy children than in the two diabetic groups.

In summary, for diabetic adolescents the maximal power developed during the exercise and the maximal oxygen consumption are decreased. The PWC increases as metabolic control of the diabetes improves. This is in accord with the work of Ludvigsson (1980), who observed a relationship between PWC and the degree of control estimated by indirect clinical criteria. If the diabetic is to reach the same level of physical performance as the non-diabetic, he or she must have an optimal degree of control.

In neuropathy of the autonomic nervous system, PWC of the diabetic is decreased (Hilsted et al., 1982; Kahn et al., 1986).

Recommendations

For detailed discussion, the reader is referred to Bar-Or (1983), Czernichow and Dorchy (1989), Dorchy and Poortmans (1989, 1991), Gillet and François (1984), Horton (1988, 1991), Jandrain et al. (1988), Kemmer and Berger (1983, 1992), Koivisto (1991), Larsson (1984), Vignati and Cunningham (1985) and Zinman (1990).

Table 30.2 Cardiorespiratory parameters measured at rest and during exhaustive exercise ($\pm$ SEM) in 17 control subjects and 17 adolescent diabetic patients subdivided into two groups according to total glycosylated haemoglobin level (HbA$_1$). Adapted from Poortmans et al. (1986).

Parameter	Phase	Control	Diabetic HbA$_1 < 8.5\%$ ($n = 9$)	Diabetic HbA$_1 > 8.5\%$ ($n = 8$)
Maximal power (W·kg^{-1})	Exercise	3.20 ± 0.08	2.80 ± 0.05†	2.56 ± 0.12‡
Heart rate (beats·min^{-1})	Rest	88 ± 3	95 ± 3	86 ± 5
	Exercise	192 ± 2	188 ± 3	$184 \pm 5^*$
Pulmonary ventilation (l·min^{-1})	Rest	12.8 ± 0.7	11.1 ± 0.7	9.7 ± 0.7†
	Exercise	78.3 ± 4.4	71.8 ± 4.7	64.1 ± 4.5
Oxygen consumption (ml·kg^{-1}·min^{-1})	Rest	6.3 ± 0.1	5.4 ± 0.3	5.4 ± 0.2
	Exercise	46.8 ± 2.7	40.6 ± 1.8†	38.8 ± 1.0‡
Respiratory quotient	Rest	0.85 ± 0.03	0.90 ± 0.03	0.92 ± 0.04
	Exercise	1.03 ± 0.01	1.07 ± 0.02	1.09 ± 0.03

Significance versus control: $^*P < 0.05$; †$P \pm 0.01$; ‡$P \pm 0.001$ (Wilcoxon test).

Roles of glucose and insulin

NON-DIABETIC

Figures 30.10–30.12 show the roles of muscle and liver glycogen and insulin during and after exercise in healthy subjects. At rest, the muscles and liver contain much glycogen — little glucose is utilized (Fig. 30.10). A means by which the reserves of glycogen can be increased is to consume complex carbohydrates (whole bread, rice, pasta, etc.) a few hours before intense physical activity (Nelson, 1982). During the exercise, muscle glycogen serves as a source

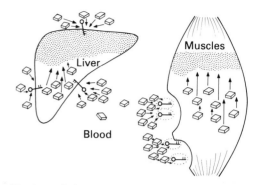

Fig. 30.12 In healthy subjects after exercise the liver and muscles assimilate blood glucose in order to replenish the glycogen reserves. This process continues for hours after termination of physical activity. Symbols as in Fig. 30.10.

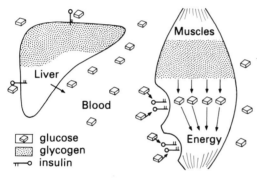

glucose
glycogen
insulin

Fig. 30.10 In healthy subjects at rest the muscles and liver contain a lot of glycogen; little glucose is consumed.

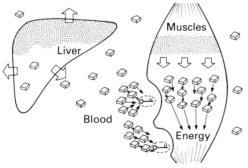

Fig. 30.11 In healthy subjects during exercise all of the muscle glycogen is broken down to glucose. In the liver, the glycogen is also converted to glucose, liberated into the blood, and circulated to the muscle. The muscles consume large amounts of glucose. Insulin is required for the transport of glucose into muscles even if the blood insulin levels is decreasing. Symbols as in Fig. 30.10.

of energy during the first few minutes, then liver glycogen is broken down to glucose and liberated into the blood, where it eventually arrives at the level of the muscle (Fig. 30.11). The circulating insulin level decreases, which allows the liver to liberate sufficient amounts of glucose necessary for muscle contraction; but the binding of insulin to the muscle membrane receptors is increased which in turn favours the uptake of glucose into the muscle during exercise. It is necessary to consume carbohydrate-rich foods or drink liquids high in glucose during prolonged activity. During the hours following exercise the body replenishes the glycogen stores from blood glucose, first in the muscles, and then in the liver (Fig. 30.12). Thus the ingestion of carbohydrates is important after exercise.

YOUNG DIABETIC

It must be pointed out that in the young diabetic, unlike the non-diabetic whose blood insulin levels drop physiologically during exercise, the effects of the exercise can be beneficial or harmful depending on the quantity of exogenous insulin received:
1 In the case of insulin overdose, or accelerated release of injected insulin near the active muscle, the hyperinsulinism blocks glucose

production by the liver and fatty acid release from adipose tissue, while at the same time increasing glucose uptake by the muscle. The consequence of this is a hypoglycaemic episode during the activity as well as during the recovery period. Severe hypoglycaemia can occur several hours after the physical activity is terminated (MacDonald, 1987; Annuzzi et al., 1991).

2 In the case of insulin underdose, the glycaemia will also increase because of stimulation of hepatic glucose production and decreased utilization at the periphery. The liberation of lipolytic hormones increases ketogenesis. The young diabetic should also be aware that physical performance is a function of the degree of metabolic control (Poortmans et al. 1986).

During physical activity

If a diabetic child or adolescent is well controlled metabolically, he or she can perform the same physical activity as a young non-diabetic. There are, however, certain precautions if a hyperglycaemic episode is to be avoided, particularly concerning nutrition and insulin injections (Table 30.3). Recommendations for management must be tailored individually.

NUTRITION

As in the case of the non-diabetic, it is useful to increase the glycogen stores by consuming complex carbohydrates during the 3 h preceding physical activity, without eating too heavily just before the activity. In the case of prolonged activity, the diabetic should drink glucose-sweetened water (4–8%), or eat fruit pastes or chocolate for example, just before or during the exercise. Glucose supplements should be taken at the end of the exercise, even a few hours later. Regular sodas are less suitable because they contain about 12% or more carbohydrate which can lead to stomach cramping, nausea, diarrhoea, bloating and discomfort.

For each hour of moderate exercise, such as swimming, tennis, jogging or cycling, 20–40 g

Table 30.3 Recommendations for physical activity in young diabetics.

Arrive at a good level of metabolic control: neither hyperglycaemia (> 300 mg · dl^{-1}), nor ketonuria. Eventually measure blood glucose concentration before the activity

Always carry some sugar

Increase the intensity and duration of the activity in a progressive fashion

In the few hours preceding the exercise, ingest slowly absorbing carbohydrates in order to replete the liver and muscle glycogen reserves

In the case of unforeseen physical activity, increase glucose consumption immediately before, during and after the activity

In the case of foreseen activity, decrease the insulin dose during and after intense muscular activity. This decrease can vary from 10 to 50% depending on the intensity of the exercise

Do not inject the insulin at a site that will be heavily involved in the muscular activity

Avoid physical exercise at the time of the peak action of insulin

If the activity is of the prolonged endurance type, be certain to ingest glucose-sweetened water or carbohydrates just before, during (every 35 to 40 min) and after the exercise

Measure the blood glucose before retiring on the evening after major physical activity, in order to avoid hypoglycaemia during the night

Evaluate the effect after every modification in insulin dose and every change in nutritional status

Make the people accompanying you aware of the procedures and treatment of severe hypoglycaemia (glucagon injection)

of carbohydrate can be planned as a snack before exercise, or during prolonged exercise, every hour. For very intensive or competitive activities, diabetic athletes may need 20–40 g of carbohydrate every 30 min. Of course, the need for carbohydrate also depends on the size of the child.

It would be unusual for diabetic athletes to have a vitamin or mineral deficiency. Proper hydration during physical exercise follows the same recommendations as those for non-diabetic individuals. Nutritional adaptations are the only possible measures in the case of unforeseen activity.

INSULIN

Insulin must be injected away from the working muscle groups used during the activity (Koivisto & Felig, 1978) (e.g. a cyclist would not use the thigh; a skier would choose the abdomen). Each injection site should be tested individually because the resorption of insulin varies from one site to another (e.g. it is faster from the abdomen than from the arms, thigh or buttock).

Adaptation of insulin dose is equally strictly individual, and will become optimum when modified based on previous experience. Obviously, the decrease in insulin dose will not only depend on the intensity and duration of the anticipated activity, but also on the level of training and nutritional status. It can vary from 10% (non-competitive swimming) to 50% (intense skiing) of the previous normal dose.

The choice of insulin modification depends on the insulin regimen and on the timing of the activity. In the case of insulin therapy consisting of two daily injections of a mixture of rapid-acting (type 1) and intermediate-acting (type 2) insulin, the young diabetic should reduce type 1 insulin of the first injection if the activity is held in the morning, type 2 insulin of the first injection if the activity is held in the afternoon, and type 1 insulin, sometimes type 2, of the second injection when the sport is to be held in the evening. Certain computers (the insulin dosage computer by Becton-Dickinson, New Jersey, USA) use programmed algorithms to calculate dosages when certain activities, rated on an intensity scale, are anticipated.

In the case of basal-prandial insulin therapy by pen injector, one should reduce (10–50%) rapid-acting insulin injected before the meal preceding exercise. However, it is sometimes necessary to reduce basal insulin for exercise expected to be of several hours duration. For patients using an insulin pump, during intense exercise in the postprandial period, the insulin delivery should be adjusted to the basal level (Koivisto & Tronier, 1983). If the exercise is very prolonged, the basal delivery should be reduced by 30–50%, and even stopped when exercising hard, which is also valuable with the basal-prandial system with the pen injector. In this case, in order to avoid the risk of late-onset hypoglycaemia, reduction of the basal insulin by 25% for several hours after the exercise period appears to be an appropriate measure (Sonnenberg et al., 1990).

Selection of sports

In principle, if the insulin dose is correctly adjusted, the injection site correctly chosen and all the nutritional precautions are accounted for, there is no limit to the choice of sporting activities for the young diabetic. The effect of the exercise is all the more favourable if the activity is carried out on a regular basis, perhaps several times per week.

It is encouraging for young diabetics to note the championship performances of many diabetic athletes including William Tabert, Hamilton Richardson and Lennart Bergelin (tennis during the 1950s), Roger Mills and David Catterrall (badminton during the 1970s), Gary Mabbutt (soccer during the early 1980s) and Dominique Garde (Tour de France cyclist, 1987). In Belgium in 1993, the best soccer player was Pär Zetterberg who is diabetic and uses the basal-prandial insulin therapy with a pen injector; his glycosylated haemoglobin is always within the normal range (Fig. 30.13).

The sports that are the most difficult for the diabetic to adapt to are those that require short explosive bursts of muscular activity. When the physical effort is progressive and spread out over several hours (bicycle touring, walking, cross-country skiing, etc.), the diabetic can easily adjust the glucose equilibrium.

The only prohibited activities are those which constitute a danger to the diabetic by provoking an eventual hypoglycaemic episode, and those which are also dangerous for the non-diabetic (e.g. sky diving, mountaineering, scuba diving, motorcycle racing, hang-gliding or windsurfing). It is preferable for diabetics not to practice any sport alone.

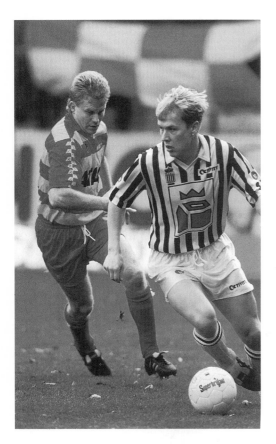

Fig. 30.13 Pär Zetterberg (*right*), who became diabetic during adolescence, was in 1993 the best footballer in Belgium. He uses the basal-prandial insulin therapy with a pen-injector. Courtesy of Bernard Delentrée (*La Nouvelle Gazette*).

In the case of diabetics who demonstrate vascular (atherosclerosis), cardiac (cardiomyopathy) or nervous (autonomic neuropathy) problems, the opportunity for sporting activities is limited; however, this is often not a paediatric problem (Hilsted *et al.*, 1982; Kahn *et al.*, 1986). However, according to Friedman *et al.* (1982), minor myocardial dysfunction is not rare, even in children. Certainly, in the case of proliferative retinopathy — which can occur any time after the age of 20 years — physical activity should be avoided because any increase in blood pressure or physical shock could cause retinal or vitreal haemorrhage. However, past and current physical activity is not associated with the prevalence of proliferative retinopathy (Cruickshanks *et al.*, 1992). Hypertension may present in diabetic adolescents and must be treated adequately, for example by angiotensin-converting enzyme inhibitors which also reduce microalbuminuria (Cook *et al.*, 1990).

Conclusion

The triad of insulin, diet and exercise has been the basis for treatment of diabetes for several decades. However, the choice of sporting activities for the young diabetic requires an understanding of the adaptation to physical activity in the healthy child and the changes caused by diabetes. Adequate insulin therapy is required to allow the full benefit of muscular activity on glucose assimilation for the child to reach the same level of physical performance as the non-diabetic. In the case of insufficient metabolic control, exercise can provoke severe hypoglycaemic episodes or produce hyperglycaemia and lead to ketoacidosis. If a diabetic child or adolescent follows individual recommendations concerning diet and insulin, he or she can engage in the same physical activity as a young non-diabetic. The choice of nutritional and insulin modifications depends on many factors such as glucose levels (usefulness of SMBG), insulin regimen and injection site, timing and intensity of the activity, training, amount and type of carbohydrates in the diet, and so on. This will require paediatric diabetologists to educate young diabetics on these principles of insulin and exercise management. The only prohibited sports are those which constitute a danger to the diabetic by provoking an eventual hypoglycaemia. The best sports are those that require progressive physical effort and are spread out over several hours.

Challenges for future research

The reader is referred to Alberti *et al.* (1992) and to Czernichow and Dorchy (1989).

• Monomeric insulin analogues. Recombinant

gene technology will lead to insulin preparations with improved pharmacokinetic properties that will enable better metabolic control, namely by a faster absorption after subcutaneous injection mimicking the meal-related insulin profile seen in non-diabetic individuals. Insulin analogues could restore a more physiologically normal insulin level and simplify adjustments of treatment for physical exercise (Tuominen *et al.*, 1995).

• Nasal or oral insulin. A nasal insulin spray allows more rapid blood levels of insulin which is useful for diabetic athletes. However, many clinical questions remain, such as the reproducibility of action and toxicity for the nasal mucosa. Protection of insulin from digestive substances is not yet totally solved.

• Blood glucose measurement without pricking. Prototypes of meters exist that measure blood glucose by directing a beam of infrared light through the skin. A miniature computer calculates blood glucose levels based on how much light is absorbed. Tests are presently being performed to determine the meter's accuracy. With such a painless device, the diabetic sportsperson will be able to measure his or her glycaemia many times daily, which will facilitate insulin-dose alteration and prevention of hypoglycaemic manifestations.

• Islet transplantation. Transplantation of pancreatic islets may represent an attractive alternative to exogenous insulin administration. Cells from donated pancreas are injected, for example, into the portal vein in the abdomen, and lodge in the liver where they produce insulin. However, provided that sufficient mass of viable β-cells are injected, islet graft rejection would anyhow interdict success of this treatment, even if immunosuppressive — and toxic — agents are used.

Researchers are now seeking ways to achieve islet transplantation without the need for continuous immune suppression. One approach is to envelop islets within selective permeable and biocompatible microcapsules or within hollow fibres, so that insulin escapes to the body and islets are protected from the immune attack. Unfortunately, until now, a wall of fibrous tissue surrounds the capsule and obstructs the insulin. Transplantation of microencapsulated islets with a new formula will be tested in humans in the near future.

Other techniques such as immunoalteration, for example by oxygen and ultraviolet treatment, are being studied. These methods would allow transplantation of islets without immunosuppressive drugs, so that the organism does not consider the new cells as foreign bodies.

The ultimate goal of islet transplantation, without immunosuppression, is to use animal islets in order to resolve the problem of availability of islet tissue for transplantation. This will be the best and permanent solution for the diabetic athlete in the future.

Acknowledgements

Several parts of this chapter have been adapted and updated from our previous review on 'Sport and the diabetic child', published in 1989 in *Sports Medicine* 7, 248–62, with permission of the editor.

References

Alberti, K.G.M.M., DeFronzo, R.A., Keen, H. & Zimmet, P. (1992) *International Textbook of Diabetes Mellitus*. Wiley, Chichester.

Annuzzi, G., Riccardi, G., Capaldo, B. & Kaijser, L. (1991) Increased insulin-stimulated glucose uptake by exercised human muscles one day after prolonged physical exercise. *Eur. J. Clin. Invest.* **21**, 6–12.

Arslanian, S., Nixon, P.A., Becker, D. & Drash, A.L. (1990) Impact of physical fitness and glycemic control on *in vivo* insulin action in adolescents with IDDM. *Diabetes Care* **13**, 9–15.

Austin, A., Warty, V., Janosky, J. & Arslanian, S. (1993) The relationship of physical fitness to lipid and lipoprotein (a) levels in adolescents with IDDM. *Diabetes Care* **16**, 421–5.

Baevre, H., Sovik, O., Wisness, A. & Heirvang, E. (1985) Metabolic responses to physical training in young insulin-dependent diabetics. *Scand. J. Clin. Lab. Invest.* **45**, 109–14.

Bar-Or, O. (1983) *Pediatric Sports Medicine for the Practitioner: From Physiologic Principles to Clinical Application*. Springer-Verlag, New York.

Baran, D. & Dorchy, H. (1982) Aptitude physique de l'adolescent diabétique. *Bull. Eur. Phys. Respir.* **18**, 51–8.

Berger, M., Berchtold, P., Cuppers, H.J., Drost, H., Kley, H.K. & Muller, W.A. (1977) Metabolic and hormonal effects of muscular exercise in juvenile type diabetics. *Diabetologia* **13**, 355–65.

Bolli, G.B., De Feo, P., De Cosmo, S., Perriello, G. & Ventura, M.M. (1984) A reliable and reproducible test for adequate glucose counterregulation in type I diabetes mellitus. *Diabetes* **33**, 732–7.

Bonadonna, R.C., Saccomani, M.P., Seely, L. *et al.* (1993) Glucose transport in human skeletal muscle. The *in vivo* response to insulin. *Diabetes* **42**, 191–8.

Bonen, A., Tan, M.H., Clune, P. & Kirby, R.L. (1985) Effects of exercise on insulin binding to human muscle. *Am. J. Physiol.* **248**, 403–8.

Bougnères, P.F., Jos, J. & Chaussain, J.L. (1990) *Le Diabète de l'Enfant*. Flammarion, Paris.

Burstein, R., Polychronakos, C., Toews, C.J., MacDougall, J.D. & Ventura, M.M. (1985) Acute reversal of the enhanced insulin action in trained athletes: association with insulin receptor changes. *Diabetes* **34**, 756–60.

Calles-Escandon, J. & Horton, E.S. (1992) The thermogenic role of exercise in the treatment of morbid obesity: a critical evaluation. *Am. J. Clin. Nutr.* **55**, 533S–37.

Campaigne, B.N., Gilliam, T.B., Spencer, M.L., Lampman, R.M. & Schork, M.A. (1984) Effects of a physical activity program on metabolic control and cardiovascular fitness in children with insulin-dependent diabetes mellitus. *Diabetes Care* **7**, 57–62.

Chase, H.P., Garg, S.K., Harris, S., Marshall, G. & Hoops, S. (1992) Elevation of resting and exercise blood pressures in subjects with type I diabetes and relation to albuminuria. *J. Diabetes Comp.* **6**, 138–42.

Cook, J., Daneman, D., Spino, M., Sockett, E., Perlman, K. & Balfe, J.W. (1990) Angiotensin converting enzyme inhibitor therapy to decrease microalbuminuria in normotensive children with insulin-dependent diabetes. *J. Pediatr.* **117**, 39–45.

Cook, T.C., Laporte, R.E., Washburn, R.A., Traven, N.D. & Slemenda, C.W. (1986) Chronic low level physical activity as a determinant of high density lipoprotein cholesterol and subfractions. *Med. Sci. Sports Exerc.* **18**, 653–65.

Costill, D.L., Cleary, P., Fink, W.J., Foster, C., Ivy, J.L. & Witzman, F. (1979) Training adaptations in skeletal muscle of juvenile diabetics. *Diabetes* **28**, 818–22.

Couturier, E., Rasio, E. & Connard, V. (1971) Insulin in plasma and lymph and glucose tissue uptake in the exercising hind limb of the dog. *Horm. Metab. Res.* **3**, 382–6.

Cruickshanks, K., Moss, S.E., Klein, R. & Klein, B.E.K. (1992) Physical activity and proliferative retinopathy in people diagnosed with diabetes before age 30 years. *Diabetes Care* **15**, 1267–72.

Czernichow, P. & Dorchy, H. (1989) *Diabétologie Pédiatrique*. Doin, Paris.

Dahl-Jorgensen, K., Meen, H.D., Hanssen, K.F. & Aagenaes, O. (1980) The effect of exercise on diabetic control and hemoglobin A₁ (HbA₁) in children. *Acta Paediatr. Scand.* **283** (Suppl.), 53–6.

Dietze, G. (1982) Modulation of the action of insulin in relation to the energy state in skeletal muscle tissue: possible involvement of kinins and prostaglandins. *Mol. Cell. Endocrinol.* **25**, 127–49.

Dorchy, H. (1988) Le stylo-injecteur d'insuline chez le jeune diabétique. Liberté et prise pondérale excessive. *Pédiatrie* **43**, 697–702.

Dorchy, H. (1994) Quel contrôle glycémique peut être obtenu chez des jeunes diabétiques sans sécrétion résiduelle d'insuline endogène? Quelle est la fréquence des hypoglycémies sévères et des complications subcliniques? *Arch. Pediatr.* **1**, 970–81.

Dorchy, H., Despontin, M., Haumont, D. & Loeb, H. (1982) Sécrétion résiduelle d'insuline chez les jeunes diabétiques. Relations avec la durée du diabète, le contrôle métabolique et la rétinopathie. *Arch. Franç. Pédiatr.* **29**, 145–48.

Dorchy, H., Ego, F., Baran, D. & Loeb, H. (1976) Effect of exercise on glucose uptake in diabetic adolescents. *Acta Paediatr. Belg.* **29**, 83–5.

Dorchy, H. & Ernould, Chr. (1990) Les colonies de vacances pour enfants et adolescents diabétiques. *Diabète Métab.* (Paris) **16**, 513–21.

Dorchy, H., Haumont, D., Loeb, H., Jennes, M., Niset, G. & Poortmans, J.R. (1980) Decline of blood glucose concentration after muscular effort in diabetic children. *Acta Paediatr Belg.* **33**, 105–9.

Dorchy, H., Niset, G., Ooms, H., Poortmans, J.R. & Baran, D. (1977a) Study of the coefficient of glucose assimilation during muscular exercise in diabetic adolescents deprived of insulin. *Diabète Métab.* (Paris) **3**, 31–4.

Dorchy, H. & Poortmans, J.R. (1989) Sport and the diabetic child. *Sports Med.* **7**, 248–62.

Dorchy, H. & Poortmans, J.R. (1991) Sport et diabète de l'enfant et de l'adolescent. *Ann. Pédiatr.* **38**, 217–23.

Dorchy, H., Roelandt, G., Baran, D. & Loeb, H. (1977b) Adolescents diabétique sous insuline quotidienne: influence de l'effort physique sur le coefficient d'assimilation glucidique. *Méd. Sport* (Paris) **51**, 368–72.

Dorchy, H., Van Vliet, G., Toussaint, D., Ketelbant-Balasse, P. & Loeb, H. (1979) Mauriac syndrome. *Diabète Métab.* (Paris) **5**, 195–200.

Dorchy, H., Vandewalle, C., Decraene, T., Nagy, Z.P., Schuit, F. & Gorus, F. (1993) Genetic and immunological markers in European Caucasians and mograbin Caucasians with type 1 (insulin-dependent) diabetes residing in Belgium. *Pediatr. Adolesc. Endocrinol.* **23**, 71−5.

Ebeling, P., Tuominen, J.A., Bourey, R., Koranyi, L. & Koivisto, V.A. (1995) Athletes with IDDM exhibit impaired metabolic control and increased lipid utilization with no increase in insulin sensitivity. *Diabetes* **44**, 471−5.

Elo, O., Hirvonen, L., Peltonen, T. & Valimaki, K. (1965) Physical working capacity of normal and diabetic children. *Ann. Paediatr. Fenn.* **11**, 25−31.

Frid, A., Ostman, J. & Linde, B. (1990) Hypoglycemia risk during exercise after intramuscular injection of insulin in thigh in IDDM. *Diabetes Care* **13**, 473−7.

Friedman, N.E., Levitsky, L, Edidin, D., Vitullo, D.A. & Lacina, S.J. (1982) Echocardiographic evidence for impaired myocardial performance in children with type I diabetes mellitus. *Am. J. Med.* **73**, 846−50.

Garratt, C.J., Butterfield, W.J., Abrams, R.E., Sterky, G. & Wichelow, M.J. (1972) Effect of exercise on peripheral uptake of ^{131}I-insulin and glucose in non-diabetics. *Metabolism* **21**, 36−47.

Gillet, P. & François, R. (1984) Diabète et sport. In R. Guillet, J. Genéty & E. Brunet-Guedj (eds) *Médecine du Sport*, pp. 325−34. Masson, Paris.

Goldberg, R.D. (1981) Lipid disorders in diabetes. *Diabetes Care* **4**, 561−72.

Goodyear, L.J., Hirshman, M.F., Valyou, P.M. & Horton, E.S. (1992) Glucose transporter number, function, and subcellular distribution in rat skeletal muscle after exercise training. *Diabetes* **41**, 1091−9.

Greene, S. (1992) Complications of hypoglycemia. *Diabetes Young* **28**, 8−10.

Hagan, R.D., Marks, J.F. & Warren, P.A. (1979) Physiologic responses of juvenile-onset diabetic boys to muscular work. *Diabetes* **28**, 1114−19.

Hagg, S.A., Taylor, S.I. & Ruderman, N.B. (1976) Glucose metabolism in perfused skeletal muscle: pyruvate dehydrogenase activity in starvation, diabetes and exercise. *Biochem. J.* **158**, 203−10.

Handberg, A., Vaag, A., Beck-Nielsen, H. & Vinten, J. (1992) Peripheral glucose uptake and skeletal muscle GLUT 4 content in man: effect of insulin and free fatty acids. *Diabetic Med.* **9**, 605−10.

Hebbelinck, M., Loeb, H. & Meersseman, H. (1974) Physical development and performance capacity in a group of diabetic children and adolescents. *Acta Paediatr. Belg.* **28** (Suppl.), 151−61.

Heller, S.R., Herbert, M., MacDonald, I.A. & Tattersall, R.R. (1987) Influence of sympathetic nervous system on hypoglycaemic warning symptoms. *Lancet* **ii**, 359−63.

Hespel, H., Vergauwen, L., Vandenberghe, K. & Richter, E.A. (1995) Important role of insulin and flow in stimulating glucose uptake in contracting skeletal muscle. *Diabetes* **44**, 210−15.

Hilsted, J., Galbo, H., Christensen, N.J., Parving, H.H. & Benn, J. (1982) Haemodynamic changes during graded exercise in patients with diabetic autonomic neuropathy. *Diabetologia* **22**, 318−23.

Horton, E.S. (1988) Role and management of exercise in diabetes mellitus. *Diabetes Care* **11**, 201−11.

Horton, E.S. (1991) Prescription for exercise. *Diabetes Spect.* **4**, 250−7.

Hughes, R.A., Thorland, W.G., Housh, T.J. & Johnson, G.O. (1990) The effect of exercise intensity on serum lipoprotein responses. *J. Sports Med. Phys. Fitness* **30**, 254−60.

Huttunen, N.-P., Lankela, S.-L., Knip, M. *et al.* (1989) Effect of once-a-week training program on physical fitness and metabolic control in children with IDDM. *Diabetes Care* **12**, 737−40.

Inkeles, S. & Eisenberg, D. (1981) Hyperlipidemia and coronary atherosclerosis: a review. *Medicine* **60**, 110−23.

Jakober, B., Schmulling, R.M. & Engstein, M. (1983) Carbohydrate and lipid metabolism in type I diabetics during exhaustive exercise. *Int. J. Sports Med.* **4**, 104−8.

Jandrain, B., Pirnay, F., Scheen, A. & Lefèbvre, P. (1988) Adaptation au sport du diabétique traité par insuline. *Diabète Métab.* (Paris) **14**, 127−35.

Johansson, B.-L., Berg, U., Bohlin, A.-B., Lefvert, A.-K. & Freyschuss, U. (1987) Exercise-induced changes in renal function and their relation to plasma noradrenaline in insulin-dependent diabetic children and adolescents. *Clin. Sci.* **72**, 611−20.

Johansson, B.-L., Linde, B. & Wahren, J. (1992) Effect of C-peptide on blood flow, capillary diffusion capacity and glucose utilization in the exercising forearm of type 1 (insulin-dependent) diabetic patients. *Diabetologia* **23**, 1151−8.

Jos, J., Thevenin, M., Dumont, G. & Beyne, P. (1985) Effet du contrôle métabolique sur les lipides et les lipoprotéines plasmatiques dans le diabète insulino-dépendant de l'enfant et de l'adolescent. *Diabète Métab.* (Paris) **11**, 174−80.

Kahn, B.B. (1992) Alterations in glucose transporter expression and function in diabetes: mechanisms for insulin resistance. *J. Cell. Biochem.* **48**, 122−8.

Kahn, J.K., Zola, B., Juni, J.E. & Vinik, A.I. (1986) Decreased exercise heart rate and blood pressure response in diabetic subjects with cardiac autonomic neuropathy. *Diabetes Care* **9**, 389−94.

Karjalainem, J., Martin, J.M., Knip, M. *et al.* A bovine albumin peptide as a possible trigger of insulin-dependent diabetes mellitus. *New Engl. J. Med.* **327**, 302−7.

Kelner, C.J.H. (1995) *Childhood and Adolescent Diabetes.* Chapman & Hall Medical, London.

Kemmer, F.W., Berchtold, P., Berger, M., Starke, A. &

Cuppers, H.J. (1979) Exercise induced fall of blood glucose in insulin-treated diabetes unrelated to alteration of insulin mobilization. *Diabetes* **28**, 1131–7.

Kemmer, F.W. & Berger, M. (1983) Exercise and diabetes mellitus: physical activity as a part of daily life and its role in the treatment of diabetic patients. *Int. J. Sports Med.* **4**, 77–88.

Kemmer, F.W. & Berger, M. (1992) Exercise. In K.G.M.M. Alberti, R.A. DeFronzo, H. Keen & P. Zimmet (eds) *International Textbook of Diabetes Mellitus*, pp. 725–43. Wiley, Chichester.

Kleinbaum, J. & Shamoon, H. (1983) Impaired counterregulation of hypoglycemia in insulin-dependent diabetes mellitus. *Diabetes* **32**, 79–83.

Koivisto, V. (1991) Diabetes and exercise. In K.G.M.M. & L.P. Krall (eds) *Diabetes Annual*, Vol. 6, pp. 169–84. Elsevier Science, Amsterdam.

Koivisto, V. & Felig, P. (1978) Effects of leg exercise on insulin absorption in diabetic patients. *New Engl. J. Med.* **298**, 79–83.

Koivisto, V. & Tronier, B. (1983) Postprandial blood glucose response to exercise in type I diabetes: comparison between pump and injection therapy. *Diabetes Care* **6**, 436–40.

Krentowski, G., Pirnay, F., Pallakarakis, N., Luyckx, A.S. & Lacroix, M. (1981) Glucose utilization during exercise in normal and diabetic subjects: the role of insulin. *Diabetes* **30**, 883–9.

Landt, K.W., Campaigne, B.N., James, F.W. & Sperling, M.A. (1985) Effects of exercise training on insulin sensitivity in adolescents with type I diabetes. *Diabetes Care* **8**, 461–5.

Larsson, Y. (1984) The role of exercise in the metabolic control of juvenile diabetes. *Acta Paedr. Jap.* **26**, 331–9.

Larsson, Y., Persson, B., Sterky, G. & Thoren, C. (1964) Functional adaptation to rigorous training and exercise in diabetic and non-diabetic adolescents. *J. Appl. Physiol.* **19**, 629–35.

Larsson, Y., Sterkey, G., Ekengren, K. & Maller, T. (1962) Physical fitness and the influence of training in diabetic adolescent girls. *Diabetes* **11**, 109–17.

Ludvigsson, J. (1980) Physical exercise in relation to degree of metabolic control in juvenile diabetics. *Acta Paediatr. Scand.* **283** (Suppl.), 45–8.

MacDonald, M.J. (1987) Post-exercise late-onset hypoglycemia in insulin-dependent diabetic patients. *Diabetes Care* **10**, 584–8.

McNiven Temple, M.Y., Bar-Or, O. & Riddell, M.C. (1995) The reliability and repeatability of the blood glucose response to prolonged exercise in adolescent boys with IDDM. *Diabetes Care* **18**, 326–32.

Maehlum, S. (1979) *Post-exercise Carbohydrate Metabolism in Diabetic and Non-diabetic Subjects*. Lie and Co.s Boktrykkeri, Oslo.

Mogensen, S.E. & Vittinghus, E. (1975) Urinary albumin excretion during exercise in juvenile diabetics. *Scand. J. Clin. Lab. Invest.* **35**, 295–300.

Moore, C.E., Hartung, G.H., Mitchell, R.F., Kappus, C.M. & Hinderlifter, J. (1983) The relationship of exercise and diet on high-density lipoprotein cholesterol levels in man. *Metabolism* **32**, 189–93.

Mueckler, M. (1990) Family of glucose-transporter genes. Implications for glucose homeostasis and diabetes. *Diabetes* **39**, 6–11.

Nelson, R.A. (1982) Nutrition and physical performance. *Phys. Sports Med.* **10**, 54–63.

Pedersen, O., Beck-Nielsen, H. & Heding, L. (1980) Increased insulin receptors after exercise in patients with insulin-dependent diabetes mellitus. *New Engl. J. Med.* **302**, 886–92.

Persson, B. & Thoren, C. (1980) Prolonged exercise in adolescent boys with juvenile diabetes mellitus. *Acta Paediatr. Scand.* **283** (Suppl.), 62–9.

Ploug, T., Stallknecht, B.M., Pedersen, O. *et al.* (1990) Effect of endurance training on glucose transport capacity and glucose transporter expression in rat skeletal muscle. *Am. J. Physiol.* **259**, E778–86.

Poortmans, J.R. (1984) Exercise and renal function. *Sports Med.* **1**, 125–54.

Poortmans, J.R. (1990) Postexercise proteinuria in normal and diseased humans. *Jap. J. Constit. Med.* **54**, 8–18.

Poortmans, J.R., Brauman, H., Staroukine, M., Verniory, A., Decaestecker, C. & Leclercq, R. (1988a) Indirect evidence of glomerular/tubular mixed-type postexercise proteinuria in healthy humans. *Am. J. Physiol.* **254**, F277–83.

Poortmans, J.R., Dewancker, A. & Dorchy, H. (1976) Urinary excretion of total protein, albumin and β_2-microglobulin during exercise in adolescent diabetics. *Biomed. Express* **25**, 273–4.

Poortmans, J.R., Dorchy, H. & Toussaint, D. (1982) Urinary excretion of total protein, albumin and β_2-microglobulin during rest and exercise in diabetic adolescents with and without retinopathy. *Diabetes Care* **5**, 617–23.

Poortmans, J.R. & Labilloy, D. (1988) The influence of work intensity on post-exercise proteinuria. *Eur. J. Appl. Physiol.* **57**, 260–3.

Poortmans, J.R., Saerens, P., Edelman, R., Vertongen, F. & Dorchy, H. (1986) Influence of the degree of metabolic control in type I diabetic adolescents. *Int. J. Sports Med.* **7**, 232–5.

Poortmans, J.R. & Vanderstraeten, J. (1994) Kidney function during exercise in healthy and diseased humans. An update. *Sports Med.* **18**, 419–37.

Poortmans, J.R., Waterlot, B. & Dorchy, H. (1988b) Training effect on post-exercise microproteinuria in type I diabetic adolescents. *Pediatr. Adolesc. Endocrinol.* **17**, 166–72.

Poortmans, J.R., Wolfs, J.C., Rampaer, L., Niset, G. & Sellier, M. (1983) Renal protein excretion after exercise in man. *Med. Sci. Sports Exerc.* **15**, 157 (abstract).

Richard, L., Delaunay, J., Dorleac, E. & Gillet, P. (1983) Apolipoprotéines et hémoglobine glycosylée chez le jeune diabétique insulino-dépendant. *Arch. Franç. Pédiatr.* **40**, 11–14.

Rönnemaa, T. & Koivisto, V.A. (1988) Combined effect of exercise and ambient temperature on insulin absorption and postprandial glycemia in type I patients. *Diabetes Care* **11**, 769–73.

Rönnemaa, T., Marniemi, J., Leino, A., Karanko, H., Puukka, P. & Koivisto, V.A. (1991) Hormone response of diabetic patients to exercise at cool and warm temperatures. *Eur. J. Appl. Physiol.* **62**, 109–15.

Rowland, T.W., Swadba, L.A., Biggs, D.E., Borke, E.J. & Reiter, E.O. (1985) Glycemic control with physical training in insulin-dependent diabetes mellitus. *Am. J. Dis. Child.* **139**, 307–10.

Rutenfranz, J., Mocellin, R., Bauer, J. & Herzig, W. (1968) Untersuchungen über die körperlichen Leistungsfähigkeit gesunder und kranker Heranwachsender. II. Die Leistungsfähigkeit von Kindern und Jungendlichen mit Diabetes Mellitus. *Zeitschr. Kinderheilk.* **103**, 133–9.

Saltin, B., Lingarde, F., Houston, M., Horlin, R. & Nygaarde, E. (1979) Physical training and glucose tolerance in middle-aged men with chemical diabetes. *Diabetes* **28** (Suppl. 1), 30–2.

Sestoft, L., Trap-Jensen, L., Lynsooe, J., Clausen, J.P. & Holst, J.J. (1977) Regulation of gluconeogenesis during rest and exercise in diabetic subjects and normal mean. *Clin. Sci. Mol. Med.* **53**, 411–18.

Soman, V.R., Koivisto, V.A., Diebert, D., Felig, P. & DeFronzo, R.A. (1979) Increased insulin sensitivity and insulin binding to monocytes after physical training. *New Engl. J. Med.* **301**, 1200–4.

Sonnenberg, G.E., Kemer, F.W. & Berger, M. (1990) Exercise in type 1 (insulin-dependent) diabetic patients treated with continuous subcutaneous insulin infusion: prevention of exercise induced hypoglycemia. *Diabetologia* **33**, 696–703.

Sterky, G. (1963) Physical work capacity of diabetic schoolchildren. *Acta Paediatr. Scand.* **52**, 1–10.

Stratton, R., Wilson, D.P., Endres, R.K. & Goldstein, D.E. (1987) Improved glycemic control after supervised 8-week exercise program in insulin-dependent diabetic adolescents. *Diabetes Care* **10**, 589–93.

Strobl, W., Widhalm, K., Schober, E., Frisch, H. & Ollak, A. (1985) Apolipoproteins and lipoproteins in children with type I diabetes: relation to glycosylated serum protein and HbA$_1$. *Acta Paediatr. Scand.* **74**, 966–71.

Travis, L.B., Brouhard, B.H. & Schreiner, B.J. (1987) *Diabetes Mellitus in Children and Adolescents*. W.B. Saunders, Philadelphia.

Touminen, J.A., Karonen, S.L., Melamies, L., Bolli, G. & Koivisto, V.A. (1995) Exercise-induced hypoglycaemia in IDDM patients treated with a short-acting insulin analogue. *Diabetologie* **38**, 106–11.

Verougstraete, C., Toussaint, D., De Schepper, J., Haentjens, M. & Dorchy, H. (1991) First micro-angiographic abnormalities in childhood diabetes. *Graefe's Arch. Clin. Exp. Ophthalmol.* **229**, 24–32.

Vignati, L. & Cunningham, L.N. (1985) Exercise and diabetes. In A. Marble, L.P. Krall, R.F. Bradley, A.R. Christlieb & J.S. Soeldner (eds) *Joslin's Diabetes Mellitus*, 11th edn, pp. 453–64. Lea & Febiger, Philadelphia.

Wahren, J., Felig, P. & Hagenfeldt, L. (1978) Physical exercise and fuel homeostasis in diabetes mellitus. *Diabetologia* **14**, 213–23.

Wahren, J., Hagenfeldt, L. & Felig, P. (1975) Splanchnic and leg exchange of glucose, amino acids, and free fatty acids during exercise in diabetes mellitus. *J. Clin. Invest.* **55**, 1303–14.

Wallace, M.B., Moffatt, R.J., Haymes, E.M. & Green, N.R. (1991) Acute effects of resistance exercise on parameters of lipoprotein metabolism. *Med. Sci. Sports Exerc.* **23**, 199–204.

Wallberg-Henriksson, H., Gunnarsson, R., Henriksson, J., DeFronzo, R. & Felig, P. (1982) Increased peripheral insulin sensitivity and muscle mitochondrial enzymes but unchanged blood glucose control in type I diabetics after physical training. *Diabetes* **31**, 1044–50.

Wallberg-Henriksson, H., Gunnarsson, R., Rossner, S. & Wahren, J. (1983) Long-term physical training in female type I (insulin-dependent) diabetic patients: absence of significant effect on glycaemic control and lipoprotein levels. *Diabetologia* **29**, 53–7.

Wasserman, D.H., Mohr, T., Kelly, P., Lacy, D.B. & Bracy, D. (1992) Impact of insulin deficiency on glucose fluxes and muscle glucose metabolism during exercise. *Diabetes* **41**, 1229–38.

Willems, D. & Dorchy, H. (1990) Taux des lipoprotéines et des apolipoprotéines chez les jeunes diabétiques insulino-dépendants. Relations avec l'hémoglobine glycosylée et la fructosamine. *Presse Méd.* **19**, 17–20.

Yki-Jarvinen, H. & Koivisto, V.A. (1983) Effects of body composition on insulin sensitivity. *Diabetes* **32**, 965–8.

Zinman, B. (1990) Diabetes and exercise: clinical implications. In K.G.M.M. Alberti & L.P. Krall (eds) *Diabetes Annual*, Vol. 5, pp. 173–85. Elsevier Science, Amsterdam.

Zinman, B., Murray, F.T., Vranic, M. *et al.* (1977) Glucoregulation during moderate exercise in insulin treated diabetics. *J. Clin. Endocrinol. Metab.* **45**, 641–53.

Chapter 31

Adolescent Hypertension and Sports

RON A. DLIN

Introduction

Hypertension affects approximately 2–5% of the adolescent population (Fixler *et al.*, 1979; Task Force on Blood Pressure Control in Children, 1987). There is evidence to support the concept that the roots of essential hypertension extend back to childhood (Task Force on Blood Pressure Control in Children, 1987). This has implications both for those adolescents with hypertension who choose to participate in exercise at levels ranging from a casual nature to a competitive sport level, and for those in whom exercise may provide health benefits due to their elevated blood pressure.

Clinical applications of sports medicine must be a focus for the practising physician who deals with suspect, borderline or established hypertension in the adolescent age group. Implications for management, as related to physical activity in this age group, are wide reaching. In youth benefits of participation for social as well as physical reasons demand both an informed and concerned approach. It is the duty of the physician to facilitate complete and normal participation in physical activities, while safeguarding the health and well-being of the adolescent with hypertension.

It is clear that elevated blood pressure is associated with a markedly increased risk for numerous cardiovascular pathologies. Over the past 20 years, many useful antihypertensive medications have become available. While they have made a very significant contribution to the treatment of high blood pressure, drugs are not without their side-effects. This problem is often accentuated in youth, where both lifestyle differences and medication requirements are different than in adults.

There is good evidence to suggest that pharmacological treatment of adults with moderate hypertension (blood pressure in excess of 160/105 mmHg) significantly reduces cardiovascular mortality and morbidity (Veterans Administration Co-operative Study Group on Antihypertensive Agents, 1967, 1972). The benefits of drug therapy for patients with less severely elevated blood pressure are less clear (Kaplan *et al.*, 1989). Risk–benefit ratios must be a clinical consideration. This does not imply that drugs have no place in mild hypertension but that the cost–benefit ratios of non-pharmacological treatments, and specifically exercise, in terms of direct and indirect beneficial effects and compliance must be a significant consideration. Tanji (1992) in an overview of the subject has suggested that the question is no longer about whether or not chronic exercise results in a decrease in blood pressure at rest but about what sort of exercise results in blood pressure control and what the mechanisms are by which it works.

Effects of exercise on blood pressure

Prior to any discussion of the influence of exercise on blood pressure a description of the normal haemodynamics of the blood pressure response to different exercise types should be outlined. Haemodynamic responses to dynamic exercise differ somewhat from those to static exercise (Fixler *et al.*, 1979; Bar-Or, 1983; Dlin, 1986).

Dynamic exercise

Dynamic exercise is used here to refer to those types of physical activity in which various larger muscle groups undergo repetitive and continuous muscle contraction involving a change in the muscle length. These contractions induce a range of motion and are carried out over a period of minutes or longer, as in walking, running or cycling.

During acute bouts of dynamic exercise there is a steady increase in systolic blood pressure (SBP) which is proportional to the exercise intensity and metabolic level while diastolic blood pressure (DBP) does not change significantly (Dehn & Mitchell, 1979; Dlin *et al.*, 1986). Blood pressure levels are dependent primarily on the relationship of stroke volume, heart rate and total peripheral resistance (TPR). During the transition from rest to exercise, or during exercise of increasing intensity, cardiac output increases as a result of increases in both stroke volume and heart rate, blood pressure increases are offset to some degree by decreases in TPR (Keul *et al.*, 1981).

Static exercise

Static exercise is used here to refer to those types of physical activity in which muscle groups perform an action, with a change in tension but little or no change in muscle length, and which is maintained over a short period of time (seconds to minutes) (e.g. lifting weights or sustained hand grip).

During static exercise the increase in blood pressure is in proportion to the muscle tension exerted and is probably related to the muscle mass involved (Buck *et al.*, 1980; Seals *et al.*, 1983). At lower intensities, below 20% of the maximal voluntary force exerted by any given muscle, blood pressure tends to stabilize during maintenance of the contraction. At exertional levels above this, SBP and DBP increase constantly as long as the force can be sustained (Donald *et al.*, 1967). The rate and magnitude of the blood pressure increase is greater when a higher percentage of maximal voluntary force is exerted (Funderburk *et al.*, 1974; MacDougall *et al.*, 1985) and the increases in SBP and DBP are almost parallel (Funderburk *et al.*, 1974). The blood pressure changes occur without large changes in cardiac output. These changes are in part due to mechanical compression of the contracting muscle, a pressure reflex of static contraction and, during heavy exercise and valsalva manoeuvres, elevated intrathoracic pressure (Arensman *et al.*, 1989).

Postexercise period

Postexercise hypotension has been observed following both dynamic and static types of exercise (Iskandrian & Heo, 1988; Tipton, 1991). Postexercise hypotension seems to occur in both normotensives and hypertensives (Hagberg *et al.*, 1987). Reductions in adrenaline, dopamine and cortisol levels (Paulev *et al.*, 1984), as well as release of endogenous opiods and peptides from the atrium and ventricles may provide a possible mechanism for this phenomenon (Shyu & Thoren, 1986; Freud *et al.*, 1988). Other authors have concluded that inhibition of sympathetic nerve traffic is the most viable mechanism for postexercise hypotension (Floras *et al.*, 1989; Boone *et al* 1990).

Effects of chronic exercise

BLOOD PRESSURE LOWERING EFFECTS

The long-term effects of exercise on blood pressure obviously derive from the immediate effects of exercise repeated over time. It is the habitual rather than the casual exercise that will contribute to the most significant impact on elevated blood pressure and its management.

Tipton in his extensive review of the subject concluded that 'the collective effect of the epidemiological studies reviewed before and after 1984, provides a solid foundation for the concept that chronic exercise is beneficial for improving physical fitness levels that will be associated with lower resting blood pressure in younger and older populations' (Tipton, 1991).

While his statement applies to all ages there are several studies to support this concept, specifically in the younger age groups. Some studies (Fraser et al., 1983; Hofman et al., 1987; Panico et al., 1987), have shown an inverse relationship between resting blood pressure and fitness levels suggesting that higher fitness confers a lower blood pressure on the more active adolescent group. Evidence from studies in athletes suggest a lower than expected incidence of hypertension in this group (Kral et al., 1966; Lehmann & Keul, 1984). No significant differences in resting or exercise blood pressure were noted in a study of adolescent athletes training in sports with varying amounts of static, dynamic and mixed features (Dlin et al., 1986).

These studies refer to preventive applications of exercise in hypertension. While the beneficial effects of exercise in lowering blood pressure in individuals with hypertension are more extensively shown in adults, regular exercise programmes have also been shown to reduce blood pressure in youths with hypertension (Hagberg et al., 1983b, 1984; Tipton, 1984, 1991). Endurance conditioning has been shown to induce a significant reduction in SBP and DBP in adolescents with hypertension (Hagberg et al., 1983b). This group of hypertensives were placed on a weight-training programme which maintained their resting blood pressure at the lower level previously achieved by the endurance programme. This decreased blood pressure was associated with a decrease in TPR. Those adolescents not continuing in either endurance or weight-training showed a return of resting blood pressure to the preconditioning levels (Hagberg et al., 1984). The blood pressure lowering effects of exercise have also

been shown for secondary hypertension (Hagberg et al., 1983a; Cade et al., 1984; Painter et al., 1986).

It is important to note that hypertensive youths who undertook moderate static exercise (Fixler et al., 1979) or maximal dynamic exercise (Fixler et al., 1979; Falkner & Lowenthal, 1980; Nudel et al 1980) had no significant adverse electrocardiogram (ECG) or haemodynamic changes. A short-term weight-training programme in a group of adolescents with hypertension had no ill effects on resting blood pressure or cardiac dimensions (Laird et al., 1979).

Type as well as intensity of training may also have a bearing on the influence of the exercise on blood pressure. The magnitude of increase in $\dot{V}O_{2\,max}$ as a result of exercise training was not correlated to the magnitude of the reduction in blood pressure in adolescence (Hagberg et al., 1983b). Several other studies have suggested that there are probably more antihypertensive benefits from lower level training programmes (in the intensity region of 50% $\dot{V}O_{2\,max}$) than are derived from more intense training programmes (at 70% or greater $\dot{V}O_{2\,max}$) (Roman et al., 1981; Hagberg et al., 1989; Hagberg, 1990).

While there is general consensus on the beneficial antihypertensive effects of endurance exercise, the long-term results of isometric or static training are less clear-cut. As stated above, adolescents with mild systolic hypertension maintained the blood pressure reductions previously attained through an aerobic training programme while on a weight-training programme (Hagberg et al., 1984). Decreased blood pressure was also shown in older hypertensives using isometric contractions (Kievloff & Huber, 1971). One study on circuit weight-training showed a decrease in DBP but not SBP (Harris & Holberg, 1987). Keleman (1989) reported a decrease in SBP and DBP in borderline hypertensives after a combined programme of circuit weight-training and jogging.

As with aerobic training a low to moderate

intensity, 40−50% of the maximal voluntary force, is suggested (Harris & Holberg, 1987; Kelemen, 1989; Sparling & Cantwell, 1989; Tanji, 1992). Although there is no hard evidence to support these suggestions, they are based on avoiding the very marked rises in both SBP and DBP shown to occur in heavy resistance exercise (MacDougall *et al.*, 1985).

The blood pressure lowering effects of exercise training should be seen between 3 and 12 weeks of a regular programme (Nomura Roman *et al.*, 1981; Nomura *et al.*, 1984; Jennings *et al.*, 1986; Urata *et al.*, 1987). The return of pretraining blood pressure levels after cessation of regular training occurs within approximately 3 months (Roman *et al.*, 1981; Cade *et al.*, 1984).

MECHANISMS

A clear understanding of all of the mechanisms underlying the blood pressure reducing effects of exercise in individuals with hypertension is still lacking. The haemodynamic mechanisms proposed to explain some of the antihypertensive effects of exercise take into account the relationship between cardiac output, TPR and blood pressure. In order to reduce blood pressure, stroke volume, heart rate, TPR or a combination of these must be reduced. If, as a result of exercise training, resting heart rate decreases relatively more than the increases in stroke volume then cardiac output and, therefore, resting blood pressure will decrease (Hagberg *et al.*, 1983b). Nelson *et al.* (1986) found an increase in cardiac output at rest following training so that in their study the entire reduction in blood pressure following an exercise programme was due to a decrease in peripheral resistance. Although weight reduction resulting from regular exercise is beneficial in obese adolescents Hagberg (1990) has shown in an analysis of several studies that the antihypertensive effect of endurance training does not have a direct relationship with weight loss. However, overweight individuals who reduced their resting blood pressure with training also had substantial reductions in

their plasma glucose, insulin and triglyceride levels (Krotkiewski *et al.*, 1979). Reduction in blood pressure in overweight persons with essential hypertension may relate to metabolic adaptations in carbohydrate and lipid metabolism (Hagberg, 1990).

Humoral aspects may also contribute although the role is as yet unclear. Patients with low plasma renin experience a decrease in their blood pressure after training more than those with higher renin levels (Kiyonaga *et al.*, 1985; Urata *et al.*, 1987) while hypertensives with higher noradrenaline levels experienced a decrease in their post-training blood pressure more than those with normal noradrenalin levels (Duncan *et al.*, 1985; Kiyonaga *et al.*, 1985; Urata *et al.*, 1987). Mild exercise may increase prostaglandin E activity which may lower blood pressure by its vasodilatory effect (Kiyonaga *et al.*, 1985).

Antihypertensive medication and exercise

It is clear that adequate treatment of hypertension significantly reduces cardiovascular morbidity and mortality (Veterans Administration Co-operative Study Group in Antihypertensive Agents, 1967, 1972). This will necessitate pharmacological treatment in some individuals. In those involved in regular exercise and requiring drug therapy, consideration of the potential interactions are important.

Antihypertensives best suited to the exercising individual must ideally offer adequate blood pressure control without interfering with exercise performance or increasing potential drug−exercise interaction risks. The drugs should not adversely affect myocardial function, either contractility or blood flow, should not significantly interfere with muscle perfusion or metabolism, and should not alter homeostatic regulatory functions such as thermoregulation.

The major antihypertensive drug classes which require consideration are β-blockers, calcium channel blockers, angiotensin-converting enzyme (ACE) inhibitors and diuretics. Although some differences exist between antihypertensive drugs within the same class, the scope of this discussion does not allow for a detailed description. An overall view of the drug class only will be presented.

β-blockers reduce $\dot{V}o_{2\,max}$ (Lundborg et al., 1981; Chick et al., 1986; Gullestad et al., 1988; Stewart et al., 1990). Long-term administration has also been shown to reduce the anaerobic threshold (Kullmer & Kinderman, 1985; Hespel et al., 1986). Studies on the effects of β-blockade on training have shown a limitation in expected $\dot{V}o_{2}$ gains (Sable et al., 1982; Stewart et al., 1990) and lesser gains in exercise duration time following training (Lundborg et al., 1981; Stewart et al., 1990).

Despite the lower heart rate induced by β-blockade, it appears that cardiac output at submaximal levels can be maintained through increases in stroke volume (Joyner et al., 1986; Martin et al., 1989; Scruggs et al., 1991).

There are some metabolic effects of β-blockade that impair gluconeogenesis in skeletal muscle as well as lipolysis, since both are dependent on β-receptor stimulation (Chick et al., 1986). There may also be some impairment of heat dissipation during exercise in those under β-blockade (Gordon et al., 1985). β-blockade does not appear to impair strength or strength gains following training (Stewart et al., 1990). While there is no contraindication to using β-blockers in the exercising individual (Kaplan et al., 1989), the above points deserve consideration.

Calcium channel blockers appear to be a safe choice in the exercising individual. They maintain antihypertensive effect and do not significantly interfere with exercise performance (Andersen & Vik-Mo, 1984; Chick et al., 1986). Some calcium channel blockers cause small reductions in exercise heart rate and maximum heart rate with no significant changes in cardiac output (Klein et al., 1983; Petri et al., 1986). No reductions in $\dot{V}o_{2\,max}$ have been shown with calcium channel blockers (Yamakado et al.,

1983; Stewart et al., 1990). They also do not appear to limit training gains from aerobic or strength exercise (Stewart et al., 1990). Calcium channel blockers may lead to enhanced gluconeogenesis in skeletal muscle and lipolysis, thus there is no interference with substrate utilization (Chick et al., 1986).

ACE inhibitors exert an adequate antihypertensive effect during exercise (Fagard et al., 1982) and do not alter $\dot{V}o_{2\,max}$, maximal work rate or rating of perceived exertion (Leon et al., 1986; Handa et al., 1991) and are therefore a good choice in the exercising individual requiring antihypertensive drug therapy.

Diuretics may induce hypokalaemia which may be worsened during prolonged exercise in hot conditions. This with a greater possibility of dehydration may lead to a decreased muscle perfusion, rhabdomyolysis and cardiac arrhythmia (Chick et al., 1988). They should be used with caution both alone and in combination with other antihypertensives.

Precautions during exercise in the individual with hypertension

There are few, if any, absolute contraindications for participation in physical activity for the adolescent with hypertension. Secondary forms of hypertension require separate discussion which is beyond the scope of this chapter.

The Task Force IV on systemic arterial hypertension at the Sixteenth Bethesda Conference (Frolich et al., 1985) stated that there were not sufficient data to arrive at firm recommendations concerning the adolescent athlete with hypertension. Reasons cited for this lack of agreement included:

1 No clear definition of the limits of normal blood pressure in the adolescent.

2 The observation that in many adolescents with hypertension it may disappear over time.

3 Lack of evidence of any deleterious effects of participation in competitive sports in these groups.

The task force did however suggest a permissive approach should be taken to prevent 'cardiac crippling' of adolescents with hypertension. They conclude that adolescents with hypertension should be allowed to participate in all competitive athletics. Restrictions should be applied only to those with severe hypertension (resting DBP, 115 mmHg) or target organ involvement, specifically those youths showing evidence of hypertensive left ventricular changes, and renal or eye involvement. These individuals should be treated as adult patients with recommendations for participation only in low intensity competitive sports (Frolich *et al.*, 1985).

Exercise testing and the blood pressure response

Several authors have suggested that exercise testing of the adolescent with hypertension is an important part of the preparticipation and ongoing assessment (Fixler *et al.*, 1979; Bar-Or, 1983; Dlin, 1986; Podolsky, 1989; Kaplan, 1990; Dlin & Rotstein, 1991; Tanji, 1992). There are, however, no clear definitions of a normal blood pressure response to exercise. No standards for proper measurement of blood pressure during exercise exist as they do for measurement at rest. There are no consistent reference criteria for reporting blood pressure values, no universally accepted methods of testing, modes of exercise or exercise protocols, and no specific point on the continuum of the exercise test is generally agreed as the ideal time of measurement. Blood pressures are variously reported at peak exercise level (Fixler *et al.*, 1979; Alpert *et al.*, 1981), peak mechanical power (Jones *et al.*, 1985; Jones, 1988), heart rate (Dlin *et al.*, 1986), percentage of maximal heart rate and of maximal oxygen consumption (Dlin *et al.*, 1984), at an exercise intensity equivalent to 4 mmol blood lactate (Dlin *et al.*, 1984), as double product (Falkner & Lowenthal, 1980) and as regression equations over mechanical power (Heck *et al.*, 1984).

In order to make valid comparisons these factors as well as the test protocol (e.g. upright versus supine, treadmill versus cycle ergometer, arm versus leg work, static versus dynamic exercises) must be considered. It is critical that blood pressure be measured during rather than after exercise as blood pressure falls within 1 s of cessation of exercise (Holmgren, 1956).

Because absolute power loads impose a varying strain on a subject depending on the fitness level, a parameter such as heart rate is a good indicator of relative cardiovascular effort and provides a reasonable and easily accessible basis for comparison (Inbar *et al.*, 1992). Maximal exercise blood pressure measurements are often technically difficult due to muscular 'noise' at high effort so that submaximal levels may provide a more reliable measure.

A practical approach would be to use the indirect (blood pressure cuff) measurement by auscultation of upright exercise (cycle or treadmill) recorded at more than one submaximal exercise level. Blood pressure should be reported in relation to simultaneously monitored heart rate (Dlin, 1986). Thus a plot of several blood pressure points related to normal values similarly plotted would provide a readily usable, practical basis for comparison to assess an individual's blood pressure response to exercise.

Norms for blood pressure response to exercise

We reported blood pressure response to exercise in 822 competitive male athletes aged 14–18 years (Dlin *et al.*, 1986). As shown in Fig. 31.1, mean SBP is described at corresponding mean heart rate with 1 SD for each of the parameters at various submaximal exercise levels on a cycle ergometer. DBP is not shown as there were no significant changes from resting values throughout the exercise task. These data are proposed as a basis for comparison for normal blood pressure response to exercise in adolescents as they represent a large database. Figure 31.1 shows blood pressure at corresponding heart rate, measurements easily carried out in any exercise testing facility. It also provides data at several submaximal exer-

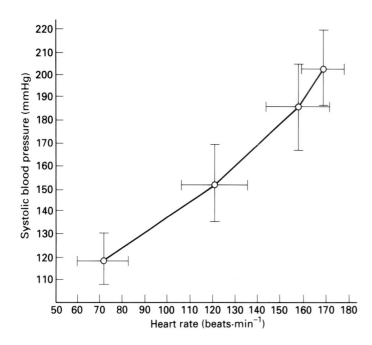

Fig. 31.1 Systolic blood pressure response plotted against heart rate of varying power loads for the study population of 822 competitive male athletes aged 14–18 years. Redrawn with permission from Dlin *et al.* (1986) © 1986 by Human Kinetics Publishers.

cise levels. These features provide for accurate and ready clinical application. Most other reports in the literature have the limitation of only providing blood pressure measurements at peak exercise measurements or at a fixed work rate (Fixler *et al.*, 1979; Riopel *et al.*, 1979; Alpert *et al.*, 1981; Heck *et al.*, 1984; Klein *et al.*, 1984; Hansen *et al.*, 1985; Jones, 1988). While the blood pressure response to exercise in this competitive athletic group is somewhat higher than that found in the literature on some groups of more sedentary youths (Dlin, 1986) it corresponds well with adult related heart rate and SBP responses reported by Jones (1988) in his text on clinical exercise testing. The peak values are below most suggested upper limits of accepted safety levels (American Academy of Pediatrics, 1977; James *et al.*, 1980, Arensman *et al.*, 1989).

Applications of the exercise blood pressure response

Use of comparative data for normal blood pressure response to exercise can be useful for identifying inappropriate blood pressure responses and for evaluating the effectiveness of drug interventions in the treatment of hypertension.

Adequate control of blood pressure with the use of medication is regularly monitored by measurement of resting levels. It would seem more than reasonable also to monitor the adolescent with hypertension requiring drug intervention using blood pressure responses during exercise. Applying standardized techniques and reference values will allow for more reliability in this type of dynamic pre- and post-treatment assessment. Tanji (1990) has suggested that it is useful to know SBP and DBP at graded increases in heart rate in persons with hypertension for the purpose of instruction during exercise.

An additional significant application of the blood pressure response to exercise may be in assessing risk for developing target organ damage from hypertension. Floras *et al.* (1981) evaluated the relationship of blood pressure measurements in the physician's office, by an ambulatory method, and during exercise testing to target organ damage in individuals with essential hypertension. They found that the group showing more target organ damage had office blood pressure values similar to the group with less target organ damage but higher ambulatory pressures. They also found that the group with higher ambulatory pressures had greater blood pressure increases with exercise testing.

Prediction of future hypertension

The significance of an abnormal SBP response during exercise in apparently normal individuals is a more complex issue. A number of studies have demonstrated that the blood pressure response during exercise may be useful in predicting the future development of hypertension in individuals with normal resting blood pressure (Franz, 1981; Wilson & Meyer, 1981; Dlin et al., 1983; Jackson et al., 1983; Benbassat & Froom, 1986; Chaney & Eyman, 1988). Wilson and Meyer (1981) and Jackson et al. (1983) studied two separate groups of middle-aged men for some years after undergoing an exercise test. Those with higher blood pressure response to exercise but similar at rest levels had a higher incidence of hypertension at the end of a follow-up period. Dlin et al. (1983) showed similar findings in two matched groups of younger individuals (mean age 25 years). Other studies (Jetté et al., 1988; Tanji et al., 1989) have shown similar findings using post-exercise blood pressure measurements. Benbassat and Froom (1986), reviewed 11 studies on the subject and found the prevalence of hypertension among normotensive subjects who showed an exaggerated exercise pressure response was 2.1–3.4 times higher than among subjects with normal exercise blood pressure responses. They point out, however, that there was a wide range of sensitivity and specificity in the studies.

While the above data suggest promise for the use of blood pressure response to exercise as a tool in the early detection of hypertension, their widespread application must be tempered

with some caution. The limitations of application relate largely to the previously cited lack of adequate standardization surrounding the blood pressure response to exercise. Tipton (1991) concludes that evidence accumulated in recent years has not been overwhelmingly convincing that acute exercise could be used as a predictor of future hypertension. Several authors (Benbassat & Froom, 1986; Dlin, 1986; Tanji, 1992) have suggested that better standardization, clear definition of a normal response and more uniform testing protocols are required for a better assessment of the possible contribution of the exercise blood pressure response in the prediction of future hypertension.

Guidelines for exercise prescription

As with other forms of treatment exercise should be regarded in terms of a prescription for the adolescent with hypertension. This prescription should include type, dose and frequency. This concept has been outlined by the American College of Sport Medicine (1990) and described in terms of exercise modality, frequency, duration and intensity.

Aerobic exercise has clearly the widest recommendations, there are, however, no general contraindications to resistance training (Frolich et al., 1985; Arensman et al., 1989; Tipton, 1991; Tanji, 1992).

There are no clear references to frequency or duration of exercise in the adolescent with hypertension. It is reasonable to follow the guidelines of the American College of Sport Medicine at three to four times per week for a duration of 20–60 min per exercise session (ACSM, 1990).

Several authors indicate the significance of exercise intensity in the exercise prescription. Most recommendations are for moderate intensity. For aerobic exercise, the suggestions are in the range of 40–70% $\dot{V}O_{2\,max}$ or 50–70% of maximal heart rate (Roman et al., 1981; Kiyonaga et al., 1985; Hagberg et al., 1989; Tipton, 1991; Tanji, 1992). For resistance training, similar light to moderate intensity is recommended. Low weight repetitions at 40–50% of maximal single repetitions are suggested (Harris & Holberg, 1987; Kelemen, 1989; Sparling & Cantwell, 1989; Tanji, 1992).

Challenges for future research

• In adolescents with resting blood pressure above the 95th percentile 33–55% will have pressures that return to normal within 2 years without any therapy (Frolich *et al.*, 1985). Could exercise blood pressure response detect those who will go on to be hypertensive? To understand better the significance of exercise blood pressure in both adolescents with normal blood pressure and those with hypertension, standard testing procedures and norms must be established. Once established, long-term follow-up and investigation of abnormal responders should be undertaken. This will allow for better understanding of these responses and their application in early detection of hypertension and usefulness as predictors of target organ involvement.

• We must continue to follow adolescents with hypertension who engage in regular physical activity as well as competitive athletics to answer better the question of beneficial and detrimental effects. These studies should include both static and dynamic exercises and the combination of the two as exists in many sports.

• There is a need for studies addressing all of the aspects of hypertension and exercise, particularly including female adolescents.

Acknowledgements

The author wishes to thank Dr Omri Inbar for his editorial assistance, Ellen Dlin for her technical assistance and Ann McKinlay for her secretarial assistance.

References

Alpert, B.S., Dover, E.V., Booker, D.L., Martin, A.M. & Strong, W.B. (1981) Blood pressure response to dynamic exercise in healthy children — black vs white. *J. Pediatr.* **3**, 556–60.

American Academy of Pediatrics (1977) *Policy Statement: Cardiovascular Evaluation for Participation in Sports*. American Academy of Pediatrics, Evanston.

American College of Sports Medicine (1990) *Guidelines for Graded Exercise Testing and Exercise Prescription*. Lea & Febiger, Philadelphia.

Anderson, K. & Vik-Moh (1984) Increased left ventricular emptying at maximal exercise after reduction in afterload. *Circulation* **69**, 492–6.

Arensman, F.W., Christiansen, J. & Strong, W.B. (1989) Juvenile hypertension and exercise. In O. Bar-Or (ed.) *Advances in Pediatric Sports Sciences*, Vol. 3. *Biological Issues*, pp. 203–21. Human Kinetics, Champaign, IL.

Bar-Or, O. (1983) *Pediatric Sports Medicine for the Practitioner. From Physiologic Principles to Clinical Applications*. New York, Springer-Verlag.

Benbassat, J. & Froom, P.F. (1986) Blood pressure response to exercise as a predictor of hypertension. *Arch. Int. Med.* **146**, 2053–5.

Boone, J.B., Levine, M., Flynn, M.G., Pizza, F.X., Kubitz, G.R. & Andres, F.F. (1990) Opioid receptor modulation of post exercise hypotension. *Med. Sci. Sports Exerc.* **22** (Suppl. II), S106.

Buck, J.A., Amundsen, L.R. & Nelson, D.H. (1980) Systolic blood pressure responses during isometric contractions of large and small muscle groups. *Med. Sci. Sports Exerc.* **12**, 145–7.

Cade, R., Mars, D., Wagemaker, H. *et al.* (1984) Effect of aerobic exercise training on patients with systemic arterial hypertension. *Am J. Med.* **77**, 785–90.

Chaney, R.H. & Eyman, K.E. (1988) Blood pressure at rest and during maximal dynamic and isometric exercise as predictor of systemic hypertension. *Am. J. Cardiol.* **62**, 1058–61.

Chick, T.W., Halperin, A.K., Jackson, J.E. & Van As, A. (1986) The effect of nifedipine on cardiopulmonary responses during exercise in normal subjects. *Chest* **89**, 641–6.

Dehn, M.M. & Mitchell, J.H. (1979) The circulatory system. In Strauss (ed.) *Sports Medicine and Physiology*, pp. 77–93. Philadelphia, W.B. Saunders.

Dlin, R.A. (1986) Blood pressure responses to dynamic exercise in healthy and hypertensive youths. *Pediatrician* **13**, 34–43.

Dlin, R.A., Dotan, R., Inbar, O., Rotstein, A., Jacobs, I. & Karlson, J. (1984) Exaggerated systolic blood pressure response to exercise in a water polo team. *Med. Sci. Sports Exerc.* **162**, 294–8.

Dlin, R.A., Hanna-Paparo, N. & Tenenbaum, G. (1986) Blood pressure response to exercise in adolescent competitive athletes. In J. Rutenfranz, R. Mocellin & F. Klimt (eds) *Children and Exercise*, Vol. XII, pp. 185–93. Human Kinetics, Champaign IL.

Dlin, R.A., Hanne, N., Silverberg, D. & Bar-Or, O. (1983) Follow-up of normotensive men with exaggerated blood pressure response to exercise. *Am. Heart J.* **106**, 316–20.

Dlin, R.A. & Rotstein, A. (1991) Rationale for pre-participation medical screening of athletes under age 30. *Harifuah (J. Israeli Med. Ass.)* **120**, 221–6.

Donald, K.W., Lind, A.R., McNicol, G.W., Humphrey, P.W., Taylor, S.H. & Stanton, H.P. (1967) Cardiovascular responses to sustained (static) contractions. *Circ. Res.* **20** (Suppl. 1), 15.

Duncan, J.J., Farr, J.E., Upton, J., Hagan, R.D., Oglesby, M.F. & Blair, S.N. (1985) The effects of aerobic exercise on plasma catecholamines and blood pressure in patients with mild essential hypertension. *JAMA* **254**, 2609–13.

Fagard, R. Lynen, P. & Amery, A. (1982) Hemodynamic responses to captopril at rest and during exercise in hypertensive subjects. *Am. J. Cardiol.* **49**, 1569–71.

Falkner, B. & Lowenthal, D.T. (1980) Dynamic exercise response in hypertensive adolescents. *Int. J. Pediatr. Nephrol.* **1**, 161–5.

Fixler, D.E., Laird, W.P., Browne, R., Fitzgerald, V., Wilson, S. & Vance, R. (1979) Response of hypertensive adolescents to dynamic and isometric exercise stress. *Pediatrics* **64**, 579–83.

Floras, J.S., Hassan, M.O., Sever, P.S., Jones, J.V., Osikowska, B. & Slight, P. (1981) Cuff and ambulatory blood pressure in subjects with essential hypertension. *Lancet* **ii**, 107–9.

Floras, J.S., Sinkey, C.A., Aylward, P.E., Seals, D.R., Thoren, P.N. & Mark, A.L. (1989) Post exercise hypotension and sympathoinhibition in borderline hypertensive men. *Hypertension* **14**, 28–35.

Franz, I.W. (1981) *Belastungsblutdruck bei Hochdruckkranken* (Blood Pressure Response to Exercise in Hypertension), pp. 81–91. Springer-Verlag, Berlin.

Fraser, G.E., Phillips, R.L. & Harris, R. (1983) Physical fitness and blood pressure in school children. *Circulation* **67**, 405–12.

Freud, B.J., Wade, C.E. & Claybaugh, J.R. (1988) Effect of exercise on atrial natriuretic factor. *Sports Med.* **6**, 346–64.

Frolich, E.D., Lowenthal, D.T., Miller, H.S., Pickering, T. & Strong, W.B. (1985) Task Force: IV. Systemic arterial hypertension. *J. Am. Coll. Cardiol.* **6**, 1218–21.

Funderburk, F.C., Hipskind, S.G., Welton, R.C. & Lind, A.R. (1974) Development of and recovery from fatigue induced by static effort at various tension. *J. Appl. Physiol.* **37**, 392.

Gordon, N.F., Krager, P.E., Van Rensburg, J.P., Van Der Linde, A., Kielblock, A.J. & Cilliers, J.F. (1985) Effect of beta-adrenoreceptor blockade on thermoregulation during prolonged exercise. *J. Appl. Physiol.* **58**, 899–906.

Gullested, L., Dolva, L.O., Sylanol, E. & Kjekshus, J. (1988) Difference between beta-l-selective and non-selective beta-blockage during continuous and intermittent exercise. *Clin. Physiol.* **8**, 487–99.

Hagberg, J.M. (1990) Exercise, fitness and hypertension. In C. Bouchard, R.J. Shephard, T. Stephens, J.R. Sutton & B.D., McPherson (eds) *Exercise Fitness and Health*, pp. 455–6. Human Kinetics, Champaign, IL.

Hagberg, J.M., Ehsani, A.A., Goldberg, D., Hernandez, A., Senacore, D.R. & Holloszy, J.O. (1984) Effect of weight training on blood pressure and hemodynamics in hypertensive adolescents. *J. Pediatr.* **104**, 147–51.

Hagberg, J.M., Goldberg, A.P., Ehsani, A.A., Heath, G.W., Delmez, J.A. & Harter, H.R. (1983) Exercise training improves hypertension in hemodialysis patients. *Am. J. Nephrol.* **3**, 209–12.

Hagberg, J.M., Goldring, D., Ehsani, A.A. *et al.* (1983b) Effect of exercise training on the blood pressure and hemodynamic features of adolescent hypertensives. *Am. J. Cardiol.* **52**, 763–8.

Hagberg, J.M., Goldring, D. & Heath, G.W. (1984) Effect of exercise on plasma catecholamines and hemodynamics during rest, submaximal exercise and orthostatic stress. *Clin. Physiol.* **4**, 117–24.

Hagberg, J.M., Montain, S.J. & Martin, W.H. (1987) Blood pressure and hemodynamic response after exercise in older hypertensives. *J. Appl. Physiol.* **63**, 270–6.

Hagberg, J.M., Montain, S.J., Martin, W.H. & Ehsani, A.A. (1989) Effect of exercise training in 60–69 year old persons with essential hypertension. *Am. J. Cardiol.* **64**, 348–53.

Handa, K., Sasaki, J., Tanaka, H. *et al.* (1991) Effects of captopril on opioid peptides during exercise and quality of life in normal subjects. *Am. Heart J.* **122**, 1389–94.

Hansen, H.S., Jorgensen, O. & Hyldebrandt, N. (1985) Blood pressure in children measured at rest and during exertion. *Acta Med. Scand.* **693** (Suppl.), 47–9.

Harris, K.A. & Holberg, R.G. (1987) Physiological

responses to circuit weight training in borderline hypertensive subjects. *Med. Sci. Sports Exerc.* **19**, 246–52.

Heck, H., Rest, R. & Hollman, W. (1984) Standard blood pressure values during ergometric bicycle tests. *Deutsche Zeitschr. Sportsmed.* **7**, 243–9.

Hespel, P., Lijnen, P., Vanhees, L. *et al.* (1986) Differentiation of exercise-induced metabolic responses during selective beta-1 and beta-2 antagonism. *Med. Sci. Sports Exerc.* **18**, 186–91.

Hofman, A., Walter, H.J., Cannelly, P.A. & Vaughan, R.D. (1987) Blood pressure and physical fitness in children. *Hypertension* **9**, 188–91.

Holmgren, A. (1956) Circulatory changes during muscular work in man. *Scand. J. Clin. Lab. Invest.* **24**, 5.

Inbar, O., Dlin, R., Sheinberg, A. & Scheinovitz, M. (1992) Response to progressive exercise in patients with cystic fibrosis and asthma. *Med. Exerc. Nutr. Health* **1**, 55–61.

Iskandrian, A.S. & Heo, J. (1988) Exaggerated systolic blood pressure response to exercise: a normal variant or a hyperdynamic phase of essential hypertension. *Int. J. Cardiol.* **18**, 207–17.

Jackson, A.S., Squires, W.G., Grimes, G. & Beard, E.F. (1983) Prediction of future resting hypertension from exercise blood pressure. *J. Cardiac Rehab.* **3**, 263–8.

James, F.W., Kaplan, S., Glueck, C.J., Tsay, J.Y., Knight, M.J.S. & Sarwar, C.J. (1980) Responses of normal children and young adults to controlled bicycle exercise. *Circulation* **61**, 902–912.

Jennings, G., Nelson, L., Nestel, P. *et al.* (1986) The effects of changes in physical activity on major cardiovascular risk factors, hemodynamics, sympathetic function and glucose utilization in man: a controlled study of four levels of activity. *Circulation* **73**, 30–40.

Jette, M.D., Landry, F., Sidney, K. & Blumchen, G. (1988) Exaggerated blood pressure response to exercise in the detection of hypertension. *J. Cardiopul. Rehab.* **8**, 171–7.

Jones, N.L. (1988) *Clinical Exercise Testing*, 3rd edn. W.B. Saunders, Philadelphia.

Jones, N.L., Makrides, L., Hitchcock, C., Chypahar, T. & McCarney, N. (1985) Normal standards for an incremental progressive cycle ergometer test. *Am. Rev. Respir. Dis.* **131**, 700–8.

Joyner, M.J., Freund, B.J., Jilka, S.M. *et al.* (1986) Effects of β-blockade on exercise capacity of trained and untrained men: a hemodynamic comparison. *J. Appl. Physiol.* **60**, 1429–34.

Kaplan, N.M., Alderman, M.H., Flamenbaum, W. *et al.* (1989) Guidelines for treatment of hypertension. *Am. J. Hypertens.* **2**, 75–7.

Kaplan, T.A. (1990) Elevated blood pressure in a high school football player: case presentation and discussion. *Pediatr. Exerc. Sci.* **2**, 299–312.

Kelemen, M.H. (1989) Resistive training safety and assessment guidelines for cardiac and coronary prone patients. *Med. Sci. Sports Exerc.* **21**, 675–7.

Keul, J., Dickhuth, H.H., Simon, G. & Lehmann, N. (1981) Effect of static and dynamic exercise on heart volume, contractility and left ventricular dimensions. *Circ. Res.* **48** (Suppl. 1) 161–70.

Kievloff, B. & Huber, O. (1971) Brief maximal isometric exercise in hypertension. *J. Am. Geriatr. Soc.* **19**, 1006–9.

Kiyonaga, A., Arakawa, K., Tanaka, H. & Shindo, M. (1985) Blood pressure and hormonal responses to aerobic exercise. *Hypertension* **7**, 125–31.

Klein, A.A., McCrory, W.W., Engle, M.A., Rosenthal, R. & Ehlers, K.H. (1984) Sympathetic nervous system and exercise tolerance response in normotensive and hypertensive adolescents. *J. Am. Coll. Cardiol.* **3**, 381–6.

Klein, W., Brandt, D., Vrecko, K. & Harringer, M. (1983) Role of calcium antagonists in the treatment of essential hypertension. *Circ. Res.* **52** (Suppl. 1), 174–81.

Kral, J., Chrastek, J. & Adamirova, J. (1966) The hypertensive effects of physical activity. In W. Rabb. (ed.) *Prevention of Ischemic Heart Disease: Principles and Practice.* C.C. Thomas, Springfield, IL.

Krotkiewski, M.K., Mandroukas, L., Sjöstrom, L., Sullivan, L., Wetterquist, H. & Bjontrop, P. (1979) Effects of long-term physical training on body fat, metabolism, and blood pressure in obesity. *Metabolism* **28**, 450–8.

Kullmer, T. & Kinderman, W. (1985) Physical performance and serum potassium under chronic beta-blockade. *J. Appl. Physiol.* **54**, 350–4.

Laird, W.P., Fixler, D.E. & Swanbom, C.D. (1979) Cardiovascular effects of weight training in hypertensive adolescents. *Med. Sci. Sports Exerc.* **11**, 78 (abstract).

Lehmann, M. & Keul, J. (1984) Häufigkeit der hypertonic bei 810 Mannlichen Sportlern (Frequency of hypertension in 810 male athletes). *Zeitschr. Kardiol* **73**, 137–41.

Leon, A.S., McNally, C. & Casal, D. (1986) Enalapril alone and in combination with hydrochlorothiazide in the treatment of hypertension: effect on treadmill exercise performance. *J. Cardiopul. Rehab.* **6**, 251–6.

Lundborg, P., Astrom, H., Bengtsson, C. *et al.* (1981) Effect of β-adrenoreceptor blockade on exercise performance and metabolism. *Clin. Sci.* **61**, 229–305.

MacDougall, J.D., Tuxen, D., Sale, D.G., Morog, J.R. & Sutton, J.R. (1985) Arterial blood pressure response to heavy resistance exercise. *J. Appl. Physiol.* **58**, 785–90.

Martin, N.B., Broeder, C.E., Thomas, E.L. *et al.* (1989) Comparison of the effects of pindolol and propranolol on exercise performance in young men with systemic hypertension. *Am. J. Cardiol.* **64**, 343–7.

Nelson, L., Esler, M.D., Jennings, G.L. & Korner, P.I. (1986) Effect of changing levels of physical activity on blood pressure and hemodynamics in essential hypertension. *Lancet* **ii**, 473–6.

Nudel, D.B., Gootman, N., Brunson, S.C., Stengler, A., Shenker, R. & Gauthier, B.G. (1980) Exercise performance of adolescent hypertensives. *Pediatrics* **65**, 1073–8.

Painter, P.L., Nelson–Worrel, J.N., Hill, M.M. *et al.* (1986) Effects of exercise training during hemodialysis. *Nephron* **43**, 87–92.

Panico, S., Celentano, E., Krogh, V. *et al.* (1987) Physical activity and its relationship to blood pressure in school children. *J. Chron. Dis.* **40**, 925–30.

Paulev, P.E., Jordal, R., Kristensen, O. & Ladefoged, J. (1984) Therapeutic effects of exercise on hypertension. *Eur. J. Appl. Physiol.* **53**, 180–5.

Petri, H., Arends, B.B. & Van Baak, M.A. (1986) The effect of verapamil on cardiovascular and metabolic responses to exercise. *Eur. J. Appl. Physiol.* **55**, 499–502.

Podolsky, M.L. (1989) Don't rule out sports for hypertensive children. *Phys. Sports Med.* **17**, 164–70.

Riopel, D.A., Taylor, A.B. & Hohn, A.R. (1979) Blood pressure, heart rate pressure, rate product, and electrocardiographic changes in healthy children during treadmill exercise. *Am. J. Cardiol.* **44**, 697–704.

Rocchini, A.P., Katch, V., Anderson, J. *et al.* (1988) Blood pressure in obese adolescents. Effect of weight loss. *Pediatrics* **82**, 16–23.

Roman, O., Camuzu, A.L. Villalon, E. & Klenner, C. (1981) Physical training program in arterial hypertension: a long term prospective follow up. *Cardiology* **67**, 230–43.

Sable, D.L., Bramwell, H.L., Sheehan, M.W., Nies, A.S., Gerber, J. & Horwitz, L.D. (1982) Attenuation of exercise conditioning by beta-adrenergic blockade. *Circulation* **65**, 679–84.

Scruggs, K.D., Martin, N.B., Broeder, C.E. *et al.* (1991) Stroke volume during submaximal exercise in endurance trained normotensive subjects and in untrained hypertensive subjects with beta blockade (propranolol and pindolol). *Am. J. Cardiol.* **15**, 416–21.

Seals, D.R., Washburn, R.A., Hanson, P.G., Painter, P.L. & Nagler, F.J. (1983) Increased cardiovascular response to static contraction of larger muscle groups. *J. Appl. Physiol.* **54**, 434–7.

Shyu, B.C. & Thoren, P. (1986) Circulatory events following spontaneous muscle exercise in normotensive and hypertensive rats. *Acta Physiol. Scand.* **128**, 515–24.

Sparling, P.B. & Cantwell, J.D. (1989) Strength training guidelines for cardiac patients. *Phys. Sports Med.* **17**, 191–4.

Stewart, K.J., Effron, M.B., Valenti, S.A. & Kelemen, M.H. (1990) Effects of diltiazem or propranolol during exercise training of hypertensive men. *Med. Sci. Sports Exerc.* **22**, 171–7.

Tanji, J.L. (1990) Hypertension: how exercise helps. *Phys. Sports Med.* **18**, 77–82.

Tanji, J.L. (1992) Exercise and the hypertensive athlete. *Clin. Sports Med.* **11**, 291–302.

Tanji, J.L., Champlain, J.J., Wong, G.Y., Lew, E.Y., Brown, T.C. & Amsterdam, E.A. (1989) Blood pressure recovery curves after submaximal exercise; a predictor for hypertension at ten year follow up. *Am. J. Hypertens.* **2**, 135–8.

Task Force on Blood Pressure Control in Children (1987) Task force on blood pressure control in children. *Pediatrics* **79**, 1–25.

Tipton, C.M. (1984) Exercise training and hypertension. *Exerc. Sport Sci. Rev.* **12**, 245–06.

Tipton, C.M. (1991) Exercise training and hypertension. An update. *Exerc. Sport. Sci. Rev.* **19**, 447–505.

Urata, H., Tanabe, Y., Kiyonaga, A. *et al.* (1987) Antihypertensive and volume depleting effects of mild exercise on essential hypertension. *Hypertension* **9**, 245–52.

Veterans Administration Co-operative Study Group on Antihypertensive Agents (1967) Effects of treatment on morbidity in hypertension. Results in patients with diastolic blood pressure averaging 115 through 129 mmHg. *JAMA* **202**, 116–22.

Veterans Administration Co-operative Study Group in Antihypertensive Agents (1972) Effects of treatment on mortality in hypertension: III. Influence of age, diastolic pressure and prior cardiovascular disease: further analysis of side effects. *Circulation* **45**, 991–1004.

Wilson, N.V. & Meyer, B. (1981) Early prediction of hypertension using exercise blood pressure. *Prev. Med.* **10**, 62–8.

Yamakado, T., Oonishi, N., Kondos, Noziri, A.,

Nakano, T. & Takezewa, H. (1983) Effects of diltiazem on cardiovascular responses during exercise in systemic hypertension and comparison with propranolol. *Am. J. Cardiol.* **52**, 1023–7.

Chapter 32

The Young Athlete with a Motor Disability

ROBERT D. STEADWARD AND GARRY D. WHEELER

Introduction

Historically, the opportunity to participate in sports programmes has been the option of people without disabilities. Persons with disabilities often did not have the physical education background that develops sports skills and enables a person to follow an active lifestyle (Eichstaedt & Kalakian, 1993). Recently, this situation has altered dramatically. It is estimated that there are 2–3 million persons with a disability in the USA competing in recreational and organized sports (Ferrara *et al.*, 1992). With the increasing prominence of international athletes with disabilities, particularly wheelchair road racers, and the development of sanctioned international performance theatres such as the Paralympic Games, an increasing number of opportunities have arisen for young people with disabilities to become involved in the sport environment. Also, high performance role models exist for young children with a disability. It is therefore, hardly surprising that many more youngsters with a disability are joining sports organizations. In turn, this has resulted in increased demand for volunteers to take on the challenge of coaching these athletes and for improvements in school-based programmes. Despite these advances, there is a growing concern among physicians and psychologists with regard to the nature of the competitive environment for children, the overemphasis on winning, potential for overuse injuries and the use of performance-enhancing drugs in child

athletes. Little is known regarding the effects of early competitive experiences on the young athlete with a disability.

The foregoing discussion is written from a philosophical viewpoint that recognizes both positive and potentially negative aspects of the sports environment. This discussion is based on a firm belief in the value of sports participation for enhancing the quality of life of young persons with disabilities, yet, equally recognizes that participation and competition must be weighed carefully against the pressures of success and/or failures and potential for overuse injury.

It would be unrealistic to attempt to cover the entire spectrum of motor disabilities in a chapter of this length. Therefore this discussion will be confined to the common congenital disabilities, progressive degenerative and neuromuscular disorders and traumatic injury. Included in these categories are cerebral palsy (CP), Duchenne-type muscular dystrophy (MD), osteogenesis imperfecta (OI), spinal cord injury (SCI), amputations and scoliosis.

This chapter is also written from the perspective that various factors will influence athletes in a functionally integrated sports environment. This is consistent with a movement away from the traditional medical classification model. Finally, this chapter covers the young athlete up to the age of 16 years.

Motor disability is a difficult construct to define since many congenital and acquired impairments should be included. In addition, the definition must include disabilities that are classified as acute or chronic. It is the purpose of this discussion to examine a series of permanent disabilities, how they affect a child's abilities to perform and the level at which he or she may perform in a sport environment. Hence, for the purpose of this chapter, we will consider a motor disability as temporary or permanent decrements in physical performance, motor capabilities and/or potential due to congenital factors, chronic degenerative disease or traumatic injury.

Historical background: involvement of children in sport

A brief history: from Stoke to Atlanta

Until recently, young children with a disability have been involved in competitive sports to a limited degree and the sports movement for people with physical disabilities has been slow to develop. This is in contrast to Special Olympics International, which has served mentally handicapped children and adults since 1968 (Sherrill et al., 1990). This has been due to a variety of factors, including underdeveloped school-based programmes of physical activity and the reluctance of the medical profession to promote strenuous activities for those with a physical disability. Prior to the mid-nineteenth century there were few, if any, opportunities for participation in sports activities for persons with a disability. Those with CP and progressive congenital disorders were considered too fragile for involvement in physical activity and sports and, up until the end of World War II, those with an SCI were not expected to live for more than 2 years, let alone take part in sports programmes. Despite the inception of the Sport Organization for the Deaf (Comité International des Sports des Sourds, CISS) in 1924 and the appearance of wheelchair basketball in the USA in 1945, it was not until 1948, with the birth of the Stoke Mandeville Games and the development of the International Stoke Mandeville Wheelchair Sports Federation (ISMWSF) in 1952

that sports for persons with physical disabilities began to develop in earnest.

Since the organization of the first Stoke Mandeville Games in 1948, at which 16 athletes competed, participation has risen to 3000 athletes attending the event in Seoul, Korea (1988) and over 4000 in Barcelona, Spain at the 1992 Summer Paralympics. Recently, over 600 athletes from 33 countries took part in the Sixth Winter Paralympics in Lillehammer, Norway and an estimated 5000 athletes will take part in the Tenth Summer Paralympic Games in Atlanta in 1996.

Development of organizations for persons with physical disabilities

Since the ISMWSF was founded, other organizations such as the International Sport Organization for the Disabled (ISOD) (1964), the CP International Sport and Recreation Association (CP-ISRA) (1978), the International Blind Sport Association (IBSA) (1981) and the International Sport Association for the Mentally Handicapped (INAS-FMH) (1986) have been founded. These organizations have all developed mandates of sports excellence, yet jealous guarding of territory and diversification of policies has led to the International Olympic Committee (IOC) expressing a need for one organization with which it could interact on a policy level. To this end the International Coordinating Committee (ICC) was founded in 1983 and later, in 1989, the International Paralympic Committee (IPC) was formed as the sole organization for sport for athletes with a disability, with the right to organize paralympic games and multidisciplinary championships and games. Finally, a united organizational front of the IPC was presented to the IOC in the movement towards integration into the Olympic Games.

Sports for children

These developments have mostly been associated primarily with adult sports. Despite the innovation and vision of individuals such as Rinda Neilsen in 1943 (Society and Home for

Crippled Children, Denmark) who emphasized the development of physical activity and sports experiences for children with rule structures as similar as possible to young athletes without disabilities, sports opportunities for children with a disability have been slow to develop.

BARRIERS TO INVOLVEMENT IN SPORTS AND PHYSICAL ACTIVITY PROGRAMMES

Schools and school physical education programmes

The role of the school is of particular importance in the discussion of sport for children. Over-stressed, inexperienced and reluctant teachers are often given added responsibility of providing meaningful movement experiences, not only for able-bodied children, but also for children with a disability during critical developmental stages. In the light of this, recent cuts in educational systems in Canada and, particularly, in adapted physical education give rise to concern. In addition, the costs associated with making older school facilities accessible for children with severe disabilities are prohibitive and accessibility remains an issue. The result is limited or no access to physical activity programmes.

Although the primary goals of physical education programmes have been skill acquisition, physical fitness and active participation, such objectives have received scant attention and programmes proceed without evaluation of movement outcomes (Watkinson, 1988). In addition to a lack of programme and outcome evaluation there is also concern with regard to professional preparation of teaching staff. A recent Canadian Association for Health, Physical Education and Recreation (CAHPER) survey suggested that only 50% of the physical educators in the area of adapted physical education had a degree and that of these, 19% had course credit in adapted physical education (Evans, 1988).

In addition to requirements of teacher training, there is a need for a continuum of programming options for modified or regular programmes and placement bases on reliable and valid assessment and, finally, adequate preparation for practising teachers (Goodwin, 1988). Dickenson (1988) has suggested the need for a review of the compulsory curriculum, financial assistance for equality of access for physical activity opportunities and higher profile for staff training.

There is unquestionably a need for a focus on school-based programmes and opportunities for young people with a disability if they are to have equal access to involvement and success in school and community-based sports and physical activity programmes.

Discrimination in the school system

Until recently, many children with a disability have been denied the right to participate in school sport. Several key court actions have helped to improve this situation. In *Grube* v. *Bethlehem Area School District 550* (1982) and *Hollonbeck* v. *Board of Education of Rochelle Township* (1988) two children with a kidney disorder and a spinal cord injury, respectively, gained the right to participate in school sport having previously been excluded. In the latter case, the judge ruled that the child's civil rights had been violated.

Medical profession and overprotection

Traditionally, the medical profession has been reluctant to recommend vigorous school-based physical education and/or community sports programmes for children. Physicians have been concerned about the risks of exacerbation of existing physical conditions and the *real* risks of litigation. Alberts (1984) states that the American Medical Association guidelines for student athletes discriminate against persons with a disability. On the issue of limiting access to physical activity, the American Academy of Pediatrics has stated that 'the list is becoming increasingly obsolete due to changes in both safety equipment and in society attitudes toward the rights of athletes to compete despite a medical condition that may increase the risk of straining and injury or aggravating a pre-existing medical condition' (American Academy of Pediatrics, 1988). However, physicians are beginning to recognize the true value of sport participation and it is suggested that physical activity and sport should be promoted, if not prescribed, rather than inhibited by physicians (de Mondenard, 1991). Overprotection is also a factor in the home and school environment by parents, teachers, principles and the child himself or herself. Others suggest that increasing knowledge of medical difficulties associated with sports participation including drug interactions will assist in removing medical barriers to participation (Peck & McKeag, 1994).

Public knowledge and attitudes: the 'fear' question

The concept of children with physical disabilities being integrated into community sports programmes is often daunting and prohibitive for the volunteers that manage these programmes. Traditional fears regarding persons with a disability may discourage many from volunteering. Recently, some efforts have been made by coaching organizations to educate volunteers and would-be coaches.

Physical disability as a barrier

The physical disability of the child is in itself a barrier to involvement in sports programmes. Without the assistance of volunteers and communities many individuals are unable to participate in the sports arena. Other issues include:
1 Declining physical strength in progressive neuromuscular disorders.
2 Cognitive difficulties and brain injury.
3 Mobility problems, contractures and deformities due to paralysis and impaired motor control associated with CP.

Knowledge of volunteers and coaches

Assisting with and developing appropriate sports and training programmes demands at least a basic knowledge of the disability in question and the implications for performance. Traditionally, volunteer coaches have had little training and that which is available to the coach deals mainly with able-bodied children. Although some sports organizations, in Canada for example, have adopted the Canadian National Coaching Certification Program for coaches of children with a disability, e.g. basketball, athletics and swimming; much remains to be done in this regard.

Availability of community sports programmes

Relatively few programmes are available at the community level. Many existing programmes cater mainly for adults although considerable progress is being made in this regard.

Availability and accessibility of facilities

Catering for children with a disability is an expensive proposition since costly adaptations are required; wheelchair access is an example. However, considerable progress has been made in this area.

Congenital or acquired disability

Disability that is acquired or congenital, together with the age of the child, represent complicating factors in the initiation and/or continuation of involvement in sport.

Motor disabilities: implications for performance, training and assessment

Fitness levels of children with motor disabilities

A variety of factors affect the overall fitness levels of children with a disability including:
1 The nature of the disability.
2 The severity of the disability.
3 Overprotection and hypokinesis associated with sociocultural factors (Bar-Or, 1986; Shephard, 1992).

Furthermore, Shephard (1992) has observed that school physical education programmes all too frequently engender negative attitudes towards physical activity. It has even been suggested that 'students rush to cease exercising once the physical activity requirement has been removed' (Ilmarinen & Rutenfranz, 1980). Bar-Or (1986) suggests that children with a disability and sick children display abnormal exercise capacity due to two main causes: (i) hypoactivity leading to detraining; and (ii) specific pathophysiological factors limiting one or more exercise-related functions.

Illness and disease and their resulting disability can lead to hypoactivity due to loss of function in severe arthritis, advanced MD, limb paralysis, extreme malnutrition (including feeding problems in CP), respiratory failure and/or cardiac failure. It is important to realize that the hypoactive unfit child, irrespective of the initial cause of hypoactivity, often enters a vicious circle of further hypoactivity and detraining. While the mechanisms of detraining as a result of hypoactivity have not been systematically studied in children it can be assumed that these are similar to those found in adults (Bar-Or, 1986).

General implications of disability on fitness and trainability

The major effects of disability and/or illness and hypoactivity are:

1 Low maximal aerobic power.
2 High submaximal oxygen cost of daily activity and submaximal exercise.
3 Low muscle strength and endurance (Bar-Or, 1986).

LOW MAXIMAL AEROBIC POWER

Aerobic power is reduced in children with MD, scoliosis, SCI, CP, amputations and OI compared to those without a disability. Bar-Or (1986) suggests that respiratory muscle weakness, impaired oxygen extraction, muscle blood flow and mechanical inefficiencies affect levels of aerobic capacity (oxygen uptake) in children with a motor disability.

Low arterial oxygen content of blood due to insufficient oxygenation and respiratory muscle weakness may affect children with scoliosis where maximum breathing is affected at high exercise intensity levels (Bar-Or, 1986). Decreased static and dynamic lung volume, stiffening of the rib cage and increased energy cost of breathing contributes to decreased aerobic power in CP. Also, small lung volume resulting in restriction of vascular beds, pulmonary hypertension and long periods of inactivity associated with circulatory insufficiency contributes to low fitness levels (Bjure, et al., 1969). The degree of scoliosis is important since aerobic power is reduced in severe cases due to impaired ventilatory function, hypoactivity and detraining, but is normal in moderate scoliosis (Shephard, 1990).

When oxygen extraction in working muscle or muscle blood flow is impaired, mixed venous content is high and maximal aerobic power is low. This may occur when muscle is atrophied in Duchenne's MD, spina bifida and SCI (Bar-Or, 1986).

A high oxygen cost of an absolute workload may limit endurance during a task. This may occur in both upper and lower extremity disorders when the energy cost of walking, running, cycling or wheelchair propulsion is high (Bar-Or, 1986). Conditions in which oxygen cost of an absolute work load is increased include: CP, amputations, scoliosis and MD (Bar-Or, 1986). Bar-Or et al. (1976) reported decreased mechanical efficiency in both trained and untrained children with CP despite improvements in aerobic capacity in a training group. Adolescents with CP are less willing to be ambulatory which may reflect the high energy cost of ambulation (Molbech, 1966) and may result in reduced aerobic capacity or power.

A combination of factors including level of the lesion, loss of vascular tone, decreased venous return and decreased functional muscle mass result in lower absolute oxygen uptakes in SCI children (Bale, 1992; Shepard, 1992).

Aerobic capacity in SCI is affected by level of the lesion (i.e. severity of disability) (Shephard, 1990) although aerobic power of trained SCI may be marginally less (Zwiren et al., 1973; Zwiren & Bar-Or, 1975) or even surpass individuals without a disability (Shephard, 1990). Aerobic power and capacity is limited in young children with CP as a function of impaired involvement in sport due to muscle spasms, athetoid movements, rigidity, lack of coordination, tremor or general lack of muscle tone (Shephard, 1990). Lundberg (1978) reported decreased aerobic capacity in children, 11−12 years of age with spastic diplegia as well as 50% reductions in physical working capacity and decreased peak postexercise lactic acid levels. Aerobic capacity of adults with CP may be 10−30% below 'normal' (Bar-Or et al., 1976), although Bar-Or et al. (1976) reported decreased submaximal exercise heart rates and 8% increase in aerobic power in a group of CP and poliomyelitic adolescents following a 12-month training programme. Although aerobic power may be reduced by 40% in adults with scoliosis (Stoboy, 1985), very little data is available in children. Peak aerobic power is poor in adults with neuromuscular disorders (Carroll et al., 1979) reflecting decreased perfusion of active tissue (Kay & Shephard, 1969) and decreased cardiopulmonary function (Inkley et al., 1974). In both amputees and MD, there has been a paucity of work in children.

HIGH SUBMAXIMAL ENERGY COST OF PHYSICAL ACTIVITY: DECREASED MECHANICAL EFFICIENCY

Inability to sustain a physical task may result from high metabolic cost of performing this task. In some disabilities (diseases) this is manifested by a high metabolic cost during running or walking but can also occur during arm cranking, propelling of a wheelchair or performing other movements (Bar-Or, 1986). Above normal oxygen consumption during submaximal tasks occurs in CP (Berg & Bjure, 1970; Lundberg, 1975, 1976, 1978; Bar-Or et al., 1976), amputees (Bard & Ralston, 1959; Molbech, 1966), advanced

scoliosis (Lindh, 1978) and neuromuscular diseases (Carroll et al., 1979).

LOW MUSCLE STRENGTH

Muscle strength is reduced in children with CP, MD, scoliosis, OI, SCI and amputations (Bar-Or, 1986). In Duchenne MD the strength of the affected child declines with age (de Lateur & Giaconi, 1979) and is as low as the 5th percentile by the age of 7−8 years and may be 2 SD below normal levels (Hosking et al., 1976). Hosking et al. (1976) examined grip strength in 61 children with neuromuscular disorders and reported grip strength values below the 5th percentile compared to normal children. Only 8% of their sample achieved muscle strength scores at the minimal expected values for their age. Further impairment in strength is likely due to peripheral nerve degeneration (Chretien et al., 1987). Asymmetry of muscle deterioration leads to contractures, deformities and loss of balance leading to hypoactivity which exacerbates atrophy. For example, asymmetrical shortening of the triceps surae results in preferential limb loading on the superior flexing foot, preventing knee flexion contracture on that side. The opposite knee develops fixed flexion resulting in unbalanced gait as strength declines asymmetrically (Bowker & Halpin, 1978).

In CP, low strength probably reflects alterations in muscle fibre characteristics towards a higher percentage of fast-twitch fibres (Castle et al., 1979). In scoliosis, muscle strength and endurance falls below normal due to the high energy cost of ambulation and hypoactivity associated with embarrassment (Shepard, 1990).

In SCI, muscle strength differences among paraplegics and quadriplegics are not highly correlated with disability classification (Kofsky et al., 1983; Shephard, 1990). Paraplegics, as a group, showed increased strength versus those without a disability (Cameron et al., 1978; Grimby, 1980) and Stoboy and Wilson-Rich (1971) and Nakamura (1973) have shown increased elbow strength of older adults with a disability versus young people without a disability. Strength differences among spinally injured athletes may also be dependent on the type of test protocols used, including isometric and isokinetic tests and hand grip strength (Shephard, 1990). Increased strength with age has been demonstrated in wheelchair-dependent adults (Stoboy & Wilson-Rich, 1971). Most investigations of strength in wheelchair users has been conducted in adults although low hand grip strength has been demonstrated in 141 paraplegic children and adolescents (Winnick & Short, 1984).

LOW MUSCLE ENDURANCE AND PEAK POWER

Muscle endurance is also reduced in children with MD, CP, OI and scoliosis and may reflect the high energy cost of ambulation and resultant hypoactivity. In MD, limitations on physical capacities are due to muscle endurance factors rather than due to deficiencies in the oxygen transport system (Bar-Or, 1986). Mean anaerobic power is reduced by as much as $2-4$ SD below the mean (Bar-Or, 1983) and there is a reduced 'metabolic index' (ratio of peak anaerobic to peak aerobic power) (Bar-Or, 1983) in children with Duchenne's MD. Hosking *et al.* (1976) also reported reduced muscle endurance as measured by 45° head and leg lift in children with MD. In a study of 61 children with neuromuscular disorders the authors reported that 89% failed to meet a minimum timed muscle endurance head elevation standard and 76% failed to reach a minimum leg elevation standard (5th percentile). Winnick and Short (1984) have demonstrated decreased muscle endurance in children and adolescents with paraplegia due to SCI as indicated by flexed arm hang and pull-ups scores.

Both peak and mean power output as assessed by the Wingate anaerobic test are subnormal in children with MD (Bar-Or, 1983, 1986). Anaerobic power and endurance in children 6–14 years of age was significantly reduced on the Wingate anaerobic test when corrected for body weight (Parker *et al.*, 1992). Peak and mean power output was $3-4$ SD below normal in

moderate to severe CP. Anaerobic power is limited due to severely compromised ability to 'spin' on a cycle or arm ergometer (Parker *et al.*, 1992) and associated with failure of normal reciprocal inhibition (Berbayer & Ashby, 1990; Parker *et al.*, 1992). Low muscle mass in CP (Lundberg, 1978) as a function of chronic shortening due to spasticity and contractures limiting muscle growth (Nash *et al.*, 1989) may also serve to limit anaerobic power in CP.

PAUCITY OF DATA

Most work reported on fitness levels of persons with a disability is based on adults. Relatively few controlled investigations have been computed on children (Shephard, 1990, 1992), due to logistical and ethical constraints making it less feasible to perform well-designed intervention studies with sick (disabled) children (Bar-Or, 1990). What is clear is that exercise and training can improve their fitness levels. Recent investigations suggest that carefully controlled training programmes can result in significant improvements in aerobic power in preadolescent children (Shephard, 1992). Although it is difficult to equate adult and child programmes on workload, there is no immediate evidence that the training responses of the prepubescent child is any less than that of an older person. For example, in CP small changes in aerobic power and 20–30% improvement in walking speed were reported following a twice weekly, 2-year training programme (Spira & Bar-Or, 1975; Bar-Or *et al.*, 1976). Others have also reported training changes in children with CP (Berg, 1970). Dresen *et al.* (1985) reported a 10% decrease in oxygen uptake in CP at submaximal workloads following a 10-week programme. Bjure *et al.* (1969) reported that 3 months of training three times a week on circuit-type activities resulted in decreased heart rate at submaximal workloads and a 22% increase in aerobic power in 16–27-year-old girls with scoliosis.

Disability-specific effects on physiological systems

Effects of specific motor disabilities on physiological systems and fitness are summarized in Table 32.1.

Implications of disability on participation in sport and the design of training programmes

Implications for performance and considerations in the design of training programmes may be considered under three main headings: (i) physiological; (ii) psychological; and (iii) ethical factors. A brief discussion on specific training considerations is presented below and a general summary of considerations in the design of training programmes is presented in Table 32.2.

PHYSIOLOGICAL CONSIDERATIONS

Decreased mechanical and metabolic efficiency

Activities to improve mechanical efficiency are important considerations in the design of training programmes for young athletes. The use of different types of prostheses in amputees is an important consideration. The use of the Flex foot over the SACH foot increases energy return and efficiency in below-knee amputees (Schneidier *et al.*, 1993). Frobose (1989, 1992) reported improved dynamic gait in children with CP after 6 months of an intensive movement and sports therapy programme. Butler *et al.* (1992) reported improvements in the walking performance of six children with CP after 4–6 months of ankle–foot orthosis training. Following training, balance and posture was improved and knee–ankle movements approached 'normal' patterns.

Weak hip extensors contribute to walking problems in CP and should be addressed in the design of training programmes. Ten weeks of hip extensor training using a tricycle produced improved gait without increased hip strength in children with CP (King *et al.*, 1993). Carmick

(1993) utilized a combination of functional electrical stimulation (FES) and motor learning tasks and produced significant improvements in locomotor efficiency in three males under 10 years of age. The physiological cost index was improved fourfold in one child and twofold in another. This suggests that FES might be a useful adjunct in physical therapy programmes for improving function in children with CP.

Water-based training programmes are also a worthwhile consideration. Ishida *et al.* (1989) compared the energy cost of walking in air and water in children with CP. Walking in water decreased energy cost of movement for children with crouched posture and spasticity and may be a useful adjunct in training regimens. Other factors which may improve mechanical efficiency of athletes during performance include advances in the design of wheelchairs.

Thermoregulation

A critical consideration in the design of training programmes and during competition is thermoregulation. Thermoregulatory dysfunction is a problem in SCI (Bloomquist, 1986) and may be exacerbated by physical activity, training and/or competition. Thermoregulatory problems may present as hypothermia or hyperthermia even in relatively mild temperatures (10–15.5°C or 50–60°F). The athlete should take in adequate amounts of water and, at the first sign of heat or cold injury should be removed from the environment and treatment sought promptly (Peck & McKeag, 1994).

Drug interactions

Combining exercise, training and medications can have serious consequences for athletes. Physicians should be aware of potential side-effects of drugs including dizziness, nausea, vomiting, fatigue, stomach ulcers, weakness and loss of appetite (Peck & McKeag, 1994). For example, Peck and McKeag (1994) note that concomitant use of theophylline (asthma control) and erythromycin can increase theophylline to toxic levels. Seizure medications may cause feelings of sedation. Physicians and coaches should be aware of side-effects and physician-directed dose changes should be implemented if the young athlete shows side-effects.

Risk for injury

Overuse conditions and psychological factors are an increasing concern among sport medicine experts although scant attention has been paid to this area regarding young athletes.

Recent reports have suggested frequent and consistent patterns of injuries in disability sport. Injuries most commonly reported by athletes are lacerations, contusions, sprains, strains and abrasions (Stewart, 1983; Monohan, 1986; Martinez, 1989; Ferrara & Davis, 1990; Hoeberigs *et al.*, 1990). According to Burnham *et al.* (1991), injuries among members of the Canadian Paralympic Team could be classified as musculoskeletal, general medical and disability-related. Richter *et al.* (1991) found that 60% of athletes with CP at the Paralympic Games in 1988 reported injuries and illness while Ferrara *et al.* (1992) found an injury rate of 32% among different disability groups in his study. In contrast very little work has been done on injury rates among paediatric athletes. Wilson and Washington (1993) surveyed 247 competitors at the 1990 Junior National Wheelchair Games (USA) and reported that of respondents to an injury survey, 97% of track athletes, 22% of field participants and 91% of swimming competitors reported injuries. Incidence of shoulder injuries was high in track and swimming, which supported work done in sport for adults. Risk factors associated with childhood injuries can be divided into intrinsic and extrinsic factors.

Anatomical considerations. Growing cartilage surfaces and joint alignment are critical intrinsic factors. This is particularly important when considering the child with a disability. Where gait is affected such as in CP, scoliosis, MD and amputees, joint alignment is likely to be compromised. This increases the risk of joint damage

due to repetitive impact trauma in events such as running. In children who use wheelchairs, the shoulder, elbow and hand are particularly susceptible due to damage to growing joint surfaces. A high incidence of shoulder injuries was reported in adult wheelchair basketball (Burnham *et al.*, 1994) although there is little information on child athletes. In sports such as swimming, awkward movements leading to imperfect swimming strokes, produce excessive stresses on the shoulder joint. And in young children with OI, excessive stress of bone and joint surfaces may exacerbate the existing condition.

Adolescent growth factors. These are important intrinsic factors. During the adolescent growth spurt unequal growth of bones, tendons, ligaments and musculature result in problems such as Osgood−Schlatter disease, Sever's disease and patellofemoral pain syndrome. In addition, decreased flexibility results in excessive localized stresses on bone and joint surfaces (Dalton, 1992). Alterations in growth rate may exaggerate already impaired movement patterns of limbs and therefore add to the risk of injury. In amputees, running style may be altered and shoulder rotation patterns may be affected for children using wheelchairs in their sports.

Physiological factors. The effects of exercise and possible dietary abuses on the development of bone (as discussed in Chapter 9) raises serious questions with regard to excessive training practices in young children with joint misalignment and gait problems. These can be important intrinsic factors. It is of particular concern in children with degenerative bone disorders and those who are engaged in repetitive training regimens involving the upper extremities.

Psychological factors. Risk-taking behaviours may be an important intrinsic factor in the development of sport injuries in young children. Our work with SCI suggests that risk taking is a particularly strong trait in this group

Table 32.1 Disability-specific effects on physiological systems in young children.

Disability	Affected system or function							Comments
	Cardiovascular	Respiratory	$\dot{V}o_{2\,max}$	Oxygen cost of movement (efficiency)	Peak anaerobic power	Muscular strength	Muscular endurance	
SCI	X	X	X	X	X	X	X	Deficit depends on level of lesion. Paraplegics generally fitter than quadriplegics. Most work completed on adults. Generally high active SCI are fitter than inactive SCI and may have higher fitness levels than able bodied. Thermoregulatory problems: heat gain and dissipation a concern during training and competition
CP	X	X	X	X	X	X	X	Depends on limbs affected and degree of spasticity and CP classification. Address losses of muscular strength and endurance as a priority during training. Functional electrical stimulation and swimming may increase metabolic efficiency of ambulation (running and walking)
Amputees	?X	?X	X?	X	?X	?X	?X	Virtually no controlled experimental work done. Potential for low fitness due to post-trauma hypoactivity. Energy cost of movement affected by prosthesis design

MD	X	X	X	X	X	Loss of functional muscle mass results in hypoactivity and declining cardiovascular fitness, strength and endurance levels. Very little work done in children
OI	?X	?X	?X	?X	?X	Concern for spontaneous fracturing during training and competition may limit opportunity. No work in this area regarding children
Scoliosis	X	X	X	?	X	Effects on fitness parameters depend on severity of scoliosis. Effects mentioned refer to severe scoliosis. Limitations in aerobic fitness a function of postural problems versus cardiac function

X, system affected; ?, lack of published information; ?X, no data available (in theory system may be affected). CP, cerebral palsy; MD, muscular dystrophy; OI, osteogenesis imperfecta; SCI, spinal cord injury.

Table 32.2 Disability-specific considerations in the design of training programmes and for competition in young children.

Training factor	SCI	CP	Scoliosis	Amputees	MD	OI
Aerobic power	Aerobic capacity varies according to lesion level and degree of hypoactivity. Trainability will depend on lesion level. Hypotension at high workloads. Overuse injuries in shoulder with repetitive training regimens. Progressive overload principle. Consider thermoregulatory difficulties during prolonged work-outs	Low levels of aerobic power associated with hypoactivity due to athetoid movements and spasticity. Trainability dependent on degree of spasticity. High energy cost of activity limits endurance in tasks. Consider water-based training and cycling. Attend to aerobic power secondary to remedial strength work	Low levels of aerobic power associated with hypoactivity, energy cost of ambulation, chest deformity, pulmonary and ventilatory function. Balance remediation of aerobic training with potential for exacerbating condition (e.g. impact stress). Consider cycling and swimming exercise as alternatives for maintaining/developing aerobic base	Low levels of aerobic fitness due to hypoactivity. Important to maintain activity levels and aerobic capacity following amputation. Improvements in aerobic power may be influenced by choice and suitability of prosthesis (see mechanical efficiency)	Duration of the disorder will affect the degree of muscle atrophy and subsequent losses of aerobic fitness and muscular strength and endurance. Avoid exacerbation of condition due to chronic fatigue	Low cardiovascular fitness reflecting overprotection. Care in selection of aerobic activities that may result in serious falls. Swimming and cycling as low impact adjuncts to training regimens.
Muscle strength and endurance	Limitations in available muscle mass a function of lesion level. Choice of activity and equipment should reflect considerations regarding trunk stability. Safety issues with free weights must be addressed. Innovations such as the 'Equalizer' gym are excellent adjuncts to training systems. Consider use of 'tubing' as a means of education regarding principles of strength training. Check for hypertension if using tubing	Limited muscular strength and endurance secondary to hypoactivity. Consider effects of increased muscular strength on tremor and spasms. Careful evaluation of strength and plan to remediate weaknesses. Attend to severe losses of strength and endurance as a priority prior to training for aerobic capacity. Rehabilitate weak hip extensors. Initiate strengthening early in life to allow for maintaining aerobic fitness levels	Decreased muscular strength and endurance due to hypoactivity and high energy cost of ambulation. Balance strengthening activities against potential for asymmetrical muscle development and possible exacerbation of condition. Use of surgical tubing for technique development as well as strength training. Water training for resistance training regimens an excellent adjunct to training regimens	Decreased functional muscle mass. Decreased ability to exert maximal effort due ambulatory inefficiencies, balance and gait problems. Careful choice of activities with consideration re: balance and control during resistance training. Consider surgical tubing as a training option and for developing technique	Loss of strength and endurance dependent on duration of disability and degree of neural impairment and muscle atrophy. Muscle strength declines with age. Muscle strength gains masked by progressive decline in muscle strength. Surgical tubing may be successfully employed for resistance training from a wheelchair	Decreased muscular strength and endurance a function of hypoactivity and 'overprotection'. Care with strengthening activities since it is unclear regarding fracture thresholds of bones in these children. Care with any resistance training in which children may lose control and drop weights

Mechanical efficiency	High energy cost of wheelchair propulsion in untrained state. Gradual increases in training intensity and volume	High energy cost of ambulation produces reluctance in physical activity. Water training useful	Energy cost of activity increased by awkward gait. Cycling and swimming decrease energy cost of ambulation and provide support for limbs	Increased energy cost of ambulation due to lower limb loss consider type of prosthesis utilized. Flex foot more 'efficient' than SACH foot	Decreased mechanical efficiency as muscle function deteriorates	No information published. Unlikely to be affected in this group
Balance and gait	Lesion level and trunk stability should be considered in setting up programmes. Seating position for wheelchair and weight/resistance training	Balance is limited. Awkward gait. Care with unassisted activities — free weights	Awkward gait and high energy costs of ambulation	Awkward gait with amputation. Gait dependent on prosthesis	Contractures affect balance. Care with activities involving weights	Care with activities in which child may lose balance and fall (cycling)
Flexibility	Consider shoulder range of motion to avoid overuse conditions. Adequate warm-up and stretching programme for shoulder musculature should always precede training sessions. Partner-assisted (static passive) stretching should be employed but monitored carefully	Muscle spasms, athetoid movements, rigidity, lack of coordination, tremor and lack of muscle tone limits flexibility. Develop a progressive flexibility programme. Use partner-assisted exercises under supervision. Consistent warm-up and stretching activities prior to activity	Careful selection of flexibility exercises to avoid exacerbation of condition. Important to maintain flexibility in unaffected joints	Develop regular progressive flexibility training programme. Use of partner-assisted programmes and PNF type stretching acceptable. Monitor any partner-assisted stretching carefully especially with younger athletes	Maintain flexibility to ameliorate/overcome effects of contractures. Partner stretching important — static passive and PNF. Careful monitoring of partner-assisted stretching regimens. Natural progression of deterioration may be slowed by vigorous and persistent stretching of triceps surae, hamstrings, posterior tibial muscles and iliotibial tracts	Develop static active flexibility training programme. Particular care with partner-assisted stretching program (static passive or PNF stretching)
Overuse conditions	Volume of training must take into account limited muscle mass. Effects of chronic repetitive strain on shoulder joint. Proper seat fit, frequent pressure releases and padding to avoid pressure sores. Use of hand protection to avoid carpal tunnel syndrome	Effects of chronic repetitive training and awkward gait on joint integrity	Potential for overuse injury in joints due to awkward gait	Potential for overuse conditions in non-prosthetic limb due to gait problems. Choice of prosthesis and careful control of training volume	Main problem is fatigue due to declining functional muscle mass. May be partly ameliorated through physical activity and training	Chronic repetitive stress may result in fractures of long bones. Essential that diet is maintained — adequate dietary calcium. Consider regular physical check-ups and respond to any localized limb pain

Continued

Table 32.2 (Continued).

Training factor	SCI	CP	Scoliosis	Amputees	MD	OI
Training principles	As per able-bodied children (frequency, intensity, duration, overload and progression)	As per able-bodied children	As per able-bodied children	As per able-bodied children	As per able-bodied children	As per able-bodied children
Psychological factors	Hypokinesis associated with a new injury — a loss of hope. Motivation may be poor at outset of training programme	Self-concept affected by disability. Self-concept of CP athletes comparable to able-bodied youth	Low self-esteem and poor body image due to appearance. May also affect involvement in activity	Initial effects of loss of limb may affect motivation to become or stay involved in physical activity/ training	Psychological consequences of a decline in function despite remedial — training efforts on part of the child	Fear of spontaneous fracturing may affect willingness to participate in sport
Particular concerns	Osteopenia (bone loss) and risk for minimal trauma fracture — care with transfers and weight training. Thermoregulatory problems in hot or cold environments. Be alert for use of autonomic dysreflexia for improving performance	Limitations in motor performance and fine motor control due to spasticity, athetoid movements, rigidity, tremors and lack of coordination. Care with activity selection	Care with exacerbation of existing conditions. Problems depend on degree of scoliosis — care with severe cases	Potential for overuse of non-prosthetic limb. Careful selection of type of prosthesis may enhance performance potential. Some children may be significantly overweight	Coach or trainer must take into account declining physical functioning in spite of training for maintaining a safe training environment	Coach or trainer must provide a safe environment and be constantly alert for potential falls or contacts. Contact sports are contraindicated
Nutritional considerations	High carbohydrate diet. Adequate fluid intake during training and prolonged events. Vigilance for use of illegal ergogenic aids. Nutritional supplementation should be discussed with a dietician/ medical professional	As per SCI	As per SCI	As per SCI	As per SCI	As per SCI

CP, cerebral palsy; MD, muscular dystrophy; OI, osteogenesis imperfecta; PNF, proprioceptive neuromuscular facilitation; SCI, spinal cord injury.

and is often a causal factor in the original injury (Wheeler *et al.*, 1993a,b). In addition, these athletes may show particular determination to succeed in a sports environment and render themselves likely to injuries due to carelessness. Lathen *et al.* (1988) reported that 63.6% of a group of individuals with a disability chose high risk sports such as white water rafting as sports they would most like to attempt. Desire to participate in high risk sport was highly related to past participation in risk sports.

Training programmes. Probably the single most important extrinsic factor in the development of injuries in children in sports is the training programme (Dalton, 1992; see also Chapters 11 and 13). Often coach and community awareness of the dangers of excessive training is poor and excessive demands placed upon children by poorly designed programmes both in and out of season results in both acute and chronic injury. A lack of awareness of physiological limitations to training stresses, such as in SCI and structural limitations due to joint misalignment, for example, may lead to serious overuse injury if training programmes are too strenuous.

Coaching errors may also contribute to sport injury due to lack of knowledge with regards to rules and game structures. This is of particular importance for young athletes engaged in sports such as wheelchair basketball which is potentially hazardous unless the rules are followed carefully. Excessive contact, may result in damage to hands and arms trapped in wheelchair spokes. As well, regulation foot plates are essential to minimize risk for lower limb injury.

Equipment. Prostheses and wheelchairs are of additional concern to equipment directly involved in the sport and constitute an important extrinsic factor in sport injury. Safety issues regarding training equipment such as weight-training systems and wheelchair maintenance are pertinent. Also, during competition, stable positions in throwing events must be ensured as well as the integrity of other competition-associated equipment. It is extremely important that the coach is aware of the need for bracing and protective clothing in certain disabilities. Also, routine equipment checks should be conducted by coaches and athletes.

Environment. The sport environment is a critical extrinsic factor in the occurrence of injuries in child athletes. For example, glass-contaminated playing surfaces, poorly prepared baseball diamonds or debris on a basketball court all increase risk for injury. The rules of a safe sport environment do not differ whether the sport is for children with or without disabilities.

Overtraining concerns. These constitute extrinsic factors for injury. Motor disabilities often result in either excessive use of a dominant or non-prosthetic limb or the use of alternative limbs for ambulation. Alterations in gait and mechanical efficiency of ambulation may increase the likelihood of overuse conditions in children with motor disabilities. In SCI, overuse injuries in the shoulder are a concern for young athletes. In CP and amputees, the effects of chronic gait alterations may cause stress and deterioration in joint articular surfaces. Several investigations have demonstrated the importance of type of prosthetic limb and effects on impact stress and gait in amputees. Ensberg *et al.* (1993a,b) demonstrated asymmetrical loading of the non-prosthetic limb and altered gait patterns in below-knee amputees versus children without a disability during running and walking. Schneider *et al.* (1993) analysed gait kinematics and dynamics during self-selected comfortable and fast speeds in 6–16-year-old children using the SACH and energy storing Flex foot and reported that the Flex foot had a greater potential for reducing the energy cost of walking at comfortable and fast speeds. Improvements in gait and decreased energy cost of ambulation are important in the prevention of overuse conditions. The effects of high impact stress in cases of severe scoliosis must be considered as well as the effects of awkward gait on the integrity of joint surfaces. In OI, the effects of decreased bone strength must be considered along with the chronic stresses that are applied to bone, for example, during strengthening regimens.

PSYCHOLOGICAL CONSIDERATIONS

Benefits of sports participation

Very little work has been completed regarding the psychology of the young athlete (Sherrill et al., 1990). The assumption has been that since there are parallels in constructs between adult athletes without a disability and athletes with a disability, both will follow a similar trend in terms of the psychological outcomes of sports participation.

Varni and Setoguchi (1991) examined perceived physical appearance of children with acquired and congenital limb deficiencies. Higher classmate approval and teacher and social support were predictive of higher perceived physical appearance. High peer acceptance, scholastic competence and athletic competence were also predictive of perceived physical appearance. Harter (1987) noted that perceived physical appearance was one of the highest predictors of self-esteem and that perceived social worth is intimately tied to cultural values with regard to physical appearance. Sherrill et al. (1990) examined the self-concept of youth at the Pan-American Victory Games for Disabled Youth and reported self-concept scores in the range for youths without a disability in a group of CP, amputees, SCI, dwarfs and Les Autrés.

As a group, children with a disability have been found to be at risk for psychological problems (Cadman et al., 1987; Wallander et al., 1988) which may increase due to societal attitudes towards physical disability and physical appearance (Richardson, 1970). Therefore, physical activity plays an important role in self and social acceptance. Since children acquire their version of normalcy from adults and the media (Varni and Setoguchi, 1991), the deification of the perfect body form, as represented in many magazines and health publications, presents a significant threat to their body image. The role of sport in the life of the young child, particularly during adolescence, may well be crucial in terms of contributing to a healthy self-esteem and body image.

Type of disability

A factor that should be kept in mind by the coach or trainer is that of disability type, i.e. whether the disability is congenital or acquired. A child who has previously been active in sports and acquires SCI must learn to adjust to new levels of capabilities and may face retraining. This young athlete must also adjust to arms as a primary means of propulsion rather than legs. The young athlete who has grown up with a disability faces different challenges. At a time when participation and success in sport becomes important, the young prepubescent athlete with MD, faces declining function in spite of training and the child with CP, scoliosis or an amputation must overcome factors such as mechanical inefficiency, balance and gait problems during their development as athletes. The coach or trainer must therefore be sensitive to a variety of frustrations that such young athletes may experience including general and disability-specific issues.

Consequences of overuse conditions

Perhaps the most serious consequences of excessive training regimens and involvement in high stress competition situations among children, are those of a psychological nature. The effects of a 'secondary' disability brought about by overuse, such as a shoulder injury in a wheelchair athlete could conceivably have disastrous consequences for the young athlete whose life was tied to athletics. Work completed at the Rick Hansen Centre (Wheeler et al., 1993b) strongly supports the notion that participation in sport represents an important part of the coping and adjustment process to a traumatic injury and the 'losses' associated with it. Furthermore, athletes expressed some degree of fear of life after sport was over. The psychological effects of debilitating injuries which seriously interrupt or terminate athletic participation in child athletes have yet to be examined.

Eating disorders

Recent evidence suggests an increase in the incidence of eating disorders and an association of eating disorders with the sport environment for those without a disability, including runners, ballet dancers and figure skaters (Frisch *et al.*, 1980; Smith, 1980; Yates *et al.*, 1983; Warren, 1985, 1988). Current theoretical perspectives consider that aetiological and maintenance factors transcend the boundaries of social learning theory, behavioural psychology, physiology and phylogeny (e.g. Epling & Pierce, 1988). The coach must be aware that there are often complicating factors affecting dietary behaviours in those with physical/motor disabilities. These factors are superimposed on normal cultural and social pressures upon young athletes to achieve ideal body shapes.

In CP, in particular, there are often mechanical feeding problems which contribute to lower mean weights and heights in children (Thommessen *et al.*, 1991a,b). A relationship is suggested between feeding problems and growth in children with CP (Ruby & Matheny, 1961). Feeding problems such as delayed self-feeding, oral motor dysfunction, poor appetite and meal time tantrums are frequent in children with various disabilities (Palmer, 1978; Webb, 1980; Howard, 1981; Rice, 1981). The prevalence of feeding problems and growth ranges from 13 to 33% (Kraemer *et al.*, 1978; Gingell *et al.*, 1981).

Therefore, it is extremely important for coaches and teachers to evaluate risk factors for inadequate nutrition. Furthermore, coaches should recognize that the child with a disability may face a triple jeopardy regarding dietary behaviours.

1 The impact of physical activity *per se* on eating behaviours.

2 The role of culture on eating behaviours.

3 Disability-specific implications for feeding problems.

Coaches of athletes with a disability have a duty to be aware of the pressures regarding food intake in young children and should not promote dietary practices of a questionable nature or encourage weight control or reduction via self-starvation. Coaches must also be able to discriminate between disability-specific eating behaviours and disordered eating patterns associated with activity and/or sociocultural origins. Education of athletes in proper dietary practices is an essential part of development in the sports environment. At present we simply do not know the incidence of disordered eating patterns in athletes with a disability and susceptibility of these young athletes to exercise-associated eating disorders has not been investigated.

ETHICAL CONSIDERATIONS

Children in competition

Concerns have been discussed above regarding the competitive environment for the young athlete. In response to problems associated with underreporting of drop-out rates in many young athletes, Rutenfranz (1985) has suggested that we have a duty to protect young athletes and suggests a code of ethics regarding the treatment of young athletes in the competitive environment. Such a code would apply to the young athlete with a disability and is particularly pertinent given the rapid advancement of sport for athletes and the increased involvement of children in the athletic environment.

1 Use of the declarations of Helsinki and Tokyo in connection with human experiments in athletic training, respectively.

2 Athletes should give informed consent acknowledging the risks of sport.

3 Special health-care and prophylactic measures should be performed by physicians whose professional reputations are not dependent on the records of special young athletes.

4 Establishment of ethics commissions in the national sports organizations that are open to questions by children and their parents. Commissions should be independent with special experience in education, paediatrics, law and ethics and should discuss the control of risks of training methods for children.

5 Commissions should fix age limits for performance at the Olympic, national and international levels.

Performance enhancement

A most controversial area in sport for children is that of performance enhancement practices, including the use of androgenic anabolic steroids. The dilemma here is, perhaps, not if but when drug usage will enter the world of sports for children with a disability. As this practice has filtered down to young able-bodied athletes from the élite able-bodied athletic community, it is likely to encroach on the world of the young athlete with a disability. Athletics for the athlete with disabilities is no longer free from issues such as drug use (Peck & McKeag, 1994).

Since 1986, all first place finishers at the Stoke Mandeville Games have been tested for illegal use of banned drugs. Though no positive tests have occurred rumours abound regarding drug use in weight-lifters and power sports (Peck & McKeag, 1994). Other concerns expressed the potential for use of blood doping, erythropoietin and β-blocker abuse (Peck & McKeag, 1994). Early signs of performance-enhancing drugs and practices infiltrating sports for persons with a disability are clearly indicated by recent disciplinary action against two weight-lifters in 1991 and the detection of illegal substances in Paralympic athletes in the 1992 Barcelona Games. In addition, we have observed the use of questionable, if not highly dangerous, practices of 'boosting' (the use of autonomic dysreflexia) in wheelchair athletes in order to enhance performance (Burnham *et al.*, 1994).

For those who are sceptical that steroids are likely to become an issue in paediatric sport, the evidence is chilling. It has been estimated that between 4.4 and 20% of high school student and collegiate athletes in the USA have used anabolic steroids (Buckley *et al.*, 1988; Smith & Perry, 1992). A recent Canadian investigation suggested that there are up to 83 000 young persons in Canada indulging in anabolic steroids. There is currently no data available regarding child athletes with a disability. What would be the motivation for a child or adolescent to utilize performance-enhancing drugs such as anabolic steroids and will these athletes resort to this?

The use of such drugs would be highly desirable in terms of offsetting the effects of disability-induced atrophy and to enhance shoulder and arm strength for wheelchair sports, such as basketball, track-and-field events and weight-lifting. It would be naive to expect young athletes, who receive the same messages about success in sports and see the results of performance-enhancing drugs, to ignore the lure of these substances. The use of such substances may have additional deleterious effects on young athletes with a disability. The potential side-effects are like those in athletes without a disability and include a variety of alterations in secondary sex characteristics and inoperable cancers. In addition, the use of these drugs may produce significant mood changes and exacerbate periods of spasticity (due to increased muscle strength) in athletes with paralysis.

Intentional induction of autonomic dysreflexia for performance enhancement

A unique international conference in Jasper, Canada ('Vista '93') marked the first time that the issue of intentional induction of autonomic dysreflexia for performance enhancement was raised in public. Ironically, anecdotal evidence suggests that the practice is well known among élite wheelchair athletes and widely practised. News of this practice among wheelchair athletes with high lesion SCI has raised a moral and ethical dilemma for the International Sports Federations and the IPC.

Autonomic dysreflexia is a naturally occurring condition peculiar to quadriplegics and paraplegics with high lesions and traditionally had been considered a medical emergency. Noxious stimuli (e.g. fractures, full bladder and urinary tract infection) below the lesion level result in mass activation of the sympathetic nervous system with peripheral and splanchnic vasoconstriction and concomitant increases in blood pressure. Blood pressure rises unchecked, as ascending sympathetic messages cannot traverse the spinal cord lesion, therefore, the risk for a variety of aneurysms is great. Eventually, the baroreceptors in the aortic arch and carotid area mediate a parasympathetic response via the vagus nerve. Above the level of the lesion, there is marked vasodilation and facial flushing with sweating. The parasympathetic effect does not traverse the lesion, therefore systolic blood pressure may continue to rise (Burnham *et al.*, 1994).

Athletes have found that intentional induction of this condition enhances wheelchair racing performance and deliberately induce the condition by drinking large amounts of fluid before competition, clamping urinary catheters or strapping legs very tightly. Deliberate self-induced lower limb fractures are also rumoured to have been used. Unfortunately, the perception of performance benefits are accurate and a recent study (Burnham *et al.*, 1994) has demonstrated significantly improved wheelchair racing performance (9.7% improvements) as a result of this 'technique'. However, dangerously high blood pressure levels accompany these performance benefits. The 'technique' likely enhances performance by promoting preferential blood flow to working tissue as well as by a glycogen saving effect due to catecholamine-mediated increases in fat metabolism (Burnham *et al.*, 1994).

The dilemma facing the sport fraternity is how to identify the condition and, perhaps most difficult, how to legislate against a naturally occurring phenomenon. It is hoped that common sense will prevail before there is a tragedy in a young athlete mimicking the élite athlete.

This practice may be one of the most serious threats to the integrity of wheelchair sports.

Legal liability

Lubell (1987) has stated that, 'Rising insurance costs and huge liability awards are threatening the very existence of some sports and recreation programs. Only imaginative risk management will keep programs alive and help, physicians, athletic trainers and coaches avoid litigation'.

With increased potential for litigation, implications for sport are serious. Coaches and/or volunteers are unlikely to flock to sports for persons with a disability knowing the lawsuits for acts of negligence are on the increase. What constitutes reasonable practice in sport for those without a disability may not always be appropriate for an athlete with a disability. For example, given the dramatic loss of bone mass in the lower limbs of SCI, are high risk outdoor sports such a white water rafting and parachuting reasonable activities? Does encouragement of such 'risky' activity constitute reasonable behaviour? As younger athletes enter the foray of élite sports, issues of sport and legal liability are unlikely to diminish in the near future.

Integration, segregation and/or specialization and equity issues

A current movement in adapted physical education is towards integration of athletes into community programmes and into élite level competition. Thus integration was a major topic at the IPC General Assembly in Berlin in September of 1993 and, more recently, at a joint IPC Sports Science Committee and International Federation of Adapted Physical Activity joint working group held in Berlin in April, 1994. Integration may be considered as athletes being 'themselves as [athletes] among other [athletes] — to have their integrity as disabled athletes respected and as such allowed full opportunities to perform in competition' (Lindström, 1992). Ethically and morally, the child with a disability should not be denied access to any programmes. However, as previously mentioned, societal attitudes remain a major obstacle (Lindström, 1992). However, one must consider, that although there is a moral responsibility to include children in sports for able-bodied persons, it would be unethical to force a child to take part in a sport environment if he or she did not wish it. Some children may prefer not to be integrated into mainstream sport environments and these wishes must be respected.

A further issue of integration is the concept of integration of athletes with different disabilities into the same class in terms of athletic participation; the so-called integrated functional classification system, as opposed to the medical or disability-based systems.

Finally, the issue of integration and gender equity must be considered. We are presently examining gender issues and disability as it pertains to involvement of women with a disability in the élite sport environment. Despite the fact that approximately 50% of individuals with a disability in Canada are women, less than a third of athletes are women. It is unclear as to why this situation exists. However, what is abundantly clear, is that these young women and girls have fewer role models in élite sport which may result in less motivation to participate.

Retirement

As younger athletes take part in élite sport, so the potential retirement age has fallen. As young athletes participate at higher levels at earlier ages then so they retire voluntarily or are forced into retirement by injury. This area has not been investigated to date. Nonetheless, coaches must consider preparing the athlete for the postcompetition phase of his or her life. Given the importance of physical activity and competitive sport as part of the coping and adjustment process in SCI, for example (Wheeler *et al.*, 1993a), this is an essential consideration. The IPC Sports Science Committee, Berlin (1994)

recently identified retirement as one of the key issues for future research in the area of disability sport.

At present we are conducting an investigation on the implications of retirement from disability sport among a group of ex-athletes as well as athletes presently competing. Our initial findings suggest that the rise to 'fame' is often meteoric and that the experience of success is associated with a variety of positive factors including improved self-esteem, improved social network and the motivation to excel in other areas. What is clear, is that the athletes are often not prepared for the impact of retirement and experience significant losses in their lives as a result (Wheeler *et al.*, 1995). Given the move towards early participation, youth excellence, and early retirement and the importance of lifelong physical activity for health maintenance, the implications of cessation of activity due to injury of disillusionment are serious.

Fitness assessment in young athletes

In considering physiological testing of the child athlete, physiologists and/or coaches and trainers should consider that children respond differently to acute and chronic exercise stress than adults and that adult protocols may not be suitable due to differences in physical size, mental capacity and ability to comprehend instructions, attention span, emotional maturity or ethical constraints (Bar-Or, 1993). In principle, adult protocols and apparatus may be adapted to use for child athlete testing with certain modifications and considerations for physical and psychological needs of the child (Bar-Or, 1993). Also, prior to subjecting any child athlete to rigorous laboratory testing procedures coaches should consider: (i) why they are doing the tests; (ii) how valuable the information will be (predictive of performance); (iii) whether repeat testing is in the budget (single test batteries are of limited use); and (iv) most importantly will the athlete be safe?

Traditionally, clinical and laboratory exercise testing of children has focused on the cardiovascular system. Most measurements have focused on maximum aerobic power and capacity and fitness testng itself has become synonymous with the testing of aerobic fitness (Shephard, 1990; Bar-Or, 1993). Several authors have described tests of maximal aerobic power in children and adults with neuromuscular disabilities (Sokolov et al., 1977; Carroll et al., 1979; Haller et al., 1983). Muscle endurance and strength have often been ignored in most exercise laboratories probably due to a lack of standardized test procedures although assessments of strength have been completed in populations with neuromuscular disorders (Edwards, 1980). Others have assessed components of arm and leg anaerobic power by ergometry and a modified Wingate 30-s procedure (Tirosh et al., 1990).

Testing the young athlete

AEROBIC CAPACITY AND POWER

Aerobic capacity (time to exhaustion at submaximal workloads) and aerobic power — peak rate of oxygen uptake in $ml \cdot kg^{-1} \cdot min^{-1}$ (relative) or $l \cdot min^{-1}$ (absolute) — may be assessed by either leg or arm ergometry depending on disability. Single or double leg protocols are suitable for CP, amputees, OI, MD while single or double arm ergometry may be used for CP, amputees, MD, OI, SCI and scoliosis.

Various protocols for assessing fitness in athletes using a wheelchair have been designed and described. A free wheeling protocols on a flat surface is described by Crews et al. (1982). Brattgard et al. (1970) described a protocol utilizing a wheelchair attached to a cycle ergometer and flywheel by a system of gears. Others have described wheelchairs mounted on a treadmill with safety supports (Gass et al., 1981; Horvat et al., 1984). The Gass et al. (1981) design incorporated a wheelchair integrated with a treadmill and the use of a graded speed and elevation maximal aerobic capacity test. Low

friction roller systems have also been described (Gandee et al., 1980; Lundberg, 1980; Bhambhani et al., 1991). Several wheelchair ergometers are wheelchair-type devices, for example, a wheelchair frame mounted on a base and attached to weighted flywheels with adjustable and calibrated torque featues (Whiting et al., 1984). Wicks et al. (1983) described a fixed wheelchair attached to a Monark cycle ergometer by a system of flywheels. The mechanical efficiency of systems varies (Dreisinger & Londeree, 1982).

Arm ergometry protocols are claimed to be readily standardized non-specific measures of cardiopulmonary fitness (Bergh et al., 1976; Hjeltness, 1977; Shephard, 1990). Mechanical efficiency is also higher than for a wheelchair ergometer (Brattgard et al., 1970). Although most are alternate arm designs, bilateral crank devices have been described (Cummings & Gladden, 1983). Others have suggested the use of the tethered swim protocol as a measure of maximum aerobic power (DiRocco, 1986). Shephard (1990) considers that such a protocol may better reflect overall cardiovascular function than assessments of aerobic power conducted in an upright position in a wheelchair.

PROTOCOLS

Bar-Or (1993) suggests that treadmill, cycle or step protocols are suitable for children over 8 years of age, although a treadmill protocol is best for children less than 8 years of age, as local muscle fatigue and inability to keep a metronome rhythm are limiting factors in cycle protocols.

Test of maximal aerobic power should last at least 6 min and ideally no more than 10 min with progressive protocols being more preferable than single stage protocols. Suggested maximums are 1- or 2-min stages, in the interests of attention maintenance (Bar-Or, 1993). For a treadmill protocol for 6−15-year-old children, initial speeds of $4−6 km \cdot h^{-1}$ at an initial slope of 10% with 2.5% increments in slope every 2 min are suggested. Slope is kept constant after 22.5% and speed is then increased by $1\,km \cdot h^{-1}$ with each consecutive stage (Bar-Or, 1993). For arm ergometer tests, Sawka *et al.* (1982) support use of higher crank rates producing higher maximal aerobic power levels. Generally, the rate of load increase during an arm ergometer test should not exceed $17-25\,W$ per stage.

Predictive tests of aerobic power or capacity rely on the linear relationship of heart rate, workload and oxygen consumption. Predictive tests may therefore be affected by limitations in peak heart rate responses to exercise in MD or SCI (Bar-Or, 1993). In addition, the use of medications (e.g. propanolol) which affect heart rate are contraindications to the use of predictive test procedures. Prediction procedures work well for amputees and paraplegics with lesions below the sympathetic outflow (Shephard, 1990). Kavanagh and Shephard (1973) applied the Åstrand nomogram to data for eight amputees and reported a good correlation between directly measured peak aerobic power and corresponding predicted levels. Also, Kofsky *et al.* (1983) satisfactorily predicted peak aerobic power from submaximal heart rate in a group of adults. Rhodes *et al.* (1981) have suggested a wheelchair analogue of the Cooper 12-min run while Gairdner (1983) has proposed a 6-min wheelchair endurance test as an indirect assessment of aerobic power and capacity.

ANAEROBIC THRESHOLD

Criteria for attainment of anaerobic threshold (AT) whether based on ventilatory changes or on blood lactate levels are similar in children and adults (Bar-Or, 1993) although it has been suggested that the $4\,mmol \cdot l^{-1}$ blood lactate level may be too high for many children (Rotstein *et al.*, 1986), since blood lactate levels are lower at all exercise intensities.

Protocols

To assess AT by expired gas analysis, a 'ramp' protocol during which power increased by $10-20\,W \cdot min^{-1}$ has been found to be satisfactory in establishing ventilatory threshold in 6–17-year-old boys and girls (Cooper *et al.*, 1984). Generally, the younger the child the slower the rate of increase in power (Bar-Or, 1993). If using blood lactate levels as an indicator of AT, stages should be extended to 2–4 min (Rotstein *et al.*, 1986). Lakomy *et al.*, (1987) reported lactate threshold as an adequate prediction of 5-km wheelchair race times.

FIELD TESTS

Field or performance-based tests are an option for testing young athletes and, although subject to error due to measurement and motivation, they are often a useful compromise between the dilemma of expensive laboratory tests and the need to measure fitness status and progress. If the coach of the young athlete uses field tests, it is essential that tests fulfil the following criteria.

1 They must be well documented with adequate instructions.

2 They must be carried out precisely according to instructions on a pre- and postprogramme basis.

3 Learning effects must be eradicated from initial measurements by repeat testing.

ANAEROBIC POWER

Tirosh *et al.* (1990) describe a 30-s all-out arm ergometer anaerobic power test (the Wingate anaerobic power test) to assess peak and mean anaerobic power in children and adolescents with a wide range of neuromuscular disabilities. The test may be utilized in either an upper or lower extremity format and the authors suggest that the test has good reliability and criterion validity and may be administered to children as young as 5 years. Optimal loads for girls are $3.92\,J \cdot rev^{-1} \cdot kg^{-1}$ body weight for legs and $2.6\,J \cdot rev^{-1} \cdot kg^{-1}$ for arms and for boys, $4.13\,J \cdot rev^{-1} \cdot kg^{-1}$ for legs and $2.89\,J \cdot rev^{-1} \cdot kg^{-1}$ for arms (Dotan & Bar-Or, 1983). A feasibility study suggested a 95% feasibility rate for 5 years of age and 61% for 18 years of age (Tirosh *et al.*, 1990).

In assessing anaerobic power in athletes with CP it should be recognized that the requirement of fast, smooth, arm or leg spinning is severely compromised due to failure of normal reciprocal relationships between agonists and antagonists (Parker *et al.*, 1992). This is consistent with reports of failure of the normal/antagonist reciprocal relationship in CP (Berbayer & Ashby, 1990) and reports that smooth contractions only occur at low frequencies of muscle contractions (Neilson *et al.*, 1990). In addition, during leg protocols problems with foot pronation typical of high extensor tone in spastic CP may cause pedalling difficulties (Parker *et al.*, 1992).

MUSCLE STRENGTH

Muscle strength in SCI is often measured by hand grip dynamometry (Jackson *et al.*, 1981; Davis *et al.*, 1984). Significant correlations have been reported between dominant hand grip force and total upper body isometric strength although there is a lack of information regarding strength assessment in young athletes with a disability.

SPECIFIC CONSIDERATIONS FOR
YOUNG ATHLETES

Disability-specific considerations include:

1 Utility and feasibility issues associated with testing. What value will testing be and can it be repeated?

2 Use of one arm or two arm protocols for amputees and CP.

3 Problems with spasticity in children with CP.

4 Trunk stabilization during anaerobic assessment in SCI.

5 Exacerbation of weakness in MD and problem of declining muscle function masking training improvements. This may prove psychologically damaging to the young MD athlete.

6 Potential harmful effects of all out protocols

in testing OI (e.g. fractures).

7 Limitations in predictive tests when maximal heart rate is affected by disability and/or medications, and more generally.

8 Modality of testing: the problem of local muscle fatigue in lower limb assessments on the cycle ergometer versus treadmill.

9 Motivational problems associated with maximal field test performance.

10 Fear and anxiety in athletes unfamiliar with protocols, wheelchair design differences, experience in fast wheeling and arm cranking and knowledge of pacing in field tasks.

Challenges for future research

• Physical and psychological effects of disability on involvement in sport. In what ways do congenital and acquired disabilities affect participation in sport?

• Effects of sports on psychological profiles, coping and adjustment. How does involvement in physical activity and sport affect coping and adjustment to a traumatic injury? How does involvement in sport affect dealing with puberty in individuals with congenital disabilities?

• Effects of sports participation on eating behaviours and the incidence of eating disorders, especially in élite athletes. Evidence suggests that disordered eating patterns are on the increase in athletes without a disability. Do similar problems exist in young athletes? As individuals become more widely used in advertising and media, will an 'ideal' body image arise?

• Frequency, aetiology and demography of sports injury. Sport-related injury is on the increase. For example, what effect will increased involvement in sport have in terms of shoulder and upper extremity injuries?

• Classification and developmental issues. As the potential for younger athletes increases so too does pressure on sport organizational bodies to examine issues of classification and developmental variations.

• Retirement from élite sports. What does the athlete need to consider in preparation for retirement from sport or being eliminated from participation by a 'secondary disability' (e.g. overuse injuries)? What is the psychological impact on the athlete of forced retirement, retirement due to classification issues (e.g. female athletes with CP) or voluntary retirement?

References

Alberts, C.L. (1984) Section 504 of the rehabilitation acts and the right to participate in school athletic programs. *Educ. Consid.* **11**, 23–6.

American Academy of Pediatrics (1988) Recommendations for participation on competitive sports. *Phys. Sports Med.* **16**, 165–7.

Bale, P. (1992) The functional performance of children in relation to growth, maturation and exercise. *Sports Med.* **13**, 151–9.

Bard, G. & Ralston, H.J. (1959) Measurement of energy expenditure during ambulation with special reference to evaluation of assistive devices. *Arch. Phys. Med. Rehab.* **40**, 415–20.

Bar-Or, O. (1983) *Pediatric Sports Medicine for the Practitioner: Physiologic Principles to Clinical Applications.* Springer-Verlag, New York.

Bar-Or, O. (1986) Pathophysiological factors which limit the exercise capacity of the sick child. *Med. Sci. Sports Exerc.* **18**, 276–82.

Bar-Or, O. (1990) Disease-specific benefits of training in the child with a chronic disease: what is the evidence? *Pediatr. Exerc. Sci.* **2**, 299–312.

Bar-Or, O. (1993) Noncardiopulmonary pediatric exercise tests. In T.W. Rowland (ed.) *Pediatric Laboratory Exercise Testing*, pp. 165–85. Human Kinetics, Springfield, MA.

Bar-Or, O, Inbar, O. & Spira, R. (1976) Physiological effects of a sports rehabilitation program on cerebral palsied and post-poliomyelitic adolescents. *Med. Sci. Sports Exerc.* **8**, 157–61.

Berbayer, D. & Ashby, P. (1990) Reciprocal inhibition in cerebral palsy. *Neurology* **40**, 653–6.

Berg, K. (1970) Effect of physical training in school children with cerebral palsy. *Acta Paediatr. Scand.* **204** (Suppl.), 27–33.

Berg, K. & Bjure, J. (1970) Methods for evaluation of the physical working capacity of school children with cerebral palsy. *Acta Paediatr. Scand.* **204** (Suppl.), 15–26.

Bergh, U., Kanstrup, I.L. & Ekblom, B. (1976) Maximum oxygen uptake during exercise with various combinations of arm and leg work. *J. Appl. Physiol.* **41**, 191–6.

Bhambhani, Y., Eriksson, P. & Steadward, R. (1991) Reliability of peak physiological responses during wheelchair ergometry in persons with spinal cord injury. *Arch. Phys. Med. Rehab.* **71**, 559–62.

Bjure, J., Grimby, G. & Nachmeson, A. (1969) The effect of physical training in girls with idiopathic scoliosis. *Acta Orthop. Scand.* **40**, 325–33.

Bloomquist, L.E. (1986) Injuries to athletes with physical disabilities: prevention implications. *Phys. Sports Med.* **14**, 96–105.

Bowker, J.H. & Halpin, P.J. (1978) Factors determining success in reambulation of the child with progressive muscular dystrophy. *Orthop. Clin. N. Am.* **9**, 431–6.

Brattgard, S., Grimby, G. & Hook, O. (1970) Energy expenditure and heart rate in driving a wheelchair ergometer. *Scand. J. Rehab.* **2**, 143–8.

Buckley, W.E., Yesalis, C.E., Friedl, K.E., Anderson, W.A., Streit, A.L. & Wright, J.E. (1988) Estimated prevalence of anabolic steroid use among male high school seniors. *JAMA* **260**, 3441–5.

Burnham, R., Higgins, J. & Steadward, R.D. (1994) Wheelchair basketball injuries. *Palaestra* **10**, 43–9.

Burnham, R., Newell, E. & Steadward, R. (1991) Sports medicine for the physically disabled: the Canadian team experience at the 1988 Seoul Paralympic Games. *Clin. J. Sports Med.* **1**, 193–6.

Burnham, R., Wheeler, G.D., Bhambhani, Y., Eriksson, P. & Steadward, R. (1994) Autonomic dysreflexia in wheelchair athletes. *Clin. J. Sports Med.* **4**, 1–10.

Butler, P.B., Thompson, N. & Major, R.E. (1992) Improvement in walking performance of children with cerebral palsy: preliminary results. *Dev. Med. Child Neurol.* **34**, 567–76.

Cadman, D., Boyle, M. & Szatmari, P. (1987) Chronic illness, disability and mental health and social well-being: findings of the Ontario Child Health Study. *Pediatrics* **79**, 805–13.

Cameron, B.J., Ward, G.R. & Wicks, J.R. (1978) Relationship of type of training to maximal oxygen uptake and upper limb strength in male paraplegic athletes. *Med. Sci. Sports Exerc.* **9**, 58 (abstract).

Carmick, J. (1993) Clinical use of neuromuscular electrical stimulation for children with cerebral palsy, part 1. Lower extremity. *Phys. Ther.* **73**, 505–13.

Carroll, J.E., Hagberg, J.M., Brooke, M.H. & Shumate, J.B. (1979) Bicycle ergometry and gas exchange measurements in neuromuscular disease. *Arch. Neurol.* **36**, 457–61.

Castle, M.E., Reyman, T.A. & Schneider, M.E. (1979) Pathology of spastic muscle in cerebral palsy. *Clin. Orthop.* **142**, 223–33.

Chretien, R., Simard, C.P. & Dorion, A. (1987) Effects of relaxation on the peripheral chronaxie of persons having multiple sclerosis. In M. Berridge & G. Ward (eds) *International Perspectives on Adapted Physical Activity*, pp. 65–72. Human Kinetics, Champaign, IL.

Cooper, D.M., Weiler-Ravell, D., Whipp, B.J. & Wasserman, K. (1984) Growth-related changes in oxygen uptake and heart during progressive exercise in children. *Pediatr. Res.* **18**, 845–51.

Crews, D., Purkett, L., Wells, C.L. & McKeeman, V. (1982) Cardiovascular characteristics of wheelchair marathon racers compared with marathon runners. *Int. J. Sports Med.* **3**, 64 (abstract).

Cummings, R.D. & Gladden, L.B. (1983) Responses to submaximal and maximal arm cycling above, at and below heart level. *Med. Sci. Sports Exerc.* **15**, 295–8.

Dalton, S.E. (1992) Overuse injuries in adolescent athletes. *Sports Med.* **13**, 58–70.

Davis, G.M., Jackson, R.W. & Shephard, R.J. (1984) Sports and recreation for the physically disabled. In R.H. Strauss (ed.) *Sports Medicine*, pp. 286–304. W.B. Saunders, Philadelphia.

de Lateur, B. & Giaconi, R. (1979) Effect on maximal strength of submaximal exercise in Duchenne muscular dystrophy. *Am. J. Phys. Med.* **58**, 26–36.

de Mondenard, J.P. (1991) Physical activities in sick children, sports on prescription. *Schweiz. Zatsch. Sportmed.* **39**, 21–31.

Dickenson, R. (1988) Some general recommendations for the field of adapted physical activity. In *Jasper Talks: Strategies for Change in Adapted Physical Activity in Canada*, pp. 36–37. Fitness Canada, CAHPER/ACSEPL, Ottawa.

DiRocco, P. (1986) Tethered swimming and the development of cardiopulmonary fitness for non-ambulatory individuals. *Am. Corr. Ther. J.* **40**, 43–7.

Dotan, R. & Bar-Or, O. (1983) Load optimization for the Wingate anaerobic test. *Eur. J. Appl. Physiol.* **51**, 409–17.

Dreisinger, T.E. & Londeree, B.R. (1982) Wheelchair exercise: a review. *Paraplegia* **20**, 20–34.

Dresen, M.H.W., de Groot, G., Mesa Menor, J.R. & Bouman, L.N. (1985) Aerobic energy expenditure of handicapped children after training. *Arch. Phys. Med. Rehab.* **66**, 301–6.

Edwards, R.H.T. (1980) Studies of muscular performance in normal and dystrophic subjects. *Br. Med. Bull.* **36**, 159–64.

Eichstaedt, C.B. & Kalakian, L.H. (1993) *Developmental/Adapted Physical Education: Making Ability Count.* Macmillan, New York.

Ensberg, J.R., Lee, A.G., Tedford, K.G. & Harder, J.A. (1993a) Normative ground reaction force data for able-bodied and below-knee amputee children during walking. *J. Pediatr. Orthop.* **13**, 169–73.

Ensberg, J.R., Lee, A.G., Tedford, K.G. & Harder, J.A. (1993b) Normative ground reaction force data for able-bodied and trans-tibial amputee children during running. *Prosthet. Orthot.* **17**, 83–9.

Epling, W.F. & Pierce, W.D. (1988) Activity anorexia: a biobehavioral perspective. *Int. J. Eat. Dis.* **7**, 475–85.

Evans, J.R. (1988) The role of education in the adapted physical education delivery system: a state of the art review. In *Jasper Talks: Strategies for Change in Adapted Physical Activity in Canada*, pp. 38–9. Fitness Canada, CAHPER/ACSEPL, Ottawa.

Ferrara, M.S., Buckley, W.E. & McCann, B.C. (1992) The injury experience of the competitive athlete with a disability: prevention implications. *Med. Sci. Sports Exerc.* **24**, 184–8.

Ferrara, M.S. & Davis, R.W. (1990) Injuries to élite wheelchair athletes. *Paraplegia* **28**, 335–41.

Frisch, R.E., Wyshack, G. & Vincent, L. (1980) Delayed menarche and amenorrhea in ballet dancers. *New Engl. J. Med.* **303**, 17–19.

Frobose, I. (1989) Results of treatment in a 6-month movement and sports therapy rehabilitation program of children with cerebral palsy. *Z. Orthop.* **127**, 108–10.

Frobose, I. (1992) Kinematic and dynamometric analysis of the motor behaviour of cerebral palsy children and its changes after intensive sport and exercise therapy. *Rehabilitation* **31**, 124–8.

Gairdner, J. (1983) *Fitness for the Disabled: Wheelchair Users.* Frizhenry & Whiteside, Toronto.

Gandee, R., Winningham, M., Dietchman, R. & Narraway, A. (1980) The aerobic capacity of an élite wheelchair marathon racer. *Med. Sci. Sports Exerc.* **12**, 142 (abstract).

Gass, C.G., Camp, E.M., Davis, H.A., Eager, B. & Grout, L. (1981) The effects of prolonged exercise on spinally-injured subjects. *Med. Sci. Sports Exerc.* **11**, 256–65.

Gingell, R.L., Pieroni, D.R. & Horung, M.G. (1981) Growth problems associated with congenital heart disease in infancy. In E. Lebenthal (ed.) *Textbook of Gastroenterology and Nutrition and Infancy*, pp. 853–60. Raven Press, New York.

Goodwin, D. (1988) The need for specialist training in adapted physical activity. In *Jasper Talks: Strategies for Change in Adapted Physical Activity in Canada*, p. 31. Fitness Canada, CAHPER/ACSEPL, Ottawa.

Grimby, G. (1980) Aerobic capacity, muscle strength and fibre composition in young paraplegics. In H. Natvic (ed.) *First International Medical Congress on Sports for the Disabled.* Royal Ministry for Church and Education, Oslo.

Grube v. *Bethlehem Area School District 550* (1982) Federal Supplement 418 (D. Penn).

Haller, R.G., Lewis, S.F., Cook, J.D. & Blomqvist, C.G. (1983) Hyperkinetic circulation during exercise in neuromuscular disease. *Neurology* **33**, 1283–7.

Harter, S. (1987) The determinants and mediational

role of global self-worth in children. In N. Eisenberg (ed.) *Contemporary Topics in Developmental Psychology*, pp. 219–42. Wiley, New York.

Hjeltnes, N. (1977) Oxygen uptake and cardiac output in graded arm exercise in paraplegics with low level spinal lesions. *Scand. J. Rehab. Med.* **9**, 107–13.

Hoeberigs, J.H., Debets-Eggen, H.B. & Debets, P.M. (1990) Sports medical experiences from the International Flower Marathon for Disabled Wheelers. *Am. J. Sports Med.* **18**, 418–21.

Hollonbeck v. *Board of Education* of *Rochelle Township* (1988) Disabled athlete barred from competing wins victory in New York Federal Court. *Occup. Ther. Week*, 25 August, 5–6.

Horvat, M.A., Golding, L.A., Beutel-Horvat, T. & McConnell, T.J. (1984) A treadmill modification for wheelchairs. *Res. Q.* **55**, 297–301.

Hosking, G.P., Bhat, U.S., Dubowitz, V. & Edwards, R.H.T. (1976) Measurement of muscle strength and performance in children with normal and diseased muscle. *Arch. Dis. Child.* **51**, 957–63.

Howard, R.B. (1981) Nutritional support of the developmentally disabled child. In R.M. Suskind (ed.) *Textbook of Pediatric Nutrition*, pp. 577–82. Raven Press, New York.

Ilmarinen, J. & Rutenfranz, J. (1980) Longitudinal studies of the changes in habitual physical activity of school children and working adolescents. In K. Berg & B. Erikson (eds) *Children and Exercise*, pp. 149–59. University Park Press, Baltimore.

Inkley, S.R., Oldenburg, F.C. & Vignos, P.J. (1974) Pulmonary function in Duchenne muscular dystrophy related to stages of the disease. *Am. J. Med.* **56**, 297–306.

Ishida, C., Umemoto, H., Fujita, M. & Suzuki, N. (1989) Comparison of walking exercises in air and in water in children with cerebral palsy. *No To Hattatsu* **21**, 460–4.

Jackson, R.W., Davis, G.M., Kofsky, P.R., Shephard, R.J. & Keen, G.C.R. (1981) Fitness levels in the lower limb disabled. In *Transactions of the 27th Annual Meeting, Orthopedics Research Society*, p. 6 (abstract).

Kavanagh, T. & Shephard, R.J. (1973) The application of exercise testing to the elderly amputee. *Can. Med. Ass. J.* **108**, 314–17.

Kay, L. & Shephard, R.J. (1969) On muscle strength and the threshold of anaerobic work. *Int. Zeitschr. Ange. Physiol.* **27**, 311–28.

King, E.M., Gooch, J.L., Howell, G.H., Peters, M.L., Bloswick, D.S. & Brown, D.R. (1993) Evaluation of the hip-extensor tricycle in improving gait in children with cerebral palsy. *Dev. Med. Child Neurol.* **35**, 1048–54.

Kofsky, P.R., Davis, G.M., Jackson, R.W., Keene, G.C.R. & Shephard, R.J. (1983) Field-testing — assessment of physical fitness of disabled adults. *Eur. J. Appl. Physiol.* **51**, 109–20.

Kraemer, R., Rudeberg, A., Hadorn, B. & Rosi, E. (1978) Relative underweight in cystic fibrosis and its prognostic value. *Acta Pediatr. Scand.* **67**, 33–7.

Lakomy, H.K.A., Campbell, I. & Williams, C. (1987) Treadmill performance and selected physiological characteristics of wheelchair athletes. *Br. J. Sports Med.* **21**, 130–3.

Lathen, C.W., Stoll, S.K. & Hyder, M. (1988) Physically disabled individuals desire participation in risk sports. *Palaestra* **4**, 19–23.

Lindh, M. (1978) Energy expenditure during walking in patients with scoliosis. The effect of surgical correction. *Spine* **3**, 122–34.

Lindström, H. (1992) Integration of sport for athletes with disabilities into sport programming for able-bodied athletes. *Palaestra* **8**, 28–32/58–9.

Lubell, A. (1987) Insurance, liability and the American way of sport. *Phys. Sports Med.* **15**, 192–200.

Lundberg, A. (1975) Mechanical efficiency in bicycle ergometer work of young adults with cerebral palsy. *Dev. Med. Child Neurol.* **17**, 434–9.

Lundberg, A. (1976) Oxygen consumption in relation to workload in students with cerebral palsy. *J. Appl. Physiol.* **40**, 873–5.

Lundberg, A. (1978) Maximal aerobic capacity of young people with spastic cerebral palsy. *Dev. Med. Child Neurol.* **20**, 205–10.

Lundberg, A. (1980) Wheelchair driving: evaluation of a new driving outfit. *Scand. J. Rehab. Med.* **12**, 67–72.

Martinez, S.F. (1989) Medical concerns among wheelchair road racers. *Phys. Sports Med.* **17**, 63–8.

Molbech, S. (1966) Energy cost in level walking in subjects with an abnormal gait. In K. Evang & K.L. Andersen (eds) *Physical Activity in Health and Disease*, pp. 146–55 Williams & Wilkins, Baltimore.

Monohan, T. (1986) Wheelchair athletes need special treatment — but only for injuries. *Phys. Sports Med.* **14**, 121–8.

Nakamura, Y. (1973) Working ability of the paraplegic. *Paraplegia* **11**, 182–93.

Nash, J., Neilson, P.D. & O'Dwyer, N.J. (1989) Reducing spasticity to control muscle contracture of children with cerebral palsy. *Dev. Med. Child Neurol.* **31**, 471–80.

Neilson, P.D., O'Dwyer, N.J. & Nash, J. (1990) Control of isometric activity in cerebral palsy. *Dev. Med. Child Neurol.* **32**, 778–88.

Palmer, S. (1978) Nutrition and developmental disorders: an overview. In S. Palmer & S. Ekvall (eds) *Pediatric Nutrition in Developmental Disorders*, pp. 107–29. C.C. Thomas, Springfield.

Parker, D.F., Carriere, L., Hebestreit, H. & Bar-Or, O. (1992) Anaerobic endurance and peak muscle power in children with spastic cerebral palsy. *Am. J. Dis. Child.* **146**, 1069–73.

Parker, D.F., Carriere, L., Hebestreit, H., Salsberg, A. & Bar-Or, O. (1993) Muscle performance and gross motor function of children with spastic cerebral palsy. *Dev. Med. Child Neurol.* **35**, 17–23.

Peck, D.M. & McKeag, D.B. (1994) Athletes with disabilities; removing medical barriers. *Phys. Sports Med.* **22**, 59–62.

Rhodes, E.C., McKenzie, D.C., Coutts, K.D. & Rogers, A.R. (1981) A field test for the prediction of aerobic capacity in male paraplegics and quadriplegics. *Can. J. Appl. Sport Sci.* **6**, 182–6.

Rice, B.L. (1981) Nutritional problems of developmentally disabled children. *Pediatr. Nurs.*, **7**, 15–18.

Richardson, S.A. (1970) Age and sex differences in values toward physical handicaps. *J. Health Soc. Behav.* **11**, 207–14.

Richter, K.E., Hyman, S.C. & Mushett-Adams, C.A. (1991) Injuries in world class cerebral palsy athletes at the 1988 South Korea Paralympics. *J. Osteo. Sports Med.* **5**, 15–18.

Rotstein, A., Dotan, R., Bar-Or, O. & Tenebaum, G. (1986) Effect of training on anaerobic threshold, maximal aerobic performance of preadolescent boys. *Int. J. Sports Med.* **7**, 281–6.

Ruby, D.O. & Matheny, W.D. (1961) Comments on growth of cerebral palsied. *J. Am. Diet. Ass.* **40**, 525–7.

Rutenfranz, J. (1985) Long-term effects of excessive training procedures on young athletes. In R.A. Binkhorst, C.G. Kemper & W.H.M. Saris (eds) *Children and Exercise: International Series on Sports Sciences*, pp. 354–7. Human Kinetics, Champaign, IL.

Sawka, M.N., Miles, D.S., Petrofsky, J.S., Wilde, S.W. & Glaser, R.M. (1982) Ventilation and acid–base equilibrium for upper body and lower body exercise. *Aviat. Space Environ. Med.* **53**, 354–9.

Schneider, K., Hart, T., Zernicke, R.F., Setoguchi, Y. & Oppenheim, W. (1993) Dynamics of below-knee child amputee gait: SACH foot versus Flex foot. *J. Biomech.* **26**, 1191–204.

Shephard, R.J. (1990) *Fitness in Special Populations*. Human Kinetics, Champaign, IL.

Shephard, R.J. (1992) Effectiveness of training programs for prepubescent children. *Sports Med.* **13**, 194–213.

Sherrill, C., Hinson, M., Gench, B., Kennedy, S.O. & Low, L. (1990) Self-concepts of disabled young athletes. *Percept. Motor Skills* **70**, 1093–8.

Smith, D.A. & Perry, P.J. (1992) The efficacy of ergogenic agents in athletic competition: part I. Androgenic-anabolic steroids. *Ann. Pharmacol.* **26**, 520–8.

Smith, N.D. (1980) Excessive weight loss and food aversion in athletes simulating anorexia nervosa. *Pediatrics* **66**, 139–42.

Sokolov, R., Irwin, B., Dressendorfer, R.H. & Bernauer, E.M. (1977) Exercise performance in 6 to 11 year old boys with Duchenne muscular dystrophy. *Arch. Phys. Med. Rehab.* **58**, 195–201.

Spira, R. & Bar-Or, O. (1975) *An Investigation of the Ambulation Problems with Severe Motor Paralysis in Adolescents: Influence of Physical Conditioning and Adapted Sports Activities*. Research Report, Dept. HEW/SRS, Washington DC.

Stewart, M.J. (1983) The handicapped in sports. *Clin. Sports Med.* **1**, 183–90.

Stoboy, H. (1985) Effort tolerance in scoliosis. In P. Welsh & R.J. Shephard (eds) *Current Therapy in Sports Medicine 1985–1986*, pp. 114–16. Decker, Burlington, ON.

Stoboy, J. & Wilson-Rich, B. (1971) Muscle strength and electrical activity, heart rate and energy cost during isometric contractions in disabled and non-disabled. *Paraplegia* **8**, 217–22.

Thommessen, M., Heiberg, A., Kase, B.F., Larsen, S. & Riis, G. (1991a) Feeding problems, height and weight in different groups of disabled children. *Acta Pediatr. Scand.* **80**, 527–33.

Thommessen, M., Kase, B.F., Riis, G. & Heiberg, A. (1991b) The impact of feeding problems on growth and energy intake in children with cerebral palsy. *Eur. J. Clin. Health* **45**, 479–87.

Tirosh, E., Bar-Or, O. & Rosenbaum, P. (1990) New muscle power test in neuromuscular disease. *Am. J. Dis. Child.* **144**, 1083–7.

Varni, J.W. & Setoguchi, Y. (1991) Correlates of perceived physical appearance in children with congenital/acquired limb deficiencies. *Dev. Behav. Pediatr.* **12**, 171–6.

Wallander, J.L., Varni, J.W. & Babani, L. (1988) Children with chronic physical disorders: maternal reports of their psychological adjustment. *J. Pediat. Psychol.* **13**, 197–212.

Warren, M.P. (1985) The effect of exercise and physical training on menarche. *Sem. Reprod. Endocrinol.* **3**, 17–26.

Warren, M.P. (1988) Delayed menarche in athletes: the role of low energy intake and eating disorders and their relation to bone density. In *International Symposium on Hormones and Sport*, Dubrovnik, Yugoslavia, 1988.

Watkinson, J. (1988) Adapted physical activity: the development and evaluation of integrated programs. In *Jasper Talks: Strategies for Change in Adapted Physical Activity in Canada*, pp. 16–17. Fitness Canada, CAHPER/ACSEPL, Ottawa.

Webb, Y. (1980) Feeding and nutrition problems of physically and mentally handicapped children in Britain: A report. *J. Hum. Nutr.* **34**, 281–5.

Wheeler, G.D., Krausher, R., Cumming, D.C., Cumming, C. & Steadward, R.D. (1993a) Adjusting to spinal cord injury: a qualitative comparison of athletes and non-athletes. Presented at the Ninth International Symposium of Adapted Physical Activity, Yokohama, Japan, 4–7 August 1993 (abstract).

Wheeler, G.D., Krausher, R., Cumming, D.C., Cumming, C. & Steadward, R.D. (1993b) Personal styles and ways of coping in wheelchair users: a comparison of athletes and non-athletes. (Unpublished)

Wheeler, G.D., Malone, L., Van Vlack, S. & Steadward, R.D. (1995) Retirement experiences of athletes with a disability (Submitted).

Whiting, R.B., Dreisinger, T.E. & Hayden, T. (1984) Wheelchair exercise testing: a comparison of continuous and discontinuous exercise. *Paraplegia* **22**, 92–8.

Wicks, J., Oldridge, N.B., Cameron, N.B. & Jones, N.L. (1983) Arm cranking and wheelchair ergometry in élite spinal cord injured athletes. *Med. Sci. Sports Exerc.* **15**, 224–31.

Winnick, J.P. & Short, F.X. (1984) The physical fitness of youngsters with spinal neuromuscular conditions. *Adapted Phys. Act. Q.* **1**, 37–41.

Wilson, P.E. & Washington, R.L. (1993) Pediatric wheelchair athletics: sports injuries and prevention. *Paraplegia* **31**, 330–7.

Yates, E., Leehay, K. & Shisslak, C. (1983) Running: an analogue of anorexia nervosa? *New Engl. J. Med.* **308**, 251–5.

Zwiren, L. & Bar-Or, O. (1975) Responses to exercise of paraplegics who differ in conditioning level. *Med. Sci. Sports Exerc.* **7**, 94–8.

Zwiren, L., Huberman, G. & Bar-Or, O. (1973) Cardiopulmonary functions of sedentary and highly active paraplegics. *Med. Sci. Sports Exerc.* **5**, 63 (abstract).

PART 7

METHODOLOGY

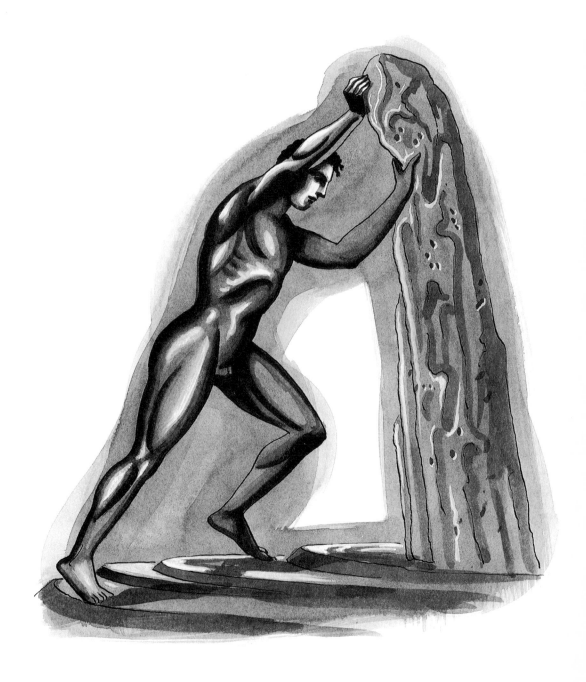

Chapter 33

Body Composition Assessment in Children and Youths

RICHARD A. BOILEAU

Introduction

The most general conceptualization of body composition is the characterization of body weight in terms of absolute and relative amounts of fat and fat-free body (FFB). The measurement and evaluation of fat and FFB is a vital aspect of assessing health, fitness and nutritional status. Obesity, a disease that can be traced to nutritional, hypokinetic and metabolic abnormalities, is a primary health concern in developed countries. While the prevalence of obesity in children and youth is not well established, estimates have ranged from 5 to 30% in various samples (Ylitalo, 1981; Coates et al., 1982; Lohman et al., 1989). On the other hand, undernutrition in terms of protein-calorie availability and intake is often a primary concern in developing countries. Body composition assessment can be a valuable tool in evaluating nutritional status and also in tracking changes due to intervention programmes.

Another use of body composition measurement is to provide information about appropriate ratios of fat and FFB for optimizing physical performance related to sports and for determination of physical fitness status. The influence of these components on physical performance is well documented (Boileau et al., 1989). Specifically, research has demonstrated an inverse relationship between body fat and performance in physical tasks requiring either vertical or horizontal displacement of body weight, and particularly in endurance perform-

ance. Moreover, a high absolute FFB mass may be essential to perform optimally activities in which force must be applied against external objects, e.g. strength events. Furthermore, in youth sports which have weight classification systems, body composition measurements can be used to provide information regarding minimal, ideal and maximal weight to assist in assuring maintenance of normal growth and maturation of the athlete (Thorland et al., 1991; Lohman, 1992).

In vivo measurements of body composition developed out of research conducted in the 1940s and 1950s in which conceptualizations and assumptions were established based on fundamental work in densitometry and hydrometry (Behnke et al., 1942; Keys & Brozek, 1953; Siri, 1961; Brozek et al., 1963) and whole-body chemical cadaver analysis (Mitchell et al., 1945; Forbes et al., 1953, 1956). Out of this early work, models of adult body composition were established which continue to form the basis of current methodology. Unfortunately, these models were assumed to be applicable to all individuals without regard to age, race, maturation status or physical development. Considerable evidence now exists that adult models developed out of earlier work cannot be universally applied. In particular, it has become apparent that the use of adult models for children and youth are inappropriate and must be adjusted based on growth and maturation of the components of the FFB (Boileau et al., 1985).

In this chapter, a brief review of recent developments in body composition methodology for children and youth will be presented. Additionally, special emphasis will be given to body composition methodology which can be applied to field testing and the clinical setting.

Methods for assessing body composition

Recent review articles have described various body composition assessment methods including densitometry, hydrometry, body potassium, neutron activation analysis, creatinine excretion and other muscle metabolites, basal metabolic rate and anthropometry (Lohman, 1984; Buskirk, 1987; Lukaski, 1987). In addition to the above established methods, new and emerging technologies such as bioelectric impedance (Lukaski et al., 1985) and conductivity (Boileau, 1988), photon absorptiometry (Mazess et al., 1981), infrared interactance (Conway et al., 1984), magnetic resonance imaging (MRI) and computerized tomography (CT) scanning (Seidell et al., 1990) have been developed. Many of these methods have been utilized for assessing body composition of children and youth. However, because much of the past and present paediatric research is based on densitometry and because most of the field/clinical techniques are validated and calibrated by densitometry, discussion will focus primarily on this method.

Densitometry

Body density is the ratio of body weight to body volume. Total body volume is normally measured by hydrostatic weighing (Akers & Buskirk, 1969) with correction for pulmonary residual volume (Wilmore, 1969). To interpret body density however, it must be transformed into the components of fat and FFB.

FOUR-COMPONENT APPROACH

Conceptually, total body density (D_B) can be represented as four components including fat, and the FFB consisting of water, mineral and residual components. The residual component, while computed by difference and not directly measured, consists mostly of protein, and thus, will be referred to as protein hereafter. Therefore, D_B can be represented by the proportions and densities of its parts in terms of four components as follows:

$$D_B = 1/(f/d_f + w/d_w + m/d_m + p/d_p). \quad (33.1)$$

The whole body is assumed to be equal to unity (eqn 33.1); thus, the sum of the parts can be represented as fractions of the whole accordingly:

$$1 = f + w + m + p.$$

The lower case letters (f, w, m and p) represent the fractions of fat, water, mineral and protein, respectively, and lower case letter d with its subscripts indicates the densities of these components. Total body mineral (TBM) is often considered as two components, bone mineral and non-osseous mineral, the latter estimated as a fraction of TBM (Heymsfield et al., 1989). The densities of the components have previously been determined (Brozek et al., 1963) and at 36°C are assumed to be:
- fat = 0.9007 g · cm³;
- water = 0.9937 g · cm³;
- bone mineral = 2.982 g · cm³;
- non-osseous mineral = 3.317 g · cm³;
- protein = 1.34 g · cm³.

Since the protein fraction cannot be directly measured, it is estimated indirectly as follows:

$$p = 1 - f - w - bm - nm$$

where bm = bone mineral and nm = non-osseous mineral. Using the above relationship of D_B to its components expressed in terms of fractions and densities, it is possible to derive a multicomponent equation to solve for the fraction of body weight that is fat (f) accordingly (Selinger, 1977):

$$f = (2.747/D_B) - 0.714(w) + 1.129(bm)$$
$$+ 1.222(nm) - 2.0503. \quad (33.2)$$

FFB weight is calculated as:

$$\text{FFB (kg)} = \text{BW} - \text{BW}(f) \qquad (33.3)$$

where BW = body weight. Derivation of this equation makes no assumptions about the proportions of w, m or p but does assume that the densities of the components are known, stable and constant. This assumption appears to be justified during growth and development.

TWO-COMPONENT APPROACH

The two-component model, consisting of fat and FFB, is more commonly used and several equations have been developed based on theoretical and empirical models of body composition. The Siri (1961) and Brozek et al. (1963) equations are prominent examples. These equations have primarily been developed from adult cadaver data and are based on adult constants for the densities of fat (D_f) and FFB (D_{FFB}). In spite of concern about the applicability of these equations to children and youth (Parizkova, 1961; Wilmore & McNamara, 1974; Boileau et al., 1981; Lohman, 1981), the Siri and Brozek equations have nevertheless been universally utilized. In general, use of either equation results in an overestimation of body fat and an underestimation of FFB in paediatric samples. The underlying problem associated with the use of these equations for children is that the density of the FFB is substantially lower than the assumed adult value of $1.1\,\text{g} \cdot \text{cm}^3$ (Boileau et al., 1985; Lohman, 1986).

To estimate relative body fatness percentage of fat from densitometry using the two-component model, one must make assumptions about the densities of not only fat but also of FFB. Since fat is a solitary component, it is reasonable to assume that the density of fat, $0.9\,\text{g} \cdot \text{cm}^3$ is somewhat constant. However, since FFB consists of several components of diverse densities, its stability, particularly during growth and development is less likely. Indeed, while not widely acknowledged, there is evidence in earlier literature that the relative content of FFB components varies significantly in

children from that assumed in adult model (Lohman et al., 1984a). Yet, much of the paediatric body composition literature contains estimates based on the Siri (1961) equation derived by assuming the chemically mature constants for the densities of fat and FFB of 0.9 and $1.1\,\text{g} \cdot \text{cm}^3$, respectively, using the following general equation:

$$f = 1/D_B\,[(D_f \times D_{FFB})/(D_{FFB} - D_f)] \\ - [D_f/(D_{FFB} - D_f)]. \qquad (33.4)$$

To utilize the appropriate equation for estimating the percentage of fat from D_B, the D_{FFB} representative of the growth and maturation status must be known to derive an equation to compute accurate body composition estimates. D_{FFB} can be calculated as a function of its components accordingly:

$$D_{FFB} = 1/(w/d_w + m/d_m + p/d_p). \qquad (33.5)$$

By employing a multicomponent estimate of FFB (eqns 33.2 and 33.3), it is possible to express water, mineral and protein as fractions of the whole FFB, thus providing an estimate of D_{FFB} with equation 33.5. Utilizing deuterium oxide dilution to measure total body water (TBW), the water content (w) of the FFB can be estimated as the ratio TBW : FFB. Similarly, the TBM of the FFB can be measured from total body dual energy radiographic scanning and the mineral content (m) estimated as the ratio TBM : FFB. Since direct measurements of protein are typically not made, the protein content (p) of FFB is estimated by difference as:

$$p = 1 - w - m. \qquad (33.6)$$

While there are few studies which have utilized this approach to document the variability in FFB during growth and development, there appears to be a consensus emerging that D_{FFB} at various stages of growth needs to be identified and utilized in the development of equations for estimating body composition from D_B. Several review papers have summarized the available data pertaining to variability in D_{FFB} during growth and development (Boileau et al., 1985; Lohman, 1986, 1989).

To establish the change in D_{FFB}, the FFB components must be measured and expressed as a fraction of the FFB estimated from the multicomponent approach (eqns 33.2 and 33.3) and applied to the general equation (eqn 33.4) for deriving an equation to estimate the fat fraction from D_B. Using the data presented in Boileau et al. (1988) on 211 children and youth and 81 young adults, the pattern of change in D_{FFB} with age (Fig. 33.1) is associated with a decrease in FFB water content (Fig. 33.2) and an increase in FFB mineral content (Fig. 33.3). Moreover, calculations of changes in FFB protein content, based on body potassium data, indicate an increase in this component from 19% in the prepubescent boy to 20.3% in the adolescent male (Fomon et al., 1982).

However, using this estimate (body potassium) of FFB protein may not be appropriate because one must assume a constant nitrogen to potassium ratio (Lohman, 1986). By extra-polating from the available data on change in FFB water and mineral content data (Fomon et al., 1982; Haschke, 1983; Boileau et al., 1984; Lohman et al., 1984b), Lohman (1986) presented the change in FFB density, water, mineral and potassium as a function of age (Table 33.1). Using the D_{FFB} from Table 33.1 as representative of age and gender groups, specific constants can be computed for each group to derive equations to estimate percentage of fat from D_B (Table 33.2). The effect of using the Siri equation, which assumes chemical maturity (adult model), for a hypothetical child at ages 8, 12 and 16 years, whose D_B remains constant, is shown in Table 33.3. The error, represented by the difference between the Siri equation estimate and the D_{FFB} age-adjusted equation, decreases from 7.1 to 1% fat as the child develops and becomes more chemically mature with increasing age.

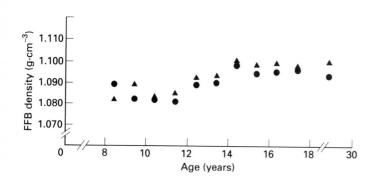

Fig. 33.1 Mean fat-free body (FFB) density values for children and youths (8–17 years of age) and adults (18–30 years of age). These values were computed from data presented by Boileau et al. (1984) and Lohman et al. (1984b). ▲, males ($n = 112$ for children; $n = 45$ for adults); ●, females ($n = 99$ for children, $n = 36$ for adults). Redrawn with permission from Boileau et al. (1988) © 1988 by Human Kinetics.

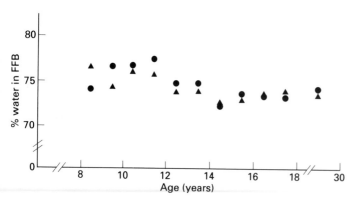

Fig. 33.2 Mean percentage fat-free body (FFB) water values for children and youths (8–17 years of age) and adults (18–30 years of age). ▲, males ($n = 112$ for children, $n = 45$ for adults); ●, females ($n = 99$ for children, $n = 36$ for adults). Redrawn with permission from Boileau et al. (1988) © 1988 by Human Kinetics.

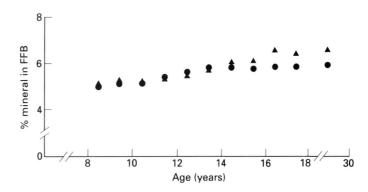

Fig. 33.3 Mean percentage fat-free body (FFB) mineral values for children and youths (8–17 years of age) and adults (18–30 years of age). ▲, males ($n = 112$ for children, $n = 45$ for adults); ●, females ($n = 99$ for children, $n = 36$ for adults). Redrawn with permission from Boileau *et al.* (1988) © 1988 by Human Kinetics.

Application to other methods

The concept of chemical maturity relative to measurement of body composition in children and youth must also be applied to other reference methods. As an example, the use of TBW to estimate body composition assumes a constant hydration of FFB of 73.8% (Brozek *et al.*, 1963). However, in prepubescent children the FFB hydration level (see Table 33.1) appears to be as high as 76–77% (Lohman, 1986). Therefore, by using the adult constant a lower than actual percentage of fat estimate is computed. Likewise, implicit in the use of body potassium to estimate body composition is that the potassium content of the FFB is known and constant. However, the potassium content $(g \cdot kg^{-1}$

FFB) appears to increase with age and maturation (Boileau *et al.*, 1985). While the direction of change in the FFB components appears to be known, more data on the magnitude of change in FFB water, mineral and protein content are needed to develop more accurate models and equations for estimating body composition in children and youth.

It is likely that different equations based on age and maturation status, such as shown in Table 33.2, will be needed to address this problem, the resolution of which will also enable more effective validation and calibration of newer techniques such as dual energy radiography and total body electrical conductivity.

Another related issue is the appropriate calibration of techniques which rely on the

Table 33.1 Age- and gender-specific constants for conversion of body density, water and potassium to percentage of fat in children and youth. These estimates are based on the following: Boileau *et al.* (1984, 1985), Fomon *et al.* (1982), Haschke (1983) and Lohman *et al.* (1984a,b). Adapted with permission from Lohman *et al.* (1986).

Age (year)	Density FFB		Water FFB		Potassium FFB		Mineral FFB	
	Male	Female	Male	Female	Male	Female	Male	Female
7–9	1.081	1.079	76.8	77.6	2.40	2.32	5.1	4.9
9–11	1.084	1.082	76.2	77.0	2.45	2.34	5.4	5.2
11–13	1.087	1.086	75.4	76.6	2.52	2.36	5.7	5.5
13–15	1.094	1.092	74.7	75.5	2.56	2.38	6.2	5.9
15–17	1.096	1.094	74.2	75.0	2.61	2.40	6.5	6.1
17–20	1.0985	1.095	74.0	74.8	2.63	2.41	6.6	6.0
20–25	1.100	1.096	73.8	74.5	2.66	2.42	6.8	6.2

FFB, fat-free body.

Table 33.2 Constants for equations to estimate percentage of fat of body density from the densities of fat and fat-free body. (The density of fat was assumed to be $0.9\,g \cdot cm^3$; the D_{FFB} was obtained from Table 33.1.)

Age (years)	Males		Females	
	$k_1{}^*$	$k_2{}^*$	$k_1{}^*$	$k_2{}^*$
7–9	5.375	4.972	5.425	5.028
9–11	5.302	4.891	5.351	4.945
11–13	5.232	4.813	5.255	4.839
13–15	5.075	4.639	5.119	4.688
15–17	5.033	4.592	5.075	4.639
17–20	4.981	4.534	5.054	4.615
20–25	4.95	4.5	5.033	4.592

* The above constants are used in the general equation:

% fat = $[(k_1/D_B) - k_2] \times 100$.

Example: for a girl, age 12 years with a measured $D_B = 1.04\,g \cdot cm^3$

% fat = $[(5.255/1.04) - 4.839] \times 100 = 21.4\%$.

Table 33.3 Effect of assuming a chemically mature fat-free body (FFB) density for estimating percentage of fat (%fat) in maturing youngsters (hypothetical male child). Assumed percentage of fat was calculated from the Siri (1961) equation.

Variable	Age (years)		
	8	12	16
Body density (g·cm³)	1.050	1.050	1.050
Actual D_{FFB} (g·cm³)	1.080	1.090	1.097
Actual %fat	14.3	18.0	20.4
Assumed D_{FFB} (g·cm³)	1.100	1.100	1.100
Assumed %fat	21.4	21.4	21.4
%fat difference (assumed−actual)	7.1	3.4	1.0

prediction of reference method values. An example is the use of skinfold thickness values or bioelectric measures to predict density and/or fat percentage and FFB estimated from densitometry. In earlier studies, it was common

practice to use equations developed for children to predict density, and then to estimate percentage of fat from that density value using the Siri or Brozek equations. This procedure now appears to be inappropriate and has been shown to produce inaccuracies similar to those cited above for densitometry.

Clinical methods for assessing body composition

While the traditional and newer body composition methods generally offer better accuracy and precision, their application is normally restricted to a laboratory setting and requires expensive technology. Additionally, these measurements may require extensive subject cooperation and/or a lengthy measurement process, both of which can be problematic with children. Methods which provide rapid, safe, inexpensive, accurate and precise body composition measurements are needed for clinical and field testing. In this context, the three most frequently utilized methods are the body mass index (BMI), anthropometry and bioelectric impedance analysis (BIA).

Body mass index

While BMI cannot be technically classified as a body composition measurement, it has received widespread use with adults in clinical and epidemiological assessments. BMI only requires measurement of height and body weight. It is defined as body weight/height^2 and expressed as $kg \cdot m^2$. The development of BMI norms from large databases permits the classification of individuals into categories such as normal, overweight and obese. Use of BMI has been criticized on the grounds that the numerator, body weight, is not only influenced by fat but also by various components of the non-fat mass. Indeed, it can be shown that most heavy weight athletes (e.g. weight-lifters, football linemen, shot putters) are classified as overweight if not as obese by this index. Furthermore, Garn et al. (1986) have demonstrated that body structure is a consideration since individuals with shorter legs have a higher BMI. In adults BMI appears to be independent of height (Forbes, 1987), but in children there is typically a significant correlation suggesting that the BMI is influenced by growth.

Using national health and examination survey data, Lohman (1992) has shown that it is difficult to interpret BMI values in terms of body composition in children and youth. As an example, he demonstrated (Table 33.4) that at the 50th percentile, the BMI ranges from 15.4 for the 6-year-old male to 21.5 for the 17-year-old male, while the sum of the triceps and subscapular skinfolds only ranges from 12 to 15 mm across the same age span. Thus, while Table 33.4 provides normative data for use of BMI in children, it is doubtful that it can be applied to make a meaningful evaluation of body composition status. Conversely, the use of height and weight indices to detect acute (weight for height) and chronic (height for age) malnutrition will continue to be useful in the context of nutritional anthropometry for broad classification purposes when employed with appropriate reference standards (Anjos *et al.*, 1992).

Anthropometry

Anthropometry, specifically measures of skinfold thickness, is the most frequently employed method to estimate body composition. Like BMI, skinfolds are relatively easy and inexpensive to obtain. Standardization of skinfold sites and techniques is described in Lohman *et al.* (1988). Subcutaneous fat, in theory, is believed to make a major contribution to the prediction of body fat since it comprises about 5% of the total body fat. Skinfold equations have been developed in several samples of children and youth to predict either D_B and/or fat percentage (Parizkova, 1961; Durnin & Rahaman, 1967; Young *et al.*, 1968; Cureton *et al.*, 1975; Boileau *et al.*, 1981; Slaughter *et al.*, 1984, 1988) and FFB (Lohman *et al.*, 1975). The SE of estimate for D_B derived from stepwise regression analysis of multiple skinfold sites are generally similar to those observed for adults (Lohman, 1981). Thus, the

Table 33.4 Body mass index (BMI) and the sum of the triceps and subscapular skinfolds by age and gender for selected percentiles. Calculations were derived using National Health and Examination Survey norms (1963–68). Adapted with permission from Lohman (1992) © 1992 by T.G. Lohman.

	BMI						Sum of two skinfolds					
	50th		85th		95th		50th		85th		95th	
Age (years)	M	F	M	F	M	F	M	F	M	F	M	F
6	15.4	15.2	16.8	17.1	18.2	18.5	12	14	16	19	20	27
7	15.6	15.4	17.1	17.6	18.9	19.6	12	15	17	22	24	28
8	16.0	15.9	18.1	18.6	20.2	21.1	13	16	19	25	28	36
9	16.2	16.3	19.0	19.5	22.4	22.9	14	17	23	29	34	41
10	16.5	16.9	19.2	20.6	21.8	23.6	14	18	24	32	33	43
11	17.2	17.5	20.9	21.7	24.2	24.8	15	19	28	31	39	43
12	17.8	18.6	21.4	22.6	24.1	26.2	15	20	24	34	44	47
13	18.7	19.4	22.6	23.4	26.6	26.8	15	21	28	39	46	52
14	19.6	20.2	23.2	24.1	26.7	26.5	14	24	27	37	39	53
15	20.4	20.7	24.0	24.7	27.8	29.4	14	25	25	41	40	56
16	20.8	20.9	24.0	24.9	26.9	29.6	14	26	24	42	39	58
17	21.5	21.0	24.9	24.3	28.5	29.3	15	27	26	42	41	59

F, female; M, male.

potential to use skinfolds to estimate body fat in children and youth appears promising.

However, there are major limitations to accurate estimation of body fatness from skinfolds in children and youth. First, many of the equations developed for paediatric samples have not been cross-validated and thus, their application to other normal samples, and such samples as the obese, racial groups and children at different pubertal stages is generally unknown.

A second problem in using skinfold equations concerns the estimated reference value of fat or FFB. Most equations use the dependent variables, D_B or percentage of fat derived from D_B, however, the problem of chemical immaturity has largely been ignored or at least not considered when predicting the dependent variables. Thus, most equations are based on the adult model using either the Siri or Brozek equation to estimate body fat and as a consequence overestimate percentage of fat from 1 to 7% (Table 33.5). It is noteworthy that the data of Harsha et al. (1978) provided in Table 33.5 underestimates percentage of fat by 0.5 and 2% for Black males and females, respectively, as opposed to the general overestimation shown for white subjects. This suggests that chemical maturation of the FFB may proceed differently in the Black than in the white population. The general problem of failing to consider the variability in chemical maturity of children and youth confounds attempts to estimate the prevalence of obesity (Lohman et al., 1989) and may result in an underestimation of minimal weight for application in sport (Boileau et al., 1985).

A third problem relates to the relationship

Table 33.5 Comparison of skinfold equations developed in children and youth. Adapted with permission from Boileau et al. (1985).

Sex	Age (a)	Sum of two skinfolds	%fat*	%fat†	Difference (%)	Reference
M	9–12	16.5	22.3	14.6	7.7	Parizkova (1961)
F	9–12	21.5	26.0	21.1	4.9	
M	13–16	15.5	17.0	13.6	3.4	
F	13–16	19.5	22.8	19.4	3.4	
F_a	—	22.0	27.3	21.5	5.8	Young et al. (1968)
F_m	—	28.1	27.3	26.1	1.2	
M	7.9	15.3	20.4	13.4	7.0	Lohman et al. (1975)
M	9.1	15.9	17.4	14.0	3.4	
M	10.1	19.1	21.6	17.0	4.6	
M	11.0	19.8	22.0	17.6	4.4	
M_w	6–16	22.8	23.5	20.1	3.4	Harsha et al. (1978)
M_b	6–16	22.5	19.4	19.9	−0.5	
F_w	6–16	29.5	29.1	27.0	2.1	
F_b	6–16	30.7	25.7	27.7	−2.0	
M_i	8–11	17.2	20.5	15.3	5.2	Boileau et al. (1981)
M_c	8–11	18.3	18.7	16.3	2.4	

* Estimated from density (hydrostatic weighing) or ^{40}K spectroscopy.
† Percentage of fat (%fat) was estimated from sum of two skinfolds (triceps and subscapular) using the following equation. Males: %fat = 1.35 (sum of two skinfolds – 0.012 (sum of two skinfolds)^2 – 4.4; females: %fat = 1.35 (sum of two skinfolds) – 0.012 (sum of two skinfolds)^2 – 2.4.
b, Black; c, California sample; F, female; i, Illinois sample; M, male; m, menarchal; n, non-menarchal; w, White; %fat, percentage of fat.

of skinfolds to density. Slaughter *et al.* (1984) have shown that this relationship varies with maturity (Fig. 33.4) with prepubescent and pubescent males and females having a significantly different relationship than adults. Part of the variability in this relationship can be attributed to variability in the D_{FFB} during growth and maturation as described above. However, maturity-related variability in the distribution of subcutaneous fat at various sites (Baumgartner *et al.*, 1986) and the ratio of internal to external fat stores must also be considered in explaining the difference in the relationship of skinfolds to D_B with maturation.

Recent progress has been made in resolving many of the problems associated with use of skinfolds to estimate body composition in children and youth. The work of Slaughter *et al.* (1984, 1988) has provided generalized equations which account for variability in chemical maturity, based on maturation, gender and race (Table 33.6). This work, based on a large paediatric sample ($n = 310$), provides prediction equations for the sum of two skinfold combinations, either triceps–subscapular or triceps–calf. These equations estimate per-

centage of fat derived from equation 33.2 above in which density, water and bone mineral measurements were employed. Furthermore, this approach has been cross-validated with several independent paediatric samples and appears to provide the most useful equations available (Slaughter *et al.*, 1988).

Bioelectric impedance analysis

A third approach which meets the requirements for clinical and field setting measurements is the BIA method. This method is based on the principle that there is a differential impedance to the flow of an oscillating electrical current in tissues of high and low water and electrolyte content. Since FFB has high water and electrolyte contents, particularly in the mineral-free FFB, the impedance to the flow of current is low, whereas fat has a substantially higher impedance to current flow because it is relatively low in water and electrolyte content (Pethig, 1979). Recent publications have extensively provided the fundamental theory, principles and applications for the use of BIA (Baumgartner *et al.*, 1990; Kushner, 1992). There

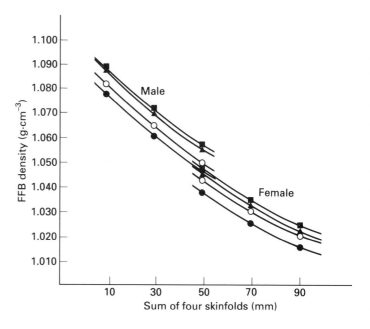

Fig. 33.4 Relation between skinfolds (of the triceps, calf, abdomen and thigh) and fat free body (FFB) density in four maturation groups for males and females. ●, prepubescent; ○, pubescent; ■, postpubescent; ▲, adult. Redrawn with permission from Slaughter *et al.* (1984).

Table 33.6 Prediction equations of percentage of fat from triceps and calf and from triceps and subscapular skinfolds (SF) in children and youth for males and females. Calculations were derived using Slaughter *et al.* (1988) equation. Adapted with permission from Lohman (1992) © 1992 by T.G. Lohman.

Triceps and calf SF
   %fat = 0.735 ΣSF + 1 M, all ages
   %fat = 0.610 ΣSF + 5 F, all ages

Triceps and subscapular SF (> 35 min)
   %fat = 0.783 ΣSF + I M
   %fat = 0.546 ΣSF + 9.7 F

Triceps and subscapular SF (< 35 mm)*
   %fat = 1.21 (ΣSF) − 0.008 (ΣSF)^2 + I M
   %fat = 1.33 (ΣSF) − 0.013 (ΣSF)^2 + 2.5 F (2 Black, 3 White)

I = Intercept varies with maturation level and racial group for M as follows:

Age	Black	White
Prepubescent	−3.5	−1.7
Pubescent	−5.2	−3.4
Postpubescent	−6.8	−5.5
Adult	−6.8	−5.5

* Thus for a white pubescent male with a triceps of 15 and a subscapular of 12, the %fat would be:

%fat = 1.21 (27) − 0.008 (27)^2 − 3.4
   = 23.4%.

F, female; M, male; %fat, percentage of fat.

are now numerous studies which have validated the use of this method to estimate the FFB in children and adults. While impedance is a function of two electrical properties, resistance (*R*) and reactance, *R* has been found to be the most useful variable of the two for the estimation of body composition (Van Loan *et al.*, 1990). Furthermore, since the length of the conductor is related to the conducting volume/mass, height (*H*) is used as an index of *R* expressed as follows:

H^2/R.

Most BIA prediction equations estimate FFB from a combination of variables including the H^2/R, and body weight. The H^2/R variable can

be shown to be related to the conductor volume and hence is related to the volume of FFB and TBW (Baumgartner *et al.*, 1990). Since body weight is highly related to FFB, including weight in the equation substantially lowers the predictive error, however in most studies H^2/R dominates the prediction of FFB. Using H^2/R and body weight as predictor variables, the relative error for estimating TBW and FFB has ranged from 3 to 8% and 3.5 to 6%, respectively. Table 33.7 presents a summary of the absolute error in estimating FFB reported in several studies conducted on children (Kushner, 1992). This error tends to be lower than observed for the skinfold method. However, it must be noted that validation studies are normally conducted under laboratory conditions where standardization of measurement procedures and subject status are carefully monitored.

We have recently analysed BIA data on a sample of 129 white males and females, aged 8–16 years, utilizing both the RJL model BIA-101 (RJL Systems, Detroit, Michigan, USA) and Valhalla model 1990B (Valhalla Scientific, San Diego, California, USA) impedance analysers to estimate TBW and FFB. FFB was computed from density, water and bone mineral measurements (eqn 33.2). The analysis was carried out utilizing H^2/R, body weight and gender as independent variables. As expected, the precision of estimating FFB was similar for both instruments, with slight variation noted in the actual prediction equations as indicated below:

FFB (RJL) = 3.919 + 0.637(H^2/R) + 0.170(BW)
         − 0.133(gender*)   (33.7)

FFB (Valhalla) = 4.138 + 0.657(H^2/R)
              + 0.16(BW) − 0.131(gender*)
                                    (33.8)

where BW = body weight, SEE (standard error of estimate) = 1.75 kg and CV (coefficient of variation) = 4.5%. *A categorical coding for gender is used: +1 = male; −1 = female. The relationship of FFB to the predicted FFB for the RJL instrument is presented in Fig. 33.5. Additionally, the relationship of TBW measured by deuterium oxide dilution to its predicted

Table 33.7 Validation studies in children for the estimation of fat-free body (FFB) weight from bioelectric impedance analysis. Adapted with permission from Kushner (1992).

n (M/F)	Age (years)	Reference method	Variable	R^2	SEE (kg)	Reference
30 (14/16)	9–14	D_BFFB	H^2/R	0.69	4.08	Cordain *et al.* (1988)
73 (33/41)	8–11	D_BFFB	H^2/R, BW, G	0.89	1.31	Deurenberg *et al.* (1989)
94 (53/41)	10–14	D_BFFB, TBW	H^2/R, BW	0.92	2	Houtkooper *et al.* (1989)
39 (18/21)	7–9	D_BFFB	H^2/R	0.85	1.07	Deurenberg *et al.* (1990)
91 (71/20)	10–15	D_BFFB	H^2/R, BW, H	0.96	1.87	
116 (41/75)	13–25	D_BFFB	H^2/R, BW, G, H	0.94	2.55	
166	7–15	D_BFFB,	H^2/R, BW, G, H	0.97	1.68	Deurenberg *et al.* (1991)
129 (69/60)	7–16	D_BFFB, TBW, bone	H^2/R, BW, G	0.97	1.75	Present study

BW, body weight; D_B, total body density; F, female; G, gender; H, height; M, male; R, resistance; SEE, standard error of estimate; TBW, total body water.

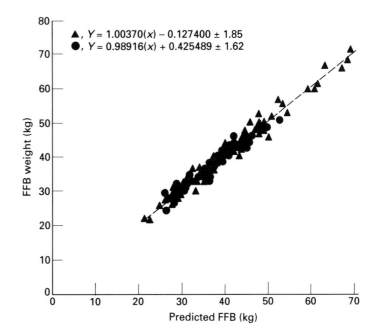

Fig. 33.5 Relationship of the fat-free body (FFB) estimated from density, water and bone mineral measurements with the predicted FFB estimated from the bioelectric impedance (RJL) in children (see text for the prediction equation). ▲, males; ●, females.

values is shown in Fig. 33.6. The relative error for FFB (4.5%) and TBW (4.9%) are within the range of values presented by Kushner (1992).

Challenges for future research

Significant progress has been made in our understanding of body composition changes during growth and maturation. However, the amount of data available on children is relatively limited in scope making definitive conclusions extremely tentative.

• The development of new techniques to measure body composition and/or its components provides improved opportunities to study larger and more diverse samples. In particular, more research is needed to further define changes in body composition components, particularly those components associated with the FFB, since correctly accounting for variability in these components is crucial to accurately assessing growth and maturity changes. Moreover, it is essential that recently developed models of body composition be tested in various racial/ethnic groups and during changes in nutritional status and physical training. There is evidence for differences in body composition among races, however,

timing of changes in body composition components is not well understood. This will necessitate multicomponent measurements of large racially and maturationally diverse samples. Expanding the current database with this in mind will provide the opportunity to define more appropriately the reference body composition of children at various ages within gender and racial groups. Conceptually, the reference body can assist in the better definition of standards for minimal body weight and obesity. The concept and measurement of minimal body weight, which is defined by FFB and essential fat, is important for the evaluation of nutritional status and for application in sports such as wrestling in which weight classification systems are used.

• The emergence of new and more precise techniques to measure both total body composition and its components offers the opportunity in future research to verify independently the validity of the multicomponent densitometric approach presented earlier. In particular, dual energy radiography has the potential of providing assessment of a three-component model made up of TBM, fat and a mineral-free lean component which is largely made up of muscle. While the validity of this approach

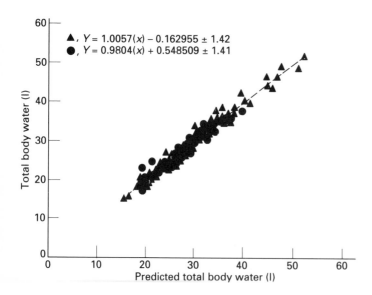

Fig. 33.6 Association of total body water (TBW) measured by deuterium oxide dilution with the predicted TBW estimated from bioelectric impedance (RJL) in children. The prediction equation is: $TBW(l) = 2.147 + 0.47 (H^2/R) + 0.145 (BW) - 0.123$ (gender); SEE = 1.42 l, CV = 4.9%. ▲, males; ●, females.

needs to be more firmly established, this technique not only offers the potential to verify the multicomponent densitometric model but also makes possible regional body composition estimates of bone, fat and muscle.

• Finally, additional research is needed to further define the accuracy and precision of clinical methods. Such methods need to be validated in diverse racial/ethnic samples. To date, few data are available for samples other than white Caucasians and the form of validation has been mostly restricted to using the two-component densitometric model. The only exceptions are the studies of Slaughter *et al.* (1984, 1988) for estimating fat and FFB from skinfolds and the data presented in this chapter for BIA. Future validation studies of clinical methods should be conducted with a multi-component method and in racially/ethnically diverse samples.

References

Akers, R. & Buskirk, E.R. (1969) An underwater weighing system utilizing 'force cube' transducers. *J. Appl. Physiol.* **26**, 649–52.

Anjos, L.A., Boileau, R.A. & Misner, J.E. (1992) Maximal mechanical aerobic and anaerobic power output of low-income Brazilian schoolchildren as a function of growth. *Am. J. Hum. Biol.* **4**, 647–56.

Baumgartner, R.N., Chumlea, W.C. & Roche, A.F. (1990) Bioelectric impedance for body composition. In K.B. Pandolf & J.O. Holloszy (eds) *Exercise and Sports Sciences Reviews*, Vol. 18, pp. 193–224. Williams & Wilkins, Baltimore.

Baumgartner, R.N., Roche, A.F., Guo, S., Lohman, T., Boileau, R.A. & Slaughter, M.H. (1986) Adipose tissue distribution: the stability of principal components by sex, ethnicity, and maturation stage. *Hum. Biol.* **58**, 719–35.

Behnke, A.R., Feen, B.G. & Welham, W.C. (1942) The specific gravity of healthy men. *JAMA* **118**, 495–8.

Boileau, R.A. (1988) Utilization of total body electrical conductivity in determining body composition. In National Academy of Sciences (eds) *Designing Foods: Animal Product Options in the Marketplace*, pp. 251–7. National Research Council/National Academy of Sciences, Washington, D.C.

Boileau, R.A., Horswill, C.A. & Slaughter, M.H. (1989) Body composition and the young athlete. In W.J. Klish & N. Kretchmer (eds) *Report of the 98th Ross Conference on Pediatric Research: Body Composition*

Measurements in Infants and Children, pp. 104–111. Ross Laboratories, Columbus, OH.

Boileau, R.A., Lohman, T.G. & Slaughter, M.H. (1985) Exercise and body composition in children and youth. *Scand. J. Sport Sci.* **7**, 17–27.

Boileau, R.A., Lohman, T.G., Slaughter, M.H., Ball, T.E., Going, S.B. & Hendrix, M.K. (1984) Hydration of the fat-free body in children during maturation. *Hum. Biol.* **56**, 651–66.

Boileau, R.A., Lohman, T.G., Slaughter, M.H., Horswill, C.A. & Stillman, R.J. (1988) Problems associated with determining body composition in maturing youngsters. In E.W. Brown & C.F. Branta (eds) *Competitive Sports for Children and Youth: An Overview of Research Issues*, pp. 3–16. Human Kinetics, Champaign, IL.

Boileau, R.A., Wilmore, J.H., Lohman, T.G., Slaughter, M.H. & Riner, W.F. (1981) Estimation of body density from skinfold thicknesses, body circumferences and skeletal widths in boys age 8 to 11 years: comparisons of two samples. *Hum. Biol.* **53**, 575–92.

Brozek, J., Grande, F., Anderson, J.T. & Keys, A. (1963) Densitometric analysis of body composition, revision of some quantitative assumptions. *Ann. N. Y. Acad. Sci.* **110**, 113–40.

Buskirk, E.R. (1987) Body composition analysis: the past, present and future. *Res. Q. Exerc. Sport* **58**, 1–10.

Coates, T., Killen, J. & Slinkard, L. (1982) Parent participation in a treatment program for overweight adolescents. *Int. J. Eat. Dis.* **1**, 37–48.

Conway, J.M., Norris, K.H. & Bodwell, C.E. (1984) A new approach for the estimation of body composition: infrared interactance. *Am. J. Clin. Nutr.* **40**, 1123–30.

Cordain, L., Whicker, R.E. & Johnson, J.E. (1988) Body composition determination in children using bioelectrical impedance. *Growth, Devel. Aging* **52**, 37–40.

Cureton, K.J., Boileau, R.A. & Lohman, T.G. (1975) Relationship between body composition measures and AAHPER test performances in boys. *Res. Q.* **46**, 218–29.

Deurenberg, P., Kusters, C.S.L. & Smit, H.E. (1990) Assessment of body composition by bioelectrical impedance in children and young adults is strongly age-dependent. *Eur. J. Clin. Nutr.* **44**, 261–8.

Deurenberg, P., van der Kooy, K., Leenen, R., Weststrate, J.A. & Seidell, J.C. (1991) Sex and age specific prediction formulas for estimating body composition from bioelectrical impedance: a cross-validation study. *Int. J. Obes.* **15**, 17–25.

Deurenberg, P., van der Kooy, K., Paling, A. & Withagen, P. (1989) Assessment of body composition in 8–11 year old children by bioelectrical impedance. *Eur. J. Clin. Nutr.* **43**, 623–9.

Durnin, J.V.G.A. & Rahaman (1967) The assessment of the amount of fat in the human body from measurement of skinfold thickness. *Br. J. Nutr.* **21**, 681−9.

Fomon, S.J., Haschke, F., Ziegler, E.E. & Nelson, S.E. (1982) Body composition of reference children from birth to age 10 years. *Am. J. Clin. Nutr.* **35**, 1169−75.

Forbes, G.B. (1987) *Human Body Composition: Growth, Aging, Nutrition and Activity*, pp. 85−7. Springer-Verlag, New York.

Forbes, R.M., Cooper, A.R. & Mitchell, H.H. (1953) The chemical composition of the adult human body as determined by chemical analysis. *J. Biol. Chem.* **203**, 359−66.

Forbes, R.M., Mitchell, H.H. & Cooper, A.R. (1956) Further studies on the gross composition and mineral elements of the adult human body. *J. Biol. Chem.* **223**, 969−75.

Garn, S.M., Leonard, W.R. & Hawthorne, V.M. (1986) Three limitations of the body mass index. *Am. J. Clin. Nutr.* **44**, 996−7.

Harsha, D.W., Frerichs, R.R. & Berenson, G.S. (1978) Densitometry and anthropometry of black and white children. *Hum. Biol.* **50**, 261−80.

Haschke, F. (1983) Body composition of adolescent males. Part II. Body composition of the male reference adolescent. *Acta Paediatr. Scand.* **307** (Suppl.), 11−23.

Heymsfield, S.B., Wang, J., Kehayias, J. & Pierson, R.N. (1989) Chemical determination of human body density *in vivo*: relevance to hydrodensitometry. *Am. J. Clin. Nutr.* **50**, 1282−9.

Houtkooper, L.B., Lohman, T.G., Going, S.B. & Hall, M.C. (1989) Validity of bioelectric impedance for body composition assessment in children. *J. Appl. Physiol.* **66**, 814−21.

Keys, A. & Brozek, J. (1953) Body fat in adult man. *Physiol. Rev.* **33**, 245−318.

Kushner, R.F. (1992) Bioelectrical impedance analysis: a review of principles and applications. *J. Am. Coll. Nutr.* **11**, 199−209.

Lohman, T.G. (1981) Skinfolds and body density and their relation to body composition: a review. *Hum. Biol.* **53**, 181−225.

Lohman, T.G. (1984) Research in progress in the validation of laboratory methods of assessing body composition. *Med. Sci. Sports Exerc.* **16**, 596−603.

Lohman, T.G. (1986) Applicability of body composition techniques and constants for children and youth. In K.B. Pandolf (ed.) *Exercise and Sport Sciences Reviews*, Vol. 14, pp. 325−57, Macmillan, New York.

Lohman, T.G. (1989) Assessment of body composition in children. *Pediatr. Exerc. Sci.* **1**, 19−30.

Lohman, T.G. (1992) *Advances in Body Composition Assessment: Current Issues in Exercise Science*. Human Kinetics, Champaign, IL.

Lohman, T.G., Boileau, R.A. & Massey, B.H. (1975) Prediction of lean body weight in young boys from skinfold thickness and body weight. *Hum. Biol.* **47**, 245−62.

Lohman, T.G., Boileau, R.A. & Slaughter, M.H. (1984a) Body composition in children and youth. In R.A. Boileau (ed.) *Advances in Pediatric Sports Sciences*, Vol. 1. *Biological Issues*, pp. 26−57. Human Kinetics, Champaign, IL.

Lohman, T.G., Going, S.B., Slaughter, M.H. & Boileau, R.A. (1989) Concept of chemical immaturity in body composition estimates: implications for estimating the prevalence of obesity in childhood and youth. *Am. J. Hum. Biol.* **1**, 201−4.

Lohman, T.G., Roche, A.F. & Martorel, R. (eds) (1988) *Anthropometric Standardization Reference Manual.* Human Kinetics, Champaign, IL.

Lohman, T.G., Slaughter, M.H., Boileau, R.A., Bunt, J. & Lussier, L. (1984b) Bone mineral measurements and their relation to body density in children, youth and adults. *Hum. Biol.* **56**, 667−80.

Lukaski, H.C. (1987) Methods for the assessment of human body composition: traditional and new. *Am. J. Clin. Nutr.* **46**, 537−56.

Lukaski, H.C., Bolonchuk, W.W., Hall, C.B. & Siders, W.A. (1985) Assessment of fat-free mass using bioelectric impedance measurements of the human body. *Am. J. Clin. Nutr.* **41**, 810−17.

Mazess, R.B., Peppler, W.W., Chestnut, C.H., Nelp, W.B. & Cohn, S.H. (1981) Total body bone mineral and lean body mass by dual photon absorptiometry. *Calc. Tiss. Int.* **33**, 361−3.

Mitchell, H.H., Hamilton, T.S., Steggerda, F.R. & Bean, H.W. (1945) Chemical composition of the adult human body and its bearing on the biochemistry of growth. *J. Biol. Chem.* **158**, 625−37.

Parizkova, J. (1961) Total body fat and skinfold thickness in children. *Metabolism* **10**, 794−809.

Pethig, R. (1979) *Dielectric and Electronic Properties of Biological Materials*, pp. 207−42. John Wiley, Chicester.

Seidell, J.C., Bakker, C.J.G. & van der Kooy, K. (1990) Imaging techniques for measuring adipose-tissue distribution − a comparison between computed tomography and 1.5-T magnetic resonance. *Am. J. Clin. Nutr.* **51**, 953−7.

Selinger, A. (1977) *The body as a three component system*. Unpublished PhD dissertation, University of Illinois, Urbana, IL.

Siri, W.E. (1961) Body composition from fluid spaces and density: analysis of methods. In J. Brozek & A. Henschel (eds) *Techniques for Measuring Body Composition*, pp. 223−44. National Academy of Sciences, Washington, DC.

Slaughter, M.H., Lohman, T.G., Boileau, R.A. *et al.*

(1984) Influence of maturation on the relationship of skinfolds to body density: a cross-sectional study. *Hum. Biol.* **56**, 681–9.

Slaughter, M.H., Lohman, T.G., Boileau, R.A. *et al.* (1988) Skinfold equations for estimation of body fatness in children youth. *Hum. Biol.* **60**, 709–23.

Thorland, W.G., Tipton, C.M., Lohman, T.G. *et al.* (1991) Midwest wrestling study: prediction of minimal weight for high school wrestlers. *Med. Sci. Sports Exerc.* **23**, 102–10.

Van Loan, M.D., Boileau, R.A., Slaughter, M.H. *et al.* (1990) Association of bioelectrical resistance with estimates of fat-free mass determined by densito-metry and hydrometry. *Am. J. Hum. Biol.* **2**, 219–26.

Wilmore, J. (1969) A simplified method for determination of residual lung volumes. *J. Appl. Physiol.* **27**, 96–100.

Wilmore, J.H. & McNamara, J.J. (1974) Prevalence of coronary heart disease risk factors in boys 8–12 years of age. *J. Pediatr.* **84**, 527–33.

Ylitalo, V. (1981) Treatment of obese school children. *Acta Paediatr. Scand.* **209** (Suppl.), 1–108.

Young, C.M., Sipin, S.S. & Roe, D.A. (1968) Body composition of preadolescent and adolescent girls: I. Density and skinfold measurements. *J. Diet. Ass.* **53**, 25–31.

Chapter 34

Anthropometry in Assessing Physique Status and Monitoring Change

WILLIAM D. ROSS

Introduction

The purpose of this chapter is to establish the basic principles and procedures for the acquisition of quality anthropometric data on children. The assessment of physique status and especially the serial monitoring of change requires precise and accurate anthropometric techniques. Children represent a special challenge to the anthropometrist and this chapter provides a few guidelines to facilitate effective data assembly, resolution and reporting.

Quality of data

Assessing individual growth status or monitoring change depends upon 'theory and process'. This emphasis is identical to that advocated by W. Edwards Deming who helped bring about a revolution in manufacturing and business in Japan. Deming believes that quality is a function of human commitment (Peters & Austin, 1983).

Measurement error

In anthropometry, quality is a generic term for 'precision' and 'accuracy'. The terms are not synonymous. Accuracy is the exactness or conformity of an obtained measure to the true score. Precision is the consistency of data that can be determined by a simple replication procedure. The comparison of repeated scores by the same measurer is also referred to as intra-observer reliability, or when compared to scores of another measurer as interobserver reliability or objectivity. Test–retest correlation coefficients are inappropriate to describe the precision of measurement although the resultant regression equation may be highly illuminating and provide for some kind of conversion (that is, correct for systematic effects). The technical error of measurement (t.e.) is a more appropriate statistic to assess quality since it takes into account both random and systematic differences (Dahlberg, 1940; Johnston et al., 1972; Mueller & Martorell, 1988; Knapp, 1992). The t.e. and per cent t.e. (%t.e.) are based on a comparison of initial scores (X_1) and replicated scores (X_2) as follows:

$$\text{t.e.} = [(\Sigma \, X_2 - X_1)/2n]^{0.5} \qquad (34.1)$$

$$\%\text{t.e.} = 100 \, (\text{St.e./mean of } X_1). \qquad (34.2)$$

Accuracy. This presupposes precision. It also requires that there is no systematic departure from the explicit definition of the measurements, landmarks and techniques used to obtain a 'true score'. One may be precise but inaccurate, never imprecise and accurate. At best accuracy can be inferred when scores of different observers agree with median values of replicated scores obtained by a criterion anthropometrist (by definition, one who has impeccable technique and does not make systematic error from the defined measurement). Guided training in standardized techniques with comparison to measurements by criterion anthropometrists is highly effective.

Technical error guideline. The %t.e. shown in Table 34.1 are typical for adults in field studies by trained anthropometrists, not from independent measures by criterion anthropometrists under the best of laboratory conditions. Replications were made from the same marked sites and do not include possible systematic error in the location of the sites. Those items with asterisks are estimates from limited observations. We did not differentiate the small differences between men and women except in listing skinfolds. The table serves only as a general guide and should not to be interpreted as precisions standards for all situations. For the same absolute t.e., the percentages will be higher in smaller size children.

Need for standardized techniques

Troika training

The use of three-person training and deployment units is common. The so-called 'troika-plan' came about by chance. Undergraduate students preparing for a pilot study in a senior's residence were advised to be prepared for multitasking — in other words, they had to be precise, accurate and versatile. The analogy was that they had to pull together as a troika (from the Russian for a three-horse carriage or sleigh). It was a strained analogy at best. The undergraduates liked the term 'troika'. It was quickly adopted as a technical term by our international colleagues for training and deployment of anthropometrists. Some insist that each troika should have at least one man and one woman as a member and that it represent a variety of professional and scientific competencies.

The advantage of 'troika training' is that it is relatively easy to organize and it is self-contained with the partners taking turns serving as subject, measurer, recorder and computer operator. Regardless of the designation or learning plan, anthropometric training has three requisites.

1 Strict adherence to the explicit definition of landmarks and techniques.
2 Adequate practice in measurement evaluated by the calculation of t.e. from replicated measures to assess intra- and interobserver reliability.
3 Overall scrutiny by a criterion anthropometrist, with comparison and correction of techniques where systematic error is suspect.

Formal training is essential

Anthropometry is deceptively simple though skilled technicians can, with formal training and persistent practice, produce accurate data. The amount of training needed varies from individual to individual, but most seem to achieve reasonable competence after triple-measurement on 100 or so subjects and spot-checking for systematic error by comparison with criterion measures. A criterion anthropometrist by definition is one who purportedly does not make systematic errors from a prescribed technique.

Replicated measurement protocol

Proforma

A well-designed anthropometric proforma is a primary and indispensable tool. It facilitates data assembly, resolution, report and recall. We provide space for four series of measurements: an original, two replications and median values from the first three.

It is often a false economy to delimit the anthropometric protocol to a few variables. Accumulated data with easy access is a valuable resource. The time involved in taking eight skinfolds rather than three is minimal. The major time expense is in marshalling the subjects and switching from instrument to instrument. The proforma should therefore be planned in terms of minimal changes of equipment and choreographed for efficient movement of the anthropometrist and subject.

An adapted proforma based on that used in

Table 34.1 Estimated technical errors of measurement expressed as a percentage of mean values obtained in field studies. Percentage technical errors in samples of smaller size children would be proportionally larger than values shown in the table.

Basic	%	Lengths	%	Breadths	%	Girths	%	Skinfolds	%
Stature (stretch)	0.2	Arm (acromiale–radiale)	0.8	Biacromial	1.0	Head	0.5*	*Male*	
Body mass	0.1	Forearm (radiale–stylion)	1.1	Bi-iliocristal	1.1	Neck	0.8*	Triceps	3.0
Sitting height	0.4	Hand (mid-stylion–dactylion)	1.2	Transverse chest	1.2	Arm relaxed	0.8	Subscapular	3.6
Span	0.3	Iliospinale to box	0.4	Anteroposterior chest depth	0.7	Arm flexed/tensed	0.9	Biceps	2.3
		Trocanterion to box	0.8	Humerus	1.0	Forearm	0.7	Iliac crest	6.2
		Thigh (trochanterion–tibiale laterale)		Wrist (bistyloid)	1.9	Wrist	1.0	Supraspinale	3.4
		Leg (tibiale laterale–box)	0.9	Hand	1.0*	Chest	0.8	Abdominal	6.2
		Tibia (tibiale mediale–sphyrion tibiale)	0.4	Femur	1.0	Waist	0.7	Front thigh	4.7
		Foot (acropodion–pternion)	0.9			Omphalion	*0.8	Medial calf	2.8
		Recumbent				Hip (gluteal)	0.7		
		Recumbent length	0.4*			Thigh (upper)	0.7	*Female*	
		Crown–rump	0.6*			Mid-thigh	0.7	Triceps	4.0
						Calf (maximal)	0.4	Subscapular	3.6
						Ankle (minimum)	0.6	Biceps	2.9
								Iliac crest	8.3
								Supraspinale	4.0
								Abdominal	8.7
								Front thigh	6.4
								Medial calf	4.5

* Based on limited observations.

the 1991 Championships in the world swimming, diving, synchronized swimming and water polo category is shown in Fig. 34.1. In field studies, it is often prudent to use non-carbon duplicating data forms: (i) an original copy for computer data entry and filling; (ii) a copy as a separate back-up file; and (iii) a copy to the individual of his or her coach for their records. For direct computer entry, normal back-up of data and separate file copies on floppy disks guards against computer errors.

Selection of a best estimate from a replicated series

From studies on skinfolds discussed by Ross and Eiben (1992) we accept that the error in one measurement is independent of the error in replicated values. Therefore, the theory for combining uncorrelated errors applies (see Beers, 1957). Thus, taking the mean of three trials as the best estimate, t.e. is reduced to about 58% of what it would be in a single series. The median of three values further reduces t.e. as demonstrated by Ward (1988). The median is particularly effective in resisting imposed systematic error since it is unaffected by gross error. When time is limited, two trials may be taken with a third taken only when the first two disagree by some set tolerance. The mean of the closest two is then used as the truest value. In practice it is easier to take three series of measures than calculate the tolerances of two to determine if a third measurement is needed.

In building norms, or making group comparisons, single measurements of all items, including skinfolds, are appropriate. However, single measurements are inappropriate in clinical use. Accurate data is essential to ascribe individual physique status or monitor change with respect to growth, ageing, treatment, diet or exercise. As a rule, take three complete series of measurements and use medians as the best estimates of true values.

Ross and Eiben (1991) claim the technical errors of skinfolds obtained at different sites or the same site on different occasions are independent of one another.

Frequency of anthropometric assessments

Frequency of measurement depends upon the objective. In some sports daily weight records are part of the training log since the individual pattern of fluctuations is of concern in meeting weigh-in requirements. Normally, weekly measurement of body weight at some designated time in the day provides adequate monitoring. The interpretation of this data is fraught with hazards, especially if the individual or coach sets inappropriate goals about a presumed 'ideal' body weight (S.M. Garm, personal communication, 1993).

Assessment of physique status should take place as soon as feasible after injury and during recovery. Prudently one should accept that any indication of loss in muscle (decline in skinfold-corrected girths) is indicative of negative nitrogen balance. This requires a reassessment of the situation and likely change in the training and nutritional programme. The possible concomitant irreversible loss in bone mineral content is a serious health risk.

When one is concerned with both structure and function, anthropometric data should be assembled at the same time as the biomechanical or physiological test procedures. A recent proposal by Dennis Caine (personal communication, 1994) for routine monitoring of growth in young gymnasts specified daily training logs, weekly measurement of body weight, quarterly measurement of stature, sitting height and span, 10 girths and eight skinfolds, and 6-monthly measurement of all the items in a comprehensive battery of tests similar to that outlined in this chapter. Weekly shifts in body weight, particularly loss, invited scrutiny. Recent experience in a second longitudinal study by D.A. Bailey (personal communication, 1994) led him to comment on an astonishing seasonal effect that is missed entirely by annual assessment.

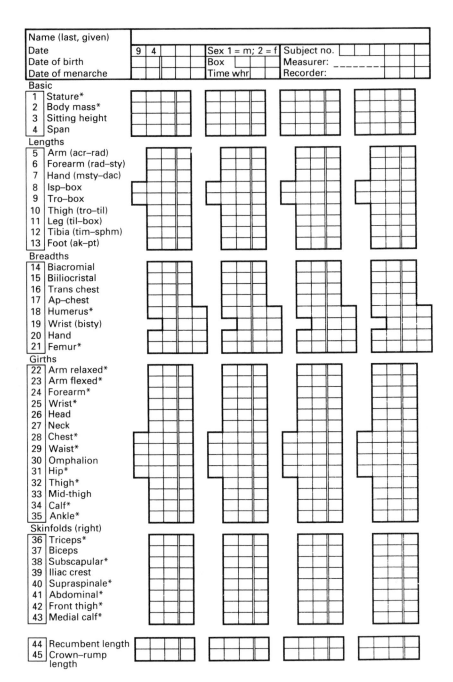

Fig. 34.1 Basic proforma for the child and adolescent athlete designed for three series of measurements and entry of median scores. * Included in the advanced O-Scale Physique Assessment System (Ward *et al.*, 1989).

Standardized procedures

Standardized anthropometry is an elusive goal. Similarly named techniques cannot be assumed to be identical. For example, the International Biological Programme (IBP) method for obtaining biacromial breadth 'when the shoulders are rounded forward' (Weiner & Lourie, 1981) is systematically larger than the classical technique advocated in this chapter where the subject stands erect. Supra-iliac skinfolds are widely misinterpreted by authors and investigators, therefore the original source must be checked. Any procedure that describes techniques without reference to explicit landmarks and exact style of measurement is suspect and invites misinterpretation and error in application.

The techniques in this chapter are mainly based on the classical definition of landmarks, by Martin (1928) and later interpretations by Stewart (1952) and Martin and Saller (1959), and most recently by Ross and Marfell-Jones (1990). The latter are similar to those used in courses sponsored by the International Society for the Advancement of Kinanthropometry (ISAK) and are generally compatible with those used in the Olympic Games studies reported by DeGaray et al. (1974), Ross et al. (1978), Borms et al. (1979) and Carter (1982, 1984). A general overview with an illustration of common landmarks is found in an International Olympic Committee (IOC) Medical Commission (Ross et al., 1988). This present chapter is based on a text prepared by the author for a proposed Barcelona Olympic Games anthropological project and used as the basis for the protocol for the successful Kinanthropometric Aquatic Sports Project. This project assembled normative data on 919 swimmers, divers, synchronized swimmers and water polo players at the 1991 World Championships in Perth, Australia (summary report in Carter & Ackland, 1994).

Right side anthropometry

The procedures in this chapter involve unilateral measurements on the right side only. This is contrary to the IBP convention to use the left side. Since kinanthropometrists and sports people are primarily interested in the most dominant side, the right is preferred. Right side measurement also facilitates the measurement of diagonal skinfolds. When there is a question of bilateral asymmetry, however, both sides should be measured. In some athletes asymmetry is an important factor in their structural appraisal. This may be of major concern in the appraisal of trauma in tennis players, runners and skaters, or in the postural assessment of growing children.

Instrumentation

The following is a listing of the equipment required for the measurements described in this chapter. One should never confuse the quality of an instrument with its cost. Invariably we select the simplest and most inexpensive instrument provided it yields as precise results as the more expensive instruments demonstrated under both laboratory and field test conditions.

Stadiometer. Ideally a wall-mounted stadiometer with digital read-out would be in place for the measurement of stretch stature and sitting height. However, either because of lack of funding or available space this is not always possible. The 1981 Canada Fitness Survey personnel successfully used a portable system for stretch stature when moving from household to household. It consisted of a retractable metric measuring tape with a homemade adapted foot piece and a simple triangular head board, a device at least 130 years old (Broca, 1865).

Anthropometric tape. Ideally, the anthropometric tape should be steel, calibrated in easy to read centimetres with millimetre gradation; 1.5–2 m long with an end tab before the zero marking, enclosed in a case and incorporating a spring for automatic retraction. One such tape is the Lufkin, Executive, Thinline 2 m W606PM (Cooper Tools, Apex, NC, USA). Other tapes may be used, though they should have the following characteristics (Ross & Eiben, 1992).

1 Non-extendibility (steel): if other materials are used, the tape must be frequently examined to ensure accurate readings.

2 Flexibility: ideally no wider than 7 mm.

3 Ease of reading: calibrated in metric units with unequivocal identification of the centimetre mark (tapes with English and metric scale on the same side are inadequate as are scales that only indicate deciles and have increments of $1-9$ rather than designate every centimetre interval).

4 A stub (at least 4 and ideally 7 or 8 cm) before the zero line to facilitate manipulation.

5 Freedom from spring or other devices ostensibly aimed at achieving a constant pressure (see section on measurement of girths).

6 Absolute accuracy of scale.

Anthropometer and segmometer. Until recently, the Martin-type classical anthropometer was the standard. A mechanical digital Harpenden model was also used. Out of necessity our colleague, Linda Blade, sought an inexpensive alternative instrument for her field studies in Nigeria. As shown in Fig. 34.2, an engineer's retractable tape was adapted using filed cotter pins as pointers as reported by Carr *et al.*

(1993). The new instrument, the so called 'segmometer', was shown to be at least as accurate for both projected and direct measures as the anthropometer that it replaces for this purpose.

With the use of a measuring box of a known height the segmometer can be used for both projected and direct measurement techniques. In the recent Kinanthropometric Aquatic Sports Project, a combination of three projected heights and five direct segmental lengths using the segmometer were included in the protocol.

Manufactured versions with a machined base and a sliding pointer in a looped tape are available from Rosscraft (Surrey, BC, Canada). The Rosscraft Segmometer 3 provides for direct and derived lengths and the Segmometer 6 additionally for limb bone breadths.

Skinfold calipers. For many years the Harpenden Caliper (British Indicators Ltd, Burgess Hill, UK) and Lamge Calipers (Cambridge Scientific Industries, Cambridge, MD, USA) were the instruments of choice. Schmidt and Carter (1990) showed the two calipers yielded small non-systematic differences. They showed the relatively inexpensive plastic Slim Guide Caliper (Creative Health Products, Plymouth, MI, USA) had similar dynamic action to the Harpenden caliper yielding slightly smaller skinfold thickness. Widely distributed by the manufacturer and Rosscraft, the Slim Guide is often used as an instrument of choice, especially in mass testing programmes where widespread

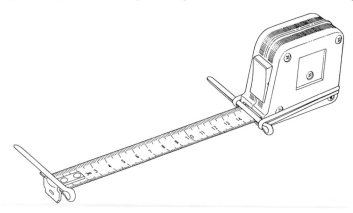

Fig. 34.2 Segmometer to replace anthropometer for projected and derived lengths. Reproduced from Carr *et al.* (1993).

professional applications are anticipated. It has larger jaw excursion accommodating skinfolds up to 80 mm. All three calipers in the hands of trained anthropometrists are roughly similar in precision, yielding a t.e. of roughly 5% for a single series replication.

Bone calipers. Adapted Mitutoyo bone calipers first described by Carter (1980) are recommended for humerus and femur widths. These calipers have extended branches with round pressure plates of 15 mm diameter. The inside diameter branches of the Mitutoyo caliper are removed and the locking device is fixed to permit easy manipulation. An electronic version based on similar design features for replication in non-specialized machine shops has been specified by Ross *et al.* (1993), however, cost for such custom calipers may be prohibitive.

A new small bone caliper based on a US patent for a double-sliding branch principle by Robert Campbell provides for a new level of precision in measuring bone breadths. The design permits firm pressure on the ends of the branches without binding. The Campbell Caliper 10, named after the inventor, is manufactured by Rosscraft under exclusive patent agreement. It has double vernier scales to permit reading in an up and down orientation.

Wide sliding calipers. Occasionally, torso and limb breaths are obtained using an anthropometer as described by Ross and Marfell-Jones (1990). The disarticulated end piece of the Siber Hegner anthropometer used as a wide sliding caliper for torso measurements is not altogether satisfactory. It tends to bind when pressure is applied to the ends of the branches instead of along the sides. The black on grey scale is somewhat difficult to read. Because of the design limitations and cost, a variety of custom anthropometers and calipers are made locally in non-specialized machine shops using various designs such as that described by Ross (1985). The double-sliding branch principle is incorporated in the Campbell Caliper 20, a wide

sliding caliper manufactured by Rosscraft. The non-binding feature permits firm pressure without binding and moderate and light pressure on others as required.

Wide spreading caliper. The large wide spreading caliper (Siber-Hegner, GPM) is the instrument of choice for anteroposterior chest depth. However, anthropometers or wide sliding calipers with recurved branches may be used as a substitute. The new Campbell Caliper 10 has optional olive-tipped pointers that attach for this purpose.

Weighing machine. Classically, the weighing machine was a balance beam scale calibrated in kilograms and tenths of kilograms. These are to be found under different brand names throughout the world. The best of them provide for calibration adjustments. In recent years, these have given way to digital scales. Most of these are converted spring-type scales with electronics to convert a digital read out. They are no more accurate that an ordinary bathroom scale.

The new generation of scales use strain gauges rather than springs. They are accurate over a long period of time. A moderately priced AND UC300 Scale (A & D Engineering, Milpitas, CA, USA) provides for simple weighing. In addition it has a tare weight option (zero with mother on the scale, given the naked baby to hold in her arms, the infant's weight may then be read directly) and other memory functions. For some studies its range of up to 125 kg is a disadvantage. The Seca 777000 (Seca, Vogel and Halke GmbH & Co., Hamburg, Germany, with regional dealers in the UK, France and USA) with AC adapter and rechargeable batteries is an accurate instrument that provides for a range of up to 200 kg. As a floor scale it is more portable than the more expensive waist-high model. Both provide an adjustment for latitude and altitude. The company also manufactures a conventional spring-type scale with a range up to 150 kg.

With access to microcomputers, simple non-linear scales that behave consistently can be calibrated and a computer algorithm used to make systematic corrections of scale values. The onus on every investigator and clinician is to calibrate weighing machines. A simple way to do this to have a set of barbell weights accurately weighed and stamped. Sometimes this is possible at a governmental agency or private company. Intermediate values can be assessed using a kit of known of weight standards of up to 2 kg.

Anthropometric box. A 50 × 40 × 30 cm box may be used for seating the subject to obtain measures such as sitting height, transverse chest breadth or humerus and femur widths. A box of known height is part of the protocol for measuring some of the projected heights in conjunction with the segmometer. The oblong box with slotted handholds enable the anthropometrist to turn the box to accommodate subjects of different size. In addition to providing a place for seating or elevating standing subjects for convenience of measurement, the box also serves as a step for the anthropometrists who may stand on it to obtain stretch stature or biacromial breadth in tall subjects.

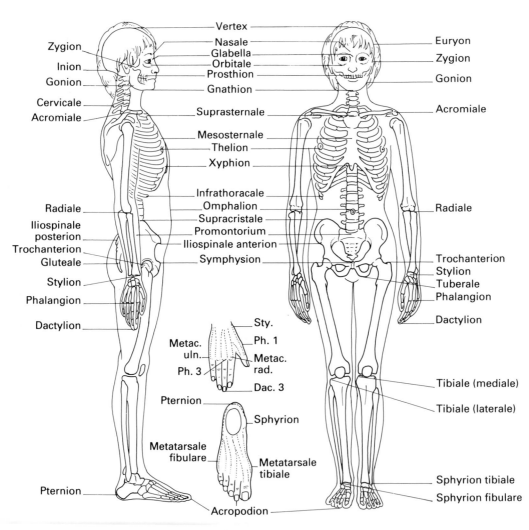

Fig. 34.3 Landmarks. Redrawn from Ross *et al.* (1983).

Measuring platform. In many field test situations, floors are not level or are uncomfortable to the barefoot subject. A useful optional piece of equipment is a 60 × 120 cm wooden five-ply platform that can be levelled by wooden shims.

Other ancillary equipment includes: screwdrivers, pliers, wrench and Allen key to service anthropometric equipment; a carpenter's spirit-level; a plumb bob; and standard weights for calibration of balance-beam weighing machine that serves, in turn, to calibrate spring scales. A simple field test calibration for skinfold calipers is to fix the instrument in a vice and suspend weights from the lower jaw. The caliper should be adjusted so that the jaws remain open in any position when the appropriate calibration weight is used (that is, $10 \, \text{g} \cdot \text{mm}^{-2}$ surface area of a caliper pressure plate for Harpenden and Slim Guide calipers).

Anthropometric technique

Precise and accurate measurement requires explicit definition of landmarks. Selected sites are illustrated in Fig. 34.3 and defined below.

Marking

Placement of instruments on the exact location of the landmarks is crucial to precise and accurate measurement. This is facilitated in some measurements by marking the skin surface of the subject in reference to the underlying skeletal structure. We prefer marking with fine-line washable felt tip pens, however, an ordinary ballpoint pen is adequate.

The general procedure for identifying a landmark is: (i) locate; (ii) release and relocate; (iii) mark; and (iv) check. The technique requires the use of the lateral nail of the thumb and distal nail of the index fingers of both hands. Cut and file the nails so that they extend only slightly when applying pressure to the fleshy portion of your own thumb and index fingers. This ensures subject comfort. Moreover, with properly groomed nails, landmarking and measuring can be done wearing rubber gloves without appreciable loss in accuracy as determined in student experiments.

With practice, landmarking can be completed unconsciously, very rapidly and accurately. The releasing, relocating and checking is automatic assuring the surface of the skin does not distort the location of the landmark. Both hands are used in the process. We have included some nuances in how to locate landmarks on atypical subjects. Do not use these except when necessary. Normally, the sequencing in landmarking is uniform with minimum manipulation and posing of the subject.

Do not innovate or teach non-standard anthropometry. If you propose an alternate procedure for location of a landmark or technique, provide the rationale and assemble the evidence. Petition the Chairman of the ISAK Working Group on Standards and Instrumentation for a considered opinion. Present the case formally, report the t.e. on your proposed procedure and the standard procedure, and show the systematic difference between median values of each. This was done for the use of the segmometer and direct length procedures in this chapter, approved on the basis of economy, ease and precision and later reported in the literature by Carr *et al.* (1993). In other instances, the proposition may be accepted as a 'nuance'. This is an occasional augmentation for problem situations such as the hip manipulation to locate the trochanterion, recumbent position for measuring abdominal skinfold and a double grasp for the measurement of front thigh skinfold.

ANTHROPOMETRIC LANDMARKS

Acromiale. Point at the most superior and external border of the acromion process of the scapula when the subject stands erect with the pendant arms by the sides.
1 Place your pencil alongside the external border of the scapula to identify the superior margin.
2 Locate the most superior lateral margin with the left side of your left thumb.

3 Release and relocate with your left index finger nail.

4 Mark with a small horizontal line.

5 Check with the left side of your left thumb nail while your right thumb nail locates the radiale.

Radiale. Point at the most superior and lateral border of the head of the radius.

1 Using your right thumb nail palpate downward in the lower portion of the lateral dimple of the elbow to locate the head of the radius.

2 Release and relocate with left index finger (a slight pronation/supination of the subject's forearm is reflected by a rotary movement of the head of the radius).

3 Mark.

4 Check using the side of the nail of your left thumb while you use the nail or your right thumb to locate the stylion.

Stylion. Most distal point on the processus syloidus radius. This is located in the so-called 'anatomical snuff-box' identified when the thumb is extended and adducted.

1 Place your right thumb nail in the box defined by the tendons (of the extensor carpi radialis longus and the adductor policus longus). Locate the stylion, the most distal tip of the radius.

2 Release and relocate with the nail of your left index finger.

3 Mark.

4 Check with the nail of the thumb of your left hand, freeing your right hand to start to locate the mesosternale.

Note: the stylion is the landmark for obtaining forearm length. We prefer a direct measure of hand length from the mid-stylion point to the dactylion using the segmometer rather than deriving hand length from projected lengths of the stylion and dactylion (Carr *et al.*, 1993).

Mesosternale. Point on the corpus sterni at the intersection of the midsagittal and horizontal planes, at the midlevel of the fourth chondrosternal articulation.

1 A two-handed palpation method provides for rapid location of the landmark. Place your index fingers on the clavicles on either side of the manubrium sternum while your thumbs locate the first costal spaces, thus encompassing the first ribs.

2 Then move your index fingers to replace the thumbs that are lowered to the second intercostal spaces to identify the second ribs.

3 Repeat the procedure for the 3rd and 4th ribs.

4 Mark the mesosternale, that is, the midpoint of the sternum at the level of the centre of the articulation of the 4th rib with the sternum.

Iliospinale. Most inferior tip of the anterior superior iliac spine. (In matters of adjusting for clothing, point to the site and tell the subject you wish to make a mark. Men usually pull down their shorts, some do not, but mostly women and children pull up on the leg of their shorts.)

1 Grasp the subject's left hip about the inguinal level with your left hand, use your thumb to palpate anteriorly to locate the undermost point of the anterior superior iliac spine. Occasionally, you will find it difficult to locate. Ask the subject to stand on his or her left foot, raise the heel of the right foot and rotate inwards and outwards on the ball of the right foot. The movement of the sartorius muscle can be traced to its origin at the site of the landmark.

2 As usual, release and relocate with the nail of the index finger.

3 Mark.

4 Check using the nail of your left thumb.

Trochanterion. Most superior point on the greater trochanter of the femur. Location of this landmark requires a persistent technique using the locate, release, relocate, mark and check procedure. The subject takes a short stride forward resting the right foot on a raised object about 15 cm high. Stand behind the subject and locate and mark the trochanterion using the following procedures.

1 Locate the landmark as follows:

   (a) stabilize the subject's left hip with your left hand;

   (b) palpate using the thenar eminence of

your right palm (i.e. the fleshy pad on the palm of your hand on the thumb side) by pushing on the lateral aspect of the subject's gluteal maximus to locate the trochanter that is on a line with the long axis of the femur;
(c) identify the uppermost part by firm downward pressure of your hand;
(d) then have the subject carefully assume the erect stance with weight equally distributed on each foot, and the toes pointing directly forward; and
(e) use the side of your right thumb as a wedge to palpate anteriorly and upward on the head of trochanter to locate the most superior point.
2 Release the pressure and reapply with the nail of your left thumb or index finger.
3 Mark the site on the relatively undistorted skin surface.
4 Check with the right thumb assuring the site is directly over the trochanterion.

Occasionally, in locating the landmark, you can ask the subject to extend his or her hip laterally, or, bend the knee and move the thigh forward and backward. When you are still doubtful, relocate the landmark when the subject is recumbent on a table lying on the left side and facing away from you.

Tibiale laterale. Most proximal point of the margo glenoidalis of the lateral border of the head of the tibia. It is often easier to locate the landmark by having the subject flex his or her leg at the knee, or sit down. The tibiale laterale is located as follows.
1 Find the depression or dimple in the knee, bounded by a triad of prominences: epicondylar femur, anterolateral portion of the head of the tibia, and the head of the fibula.
2 From this orientation, press inward using the side of your right thumb as a wedge, locate the border of the tibia, and palpate posteriorly until you locate the landmark, which is the most superior point. This is at least one-third of the anterior posterior distance.
3 Release, relocate with the nail of the index finger and mark.
4 Check pressing downward using the nail of

your right thumb. (The tibiale laterale is approximately in the same transverse plane as the tibiale mediale.)

Tibiale mediale and sphyrion tibiale. These landmarks define the length of the tibia. The subject sits and crosses the right leg over the left thigh presenting the medial side of the tibia.
1 Locate the proximal border of the tibia with the nail of your right thumb.
2 Release and relocate with the nail of your left index finger.
3 Mark.
4 Check using the nail of your left index finger pushing downward to the bony margin while searching for the sphyrion tibiale with your right thumb nail.
5 Locate the sphyrion tibiale, the most distal point on the tibia (not the lateral protuberant malleolare) with your right thumb nail.
6 Release and relocate with the nail of your left index finger.
7 Mark.
8 Check with the nail of your right thumb by pushing upwards to the designated landmark.

Mid-acromiale—radiale. A line is marked horizontal to the long axis of the humerus at the mid-acromiale—radiale distance, as determined by an anthropometric tape.
1 Wrap the anthropometric tape around the arm at the level of the mark, holding the tape with your left thumb and second digit.
2 Mark horizontal lines at the level of the mid-acomiale—radiale mark on the posterior and anterior surfaces of the surface of the arm.
3 With the subject having pendant arms with the hands along the thigh, make a vertical line at the most posterior surface to intersect with the horizontal line to mark the site where the triceps skinfold is raised.
4 With the subject very slightly rotating the hand outward, make a vertical line at the most anterior surface directly over the belly of the biceps brachii to identify the site where the biceps skinfold is raised.

Mid-stylion line. The subject flexes at the elbow

and presents the right wrist, palmar surface upward.

1 Wrap the tape around the wrist pinning it distal to the stylion ulnare and stylion radiale on the dorsal surface with your left thumb and second digit (it is not necessary to hold the case).

2 Draw a small line on the palmar surface at the proximal border of the tape in the mid-portion of the wrist.

3 Release the tape and estimate the mid-portion of the subject's wrist and make a cross on the previous line.

4 Check that the cross is in the mid-portion and in line with the dactylion, the most distal point on the terminal phalanx III when the hand is extended with the fingers together.

Mid-thigh. There are several methods for locating the mid-thigh. One is to use half the measured distance in a seated subject from the inguinal line at mid-thigh to the anterior margin of the patella. This is consistent with the technique for estimating the site for obtaining mid-thigh skinfolds. For girth measurement we prefer defining the mid-thigh as half the measured distance from the previously located trochanerion to the tibiale laterale when the subject stands erect.

1 In identifying this level you place anthropometric tape zero indicator of the marked site on the marked trochanterion and pin it there with pressure by the third digit of your left hand.

2 Let the tape hang freely and hold it to the thigh with your outstretched left thumb.

3 Extend the tape downwards and note the distance to the previously marked tibiale laterale.

4 Estimate half the distance on the tape held in place with your third finger and thumb and mark the lateral thigh at this level.

Body mass, stature, sitting height, span and recumbent lengths (Fig. 34.4)

Body mass (weight). We agree in personal communication with S.M. Garn that there is no such thing as an ideal body weight for all people for all health risks. Instead, we scale for the sum of six skinfolds and a geometrical size adjusted proportional body weight as a frame for summaries and proportional profiles with 20 other items for 46 age- and sex-specific norms by Ward *et al.* (1989). There is a need for other simple displays for assessing physique status relevant to age, sex, ethnic and activity background of individuals (see research challenges).

Ideally, body mass expressed in units of weight should be obtained on an accurately calibrated beam-type balance and recorded to the nearest 0.1 kg. The subject should be weighed nude or in clothing of known weight so a correction to nude weight can be made. The most stable values for monitoring weight change are those obtained routinely in the morning, 12 h after having ingested food, and after voiding. However, such exact control is not generally necessary for growth records. For most purposes, a calibrated spring scale with measurement made to the nearest 0.5 kg is satisfactory.

Stature (stretch). There for four general techniques for measuring stature which yield slightly different values. These are (i) free standing stature; (ii) stature against the wall; (iii) recumbent length; and (iv) stretch stature. The standard method for this chapter is stretch stature against a wall. An explicit description of the selected technique and strict adherence to it are important.

The measurement is normally made with the stadiometer, although a constructed device is not essential. The instrument can be fairly elaborate, featuring ball-bearing counter-weighted headboards and digital or electronic read-outs, or it can be little more than two wooden planes at right angles. The practice of using a wooden rectangular chalk box and pencil marks on the door jamb can yield satisfactory results. A carpenter's retractable measuring tape with footpiece can be used to measure the length from the floor to mark. Unfortunately, the typical doctor's office stadi-

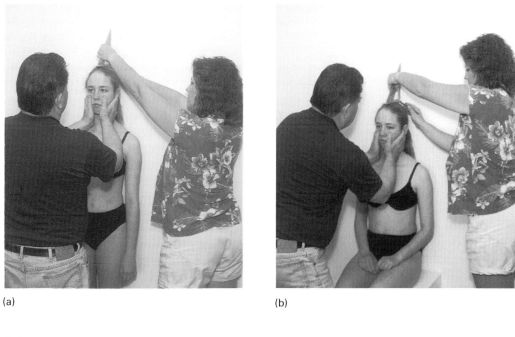

(a)   (b)

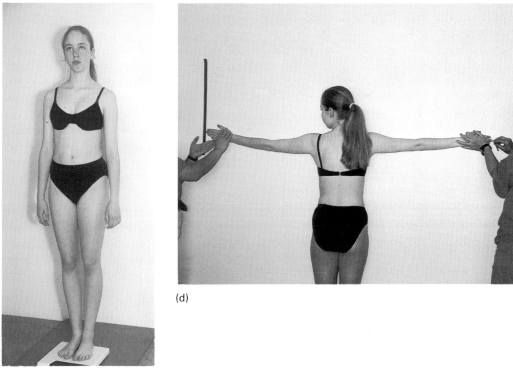

(c)

(d)

Fig. 34.4 Basic four measurements: (a) stature (stretch); (b) sitting height; (c) body mass; (d) span.

ometer attached to a beam-type scale is inadequate and should not be used for critical measurements.

Stature is the maximum distance from the floor to the vertex of the head. Technically, the vertex is defined as the highest point on the skull when the head is held in the Frankfort plane. This position is when the imaginary line joining the orbitale to the tragion is perpendicular or at right angles to the long axis of the body as shown in Fig. 34.5. The orbitale is located on

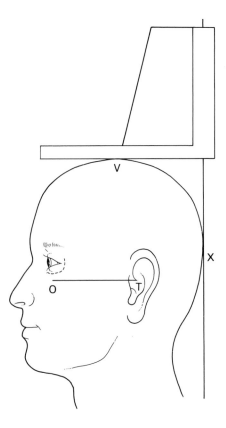

Orbitale: Lower margin of eye socket
Tragion: Notch above tragus of ear or at
  upper margin of zygomatic bone at that point
Frankfort plane: Orbitale–tragion line
  horizontal
Vertex: Highest point on skull when head is
  held in Frankfort plane

Fig. 34.5 Position of the head in the Frankfort plane. Redrawn from Ross (1977).

the lower or most inferior position on the margin of the eye socket. The tragion is the notch above or superior to the tragus or flap of the ear, at the superior aspect of the zygomatic bone. This position corresponds almost exactly to the visual axis when the subject is looking directly ahead.

In making the stature measurement, the measurer has the barefoot subject stand erect with heels together and arms hanging naturally by the sides. The heels, buttocks, upper part of the back and usually, but not necessarily, the back of the head are in contact with the vertical wall. Instruct the subject to 'look straight ahead' and 'take a deep breath', while you apply gentle traction to the mastoid processes. One technique is to do so while your thumbs are at the level of the orbitale and your index fingers are at the level of the tragion. Your assistant ensures that the subject's heels are not elevated while you apply gentle stretch force, by cupping the subject's head and applying gentle traction at the mastoid processes. Your assistant then brings the headpiece firmly down in contact with the vertex and makes a pencil mark on the paper tape level of the underside of the headpiece. The subject then steps away from the wall. Remove the headpiece and measure the vertical distance from floor to pencil mark with the retractable metal tape, or, with an anthopometric tape to the mark from an established horizontal line on the paper, e.g. 1 m high. In field test situations, the subject's name or number can be used to identify the marks to measure at a convenient time. Record the distance to the nearest 0.1 cm. The paper record identified for day and time of measurement may also be saved. You can use a similar paper on the wall marking procedure for sitting height and span.

Sitting height. Distance from the vertex to the base of the sitting surface when the seated subject is instructed to sit tall and gentle traction is applied to the mandible. This measurement is usually made when the subject is seated on the measuring box before a paper tape affixed to the wall. The feet are on the floor. Care must be taken to ensure the subject does not push with the legs. Orient the subject's head in the Frankfort plane as in stretch stature above. Instruct the subject to 'take a deep breath, look straight ahead, and sit as tall as possible' while you apply gentle traction to the mastoid processes with your cupped hands. Again, you may identify the level of the orbitale with your thumbs and the tragion with your index fingers to guide your assistant in assuring the head is in the proper position. Marking is the same as in stretch stature. A more detailed account with comparison of five sitting height techniques is found in a technical note by Carr *et al.* (1989).

Span. Distance from the left to the right dactylion of the hands when the palms are facing forward on the wall and the outstretched arms are abducted to the horizontal with the shoulders. The dactylion is the fleshy part of the most distal finger not the nail. Normally, this is obtained in a corner of a room on a wall. A paper is attached to the wall to facilitate marking. Instruct the subject to face the wall, raise the arms to the horizontal and place the hands flat on the wall and place one finger in the corner or abutment. Hold the subject's opposite wrist and encourage him or her to stretch as far as possible. Your assistant can hold the other wrist assuring the dactylion is at the abutment. Record the maximum span with a mark on the wall or paper affixed to the wall. When a series of subjects are measured, each mark on the wall can be identified with initials and measured subsequently. As for stature and sitting height, the paper with a known distance from the abutment marked on it with subject's initials can be served as confirmatory data. The distance from the abutment to the scratch line is measured subsequently to the nearest 0.1 cm.

Recumbent length and crown–rump length. In longitudinal studies, children aged 3 years should be measured using standing stature and sitting height as well as with the infant technique for recumbent and crown–rump

length which yield slightly greater values. In making these measures, you should orient the subject's head in the Frankfort plane to a fixed headboard while your assistant applies a right-angled square to the stretched feet or rump and records the distance to the nearest 0.1 cm from a tape affixed to the table top.

Projected lengths by segmometer and box (Fig. 34.6)

Based upon criticism of projected measurements using anthropometers by Day (1984, 1986) an immediate need for an inexpensive alternative resulted in the design and testing of a new instrument and restatement of techniques. These include two projected heights adding box height, one projected height from the top of the box while standing on it, and five direct segmental lengths using the segmometers described previously.

During projected measures on the upper extremity, the subject stands erect with the arms at the sides and palms against the thighs. The segmometer housing is held in the right hand by an overgrasp of the fingers. The pointer end is grasped in the left hand (index and thumb) and placed on the top of the box. The housing pointer is extended by the right hand to the designated landmark. Reading is made to the nearest 0.1 cm.

Iliospinale height. Projected height from the box to the iliospinale landmark. The subject stands with the feet together facing a corner of the box, with heels together and feet on either side of the box. Place the end pointer flush on the box with your left hand and extend the housing pointer of the segmometer vertically upward with your right hand to the marked iliospinale landmark.

Trochanterion height. Projected height from the box to the trochanterion landmark. The subject stands with the feet together and facing away from the anthropometrist with the right side of the right leg against the box. Place the end

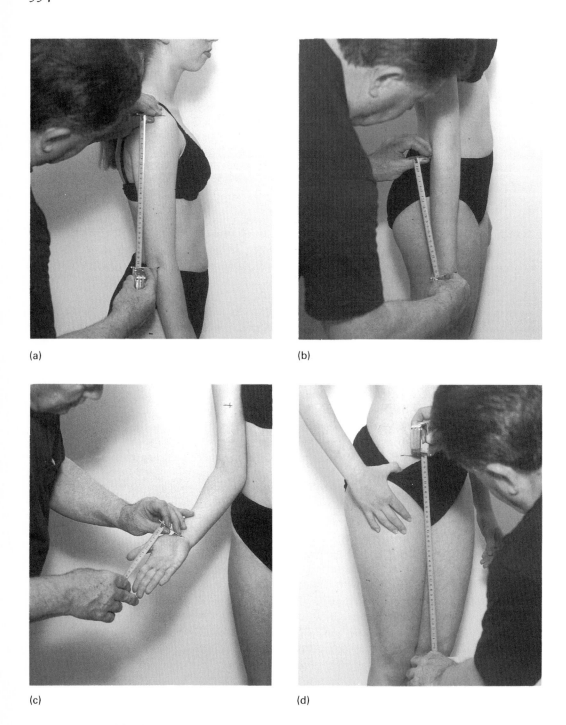

(a)

(b)

(c)

(d)

Fig. 34.6 Projected heights and segmental lengths: (a) arm (acromiale–radiale); (b) forearm (radiale–stylion); (c) hand (mid-stylion–dactylion); (d) iliospinale to box.

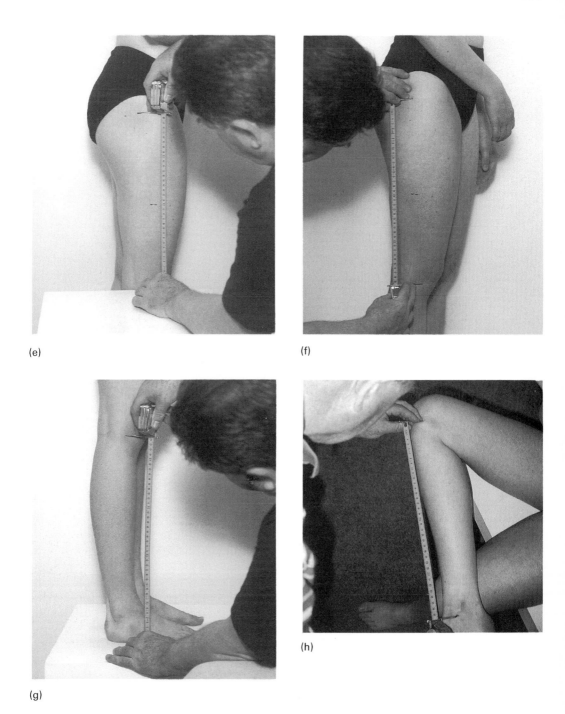

Fig. 34.6 *Continued*. (e) Trocanterion to box; (f) thigh (trochanterion–tibiale laterale); (g) leg (tibiale laterale to box); (h) tibia (tibiale mediale–sphyrion mediale).

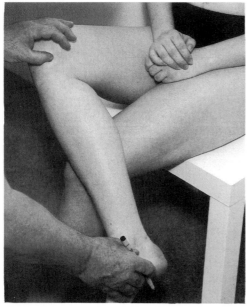

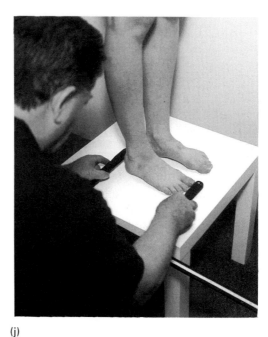

(i)   (j)

Fig. 34.6 *Continued.* (i) Position for measuring the tibia; (j) foot (acropodion—pternion).

pointers flush on the box with your left hand and extend the housing pointer of the segmometer vertically upward with your right hand to the marked trochanterion landmark.

Tibiale laterale height. Distance from the box to the tibiale laterale landmark. In measuring the tibiale laterale height, position the subject to stand on a box with feet together with his or her right leg facing you. Place the end pointer of the segmometer flush on the box with your left hand and move the housing pointer vertically upward with the right hand to the marked tibiale laterale landmark.

Direct lengths by the segmometer (Fig. 34.6)

When using the segmometer for direct lengths cradle the end pointer between your thumb and index finger of your left hand. Use the mid-finger of your left hand to anchor on the skin surface at the lower site stabilizing and protecting against penetration by the pointer that is guided by your thumb and index finger to the marked site. Extending the tape with your right hand place the housing pointer on the upper marked site. Reading is made to the nearest 0.1 cm.

Arm (acromiale—radiale length). The distance from the acromiale to the radiale. The subject stands erect with arms extended downwards and palms pressed against the side of the thigh. Place the end pointers on the acromiale and the housing pointer on the radiale keeping the segmometer parallel to the long axis of the humerus.

Forearm (radiale—stylion length). Distance from the radiale to the stylion. The subject maintains the same position as for the acromiale—radiale length. Place the end pointer on the radiale and the housing pointer on the dactylion keeping the segmometer parallel to the long axis of the radius.

Mid-stylion—hand (mid-stylion line to dactylion length). Shortest distance from the mid-stylion line to the dactylion III. The subject extends the right hand supinated (palms up), fully extending the fingers. Place the end pointer on the marked mid-stylion line and apply the housing pointer held in your right hand to the subject's dactylion, the most distal point on the fleshy surface of the third digit.

Thigh (trochanterion—tibiale laterale length). Distance from the trochanterion to the tibiale laterale. The subject stands with feet together on the box with the right leg facing you. Anchor the end pointer with your left third finger and lower the point grasped by your thumb and index finger to the site. Extend the housing pointer with your right hand to the marked tibiale laterale.

Leg (tibiale laterale height). Height of the tibiale laterale from the floor or top of a box (see projected tibiale laterale height above).

Tibia (tibiale mediale—sphyrion tibiale). Direct length from tibiale mediale to the sphyrion tibiale. The subject sits on the box and crosses the right leg over the left leg to present a horizontal medial surface of the leg. The end pointer is applied to the tibiale mediale site by firmly anchoring the left mid-finger to the proximal tibia border and using the thumb and index finger to place the end pointer on the marked site. The housing pointer is extended to the marked sphyrion tibiale, the most distal point on the sphyroid process of the tibia, anchoring the right mid-finger slightly distal to the landmark and manipulating the housing pointer to the exact site.

Foot length. Distance between the acropodion and pternion (that is, the most distal toe and posterior surface of the heel). This is usually obtained by an anthropometer used as a wide sliding caliper. The subject stands and the measurement is made from his right side. Position the caliper parallel to the long axis of the foot. Use an overgrasp of the left hand with fingers on top opposed by the thumb underneath, grasp the shaft of the caliper with the fingers of the left hand and manipulate the cursor branch with your thumb. With the Campbell caliper, hold the right branch as you do the left. Use minimal pressure to the sites. (Note that in locating the acropodian, when possible, avoid obvious bone spurs or deformities from shoe wear.) (Note: the measurement of feet is a kinanthropometric specialization advanced by Dr Michael Hawes, University of Calgary, in the design of athletic footware. Foot length is only a gross indicator of size.) In the measurement sequence, foot length usually follows torso breadth measurements and is included in the breadth station using the wide sliding calibers rather than a segmometer.

Breadths (Fig. 34.7)

The disarticulated end piece of the Siber—Hegner anthropometer is used as a large wide sliding caliper for torso breadths; and small Mitutoyo adapted caliper for bone breadths. The anthropometer must be assembled properly. The sliding branch should be on your right-hand side. When closed, the anthropometer indicator should read 0.7 mm (the small distance the branches are apart when fully closed). Both the sliding and the bone calipers are held in the same manner. Use an undergrasp, holding the branches by your thumb and index finger as you would grasp a pencil. The caliper itself rests on the backs of your hands or forearms. Use your third digits or mid-fingers to locate the landmarks. Apply firm pressure to the branches (except for the anteroposterior chest depth and foot length measurements). If there is a vernier scale on the smaller bone calipers you can read to the nearest 0.01 cm on some models and to the nearest 0.1 mm on others. Thus a typical value for the humerus might be 7.21 cm or 72.6 mm, without a vernier scale reading to the nearest 0.05 cm or 0.5 mm (thus without a vernier caliper, the last digit is either a 5 or 0).

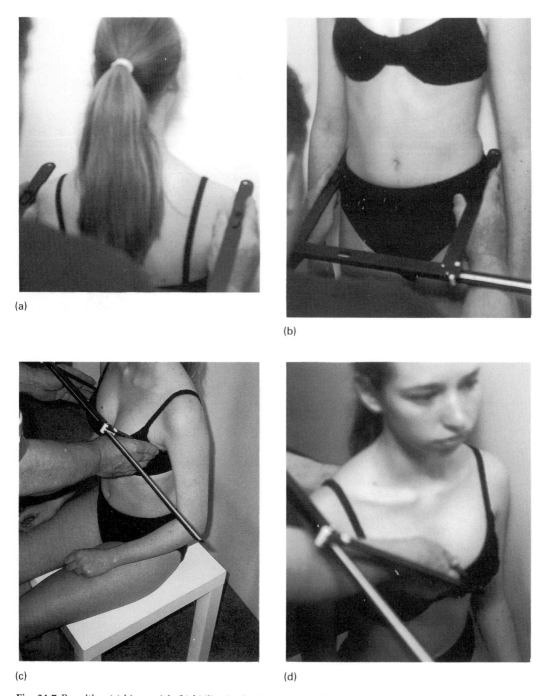

Fig. 34.7 Breadths: (a) biacromial; (b) bi-iliocristal; (c) transverse chest; (d) anteroposterior chest depth.

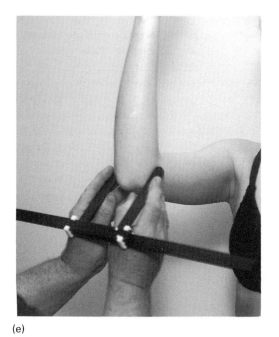

(e)

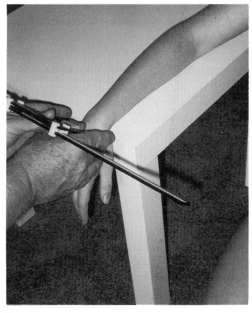

(f)

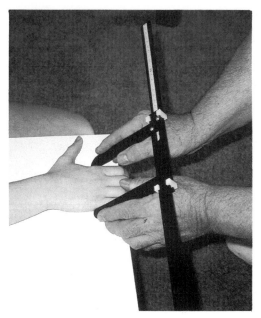

(g)

Fig. 34.7 *Continued*. (e) Humerus; (f) wrist (distal stylion); (g) hand.

Biacromial breadth. Distance between the most lateral points on the acromion processes when the subject stands erect with the arms hanging loosely at the sides. Stand behind the subject, locate the sites with your third fingers and apply the branches of the wide sliding caliper. Position the branches to point upward at an angle of about 45° from the horizontal encompassing the largest diameter between the acromial processes. Apply firm pressure to the branches over the acromial sites using your index fingers along the sides of the branches, not just at the tips.

Bi-iliocristal breadth. Distance between the most lateral points on the superior border of the iliac crest. Stand in front of the subject, locate the sites with your third digits and apply the branches of the caliper to the sites. Position the branches to point upward at an angle of about 45° from the horizontal encompassing the largest diameter between the most lateral aspects of the iliac crests. Apply firm pressure with your index finger to the branches over the iliac sites.

Transverse chest width. Distance of the most lateral aspect of the thorax. Approach the subject who sits erect facing you. From the mesosternale level apply the branches at an angle of about 30° downward from the horizontal to encompass the widest diameter avoiding both the pectoral and latissimus dorsi muscle contours. When the site is approximated, remove your thumbs from the pinch grasp of the branches slightly rotating your hands outwards and applying moderate pressure along the branches with your index fingers. Make the measurement at the end of the normal expiratory excursion (end-tidal).

Anteroposterior chest depth. Depth of the chest at mesosternale level obtained with spreading caliper or anthropometer with recurved branches used as a sliding caliper. This measure is easiest to obtain from the right side of a subject seated in an erect posture. Apply the caliper over the right shoulder in a downward direction. Anchor slightly below the mesosternale with the third digit of your right hand and manipulate the tip of the branch to the site as if you were grasping a pencil. Concurrently, locate the spinous process of the vertebra at the same level as the mesosternale with the third digit of your left hand and apply the branch as you would in holding a pencil. Use gentle pressure. Make the measurement at the end of a normal expiration (end-tidal).

Bi-epicondylar humerus width. Distance between medial and lateral epicondyles of the humerus when the arm is raised forward to the horizontal and the forearm is flexed to a right angle at the elbow. Apply the small bone caliper bisecting the right angle formed at the elbow. Palpate epicondyles using your third digits starting proximal to the sites. The measured distance is somewhat oblique since the medial epicondyle is lower than the lateral. However, with the altered plane, keep the calipers as close to horizontal as possible while ensuring the pressure plates are applied firmly to the encompassed sites.

Wrist width. Bistyloid breadth when the right forearm is resting on a table or the subject's thigh and the hand flexed at the wrist to an angle of about 90°. Apply the caliper branches to bisect the angle formed at the wrist. Palpate the styloid processes with your third digits, starting proximal to the sites. Apply firm pressure to the faces of the caliper to minimize the intervening tissue, however, not great enough to alter position of the radius with respect to the ulna.

Hand width. Distance between the metacarpale laterale and metacarpale mediale when the subject places the palm of the hand on a table. The fingers are kept together and flexed over the edge at the second and terminal phalangeal joints. The thumb is fully abducted. Apply the caliper branches pointing downwards at a 45° angle. Palpate the landmarks with your third fingers then apply the faces of the caliper with firm pressure but not to the extent of compressing the width.

Bicondylar femur width. Distance between medial and lateral of the femur when the subject is seated and the leg is flexed at the knee to form a right angle with the thigh. Apply the small bone caliper with the branches pointing downwards at a 45° angle to bisect the right angle formed at the knee. Palpated for the widest diameter starting proximal to the sites. Apply firm pressure to the caliper branches. If you have difficulty locating the most medial and lateral aspects of the condyles, use your third digits in a slightly circular motion and manipulate the caliper pressure plates to ensure that the widest diameter is encompassed.

Girths

The optimal anthropmetric tape for measuring girth is described previously. The case is held in the right hand with the 4th and 5th fingers throughout all the girth measurements. The girths are measured with the tape at right angles to the long axis of a bone or body segment. The tape is passed around the part and held so the stub end and the scale calibrations are in juxtaposition, that is, one reads to a scale mark and not across a tape space. The reading edge of the tape is manipulated to the designated level. When measuring, the tape is pulled out of its housing and around the part by the left hand, which then transfers the stub end to the right hand. The tape is then controlled by the right hand that can pull it slightly to maintain it at the designated level. The left hand then resumes control of the stub end and can make any further adjustments to the tape. The so-called 'cross-handed' technique is simply a matter of reaching across with the left hand and gripping the stub end of the tape with the thumb and index finger while the right hand similarly grasps the tape at the housing end. The tape is then brought into juxtaposition using the third digit of each hand to control or make adjustments. The aim is to obtain the perimeter distance of the part with the tape in contact with, but not depressing, the fleshy contour. The development of this light touch requires considerable practice since the pressure on the tape is not constant, but is governed by the compressibility of the fleshy contour which itself varies among individuals. Careful attention must be given to the girth specifications. The arm girth relaxed is at a designated and marked level whereas the flexed-and-tensed arm girth is obtained at the site of the greatest perimeter over volitionally contracted musculature.

In general, the thumb and index fingers are the 'snubbers' loosening and tightening the tape and the third digits are the 'levellers' assuring the tape is perpendicular to the long axis of the body part. The third digit of the left hand is also the 'anchor' and pins the tape to the designated level and carries the tape from site to site. It is very easy to distinguish skilled anthropometrists from novices or those using nondescript and asystematic techniques. Technically good anthropometrists have economy of movement and precise control of the tape. The right hand holds the case at all times, maintains pressure and occasionally holds the stub end as well. The left hand is used to adjust the tape when both ends are held in the right. It is the crossover hand and its third digit which serves as the anchor to pin at designated levels and to assist in moving the tape from site to site. Skill is achieved by persistent practice, ideally in a troika under the tutelage of a criterion anthropometrist. Videotaping and viewing with stop frame appraisal of technique can be englightening. Appendicular girths are illustrated in Fig. 34.8 and the head, neck and torso girths in Fig. 34.9.

Head girth. Maximum perimeter of the head when the tape is located immediately superior to the glabellar point (midpoint between brow ridges). The tape is located perpendicular to the long axis of the seated subject whose head is oriented in the Frankfort plane. Because of the intervening hair, the usual light touch for girths is replaced by a firmer pressure that crushes hair to minimize its influence.

Neck girth. Perimeter of the neck taken immediately superior to the larynx (Adam's apple). The tape is located perpendicular to the long axis of the neck of the seated subject when his head is oriented in the Frankfort plane. The usual light anthropometric touch is applied to the tape.

Arm girth relaxed. Perimeter distance of the right arm parallel to the long axis of the humerus when the subject is standing erect and the relaxed arm is hanging by the sides. The level of the tape is at the measured and marked mid-acromiale—radiale distance.

Arm girth flexed and tensed. Maximum circumference of the flexed and tensed right arm raised to the horizontal position. Encourage to 'make a muscle' by tensing and fully flexing his or her forearm at the elbow. In making this measurement, a preliminary flexing permits you to adjust the tape to the maximal girth that is then achieved at a second trial where the

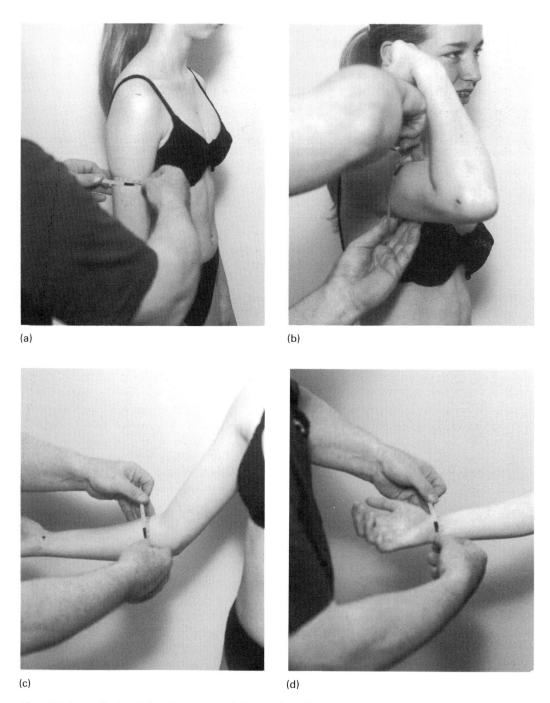

Fig. 34.8 Appendicular girths: (a) arm relaxed; (b) arm flexed/tensed; (c) forearm; (d) wrist.

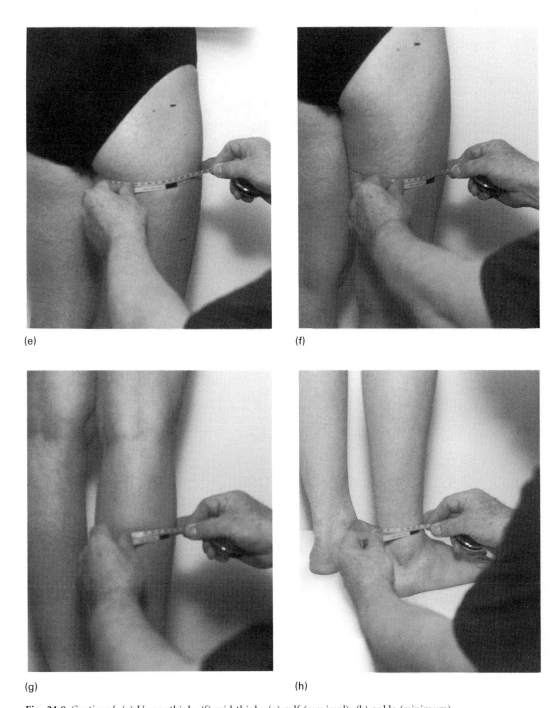

(e)

(f)

(g)

(h)

Fig. 34.8 *Continued*. (e) Upper thigh; (f) mid-thigh; (g) calf (maximal); (h) ankle (minimum).

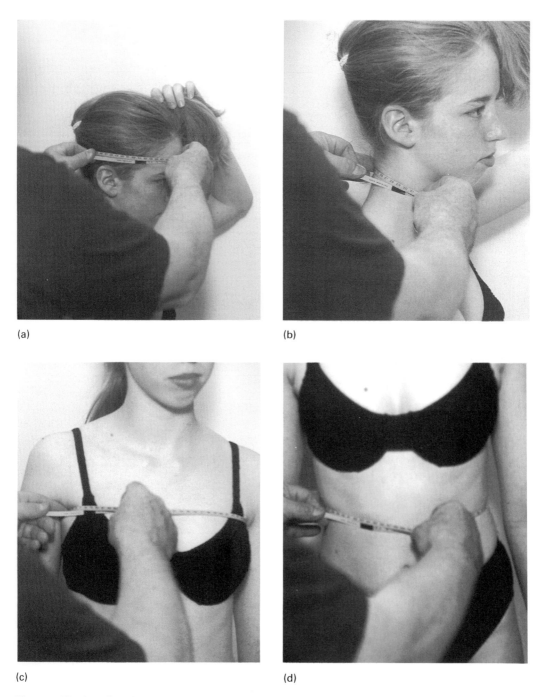

(a)

(b)

(c)

(d)

Fig. 34.9 Head, neck and torso girths: (a) head; (b) neck; (c) chest; (d) waist.

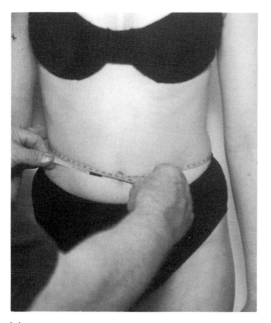
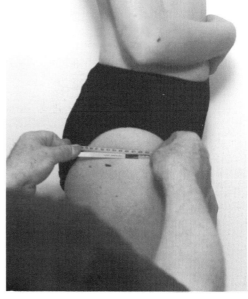

(e)   (f)

Fig. 34.9 *Continued*. (e) Omphalion; (f) hip (gluteal).

subject is encouraged verbally. When making this measurement you should stand laterally to the right of the subject.

Forearm girth. Maximal girth of the right forearm when the hand is held palm up and relaxed. The measure is made no more distally than 8 cm from the radiale. In subjects with pronounced forearm development where the belly of the muscle is more distal than normal, a 'true' maximal value will differ from the conventional forearm girth that is taken at the more proximal level.

Wrist girth. Perimeter of the right wrist taken distal to the styloid processes. The subject flexes the forearm at the elbow and presents the wrist with the hand supine. You can obtain this measure and palpate the styloid processes at the same time with your third digits.

Chest girth. End-tidal perimeter of the chest at mesosternale level. The subject slightly abducts

the arms to permit you standing obliquely to his or her right side to pass the tape behind the torso so you can reach in front and grasp it with your right hand. The stub end of the tape and housing is then held in your right hand freeing your left hand to adjust the tape at the subject's back or front to the horizontal level of the marked mesosternale. Use a cross-handed technique to put the tape scale in juxtaposition with the zero on the stub end of the tape, ideally at the right front side of the subject. (There is a comfort zone that is violated when you face, and are too close to, the subject.) The reading is obtained at the end of a normal expiration (end-tidal). It is best not to tell subjects, children particularly, to 'breathe normally' or draw attention to the normal respiratory rhythm.

Waist girth. Perimeter at the level of the noticeable waist narrowing located approximately half way between the costal border and iliac crest. In subjects where the waist is not apparent, an arbitrary waist measurement is made at this level about the lateral level of the 10th rib.

Omphalion girth (abdominal girth). Perimeter at the level of the omphalion (centre of the umbilicus, navel). In subjects with accentuated curvature at the hips, it is important to align the centre of the tape with the landmark, even though the tape does not conform to the curvature.

Gluteal girth (hip girth). Perimeter at the level of the greatest posterior protuberance and at approximately the symphysion pubis level anteriorally. The subject during this measure stands erect, feet together, without volitionally contracting the gluteal muscles. You extend the tape behind the subject with your left hand, graping it with your right hand. Reach in front of the subject using the cross-handed technique to grasp the stub end of the tape. Pull the tape and pin it at the prescribed level on the right hip with the third digit of your left hand and adjusting with your right third digit so the tape is perpendicular to the long axis of the torso.

Thigh girth. Perimeter of the right thigh which is measured when the subject stands erect, weight equally distributed on both feet, and assisting by holding clothing out of the way. Ask the subject to place the feet slightly apart, thus speading the legs to permit tape passage. Extend the tape and lay it across the calf, then reach with your right hand in front and grasp the stub end, cross over with your left hand and grasp the stub end of the tape. This cross-handed technique permits you to raise the tape so you can pin it with the third digit of your left hand 1 cm from the subject's gluteal line or arbitrary join of gluteal protuberance and the thigh. Manipulate the rest of the tape using your right third digit. Continue snubbing and levelling to assure measurement is made when the tape is perpendicular to the long axis of the femur while you maintain the level with your third digit used as an anchor.

Mid-thigh. Perimeter distance of the right thigh perpendicular to the long axis of the femur at the marked mid-trochanterion–tibiale level. Simply drop the tape from the upper thigh measurement, pin with the third left digit and use both left and right digits to assure the tape is at the marked site and perpendicular to the long axis of the femur.

Calf girth. Maximum perimeter of the calf when the subject stands with weight equally distributed on both feet. Make this measurement by manipulation of the tape taking a series of girth measurements to assure the largest value, loosening and snubbing of the tape with your thumbs and index finger grips and levelling with your third digit to ensure the measurement is obtained when the tape is perpendicular to the long axis of the leg.

Ankle girth. Perimeter of the narrowest part of the lower leg superior to the sphyrion tibiale. Viewed from the side, because of the ovoid shape of the leg, this is slightly below the visual impression of the narrowest point. The tape is manipulated by loosening and tightening to obtain the minimal girth measure. In the process, use your third digits to maintain the perpendicular orientation of the tape to the long axis of the leg.

Skinfold thicknesses (Fig. 34.10).

The objective in obtaining a skinfold measurement is to obtain a double layer of skin and the underlying adipose tissue, but not the muscle. Unlike the either handed techniques illustrated by Lohman *et al.* (1990), the caliper is always held in the right hand and the skinfold raised by the left hand. The skinfold is raised by the pinching, slightly rolling action of the left thumb and index finger. The grasp is large enough to get a complete double layer. The fold is grasped firmly and held throughout the measurement. Hold the skinfold at the designated site and apply the caliper so that the near edge of the pressure plate is 1 cm from the lateral side of the controlling thumb and index finger. Make sure you apply the calipers at right angles to the fold. Release the trigger completely and allow time for the full pressure of the caliper to take effect, but not so long that the adipose tissue becomes 'squeezed out' of the skinfold. Considerable practice is required to make this judgement for skinfolds of varying sizes and varying degrees of compressibility. Make the reading approximately 2 s after application, when the needle slows. In measuring obese subjects, you must use firm pressure of the thumb and index finger to reduce excessive movement of the indicator. When skinfold thicknesses are difficult to raise, you can force the caliper to the muscle level and then slightly withdraw while controlling the fold with your grasp. All skinfold measurements are made on the right side of the body including the abdominal skinfold (previously an exception). In training programmes, natural left handers are taught the grasping procedures first using their dominant hand, then the application of the caliper after site location has been engrained. Natural right handers are first introduced to the caliper dynamics holding it in their dominant hand. The techniques are the same, the method of teaching differs.

Triceps. Caliper distance when applied 1 cm from the left thumb and index finger raising a vertical fold at the marked mid-acromiale—radiale line on the posterior surface of the arm.

Subscapular. Caliper distance when applied 1 cm distally from the left thumb and index finger raising a fold beneath the inferior angle of the scapula in a direction running obliquely downwards at an angle determined by the natural cleavage lines of the skin (Langer's lines, see *Gray's Anatomy*, 1950).

Biceps. Caliper distance when applied 1 cm distally from the left thumb and index finger raising a vertical fold at the marked mid-acromiale—radiale line on the anterior surface of the right arm.

Iliac crest. Caliper distance when applied 1 cm anteriorly from the left thumb and index finger raising a fold immediately superior to the iliac crest at the mid-torso or auxillary line. The fold runs anteriorly downwards and usually is progressively smaller as one moves in this direction from the designated site.

Supraspinale (formerly Heath—Carter supra-iliac). Caliper distance when applied 1 cm anteriorally from the left thumb and index finger raising a fold about 7 cm above the spinale on a line to the anterior axillary border (armpit). The fold follows the natural fold lines running medially downwards at about a 45° angle from horizontal.

Abdominal. Caliper distance when applied 1 cm inferior to the left thumb and index finger raising a vertical fold which is raised 3—5 cm lateral to the right, and at the level of the omphalion (midpoint of the navel). In some subjects, this is difficult to obtain. You can occasionally have a subject flex forward slightly to accommodate the measurement. In extreme cases, make the measurement with your subject in a recumbent supine position.

Front thigh. Caliper distance when applied 1 cm distally to the left thumb and index finger raising a fold half the distance from the inguinal line and the anterior patella on the anterior of the right thigh along the long axis of the femur when the leg is flexed at an angle of 90° at the knee when the subject is either seated or stands placing a foot on a box. Apply the caliper so it faces away from the subject. In some subjects when the fold is difficult to raise, take a firm grasp, push the calipers to the muscle level and slightly retract them. You can instruct the subject to assist by supporting the underside of the leg lifting up with his or her hands. A further tactic is to have an assistant use two hands to raise the fold. You stand to the subject's right while you or your assistant on the subject's left side raises the fold with his or her right thumb and index finger at the prescribed site. You

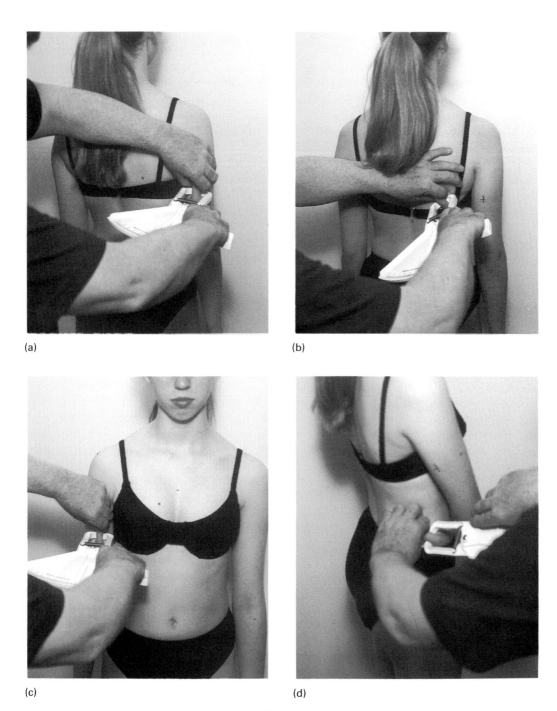

(a)

(b)

(c)

(d)

Fig. 34.10 Skinfolds: (a) triceps; (b) subscapular; (c) biceps; (d) iliac crest.

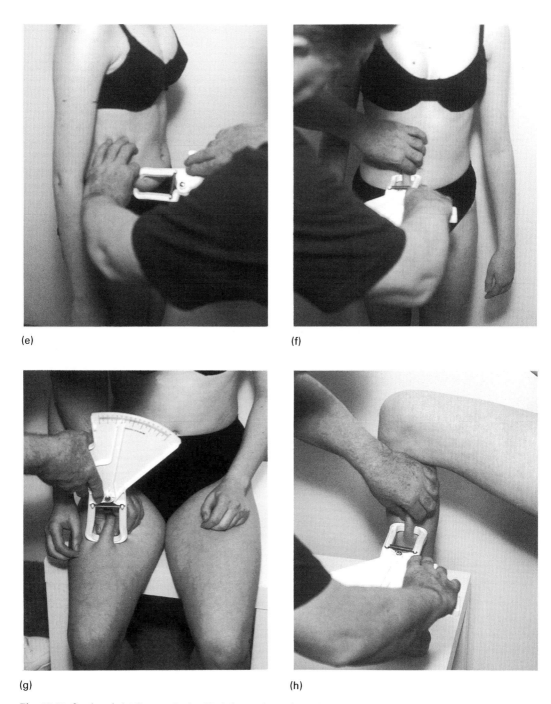

(e)

(f)

(g)

(h)

Fig. 34.10 *Continued*. (e) Supraspinale; (f) abdominal; (g) front thigh; (h) medial calf.

apply the caliper and second grasp of the fold is attempted with the assistant's right thumb and index finger 1 cm distal to the caliper. The measurement is made on the double grasped fold (the front thigh is a particularly good predictor of total adiposity despite the difficulty and need for special technique for some individuals).

Medial calf. The caliper distance when applied 1 cm distal to the left thumb and index finger raising a vertical fold on the medial right calf at the estimated greatest circumference. This is easiest to obtain when the subject's leg is flexed to an angle of 90° at the knee by placing the foot on a box.

Conclusion

Our concluding statement is the same as we made in Ross *et al.* (1988): 'Scientists and physicians should be aware of the dangers in extrapolating simplistic relationships to individual prescription. They should recognize that precision and accuracy in measurements sufficient for group comparisons and experimental designs are often inadequate for individual assessment. Moreover, they must accept that comprehensive data can and should be collected serially and that it can be managed by evolving microcomputer technology and creative use of iconometrographic techniques. For some, this means a basic re-orientation and deployment in a clinical setting'.

Challenges for future research

A major function of a society is to provide for the optimal growth and development of children and youths and to preserve health and vigour of adults throughout the lifespan.

- National research establishments in supposedly enlightened countries have not given much attention to the need for adequate normative data for the expanding ethnic diversity of their populaces. A major challenge is to address this shortcoming in both advanced and emerging nations. We need to know about human growth and the relationships of structure and function in health and disease. The support given to human biological research is miniscule compared to its importance.

- A related challenge is to construct databases for archiving and access. There are presently no systems that have an efficient method for quality control or a plan for responsible cumulative acquisition and dissemination of data. Much excellent data is simply not freely available. The late Albert R. Behnke Jr advocated an international institute for corporeal information — despite the need and the advance in electronic communication, this challenge persists.

- These first two challenges relate to the need for the initiation and update of scientific training in human biology with an emphasis on theory, technique and technology. It is only then that we can appreciate the new anatomically based medical imaging techniques and their limitations, and be able to use anthropometry in innovative ways to assess human structure, look at individual differences with respect to appropriate norms and consider the relationship between structure and performance. Anthropometry is the quantitive interface between human structure and function. Biomechanical and physiological assessments of individual performance are rarely appropriate without some explanation of size.

- Ales Hrdlicka, in his classical textbook on *Practical Anthropometry* (Stewart, 1952), defined physical anthropology as human phylogeny and comparative human anatomy and physiology. In the sexist terms of the 1930s, he stated that 'Anthropometry is a handmaiden to the study of man; it has no individuality outside of that' (Stewart, 1952). Hrdlicka's 'handmaiden' analogy was and is inappropriate. However, we appreciate, as he did, that anthropometry is the quantitative interface between human structure and function and as such makes a unique contribution to the study of the human body.

- The last and perhaps the most pressing

challenge is to make health professionals (physical educators, coaches, nutritionists, physical therapists, sport scientists and sport physicians) into both participants and witnesses in research. With the increasing availability of microcomputers, health professionals are now able to train interactively at a computer terminal to assure quality of measurement, enter data in accessible spreadsheet formats, call up appropriate norms, assess status and monitor change. They can then use models to assess theoretical and actual departures from metabolic norms or physical performance expectancies. They can also focus on individual differences and use anthropometry to foster optimal growth and development of young athletes. This will contribute to the maintenance of health and vigour of these athletes throughout their lifespan.

Acknowledgement

The photographs are courtesy of G.W. Carroll, Rosscraft.

References

Anon. (1981) *Standard Test of Fitness, Operations Manual*, 2nd edn. Fitness and Amateur Sport, Government of Canada, Ottawa.

Beers, Y. (1957) *Introduction to the Theory of Error*. Addison-Wesley, Reading.

Borms, J., Hebbelinck, M., Carter, J.E.L., Ross, W.D. & Lariviere, G. (1979) Standardization of basic anthropometry in Olympic athletes: the MOGAP procedure. In U. Novotny & S. Tittlbachova (eds) *Methods of Functional Anthropometry*, pp. 31–9. Charles University, Prague.

Broca, P. (1865) Instructions générales pour les researches et observations anthropologiques (anatomie et physiologic). In *Paris, Mém, Soc. d'Anthrop*, 2nd edn. Paris.

Carr, R.V., Blade, L., Rempel, R. & Ross, W.D. (1993) Technical note: on the measurement of direct vs. projected anthropometric lengths. *Am. J. Phys. Anthropol.* **90**, 515–17.

Car, R.V., Rempel, R.D. & Ross, W.D. (1989) Sitting height: an analysis of five measurement techniques. *Am. J. Phys. Anthropol.* **79**, 339–44.

Carter, J.E.L. (1980) *The Heath–Carter Somatotype Method*. San Diego State University Syllabus Service, San Diego.

Carter, J.E.L. (ed.) (1982) *Anthropometry of Montreal Olympic Athletes*, Part 1. *The Montreal Olympic Games Anthropological Project. Medicine and Science in Sport*, Vol. 16. Karger, Basel.

Carter, J.E.L. (ed.) (1984) *Physical Structure of Olympic Athletes*, Part II. *Kinanthropometry of Olympic athletes. Medicine and Science in Sport*, Vol. 18. Karger, Basel.

Carter, J.E.L. & Ackland, T.R. (1994) *Kinanthropometry in Aquatic Sports: A Study of World Class Athletes*. Human Kinetics, Champaign, IL.

Dahlberg, G. (1940) *Statistical Methods for Medical and Biological Students*. George Allen & Unwin, London.

Day, J.A.P. (1984) Bilateral symmetry and reliability of upper limb measurements. In J.A.P. Day (ed.) *Perspectives in Kinanthropometry*, pp. 257–61. Human Kinetics, Champaign, IL.

Day, J.A.P. (1986) The reliability and bilateral symmetry of the upper limbs: the last word. In T. Reilly, J. Watson & J. Borms (eds) *Kinanthropometry III*, pp. 109–113. E. & F.N. Spon, London.

DeGaray, A.L., Levine, L. & Carter, J.E.L. (1974) *Genetic and Anthropological Studies of Olympic Athletes*. Academic Press, New York.

Gray, H. (1950) *Anatomy of the Human Body*. Lea & Febiger, Philadelphia.

Johnston, K.E., Hamill, P.V. & Lemeshow, S. (1972) *Skinfold Thickness of Children 6–11 Years. United States Vital and Health Statistics*, Series 11, No. 120. US Government Printing Office, Washington, DC.

Knapp, T.R. (1992) Notes and comments. Technical error of measurement: a methodological critique. *Am. J. Phys. Anthropol.* **87**, 235–6.

Lohman, T.G., Roche, A.F. & Martorell (eds) (1990) *Anthropometric Standardization Reference Manual*. Human Kinetics, Champaign, IL.

Martin, R. (1928) *Lehrbuch der Anthropologie*. Gustav Fischer, Jena.

Martin, R. & Saller, K. (1959) *Lehrbuch der Anthropologie*. Fischer, Stuttgart.

Mueller, W.H. & Martorell, R. (1988) Reliability and accuracy of measurement. In T.G. Lohman, A.F. Roche & R. Martorell (eds) *Anthropometric Standardization Reference Manual*, pp. 83–6. Human Kinetics, Champaign, IL.

Peters, T.J. & Austin, N.K. (1983) *A Passion for Excellence: The Leadership Difference*. Random House, New York.

Ross, W.D. (1977) A paradox-correcting stodecimeter. In H. Lavallée & R.J. Shephard (eds) *Frontiers of Activity and Child Health*. Editions du Pélican, Quebec.

Ross, W.D. (1985) The design of a parallax-correcting anthropometer for replication in non-specialized machine shops. *Am. J. Phys. Anthropol.* **66**, 93−6.

Ross, W.D., Brown, S.R., Faulkner, R.A., Vajda, A.S. & Savage, M.V. (1976) Monitoring growth in young skaters. *Can. J. Appl. Sport Sci.* **1**, 166.

Ross, W.D. & Eiben, O.G. (1991) The sum of skinfolds and the O-scale system for physique assessment rating of adiposity. *Anthropol. Közl.* **33**, 299−303.

Ross, W.D. & Eiben, O.G. (1992) A commentary on the optimal design of an anthropometric tape. *Acta Med. Auxol.* **24**, 101−4.

Ross, W.D., Hebbelinck, M., Brown, S.A. & Faulkner, R.A. (1978) Kinanthropometric landmarks and terminology. In R.J. Shephard & H. Lavellee (eds) *Fitness Assessment*, pp. 44−50. C.C. Thomas, Springfield.

Ross, W.D. & Marfell-Jones, M.J. (1990) Kinanthropometry. In J.D. MacDougall, H.A. Wenger & H.J. Green (eds) *Physiological Testing of the High-Performance Athlete*, pp. 223−308. Human Kinetics, Champaign, IL.

Ross, W.D., Rempel, R.D., Quibell, R. & Smith, D. (1993) Technical note. An electronic caliper designed for measuring bone breadths in living subjects. *Am. J. Hum. Biol.* **90**, 373−5.

Ross, W.D., Ward, R. & DeRose, E.H. (1988) Anthropometry applied to sport medicine. In A. Dirix, H.G. Knuttgen & K. Tittel (eds) *The Encyclopaedia of sports Medicine*, Vol. 1. *The Olympic Book of Sports Medicine*, pp. 233−65. Blackwell Scientific Publications, Oxford.

Ross, W.D., Ward, R., Sigmon, B.A. & Leahy, R.M. (1983) Anthropometric concomitants of X-chromosome anenploidies. In A.V. Sandberg (ed.) *The Cytogenetics of the Mammalian X-Chromosome.* Alan R. Liss, New York.

Schmidt, P.K. & Carter, J.E.L. (1990) Static and dynamic differences among five types of skinfold calipers. *Hum. Biol.* **62**, 369−88.

Stewart, T.D. (ed.) (1952) *Hrdlicka's Practical Anthropometry.* 4th edn. Wistar, Philadelphia.

Ward, R. (1988) The O-scale system for human physical assessment. PhD thesis, Simon Fraser University.

Ward, R., Ross, W.D., Leyland, A.J. & Selbie, S. (1989) *The Advanced O-Scale Physique Assessment System.* Kinemetrix, Burnaby.

Weiner, J.S. & Lourie, J.A. (1981) *Practical Human Biology.* Academic Press, New York.

Chapter 35

Testing Aerobic Power, Capacity and Performance

DAVID DOCHERTY

Introduction

The measurement of aerobic performance in children is of importance to physical educators, coaches, physicians, paediatricians, sport scientists and auxologists. It is probably one of the most frequently reported physiological performance measures in the literature related to physical activity. The information obtained from the testing of aerobic performance is relevant to the general health and well-being of children and the monitoring of young athletes engaged in endurance activities and sports requiring short duration, high intensity and repeated effort. Tests designed to measure aerobic performance involve exercise of large muscle groups for at least several minutes at an intensity that challenges the cardiovascular and pulmonary systems to their functional limits (Rowland, 1992). However, the specific test that is selected, the mode of testing and the test protocol are dependent upon the purpose of the testing and the information that is required by the individual conducting the test.

Aerobic power and capacity

Prior to considering the different methods for measuring aerobic performance in children, a distinction should be made between the terms 'aerobic power' and 'aerobic capacity'. Aerobic power refers to the maximal rate at which energy can be produced by predominantly oxidative processes. Maximum aerobic power is, therefore, the maximum amount of oxygen that can be consumed per unit of time (Thoden, 1991). The maximum level of oxygen consumption is best determined from a progressive exercise test to exhaustion or close to exhaustion. It is usually expressed as maximum oxygen consumption ($\dot{V}_{O_2\,max}$) and represented as an absolute measure ($l \cdot min^{-1}$) or expressed relative to some measure of body size ($ml \cdot kg^{-1} \cdot min^{-1}$). Rowland (1992) suggests that absolute $\dot{V}_{O_2\,max}$ reflects cardiovascular function whereas relative $\dot{V}_{O_2\,max}$ reflects aerobic performance capabilities. The most appropriate method for expressing relative aerobic power or correcting for differences due to body size has been the topic of considerable debate (Rowland, 1991; Winter, 1992). There is little disagreement that 'scaling', or partitioning out differences in physiological variables due to size, is a necessary adjustment when testing children (Winter, 1992). The specific method for adjusting aerobic power values for size will continue to be an individual preference and dependent upon the purpose of the testing. However, until there is unanimity on the best method for adjusting variables for differences in body size it is recommended that body weight and height[2.25] be used (Mirwald & Bailey, 1986; Gaul, 1990). The use of body weight will allow for comparison of data with other studies and existing normative standards. Scaling to height[2.25] allows an adjustment for size that is generally unaffected by environmental factors and incorporates

573

the principles of allometry (Schmidt-Nielsen, 1984).

Aerobic capacity refers to the total amount of energy that can be produced by oxidative processes and is estimated to be 45 000–80 000 kJ for a 70-kg trained man. There is currently only one test that measures aerobic capacity developed by Boulay *et al.* (1984) but it takes considerable time to administer and has not been validated in children. Anaerobic threshold (AT) is considered to reflect aerobic or endurance capacity (Vago *et al.*, 1987). It is relatively easy and quick to administer and has been used with children (see Tables 35.4–35.7). AT is considered to be the level of intensity at which energy can no longer be supplied through oxidative processes, which results in anaerobiosis (Washington, 1993). Consequently, lactic acid accumulates significantly above this level which quickly produces fatigue. AT occurs at levels of intensity that are less than $\dot{V}o_{2\,max}$. It is a critical factor in determining the ability of an individual to sustain prolonged work at a high intensity and is closely related to performance in distance events (Farrell *et al.*, 1979; Sjoden & Jacobs, 1981). It has also been suggested that AT may be a more sensitive measure than $\dot{V}o_{2\,max}$ in identifying changes in the aerobic fitness of children following training programmes (Bar-Or, 1983). AT is usually expressed as a running velocity, heart rate (beats · min^{-1}), percentage of $\dot{V}o_{2\,max}$, absolute $\dot{V}o_{2\,max}$, or $\dot{V}o_{2\,max}$ normalized for body size.

Conducting maximal paediatric exercise tests

Although children respond to exercise tests similarly to adults there are several important differences. Most people are anxious and apprehensive when they are introduced to a laboratory testing situation. The environment, the equipment and the unfamiliar personnel can appear threatening. It is important to recognize these anxieties and make the child subject as relaxed and comfortable as possible.

This can be accomplished in several ways. The most important factor in reducing the stress associated with testing is the manner of the testing personnel. They must appear friendly and non-threatening. Introduction of the laboratory personnel and use of names helps in establishing rapport and putting the subject at ease. A clear explanation of the test protocols and the equipment is important, with opportunity and encouragement for the child to ask questions.

The presence of a parent or sibling can often help to reduce anxiety levels, at least for the child, but they should remain at a distance from the testing area. Many laboratories use distraction techniques, especially during the test, such as pictures, videos, monitoring heart rate and music. The technician should also engage the child in conversation explaining the test procedures and asking simple questions about school, sports programmes and recent holidays that can help to distract the child from the effort and anxiety associated with the test.

Few children will have previously exercised to a maximal effort. They generally do not have a conception of maximal exertion and need to be encouraged and cajoled to achieve it in a test. They will often wish to stop the test prior to physiological exhaustion. For adults and children, maximal effort is not a pleasant experience and is associated with short-term discomfort. Ethically, it is important to rationalize the use of maximal test protocols with children since it does subject them to physiological and psychological stress. However, it is the experience of technicians of maximal paediatric exercise tests that children quickly recover from such stress (Tomassoni, 1993). In fact it is important to familiarize children with the protocol since their performance is usually better in the second test. The use of incentives with children is important in order to attain maximal effort. Incentives can include social reinforcement (prizes) and intrinsic reinforcement (personal goals).

Testing modes

The two most commonly used exercise ergometers in the laboratory for the testing of aerobic fitness are the motor-driven treadmill and the cycle ergometer. More recently the rowing ergometer (Concept II, RRI, Mornsville, VT, USA) has been used for sport-specific testing and a weighted pulley and tethered swimming for measuring aerobic merformance of swimmers. However, neither of the latter two modes have been used with children so they will not be discussed in this section.

Treadmill ergometer testing

Bar-Or (1983) advocates the treadmill as the ergometer of choice in measuring the maximal exercise performance of children, especially children of 7 years of age and younger. The rationale is based on a number of factors. The larger muscle mass involved in locomotion (compared to cycling) enables higher loads to be placed on the cardiorespiratory and metabolic systems (Boileau *et al.*, 1977). Consequently, maximal heart rate values are higher and $\dot{V}o_{2\,max}$ values greater on treadmill tests compared to cycle ergometer tests (Cumming & Langford, 1985; Armstrong *et al.*, 1991). Walking and running are also regarded as a more natural form of exercise (Godfrey, 1974; Rowland, 1992). In using a cycle ergometer the child must maintain a pedalling cadence which requires localized muscular strength and endurance as well as a good attention span (Rowland, 1992). The treadmill forces the child to maintain the exercise power output and adjust quickly as the load is progressively increased throughout the test.

Cycle ergometer testing

The cycle ergometer has some advantages over the treadmill and the ultimate choice will depend upon the variables that the researcher wishes to measure and the age of the subjects. In comparison to treadmills, cycle ergometers are safer, easier to maintain, less noisy and physically threatening, transported more easily and considerably cheaper. In testing large numbers of subjects it is possible, even with limited metabolic equipment measurement systems, to test efficiently many subjects using different cycle ergometers for warm-up, actual testing and cool-down. The cycle ergometer also allows for precise measurement of power output and a reasonably static position for collection of other physiological data such as blood pressure and intermittent blood sampling. Rowland (1992) also contends that cycle endurance time 'may be a more valid indicator [compared to treadmill testing] of cardiovascular functional reserve'. He bases this contention on the fact that cycle exercise is not strongly affected by body fat. Endurance time, or peak mechanical power (PMP) on the cycle is closely related to absolute $\dot{V}o_{2\,max}$ (Boileau *et al.*, 1977) and therefore maximal cardiac reserve.

The standard cycle ergometer is adequate for testing most children 8 years of age and older. However, Bar-Or (1983) recommends modifications for small instead of 17.5 cm in most adult ergometers; seat height should allow for an optimal 15° angle at the knee during extension; and the handlebars lengthened or the distance between the seat and handlebars reduced by some modification. For optimal mechanical efficiency for 6–10-year-old children pedal revolutions should be 50–60 rev $\cdot$ min^{-1}.

Load protocols

Load protocols for treadmill testing

Table 35.1 shows the different testing protocols that have used the treadmill to elicit maximal oxygen consumption in children. Numerous variations can be seen in regard to velocity (60–134 m $\cdot$ min^{-1}), gradient (0–22%), time for different progressive stages (1–4 min) and the way in which the test was administered (continuous or intermittent). Several studies actually compared the different protocols

Table 35.1 $\dot{V}o_{2\,max}$ protocols for treadmill testing.

Exercise protocol	Population — n	Age (years)	Criteria	Reliability	Reference
Walk (90 m·min⁻¹ or 5.5 km·h⁻¹) Jog (110 m·min⁻¹ or 6.6 km·h⁻¹) Run (130 m·min⁻¹ or 7.9 km·h⁻¹) Initial grade at 0%; 2.5% grade increments every 2 min. In run – 6-min warm-up (0% grade; 130 m·min⁻¹)	8 M (six active in sports)	10–12	Exhaustion	0.56 >0.90 >0.90	Paterson et al. (1981)
Run/walk (110 m·min⁻¹ or 6.6 km·h⁻¹). Initial grade 0%; 2.5% grade increments every 2 min	66 M (hockey)	10	Exhaustion and plateau (<2.1 ml)	0.74 (plateau) 0.27 (no plateau)	Cunningham et al. (1977)
Walk (54 m·min⁻¹) for 6 min as warm-up. Speed increased 80 m every 2 min for next 6 min to 560 m·min⁻¹. Then grade increased 2% every 2 min	28 M 30 F (non-athletes)	10–14 10–14	Plateau (<2.1 ml) Level HR R values (<1)	Not reported	Palgi et al. (1984)
Warm-up 3 min at 93 m·min⁻¹, 7.5% grade. 4-min rest. 93 m·min⁻¹ at 10% grade increased by 2.5% every 2 min	31 M 21 F (IQ 40–114)	6–15 6–15	Exhaustion	Not reported	Skinner et al. (1971)

Protocol	Subjects	RPE	Endpoint		Reference
The same except grade was increased 2.5% every 3 min	26 M 20F (IQ 40–114)	6–15 6–15	Exhaustion	Not reported	Cumming & Langford (1985)
Same warm-up. 93 m·min⁻¹, 15% grade for 4 min. Rest 10 min and walk for 4 min at 17.5% grade. Continue with 2.5% increments	26 M 20 F (IQ 40–114)	6–15 6–15	Exhaustion	Not reported	Bruce et al. (1973) Krahenbuhl et al. (1977)
Bruce protocol: 45 m·min⁻¹ at 10% for 3 min. Grade increases by 2% and speed in standard increments each min (17–25 m·min⁻¹) depending on stage	5 M 5 F 5 M 8 F 22 M 22 F	9–10 9–10 12–13 12–13 8 8	Severe fatigue (exhaustion) Highest $\dot{V}o_2$ fatigue	Not reported	Cumming & Langford (1985)
Short Bruce protocol: as above but start at stage 3 (92 m·min⁻¹) and 14%	As above		As above	Not reported	Cumming & Langford (1985)
Carolina protocol: 93 m·min⁻¹ with grade increased 2% every min	As above		As above	Not reported	Riopel et al. (1979) Cumming & Langford (1985)
Continuous walking: 80m·min⁻¹ at 6% grade for 3 min. Grade increased 2% every 3 min	16 M	10–12	Exhaustion and plateau (rise in $\dot{V}o_2$) < mean increase per work load minus twice SD	Not reported	Sheehan et al. (1987)
Continuous running: 134 m·min⁻¹ at 0% for 3 min. Grade increased 2% every 3 min	As above		$R > 1$ (1.5 too high) MHR for age ($\pm$ 1 SD) = 208 $\pm$ 10 beats·min⁻¹)	Not reported	

Continued

Table 35.1 (*Continued*).

Exercise protocol	Population		Criteria	Reliability	Reference
	n	Age (years)			
Intermittent running: 134 m·min^{-1} at 2% grade. Grade increased 2% every 3 min. 3 min rest between stages (walk at 67 m·min^{-1})	As above			Not reported	
Continuous running holding rails: 134 m·min^{-1} on 4% grade from 3 min. Grade increased 2% every 3 min	As above			Not reported	
Running at 115 m·min^{-1} at 0% grade for 4 min. Grade increased 2.5% per min until completion	49 M 34 F	7–8 7–8	Exhaustion Peak $\dot{V}O_2 \leq 2.1$	Not reported	Krahenbuhl et al. (1978)
Run/walk at 93 m·min^{-1} at 0% grade. Grade increased 2.5% every 2 min	24 M (normal)	10–12	Exhaustion and plateau (2 ml) Plateau HR Breathlessness	Not reported	Stewart & Gutin (1976)
Walk at 60 m·min^{-1} at 0% grade. Increase speed by 60 m·min^{-1} every 3 min	M (n not specified)	9–10	Not reported		Atomi et al. (1986)

Protocol	Subjects	Age (years)	End-point	Reliability	Reference
Walk at 80 m·min⁻¹ at 0% grade. Increase speed by 80 m·min⁻¹ every 3 min until 96 m·min⁻¹ then increase grade 2.5% every min	20 M (active)	9–13	Exhaustion $R > 1$ HR 190 beats·min⁻¹	Not reported	Rowland et al. (1987)
Walk at 60 m·min⁻¹ at 12% grade for 3 min. Then 3-min periods at 14% and 92 m·min⁻¹; 18% and 137 m·min⁻¹; and 20% at 150 m·min⁻¹	48 M 52 M 27 M (grouped into sedentary, moderately active and athletic)	9–12 13–15 16–18	Exhaustion	Not reported	Cumming et al. (1980b)
Initial grade 0% and increased every 2 min by 2.5%. Speed adjusted to age: 110 m·min⁻¹ 10.8–11.8 years; 130 m·min⁻¹ 12.8–13.8 years; 160 m·min⁻¹ >14.8 years	62 M each year over 5 years (10.8–14.8 years)		Exhaustion	3.4% coefficient of variation	Cunningham & Paterson (1985)

F, female; HR, heart rate; M, male; MHR, maximal heart rate; SD, standard deviation.

in terms of maximal oxygen consumption and ease of administering the test (Skinner et al., 1971; Paterson et al., 1981; Cumming & Langford, 1985).

There appears to be two general protocols that have been used in treadmill testing to elicit maximal aerobic performance, one based on increments in speed and gradient, and the other only on increments in gradient. The Bruce protocol (Table 35.2) consists of increasing both the treadmill gradient and velocity every 3 min. Bar-Or (1983) and Cumming and Langford (1985) recommend the Bruce protocol. However, there are concerns that it may be initially too intense for unfit children, and fit children may experience localized leg fatigue prior to attaining $\dot{V}O_{2\,max}$. Cumming and Langford (1985) did use a modified protocol, starting the test at stage 3 to alleviate the problem of localized fatigue. However, the $\dot{V}O_{2\,max}$ values were similar for both protocols. In addition, the Bruce protocol has been criticized on the grounds that it changes slope and velocity at the same time (which makes adaptation difficult, especially for unfit subjects) and most exercise is performed at relatively steep slopes (Rowland, 1992). Most other treadmill tests have employed the Balke or a modified Balke testing protocol which involves a constant treadmill velocity and a change in gradient at specific time intervals. There is considerable variation in the treadmill speed (walk, jog and run), and the time increments (1–2 min). In addition, treadmill testing has been conducted with

stepwise loading, supramaximal and discontinuous protocols (Freedson & Goodman, 1993). The protocol is dependent upon the age and fitness level of the subjects, the purpose of testing ($\dot{V}O_{2\,max}$, clinical analysis or AT), and the preference of the researcher.

In general it appears that running tests produced higher $\dot{V}O_{2\,max}$ values than walking and, although values were slightly higher in the intermittent as opposed to the continuous protocol, the difference was not statistically significant. Paterson et al. (1981) found no difference in $\dot{V}O_{2\,max}$ values between running at $130\,m\cdot min^{-1}$ and jogging at $110\,m\cdot min^{-1}$. Since the jogging speed was subjectively more acceptable to the subjects they recommend the slower running speed. Sheehan et al. (1987) found no difference in $\dot{V}O_{2\,max}$ between the intermittent and continuous test protocols but recommend the latter since it is less time-consuming.

Following a review of the different protocols to assess aerobic performance of children, including a variety of subgroups, Rowland (1992) recommended a modified 2-min Balke protocol that is adjusted for age and fitness level (Table 35.3). A lower velocity (walking) and gradient increment is suggested for children who are small, obese or have low fitness levels whereas older and fitter subjects should be tested with a running protocol to reduce the testing time and avoid localized muscular fatigue at the higher treadmill gradients.

Unfortunately, no study has compared all the different protocols described in Table 35.1. At this time it not possible to identify which of the many protocols should be the standard for measuring aerobic power in children and whether or not a single protocol is appropriate for all ages. As Godfrey (1974) noted, a fixed increment of work rate will mean different things to different children because of variations in size due to growth. An increment of 20 W will represent about 10% of the maximal work capacity of a 15-year-old child but 50% of a 5-year-old child. Some researchers have varied increments of work rate based on surface area

Table 35.2 The Bruce treadmill protocol.

| Stage | Speed | | Gradient | Duration |
	$m\cdot min^{-1}$	$km\cdot h^{-1}$		
1	45	2.7	10	3
2	67	4.0	12	3
3	92	5.5	14	3
4	113	6.8	16	3
5	133	8.0	18	3
6	146	8.8	20	3
7	162	9.7	22	3

Table 35.3 The modified Balke treadmill protocol. Adapted from Rowland (1992).

Subject	Age* (years)	Speed km·h^{-1}	Speed m·min^{-1}	Initial grade (%)	Increment (%)	Stage duration (min)
Poorly fit	<10	3.0	80	6	2	2
Sedentary	<10	3.25	87	6	2	2
Active	>10	5.0	134	0	2–1.5	2
Athletic	>10	5.25	141	0	2–1.5	2

* Should be based on developmental age or maturity status.

(Goldberg et al., 1966) and body weight (Macek & Vavra, 1980). It is also possible that the stage durations in maximal testing could be 1–2 min based on the observation that children quickly reach steady-state in regard to heart rate and $\dot{V}_{O_2\,max}$ (Godfrey, 1974). Protocols determined by body size (height, weight or body surface area) appear to be more common in testing that employs cycle ergometers than treadmills. However, further research needs to be conducted to identify the optimal protocols for treadmill testing based on age, body size, fitness level, developmental age (maturity) and gender.

Load protocols for cycle ergometer testing

Table 35.4 shows the different protocols that have been used to elicit $\dot{V}_{O_2\,max}$ using the cycle ergometer. Most protocols consider body weight in setting the power output or resistance levels since smaller children will have difficulty in maintaining an optimal pedalling frequency of 50–60 rev·min^{-1} towards the end of the test due to localized muscular fatigue. Body size can be expressed as body weight (Docherty et al., 1985), height (Godfrey, 1974) or body surface area (James, 1978; Cumming & Langford, 1985).

Cumming and Langford (1985) compared six of the nine tests described in Table 35.4 and found the protocols produced similar values for $\dot{V}_{O_2\,max}$. It should be noted that Cumming and Langford inadvertently used 1-min stages for the Goldberg protocol but the $\dot{V}_{O_2\,max}$ values were among the highest reported for the

cycle ergometer tests. The values reported by Docherty et al. (1985), who also used a 1-min protocol, were equal to, or greater than, the values reported by Cumming and Langford. It would appear that, at least for cycle ergometer testing, 1-min stages are sufficient to produce maximal values for oxygen consumption in children. This could reflect the oxygen kinetics of children since they achieve an aerobic steady-state within 1 min at a specific power output (Godfrey, 1974). Such rapid adjustment has been attributed to the shorter oxygen uptake transient time of children compared to adults. As noted by Bar-Or (1983) children attain 55% of final $\dot{V}_{O_2}$ in 30 s and a steady-state within 2 min compared to adults who only reach 33% in 30 s and take 3–4 min to reach steady-state, depending upon aerobic fitness levels. However, it should be reiterated that $\dot{V}_{O_2\,max}$ values on the treadmill are generally 7.4–19% higher than those on the cycle ergometer (Ikai & Kitagaw, 1972; Boileau et al., 1977; Cumming & Langford, 1985).

Criteria for $\dot{V}_{O_2\,max}$

Maximal oxygen consumption is considered to have been attained when a plateau in oxygen consumption (or less than 2 ml·kg^{-1}·min^{-1}) has occurred as power output is increased beyond the level that first produced the maximum value (Bar-Or, 1983). Occasionally, there may even be a slight decrease in $\dot{V}_{O_2}$. Other criteria are also used to confirm or establish that the maximal value for $\dot{V}_{O_2\,max}$ has been

Table 35.4 $\dot{V}_{O_{2\,max}}$ protocols for cycle ergometer testing.

Exercise protocol	Population n	Age (years)	Criteria	Reliability	Reference
Godfrey protocol (increments based on height): <125 cm 10 W·min^{-1} 125–150 cm 15 W·min^{-1}	6 M 6 F 7 M 8 F	9–10 9–10 12–13 12–13	Exhaustion	Not reported	Cumming & Langford (1985)
<150 cm 20 W·min^{-1}			As long as possible	Not reported	Godfrey et al. (1971) Godfrey (1974)
James protocol* (increments based on BSA; each stage set at 3-min duration; load in W): <1.0 m^2: 32, 48, 80, 96, 112, 128, etc. 1.0–1.19 m^2: 32, 64, 96, 112, 128, 144, etc. >1.19 m^2: 32, 80, 128, 160, 192, 224, 256, etc. (pedal speed 60–70 rev·min^{-1})	6 M 6 F 7 M 8 F 103 (not specified)	9–10 9–10 12–13 12–13	Exhaustion HR >180 beats·min^{-1} Respiration rate ≤40·min (maximal voluntary capacity)	Not reported Not reported	Cumming & Langford (1985) James (1978)
Rapid load protocol* (increments based on BSA; each stage set at 1 min; load in W): ≤1.0 m^2: 16, 48, 80, 96, 112, 128, etc. 1.0–1.2 m^2: 16, 64, 96, 112, 144, etc. <1.2 m^2: 16, 80, 128, 160, 192, 244, etc.	6 M 6 F 7 M 8 F	9–10 9–10 12–13 12–13	Voluntary fatigue	Not reported	Cumming & Langford (1985)

Goldberg protocol as above except each stage set at 2 min intervals					Goldberg *et al.* (1986)
Power output increments increased by $8\,W \cdot kg^{-1}$. $3\,min^{-1}$*	6 M 6 F 7 M 8 F	9–10 9–10 12–13 12–13	Voluntary fatigue	Not reported	Cumming & Langford (1985)
3 min warm-up at $1\,W \cdot kg^{-1}$; 3 min at $2\,W \cdot kg^{-1}$; load increased each min until maximum (increments not reported)*	10 M	10–11	Not reported	Not reported	Macek & Vavra (1980)
2 min warm-up at 50 W; 80 W initial power output, for 1 min. Power output increased 16 W (< 45 kg) and 32 W (> 45) every min	35 M (athletic)	12–13	$R > 1.1$ Plateau (≤ 2 ml)	Not reported	Docherty *et al.* (1985)
Increase load every 3 min	9 M	11–13	Plateau	Not reported	Eriksson & Koch (1973)
1 W for 6 min, 2.1 W for 6 min then 16 W every 1 min	6 M 6 F 7 M 8 F	9–10 9–10 12–13 12–13	Exhaustion Exhaustion	Not reported	Cumming & Langford (1985)

BSA, body surface area; F, female; HR, heart rate; M, male.

attained. These include exhaustion, reaching age-predicted maximum heart rate, a respiratory exchange ratio (RER) value greater than 1, and plasma lactate concentration above 9 $mmol \cdot l^{-1}$ (Bar-Or, 1983; Thoden, 1991). Sheehan et al. (1987) used a more individualized standard in which plateau was defined as the value in which 'rise in $\dot{V}O_2$ was less than the mean increase per workload increment minus twice the standard deviation'. They also set an R value of 1.15 and a heart rate at 208 ($\pm$ 10) $beats \cdot min^{-1}$.

A $\dot{V}O_2$ plateau, as defined above, is often not reached in children (Bar-Or, 1983). Most studies report that only 40–50% of children tested actually demonstrate a plateau in $\dot{V}O_2$ (Stewart & Gutin, 1976; Cunningham et al., 1977; Cumming & Langford, 1985; Sheehan et al., 1987). However, Krahenbuhl et al. (1978) found 83 of 117 (71%) of subjects, 7–9 years of age, demonstrated a levelling criterion of $2.1 ml \cdot kg^{-1} \cdot min^{-1}$ or less and 95% in a later study (Krahenbuhl & Pangrazi, 1983). However, Rivera-Brown et al. (1992) found that only 8 and 13% of adolescent females and males met the criteria of an increase in $\dot{V}O_2$ of less than $2.1 ml \cdot kg^{-1} \cdot min^{-1}$ with an increase in work rate using a Bruce treadmill protocol to volitional fatigue. Bar-Or (1983) suggests a plateau is less likely to occur during cycle ergometry. Most of the studies referenced above used treadmill walking or running. The achievement of a plateau in $\dot{V}O_2$ is apparently more prevalent in fitter subjects, subjects with previous experience (Cunningham et al., 1977; Cumming & Langford, 1985) and in intermittent (66.7%) as opposed to continuous protocol (Sheehan et al., 1987). It should also be noted that maximal performance in children is also dependent on the motivational abilities of the individual conducting the test. Allowing children to terminate a test at 'volitional fatigue' is unlikely to produce maximal values or $\dot{V}O_2$ plateau with increased work rate. Paterson et al. (1981), based on similar $\dot{V}O_{2\,max}$ values for subjects who demonstrated a plateau compare to those who did not, suggest that $\dot{V}O_{2\,max}$ can be assumed without proof of a plateau in oxygen con-

sumption. However, if a plateau is not demonstrated other criteria should be used to determine whether or not the 'peak' $\dot{V}O_2$ can be considered $\dot{V}O_{2\,max}$. Given the difficulty in achieving the criterion of less than or equal to $2.1 ml \cdot kg^{-1} \cdot min^{-1}$ with increased power output, Armstrong et al. (1991) prefer to use the term 'peak $\dot{V}O_2$' rather than $\dot{V}O_{2\,max}$.

Several studies have found that the R values for children are generally lower than those for adults (Rowland et al., 1987; Sheehan et al., 1987). This has been associated with the lower serum lactates of children compared to adults following maximal effort. The comparatively lower R values and lactate concentration have been explained by the differences between children and adults in their response to strenuous exercise (Cunningham et al., 1977; Paterson et al., 1981). As previously noted children have limited anaerobic glycolytic capacity which results in lower R values and lactate levels at maximum power outputs (see also Chapter 3). However, Cunningham et al. (1977) found that subjects who attained a plateau in $\dot{V}O_2$ demonstrated higher R values (1 versus 0.92) and greater lactate levels (6.5 versus $5.4 mmol \cdot l^{-1}$) than subjects who did not attain a plateau in $\dot{V}O_2$. Cumming et al. (1980a) have also reported high lactate values for young children ($9.5–12.1 mmol \cdot l^{-1}$). Several studies have reported effective use of R at greater than or equal to 1 (Palgi et al., 1984; Sheehan et al., 1987) and even greater than 1.1 (Shephard, 1982; Docherty et al., 1985) as a criterion for determining $\dot{V}O_{2\,max}$ in the absence of a plateau. It does not seem unreasonable that, in the absence of a $\dot{V}O_2$ plateau, one of the criteria at least should be met before assuming $\dot{V}O_{2\,max}$ has been reached: an R value above or equal to 1, a lactate concentration over $9 mmol \cdot l^{-1}$, or a heart rate above $195 beats \cdot min^{-1}$. In order to obtain these levels of strenuous effort it is necessary to provide repeated verbal encouragement (Bar-Or, 1983).

Mechanical efficiency

Based on similar levels of aerobic power children should be able to match adults in events that demand extended effort. However, the child is less of an aerobic performer than might be expected from the high $\dot{V}_{O_2 max}$. Differences in performance have been attributed to the mechanical inefficiency of children, especially in walking and running activities. For a given task (constant metabolic load) the metabolic cost ($\dot{V}_{O_2}$) for children is higher (Rowland et al., 1987). Bar-Or (1983) has expressed this as children using a greater portion of their metabolic 'reserve' which places them at a functional disadvantage. An 8-year-old child running at $180\,m \cdot min^{-1}$ is operating at 90% of maximal aerobic power compared to a 16 year old who is only at 75% of maximum. Mechanical inefficiency is attributed to a lack of economy of motion such as a 'wasteful gait' (possibly lateral movement and a high stride cadence relative to velocity). Training helps locomotion, especially running, to become more metabolically economical as reflected by a lower $\dot{V}_{O_2}$ (Daniels et al., 1978). It should also be noted that the mechanical efficiency of cycling is similar in children, adolescents and adults (Bar-Or, 1983). These are important considerations in selecting the exercise mode for assessing the aerobic power of children, especially in longitudinal and cross-sectional studies.

Validity and reliability of $\dot{V}_{O_2 max}$

It is generally assumed that tests in which maximal oxygen consumption is 'directly' measured are valid tests of aerobic power. Frequently, they are used as the gold standard or criterion measure with which other tests, such as submaximal and field tests, are validated. Therefore, the major concern would be whether or not the test mode and protocol have produced the maximal level of oxygen consumption. As previously noted tests on the treadmill produce values 7–19% greater than those on the cycle ergometer. However, Cumming and Langford (1985) in comparing nine maximal tests of different protocols and the two modes of cycle ergometer and treadmill, concluded that the rank order of the test results showed high correlations. They proposed that any of the tests applied consistently in one laboratory may be used to measure comparative fitness for that test and comparative fitness for various groups of children.

Cunningham et al. (1977) compared the maximal oxygen uptake of 66 10-year-old ice hockey players over a 4–5-month period to determine the reliability and reproducibility of the results. They concluded that reliability was enhanced in the presence of a $\dot{V}_{O_2}$ plateau at maximum ($r = 0.74$ compared to 0.27 for those boys who did not demonstrate a plateau). The mean values were not significantly different. The time period between testing would certainly detract from the meaningfulness of these results in regard to the question of reliability. A subsequent study over 3–4 weeks, using three treadmill protocols and three tests on each protocol, found high reliability coefficients for the jog and run (0.90) and a coefficient of variation of 3–5% (Paterson et al., 1981). This was achieved even though the authors were unsuccessful in using plateau criteria to establish $\dot{V}_{O_2 max}$. In comparison the Walk test (see Table 35.1) had a lower reliability (0.56) and a higher coefficient of variation (8%).

A similar comprehensive study on the reliability and consistency of cycle ergometer tests of $\dot{V}_{O_2}$ was not found. Boileau et al. (1977) and Cumming et al. (1967) reported respective coefficients of variation of 4.4 and 4.5% for children who attained $\dot{V}_{O_2 max}$ criteria. In our laboratory we have found reliability coefficients of 0.83. The test–retest reliability will be enhanced by stipulation of pedalling rate and ensuring standardization in regard to seat and handlebar settings. Table 35.4 shows few studies that have reported reliability or recommended pedalling frequencies. For both treadmill and cycle ergometer testing, validity and reliability will be enhanced by ensuring the dead space of the valve and mouthpiece is small and does not exceed 55 ml for children under 10 years of age (Godfrey, 1974; Bar-Or, 1983).

Submaximal tests to predict aerobic power

Predictive and submaximal tests are usually based on the relationship between heart rate, power output and oxygen consumption. As Bar-Or (1983) indicates, the assumptions that heart rate is linearly related to $\dot{V}o_2$ in all individuals and individuals of the same age have equivalent maximal heart rates, do not hold true in practice. Godfrey (1974) concludes that the extrapolation procedures for estimating $\dot{V}o_{2\,max}$ in children are of very dubious validity. Cumming and Langford (1985) and Hermansen and Oseid (1971) also caution against indirect measurement of $\dot{V}o_{2\,max}$. Bar-Or (1983) offers an alternative to the often used Åstrand and Rhyming nomogram and PWC170 which he refers to as WR17. The test is based on the mechanical power or physical working capacity (PWC) the child is able to produce when the exercise is perceived to be 'hard' or '17' on the Borg category scale of physical exertion. Such an approach alleviates the problem that a heart rate of 170 beats·min^{-1} in the PWC170 test may be close to the maximal heart rate of a child or well below it. Bar-Or (1983) considers this test correlates highly with other tests of maximal aerobic power and serves as a valid fitness test for children.

Field tests to predict aerobic power

The measurement of aerobic power is best determined from a progressive test in which $\dot{V}o_{2\,max}$ is actually measured (Åstrand & Rodahl, 1977). However, the equipment is expensive and expertise required to measure $\dot{V}o_{2\,max}$ are not feasible for testing large populations or in institutional settings. A variety of distance runs have been used to estimate or reflect aerobic fitness of children. Safrit et al. (1988) examined the 'validity generalization' of the different studies that used distance runs and a criterion measure of treadmill $\dot{V}o_{2\,max}$. From an analysis of five studies for girls and eight studies for boys they concluded that validity of distance runs is generalizable for girls and boys. However, they suggest that the results should be interpreted with caution due to the small sample sizes and the shortness of the distance runs (< 1600 m). The mean 'true validity' coefficients were 0.71 and 0.78 for girls and boys, respectively.

Table 35.5 shows the test distances and the evaluation criteria for a number of studies examining the relationship between distance runs and $\dot{V}o_{2\,max}$. Validity correlation coefficients generally range from 0.70 to 0.82 with the notable exceptions of 0.22 and 0.26 for the 1200-m and 1600-m runs for 8-year-old girls (Krahenbuhl et al., 1977). There is a trend for the correlation coefficients to increase with the distance from 0.22 to 0.76, with 1600 m proving to be the strongest predictor for both boys and girls (Krahenbuhl et al., 1978). More recently, Anderson (1992) found a correlation of -0.83 between cycle $\dot{V}o_{2\,max}$ and 1600-m run time for young boys (aged 10–12 years).

The multistage 20-m shuttle run test has been proposed as a valid and reliable method for measuring functional maximal aerobic power (Legér & Lambert, 1982; Legér et al., 1984; Legér & Gadoury, 1989). Compared to distance runs the test has the advantage of being less dependent on pacing, can be administered indoors and is of relatively short duration. The test involves running back and forth as long as possible in the 20-m course. Speed starts at 7.5 km·h^{-1} and is increased every 1 min by 0.5 km·h^{-1} until the subject is unable to maintain the pace or voluntarily withdraws from the test. A validity coefficient of 0.7 with $\dot{V}o_{2\,max}$ has been reported for 188 boys and girls 8–19 years of age (Mercier et al., 1983) and a reliability coefficient of 0.89 (L. Legér & Goodbois, 1982, unpublished data). Anderson (1992) found a correlation coefficient of 0.72 between the shuttle run and cycle $\dot{V}o_{2\,max}$. However, he also found a significant difference between the measured values of $\dot{V}o_{2\,max}$ and the predicted values from the shuttle run. Similar to other researchers, Anderson also found significantly high correlations between running speed (40-m dash) and the 1600-m run and the multistage shuttle run (0.79 and −0.85, respectively). He interpreted this relationship to reflect the differences in running efficiency and/or the anaerobic contribution to both measures of aerobic fitness.

Measurement of anaerobic threshold

Lactate and ventilatory threshold

The AT is defined as the level of exercise above which aerobic energy production is supplemented by anaerobic mechanisms and blood lactate abruptly increases (Baraldi *et al.*, 1989). Consequently, blood lactate levels have been used to determine the exercise intensity at which there is a non-linear increase. The critical level of blood lactate has been defined as $2 \, mmol \cdot l^{-1}$ (Tanaka & Shindo, 1985), 4 $mmol \cdot l^{-1}$ (Sjodin & Jacobs, 1981; Rotstein *et al.*, 1986) or the breakpoint of blood lactate plotted against oxygen consumption (Atomi *et al.*, 1986). When blood lactate is used as the main criterion for determining AT it is referred to as the lactate threshold (LT). Blood lactate measurement requires some form of invasive serial sampling during a progressive exercise test. Blood samples can be extracted from peripheral venous puncture, such as a warmed finger tip or the ear lobe, and analysed using commercial lactate analysers. Table 35.6 shows the different protocols that have been used to determine LT. Because blood lactate measurement is invasive, other techniques have been used to assess AT in children. In addition, it is increasingly recognized that blood lactate concentration is influenced by numerous complex factors that limit its use as an indicator of the point at which oxygen supply is unable to meet the demands of exercising muscle (Washington, 1993).

Ventilatory and gas exchange indices have been used to determine AT. The most common ventilatory technique is referred to as the ventilation or ventilatory threshold (VT). For the purposes of this chapter VT will be used to denote the ventilatory AT. VT has been empirically defined as the point of disproportionate or non-linear increase in ventilation ($\dot{V}E$) relative to the increase in $\dot{V}O_2$ during a progressive test (Paterson *et al.*, 1987). The various protocols for establishing VT are presented in Table 35.7. The breakpoint of $\dot{V}E$ is sometimes checked by referring to the exercise intensity at which: (i) $\dot{V}CO_2$ increases non-linearly; (ii) there is an increase in $\dot{V}E/\dot{V}CO_2$ without a concomitant increase in the ventilatory equivalent of CO_2 ($\dot{V}E/\dot{V}CO_2$); (iii) there is an increase in oxygen concentration in the mixed air (F_EO_2); and (iv) there is an excess rise in RER (Weymans *et al.*, 1985). The VT shows a good correlation with the point of increase in blood lactate (Thoden, 1991) although no cause and effect relationship has been demonstrated (Neary *et al.*, 1985). Wolfe *et al.* (1986) consider VT an easily measured and reproducible method of assessing exercise performance in children and adults.

Field tests to predict anaerobic threshold

Conconi *et al.* (1982) have developed a 'field test' for determination of AT based on the relationship between running velocity and heart rate (velocity/heart rate). AT is defined as the deflection point for heart rate (HRD) plotted against work rate in W. There is a high correlation ($r = 0.99$) determined from the HRD and LT. Baraldi *et al.* (1989) found a significant correlation ($r = 0.8$) between the Conconi method and VT. Gaisl and Hofmann (1990) have recently summarized the protocols they have established for determining heart rate threshold (HRT) using a cycle ergometer, treadmill or running track (20-m shuttle run). They suggest such a test is a relatively easy and inexpensive technique to evaluate AT, which can subsequently be used in the study of cardiorespiratory fitness and setting optimal training intensities. Mahon and Vaccaro (1991) assessed the relationship between $\dot{V}O_2$ measured at VT and HRD for boys with a mean age of 10.7 (SD = 1.0) years. There was no significant

Table 35.5 Test evaluation criteria for distance runs (cardiovascular/aerobic fitness).

Test description	Test battery	Validity (population)	Age (years)	Reliability (population)	Reference
6 min	AAHPER HRFT (1980)	0.71–182 ($\dot{V}_{O_2 max}$ 22 M and 25 F)	9–11		Jackson & Coleman (1976)
		0.71–0.82 ($\dot{V}_{O_2 max}$ 38 M and F)	8		Krahenbuhl et al. (1977)
9 min	Eurofit (1988)	0.70 (with 1000 m)	11–14	0.87 (not reported)	Mechelin et al. (1986)
				0.61–0.9* (545 M and F)	Safrit & Wood (1987)
12 min	AAHPER HRFT (1980)	0.9 ($\dot{V}_{O_2 max}$ 9 M)	14	0.94 (150 M, grade 9)	Doolittle & Bigbee (1968)
		0.75 ($\dot{V}_{O_2 max}$ 15 M and F)	11		Gutin et al. (1976)
		0.71–0.82 ($\dot{V}_{O_2 max}$ 22 M and F)	9–11		Jackson & Coleman (1976)
		65 ($\dot{V}_{O_2 max}$ 17 M)	11–14	0.92 0.94 (not reported)	Maksud & Coutts (1971) Miller (1988) and Johnson & Nelson (1986)
1200 yards (1.1 km)		0.81 ($\dot{V}_{O_2 max}$ 15 M and F)	11		Gutin et al. (1976)
		0.64 ($\dot{V}_{O_2 max}$ 20 M)	8		Krahenbuhl et al. (1977)
		0.22 ($\dot{V}_{O_2 max}$ 18 F)	8		Krahenbuhl et al. (1977)
1760 yards (1.6 km)		0.76 ($\dot{V}_{O_2 max}$ 15 M and F)	11		Gutin et al. (1976)
1.6 km		0.66 ($\dot{V}_{O_2 max}$ 140 M and 56 F)	10		Cureton et al. (1977)
		0.71 ($\dot{V}_{O_2 max}$ 20 M)	8		Krahenbuhl et al. (1977)
		0.26 ($\dot{V}_{O_2 max}$ 18 F)	8		Krahenbuhl et al. (1977)

Test	Norms	Age (years)	Reliability (r)	Validity (r with $\dot{V}O_{2\,max}$)	Reference
500 m	Manitoba (1977), CAHPER (1980)	12–19	0.8–0.9 (161 F)	0.22–0.50 ($\dot{V}O_{2\,max}$, 49 M and 34 F, grade 1–3)	Beunen et al. (1977); Krahenbuhl et al. (1978)
1000 m		12–19	0.77–0.89 (174 M)		Beunen et al. (1977)
1200 m				0.23–0.47 ($\dot{V}O_{2\,max}$, 49 M and 34 F, grades 1–3)	Krahenbuhl et al. (1978)
1600 m	Manitoba (1977), Manitoba (1989), CAHPER (1980)		0.82–0.92 (120 M and F)	0.6–0.76 ($\dot{V}O_{2\,max}$, 49 M and 34 F, grades 1–3)	Krahenbuhl et al. (1978)
Shuttle run (20 m, multistage, 1 min)		6–16	0.89 (139 M and F)	0.70 ($\dot{V}O_{2\,max}$, 180 M and F)	Legér & Bodbois (1982, unpublished data); Mercier et al. (1983)
Shuttle run (20 m, multistage, 2 min)	Eurofit (1988)	8–19	0.84	0.97	Van Gerven et al. (1982)

* Two practice trials (three recommended).

AAHPER, American Association of Health, Physical Education and Recreation; CAHPER, Canadian Association of Health, Physical Education and Recreation; F, female; HRFT, health-related fitness test; M, male.

Table 35.6 Criteria for determining lactate threshold (LT) in children.

Protocol and mode	Population n	Age (years)	Criteria	Units of measure	Reliability	Reference
Level running on treadmill at 80–110 m·min⁻¹ increased by 10 m·min⁻¹ every 3 min with 1 min rest. Blood lactates from venous puncture at earlobe 3 min after $\dot{V}O_{2\,max}$ test	24 M	11–12	Prior to blood lactate accumulation	$\dot{V}O_2$ ml·kg⁻¹·min⁻¹ %$\dot{V}O_{2\,max}$	Not reported	Atomi *et al.* (1986)
Treadmill run at 1% grade for 5 min, 2–3 min rest between changes in speed. Initial speed 133 m·min⁻¹ increased by 16 m·min⁻¹ or 8 m·min⁻¹ depending upon velocity at AT. Blood lactates from finger puncture	28 M (non-athletes but active)	10.2–11.6	LA-4-*V* (running velocity at which blood lactate = 4 mmol·l⁻¹) LA-I-*V* (running velocity at which inflection point of lactate curve) % of $\dot{V}O_2$ at LA-4-*v* (LA-4-*v*%) % of $\dot{V}O_2$ at LA-I-*v* (LA-I-*v*%)		Not reported	Rotstein *et al.* (1986)

Protocol	Subjects		Method	Measured variables		Reference
Uphill running on treadmill. Velocity is increased every 4 min (details not provided)	16 (middle- and long-distance runners). Sex not given	11–16	4 m·mol⁻¹	Velocity at blood lactate concentration of 4 m·mol⁻¹	Not reported	Sjodin & Jacobs (1981)
Level running on treadmill starting at 100 m·min⁻¹ and increased 10 m·min⁻¹ every 3 min with 1 min rest. Blood lactates from earlobe	11 M	9–10	Breakpoint in blood lactate vs. $\dot{V}_{O_2}$	$\dot{V}_{O_2}$ at LT in l·min⁻¹ ml·kg⁻¹·min⁻¹ %$\dot{V}_{O_{2\,max}}$ HR	Not reported	Atomi et al. (1986)
Level running on treadmill starting at 80–100 m·min⁻¹ and increased 20 m·min⁻¹. Blood lactates from earlobe	10 M 15 M 11 M 19 M	7.2 8.8 10.9 14.6	Velocity just below 2 m·mol⁻¹ lactate. Plot lactate against running velocities (visual inspection)	Velocity just below 2 m·mol⁻¹ lactate. Velocity below lactate accumulation		Tanaka & Shindo (1985)

AT, anaerobic threshold; F, female; HR, heart rate; M, male.

Table 35.7 Criteria for determining ventilatory threshold (VT) in children.

Protocol and mode	Population n	Age (years)	Criteria	Units of measure	Reliability	Reference
Multistage treadmill: walk at 53 m·min⁻¹ for 6 min. Increase speed 13 m·min⁻¹ every 2 min until 93 m·min⁻¹. Increase grade 2% every 2 min	28 M 30 F	10–14 10–14	Non-linear increase in 2 of 3 measures plotted against $\dot{V}O_2$: $\dot{V}E$, $\dot{V}O_2$, F_EO_2	$\%\dot{V}O_{2\,max}$ $\dot{V}O_2$ at AT	Not reported	Palgi *et al.* (1984)
Multistage treadmill run: start at 0% and speed relative to age. Increase grade 2.5% every 2 min: 10–11 years: 110 m·min⁻¹; 12–13 years: 130 m·min⁻¹; 14–15 years: 160 m·min⁻¹	18 M (longitudinal study, top 25% $\dot{V}O_{2\,max}$)	11–15	Non-linear increase in $\dot{V}E$ vs. $\dot{V}O_2$ (eyed)	$\dot{V}O_2$ at AT in l·min⁻¹ m·kg⁻¹·min⁻¹ $\%\dot{V}O_{2\,max}$	Interobserver = 0.93 CV, 5.6 ± 4.7 (abs.) CV, 6.3 ± 3.8 (rel.)	Paterson *et al.* (1987)
Cycle ergometer: start with 0 resistance for 3 min at 50 rev·min⁻¹. Load increased by 24.5 W every 2 min	22	9–11	Increase in V_E for $\dot{V}O_2$, no increase in CO_2 Increase in end-tidal F_EO_2	$\dot{V}O_2$ at AT $\%\dot{V}O_{2\,max}$	Not reported	Becker & Vaccaro (1983)

Protocol	Subjects		Criteria	Measure		Reference
Treadmill warm-up for 5 min, 3-min rest. Speed set at 108 m · min⁻¹ and grade increased 2% every min	38 M 32 F	7–14 7–14	Increase in $\dot{V}_E$ for $\dot{V}_{O_2}$, no increase in V_E/V_{CO_2} Increase in work intensity exceeded HR and linearity of HR/work rate was lost (Conconi method)	Work rate equivalent (W)	Not reported	Baraldi et al. (1989)
Treadmill set at 80 m · min⁻¹ for 6 year old and 93 m · min⁻¹ above 6. Grade was increased 2% every min	7 M 9 M 10 M 5 F 7 F 14 F	6 11 14 6 11 14	Non-linear increase in $\dot{V}_E$ vs. $\dot{V}_{O_2}$; checked by non-linear increase in $\dot{V}_{CO_2}$ Increase in $V_E/\dot{V}_{O_2}$, no increase in V_E/V_{CO_2} Increase in oxygen in mixed air Excess rise in R	$\dot{V}_{O_2}$ at AT in ml · kg⁻¹ · min⁻¹ %$\dot{V}_{O_2\,max}$	Not reported	Weymans et al. (1985)
Treadmill at 80 m · min⁻¹ for 5–6 year old and 93 m · min⁻¹ for above 6 and increased 2% until HR = 170 beats · min⁻¹)	8 M 7 F	5–6 5–6	Non-linear change in V_E with increase of $\dot{V}_{O_2}$; checked by non-linear increase in $\dot{V}_{CO_2}$ Change in slope $V_E/\dot{V}_{C_2}$ Excess rise in R	$\dot{V}_{O_2}$ at VT in m$\dot{V}_{O_2}$ · kg⁻¹ · min⁻¹ %$\dot{V}_{O_2\,max}$ (predicted from PWC170)	Not reported	Reybrouck et al. (1982)
Multistage progressive treadmill test using the Bruce protocol	10 M (prepubertal distance runner)	10–13	Plotted $\dot{V}_E/\dot{V}_{O_2}$ and V_E/V_{CO_2} against time AT = first isolated upward break	$\dot{V}_{O_2}$ at AT in l · min⁻¹ %$\dot{V}_{O_2\,max}$ %exercise time %MHR	Not reported	Wolfe et al. (1986)

Continued

Table 35.7 (*Continued*).

Protocol and mode	Population		Criteria	Units of measure	Reliability	Reference
	n	Age (years)				
Treadmill at 80 m · min⁻¹ at 0% grade for 1 min. Speed increased 13.3 m · min⁻¹ until predetermined running speed reached. Then gradual increased 2.5% · min⁻¹ until $\dot{V}o_{2\,max}$	22 M (active)	8–13 (× mean age = 10.6 years)	Systematic increase in $\dot{V}E/\dot{V}o_2$, no increase in $\dot{V}E/\dot{V}co_2$ HRD point where HR flattened with increase in exercise	$\dot{V}o_2$ at VT and HRD in ml · kg⁻¹ · min⁻¹	Not reported	Mahon & Vaccaro (1991)

AT, anaerobic threshold; CV, coefficient of variance; F, female; HR, heart rate; HRD, deflection point for heart rate; M, male; MHR, maximal heart rate.

difference between the mean $\dot{V}_{O_2}$ at VT and HRD and a correlation of 0.76. They concluded that HRD can be used as a predictor of VT in most but not all children and caution should be used in interpreting the significance of HRD. It is useful in establishing group values. Table 35.8 shows the different field test protocols that have been used to determine HRD in children.

Units of measurement for anaerobic and ventilatory thresholds

Anaerobic threshold, whether determined from LT or VT, can be expressed in a number of ways. $\dot{V}_{O_2}$ at VT is often used and expressed as an absolute ($l \cdot min^{-1}$) and relative ($ml \cdot kg^{-1} \cdot min^{-1}$) measure. Many authors also express VT as a percentage of $\dot{V}_{O_{2\,max}}$ ($\%\dot{V}_{O_{2\,max}}$). Such expressions of performance are useful in comparing the VT of children to adults and monitoring change due in the metabolic mechanisms over age, especially related to metabolic acidosis. Certainly children have higher relative thresholds ($\%\dot{V}_{O_{2\,max}}$) than adults, attributed to the lower anaerobic glycolytic capacity of children (Tanaka & Shindo, 1985). However, VT expressed as $\%\dot{V}_{O_{2\,max}}$ and absolute or relative $\dot{V}_{O_{2\,max}}$ are not significant predictors of performance (Palgi et al., 1984; Wolfe et al., 1986). From a progressive multistage treadmill test Wolfe et al. (1986) found that AT was the strongest predictor of performance when expressed as a percentage of maximum heart rate $\%\dot{V}_{O_{2\,max}}$. Other authors have expressed AT as a running velocity (Rotstein et al., 1986) and work rate equivalent in W (Baraldi et al., 1989). Both expressions have a direct relationship with endurance performance. The manner in which VT or AT should be expressed is dependent upon the purpose of collecting such data. For comparison with other groups, monitoring subjects over time, or establishing training zones (McConnell et al., 1992), VT is usually expressed as $\%\dot{V}_{O_{2\,max}}$, $\dot{V}_{O_2}$ (absolute or relative) or a percentage of maximum heart rate reserve (%HRR). For prediction of performance

VT should be expressed as a specific heart rate or performance velocity (running or cycling).

Validity and reliability of anaerobic and ventilatory thresholds

The correlation between AT and $\dot{V}_{O_{2\,max}}$ is generally high (0.84) but there is considerable variation in AT between individuals with the same $\dot{V}_{O_{2\,max}}$ (Rowland & Green 1989; McConnell et al., 1992). AT has been regarded as a better measure in assessing aerobic performance, when expressed as a running velocity or a work rate equivalent, since it is less demanding on the subject and a stronger predictor of performance (Palgi et al., 1984). Palgi et al. also suggest that $\dot{V}_{O_{2\,max}}$ is dependent upon the willingness of the subject to give an 'all-out' effort and is therefore prone to underestimation and not conducive to repeat testing. However, it should be noted that $\dot{V}_{O_{2\,max}}$ has been more often used in regard to its relationship to health and well-being. AT has been shown to be a good predictor of performance but has not been studied in regard to cardiovascular health and other risk factors.

There is some problem in identifying the test protocol that provides optimal values for VT. From Tables 35.6 and 35.7 it can be seen that a variety of protocols have been used but no study has compared different protocols, especially optimal load changes and duration of exercise periods. It is also possible that different protocols produce optimal values for children of varying developmental ages. From the present it is not possible to recommend a specific test protocol.

Only one study in Tables 35.6 and 35.7 examined the question of test reliability in children. Given the subjective nature in determining the breakpoints, especially in ventilation, some authors have found that, even with adults, the reproducibility of the method on a test−retest basis, or among different investigators, is poor (Thoden, 1991). However, Paterson et al. (1987) report an inter-observer

Table 35.8 Criteria for determining heart rate deflection point (HRD).

Protocol and mode	Population		Criteria	Units of measure	Reliability	Reference
	n	Age (years)				
Conconi test Cycle ergometer: pedal rate 70 rev · min^{-1} 3 min warm-up (40 W for F and 60 W for M). Increased 10 W per min until exhaustion	Based on testing young subjects in authors' laboratory over time		HR recorded on sport tester every 5 s. Non-linear change in HR (HRT)	HRT	Not reported	Gaisl & Hofmann (1990)
Treadmill: 5 min warm-up at 6 km · h^{-1}. Initial test speed 6–8 km · h^{-1} at 5% grade. Speed increased every 200 m by 0.5 km · h^{-1} until exhaustion	Based on testing young subjects in authors' laboratory over time		HR recorded on sport tester every 5 s. Non-linear change in HR (HRT)	HRT	Not reported	
200 m shuttle run: start at 7 km · h^{-1} (100 s per 200 m. Decrease time by 2–4 s every 200 m until unable to maintain pace	Based on testing young subjects in authors' laboratory over time		HR recorded on sport tester every 5 s. Non-linear change in HR (HRT)	HRT	Not reported	

Protocol	Subjects	Age	Criteria	%$\dot{V}_{O_2 max}$ $\dot{V}_{O_2}$	Reference
Treadmill incremental test Begin walking 5 k · h^{-1} at 0%/ 3 min. Increase speed to preselected comfortable running speed 1 min. Increase slope 4% every min	16 M	10–14	15-s analysis: (1) $V_E/\dot{V}_{O_2}$ vs. time (2) V_E/V_{CO_2} vs. time (3) Pet_{O_2} and Pet_{CO_2} vs. time Criteria = systematic increase in both $V_E/\dot{V}_{CO_2}$ and Pet_{CO_2} with no corresponding increase in the others	Not reported	Mahon & Vaccaro (1989)

F, female; HR, heart rate; HRT, heart rate threshold; M, male; Pet_{CO_2}, partial pressure of end-tidal carbon dioxide; Pet_{O_2}, partial pressure of end-tidal oxygen.

correlation coefficient of 0.93 and respective coefficients of variation for absolute and relative VT to be 5.6 (4.7) and 6.3 (3.8)%. The question of reliability in regard to different protocols, developmental age and level of physical training needs further investigation.

Conclusion

It is evident from an analysis of Tables 35.1–35.8 that a variety of protocols have been used to measure the different components of paediatric aerobic performance, in particular $\dot{V}O_{2\,max}$ and VT or AT. As Rowland (1992) notes the aerobic testing of children has involved almost 'every conceivable combination of slope increments, speed increments, and stage durations'. It is difficult to find two studies that have used the same protocol. Comparison of results between studies and identification of optimal protocols is difficult, if not impossible. Part of the problem relates to the purpose of testing and the data required by the clinician or the researcher. Comparisons across studies must be done with caution and with particular attention to the variations in testing protocols, definition of terms, measurement criteria, the age of the subjects (including developmental versus chronological), and their level of training or activity. Given the many factors related to aerobic performance in children it is unrealistic, and perhaps undesirable, to expect an optimal protocol for children of all ages, sizes and different activity levels and the various purposes for testing. However, there would seem some merit in identifying recommended protocols with consideration of the above factors to at least delimit the escalation of more protocols and reduce those that are currently being used.

Challenges for future research

There are certain questions that need to be addressed in the area of paediatric exercise testing at it relates to the measurement of aerobic performance.
- Further research is needed into the effect of changes in gait or locomotion on the measurement of $\dot{V}O_{2\,max}$ and VT.
- Optimal protocols need to be identified in measuring $\dot{V}O_{2\,max}$, especially on the cycle ergometer, to reduce concerns related to localized muscular fatigue.
- There should be a common expression to normalize values for body size, especially to accommodate changes in performance due to growth.
- More research is needed to identify optimal protocols for pre- and postmenarcheal females. Currently, as in other measurement areas, there are more data for males and protocols established for males.
- Reliability needs to be established for all tests using the intraclass correlation coefficients (R) and based on age, gender and level of training.
- Normative standards need to be developed based on developmental age rather than chronological age.
- More research is needed to identify the optimal protocols for establishing HRD in children of different developmental ages.
- The physiological and metabolic events that mediate HRD need to be elucidated.
- There is a need to identify the protocols to measure VT and AT in children of different developmental ages.

References

Anderson, G.S. (1992) The 1600 m run and multistage 20 m shuttle run as predictive tests of aerobic capacity in children. *Pediatr. Exerc. Sci.* **4**, 302–11.

Armstrong, N., Williams, J., Balding, J., Gentle, P. & Kirby, B. (1991) Cardiopulmonary fitness, physical activity patterns, and selected coronary risk factor variables in 11 to 16 year olds. *Pediatr. Exerc. Sci.* **3**, 219–28.

Åstrand, P.-O. & Rodahl, K. (1977) *Textbook of Work Physiology*. McGraw-Hill, New York.

Atomi, Y., Fukunaga, T., Yamamoto, Y. & Hatta, H. (1986) Lactate threshold and $\dot{V}O_{2\,max}$ of trained and untrained boys relative to muscle mass and composition. In J. Rutenfranz, R. Mocellin & F. Klimt (eds) *Children and Exercise XII*. Human Kinetics, Champaign, IL.

Baraldi, E., Zanconato, S., Sanfuz, P.A. & Zacchello F. (1989) A comparison of two noninvasive methods in the determination of the anaerobic thresholds in children. *Int. J. Sports Med.* **10**, 132–4.

Bar-Or, O. (1983) *Pediatric Sports Medicine for the Practitioner.* Springer-Verlag, New York.

Becker, D.M. & Vaccaro, P. (1983) Anaerobic threshold alterations caused by endurance training in young children. *J. Sports Med.* **23**, 445–9.

Beunen, G., Van Gerven, D. & Vanden Eynde, B. (1977) Reliability of three cardiorespiratory field tests. In H. Lavelle & R.J. Shephard (eds) *Frontiers of Activity and Child Health*, pp. 75–81. Pelican, Quebec.

Boileau, R.A., Bonen, A., Heyward, V.H. & Massey, B. (1977) Maximal aerobic capacity on the treadmill and bicycle ergometer of boys 11–14 years of age. *J. Sports Med.* **17**, 152–62.

Boulay, M.R., Hamel, P., Simoneau, V.A., Lortie, G., Prud'homme, D. & Bouchard, C. (1984) A test of aerobic capacity: description and reliability. *Can. J. Appl. Sport Sci.* **9**, 122–6.

Bruce, R.A., Kusumi, F. & Hosmer, D. (1973) Maximal oxygen intake and nomographic assessment of functional impairment in cardiovascular disease. *Am. Heart J.* **85**, 546–62.

Conconi, F., Ferrari, M., Ziglio, P.G., Droghetti, P. & Codeca, L. (1982) Determination of the anaerobic threshold by a noninvasive field test in runners. *J. Appl. Physiol.* **52**, 869–73.

Cumming, G.R., Goodwin, A., Baggley, G. & Antel, J. (1967) Repeated measurements of aerobic capacity during a week of intensive training at a youth track camp. *Can. J. Physiol. Pharmacol.* **45**, 805–11.

Cumming, G.R., Hastman, L., McCort, J. & Mc-Cullough, S. (1980a) High serum lactates do occur in young children after maximal work. *Int. J. Sports Med.* **1**, 66–9.

Cumming, G.R. & Langford, S. (1985) Comparison of nine exercise tests used in pediatric cardiology. In R.A. Binkhorst, Kemper, H.C. & W.H. Saris (eds) *Children and Exercise XI*, pp. 58–67. Human Kinetics, Champaign, IL.

Cumming, G.R., McDonald, D. & Skrypnyk, H. (1980b) Correlations between echocardiographic dimensions, sports activity, and maximal oxygen uptake in normal boys. In H. Lavallee & R.J. Shephard (eds) *Child Growth and Development*, Proceedings of the International Symposium on Child Growth and Development, pp. 296–310. University of Quebec Press, Trois Rivières, Canada.

Cunningham, D.A., MacFarlane Van Waterschoot, B., Paterson, D.H., Lefcoe, M. & Sangal, S.P. (1977) Reliability and reproducibility of maximal oxygen uptake measurement in children. *Med. Sci. Sports* **9**, 104–8.

Cunningham, D.A. & Paterson, D.H. (1985) Age specific prediction of maximal oxygen uptake in boys. *Can. J. Appl. Sport Sci.* **10**, 75–80.

Cureton, K.L., Boileau, R.A., Lohman, T.G. & Misner, J.E. (1977) Determinants of distance running performance in children: analysis of a path model. *Res. Q.* **48**, 270–9.

Daniels, J., Oldridge, N., Nagle, F. & White, B. (1978) Changes in oxygen consumption of young boys during growth and running training. *Med. Sci. Sports* **3**, 161–5.

Docherty, D., Wenger, H.A. & Collis, M.L. (1985) The effects of resistance training on aerobic and anaerobic power of young boys. *Med. Sci. Sports Exerc.* **19**, 389–92.

Doolittle, T.L. & Bigbee, R. (1968) The twelve minute run-walk: a test of cardiorespiratory fitness of adolescent boys. *Res. Q.* **39**, 491–5.

Eriksson, B.O. & Koch, G. (1973) Effect of physical training on hemodynamic response during submaximal and maximal training. *Acta Physiol. Scand.* **87**, 27–39.

Farrell, P.A., Wilmore, J.H., Cole, E.P., Billing, J.E. & Costill, D.L. (1979) Plasma lactate accumulation and distance running performance. *Med. Sci. Sports* **11**, 338–44.

Freedson, P.S. & Goodman, T.L. (1993) Measurement of oxygen consumption. In T.W. Rowland (ed.) *Pediatric Laboratory Exercise Testing*, pp. 91–114. Human Kinetics, Champaign, IL.

Gaisl, G. & Hofmann, P. (1990) Heart rate determination of anaerobic threshold in children. *Pediatr. Exerc. Sci.* **2**, 29–36.

Gaul, K.A. (1990) *Exercise and the young female: maturational differences in the responsiveness to aerobic training.* Doctoral dissertation, University of Victoria, Canada.

Godfrey, S. (1974) *Exercise Testing in Children.* W.B. Saunders, Philadelphia.

Godfrey, S., Davies, C., Wozniak, E. & Barnes, C. (1971) Cardiorespiratory response to exercise in normal children. *Clin. Sci.* **40**, 419–31.

Goldberg, S.J., Weis, R.W. & Adams, F.H. (1966) A comparison of the maximal endurance of normal children and patients with congenital cardiac disease. *J. Pediatr.* **69**, 46–55.

Gutin, B., Fogle, R.R. & Stewart, K. (1976) Relationships among submaximal heart rate, aerobic power, and running performance. *Res. Q.* **47**, 536–40.

Hermansen, L. & Oseid, S. (1971) Direct and indirect estimation of maximal oxygen uptake in prepubertal boys. *Acta Paediatr. Scand.* **217** (Suppl.), 18–23.

Ikai, M. & Kitagawa, K. (1972) Maximal oxygen uptake in Japanese related to sex and age. *Med. Sci. Sport Exerc.* **4**, 127–31.

Jackson, A.S. & Coleman, A.E. (1976) Validation of

distance run tests for elementary school children. *Res. Q.* **47**, 87–94.

James, F.W. (1978) Exercise testing in children and young adults. An overview. *Cardiovasc. Clin.* **9**, 187–203.

Johnson, B.L. & Nelson, J.K. (1986) *Practical Measurements for Evaluation in Physical Education*, 4th edn. Burgess Publishing, Edina, MN.

Krahenbuhl, G.S. & Pangrazi, R.P. (1983) Characteristics associated with running performance in young boys. *Med. Sci. Sports Exerc.* **15**, 486–90.

Krahenbuhl, G.S., Pangrazi, R.P., Burkett, L.N., Schneider, M.J. & Petersen, G. (1977) Field estimation of $\dot{V}O_{2 max}$ in children eight years of age. *Med. Sci. Sports* **9**, 37–40.

Krahenbuhl, G.S., Pangrazi, R.P., Petersen, G.W., Burkett, L.N. & Schneider, M.J. (1978) Field testing of cardiorespiratory fitness in primary school children. *Med. Sci. Sports* **10**, 208–13.

Legér, L. & Gadoury, C. (1989) Validity of the 20 m shuttle run test with 1 min stages to predict $\dot{V}O_{2 max}$ in adults. *Can. J. Sports Sci.* **14**, 21–6.

Legér, L. & Lambert, J. (1982) A maximal 20 m shuttle run test to predict $\dot{V}O_{2 max}$. *Eur. J. Appl. Physiol.* **49**, 1–12.

Legér, L., Mercier, D., Lambert, J. & Gadboury, C. (1984) The multistage 20 meter shuttle run. (Unpublished paper.)

McConnell, T.R., Haas, J.H. & Conlin, N.C. (1992) Gas exchange anaerobic threshold: implications. *Pediatr. Exerc. Sci.* **4**, 360–66.

Macek, M. & Vavra, J. (1980) Adjustment of oxygen uptake at the onset of exercise: comparison between prepubertal boys and adults. *Int. J. Sports Med.* **1**, 70–2.

Mahon, A.D. & Vaccaro, P. (1989) Ventilatory threshold and $\dot{V}O_{2 max}$ changes in children following endurance training. *Med. Sci. Sport Exerc.* **21**, 425–31.

Mahon, A.D. & Vaccaro, P. (1991) Can the point of deflection from linearity of heart rate determine ventilatory threshold in children? *Pediatr. Exerc. Sci.* **3**, 256–62.

Maksud, M.G. & Coutts, K.D. (1971) Application of the Cooper twelve minute run–walk test to young males. *Res. Q.* **42**, 54–9.

Mechelin, W., Hlobil, H. & Kemper, H.C. (1986) Validation of two running tests as an estimate of maximal aerobic power in children. *Eur. J. Appl. Physiol.* **55**, 503–6.

Mercier, D., Legér, L. & Lambert, J. (1983) Relative efficiency and predicted $\dot{V}O_{2 max}$ in children. *Med. Sci. Sports Exerc.* **15**, 143 (abstract).

Miller, D.K. (1988) *Measurement by the Physical Educator: Why and How*. Benchmark Press, Indianapolis, IN.

Mirwald, R.L. & Bailey, D.A. (1986) *Maximal Aerobic Power*. Sports Dynamics, London.

Neary, P., MacDougall, J.D., Bachus, R. & Wenger, H.A. (1985) The relationship between lactate and ventilation thresholds: coincidental or cause and effect? *Eur. J. Appl. Physiol.* **54**, 104–8.

Palgi, Y., Gutin, B., Young, J. & Alejanaro, D. (1984) Physiologic and anthropmetric factors underlying endurance performance in children. *Int. J. Sports Med.* **5**, 67–73.

Paterson, D.H., Cunningham, D.A. & Donner, A. (1981) The effect of different treadmill speeds on the variability of $\dot{V}O_{2 max}$ in children. *Eur. J. Appl. Physiol.* **47**, 113–12.

Paterson, D.H., McLellan, R., Stella, R.S. & Cunningham, D.A. (1987) Longitudinal study of ventilation threshold and maximal oxygen uptake in athletic boys. *J. Appl. Physiol.* **62**, 2051–7.

Reybrouck, T., Weymans, M., Ghesquiere, J., Van Gerven, D. & Stijns, H. (1982) Ventilatory threshold during treadmill exercise in kindergarten children. *Eur. J. Appl. Physiol.* **50**, 79–86.

Riopel, D.A., Taylor, A.B. & Hohn, A.R. (1979) Blood pressure, heart rate, pressure-rate product and electrocardiographic changes in healthy children during treadmill exercise. *Am. J. Cardiol.* **44**, 607–704.

Rivera-Brown, A.M., Rivera, M.A. & Frontera, R. (1992) Applicability of criteria for $\dot{V}O_{2 max}$ in active adolescents. *Pediatr. Exerc. Sci.* **4**, 331–9.

Rotstein, A., Dotan, R., Bar-Or, O. & Tenenbaum, G. (1986) Effect of training on anaerobic threshold, maximal aerobic power and anaerobic performance in pre-adolescent boys. *Int. J. Sports Med.* **7**, 281–6.

Rowland, T.W. (1991) 'Normalizing' maximum oxygen uptake, or the search for the Holy Grail (per kg). *Pediatr. Exerc. Sci.* **3**, 95–102.

Rowland, T.W. (1992) *Pediatric Exercise Testing: Clinical Guidelines*. Human Kinetics, Champaign, IL.

Rowland, T.W. (1993) Aerobic exercise testing protocols. In T.W. Rowland (ed.) *Pediatric Laboratory Exercise Testing*, pp. 19–42. Human Kinetics, Champaign, IL.

Rowland, T.W., Auchinachie, J.A., Keenan, T.J. & Green, G.M. (1987) Physiologic responses to treadmill running in adult and prepubertal males. *Int. J. Sports Med.* **8**, 292–7.

Rowland, T.W. & Green, G.M. (1989) Anaerobic threshold and the determination of training target heart rates in premenarcheal girls. *Pediatr. Cardiol.* **10**, 75–9.

Safrit, M.J. & Wood, T.M. (1987) The test battery reliability of the health related fitness test. *Res. Q. Exerc. Sport* **58**, 160–7.

Safrit, M.J., Hooper, S., Ehlert, S., Costa, M. & Paterson, P. (1988) The validity generalization of distance run tests. *Can. J. Sport Sci.* **13**, 188–96.

Schmidt-Nielsen, K. (1984) *Scaling: Why is Animal Size so Important?* Cambridge University Press, Cambridge.

Sheehan, J.M., Rowland, T.W. & Burke, E.J. (1987) A comparison of four treadmill protocols for determination of maximum oxygen uptake in 10 to 12 year old boys. *Int. J. Sports Med.* **8**, 31–4.

Shephard, R. (1982) *Physical Activity and Growth.* Yearbook Medical Publishers, Chicago.

Sjodin, B. & Jacobs, I. (1981) Onset of blood lactate accumulation and marathon running performance. *Int. J. Sports Med.* **2**, 26–9.

Skinner, J.S., Bar-Or, O., Bergsteinova, V., Bell, C., Royer, D. & Buskirk, E.R. (1971) Comparison of continuous and intermittent tests determining maximal oxygen intake in children. *Acta Paediatr. Scand.* **217** (Suppl.), 24–8.

Stewart, K.J. & Gutin, B. (1976) Effects of physical training on cardiorespiratory fitness in children. *Res. Q.* **47**, 110–20.

Tanaka, H. & Shindo, M. (1985) Running velocity of blood lactate threshold of boys aged 6–15 years compared with untrained males. *Int. J. Sports Med.* **6**, 90–4.

Thoden, J. (1991) Testing aerobic power. In J.D. MacDongall, H.A. Wenger & H.J. Green (eds) *Physiological Testing of the High-Performance Athlete*, 2nd edn, pp. 107–74. Human Kinetics, Champaign, IL.

Tomassoni, T.L. (1993) Conducting the pediatric exercise test. In T.W. Rowland (ed.) *Pediatric Laboratory Exercise Testing*, pp. 1–18. Human Kinetics, Champaign, IL.

Vago, P., Mercier, J., Ramonatxo, M. & Prefaut, C. (1987) Is ventilatory anaerobic threshold a good index of endurance capacity? *Int. J. Sports Med.* **8**, 190–5.

Van Gerven, D., Beunen, G., Ostyn, M. *et al.* (1982) Reliability of a relation between two submaximal incremental bicycle ergometer tests in children. In *Cardiorespiratory Fitness in Canada: A Current View of Youth and Sports*, pp. 36–42. International Council for Physical Fitness Research XVth Meeting of ICPER (XXIst Symposium of Maglingen). Maglingen, Switzerland.

Washington, R.L. (1993) Anaerobic threshold. In T.W. Rowland (ed.) *Pediatric Laboratory Exercise Testing*, pp. 115–30. Human Kinetics, Champaign, IL.

Weymans, M., Reybrouck, T., Stigns, H. & Knops, J. (1985) Influence of age and sex on the ventilatory anaerobic threshold in children. In R.A. Binkhorst *et al.* (eds) *Children and Exercise XI*, pp. 114–18. Human Kinetics, Champaign, IL.

Winter, E.M. (1992) Scaling: partitioning out differences in size. *Pediatr. Exerc. Sci.* **4**, 296–301.

Wolfe, R.R., Washington, R., Daberkow, E., Murphy, J.R. & Brammel, H.L. (1986) Anaerobic threshold as a predictor of athletic performance in young female runners. *Am. J. Dis. Child.* **140**, 922–4.

Chapter 36

Testing Anaerobic Performance

EMMANUEL VAN PRAAGH

Introduction

In exercise and sport science the concept of physical fitness is often central to discussion among physical educators, trainers and researchers (Åstrand, 1992). However, the term is vague and may be differently defined according to age, sex or motivation (leisure or training) of the individual. Human performance-related fitness may involve activities of extremely short duration (<1 s) and short-term activities over the first 10 s to 1 min. The estimate of anaerobic power raises several theoretical questions. For instance, an individual's power output during a test depends on the muscle groups involved and the type of movement (concentric, eccentric, monoarticular, polyarticular, etc.) and the joint range of motion.

This chapter will focus on testing the capability of children and adolescents during the performance of high-intensity activities which range between 200 ms and 1 min in duration. Exercises which can be performed for several minutes will not be discussed in this chapter because the main energy production for these endeavours comes from the aerobic metabolic pathways.

Definitions

Anaerobic performance is a rather complex concept. In the literature it is often defined as synonymous with muscle power. An anaerobic task like, for example, sprinting involves a short burst of effort. Such an activity requires an immediate availability of energy to power maximum muscular activity. However, we can also consider that all short-term muscular force and work done by means of 'anaerobic' energy release can be defined as performance.

The following terms will be used in this chapter:

1 Force (mass $\times$ acceleration) is measured in newtons (N).

2 Work (force $\times$ distance) is measured in joules (J).

3 Power (work per unit of time, or force $\times$ velocity) is measured in watts (W).

4 Endurance (time for which a static force or power level involving combinations of concentric and/or eccentric muscular contractions can be maintained) is measured in seconds (s).

5 Fatigue is defined as an inability to maintain the required or expected force or power (Edwards, 1981). For further details on exercise terminology see Knuttgen and Kraemer (1987).

Measuring anaerobic performance

In adults, quantitative biochemical measurements of anaerobic energy supply during short-term exercise can be made by invasive methods. To know more about the underlying mechanisms of anaerobic ability during childhood, some authors have used biopsy techniques (Eriksson, 1980). This kind of investigation is ethically questionable in the healthy child. Therefore, in this particular population some researchers have concentrated on measuring the external work and power generated during standardized tests (Bar-Or, 1987; Sargeant, 1989; Van Praagh et al., 1990).

In numerous physical activities and sports, the child or the young athlete must activate and synchronize their motor units in order to throw a mass (e.g. shotput) or to displace their body mass against gravity (e.g. high jump). These activities need a burst of muscular contractions of a very short duration (< 1 s). Such instantaneous activity reflects the ability to transform adenosine triphosphate (ATP) breakdown into external power. High-intensity muscle power may also be sustained over a longer time period (> 1 s to 60 s). We may therefore consider: instantaneous anaerobic performance to be less than 1 s and short-term anaerobic performance to be greater than 1 s and up to 60 s.

Instantaneous power

FUNDAMENTAL CONSIDERATIONS

The measurement of maximal power output raises several methodological problems (for review see Sargeant, 1992):

1 Since power is the product of force and velocity, the external load (the load on the cycle ergometer or the body mass during jumping or running) must closely match the capability of the active muscles so that they operate at their optimal velocity (Wilkie, 1960). Clearly this is a difficult condition to fulfil or to guarantee in freely accelerating, or decelerating, cycling or running sprint efforts.

2 If 'true' peak power output is to be measured, the duration of the test must be short (< 1 s), because power output decreases rapidly as a function of time (Fig. 36.1). The measurement of 'true' peak power requires measurements of instantaneous values of force and velocity. This condition is only satisfied in tests which use a force platform, or several monoarticular force–velocity tests. In other power tests (staircase running or cycling on friction-loaded ergometers), the forces and the velocities are averaged instead of being instantaneous values (Vandewalle et al., 1987).

3 Anaerobic glycolysis and aerobic contribution are limited during instantaneous power exercises or tests. In contrast, using the 30-s Wingate test in prepubescent and adolescent boys it has been shown that the aerobic fraction, compared to young men, was fairly high (Van Praagh et al., 1991; Hebestreit et al., 1993). Lactate production starts during the first seconds of a supramaximal exercise. In adults it has been observed that the glycolytic metabolism is already involved in exercise lasting less than 10 s (Saltin et al., 1971). Therefore, only exercises lasting approximately 1 s can be considered as 'alactacid'.

4 Different results of peak power between several tests can be due to factors such as: (i) whether instantaneous or mean power is measured; (ii) the legs act simultaneously or successively; (iii) total body mass or active muscle mass is taken into account (Van Praagh et al., 1990); or (iv) peak power is measured at the beginning of exercise or after several seconds of a flying start (Vandewalle et al., 1987). However, in most peak power tests there are no objective criteria to confirm maximality and thus the researcher or the trainer must rely on the willing cooperation of the subject.

Performance tests that apparently cause maximal activation of the ATP–creatine phosphate (CP) energy system have been developed to provide field tests to evaluate the capacity of this immediate means for energy transfer. These tests are generally referred to as power tests (e.g. work done per unit time: $J \cdot s^{-1} = W$). In the laboratory, these tests can be done on several ergometric devices. Isokinetic devices (Cybex II, Lumex Inc., NY, USA) can be used for monoarticular tests of peak torque and mean power. Force platforms are also useful for the measurement of instantaneous leg power. Cycle ergometers (frictional or isokinetic) can be used for the measurement of peak and mean leg (arm) power. Finally, motorized and non-motorized treadmills can be used for short-term running tests. All these devices must

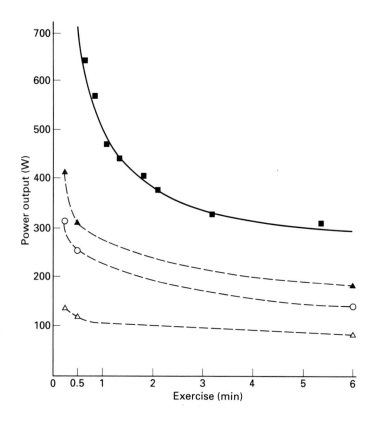

Fig. 36.1 Maximal external power as a function of exercise duration. Adult data ($n = 1$) from Wilkie (1960); children's data from Van Praagh *et al.* (1989, 1990). ■, adult; ▲, 12-year-old boys; ○, 12-year-old girls; △, 7-year-old boys. Redrawn with permission.

be carefully and regularly calibrated. Some commercially available cycle ergometers may show calibration errors of as much as 40% (Van Praagh *et al.*, 1992).

LABORATORY TESTS

Isokinetic monoarticular tests

Movement across a single joint (e.g. knee or elbow) can be measured with ergometers which control the force of movement (dynamic) or the velocity of movement (isokinetic). Few data are available for children. The aim of isokinetic testing is the measurement of peak torque and mean power. Torque expressed in $N \cdot m$ and the angular velocity in $rad \cdot s^{-1}$ yield power in W. Isokinetic dynamometer recordings are rarely generated under true constant angular velocity. The term isokinetic is therefore a misnomer, primarily due to the slow response frequency of the system (Murray & Harrison, 1986). Torque is measured throughout a range of motion at different limb velocities. Sargeant (1989) reported the difficulty in voluntarily accelerating a limb to optimal velocity for peak power output. Another methodological drawback is the lack of standardization of the torque–velocity relationship. In children, some authors have measured torque in a slow ($30° \cdot s^{-1}$) and/or fast ($300° \cdot s^{-1}$) movement. In prepubescent boys, Weltman *et al.* (1986) reported torque ($N \cdot m$) values as a function of angular velocity ($30°$ and $90° \cdot s^{-1}$) for flexion and extension at the knee and elbow joints. The results are then difficult to compare. Moreover, the commercially available dynamometers have some limitations. They cannot achieve higher angular velocity than $300° \cdot s^{-1}$. This velocity is considerably lower than that actually attained during sprinting on the flat. Children reach stride cadences exceeding 5 strides $\cdot s^{-1}$, a velocity far exceeding $300°\cdot s^{-1}$. The force–velocity relationship is highly specific and it is obvious that the torque–velocity relationship cannot be simply evaluated by an isolated movement at a markedly different velocity. Berg *et al.* (1986) concluded that sprint ability in pubescent boys was not highly related to knee torque production at $30°\cdot s^{-1}$ and $300°\cdot s^{-1}$. Because most of isokinetic dynamometers are designed for adults, modification of the equipment is required to test children.

Force platform tests

Vertical jumping. Since the early work of E.J. Marey (Marey & Demenÿ, 1885) who recorded the simultaneous measurement of force (pneumatic force platform) and displacement during a vertical jump (Fig. 36.2), numerous authors developed vertical jump protocols. Today, sophisticated instrumentation (force platform) allows the recording of the ground reaction forces and acceleration of the body centre of mass. Peak power output is derived from the product of instantaneous force exerted by the subject on the force platform and the acceleration of the body centre of mass (Davies & Young, 1984). The height of the jump (*H*) is measured according to the formula:

$$H = vt^2 \cdot 2g^{-1},$$

where vt = take-off velocity and g = acceleration due to gravity. Peak force is the recording of maximal force during the time of contact on the platform before take-off. The test is considered as the gold standard in jump power testing and has been used for validation of other anaerobic power tests. Peak power output recorded during a vertical jump on a force platform is highly correlated with that measured on an isokinetic cycle ergometer ($r = 0.95$). However, the comparison of power outputs between different forms of activities can never be mechanically exact. In fact, during jumping on the platform, peak force always precedes peak velocity, whereas during, for example, cycling peak force and velocity coincide (Davies

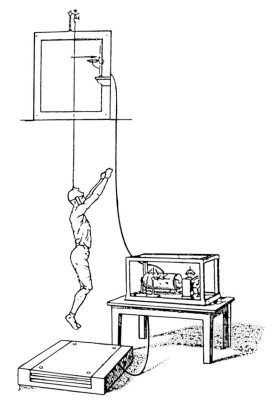

Fig. 36.2 The equipment used by E.J. Marey to record the simultaneous measurement of ground reaction force and displacement during a vertical jump. Redrawn with permission from Marey & Demenÿ (1885).

et al., 1984). This method requires an expensive force-plate technology, technical staff and is time-consuming. Davies and Young (1984) reported fairly low intrasubject variation ($\pm 7\%$).

Vertical jump performance. Komi and Bosco (1978) have conceived three different jumping situations to evaluate anaerobic leg power and muscular fatigue:

1 Squatting jump from a static position with a knee angle of $90°$.

2 Countermovement jump from a standing position with a preliminary countermovement.

3 Dropping jump when the subject drops from heights of 0.2 to 0.8 m onto the force platform with a subsequent upward jump.

In all jumping conditions the children keep their hands on hips throughout the entire jump. Each jump is recorded on magnetic tape and a vertical force–time curve produced by each jump is analysed with computerized calculations (see Komi & Bosco, 1978; Mero *et al.*, 1989). It is assumed that the 'stretch-shortening cycle' which occurs during this type of jump, allows the stored elastic energy to be utilized during positive work and thus increases the vertical jump performance. The tolerance to progressive dropping height increases from childhood up to the age of 20–25 years (Bosco & Komi, 1980). It is therefore recommended to protect the young body against high stretch loads, especially when muscles and bones have not yet reached maturity and when ossification processes are not yet achieved.

FIELD TESTS

Field tests are used for their simplicity, but they should be compared with reliable laboratory indices for validation. The problem is that only a few muscular power tests (force platform jump test or running test) can be considered as gold standards.

Sargent test

The measurement of maximal leg power by means of a vertical jump was first developed for adults by Sargent (1921). Subjects are required to jump vertically as high as they can. At the peak of the jump, the examinee marks the measuring board with chalk. The subject's ability to exert 'power' with the legs is derived from the height of the jump. The best or the average value of three jumps is generally taken as the test score. The vertical jump has been accepted as a valid measure of leg power and various vertical jump protocols have been derived from the Sargent test (e.g. jump-and-reach test, the Abalakow test) (for review see Kirby, 1991). The objectivity and reliability coefficients are high, but the validity of the test, compared with the sum of four power

events in track and field, is rather low ($r = 0.78$; Safrit, 1990). In adults, the height of a vertical jump is correlated ($0.63 < r < 0.84$) with maximal relative anaerobic power ($W \cdot kg^{-1}$) on a Monark ergometer (Varberg, Sweden). The use of the force-platform technique or the Vertec apparatus probably improves the validity of the test. Davies and Young (1984) found a high correlation ($r = 0.92$) between the height of a vertical jump and the data obtained on the force platform in children. In adults, the test–retest reliability coefficients of several vertical jump tests are high ($r = 0.92$; Glencross, 1966). The test is suitable for any subject able to perform a vertical jump. Norms are available (Safrit, 1990; Baumgartner & Jackson, 1991). When administered properly this simple field test measures one of the most important single factors in sport performance. A major weakness is the lack of standardization in test administration. For instance, a countermovement increases the vertical jump performance by approximately 15% (Bosco, 1983), probably because of the use of potential elastic energy; moreover a rapid elevation of the arms may improve the height of a vertical jump. No reliability coefficients are reported in children.

Lewis nomogram test

Because the vertical jump test has the dimension of work (force × displacement), the Lewis nomogram has been designed to be used concomitantly with the former test (Fox & Mathews, 1981). The aim is to add 'speed' to the body mass and the vertical distance performed. There are no measures of objectivity or reliability and no norms are available for the test. Recently, Harman *et al.* (1991) conducted a validation study on male adults and concluded that the Lewis formula does not provide accurate estimate of muscle leg power.

Standing broad jump test

The purpose of this test is to evaluate the ability of a subject to exert power with the legs.

The problem of field-based assessments is that the test does not reflect a single factor, power of the legs in this particular case, but also learning, coordination and maturation. The test appears to be objective as well as reliable. However, the validity of the test is questionable. The common variance this test item shares with a 'pure' power test is low ($r = 0.61$; Johnson & Nelson, 1986). The test is feasible for girls and boys from 6 years on (Eurofit, 1988). Normative data are available for both age and sex groups (American Alliance for Health, Physical Education and Recreation, 1975).

Acceleration in sprint running

Sprint running is measured by means of three adjustable photocell systems placed at hip height. Accelerations are calculated using the time recordings from the photocells placed at 0.2 and 4 m from the starting line. The subject makes a standing start and runs 10 m as fast as possible. In girls, acceleration in sprint running is independent of height, in contrast to the vertical jump which increased with height (Nielsen et al., 1980). Both in the vertical jump and in the fast stepping of a sprint start, the actual contraction times are very short (200–300 ms).

Short-term power

This kind of performance is mainly, but not exclusively, anaerobic in nature (Saltin, 1990; Van Praagh et al., 1991).

LABORATORY TESTS

Cycling ergometry

External mechanical power (W) of the legs (or arms) can be estimated on a cycle ergometer by determining the relationship between force and velocity, the so-called force–velocity test (Pérès et al., 1981; Sargeant et al., 1981; Van Praagh et al., 1989, 1990) or by measuring the speed of cycling (v) for a given braking force (N), the so-

called Wingate test (Cumming, 1973; Inbar & Bar-Or, 1986; Bar-Or, 1987).

8-s force–velocity test. In order to overcome the methodological limitations in load selection, Vandewalle et al. (1985) in adults and Van Praagh et al. (1989, 1990) in children described a new approach to this problem. A series of short sprints (8 s) are performed against a range of increasing braking forces. For each subject, the optimal braking force (F_{opt}) that elicits the peak power output is computed and subsequently used in the Wingate test. Linear force–velocity relationships and parabolic force–power (or velocity–power) relationships have generally been obtained in children with either friction-loaded ergometers (Van Praagh et al., 1989, 1990; Bedu et al., 1991) or isokinetic cycle ergometers (Sargeant & Dolan, 1986).

The force–velocity relationship can be described as:

$$v = v_0 (1 - F/F_0)$$

where v = velocity and F = force; v_0 corresponds to the extrapolation of v for zero braking force and F_0 to the extrapolation of F for zero velocity. This relationship is illustrated in Fig. 36.3. The quasi-linear relationship allows the determination of internal test validity (Sargeant, 1992). Moreover, single aberrant values within a series of experimental plots can be identified and analysed. Peak power is obtained at optimal values of force and velocity, which correspond respectively to $0.5 F_0$ and $0.5 v_0$. Peak power is thus equal to $0.25 v_0 F_0$.

The cycle ergometer must be adapted to the body dimensions of the child (crank length, frame, handlebars and saddle height). The number of pedal revolutions (rev·min^{-1}) is measured by optical sensor at the flywheel, which computes peak or mean velocities. The results of the force–velocity test depend on the protocol. For example, peak power is approximately 15% higher when the child may stand on the pedals, instead of sitting on the saddle. In children it is appropriate to express leg power corrected for active muscle (lean thigh

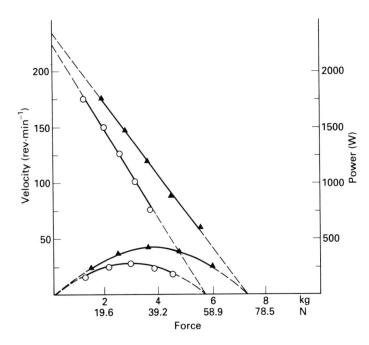

Fig. 36.3 Force–velocity (straight lines) and force–power (parabolas) relationships in 12-year-old girls (○) and boys (▲). Redrawn with permission from Van Praagh *et al.* (1990).

volume or lean leg volume) instead of total body mass (Table 36.1). In the author's laboratory, the Wingate test was compared with the force–velocity test. The peak power output standardized for lean thigh volume showed high correlations ($r = 0.93$, $P < 0.001$) between the tests, suggesting that both tests assessed the same variable (Van Praagh *et al.*, 1990).

In children and disabled populations the 30-s supramaximal test represents a strenuous effort. In our daily practice some tall and muscular adolescents experienced nausea and dizziness after the test. One way of decreasing these side-effects is to cool down after the test by cycling against a low resistance for several minutes. However, it could be demonstrated that boys recovered faster than young men after performing a Wingate test. A resting period of 2 min was found sufficient for a full recovery after a Wingate test, in healthy 9–12-year-old boys (Hebestreit *et al.*, 1993). If the aim is to measure peak power in untrained subjects, we recommended the less stressful force–velocity test. Moreover, the force–velocity test yields higher peak power output because of the shortness of the test. The

Wingate test reflects leg (or arm) muscle endurance more accurately and is relevant for fatigue studies. In children, the force–velocity test needs further validity and reliability studies (van Mil *et al.*, in press).

20-s isokinetic cycling test. As mentioned earlier, true maximal power output can only be measured if the external load is closely matched to the capability of the active muscles so that they are functioning at their optimal velocity. In freely accelerating or decelerating velocity, as achieved in friction–loaded cycle ergometers (Wingate test or force-velocity test) or running sprints (staircase running) these conditions are hard to fulfil. As Sargeant (1992) pointed out, if an exercise is sustained for more than a few seconds, power output may be reduced as a consequence of lowered optimal velocity due to fatigue. To overcome this problem, Sargeant's group developed an isokinetic cycle ergometer where velocity is maintained constant despite maximal leg extension on the pedals (Fig. 36.4).

During the course of each 20-s effort, the peak force declined from the maximum level

Table 36.1 Peak leg and arm power in children (healthy non-athletes)

	Age (years)/sex	Ergometer test	Power		Reference
			W	$W \cdot kg^{-1}$ BM	
Leg	10/F and M	Staircase	294	9.8	Margaria et al. (1966)
	12/M	Cycle (5-s Wingate test)	280*	—	Bar-Or & Inbar (1978)
	11/F and M	Cycle (isokinetic)	1283 (2 legs)	32.7	Davies & Young (1984)
	11/F and M	Force platform	711	18.1	Davies & Young (1984)
	13/M	Cycle (isokinetic)	785 (1 leg)	15.3	Sargeant et al. (1984)
	12/F	Cycle (force−velocity test)	310	7.4	Van Praagh et al. (1989)
	12/M	Cycle (force−velocity test)	415	9.7	Van Praagh et al. (1990)
	7/M	Cycle (force−velocity test)	146	5.8	Van Praagh et al. (1990)
	11/F and M	Non-motorized treadmill	261	7	Van Praagh et al. (1991, unpublished data)
				$W \cdot l^{-1}$ LTV	
	13/M	Cycle (isokinetic)	785	204	Sargeant et al. (1984)
	7/M	Cycle (frictional)	146	69	Van Praagh et al. (1989)
	12/F	Cycle (frictional)	310	53	Van Praagh et al. (1990)
	12/M	Cycle (frictional)	415	82	Van Praagh et al. (1990)
				$W \cdot l^{-1}$ LAV	
Arm	14−15/M	Cycle (3-s Wingate test)	300*	155*	Blimkie et al. (1988)
	14−15/F	Cycle (3-s Wingate test)	200*	132*	Blimkie et al. (1988)

* Calculated values.

BM, body mass; F, female; LAV, lean arm volume; LTV, lean thigh volume; M, male.

attained within the first few seconds (Fig. 36.5). The level of peak force is inversely and linearly related to crank velocity over the range studied. In studies on children, the coefficient of variation of the peak force is lower than 6% (Sargeant et al., 1984).

30-s Wingate test. This supramaximal cycling test, which is derived from Cumming's test (1973) is the most frequently used and has been studied by many authors. It measures external work during a 30-s sprint cycling test (Fig. 36.6). Peak power reflects the ability of the muscles to produce high mechanical power in a short time, whereas mean power or total work represents the endurance of these muscles, i.e. their ability to sustain high power.

Selecting the appropriate braking force for subjects, is one of the methodological problems in test protocols where a single exercise bout is performed. In fact, one cannot measure true maximal power if the same braking force (re-

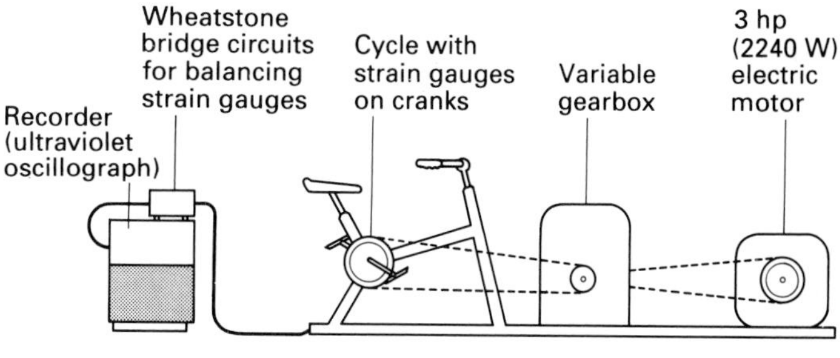

Fig. 36.4 The isokinetic cycle ergometer. Redrawn with permission from Sargeant et al. (1984).

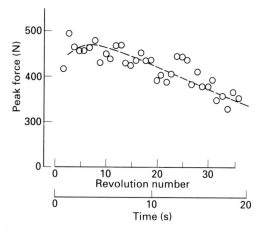

Fig. 36.5 Decrease of the peak force in each revolution as a function of crank velocity during a 20-s maximal cycling exercise, using an isokinetic ergometer. Redrawn with permission from Sargeant *et al.* (1984).

lated or not related to body mass) is used for each subject, since maximal power is obtained only when forces and velocities are optimal.

In children, maximal power output is often expressed relative to body mass (Table 36.2). This may be useful in activities that require lifting of the body mass (e.g. running or jumping), but in activities such as rowing or cycling

it seems inappropriate to standardize leg muscle power for body mass. Moreover, the normal relationship between body mass and leg muscle power may vary as a consequence of muscular atrophy, nutritional disease, obesity, growth and training (for review and discussion see Sargeant, 1989, 1992; Van Praagh *et al.*, 1990). Peak and mean power output can also be determined during arm cranking (Blimkie *et al.*, 1988). The objectivity of the test is not reported, but the test is highly reliable ($r = 0.89-0.98$) and fairly valid (r values of 0.75 or more with a variety of anaerobic tasks; Bar-Or, 1987). Norms are available (Bar-Or, 1983; Inbar & Bar-Or, 1986).

Running

Sprinting upstairs. It is difficult to measure power output during flat running. Therefore, Margaria *et al.* (1966) proposed a simple, but reliable test in which subjects (including children) after a short 2-m run on the flat, run up a flight of stairs as rapidly as possible, taking two steps at a time. The only equipment required is a timing device (switch mats or photoelectric cells) and a suitable flight of stairs

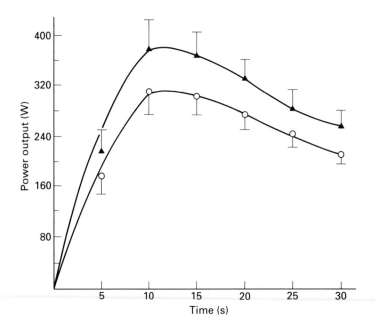

Fig. 36.6 Mean leg power output during the 30-s Wingate test in 12-year-old girls (○) and boys (▲). Redrawn with permission from Van Praagh *et al.* (1990).

Table 36.2 Mean leg power (athletes and non-athletes).

Age (years)/sex	Training state	Ergometer (test)	Leg power W	W·kg⁻¹ BM	Reference
12–17/F and M	T	Cycle (Wingate test)	335–424	—	Cumming (1973)
7–9/M	U	Cycle (Wingate test)	150*	5.5	Inbar & Bar-Or (1975)
12/M	U	Cycle (Wingate test)	255*	—	Bar-Or & Inbar (1978)
11–13/M	T	Cycle (Wingate test)	270*	7.2	Grodjinovski et al. (1980)
13.4/M	T	Cycle (Wingate test)	380	7.8	Tharpe et al. (1984)
7.4/M	U	Cycle (Wingate test)	123	4.7	Van Praagh et al. (1989)
12.7/F	U	Cycle (Wingate test)	254	5.9	Van Praagh et al. (1990)
12.9/M	U	Cycle (Wingate test)	307	7.2	Van Praagh et al. (1990)
10.8/M	U	Cycle (Wingate test)	212	5.8	Docherty & Gaul (1991)
11/F	U	Cycle (Wingate test)	194	5.0	Docherty & Gaul (1991)
8–14/F	T	Non-motorized treadmill	161–434	5.5–8.4	Fargeas et al. (1993)
9–14/M	T	Non-motorized treadmill	180–500	6.0–9.0	Van Praagh et al. (1993)

* Calculated values.
BM, body mass; F, female; M, male; T, trained; U, untrained.

(each step: 0.175 m). Knowing the body mass (kg), the total vertical distance that the body is lifted up the stairs (m) and the time to traverse four steps (s), one can calculate the external power output of the subject:

$$\begin{aligned}
\text{power (W)} &= \text{force} \times \text{velocity} \\
&= \text{body weight (N)} \times \text{vertical} \\
&\quad \text{velocity (m·s}^{-1}) \\
&= \text{body mass (kg)} \times 9.81 \times H \\
&\quad (\text{m}) \cdot t^{-1}(\text{s})
\end{aligned}$$

where H is the vertical elevation of the body centre of mass (to simplify the procedure one can measure h instead, which is the level difference between the steps), t is the time spent between the cells and 9.81 is the acceleration of gravity in m·s⁻². Maximal velocity is attained in 1.5–2 s and is maintained constant for at least 5 s. Modifications of the original protocol have been proposed. For instance, 6-m run on the flat and three steps at a time instead of two (Kalamen, 1968) (Fig. 36.7).

In the case of the latter test no data are available for children. Margaria et al. reported an increase of the maximal leg power output as a function of age. The intrasubject variation of the test is usually large (± 15%) compared to

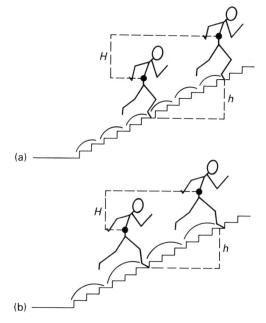

Fig. 36.7 Two different protocols of a staircase test: (a) Margaria's protocol; (b) Kalamen's protocol. Redrawn with permission from Vandewalle et al. (1987). For further details see text.

cycle or platform measurements (± 4% and 7%, respectively; Davies & Young, 1984). The validity coefficients for athletes seem significantly higher than those for untrained subjects. Norms are not reported.

Despite the statements made by Margaria *et al.* (1966), performance may be influenced by several factors including step height, leg length, stride pattern and skill of climbing stairs at maximal velocity. In young children, because of risk of injury in taking two steps at time, the tester might consider the 30-m dash with a standing start as an alternative (see p. 613).

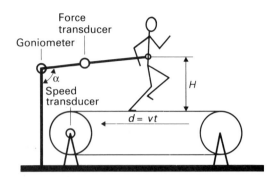

Fig. 36.8 Schematic representation of the non-motorized treadmill. *d*, distance, *H*, height; *t*, time; *v*, velocity. Redrawn with permission from Belli and Lacour (1989).

Sprint running on a non-motorized treadmill. This is a promising form of testing whole-body short-term power output. Assessment of mechanical work during distance running on the motorized treadmill is still an unresolved problem (Asmussen & Bonde-Petersen, 1974). However, attempts have been made to measure maximal velocity and power output during brief high-intensity exercise in adult populations on non-motorized treadmills (Lakomy, 1987). In our laboratory (Fargeas *et al.*, 1993; Van Praagh *et al.*, 1993) an attempt has been made to evaluate short-term power output ($<10\,s$) in untrained and trained children (see Tables 36.1 & 36.2). The subject is connected (around the waist) with a strong belt to a horizontal bar, which is attached at its other end to a joint containing a potentiometer for recording vertical displacement during running. A strain gauge system installed in the middle length of the bar records the horizontal traction force of the runner (Fig. 36.8). A constant torque motor installed in the rear wheel of the treadmill is not used to drive the treadmill belt, but to compensate for belt friction or to simulate different loads. Signals from the goniometer (vertical displacement), transducer (horizontal traction force) and from the treadmill (belt speed) are monitored by a microcomputer, which then calculates the mechanical parameters:

potential power ($m \cdot g \cdot H \cdot t^{-1}$)
+ kinetic power ($F \cdot d \cdot t^{-1}$)

where F is force and d is distance. The test seems promising for the measurement of the subject's peak and average mechanical power since the latter is a reflection of the capacity of the specific muscles engaged in the power test. Performing on a cycle ergometer is ideal for the cyclist, but it has less practical value for athletes in other sports (Saltin, 1990). In adults, the test was found reliable ($r = 0.93$; Lakomy, 1987). In children, Fargeas *et al.* (1993) observed a correlation coefficient of 0.94 ($P < 0.001$) for the absolute power values between the force–velocity cycling test and the non-motorized treadmill running test. This test has its own limitations: there is no ideal test in anaerobic testing.

Jumping

The purpose of this test is to evaluate the mechanical leg power of a subject during a series of vertical jumps. The subject stands on the Ergojump mat (Ergotest, Azur Systèmes, Grasse, France) and begins performing as many maximal vertical jumps as possible in 15 or 60 s. The equipment must include an electrical timer which starts and stops when the subject lands on the mat. The performance is derived by plugging the total flight time (*Tf*) and total number of jumps (*n*) into a formula (Bosco, 1983). The test presents a high degree of validity for evaluating power on athletic populations (basketball or volleyball players), but it lacks validity as a general power test. The reliability is high for volleyball players ($r = 0.95$). The test is suitable for males from age 16 years.

RUNNING PERFORMANCE IN THE FIELD

30–50-m sprints. It is well documented that running velocity is highly correlated with muscular power. Tests of running velocity during short distances (30–50 m) with a standing start are easy to perform and also tend to motivate most of the children. Van Praagh *et al.* (1989, 1991) compared the peak power ($W \cdot kg^{-1}$) measured by the force–velocity test and a 30-m dash in a group of 7- and 12-year-old girls and boys. Altogether, the correlation was rather high ($r = 0.80$, $P < 0.001$), but it was significantly lower when only the values of the girls' group were analysed. It was concluded that the higher fat mass of the girls was a handicap in running velocity.

30-s shuttle run test. This test was developed in order to have a simple field test for measuring average running velocity (Van Praagh, 1989). In 12-year-old girls and boys non-significant differences in peak blood lactate could be observed between the 30-s Wingate test and the 30-s shuttle run test, suggesting that the latter was also a strenuous effort for this population (Van Praagh *et al.*, 1990).

Conclusion

In children, quantitative measurements of anaerobic supply are not yet available and often not ethically justified. Therefore, the measurement of short-term external power seems a suitable alternative. However, one must keep in mind the limitations of each anaerobic power test so that the results obtained can be properly interpreted. However, the final choice of test must meet scientific (objectivity, reliability, validity) and practical (equipment, administration, age, category, suitability for research, norms) aspects. The use of the force–velocity cycling test is recommended for assessing peak power, because of the accuracy of measuring external short-term power output, the information given concerning the force and velocity components of maximal power and its easy and fairly inexpensive administration. The 30-s Wingate test is more recommended for mean power and fatigue studies.

Challenges for future research

Unlike the substantial body of results relating to the aerobic power in children and adolescents, there is a dearth of published results on anaerobic power and capacity because of methodological and ethical constraints. Because of its fundamental importance in exercise and sports events the following suggestions for short-term research are proposed.

• In children, a worldwide accepted method to measure a subject's anaerobic power and capacity is not yet available. However, the recent method of maximal accumulated oxygen deficit as described in adults by Medbø *et al.* (1988) seems also promising in children (Carlsson & Naughton, 1992). Further investigations are necessary.

• A better understanding of the low anaerobic ability of children requires invasive techniques which are not ethically justified. New technologies (e.g. nuclear magnetic resonance studies or linking of these with Cybex ergometer; for discussion see Chance *et al.*, 1983) may provide more insight into the underlying mechanism of anaerobic power output in a non-destructive way.

• Astonishingly few results in young girls are available. More research in this area will help to understand causes for interindividual differences.

• Most of the published reports are concerned with the assessment of anaerobic leg power. In children and adolescents there is a lack of short-term arm crank ergometry.

• The use of the non-motorized treadmill seems promising in the study of short-term human locomotion patterns.

• The trainability of anaerobic power in adolescent populations needs further investigation.

References

American Alliance for Health, Physical Education and Recreation (1975) *Youth Fitness Test Manual*. AAHPER, Washington, DC.

Asmussen, E. & Bonde-Petersen, F. (1974) Storage of elastic energy in skeletal muscle in man. *Acta Physiol. Scand.* **91**, 385–92.

Åstrand, P.-O. (1992) Children and adolescents: performance, measurements, education. In J. Coudert & E. Van Praagh (eds) *Pediatric Work Physiology*, Vol. XVI. *Children and Exercise*, pp. 3–7. Masson, Paris.

Bar-Or, O. (1983) *Pediatric Sports Medicine For the Practitioner: From Physiologic Principles to Clinical Applications*. Springer-Verlag, New York.

Bar-Or, O. (1987) The Wingate anaerobic test, an update on methodology, reliability and validity. *Sports Med. N. Zeal.* **4**, 381–94.

Bar-Or, O. & Inbar, O. (1978) Relationships among anaerobic capacity, sprint and middle distance running of school children. In R.J. Shephard & H. Lavallée (eds) *Physical Fitness Assessment*, pp. 142–7. C.C. Thomas, Springfield, IL.

Baumgartner, T. & Jackson, A. (1991) *Measurement for Evaluation in Physical Education and Exercise Science*. William C. Brown, Dubuque, IL.

Bedu, M., Fellmann, N., Spielvogel, H., Falgairette, G., Van Praagh, E. & Coudert, J. (1991) Force–velocity and 30-s Wingate tests in boys at high and low altitudes. *J. Appl. Physiol.* **70**, 1031–7.

Belli, A. & Lacour, J.R. (1989) Treadmill ergometer for power output measurement during sprint running. In *Twelfth International Congress of Biomechanics*, p. 391 (abstract). University of California, Los Angeles.

Berg, K., Miller, M. & Stephens, L. (1986) Determinants of 30-meter sprint time in pubescent males. *J. Sports Med.* **26**, 225–31.

Blimkie, C.J.R., Roache, P., Hay, J.T. & Bar-Or, O. (1988) Anaerobic power of arms in teenage boys and girls: relationship to lean tissue. *Eur. J. Appl. Physiol.* **57**, 677–83.

Bosco, C. (1983) A simple method for measurement of mechanical power in jumping. *Eur. J. Appl. Physiol.* **50**, 273–82.

Bosco, C. & Komi, P.V. (1980) Influence of aging on the mechanical behavior of leg extensor muscles. *Eur. J. Appl. Physiol.* **45**, 209–19.

Carlson, J.S. & Naughton, G.A. (1992) Determination of the maximal accumulated oxygen deficit in male children. In J. Coudert & E. Van Praagh (eds) *Pediatric Work Physiology*, Vol. XVI. *Children and Exercise*, pp. 23–5. Masson, Paris.

Chance, B., Sapega, A., Sokolow, D. *et al.* (1983) Fatigue in retrospect and prospect: 31P NMR studies of exercise performance. In H.G. Knuttgen & J. Poortmans (eds) *Biochemistry of Exercise*, Vol. 13, pp. 895–908. Human Kinetics, Champaign, IL.

Cumming, G.R. (1973) Correlation of athletic performance and aerobic power in 12–17-year-old children with bone age, calf muscle, total body potassium, heart volume and two indices of anaerobic power. In O. Bar-Or (ed.) *Pediatric Work Physiology*, pp. 109–34. Wingate Institute, Natanya, Israel.

Davies, C.T.M., Wemyss-Holden, J. & Young, K. (1984) Measurement of short term power output: comparison between cycling and jumping. *Ergonomics* **3**, 285–96.

Davies, C.T.M. & Young, K. (1984) Effects of external loading on short-term power output in children and young male adults. *Eur. J. Appl. Physiol.* **52**, 351–4.

Docherty, D. & Gaul, C.A. (1991) Relationship of body size, physique, and composition to physical performance in young boys and girls. *Int. J. Sports Med.* **12**, 525–32.

Edwards, R.H.T. (1981) Human muscle function and fatigue. In R. Porter & J. Whelan (eds) *Human Muscle Fatigue: Physiological Mechanisms*, pp. 1–18. Ciba Foundation Symposium, Pitman, London.

Eriksson, B.O. (1980) Muscle metabolism in children: a review. *Acta Paediatr. Scand.* **283** (Suppl.), 20–7.

Eurofit (1988) *Handbook for the Eurofit Tests of Physical Fitness*. Council of Europe, Strasberg.

Fargeas, M.A., Lauron, B., Léger, L. & Van Praagh, E. (1993) A computerized treadmill ergometer to measure short-term power output. In *Fourteenth International Congress of Biomechanics*, pp. 394–5 (abstract). International Society of Biomechanics, Paris.

Fargeas, M.A., Van Praagh, E., Léger, L., Fellman, N. & Coudert, J. (1993) Comparison of cycling and running power outputs in trained children. *Pediatr. Exerc. Sci.* **5**, 415 (abstract).

Fox, E.L. & Mathews, D.K. (1981) *The Physiological basis of Physical Education and Athletics*. W.B. Saunders, Philadelphia.

Glencross, D.J. (1966) The nature of the vertical jump test and the standing broad jump. *Res. Q.* **37**, 353–9.

Grodjinovsky, A., Inbar, O., Dotan, R. & Bar-Or, O. (1980) Training effect on the anaerobic performance of children as measured by the Wingate anaerobic test. In K. Berg & B.O. Eriksson (eds) *Children and Exercise*, Vol. IX, pp. 139–45. University Park Press, Baltimore.

Harman, E.A., Rosenstein, M.T., Frykman, P.N., Rosenstein, R.M. & Kraemer, W.J. (1991) Estimation of human power output from vertical jump. *J. Appl. Sport Sci. Res.* **3**, 116–20.

Hebestreit, H., Mimura, K. & Bar-Or, O. (1993) Recovery of muscle power after high-intensity short-term exercise: comparing boys and men. *J. Appl. Physiol.* **74**, 2875–80.

Inbar, O. & Bar-Or, O. (1975) The effects of intermittent warm-up on 7–9-year-old boys. *Eur. J. Appl. Physiol.* **34**, 81–9.

Inbar, O. & Bar-Or, O. (1986) Anaerobic characteristics in male children and adolescents. *Med. Sci. Sports Exerc.* **3**, 264–9.

Johnson, B.L. & Nelson, J.K. (1986) *Practical Measurements for Evaluation in Physical Education.* Burgess, Edina, MN.

Kalamen, J. (1968) *Measurement of maximum muscular power in man.* Unpublished doctoral thesis, Ohio State University, Columbus, Ohio, USA.

Kirby, R.F. (1991) *Kirby's Guide for Fitness and Motor Performance Tests.* BenOak, Cape Girardeau. MI.

Knuttgen, H.G. & Kraemer, W.J. (1987) Terminology and measurement in exercise performance. *J. Appl. Sport Sci. Res.* **1**, 1–10.

Komi, P.V. & Bosco, C. (1978) Utilization of stored elastic energy in men and women. *Med. Sci. Sport* **10**, 261–5.

Lakomy, H. (1987) The use of a non-motorized treadmill for analysing sprint performance. *Ergonomics* **30**, 627–38.

Marey, E.J. & Demenÿ, G. (1885) Locomotion humaine; mécanisme du saut (Human locomotion: the mechanism of jumping). *Compte Rendu Séances Acad. Sci.* 489–94.

Margaria, R., Aghemo, P. & Rovelli, E. (1966) Measurement of muscular power (anaerobic) in man. *J. Appl. Physiol.* **21**, 1662–4.

Medbø, J.I., Mohn, A.C., Tabata, I., Bahr, R., Vaage, O. & Sejersted, O.M. (1988) Anaerobic capacity determined by maximal accumulated oxygen deficit. *J. Appl. Physiol.* **64**, 50–60.

Mero, A., Häkkinen, K. & Kauhanen, H. (1989) Hormonal profile and strength development in young weight lifters. *J. Hum. Move. Studies* **16**, 255–66.

Murray, D.A. & Harrison, E. (1986) Constant velocity dynamometer: an appraisal using mechanical loading. *Med. Sci. Sports Exerc.* **6**, 612–24.

Nielsen, B., Nielsen, K., Behrendt Hansen, M. & Asmussen, E. (1980) Training of 'functional muscle strength' in girls 7–19 years old. In K. Berg & B.O. Eriksson (eds) *Children and Exercise*, Vol. IX, pp. 69–78. University Park Press, Baltimore.

Pérès, G., Vandewalle, H. & Monod, H. (1981) Aspect particulier de la relation charge-vitesse lors du pédalage sur cycloergomètre (Particular aspect of the load–velocity relationship during pedalling on the cycle ergometer). *J. Physiol.* (Paris) **77**, 10A (abstract).

Safrit, M.J. (1990) *Introduction to Measurement in Physical Education and Exercise Science.* Times Mirror/Mosby, St Louis.

Saltin, B. (1990) Anaerobic capacity: past, present, and prospective. In A.W. Taylor, P.D. Gollnick, H.J. Green *et al.* (eds) *Biochemistry of Exercise*, Vol. VII, pp. 387–412. Human Kinetics, Champaign, IL.

Saltin, B., Gollnick, P.D., Eriksson, B.O. & Piehl, K. (1971) Metabolic and circulatory adjustments at onset of work. In A. Gilbert & P. Guille (eds) *Proceedings from Meeting on Physiological Changes at Onset of Work*, pp. 46–58. Toulouse, France.

Sargeant, A.J. (1989) Short-term muscle power in children and adolescents. In O. Bar-Or (ed.) *Advances in Pediatric Sports Sciences*, Vol. 3. *Biological Issues*, pp. 41–63. Human Kinetics, Champaign, IL.

Sargeant, A.J. (1992) Problems in, and approaches to, the measurement of short term power output in children and adolescents. In J. Coudert & E. Van Praagh (eds) *Pediatric Work Physiology*, Vol. XVI *Children and Exercise*, pp. 11–17. Masson, Paris.

Sergeant, A.J. & Dolan, P. (1986) Optimal velocity of muscle contraction for short-term power output in children and adults. In J. Rutenfranz, R. Mocellin & F. Klimt (eds) *Children and Exercise*, Vol. XII, pp. 39–42. Human Kinetics, Champaign, IL.

Sargeant, A.J., Dolan, P. & Thorne, A. (1984) Isokinetic measurement of maximal leg force and anaerobic power output in children. In. J. Ilmarinen & I. Välimäki (eds) *Children and Sport*, pp. 93–8. Springer-Verlag, Berlin.

Sargeant, A.J., Hoinville, E. & Young, A. (1981) Maximum leg force and power output during short-term dynamic exercise. *J. Appl. Physiol.* **51**, 1175–82.

Sargent, D.A. (1921) The physical test of a man. *Am. Phys. Educ. Rev.* **26**, 188–94.

Tharpe, G.D., Johnson, G.O. & Thorland, W.G. (1984) Measurement of anaerobic power and capacity in élite young track athletes using the Wingate test. *J. Sports Med.* **24**, 100–6.

van Mil, G.A.H., Schoeber, N., Calvert, R. & Bar-Or O. (in press) Optimization of braking force in the Wingate test for children and adolescents with a neuromuscular disease. *Med. Sci. Sports Exerc.* (in press).

Van Praagh, E., Falgairette, G., Bedu, M., Fellmann, N. & Coudert, J. (1989) Laboratory and field tests in 7-year-old boys. In S. Oseid & K-H. Carlsen (eds) *Children and Exercise*, Vol. XIII, pp. 11–17. Human Kinetics, Champaign, IL.

Van Praagh, E., Bedu, M., Falgairette, G., Fellmann, N. & Coudert, J. (1991) Oxygen uptake during a 30-s supramaximal exercise in 7 to 15 year old boys. In R. Frenkl & I. Szmodis (eds) *Children and Exercise*, Vol. XV, pp. 281–7. Nevi, Budapest.

Van Praagh, E., Bedu, M., Roddier, P. & Coudert, J. (1992) A simple calibration method for mechanically braked cycle ergometers. *Int. J. Sports Med.* **13**, 27–30.

Van Praagh, E., Fargeas, M.A., Léger, L., Fellmann, N. & Coudert, J. (1993) Short-term power output in children measured on a computerized treadmill ergometer. *Pediatr. Exerc. Sci.* **5**, 482 (abstract).

Van Praagh, E., Fellmann, N., Bedu, M., Falgairette, G. & Coudert, J. (1990) Gender difference in the relationship of anaerobic power output to body composition in children. *Pediatr. Exerc. Sci.* **2**, 336–48.

Vandewalle, H., Pérès, G., Heller, J. & Monod, H. (1985) All out anaerobic capacity test on cycle ergometers. *Eur. J. Appl. Physiol.* **54**, 222–9.

Vandewalle, H., Pérès, G., Heller, J. & Monod, H. (1987) Standard anaerobic exercise tests. *Sports Med. N. Zeal.* **4**, 268–89.

Weltman, A., Janney, C., Rians, C.B. *et al.* (1986) The effects of hydraulic resistance strength training in pre-pubertal males. *Med. Sci. Sports Exerc.* **18**, 629–38.

Wilkie, D.R. (1960) Man as a source of mechanical power. *Ergonomics* **3**, 1–8.

Chapter 37

Longitudinal Studies during Growth and Training: Importance and Principles

HAN C.G. KEMPER

Introduction

Individual changes in growth, development and fitness can only be studied if the same individuals are measured repeatedly over a period of time. This is called a longitudinal study. Two types of longitudinal research can be distinguished:

1 In the non-interventive research, early characteristics are noted and changes over time analysed on individual basis. Most of this prospective longitudinal research is descriptive and from such non-interventive research there can be no attempt made to establish causal relationships (Mednick & Baert, 1981).

2 If one is interested in the effects of a training programme on sporting youth, one has to take on longitudinal research with an interventive nature. This is called manipulative or experimental longitudinal research. Assuming that proper controls (e.g. no training) and research designs are used, certain causal statements can be made concerning the conclusions of such research.

The great need for experimental longitudinal research in the child and adolescent athlete is because:

1 Children and adolescents are in a phase of continuous growth and development. Their morphological, physiological and psychological characteristics keep changing over the years and these changes are similar to training effects. For example, during growth and maturation children increase their muscle force, aerobic power and motor coordination. Without control groups of children who do not train, the effects of sport cannot be evaluated.

2 Non-interventive comparisons of children who train against those who do not train cannot discern the effects of sports training over a period of time. Self-selection is a serious problem in comparing sporting with non-sporting groups. It can be assumed that the sporting children are different from the non-sporting group because they are genetically better suited for sport performances than their non-sporting counterparts.

So, only an interventive longitudinal study in which the experimental and control group are randomly chosen and are compared over a period of time can give solid conclusions about the effects of participation in sport and training in growing youth. In this chapter the importance of longitudinal training studies will be discussed including the disadvantages of longitudinal designs such as testing and drop-out effects. Moreover, a review will be given of longitudinal studies in children and adolescents in which the effects of physical activity, sports participation and training are evaluated.

Due to the lack of studies in which girls have been tested using true experimental designs, this type of experiment needs further research with regard to gender.

Longitudinal studies

In the literature there is a large number of

studies which evaluate the effects of sports training on youngsters by measuring at one point in time one or more performance characteristics in a physically active or sporting group and comparing the outcomes with a comparable non-physically active or non-sport group. The differences have been attributed to the different physical activity or sport pattern in both groups. However, this cross-sectional design is seriously invalidated by numerous confounding effects (Cook & Campbell, 1979). Because only group comparisons can be made at one point of time, it is not possible to evaluate individual changes over time.

Practical problems

The most common practical problems are as follows.

1 Long-term financial commitment. The period of repeated (e.g. annual) measurements must be preceded by an expensive training period for the staff. All the investigators must be hired before the start of the first measurements. Because there is no loss of subjects in the initial stage, there is a high cost of staff commitment.

2 Long-term commitment of staff members and subjects. The longer the duration of the study, the more chance there is that a large percentage of individuals will drop out, and if this drop out is selective the population will no longer be representative. The same holds true when staff members leave and new investigators join the study. This may cause a test leader bias. Sometimes the original purposes of the longitudinal research are modified by new ideas and interests.

3 Techniques that become obsolete. Although measures and techniques are thoroughly investigated at the start, they may be out of date several years later. Apparatus can fail over the years and new apparatus with other specifications can seriously disturb the individual curves. Likewise, new techniques that appear later cannot be included in the follow-up. It is also advisable to record the raw data rather then complex derivatives. Any new techniques

of analysis and changes of interest during the project can be used on these raw data afterwards.

4 Adherence of subjects. To recruit subjects for repeated measurements over a longer period is a serious problem. During the first measurements all subjects are curious and eager to participate. Keeping their interest in the following years is a major challenge. Therefore the subjects have to be informed and stimulated by special measures, that are extrinsic to the research such as information sessions, general explanatory texts, personal reports with update of their own result and in the case of children, gifts (photographs, T-shirts, etc.).

5 Final analysis and publication. Only when the final measurements are completed can analysis begin and results published. The database will be large and the longitudinal analyses complicated, taking up considerable time and money.

6 The importance of the final stage in a longitudinal study cannot be underestimated. It therefore needs to be thoroughly planned.

Individual changes

During youth children and adolescents grow and develop to maturity at different paces. Children who grow fast and reach full maturity at an early chronological age are called early maturers in contrast with late maturers, who reach full maturity at a later chronological age. Both types of subjects are involved in longitudinal studies. Grouped data of children of the same chronological age are composed of a mixture of subjects with different states of biological maturation. The effects of a training or sport programme may be different depending on the state of maturation (Vrijens, 1978).

Moreover, changes that are related to biological development can be measured. In growth studies height and weight are measured with intervals of 2–6 months in order to calculate their velocities (i.e. change over time) (for example height velocity in cm · year^{-1}). These velocities can be used as indicators for the biological age of the growing child. During puberty an increase in height occurs in both boys and girls and the peak height velocity (PHV) correlates well with other parameters of biological maturation such as sexual maturation, menarche and breast development in girls, and penis or testis development in boys. This is the case in both sexes with axillary and pubic hair development (Falkner & Tanner, 1978).

Using longitudinal data, the changes in dependent variables such as aerobic power or muscle power can be related not only to chronological age but also to other age scales that may be more relevant to the effects of physical activity on the human body. In the literature, age relative to PHV and skeletal age (Kemper, 1985) are used. Beunen and Malina (1988) also used different functional parameters such as peak muscle force velocity as age-related parameters (see Chapter 1 for details).

In Fig. 37.1 12-min endurance run performances are related both to skeletal age and chronological age of a group of boys and girls. In Fig. 37.2 maximal arm pull muscle force is related to PHV-age and to chronological age in the same group of boys and girls as in Fig. 37.1.

Principles of longitudinal designs

In almost every study of growth, development and training confounding effects will occur, no matter which design has been used. Three classical designs have been most in use: (i) the cross-sectional design; (ii) the time-lag design; and (iii) the longitudinal design (Fig. 37.3). Each measurement taken on a subject at a particular point of time is influenced by three factors:

1 Chronological age of the subject, defined as the period which elapses between birth and time of measurement. Age effects produce the mean growth curve.

2 Birth cohort to which the subject belongs. This is defined as the group of individuals born in the same year. Cohort effects can be used to study secular trends.

3 Time of measurement, i.e. the moment at which the measurement is taken. Time of measurement effects are related to changes in environmental conditions that can occur over a period of time (such as changes in the methods of measuring in circumstances).

The three different designs are characterized in the following ways. In a cross-sectional study

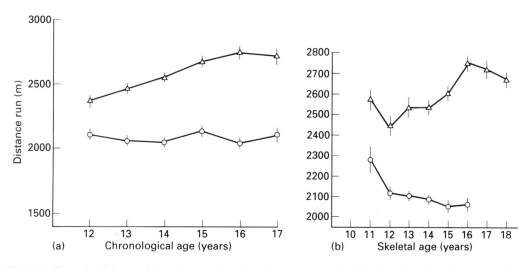

Fig. 37.1 Example of the aerobic endurance (12-min endurance run test) related to chronological age (a) and skeletal age (b). △, males; ○, females. Redrawn with permission from Kemper (1985).

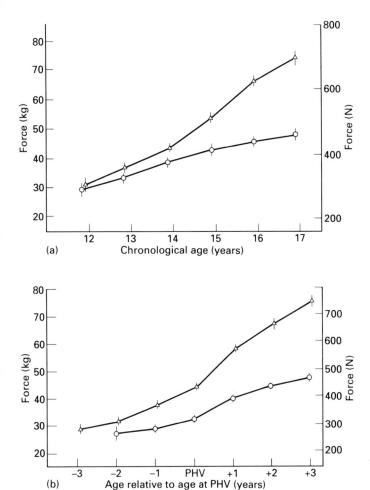

(a)
Chronological age (years)

(b)
Age relative to age at PHV (years)

Fig. 37.2 Example of static arm strength (arm pull test) related to chronological age (a) and peak height velocity (PHV) age (b). Redrawn with permission from Kemper (1985).

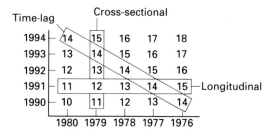

Fig. 37.3 Graphical representation of the three classical research designs: cross-sectional, time-lag and longitudinal.

the time of measurement is kept constant (cohort and age being varied), i.e. different groups are measured at the same point of time (the vertical bar in Fig. 37.3). Conversely, in a time-lag study different groups of the same age are measured at different points of time, thus age is kept constant (cohort and time of measurement being varied) (the diagonal bar in Fig. 37.3). In a longitudinal study information is gathered from one cohort at different moments, thus at different ages. Since the cohort is kept constant (age and time of measurement being varied) the same group is measured repeatedly (the horizontal bar in Fig. 37.3). None of these designs allows all three effects (age, time of measurement and cohort) to be isolated (Schaie, 1965).

Multiple longitudinal design

In the literature descriptions can be found of several designs which try to overcome the confounding effects (Tanner, 1962; Rao & Rao, 1966; Kowalski & Prahl-Andersen, 1979). The 'multiple longitudinal' design uses repeated measurements on more than one cohort (Kemper & Van 't Hof, 1978), with overlapping ages during the study. This has the advantage of isolating the main effect, e.g. the age effect, from interfering effects such as time of measurement and cohort.

In Fig. 37.4 an example is given of a multiple longitudinal design using three birth cohorts (1980, 1981 and 1982) that will be measured during four consecutive years (1993–1996). Because there is an overlap in age, the cohorts can be compared with each other at different ages (horizontal comparisons in Fig. 37.4). A systematic difference between the cohorts at these ages is called a 'cohort effect'. At the same time, it is possible to distinguish another con-

founding factor in a longitudinal study, namely the factor of time of measurement (Veling & Van 't Hof, 1980). If there are no cohort effects, the time of measurement is blamed for a possible difference between the two groups. If it appears that there is no time of measurement effect and no cohort effect either, then the data of all cohorts at all points of time can be arranged in age groups and a real developmental pattern can be discerned (Bell, 1954).

This pattern is illustrated in Fig. 37.5 with a data set from the Amsterdam Growth and Health Study. In this multiple longitudinal study three birth cohorts (1962, 1963 and 1964) are used to measure $\dot{V}o_{2\,max}$ five times. Due to the overlap in age groups at the age of 13, 14, 15 and 16 the mean values of the cohorts can be combined (if there are no significant cohort effects) to construct the mean age curve. Another advantage of a multiple design is that in four yearly measurement periods a 5-year developmental pattern can be estimated (in Fig. 37.5: from 12 to 17 years).

Testing or learning effects

Another problem with repeated measurements is a testing or learning effect. Many variables, physical as well as psychological, require a certain motivation or habituation of the subject while being measured. This introduces differences between periods of measurement that are solely due to the changes in attitude towards the measurement procedure itself. Such testing effects may be positive (i.e. when habituation or learning is important) or negative (i.e. when motivation decreases). Physical performance tests, where maximal motivation is needed, are particularly threatened by these effects. Repeated measurements may therefore have a disturbing influence on the quantity measured and diminish the external validity of the results.

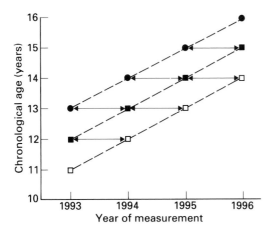

Fig. 37.4 Example of a multiple longitudinal design with three birth cohorts (□, 1982; ■, 1981; ●, 1980) that will be measured in 4 consecutive years (1993, 1994, 1995 and 1996). Horizontal arrows indicate possible comparisons of different cohorts of the same age groups at different times of measurement.

Systematic testing effects can be estimated if the design also includes a control group in which repeated measurements are not made. Cross-sectional data gathered from an identical population can be compared with those of the

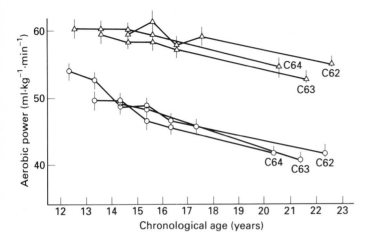

Fig. 37.5 Mean and SE of maximal aerobic power, measured in the Amsterdam growth and health study in males ($\triangle$) and females ($\circ$) from three birth cohorts (C62, C63 and C64).

longitudinally measured population, except that they were not repeated measurements but derived from independent samples. In this design, when comparing data from both populations, systematic divergence of mean values in the course of the study is an indication of testing effect (Fig. 37.6).

Cohort effect, as well as time of measurement and testing effects, if established for a certain characteristic, will seriously hinder the interpretation of individual and mean growth curves. If neither cohort, time of measurement nor testing effects can be found, the data of the different cohorts can simply be averaged and arranged in age groups to study the overall changes.

Longitudinal studies in growth, development and physical fitness

In *A History of the Study of Human Growth*, Tanner (1981) reviewed the well-established growth studies since 1900. This section will focus on longitudinal studies in children and adolescents that include physical performance and fitness measurements over a period of more than 3 years.

Most of the major growth studies in the USA (e.g. the Harvard, Fels and Denver studies) and in Europe [e.g. Harpenden study (Tanner *et al.*, 1976) and several studies coordinated by the International Children's Centre (ICC)] are not reviewed because they did not include physical

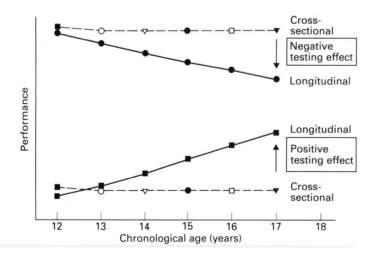

Fig. 37.6 Negative and/or positive testing effects can be studied by comparing cross-sectional data with longitudinal data: the same symbols represent mean values of same subjects, different symbols represent the mean of different subjects.

performance measurements and/or a physical activity component. In this chapter the studies are divided into five periods, each period summarized in a table with the most important figures of each study (Kemper, 1988). In order to facilitate comparison between the studies, we arranged all possible measurements into six categories:

1 Anthropometric (height, weight, circumferences, skinfolds and breadth).
2 Maturation (i.e. skeletal age, sexual development, age relative to PHV).
3 Physical performances [i.e. speed, strength, aerobic power ($\dot{V}o_{2\,max}$), anaerobic power, endurance, flexibility and balance].
4 Psychosocial and/or mental tests.
5 Physical activity pattern.
6 Nutritional habits.

The last two categories of measurement are important aspects concerning the influence of lifestyle on growth, development and physical fitness.

First longitudinal approaches: USA 1920–40
(Table 37.1)

The first longitudinal approaches to growth studies were initiated in the USA by Baldwin (1921) who designed a mixed longitudinal study. This means that in the course of the study new subjects were recruited periodically and subsequently followed. He introduced a method of measuring standing height with a wall meter and initiated the measurement of height, weight, width, circumferences, vital capacity and strength in Iowa children. After his death the work was continued by McCloy (1936) who introduced the first skinfold measurements and Meredith (1935) who is well known for introducing accurate measurement procedures into anthropometrics.

The Berkeley growth study began in 1928 at the Institute of Child Welfare and was the first growth study at the University of California. Bayley (1940) started with 31 boys and 30 girls recruited at birth from two Berkeley hospitals. Nearly 70% of them were followed successfully until maturity. This is a high percentage over a period of 18 years. Data were collected on physical and intellectual development. Photographs and radiographs of the hand and wrist were taken as a measure of a skeletal maturation.

The adolescent growth study at the University of California, started in 1932 with 120 boys and girls, ended 7 years later with 60 subjects of each sex. This study is important for its orientation towards physiological changes at puberty. Blood pressure, basal oxygen consumption, heart rate and strength (Jones, 1949) as well as skeletal maturation were measured at 6-month intervals. The results of motor performance tests on the same children were reported by Espenschade (1947). This growth study demonstrated for the first time that there was no pubertal period during which strength or motor performance declined.

Second period: Europe, 1940 to present
(Table 37.2)

Before 1940 the important longitudinal studies came predominantly from North America. After 1940 the European countries dominated in this field of growth research. Coordinated by the ICC, a group of representatives from different European research centres formulated a common baseline for measures, sampling procedures and design in longitudinal studies on child growth (Falkner, 1954).

The first two ICC growth studies were initiated by Moncrieff and Debré in Paris, who agreed that exactly the same somatic and psychological methods should be used in the same cohorts of their London (Moore et al., 1954) and Paris growth studies (Falkner, 1954). Other international child health centres showed an interest in coordinated longitudinal growth study research and soon the ICC studies were extended with growth studies in Stockholm/Götheborg by Wallgren, in Zürich by Franconi, in Brussels by Graffar and Courbier (1966) and also some workers from outside Europe joined the group (from Dakar, Kampala and Louisville). An overview of 25 years of internationally

Table 37.1 Longitudinal approaches in the USA between 1920 and 1940 (first period).

Name of the study, institute, country	Founder and period	Number of children		Sex	Age (years)	Design	Anthropometrics	Maturation	Nutrition	Activity	Physical performance	Psychosocial/mental
		Start	End									
Iowa growth studies, USA	Baldwin, McCloy and Mereclith 1920s	?	?	M, F	0–25	Mixed Longit.	+					+
Berkeley growth study, University of California, USA	Bayley, 1928–1940	30 31	47	M, F	0–20	Longit.	+	+			+	+
Adolescent growth study, University of California, USA	Stolz, 1932–1939	120 120	60 60	F M	11–18	Longit.	+	+			+	+

F, female; M, male.

Table 37.2 Longitudinal approaches in Europe between 1940 and present (second period).

Name of the study, institute, country	Founder and period	Number of children		Sex	Age (years)	Design	Anthropometrics	Maturation	Nutrition	Activity	Physical performance	Psychosocial/mental
		Start	End									
ICC, Paris Study, Centre International de l'Enfance, Paris, France	Debré, 1953–1975	237 260	18 25	F M	0–18	Longit.	+	+	+		+	+
ICC, Stockholm/Götheborg Study, University of Götheborg, Sweden	Wallgren, 1955–?	90 122	74 100	F M	0–18	Longit.	+	+	+		+	+

F, female; M, male.

coordinated research was published containing a selection of the teams, their present status and a bibliography (Falkner, 1980).

In all ICC studies the investigations began with 3-month measurements in the first year after birth. During the second year there were 6-month measurements. The measurements were continued thereafter at yearly intervals until maturity. In the Zürich study 6-month intervals were used during puberty (Largo et al., 1978). The baseline anthropometric measurements and radiographs of the hand and wrist were based on the Harpenden growth study techniques. Only the Paris and Stockholm/Götheborg studies added activity histories and physical fitness measurements and are therefore included in Table 37.2. Sample sizes differed quite considerably from one centre to another, the smallest sample being the Stockholm/Götheborg study with 90 girls and 122 boys (Karlberg et al., 1976) and the largest in the Paris study with 237 girls and 260 boys (Roy-Pernot et al., 1976). However, the selective drop-out from the original samples was considerable, particularly in the Paris study: out of 497 babies, only 43 remained in the study until the age of 18.

Third period: North America and Europe
(Table 37.3)

The initial objective for the Medford boys growth study was to investigate whether training practices pertaining to interschool competitive athletics among elementary schoolboys were harmful to the physical and emotional welfare of the participants. In this North American mixed longitudinal growth study annual testing of strength and motor performances was conducted for 12 years from 1956 to 1968 (Clarke, 1971), starting with children aged 7, 9, 12 and 15 years. The same boys were tested annually within 2 months of their birthdays until the age of 18.

The Prague growth study (Parízková, 1974; Sprynarova, 1974) was initiated in 1961. 143 boys with complete data were subdivided into two activity groups according to overall time spent on physical activity. Inspired by the World Health Organization Lange Andersen, Seliger and Rutenfranz coordinated during the 1970s a longitudinal study of children in Norway and the former German Federal Republic. Two small rural communities were chosen (Lom and Fredeburg). The children were followed from the age of 8 to 16. Measurements included $\dot{V}O_{2\,max}$ (Lange Andersen et al., 1974c), heart rate and oxygen pulse during submaximal and maximal exercise (Lange Andersen et al., 1974a), respiratory response (Lange Andersen et al., 1974b) and influence of physical education (Lange Andersen et al., 1976).

In former Czechoslovakia (Bratislava) Placheta (1980) performed a complex 3-year longitudinal examination of several groups of boys aged 12−15 years who were skilled at different motor activities including cyclists, rowers and ice-hockey players, plus a control group. To assess the influence of motor activity on development, the state of health, physique, physical fitness, blood chemistry and lung functions were measured.

The Canadian stream (Table 37.4)

The Saskatchewan Growth and Development Study (Bailey, 1968), began in 1964 with a group of 7-year-old boys. In 1965 7-year-old girls were added with the objective of following both groups for a period of 15 years. However, after 10 years of data collection for the boys, and 9 years for the girls, financial support was withdrawn. Although preliminary results in boys have been published (Carron & Bailey 1974; Mirwald, 1980) a considerable amount of data remained unanalysed. This study and the one in Prague were the first to produce longitudinal data on the maximal oxygen uptake of the same subjects over a considerable period of time.

Cunningham et al. (1977, 1981) completed a 5-year longitudinal study on 81 boys recruited from participants in organized ice hockey (aged 10−15 years). This study included yearly tests

Table 37.3 Third period with longitudinal studies in North America and Europe.

Name of the study, institute, country	Founder and period	Number of children Start	Number of children End	Sex	Age (years)	Design	Anthropometrics	Maturation	Nutrition	Activity	Physical performance	Psychosocial/mental
Medford boys growth study, University of Oregon, USA	Clarke, 1956–1968	109	42	M	7–9/12–18	Mixed, longit.	+	+			+	+
Prague growth study, Charles University Prague, CSSR	Pařízková, 1961–1968	139	39	M	11–18	Longit.	+	+		+		
Two-countries study, Norway and Former Federal Republic of Germany	Lange Andersen, Rutenfranz and Seliger, 1969–1978	30	–	M	8–16	Longit.	+			+	+	
Youth and physical activity, Purkyne University, Brno, CSSR	Placheta, 1972–1975	127	103	M	12–15	Longit.	+	+	+	+	+	+

Table 37.4 A Canadian stream: three longitudinal studies.

Name of the study, institute, country	Founder and period	Number of children Start	Number of children End	Sex	Age (years)	Design	Anthropometrics	Maturation	Nutrition	Activity	Physical performance	Psychosocial/mental
Saskatchewan growth and development study, University of Saskatchewan, Saskatoon	Bailey, 1964–1973	207 / ?	131 / ?	M / F	7–16 / 7–15	Longit.	+	+		+	+	+
Canada growth and development study, University of Western Ontario, Canada	Cunningham, 1975–1979	?	181	M	10–15	Longit.	+	+		+	+	+
Trois Rivières regional study, University of Québec, Canada	Lavallée, 1969–1977	546	400	M, F	6–12	Mixed, longit.	+			+	+	

F, female; M, male.

of maximal oxygen uptake on a treadmill. Maturation level was determined by a hand–wrist X-ray at age 10 and 14. The intent of the Canadian longitudinal study in the Trois Rivères region (Jécquier et al., 1977) was not only to measure the physical and psychological development of French Canadian schoolchildren, but also to study the effect of additional physical education upon their development between the ages of 5 and 12 (the usual one lesson per week was changed to five). Over the 8 years of annual observation, almost 30% of the original sample was lost to the study. In the presence of many interfering factors such as experimental versus control groups, urban versus rural localities, it was not easy to evaluate the research hypotheses in this study (Shephard et al., 1980).

Benelux studies (Table 37.5)

The Leuven growth study of Belgian boys was designed to provide information on the physical fitness of normal boys from 12 to 20 years of age. In the Leuven study, children from entire classes of 59 schools were measured at yearly intervals at the same time of the year. Due to the design of the study it is understandable that from the original sample of 4278 boys observed for the first time in 1969 only 587 were followed throughout the 6-year period (Ostyn et al., 1980). In 1990 results were also published on the fitness of girls, but this was a cross-sectional design (Simons et al., 1990).

A second Leuven study was initiated in 1969 – the Leuven longitudinal experimental growth study. This multidisciplinary study included children from 3 to 15 years of age (Hebbelinck et al., 1980). The Nijmegen growth study of the Netherlands was a large-scale interdisciplinary study, which has been limited to the 4–14 year age range. By stopping at 14 years of age, some valuable information was undoubtedly missed concerning the developmental processes of boys and girls during puberty (Prahl-Andersen et al., 1979).

While the ICC studies and most of the North American studies used one single longitudinal cohort (except the Medford study), and the Harpenden, Leuven and Trois Rivières studies used mixed longitudinal designs, the Nijmegen study used a multiple longitudinal design. This design is a sophisticated compromise between the more traditional approaches to the study of development, namely cross-sectional, longitudinal and time-lag designs, described above. The Amsterdam growth and health study is also a multiple longitudinal study. It started with three birth cohorts of boys and girls (from the first and second forms of a secondary school) in 1977 who were followed for 4 years (between 12 and 17 years of age) and measured again in 1985 (22–22 years of age) and 1991 (26–28 years of age), covering an age range of almost 15 years.

Most of the reviewed longitudinal studies are only descriptive and of a non-interventive type. A step further in the development of knowledge about training effects is to set up more experimental research; interventive longitudinal studies can be useful in revealing the influence of different types of training upon the health and performance of young people.

Longitudinal training studies in the child and adolescent

Longitudinal studies in children that aim to analyse the effects of training can be divided in two major types. In the first type, children are followed over a period of time. During that period some remain or become more physically active (called athletes) and the others remain or become inactive (called non-athletes). At the end of the study based on a retrospective determination, subgroups are made of children with differences in the observed or measured levels of physical activity. Children that showed a relatively high level of activity during the observation period are contrasted with children of the same sex, age and other relevant characteristics that showed a relatively low level of activity, during the same observation period. In four of the afore-mentioned studies (the

Table 37.5 Studies from Benelux (Belgium, the Netherlands and Luxembourg).

Name of the study, institute, country	Founder and period	Number of children Start	End	Sex	Age (years)	Design	Anthropometrics	Maturation	Nutrition	Activity	Physical performance	Psychosocial/mental
Leuven boys growth study, University of Leuven, Belgium	Simons, 1969–1974	4278	587	M	12–20	Mixed, longit.	+	+		+	+	+
Leuven longitudinal experimental growth study, Free University of Brussels, Belgium	Hebbelinck, 1969–1982	255 270	– –	F M	3–15	Longit.	+	+		+	+	+
Nijmegen Growth Study, University of Nijmegen, the Netherlands	van der Linden, 1970–1976	254 232	187 151	F M	4–14	Mult. longit.	+	+			+	+
Amsterdam growth and health study, the Netherlands	Kemper 1976–1991	159 148	100 82	F M	13–28	Mult. Longit.	+	+	+	+	+	+

F, female; M, male.

Saskatchewan growth and development study, Prague growth study, youth and physical activity Bratislava and Amsterdam growth health and fitness) the following tracking procedure was taken: subjects were divided into high activity (athletes) and low activity (non-athletes) groups as relative high active (athletes) and relative low active (non-athletes) on the base of their longitudinally collected data. In all these comparisons active children demonstrated higher physiological characteristics than the less active children. However, these results are not conclusive about the effects of physical activity: because the children made their own decisions about being active or not, self-selection may have influenced the results. Kemper *et al.* (1986) showed for example that the aerobic power of adolescent boys and girls is significantly higher in the active ones but the differences remain the same between 12 and 18 year olds as should be expected as a result of higher training stimuli throughout the years. Therefore the author concluded that the differences in $\dot{V}_{O_2\,max}$ were not only caused by training but also by heredity: active adolescents are more active because they have a higher aerobic power at their disposal.

The second type of training studies utilizes the school environment: a change is initiated in the school curriculum by adding physical education (PE) lessons as extra or as a replacement for other school subjects. Comparisons are made before and after the change with control classes that did not have curriculum modifications. Kemper (1976) reviewed these and found in general no effects in physical fitness before puberty. The main reasons are:

1 High training status of prepubertal children.

2 Low intensity of PE classes.

3 Small number of extra PE lessons.

4 Non-homogeneity of maturation between subjects.

5 Low specificity of training stimulus: most of the PE lessons are devoted to motor coordination improvement and less to endurance and resistance training.

This is reflected by the fact that in most of the studies motor coordination increased significantly in the experimental groups compared to control groups but not $\dot{V}_{O_2\,max}$ and maximal muscle force (F_{max}).

The only long-term intervention study (6 years) is the Trois Rivières regional study in Canada (Shephard, 1982): children enrolled in the experimental programme received five 40-min PE lessons per week integrated into the normal primary school curriculum. Control subjects received the usual one lesson of PE per week. This experiment followed boys and girls from 6 to 12 years of age. $\dot{V}_{O_2\,max}$ and other physical fitness characteristics increased significantly more in the experimental classes than in the control classes in the last 3 years, from age 8 to 11 years.

Aerobic training

Several critical reviews have been written about aerobic training effects in children. Sady (1986) reviewed more than 20 training studies. Only those studies were selected that made use of comparable control groups of children who were not trained. The increse in $\dot{V}_{O_2\,max} \cdot kg^{-1}$ body weight appears to vary considerably and there seem to be no differences in trainability between pubescent and postpubescent children. In Fig. 37.7 the per cent increase of $\dot{V}_{O_2\,max} \cdot kg^{-1}$ body weight in the training group with respect to the increase in the control group is plotted for 27 studies against the duration of the aerobic training period: short term (≤ 6 months) and long term (> 6 months) were distinguished. The results show that in training studies with a duration between 4 and 15 weeks, effects vary between -2% (in two studies detraining was measured) and $+20\%$ of baseline $\dot{V}_{O_2\,max} \cdot kg^{-1}$ body weight. In training studies with a duration between 0.5 and 5 years the effects vary from -10 to $+10\%$ of baseline $\dot{V}_{O_2\,max} \cdot kg^{-1}$ body weight.

Rowland (1985) stated that, when training programmes in children are examined, those regimens failing to demonstrate a beneficial effect on aerobic fitness, also do not comply

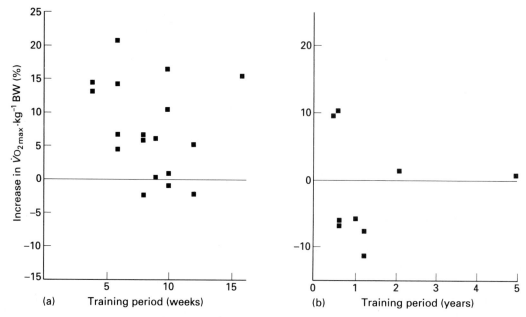

Fig. 37.7 Percentage increase of $\dot{V}_{O_2\,max} \cdot kg^{-1}$ body weight (BW) in training group with respect to control group of 27 training studies of different duration ranging from 4 weeks to 5 years. (a) Short-term training ($\leqslant 6$ months) and (b) long-term training (> 6 months).

with adult standards formulated by the American College of Sports Medicine (1990). Pate and Ward (1990) also concluded from 14 well-designed studies that both pre- and post-pubertal children are physiologically adaptive to endurance exercise training as demonstrated by statistically significant increases in $\dot{V}_{O_2\,max}$ body weight in the training groups compared to the non-training groups. Although it is possible that a critical age exists before which the child is less trainable (before PHV-age) (Kobayashi *et al.*, 1978; Mirwald & Bailey, 1985) other authors (Weber *et al.*, 1976; Cunningham *et al.*, 1984; Froberg *et al.*, 1991) cast considerable doubt on the hypothesis that greater training effects may be gained by exercise training during PHV-age. Vaccaro and Mahon (1987) stated that the critical stage of maturity during which endurance training has its greatest influence on the cardiorespiratory system is still speculative. The degree of trainability seems to be dependent on (i) motivation (pre-pubescents are less trainable); and (ii) from

pretraining levels (children can be very active even when not taking part in programmed sports training). Although in some studies no training effect or even a negative effect was shown in $\dot{V}_{O_2\,max} \cdot kg^{-1}$ body weight (Fig. 37.7) performance measures such as running time are always improved. Possible explanations for this apparent discrepancy are that training induces a higher mechanical efficiency and that $\dot{V}_{O_2\,max}$ does not reflect well the $\dot{V}_{O_2\,max}$ of children (Bar-Or, 1989).

Strength training

Fewer studies have been performed on the effect of strength training than on aerobic training in children. While some authors have reported a small degree of trainability before puberty (Vrijens, 1978), more recent studies (Weltman, 1984) demonstrated a significant increase in 6–11-year-old boys following a period of strength training. The discrepancy can be explained by the way the strength effects

were evaluated: Vrijens used non-specific testing by training with dynamic exercises and
testing the effects isometrically. In contrast,
Weltman trained and tested the effects iso-
kinetically. The results of Weltman and of others
(Sewall & Micheli, 1986; Pfeiffer & Francis,
1986) confirm that increases in muscle strength
are possible before puberty in boys and girls
and are not related to spelling or maturity
levels. Such increases are reached without the
risk of musculoskeletal injuries. It has been
recommended that strength training be used
for prepubescent children only (i) when it is
indicated for well-defined athletic or rehabilitation purposes (Bar-Or, 1989); (ii) under the
supervision of qualified instructors; and (iii)
using loads that can be repeated more than
seven to 10 times.

Anaerobic muscle performances, such as the
Margaria stair-running test (Margaria *et al.*,
1966) and the Wingate 30-cycle test (Bar-Or,
1987) can also be improved during childhood
and adolescence regardless of maturation level.

Challenges for future research

Longitudinal research covering the whole
period of puberty is relatively scarce. Therefore,
in early or late maturing children it is not
always possible to detect PHV, which is a
yardstick of pubertal maturation. Comparison
of the different longitudinal studies stresses
the need for further standardization in sampling
procedures, frequency of measurements and
measurement methods.

Most of the growth and training studies have
used boys as subjects. Longitudinal growth
and training studies have to be designed in
which both sexes are included. Much knowledge is still lacking about the trainability of
children. To achieve a better understanding of
trainability during growth and development
the following research questions need to be
resolved.
- What are the best guidelines for adequate
training stimuli in boys and girls?
- What is the impact of biological age on the

training effects and is there any biological age
where trainability is minimal or maximal?
- To what extent do aerobic power, anaerobic
power and strength track into adulthood?
- Will adequate training started in early
childhood lead to higher performance levels in
adulthood?
- Will intensive training during childhood and
adolescence have detrimental effects on health?

References

American College of Sports Medicine (1990) The
recommended quantity and quality of exercise for
developing and maintaining cardiorespiratory fitness and muscular fitness in healthy adults. *Med.
Sci. Sports Exerc.* **22**, 265–74.

Bailey, D.A. (1968) *Saskatchewan Growth and Development Study*. Report of the College of Physical
Education. University of Saskatchewan, Canada.

Baldwin, B.T. (1921) *The Physical Growth of Children
from Birth to Maturity*. University of Iowa Studies
in Child Welfare, Vol. 1, No. 1. University of Iowa,
Iowa.

Bar-Or, O. (1989) Trainability of the prepubescent
child. *Phys. Sports Med.* **17**(5), 65–82.

Bar-Or, O. (1987) The Wingate anaerobic test. An
update on methodology, reliability an validity.
Sports Med. **4**, 381–94.

Bar-Or, O. (1989) Trainability of the prepubescent
child. *Phys. Sports Med.* **17**(5), 65–82.

Bayley, N. (1940) *Studies in the Development of Young
Children*. University of California Press, Berkeley.

Bell, R.Q. (1954) An experimental test of the accelerated longitudinal approach. *Child Dev.* **25**, 281–6.

Beunen, G. & Malina, B. (1988) Growth an physical
performance relative to the timing of the adolescent
growth sport. *Exerc. Sport Sci. Rev.* **16**, 503–41.

Carron, A.V. & Bailey, D.A. (1974) Strength development in boys from 10 through 16 years. *Monogr.
Soc. Res. Child Dev.* **39** (Serial No. 157), 4.

Clarke, H.H. (1971) *Physical and Motor Tests in
the Medford Boys' Growth Study*. Prentice Hall,
Englewood Cliffs, NJ.

Cook, T.H. & Campbell, D.T. (1979) *Quasi Experimen-
tation*. Rand McNally, Chicago.

Cunningham, D.A., Paterson, D.H. & Blimkie, C.J.R.
(1984) The development of the cardiorespiratory
system with growth and physical activity. In R.A.
Boileau (ed.) *Advances in Pediatric Sport Sciences*,
pp. 85–116. Human Kinetics, Champaign, IL.

Cunningham, D.A., Stapleton, J.J., MacDonald, I.C. &
Paterson, D.H. (1981) Daily expenditure of young
boys as related to maximal aerobic power. *Can. J.*

Appl. Sport Sci. **6**, 207–11.

Cunningham, D.A., van Waterschoot, B.M., Paterson, D.H., Lefcoe, M. & Sangal S.P. (1977) Reliability and reproducibility of maximal oxygen uptake measurement in children. *Med. Sci. Sport Exerc.* **9**, 104–8.

Espenschade, A. (1947) Development of motor coordination in boys and girls. *Res. Q.* **18**, 13–40.

Falkner, F. (1954) Measurement of somatic growth and development in children. *Courrier CIE* **4**, 169–81.

Falkner, F. (ed.) (1980) *Twenty-five Years of Internationally Coordinated Research: Longitudinal Studies in Growth and Development*. International Children's Centre, Courrier, Montreux, Switzerland.

Falkner, F. & Tanner, J.M. (ed.) (1978) *Human Growth*, Vol. 2. *Postnatal Growth*. Plenum Press, New York.

Froberg, K., Andersen, B. & Lammert, O. (1991) Maximal oxygen intake and respiratory functions during puberty in boy groups of different physical activity. In R. Frenkl & I. Szmodis (eds) *Children and Exercise, Pediatric Work Physiology XV*, pp. 265–80. NEVI Budapest.

Graffar, M. & Courbier, J. (1966) Contribution à l'étude de l'influence des conditions socio-économiques sur la croissance et le développement (Contribution to the study of the effects of socio-economic status on growth and development). *Courrier CIE* **16**, 1–25.

Hebbelinck, M., Blommaert, M., Borms, J., Duquet, W., Vajda, A. & Meer, J. van der (1980) A multidisciplinary longitudinal growth study – introduction of the project 'LLEGS'. In M. Ostyn, G. Beunen & J. Simons (eds) *Kinanthropometry II. International Series of Sport Sciences*, Vol. 9, pp. 317–25. University Park Press, Baltimore.

Jéquier, J., Lavallée, H., Rajic, M., Beaucage, C., Shephard, R.J. & Labarre, R. (1977) *The Longitudinal Examination of Growth and Development: History and Protocol of the Trois Rivières Regional Study in Lavallée, Shephard, Frontiers of Activity and Child Health*, pp. 49–54. Pelican, Ottawa.

Jones, H.E. (1949) *Motor Performance and Growth. A Developmental Study of Static Dynamometric Strength*. University of California Press, Berkeley.

Karlberg, P., Taranger, J., Engström, I. *et al.* (1976) The somatic development of children in a Swedish urban community: a prospective longitudinal study. I. Physical growth from birth to 16 years and longitudinal outcome of the study during the same period. *Acta Paediatr. Scand.* **258** (Suppl.), 7–76.

Kemper, H.C.G. (ed.) (1985) *Growth, Health and Fitness of Teenagers: Longitudinal Research in International Perspective*. Medicine and Sport Sciences, Vol. 20. Karger, Basel.

Kemper, H.C.G. (1986) Longitudinal studies on the development of health and fitness and the interaction with physical activity of teenagers. *Pediatrician* **13**, 52–9.

Kemper, H.C.G. (1988) Longitudinal studies in the development of physical fitness in teenagers. In R.M. Malina (ed.) *Young Athletes, Biological, Psychological and Educational Perspectives*, pp. 3–17. Human Kinetics, Champaign, IL.

Kemper, H.C.G. & van 't Hof, M.A. (1978) Design of a multiple longitudinal study of growth and health in teenagers. *Eur. J. Pediatr.* **129**, 147–55.

Kemper, H.C.G., Verschuur, R., Ras, J.G.A., Snel, J., Splinter, P.G. & Tavecchio, I.W.C. (1976) Effect of 5 versus 3 lessons a week of physical education upon the physical development of 12 and 13 year old schoolboys. *J. Sports Med. Phys. Fitness* **16**, 319–26.

Kobayashi, K., Kitamure, K., Miura, M. *et al.* (1978) Aerobic power as related to body growth and training in Japanese boys: a longitudinal study. *J. Appl. Physiol.* **44**, 666–72.

Kowalski, C.J., Prahl-Andersen, B. (1979) General considerations in the design of studies of growth and development. In C.J. Kowalski, B. Prahl-Andersen & P. Heyendael (eds) *A Mixed Longitudinal Interdisciplinary Study of Growth and Development*, pp. 3–13. Academic Press, New York.

Lange Andersen, K., Seliger, V., Rutenfranz, J. & Berndt, I. (1974a) Physical performance capacity of children in Norway: Part II. Heart rate and oxygen pulse in submaximal and maximal exercises. Population parameters in a rural community. *Eur. J. Appl. Physiol.* **33**, 197–206.

Lange Andersen, K., Seliger, V., Rutenfranz, J. & Messel, S. (1974b) Physical performance capacity of children in Norway: Part III. Respiratory response to graded exercise loadings. Population parameters in a rural community. *Eur. J. Appl. Physiol.* **33**, 265–76.

Lange Andersen, K., Seliger, V., Rutenfranz, J. & Mocellin, R. (1974c) Physical performance capacity of children in Norway: Part I. Population parameters in a rural inland community with regard to maximal aerobic power. *Eur. J. Appl. Physiol.* **33**, 177–95.

Lange Andersen, K., Seliger, V., Rutenfranz, J. & Skrobak Kacyznski, J. (1976) Physical performance capacity of children in Norway: Part IV. The rate of growth in maximal aerobic power and the influence of improved physical education of children in a rural community. Population parameters in a rural community. *Eur. J. Appl. Physiol.* **35**, 49–58.

Largo, R.H., Gasser, T., Prader, A., Stuetzle, W. & Humber, P.J. (1978) Analysis of the adolescent growth spurt, using smoothing spline functions. *Ann. Hum. Biol.* 421–34.

McCloy, C.H. (1936) *Appraising Physical Status. The Selection of Measurements.* University of Iowa Studies in Child Welfare, Vol. XII, No. 2. University of Iowa, Iowa.

Margaria, R., Aghemo, P. & Rovelli, E. (1966) Measurement of muscular power (anaerobic) in man. *J. Appl. Physiol.* **21**, 1662–3.

Mednick, J.A. & Baert, A.E. (eds) (1981) *Prospective Longitudinal Research: An Empirical Basis for the Primary Prevention of Psychosocial Disorders.* Oxford University Press, Oxford.

Meredith, H.V. (1935) *The Rhythm of Physical Growth.* University of Iowa Studies in Child Welfare, Vol. XI, No. 3. University of Iowa, Iowa.

Mirwald, R.L. (1980) Saskatchewan growth and development study. In M. Ostyn, G. Beunen & J. Simons (eds) *Kinanthropometry II. International Series of Sports Science*, Vol. 9, pp. 289–305. University Park Press, Baltimore.

Mirwald, R.L. & Bailey, D.A. (1985) *Longitudinal Analyses of Maximal Aerobic Power in Boys and Girls by Chronological Age, Maturity and Physical Activity.* University of Saskatchewan, Saskatoon.

Moore, T., Hindley, G.B. & Falkner, F. (1954) A longitudinal research in child development and some of its problems. *Br. Med. J.* **ii**, 1132–7.

Ostyn, M., Simons, J., Beunen, G., Renson, R. & Gerven, D. van. (1980) *Somatic and Motor Development of Belgian Secondary Schoolboys: Norms and Standards.* University Press, Leuven.

Parízková, J. (1974) Particularities of lean body mass and fat development in growing boys as related to their motor activity. *Acta Paediatr. Belg.* **28** (Suppl.), 233–43.

Pate, R.R. & Ward, D.S. (1990) Endurance exercise trainability in children and youth. In W.A. Grano, J.A. Lombardo, B.J. Sharkey & J.A. Stone (eds) *Advances in Sports Medicine and Fitness*, Vol. 3, pp. 37–55. Year Book Medical Publishers, Chicago.

Pfeiffer, R. & Francis, R.S. (1986) Effects of strength training on muscle development in prepubescent, pubescent and postpubescent males. *Phys. Sports Med.* **14**, 137–43.

Placheta, Z. (1980) *Youth and physical activity.* University of Purkyne, Brno, CSSR.

Prahl-Andersen, B., Kowalski, C.J. & Heydendael, P. (1979) *A Mixed Longitudinal Interdisciplinary Study of Growth and Development.* Academic Press, New York.

Rao, M.N. & Rao, C.R. (1966) Linked cross-sectional study for determining norms and growth rates — a pilot survey of Indian school-going boys. *Saykgya* **68**, 237–58.

Rowland, T.W. (1985) Aerobic response to endurance training in prepubescent children: a critical analysis. *Med. Sci. Sports Exerc.* **17**, 493–7.

Roy-Pernot, M.P., Sempé, M. & Filliozat, A.M. (1976) *Rapport d'Activité Terminal de l'Équipe Française. Compte Rendu de la 13-ème Réunion des Équipes Chargées des Études sur la Croissance et le Développement de l'Enfant Normal* (Final report of the French group. Proceedings of the 13th conference of the groups involved with the growth and development of normal children). Centre International de l'Enfance, Paris.

Sady, S.P. (1986) Cardiorespiratory exercise training in children. *Clin. Sports Med.* **5**, 493–514.

Schaie, K.W. (1965) A general model for the study of development problems. *Psychol. Bull.* **64**, 92–107.

Sewall, L. & Micheli, L.J. (1984) Strength training for children. *J. Pediatr. Orthop.* **6**, 143–6.

Shephard, K. (1982) *Physical Activity and Growth.* Medical Publishers, Chicago.

Shephard, R.J., Lavallée, H., Jequier, J., Rajic, M. & Labarre, R. (1980) Additional physical education in the primary school. A preliminary analysis of the Trois Rivières regional experiment. In M. Ostyn, G. Beunen & G. Simons (eds) *Kinanthropometry II. International Series of Sports Science*, Vol. 9, pp. 306–16. University Park Press, Baltimore.

Simons, J., Beunen, G.P., Renson Claessen, A.L.M., Reusel, B. van & Lefèvre, J.A.V. (1990) Growth and fitness of Flemish girls. The Leuven Growth Study HKP. In *Sport Science Monograph Series*, Vol. 3. Human Kinetics, Champaign, IL.

Sprynarova, S. (1974) Longitudinal study of the influence of different activity on functional capacity or boys from 11–18 years. *Acta Paediatr. Belg.* **29** (Suppl.), 204–13.

Tanner, J.M. (1962) *Growth at Adolescence.* Blackwell Scientific Publications, Oxford.

Tanner, J.M. (1981) *A History of the Study of Human Growth.* Cambridge University Press, London.

Tanner, J.M., Whitehouse, R.H., Marubini, E. & Rescle, L. (1976) The adolescent growth spurt of boys and girls of the Harpenden Growth Study. *Ann. Human Biol.* **3**, 109–26.

Vaccaro, P. & Mahon, A. (1987) Cardiorespiratory response to endurance training in children. *Sports Med.* **4**, 352–63.

Veling, S.H.S. & van't Hof, M.A. (1980) Data quality control methods in longitudinal studies. In M. Ostyn, G. Beunen & J. Simons (eds) *Kinanthropometry II. International Series of Sports Science*, Vol. 9, pp. 436–42. University Park Press, Baltimore.

Vrijens, J. (1978) Muscle strength development in the pre- and post pubescent ages. *Med. Sport* **11**, 152–8.

Weber, G., Kartodihardjo, W. & Klissouras, V. (1976) Growth and physical training with reference to heredity. *J. Appl. Physiol.* **40**, 211–15.

Weltman, A. (1984) Weight training in prepuberal children. Physiologic benefit and potential damage. In O. Bar-Or (ed.) *Advances in Pediatric Sports Sciences*, Vol. 3. Human Kinetics, Champaign, IL.

Chapter 38

Assessment of Energy Expenditure and Daily Physical Activity

WIM H.M. SARIS

Introduction

Physical activity is a prerequisite for optimal growth and development of children and to maintain health over the years. In an increasing number of chronic diseases such as cardiovascular disease, obesity, diabetes and even in certain types of cancer such as colonic cancer, evidence is available that the daily level of physical activity plays an important role. Furthermore, in relation to athletic performance the level of training intensity and length will affect energy turnover besides the daily physical activity.

It is particularly important to have information about daily physical activity under conditions of extreme endurance training, or in some groups of élite athletes where dieting is a common habit in order to keep body weight within certain limits, such as is seen in gymnastics (Van Erp-Baart et al., 1989) (see also Chapter 20). Therefore, the measurement of physical activity has become a field of interest for epidemiologists, exercise physiologists and clinicians specializing in the treatment of hypokinetic diseases.

While the foundation of much of the present theory and methodology in the assessment of habitual physical activity was established at least 100 years ago, most of the progress in this area has taken place in the last 20 years. This chapter focuses on the methodological constraints on these measurement and special attention will be given to those techniques that best fit the different young athletic groups to be measured.

Components of energy turnover

The main component of the daily energy turnover is the energy expenditure for maintaining process, called resting energy expenditure (REE) or resting metabolic rate. This is the energy expenditure used in the ongoing processes of the body in the resting state when no food is digested. REE is normally measured in the morning after waking up without moderate or intense physical activity before the measurement is taken. The measurement has to be done after an overnight fast, in a thermoneutral environment in the supine position. If appropriate equipment is not available the REE can be calculated with the use of prediction formulae which are adjusted for the different age ranges (FAO/WHO/UNU, 1985). Table 38.1 shows different formulae, including the correlation coefficients and residual standard deviation.

The second component of the daily energy turnover is the diet-induced energy expenditure (DEE) or diet-induced thermogenesis, normally measured over a period of 3–4 h after a standardized meal. DEE values reflect the energy needed for digestion and storage of the ingested nutrients.

Finally, there is the energy turnover of activities, called exercise-induced energy expenditure (EEE), which is the subject of this chapter and is the most variable component of the

Table 38.1 Equations for predicting resting energy expenditure from body weight (BW) in kg.

Age range (years)	kcal·day^{-1}	Correlation coefficient	SD*	mJ·day^{-1}	Correlation coefficient	SD*
Males						
0–3	$60.9 \times BW - 54$	0.97	53	$0.2550\,BW - 0.226$	0.97	0.222
3–10	$22.7 \times BW + 495$	0.86	62	$0.0949\,BW + 2.07$	0.86	0.259
10–18	$17.5 \times BW + 651$	0.90	100	$0.0732\,BW + 2.72$	0.90	0.418
18–30	$15.3 \times BW + 679$	0.65	151	$0.0640\,BW + 2.84$	0.65	0.632
30–60	$11.6 \times BW + 879$	0.60	164	$0.0485\,BW + 3.67$	0.60	0.686
>60	$13.5 \times BW + 487$	0.79	148	$0.0565\,BW + 2.04$	0.79	0.619
Females						
0–3	$61.0 \times BW - 51$	0.97	61	$0.2550\,BW - 0.214$	0.97	0.255
3–10	$22.5 \times BW + 499$	0.85	63	$0.0941\,BW + 2.09$	0.85	0.264
10–18	$12.2 \times BW + 746$	0.75	117	$0.0510\,BW + 3.12$	0.75	0.489
18–30	$14.7 \times BW + 496$	0.72	121	$0.0615\,BW + 2.08$	0.72	0.506
30–60	$8.7 \times BW + 829$	0.70	108	$0.0364\,BW + 3.47$	0.70	0.452
>60	$10.5 \times BW + 596$	0.74	108	$0.0439\,BW + 2.49$	0.74	0.452

* Standard deviation of differences between actual basal metabolic rate and predicted estimate.

energy turnover. It ranges between an average value of 25–30% of total energy expenditure, and up to 75% in extreme situation during heavy sustained exercise. In addition to these three components, the human body can adapt energy expenditure (adaptive energy expenditure, AEE) under certain conditions such as in the cold or heat or during starvation when energy expenditure is decreased.

In order to classify the energy turnover of specific activities including sport activities, or to specify the level of daily physical activity in relation to the total energy turnover, the MET (metabolic units) rating has been introduced. The MET value is the ratio of the energy cost of an activity divided by REE. This MET value is approximately equal to the energy cost of the activity expressed as kcal·h^{-1}·kg^{-1} body weight since REE for adults is roughly 1 kcal·h^{-1}·kg^{-1} or 4.2 kJ·h^{-1}·kg^{-1}.

Recently, an extensive list of MET values has been published (Ainsworth *et al.*, 1993). Much of the data in this list are derived from actual measurements by indirect calorimetry. However, when data were not available the figures were based upon educated guesses. For some activities the values are not those obtained during the actual execution of the activities.

For instance, the gymnastic activities require higher energy expenditure values than the mean value that is shown. However, in 1 h of gymnastics considerable time is spent standing, receiving directions and so on (Van Erp-Baart *et al.*, 1985). So the value shown by Ainsworth *et al.* represents the average for approximately 1 h. Conversely, cycling is done continuously, so these values represent the actual energy cost of doing the activity.

In almost all the metabolic costs of activities that have been reported, young adults served as subjects. There are little data based on children and elderly people. The energy expended by children in kJ·kg^{-1} body weight is significantly higher compared to the same activities executed by adults (Montoye, 1982). This is probably because of the greater surface area to body weight ratio and poorer coordination in children. Sallis *et al.* (1991) calculated on the basis of energy costs of treadmill walking and running in five studies child to adult ratios ranging from 1.35 at the age of 5 years to about 1 at the age of 18 years. However, the REE per unit of body weight is also considerably higher in children as a result of the proportional differences in the increase of energy expenditure so that the MET values are a little lower in children.

Table 38.2 MET values of various activities in children aged 9–12 years.

Sitting	
quietly	1.1
reading	1.2
watching television	1.3
doing puzzles	1.5
Standing	
quietly	1.5
singing	1.8
Dressing	2.6
Eating	1.4
Walking	
slow pace	2.8
firm pace	3.5
Bicycling	
slow	2.5
firm	5.0
Running	8.3
Playing outdoors	4.5
Ballet	4.4
Gymnastics	5.0
Judo	6.3
Roller skating	7.5
Soccer	6.0

In Table 38.2 a limited number of MET values are given for children based on available data in the literature.

Besides the use of MET values to indicate the intensity level of specific activities, one can calculate the MET value over the total daily activities based on the measured total energy expenditure (TEE), as described in detail below, and REE. Normally this ratio TEE to REE is called the activity factor (AF). For sedentary subjects the AF is around 1.5 and this value can increase to around 3.5–4.5, as found in extreme endurance exercise such as professional cycle racing (Saris *et al.*, 1989). It has been suggested from animal studies that 4–5 is the ceiling of AF over weeks for humans to perform without life-threatening effects.

Procedures for measuring oxygen consumption (indirect calorimetry)

It is possible to measure energy expenditure by

determination of oxygen consumption, assuming that physical exercise throughout the day is almost entirely aerobic. The approach requires the use of an open respiratory circuit system, in which the expired gas volume is measured and a gas sample is taken for analysis of oxygen and carbon dioxide by a Haldane or micro Scholander apparatus, or by means of an electronic analyser. Furthermore, ambient temperature (°C), barometric pressure and relative humidity are recorded. The recorded data are then substituted in an appropriate formula to calculate oxygen consumption. Croonen and Binkhorst (1974) showed that, on the basis of volume and the fraction of oxygen, energy expenditure can be calculated with an accuracy of −2 to +4%, depending on whether the value of the respiratory quotient (RQ) is low or high.

The classical method uses a Douglas bag fixed on the subject's back, in which expired air is collected. More sophisticated devices were already developed at the end of the nineteenth century. The well-known Kofrany–Michaelis respirometer was developed in the 1940s. Modern versions of this equipment are the Oxylog, the Miser and the recently developed portable K-3 monitor and metabolic cart. Although the accuracy of the measurements is high, the application to the measurement of daily physical activity is limited, especially in children. This is because of the necessity of wearing a face mask or mouthpiece with a nose clamp during a period of 5–20 min. Especially in young children, this interference with normal activities is unacceptable.

An alternative method has been described by Durnin and Passmore (1967), in which oxygen consumption is measured for a few characteristic activities and an activity diary is kept as well. The daily energy expenditure is predicted from these data. A disadvantage of the method is that the accuracy is dependent upon the cooperation of the subject, who must record his or her activities. Furthermore, only a limited number of values generated by Durnin and Passmore (1967), are based on data with children.

The doubly labelled water (DLW) technique

The most accurate and applicable field technique is the use of the stable isotopes deuterium and oxygen ^{18}O. It bridges the gap between the very accurate but restrictive indirect calorimetry in respiration chambers, or with Douglas bags, and other field techniques to be discussed, each of which has its disadvantages with respect to validity and accuracy.

Since the oxygen atoms of expired carbon dioxide are in isotopic equilibrium with body water, the kinetics of water elimination and respiration are interdependent. When a subject is given $^2H_2^{18}O$, the ^{18}O is eliminated from the body carbon dioxide and water while ^2H is eliminated only as water. Hence the decrease of $^2H_2^{18}O$ is a measure of water plus carbon dioxide flux. From the difference between both elimination rates, carbon dioxide production can be calculated and from this energy expenditure can be calculated using an estimated RQ value. Both markers, ^{18}O and ^2H, are stable isotopes which occur naturally in the body water at a level around 2000 and 150 p.p.m., respectively. The enrichment needed to detect the decrease accurately is about 200–400 p.p.m. These levels do not have any measurable health effects. In practice, an observation starts with a baseline sample in order to detect the natural abundance. Such a baseline sample is needed because there is a variation of both isotopes in different environmental situations including food. Also control values are needed during the observation period in those situations where a change in the natural enrichment is expected, for instance at different altitudes during climbing. After the collection of the baseline sample a weighted dose is administered. After an equilibration time in the body which takes normally 4–8 h, an initial sample of the body fluid (e.g. blood, urine or saliva) is taken in order to calculate the disappearance rate of both isotopes, respectively K_O and K_H. Body water samples are collected at regular intervals (Westerterp et al., 1995). The optimal observation period is 1–3 biological half-lives of the isotopes. Calculating the carbon dioxide production from the difference between K_O and K_H one has to correct for isotope fractionation and incorporation in compartments other than water. Because fractionation is a function of mass, ^2H and ^{18}O are more abundant in liquid water than in water vapour and ^{18}O is more abundant in carbon dioxide than in water. These fractionation factors f_1, f_2 and f_3 are 0.941, 0.992 and 1.039, respectively. Based on these assumptions one can calculate the carbon dioxide production with the proposed equation from Schoeller et al. (1986):

$$rCO_2 = (K_O \cdot D_O \cdot K_H \cdot D_H) \cdot (f_2 - f_1) \cdot rGf$$
$$\frac{}{2f_3} \qquad \frac{}{2f_3}$$

where K_O, D_O, K_H and D_H are elimination rates and dilution spaces for ^{18}O and ^2H, respectively. Factor f_1, f_2 and f_3 are for fractionation of ^2H in water vapour, ^{18}O in water vapour and ^{18}O in carbon dioxide, respectively. rGf is the rate of isotopical fractionated gaseous water loss. Assuming that breath is saturated with water and contains 3.5% carbon dioxide, knowing that incorporation of the isotopes has been estimated for ^{18}O and ^2H on 1 and 4% respectively, and transcutaneous fractionated (non-sweat) water loss amounts to about 50% of breath water, then

$$rCO_2 = 0.455 \, N \, (1.01 \, K_O - 1.04 \, KH).$$

Recently, the method and calculations for its use in humans was discussed extensively in a workshop (Prentice, 1990). Several assumptions must be taken into account:

1 Total body water pool remains constant.
2 Rates of water influx and water and carbon dioxide efflux are constant.
3 Isotopes label only the water and carbon dioxide in the body.
4 Isotopes leave the body only as water and carbon dioxide.
5 Concentrations of isotopes in water and carbon dioxide leaving the body are the same as those in body water (no isotopic fractionation).
6 Natural abundance or background levels isotopes are constant.
7 No isotopes that have left the body re-enter.

Sources of error are analytical errors in the mass spectrometric determination of isotopic enrichments, calculation of total body water, evaporative water loss, biological variation in the isotopic enrichments and the heat equivalent per mol of expired carbon dioxide on the basis of the estimated RQ.

To convert carbon dioxide to energy expenditure information is needed on the metabolic fuel source in order to calculate the energy equivalent of carbon dioxide. One option is the calculation of the food quotient (FQ) from the macronutrient composition of the diet. In energy balance the value of the FQ equals the RQ. For each 0.01 unit deviation in RQ an error of 1% is introduced in the calculation of TEE.

In recent years studies have compared the method with respirometry in five laboratories. In Table 38.3 the results of these studies are shown. The data resulted in an accuracy of 1–3% with a precision of 2–8%. Therefore, the DLW can now be considered as the gold standard for the measurements of energy expenditure under field conditions. The method has been applied in subjects from infancy to old age with extreme differences in physical activity

levels (e.g. hospitalized patients to professional cyclists in the Tour de France or climbers of Mount Everest). Disadvantage of the method is the lack of information about the pattern of energy expenditure during the observation period. Furthermore, the costs for ^{18}O are extremely high for one observation (child about \$US300) and expertise is needed to analyse the sample on a high precision isotope ratio mass spectrometer.

Heart rate (HR) recording and daily physical activity

Of all physiological variables, HR is one of the easiest to register with the least encumbrance to the subject. Therefore it has gained popularity as a method for assessment of daily physical activity. The advances in microelectronics have made it possible to detect and store heart pulses reliably over long periods of time, using small equipment. Therefore monitoring the HR has become one of the most commonly employed methods in children and adolescence (Fig. 38.1).

In the athletic world the measurement of HR has become part of the professional training

Table 38.3 Doubly labelled water technique compared to other measures of total energy exchange.

Subjects	n	Error (%)	±SD	Ref. method	Reference*
Adults	4	−0.4	±5.6	I/B	Schoeller & Van Santen (1982)
Adults	1	−4.6	−	RGE	Klein et al. (1984)
Adults	5	+1.5	±7.6	RGE	Schoeller & Webb (1984)
Adults	4	+1.9	±2.0	RGE	Coward & Prentice (1984)
Exercising adults	2	−2.5	±4.9	RGE	Westerterp et al. (1984)
Premature infants	4	−0.3	±2.6	RGE	Roberts et al. (1986)
Adults on TPN	5	+3.3	±5.9	I/B	Schoeller et al. (1986a)
Adults	9	+1.4	±7.7	RGE	Schoeller et al. (1986b)
Postsurgery infants	9	−0.9	±6.2	RGE	Jones et al. (1987)
Adults	5	+1.4	±3.9	RGE	Westerterp et al. (1988)
Exercising adults	4 × 2	−1.0	±7.0	RGE	Westerterp et al. (1988)
Lean/obese adults	12	−2.5	±5.8	RGE	Ravussin et al. (1991)
Preterm infants	8	−5.1	±5.7	RGE	Westerterp et al. (1991)
Weighted mean ± SD	76	0.2	±6.2		

* For details of references see Prentice (1990); Ravussin et al. (1991); Westerterp et al. (1991).
I/B, intake plus change in body mass; RGE, respiratory gas exchange; TPN, total parenteral nutrition.

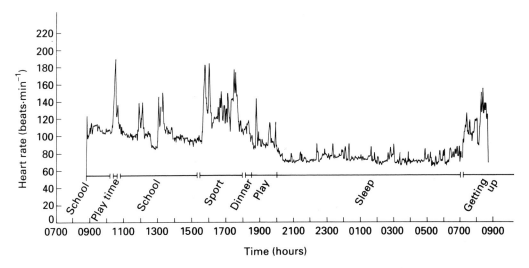

Fig. 38.1 Twenty-four hour profile of an 8-year-old boy during a normal schoolday.

programme. Determination of HR at the aerobic threshold is routine in order to increase performance. This interest has boosted the development of reliable HR recorders with minimal weight and size and maximal storage capacity.

The method is based on the relationship between HR and oxygen consumption. Different mathematical approaches such as the use of several linear regression equations or an exponential relationship, have been suggested in order to make the prediction as accurate as possible. It has been suggested that a two-linear relationship of the individual HR versus $\dot{V}_{O_2}$ based on a HR (transition HR) that discriminated between resting and exercising HR is the best predictor of TEE.

In general, one of the major problems is the low HR during normal activities with possible confounding stimuli, such as emotional stress or small movements without concomitant changes in $\dot{V}_{O_2}$. The relation between HR and $\dot{V}_{O_2}$ depends upon the type of exercise. Especially dynamic leg exercise prevents pooling of the blood in the legs due to the active muscle contractions. The HR while standing proved to be a reasonable indicator for the transition point or flex point from the resting type of activities, such as sitting, to dynamic activities,

such as walking (Fig. 38.2). Rather, it is the determination of this transition point where the weakness of the HR method lies in predicting TEE, since a considerable part of the HR values is recorded in this heart beat range. Recently, Hebestreit *et al.* (1933) designed a nomogram for the correction of HR depending on climatic heat stress in order to improve the estimation of TEE (Fig. 38.3). Normally, the individual HR $\dot{V}_{O_2}$ regression equations are determined under standardized climatological conditions in the laboratory (22°C, 50% humidity). Especially in children climatic heat stress will increase HR for the same $\dot{V}_{O_2}$. Correction will reduce the error of overestimating the TEE in a hot climate.

Two studies have been published in adults on the validation of the HR method versus DLW. The percentage difference with the DLW method was +2% ± 17.9 ranging from − 22 to +52%, with nine out of the 14 values lying within ±10% of DLW TEE estimates in the study of Livingstone *et al.* (1990). Schultz *et al.* (1989) found with a HR/$\dot{V}_{O_2}$ linear regression approach in nine subjects a percentage difference of +9.8 ± 20.3 ranging from − 20.7 to +47.7%, with four out of the nine values lying within ±10% of the DLW TEE estimates. Other

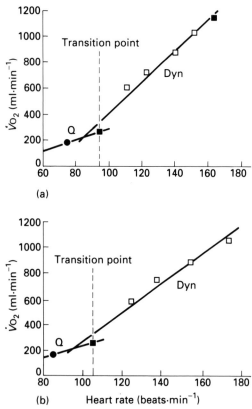

(a)

(b) Heart rate (beats·min^{-1})

Fig. 38.2 Example of the mathematical approach to calculate TEE from HR. Mean oxygen uptake ($\dot{V}_{O_2}$) as a function of HR (f_c) during quiet activities (Q, sleeping and standing) and dynamic activities (Dyn, five submaximal exercise intensities on a treadmill) in (a) boys ($n = 9$), and (b) girls ($n = 10$).
Boys $f_{c,EqQ}$: $\dot{V}_{O_2} = 4.663 f_c - 169.837$;
  $f_{c,EqQ}$: $\dot{V}_{O_2} = 12.439 f_c - 829.985$ $r^2 = 0.977$.
Girls $f_{c,EqQ}$: $\dot{V}_{O_2} = 5.38 f_c - 286.2$;
  $f_{c,EqQ}$: $\dot{V}_{O_2} = 11.72 f_c - 896.358$ $r^2 = 0.978$.
Redrawn with permission from Emons *et al.* (1992).

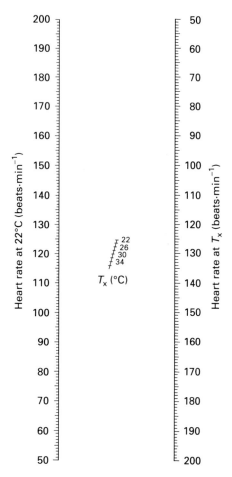

Fig. 38.3 Nomogram for the correction of HR at temperature T_x to an ISO-$\dot{V}_{O_2}$ heart rate at 22°C in children. Redrawn with permission from Hebestreit *et al.* (1993).

procedures such as second order regressions between HR and $\dot{V}_{O_2}$ or two linear regressions such as the transition point order regressions did not yield better results.

In both studies it became clear that the principal challenge to the integrity of the HR method lies in predicting the energy expenditure of mainly sedentary subjects. The results in adults do not give a conclusive answer about which mathematical equation is preferred. Interesting

was the observation by Livingstone *et al.* (1990) that the calculated AF (TEE$_{DLW}$/REE) highly correlated with percentage daytime HR above transition point ($r = 0.95$). This indicates that perhaps the HR method can be improved by using only the activity part of the HR profile in order to estimate physical activity. Unfortunately, this implies that the aim of using the HR method to estimate TEE is not realistic. Saris *et al.* (1986) proposed a similar use of the method. They calculated on the basis of individual aerobic power, the energy expenditure spent above 50% of aerobic power, using an individual linear regression equation between $\dot{V}o_2$ and HR.

Recently, a validation study in 8–11-year-old children was published (Emons *et al.*, 1992). The best prediction of TEE was found with a linear regression for five boys and four girls (aged 10 years). The differences were +13.9% ± 20.1 and +6.3% ± 12.5, respectively, ranging from −12% to +42% with values for five out of nine children lying within 10% of the TEE DLW estimates. These values are not markedly different from those in adults. It was speculated that, based on the fact that in general children are more active, the HR method would predict TEE more accurately. The results of the Emons *et al.* (1992) study do not give any evidence for this hypothesis. In all three studies TEE is overestimated by the HR method. This is in agreement with an earlier observation based on the respiratory gas exchange method (Saris, 1986). This consistent finding may be explained by the slower return of the HR to baseline values after exercise in contrast to oxygen consumption.

As an example of the use of the HR method in an athletic population, the results from a study in female gymnastics are given (Van Erp-Baart *et al.*, 1985). Food intake in 11 élite female gymnasts (mean age 15.4 years) revealed a 24-h energy intake of 7.3 mJ. In order to determine whether this group tended to be nutritionally imbalanced information was collected about energy expenditure during training using the observation technique and direct measurement of oxygen consumption of specific activities such as balance beam and parallel bars. To have an idea about 24-h energy turnover, the HR method was used and REE was measured. Mean time spent on a training session was 3 h and 15 min. The intensity of the training was on average 15% heavy, 8% moderate and 77% light with an average MET value of 4. Total 24-h energy turnover was 9.1 mJ and REE 5.3 mJ. The calculated activity factor was 1.72 based on the HR recordings and 1.38 based on food intake recordings. It was concluded that at least a number of these gymnasts had a real energy deficit which could lead to an impairment in performance.

In conclusion, the HR method provides a fair estimation of the daily energy turnover of groups. However, the value of the method on an individual level is limited due to the large variation in estimation. The possibility of dissociating the activity component from daily energy turnover looks promising to evaluate daily physical activity.

Movement counters

Almost all forms of physical activity require movement of the trunk or extremities. Therefore it is not surprising that many ingenious devices have been proposed and have sometimes been used to obtain an objective estimation of the movement of the body over a certain period of time. In fact, Leonardo da Vinci had already designed a pedometer to measure distance by counting steps. The pedometer records the acceleration and deceleration of the waist in the vertical direction. The functional principle is that an arm balanced by a delicate spring is displaced downwards by slight jolts in the direction of suspension. This method does not record intensity of movement. Saris and Binkhorst (1977) showed in their study with children and adults that the pedometer does not accurately reflect differences in energy expenditure level at different speeds of walking and running, and during cycling no counts are registered. In addition, the commercially available brands are not reliable enough to use in research on physical activity.

Over the years several electronic devices have been developed based on the principle of counting steps or motion. Although some of them are more reliable than others, they all do not take intensity of the movement into account and thus do not reflect the forces and energy turnover well. These types of movement counters yield a total number of movements and do not make distinctions between the intensity of the movements. Moreover typical movements, such as cycling are not counted.

A better reflection of daily physical activity is given by portable accelerometers also called actometer. When a person moves, the limbs and body are accelerated and decelerated. Measurements with force–platform in a respiration chamber showed good agreement with energy turnover. The first accelerometers were based on a modified automatic wrist watch in which the rotor was directly connected to the hands. The stronger the movement the faster the turning of the rotor. For accelerometers worn on the ankle, readings do reflect the differences in energy turnover during walking and running in children with reasonable accuracy (Saris & Binkhorst, 1977). Several accelerometers have been developed and are commercially available.

Meijer et al. (1991b) described an accelerometer based on a piezo-electrical ceramic element worn in a belt on the back at the L4–5 level. They argued that movements recorded at this position represent the larger movements of the body (e.g. walking, running) which have the greatest impact on daily physical activity. They compared the results of this accelerometer over a 7-day period with the AF index obtained from the DLW and REE measurement in 21 adults (Meijer et al., 1990). Although technical problems still hamper this technique, the results were encouraging. A strong relationship was observed, both with the absolute value of the energy compartment TEE-REE ($r = 0.88$; $P < 0.001$) and with the AF index ($r = 0.71$; $P < 0.001$), provided corrections were made for the individual energy expenditure and accelerometer counts for the same activity. If not corrected for these individual differences, the accelerometer values still correlated significantly with the AF index ($r = 0.64$; $P < 0.001$). Using both techniques in a study on the effects of a 5-month endurance training programme, Meijer et al. (1991d) observed a significant correlation between accelerometer counts during the running periods and the increase in TEE-REE ($r = 0.78$; $P < 0.01$; $n = 14$), suggesting that the accelerometer results reflect changes in daily physical activity accurately.

Another extensively studied accelerometer is the so-called Caltrac. A field study correlating Caltrac values with the DLW method showed a significant correlation with energy turnover ($r = 0.54$) (Gretebeck et al., 1991). Results from a respiration chamber study showed even better results ($r = 0.92$) (Schutz et al., 1988). In over 25 studies using different techniques ranging from HR recording to questionnaire to validate the Caltrac, that the interinstrument variability of the instrument was low and its validity was good under controlled laboratory conditions. Initial results with the use of triaxial accelerometer instead of the single-plane instruments suggest a little better estimate of daily energy turnover.

In conclusion, the results on the validation of the movement counter based on the acceleration principle are much better than was expected from results of earlier observation. Because this method is the best approach in large-scale studies (Saris, 1986), it gives excellent opportunities for further research on the relation between physical activity and health. An extra advantage of this method is the availability of information on physical activity pattern over the day. However, there are still problems regarding the technical reliability of the available devices.

Retrospective activity surveys, diaries and time–motion analysis

Due to the cost of equipment and major demand on labour in the above methods, questionnaires are very popular in large-scale epidemiological studies. However, a naive investigator may become confused by the proliferation of questionnaires in the past three decades.

Several survey procedures have been developed and extensively analysed (Lange Anderssen et al., 1978). In their review La Porte et al. (1985) differentiated four types of surveys: (i) short-term diary (less than 24 h); (ii) recall surveys of the past 1–7 days; (iii) a quantitative history over the past 1–5 years; and (iv) general survey regardless of time frame of reference. The use of these procedures, however, in the child population is very limited. There are only a few validation reports available concerning the use of physical activity surveys in children. Under the age of 10–12 years children can only give limited information about their activity pattern. The validity of a self-kept log is questionable, and the questionnaires have to be limited to simple questions like 'How do you go to school?' or the type of sports club activity the child is involved in. Moreover, the information of parents is often secondary, especially when it concerns outdoor playing activities.

Validity of the different types of questionnaires is difficult to determine because of inadequate criteria. DLW is a criterion but this is limited to an average energy turnover over a 2-week period. Careful observation, energy intake with food analyser or at least indirect calorimetry of distinct activities and diaries might also serve as criteria. Saris et al. (1980) constructed an eight-item physical activity index for children to be filled in by the parents (PA_1 index) or the teacher (PA_2 index) and recall over the previous day (PA_3 index) according to the Edholm scale (Lange Anderssen et al., 1978). Significant differences for PA_1 and PA_2 were found between children with a high or low performance capacity in two age groups (4–6 and 8–12 years, respectively). The high performance groups had significantly higher values for PA_1 and PA_2 (respectively, 63.2 and 70.2% compared to 53.3 and 40.1% for the 4–6-year-old age group, and 62.5 and 64.7% compared to 47.6 and 54.6% in the 8–12-year-old age group). No differences were found for the PA_3 index. This is in agreement with the data from Telama et al. (1985). In this study information about physical activity of 3- and 6-year-old children was based on a questionnaire addressed to the parents and, from the age of 8 years, to the child. The best reliable values were obtained from questionnaires about participation in sport, which may be due to the regular character of this type of activity. Reliability showed a consistent improvement with increasing age. Furthermore, the reliability of the estimations of parents was rather low.

Below the age of 10–12 years, the amount of time spent at a certain level of activity is difficult to recall. Baranowski (1988) demonstrated in children that if context-specific times such as before school, during school and after school were probed, the results improved compared with direct observation. More objective data are obtained when direct observations are made by an investigator. McKenzie et al. (1991) used 1-min intervals for observatory sampling of the physical activity of 4–9-year-old children and were able to show a significant correlation with HR recordings. However, this procedure is limited as a field method, because the observation area is restricted. The playground at school or summer campground is suitable in this respect, although in this situation, too, children may disappear within a few seconds. Another problem in the time and motion analysis of playing children is the frequent change in activity. Stop watches and recording pads are often inadequate, as is the standard coding list of activities. If observations are to be expressed in terms of energy expenditure, values must be estimated from tables with limited information about children. Time and motion studies are most appropriate when energy expenditure is required in steady-state activities as in an occupational setting. One may question the reliability of the calculated energy expenditure when there is a frequent change in activity without reaching the steady-state values for energy expenditure as given by the tables. Therefore in children the end-product of this method is often descriptive rather than quantitative.

Conclusion

As mentioned above, habitual physical activity is a complex behaviour and can be expressed in different dimensions. Hence the large variety of methods: La Porte et al. (1985) mentioned more than 30 different techniques. However, too often well-known but inaccurate techniques are defended because 'something is better than nothing'. This is especially true in studies with children, because the problems encountered obtaining valid data are numerous in comparison with the adult population. In the last decade progress has been made in bolstering established techniques with information on validity, reliability and practical implications for the child population.

With the introduction of the DLW technique a 'gold standard' for research on physical activity became available. Not only is the advantage of good validity important, but also the ideal situation that the daily physical activity is not hindered by the technique, makes the DLW method even more valuable.

Introduction of the AF also gives insight to the activity component of total energy turnover. The available studies using DLW as a gold standard to evaluate the more traditional methods such as HR and movement counter, offer new insight to the validity of those methods.

For very small groups a direct measurement of oxygen uptake or DLW technique has to be preferred. For larger groups HR recording combined with accelerometers appears to be the most favourable technique. In a large-scale population design, only survey procedures are currently applied. However, the application of validated accelerometers should be strongly encouraged, because of possible inaccurate information from questionnaires.

Furthermore it is suggested that different techniques can be combined. This approach would lead to a more accurate and detailed estimation of physical activity. Especially when a specific analysis is needed, for instance in athletic groups with regard to training load, combinations of overall measurement of energy turnover by DLW and HR and specific training-related information by observation, diary or HR can reveal possible undesirable effects of the training programme on performance.

Challenges for future research

With the increasing involvement of children and adolescents in advanced levels of athletics it is necessary to be informed in detail about the intensity of the training hours and, moreover, about the overall daily energy turnover. At a number of points the available techniques do not fulfil this demand. Therefore, further research is needed, especially directed to the younger age group.

• Until recently the DLW method has not been used in young athletic age groups that have problems related to energy balance such as gymnastics or swimming (intensive endurance training). Valid information about energy turnover and levels of training intensity is needed.

• Although detailed information about energy expenditure of specific activities is available for adults, data for children and adolescents are lacking. Besides this, information of modern sport activities like roller skating, skate-boarding and snow-boarding, surfing and so on is missing for all age groups. Comparable with the development of an updated food table with continuous input of nutrient analysis of new food products, we also need an update activity list including data for children and elderly people.

• With progress in data storage and electronics it is a challenge to develop sophisticated devices, the size of a wristwatch, to record simultaneously physiological functions such as HR and triaxial acceleration over longer periods of time (days or weeks). Adjustment of the HR-oxygen uptake relation based on the triaxial accelerometer input can lead to an improvement of the prediction of energy turnover on bases of the HR recordings.

• Until recently questionnaires regarding daily physical activity have been poorly validated. This is especially true for those developed for the younger age group. Validation studies are urgently needed. In this way a certain level of standardization in questionnaires needs to be developed.

• Application of the different techniques to

groups of children with an expected low or high level of energy turnover, e.g. children with muscular dystrophy and athletes during an intensive training programme, will give more insight to the techniques that measure the level of daily physical activity in children.

References

Ainsworth, B.E., Haskell, W.L., Leon, A.S. *et al.* (1993) Compendium of physical activities: classification of energy costs of human physical activities. *Med. Sci. Sports Exerc.* **25**, 71–80.

Baranowski, T. (1988) Validity and reliability of self report measures of physical activity: an information-processing perspective. *Res. Q. Exerc. Sport* **59**, 314–27.

Croonen, F. & Binkhorst, R.A. (1974) Oxygen uptake calculated from expiratory volume and oxygen analysis only. *Ergonomics* **17**, 113–18.

Durnin, J.V.G.A. & Passmore, R. (1967) *Energy, Work, and Leisure*, pp. 96–105. Heinemann Educational, London.

Emons, H.J.G., Groenenboom, D.C., Westerterp, K.R. & Saris, W.H.M. (1992) Comparison of heart rate monitoring with indirect calorimetry and the doubly labeled water method for the measurement of energy expenditure in children. *Eur. J. Appl. Physiol.* **65**, 99–103.

FAO/WHO/UNU (Food and Agriculture Organization/World Health Organization/United Nations) (1985) *Energy and Protein Requirements*. Technical Report Series No. 724. WHO, Geneva, Switzerland.

Gretebeck, R., Montoye, H.J. & Porter, W. (1991) Comparison of doubly labeled water method for measuring energy expenditure with Caltrac accelerometer recordings. *Med. Sci. Sports Exerc.* **23**, S60 (abstract).

Hebestreit, H., Zehr, P., McKintey, C., Riddel, M. & Bar-Or, O. (1993) Correcting children's heart rate for the influence of climatic heat stress: equation for an improved estimation of energy expenditure. *Pediatr. Exerc. Sci.* **5**, 428 (abstract).

La Porte, R.E., Montoye, H.J. & Caspersen, C.J. (1985) Assessment of physical activity in epidemiologic research: problems and prospects. *Publ. Health Rep.* **100**, 131–46.

Lange Anderssen, K., Rutenfranz, J., Masironi, R. & Seliger, V. (1978) *Habitual Physical Activity and Health*, pp. 105–59. WHO Regional Publications European Series No. 6. WHO, Copenhagen.

Livingstone, M.B.E., Prentice, A.M., Coward, W.A. *et al.* (1990) Simultaneous measurement of free living energy expenditure by the doubly labeled water method and heart rate monitoring. *Am. J. Clin. Nutr.* **52**, 59–65.

McKenzie, T., Sallis, J., Patterson, T. & Elder, J. (1991) BEACHES: an observational system for assessing children's eating and physical activity behaviors and associated events. *J. Appl. Behav. Anal.* **24**, 1–13.

Meijer, G.A.L., Janssen, G.M.E., Westerterp, K.R., Verhoeven, F.M.H., Saris, W.H.M. & Ten Hoor, F. (1991a) The effect of a 5 month endurance training programme on physical activity: evidence for a sex difference in the metabolic response to exercise. *Eur. J. Appl. Physiol.* **62**, 11–17.

Meijer, G.A.L., Westerterp, K.R., Verhoeven, F.M.H., Koper, H.B.M. & Ten Hoor, F. (1991b) Methods to assess physical activity with special references to motion sensors and accelerometers. *IEEE Trans. Biomed. Eng.* **38**, 221–9.

Meijer, G.A.L., Westerterp, K.R., Wouters, L. & Ten Hoor, F. (1990) Validity of the accelerometer in the field: a comparison with the doubly labeled water technique. In G.A.L. Meijer *Physical activity implications for human energy metabolism*, pp. 51–61. Thesis, University of Limburg, Maastricht.

Montoye, H.J. (1982) Age and oxygen utilization during submaximal treadmill exercise in males. *J. Gerontol.* **37**, 396–402.

Prentice, A.M. (ed.) (1990) *The Doubly Labeled Water Method for Measuring Energy Expenditure, Technical Recommendations for Use in Humans*. A consensus report by the IDECG working group. International Atomic Energy Agency, Vienna.

Ravussin, E., Harper, I.T., Rising, R. & Bogardus, L. (1991) Energy expenditure by doubly labeled water: validation in lean and obese subjects. *Am. J. Physiol.* **261**, E402–E409.

Sallis, J.F., Buono, K.J. & Freedson, P.S. (1991) Bias in estimating caloric expenditure from physical activity in children. *Sports Med.* **4**, 203–9.

Saris, W.H.M. (1986) Habitual physical activity in children: methodology and findings in health and disease. *Med. Sci. Sports Exerc.* **18**, 253–63.

Saris, W.H.M. & Binkhorst, R.A. (1977) The use of pedometer and actometer in studying daily physical activity in man. Part I. Reliability of pedometer and actometer. *Eur. J. Appl. Physiol.* **37**, 219–28.

Saris, W.H.M., Binkhorst, R.A., Cramwinckel, B.A., Waesberghe, F. & Veen-Hezemans, A.M. (1980) The relationship between working performance, daily physical activity, fitness, blood lipids and nutrition in schoolchildren. In K. Berg & B.O. Eriksson (eds) *Children and Exercise*, Vol. IX, pp. 166–74. University Park Press, Baltimore.

Saris, W.H.M., Elvers, J.W.H., van't Hoff, M. & Binkhorst, R.A. (1986) Changes in physical activity profiles of children aged 6 to 12 years. In J.

Rutenfranz, R. Mocellin & F. Klimt (eds) *Children and Exercise*, Vol. IXX, pp. 121–30. Human Kinetics, Champaign IL.

Saris, W.H.M., Van Erp, M.A., Brouns, F., Westerterp, K.R. & Ten Hoor, F. (1989) Study on food intake and energy expenditure during extreme sustained exercise: the Tour de France. *Int. J. Sports Med.* **10** (Suppl. 1), S26–31.

Schoeller, D.A., Ravussin, E., Schutz, Y., Acheson, K.J., Baertsch, P. & Jequier, E. (1986) Energy expenditure by doubly labeled water validation in humans and proposed calculation. *Am. J. Physiol.* **250**, R823–30.

Schultz, S., Westerterp, K.R. & Brück, K. (1989) Comparison of energy expenditure by the doubly labeled water technique with energy intake, heart rate and activity recording in man. *Am. J. Clin. Nutr.* **49**, 1146–54.

Schutz, Y., Froideraux, F. & Jequier, E. (1988) Estimation of 24 h energy expenditure by a portable accelerometer. *Proc. Nutr. Soc.* **47A**, 23 (abstract).

Telama, R., Viikari, J. & Välimäki, I. (1985) Arthrosclerosis precursors in Finnish children and adolescents. I. Leisure-time physical activity. *Acta Paediatr. Scand.* **318** (Suppl.) 169–80.

Van Erp-Baart, M.A., Saris, W.H.M., Binkhorst, R.A., Vos, J.A. & Elvers, J.W.H. (1989) Nation wide survey on nutritional habits in élite athletes. Part I. Energy carbohydrate protein and fat intake. *Int. J. Sports Med.* **10** (Suppl. 1), S3–S10.

Van Erp-Baart, M.A., Frederix, L.W.H.M., Lavaleye, T.C.I., Vergouwen, P.C.J. & Saris, W.H.M. (1985) Energy intake and energy expenditure in top female gymnasts. In R.A. Binkhorst, H.C.G. Kemper & W.H.M. Saris (eds) *Children and Exercise*, pp. 218–23. Human Kinetics, Champaign, IL.

Westerterp, K.R., Lafeber, H.N., Sulkers, E.J. & Sauer, P.J. (1991) Comparison of short term indirect calorimetry and doubly labeled water method for flu assessment of energy expenditure in preterm infants. *Biol. Neonate* **60**, 75–82.

Westerterp, K.R., Wouters, L. & Van Marten, L. (1995) The Maastricht protocol for the measurement of body composition and energy expenditure with labelled water. *Obesity Res.* **3**, 49–57.

Chapter 39

Monitoring of Growth and Maturation

ROBERT M. MALINA AND GASTON BEUNEN

Introduction

Growth and maturation are related concepts. Growth refers to the increase in size of the body as a whole or in the size specific parts or segments of the body from conception to adulthood. Maturation, on the other hand, refers to the tempo and timing of progress towards the mature biological state. Growth and maturation are target-seeking; the target is the adult state.

Growth and maturation are important indicators of the health and nutritional status of an individual and the community. The processes underlying growth and maturation are quite plastic and respond to a variety of conditions in the environments in which children are reared.

There is considerable interest in the growth and maturation of children and youths involved in sport. This interest stems from (i) claims of both positive and negative influences of regular training for sport on the growing and maturing individual; (ii) interest in characteristics associated with success in some sports at an early age; (iii) interest in identifying potentially successful athletes at a young age; and (iv) interest in the trainability of children and youths. Conversely, current concerns for the state of fitness or unfitness of children and youths often overlook changes in fitness which accompany normal growth and maturation, and the influence of variation in growth and maturation on measures of fitness.

This chapter presents an overview of pro-cedures of monitoring the growth and maturation of children and youths. The discussion of growth is limited to stature and weight, while that of maturation focuses on the assessment of skeletal, sexual and somatic maturation.

Growth

Overall body size

The monitoring of growth in children and youths in the context of sport is most often limited to weight and stature. Body weight is a measure of body mass, which is a composite of independently varying tissues. Stature or standing height is a linear measurement of the distance from the floor or standing surface to the top (vertex) of the skull. It is a composite of linear dimensions contributed by the lower extremities, trunk, neck and head. Both stature and weight show diurnal variation, which refers to variation in the dimension during the course of a day. This can be a problem in short-term longitudinal studies, in which apparent changes might simply reflect variations in the time of the day at which the measurement was taken.

Measurements of stature and weight indicate size attained or growth status at a given chronological age (CA). Hence, it is imperative to have accurate birth dates. The size of a child or a group of children is ordinarily compared to corresponding data derived from a large sample of children free from overt disease. These data, commonly referred to as growth charts, are reference data, i.e. they are the reference of comparison in evaluating the growth status of a child or group of children. Reference data for statures and weights of a nationally representative sample of American children and youths are presented as smoothed percentiles in Tables 39.1 and 39.2. These data have been recommended for international studies of the nutritional status of children under 10 years of age (Waterlow et al., 1977), and are widely used in evaluating the growth status of children.

Measuring the same child or children at regular intervals over time provides an estimate of growth rate or velocity, i.e. $cm \cdot year^{-1}$ or $kg \cdot year^{-1}$. Rates of growth vary considerably among children and with the season of the year. They are also influenced by the interval between observations.

Butler et al. (1990) have suggested that the overall pattern of statural growth during childhood is somewhat cyclical with a mean peak interval of about 2 years in boys and girls.

Cycles continue until interrupted by the onset of the adolescent spurt (discussed below). More recently, Lampl et al. (1992) have shown that over very short periods of time (days or weeks), there is much variation in growth velocity. During the first 2 years of life, growth in length apparently proceeds in a 'saltatory' manner with series of stepwise increases or jumps separated by variable periods of no growth (stasis). When weekly measurements are made, the periods of stasis vary in length from 7 to 63 days.

The use of increments between adjacent ages must thus be used with care. The continuous growth process is overlooked by simply connecting adjacent points and two measurement errors are involved. Distributions of increments also tend to be skewed. In addition, successive increments are negatively related (van't Hof et al., 1976).

Although the use of increments has limitations, when used carefully, they can provide useful information on growth rates. Percentiles

Table 39.1 Smooth percentiles of stature (cm) for American children and youths. Data are from the US National Center for Health Statistics (Hamill et al., 1977). Percentiles were smoothed by cubic spline approximation. Age intervals are 6 months, e.g. 2.5 years = 2.26 − 2.75.

Age (years)	Smoothed percentile						
	5th	10th	25th	50th	75th	90th	95th
Males							
2.5	85.4	86.5	88.5	90.4	92.9	95.6	97.8
3.0	89.0	90.3	92.6	94.9	97.5	100.1	102.0
3.5	92.5	93.9	96.4	99.1	101.7	104.3	106.1
4.0	95.8	97.3	100.0	102.9	105.7	108.2	109.9
4.5	98.9	100.6	103.4	106.6	109.4	111.9	113.5
5.0	102.0	103.7	106.5	109.9	112.8	115.4	117.0
5.5	104.9	106.7	109.6	113.1	116.1	118.7	120.3
6.0	107.7	109.6	112.5	116.1	119.2	121.9	123.5
6.5	110.4	112.3	115.3	119.0	122.2	124.9	126.6
7.0	113.0	115.0	118.0	121.7	125.0	127.9	129.7
7.5	115.6	117.6	120.6	124.4	127.8	130.8	132.7
8.0	118.1	120.2	123.2	127.0	130.5	133.6	135.7
8.5	120.5	122.7	125.7	129.6	133.2	136.5	138.8
9.0	122.9	125.2	128.2	132.2	136.0	139.4	141.8
9.5	125.3	127.6	130.8	134.8	138.8	142.4	144.9
10.0	127.7	130.1	133.4	137.5	141.6	145.5	148.1
10.5	130.1	132.6	136.0	140.3	144.6	148.7	151.5

Continued

Table 39.1 (*Continued*).

Age (years)	Smoothed percentile						
	5th	10th	25th	50th	75th	90th	95th
11.0	132.6	135.1	138.7	143.3	147.8	152.1	154.9
11.5	135.0	137.7	141.5	146.4	151.1	155.6	158.5
12.0	137.6	140.3	144.4	149.7	154.6	159.4	162.3
12.5	140.2	143.0	147.4	153.0	158.2	163.2	166.1
13.0	142.9	145.8	150.5	156.5	161.8	167.0	169.8
13.5	145.7	148.7	153.6	159.9	165.3	170.5	173.4
14.0	148.8	151.8	156.9	163.1	168.5	173.8	176.7
14.5	152.0	155.0	160.1	166.2	171.5	176.6	179.5
15.0	155.2	158.2	163.3	169.0	174.1	178.9	181.9
15.5	158.3	161.2	166.2	171.5	176.3	180.8	183.9
16.0	161.1	163.9	168.7	173.5	178.1	182.4	185.4
16.5	163.4	166.1	170.6	175.2	179.5	183.6	186.6
17.0	164.9	167.7	171.9	176.2	180.5	184.4	187.3
17.5	165.6	168.5	172.4	176.7	181.0	185.0	187.6
18.0	165.7	168.7	172.3	176.8	181.2	185.3	187.6
Females							
2.5	84.6	85.3	87.3	90.0	92.5	95.0	96.6
3.0	88.3	89.3	91.4	94.1	96.6	99.0	100.6
3.5	91.7	93.0	95.2	97.9	100.5	102.8	104.5
4.0	95.0	96.4	98.8	101.6	104.3	106.6	108.3
4.5	98.1	99.7	102.2	105.0	107.9	110.2	112.0
5.0	101.1	102.7	105.4	108.4	111.4	113.8	115.6
5.5	103.9	105.6	108.4	111.6	114.8	117.4	119.2
6.0	106.6	108.4	111.3	114.6	118.1	120.8	122.7
6.5	109.2	111.0	114.1	117.6	121.3	124.2	126.1
7.0	111.8	113.6	116.8	120.6	124.4	127.6	129.5
7.5	114.4	116.2	119.5	123.5	127.5	130.9	132.9
8.0	116.9	118.7	122.2	126.4	130.6	134.2	136.2
8.5	119.5	121.3	124.9	129.3	133.6	137.4	139.6
9.0	122.1	123.9	127.7	132.2	136.7	140.7	142.9
9.5	124.8	126.6	130.6	135.2	139.8	143.9	146.2
10.0	127.5	129.5	133.6	138.3	142.9	147.2	149.5
10.5	130.4	132.5	136.7	141.5	146.1	150.4	152.8
11.0	133.5	135.6	140.0	144.8	149.3	153.7	156.2
11.5	136.6	139.0	143.5	148.2	152.6	156.9	159.5
12.0	139.8	142.3	147.0	151.5	155.8	160.0	162.7
12.5	142.7	145.4	150.1	154.6	158.8	162.9	165.6
13.0	145.2	148.0	152.8	157.1	161.3	165.3	168.1
13.5	147.2	150.0	154.7	159.0	163.2	167.3	170.0
14.0	148.7	151.5	155.9	160.4	164.6	168.7	171.3
14.5	149.7	152.5	156.8	161.2	165.6	169.8	172.2
15.0	150.5	153.2	157.2	161.8	166.3	170.5	172.8
15.5	151.1	153.6	157.5	162.1	166.7	170.9	173.1
16.0	151.6	154.1	157.8	162.4	166.9	171.1	173.3
16.5	152.2	154.6	158.2	162.7	167.1	171.2	173.4
17.0	152.7	155.1	158.7	163.1	167.3	171.2	173.5
17.5	153.2	155.6	159.1	163.4	167.5	171.1	173.5
18.0	153.6	156.0	159.6	163.7	167.6	171.0	173.6

Table 39.2 Smooth percentiles of body weight (kg) for American children and youths. Data are from the US National Center for Health Statistics (Hamill *et al.*, 1977). Percentiles were smoothed by cubic spline approximation. Age intervals are 6 months, e.g. 2.5 years = 2.26 − 2.75.

Age (years)	Smoothed percentile						
	5th	10th	25th	50th	75th	90th	95th
Males							
2.5	11.27	11.77	12.55	13.52	14.61	15.71	16.61
3.0	12.05	12.58	13.52	14.62	15.78	16.95	17.77
3.5	12.84	13.41	14.46	15.58	16.90	18.15	18.98
4.0	13.64	14.24	15.39	16.69	17.99	19.32	20.27
4.5	14.45	15.10	16.30	17.69	19.06	20.50	21.63
5.0	15.27	15.96	17.22	18.67	20.14	21.70	23.09
5.5	16.09	16.83	18.14	19.67	21.25	22.96	24.66
6.0	16.93	17.72	19.07	20.69	22.40	24.31	26.34
6.5	17.78	18.62	20.02	21.74	23.62	25.76	28.16
7.0	18.64	19.53	21.00	22.85	24.94	27.36	30.12
7.5	19.52	20.45	22.02	24.03	26.36	29.11	32.73
8.0	20.40	21.39	23.09	25.30	27.91	31.06	34.51
8.5	21.31	22.34	24.21	26.66	29.61	33.22	36.96
9.0	22.25	23.33	25.40	28.13	31.46	35.57	39.58
9.5	23.25	24.38	26.68	29.73	33.46	38.11	42.35
10.0	24.33	25.52	28.07	31.44	35.61	40.80	45.27
10.5	25.51	26.78	29.59	33.30	37.92	43.63	48.31
11.0	26.80	28.17	31.25	35.30	40.38	46.57	51.47
11.5	28.24	29.72	33.08	37.46	43.00	49.61	54.73
12.0	29.85	31.46	35.09	39.78	45.77	52.73	58.09
12.5	31.64	33.41	37.31	42.27	48.70	55.91	61.52
13.0	33.64	35.60	39.74	44.95	51.79	59.12	65.02
13.5	35.85	38.03	42.40	47.81	55.02	62.35	68.51
14.0	38.22	40.64	45.21	50.77	58.31	65.57	72.13
14.5	40.66	43.34	48.08	53.76	61.58	68.76	75.66
15.0	43.11	46.06	50.92	56.71	64.72	71.91	79.12
15.5	45.50	48.69	53.64	59.51	67.64	74.98	82.45
16.0	47.74	51.16	56.16	62.10	70.26	77.97	85.62
16.5	49.76	53.39	58.38	64.39	72.46	80.84	88.59
17.0	51.50	55.28	60.22	66.31	74.17	83.58	91.31
17.5	52.89	56.78	61.61	67.78	75.32	86.14	93.73
18.0	53.97	57.89	62.61	68.88	76.04	88.41	95.76
Females							
2.5	10.80	11.35	12.11	13.03	14.23	15.16	15.76
3.0	11.61	12.26	13.11	14.10	15.50	16.54	17.22
3.5	12.37	13.08	14.00	15.07	16.59	17.77	18.59
4.0	13.11	13.84	14.80	15.96	17.56	18.93	19.91
4.5	13.83	14.56	15.55	16.81	18.48	20.06	21.24
5.0	14.55	15.26	16.29	17.66	19.39	21.23	22.62
5.5	15.29	15.97	17.05	18.56	20.36	22.48	24.11
6.0	16.05	16.72	17.86	19.52	21.44	23.89	25.75
6.5	16.85	17.51	18.76	20.61	22.68	25.50	27.59
7.0	17.71	18.39	19.78	21.84	24.16	27.39	29.68
7.5	18.62	19.37	20.95	23.26	25.90	29.57	32.07
8.0	19.62	20.45	22.26	24.84	27.88	32.04	34.71
8.5	20.68	21.64	23.70	26.58	30.08	34.73	37.58
9.0	21.82	22.92	25.27	28.46	32.44	37.60	40.64

Continued

Table 39.2 (*Continued*).

Age (years)	Smoothed percentile						
	5th	10th	25th	50th	75th	90th	95th
9.5	23.05	24.29	26.94	30.45	34.94	40.61	43.85
10.0	24.36	25.76	28.71	32.55	37.53	43.70	47.17
10.5	25.75	27.32	30.57	34.72	40.17	46.84	50.57
11.0	27.24	28.97	32.49	36.95	42.84	49.96	54.00
11.5	28.83	30.71	34.48	39.23	45.48	53.03	57.42
12.0	30.52	32.53	36.52	41.53	48.07	55.99	60.81
12.5	32.30	34.42	38.59	43.84	50.56	58.81	64.12
13.0	34.14	36.35	40.65	46.10	52.91	61.45	67.30
13.5	35.98	38.26	42.65	48.26	55.11	63.87	70.30
14.0	37.76	40.11	44.54	50.28	57.09	66.04	73.08
14.5	39.45	41.83	46.28	52.10	58.84	67.95	75.59
15.0	40.99	43.38	47.82	53.68	60.32	69.54	77.78
15.5	42.32	44.72	49.10	54.96	61.48	70.79	79.59
16.0	43.41	45.78	50.09	55.89	62.29	71.68	80.99
16.5	44.20	46.54	50.75	56.44	62.75	72.18	81.93
17.0	44.74	47.04	51.14	56.69	62.91	72.38	82.46
17.5	45.08	47.33	51.33	56.71	62.89	72.37	82.62
18.0	45.26	47.47	51.39	56.62	62.78	72.25	82.47

for 6-monthly increments in stature and weight of American children from the Fels longitudinal study (Baumgartner *et al.*, 1986), and for annual velocities for stature and weight of Swiss children from the first Zurich longitudinal study (Prader *et al.*, 1989) are presented in Tables 39.3–39.6.

The pattern of change in stature and weight is generally similar in all children. However, size attained at a given age, rates of growth and the timing of the adolescent growth spurt vary considerably among children. The timing of the adolescent spurt is considered with indicators of maturation.

Other body dimensions

Much of the variation in human morphology during growth and maturation relates to the development of skeletal, muscle and adipose tissues, as well as the viscera. Thus, in addition to stature and weight, other dimensions taken in the monitoring of growth often focus on bone, muscle and fat. Skeletal breadth measurements are taken across specific bone landmarks, and therefore, provide an indication of

the robustness or sturdiness of the skeleton. Skeletal length measurements are also taken between specific landmarks, but the most commonly used length measurement, leg length, is ordinarily estimated by subtracting sitting height from stature. Limb circumferences are indicators of relative muscularity. A circumference, of course, includes bone, surrounded by a mass of muscle tissue, which is ringed by a layer of subcutaneous fat. Thus, they do not provide measures of muscle tissue *per se*; however, since muscle is the major tissue comprising the circumference, limb circumferences indicate relative muscular development. Skinfold thicknesses are indicators of subcutaneous fat and are measured as a double fold of skin and underlying subcutaneous tissue.

Dimensions selected for measurement in a sample of children and youths depend upon the purpose of the study, i.e. the specific question(s) under consideration. Thus, no single battery of measurements will meet the needs of every study. In addition, measurements used in field studies (i.e. studies not performed in a clinical setting) are often selected

Table 39.3 Percentiles of 6-month increments in stature (cm per 6 months) from the Fels longitudinal study. Adapted from Baumgartner *et al.* (1986).

Age at end of interval (years)	Percentiles for males (cm per 6 months)							Age at end of interval (years)	Percentiles for females (cm per 6 months)						
	5	10	25	50	75	90	95		5	10	25	50	75	90	95
6.0	2.07	2.43	2.93	3.35	3.67	4.10	4.23	6.0	2.23	2.46	2.84	3.30	3.75	4.10	4.49
6.5	2.07	2.31	2.76	3.21	3.60	3.96	4.22	6.5	1.93	2.20	2.60	3.11	3.49	3.94	4.29
7.0	2.24	2.45	2.70	3.19	3.53	3.93	4.11	7.0	2.11	2.36	2.66	3.08	3.50	3.81	3.98
7.5	2.01	2.20	2.62	2.99	3.45	3.88	4.11	7.5	1.98	2.23	2.64	3.07	3.39	3.67	4.03
8.0	1.86	2.18	2.51	3.02	3.45	3.75	3.90	8.0	1.82	2.17	2.56	3.01	3.35	3.85	4.07
8.5	2.01	2.23	2.59	2.96	3.21	3.56	3.79	8.5	1.86	1.99	2.41	2.88	3.27	3.68	3.90
9.0	1.89	2.11	2.45	2.84	3.21	3.52	3.67	9.0	1.93	2.13	2.47	2.84	3.22	3.53	3.77
9.5	1.61	1.83	2.28	2.67	2.96	3.36	3.64	9.5	1.78	1.95	2.36	2.80	3.29	3.58	3.92
10.0	1.89	2.06	2.35	2.70	3.06	3.44	3.69	10.0	1.70	1.99	2.38	2.91	3.28	3.83	4.38
10.5	1.56	1.83	2.14	2.56	2.93	3.38	3.67	10.5	1.64	1.99	2.37	2.82	3.56	4.21	4.70
11.0	1.68	1.87	2.22	2.52	2.96	3.43	3.74	11.0	1.87	2.08	2.53	3.06	3.74	4.33	4.76
11.5	1.69	1.86	2.20	2.57	3.06	3.70	4.00	11.5	1.84	2.09	2.54	3.34	4.02	4.63	4.84
12.0	1.60	1.86	2.24	2.73	3.27	4.07	4.68	12.0	1.60	1.98	2.65	3.32	3.98	4.52	4.86
12.5	1.49	1.83	2.20	2.77	3.53	4.93	5.44	12.5	1.11	1.61	2.41	3.19	3.87	4.38	4.58
13.0	1.87	2.10	2.55	3.29	4.45	5.22	5.75	13.0	0.52	1.05	1.99	2.76	3.46	4.09	4.21
13.5	1.55	2.19	2.75	3.49	4.41	5.03	5.31	13.5	0.35	0.57	1.20	1.98	2.90	3.56	3.92
14.0	1.84	2.15	2.93	4.01	4.64	5.21	5.49	14.0	−0.09	0.28	0.78	1.33	2.35	3.11	3.66
14.5	1.51	1.75	2.60	3.59	4.54	5.26	5.48	14.5	−0.21	0.04	0.47	0.88	1.65	2.77	2.97
15.0	0.90	1.42	2.26	3.19	4.01	4.66	5.11	15.0	−0.47	−0.16	0.24	0.68	1.24	1.75	2.33
15.5	0.32	0.66	1.24	2.05	3.26	4.28	4.66	15.5	−0.67	−0.43	0.07	0.49	0.83	1.27	1.62
16.0	0.12	0.60	0.94	1.56	2.48	3.57	3.91	16.0	−0.48	−0.33	0.04	0.46	0.75	1.08	1.42
16.5	−0.50	0.03	0.44	0.94	1.50	2.44	2.98	16.5	−0.61	−0.37	−0.05	0.23	0.63	0.91	1.02
17.0	−0.55	−0.16	0.25	0.83	1.33	1.94	2.85	17.0	−0.84	−0.65	−0.13	0.19	0.56	0.81	0.94
17.5	−0.66	−0.37	0.12	0.41	1.00	1.43	1.73	17.5	−0.74	−0.51	−0.21	0.04	0.38	0.97	1.25
18.0	−0.55	−0.33	−0.03	0.32	0.72	1.01	1.45	18.0	−0.78	−0.64	−0.15	0.09	0.46	0.83	1.05

on the basis of site location and accessibility, although local cultural preferences may limit the accessibility of some measurements, e.g. chest circumference or some trunk skinfolds in adolescent girls. Procedures for taking a variety of measurements, based on discussions at a standardization conference, are described in Lohman *et al.* (1988), and are also described in Chapter 34.

Most body dimensions, with the exception of subcutaneous fat and dimensions of the head and face, follow the same general pattern of growth in size attained and rate as do stature and weight. Reference and comparative data for a variety of anthropometric dimensions of North American children and youths, including the nationally representative sample of

American children, have been compiled by Roche and Malina (1983) and Malina and Roche (1983).

Measurement variability

Implicit in studies utilizing body measurements is the assumption that every effort is made to ensure reliability, accuracy of measurement and standardization of technique. It is assumed that measurements are made by trained observers. This is essential to obtain reliable and accurate data, and to enhance the usefulness of the data from the comparative perspective. Furthermore, reliable and accurate data are particularly critical in serial studies, short or long term, in which the definition of

Table 39.4 Percentiles of 6-month increments in body weight (kg per 6 months) from the Fels longitudinal study. Adapted from Baumgartner *et al.* (1986).

Age at end of interval (years)	Percentiles for males (kg per 6 months)							Age at end of interval (years)	Percentiles for females (kg per 6 months)						
	5	10	25	50	75	90	95		5	10	25	50	75	90	95
6.0	0.24	0.45	0.82	1.18	1.54	2.01	2.23	6.0	0.23	0.44	0.78	1.12	1.44	1.97	2.49
6.5	0.21	0.51	0.90	1.16	1.54	2.07	2.34	6.5	0.28	0.48	0.83	1.19	1.63	2.00	2.54
7.0	0.33	0.49	0.88	1.26	1.75	2.25	2.53	7.0	0.28	0.44	0.80	1.18	1.59	2.27	2.52
7.5	0.40	0.60	0.92	1.38	1.79	2.40	2.87	7.5	0.36	0.61	0.95	1.32	1.81	2.47	3.03
8.0	0.34	0.63	1.00	1.52	1.93	2.54	3.23	8.0	0.14	0.39	0.92	1.36	1.98	2.73	3.21
8.5	0.28	0.45	1.01	1.43	2.07	2.77	3.35	8.5	0.26	0.53	1.00	1.48	2.06	2.87	3.36
9.0	0.02	0.50	0.95	1.56	2.28	2.95	3.58	9.0	0.31	0.62	1.02	1.47	2.20	2.97	3.51
9.5	0.21	0.51	0.96	1.54	2.26	3.05	3.60	9.5	0.37	0.58	1.02	1.53	2.48	3.27	3.90
10.0	0.08	0.38	1.18	1.70	2.38	3.14	3.92	10.0	0.14	0.44	1.05	1.57	2.36	3.48	4.35
10.5	0.22	0.56	1.09	1.61	2.65	3.63	4.30	10.5	0.23	0.53	1.17	1.96	2.87	4.04	4.80
11.0	0.20	0.53	1.01	1.73	2.46	3.51	4.01	11.0	−0.12	0.70	1.28	2.01	3.22	3.94	4.63
11.5	0.34	0.66	1.24	1.91	3.03	4.33	4.99	11.5	0.28	0.88	1.39	2.48	3.44	4.39	4.97
12.0	−0.21	0.54	1.30	2.00	3.27	4.24	4.85	12.0	0.31	0.68	1.68	2.74	3.90	5.11	5.47
12.5	−0.01	0.60	1.35	2.45	3.47	4.79	5.36	12.5	−0.09	0.51	1.43	2.76	3.69	4.79	5.63
13.0	0.54	0.94	1.71	2.81	3.92	5.29	6.17	13.0	−0.78	−0.03	1.40	2.15	3.26	4.15	4.76
13.5	0.37	0.62	1.73	3.06	4.20	5.31	5.81	13.5	−0.40	0.47	1.28	2.31	3.48	4.64	5.14
14.0	−0.06	0.95	2.20	3.33	4.23	5.71	6.56	14.0	−1.52	−0.61	0.51	1.83	3.11	4.13	4.61
14.5	−0.06	1.08	2.60	3.67	4.57	5.72	6.41	14.5	−2.15	−1.12	0.41	1.50	2.51	3.67	3.94
15.0	−0.72	0.44	1.87	3.24	4.48	5.73	6.34	15.0	−1.94	−0.92	−0.01	1.00	2.33	3.45	3.91
15.5	−1.25	0.10	1.46	2.59	3.79	5.34	6.26	15.5	−2.01	−1.23	−0.01	0.92	2.00	2.92	3.73
16.0	−1.36	−0.33	1.03	2.18	3.54	5.07	6.18	16.0	−2.85	−2.10	−0.76	0.37	1.27	2.08	2.96
16.5	−1.68	−0.73	0.45	1.69	2.97	3.85	5.18	16.5	−2.48	−1.60	−0.20	0.75	1.66	2.82	3.44
17.0	−2.32	−1.63	−0.17	1.21	2.54	3.57	4.37	17.0	−2.51	−1.96	−0.59	0.64	1.46	2.54	3.00
17.5	−2.57	−1.21	−0.00	1.09	2.52	3.99	5.43	17.5	−2.52	−1.75	−0.86	0.40	1.32	2.45	3.08
18.0	−3.05	−2.04	−0.58	0.77	2.24	3.82	4.97	18.0	−3.11	−1.41	−0.72	0.47	1.55	2.93	3.68

rather small changes is necessary and errors of measurement can mask the true changes. Therefore, quality control and careful monitoring of the measurement process are essential. Duplicate measurements taken independently on the same individual by either the same technician or by two different technicians can be used to estimate interobserver and intra-observer measurement error.

The technical error of measurement (G_e) is a widely used measure of replicability. It is the square root of the sum of the squared differences of replicates divided by twice the number of pairs, i.e. the intrasubject variance (Malina *et al.*, 1973):

$$G_e = \sqrt{(\Sigma d^2 / 2n)}$$

where d is the difference between replicate measurements, and n is the number of pairs of replicates.

The statistic assumes that the distribution of replicate differences is normal and that errors of all pairs can be pooled. It indicates that about two-thirds of the time, the measurement in question should fall within $\pm G_e$ (see Mueller & Martorell, 1988 and Marks *et al.*, 1989 for more comprehensive discussions of measurement variability and quality). Examples of intra-observer and interobserver G_e are summarized in Malina (1995).

Ratios and proportions

In addition to providing specific information in their own right, measurements can be related

Table 39.5 Percentiles for cross-sectional stature velocities (cm · year^{-1}) from the first Zurich longitudinal study of growth and development. Adapted from Prader *et al.* (1989).

Age (years)	Smoothed centiles for males (cm · year^{-1})							Age (years)	Smoothed centiles for females (cm · year^{-1})						
	3	10	25	50	75	90	97		3	10	25	50	75	90	97
6.50	4.6	5.3	5.6	6.2	6.7	7.3	7.7	6.50	4.4	5.0	5.5	6.1	6.6	7.0	7.5
7.50	4.6	5.0	5.4	6.0	6.5	7.2	7.5	7.50	4.6	4.9	5.3	5.9	6.4	6.8	7.2
8.50	4.2	4.6	5.0	5.5	6.1	6.5	6.8	8.50	4.0	4.5	5.0	5.5	5.9	6.5	7.1
9.50	3.4	4.0	4.5	4.9	5.4	6.0	6.6	9.25	3.1	3.9	4.4	5.0	5.7	6.5	7.5
10.25	2.5	3.4	4.1	4.8	5.8	6.4	7.1	9.50	2.9	3.7	4.3	5.0	5.8	6.6	7.7
10.75	2.2	3.2	3.9	4.8	5.8	6.4	7.1	9.75	2.7	3.6	4.2	5.0	5.9	6.8	7.9
11.25	2.1	3.0	3.9	4.7	5.5	6.2	7.4	10.25	2.4	3.5	4.2	5.3	6.3	7.3	8.5
11.75	2.3	3.1	4.1	4.9	5.9	7.1	8.8	10.75	2.4	3.6	4.5	5.7	6.8	7.8	8.9
12.25	2.5	3.4	4.3	5.2	6.7	8.4	10.3	11.25	2.7	3.8	4.8	6.1	7.2	8.2	9.3
12.75	2.7	3.7	4.8	5.8	7.9	9.6	11.4	11.75	2.9	3.9	4.9	6.3	7.5	8.5	9.5
13.25	2.8	3.9	5.2	6.6	8.8	10.1	11.9	12.25	2.6	3.6	4.7	6.1	7.5	8.5	9.4
13.75	2.6	4.0	5.4	7.0	9.1	10.4	11.9	12.75	1.9	3.0	4.1	5.5	7.1	8.1	9.1
14.25	2.2	3.6	5.0	6.9	9.0	10.3	11.6	13.25	1.0	2.1	3.3	4.6	6.5	7.5	8.5
14.75	1.6	2.8	4.2	6.2	8.4	9.8	11.0	13.75	0.4	1.3	2.3	3.5	5.5	6.6	7.7
15.25	0.9	1.8	3.0	4.9	7.2	8.8	9.9	14.25	0.1	0.6	1.5	2.5	4.3	5.4	6.7
15.50	0.7	1.4	2.5	4.3	6.4	8.1	9.2	14.75	0.0	0.2	0.9	1.7	3.2	4.2	5.7
15.75	0.4	1.0	2.0	3.6	5.5	7.3	8.5	15.25		0.0	0.1	1.1	2.1	3.1	4.6
16.25	0.1	0.5	1.2	2.3	3.8	5.4	6.8	15.50			0.4	0.9	1.7	2.6	4.0
16.50	0.0	0.3	0.9	1.8	3.0	4.4	6.0	15.75			0.3	0.8	1.4	2.2	3.5
16.75		0.2	0.7	1.4	2.4	3.6	5.2	16.50			0.1	0.5	0.8	1.3	2.0
17.50		0.0	0.2	0.6	1.2	1.9	3.1	17.50			0.0	0.1	0.4	0.7	1.0
18.50			0.1	0.4	0.7	1.3	1.9	18.50				0.0	0.3	0.6	0.8
19.50			0.0	0.0	0.5	1.0	1.2	19.50					0.0	0.2	0.6

to each other in the form of indices or ratios. Ratios thus provide information on body shape and proportions. Two commonly used ratios are described, although any two measurements can be related to each other.

The relationship between weight and stature is commonly expressed as the body mass index:

weight/stature^2

where weight is in kilograms and stature is in metres. Although the body mass index grades reasonably well on total body fatness and finds wide use in studies of the overweight and obesity, its utility in childhood, in adolescent males and with young athletes is questionable.

The ratio of sitting height to stature,

$$\frac{\text{sitting height}}{\text{stature}} \times 100$$

provides an estimate of relative trunk length, and conversely relative leg length. It basically asks what percentage height while standing is accounted for by height while sitting. By subtraction, the remaining percentage is accounted for by the lower extremities. The ratio decreases from infancy to adolescence, and then increases slightly in late adolescence. It is useful in studies of population variation in the proportional contribution of lower extremity length to stature (Malina & Bouchard, 1991).

Maturation

Maturation varies according to the biological system used, but the more commonly used maturity indicators in growth studies are reasonably well related. They include maturation of the skeleton, sexual maturation, timing of the adolescent growth spurt and percentage

Table 39.6 Percentiles for cross-sectional body weight velocities (kg·year^{-1}) from the first Zurich longitudinal study of growth and development. Adapted from Prader *et al.* (1989).

Age (years)	Smoothed centiles for males (kg·year^{-1})							Age (years)	Smoothed centiles for females (kg·year^{-1})						
	3	10	25	50	75	90	97		3	10	25	50	75	90	97
6.50	0.88	1.35	1.68	2.27	2.80	3.55	4.44	6.50	0.85	1.38	1.85	2.41	2.84	3.48	4.58
7.50	0.78	1.37	1.83	2.58	3.00	3.82	4.69	7.50	0.84	1.43	1.89	2.40	3.11	4.01	5.07
8.50	0.63	1.59	2.19	2.69	3.19	4.02	4.88	8.50	0.71	1.41	2.03	2.77	3.59	4.80	6.15
9.50	0.41	1.51	2.23	2.69	3.52	4.39	5.78	9.25	0.43	1.23	2.06	3.03	4.22	5.64	7.51
10.25	0.21	1.02	1.90	2.76	4.12	5.22	7.23	9.50	0.31	1.15	2.06	3.08	4.45	5.94	8.00
10.75	0.05	0.79	1.82	2.94	4.46	5.82	8.28	9.75	0.18	1.07	2.08	3.11	4.70	6.25	8.49
11.25	−0.11	0.72	1.85	3.21	4.74	6.49	9.23	10.25	−0.08	0.99	2.18	3.29	5.23	6.87	9.43
11.75	−0.29	0.83	2.00	3.58	4.95	7.25	10.07	10.75	−0.32	1.05	2.36	3.69	5.83	7.46	10.27
12.25	−0.47	1.08	2.31	4.10	5.44	8.15	10.80	11.25	−0.55	1.15	2.55	4.23	6.40	7.95	10.91
12.75	−0.66	1.41	2.80	4.71	6.47	9.10	11.41	11.75	−0.81	1.15	2.66	4.72	6.84	8.30	11.27
13.25	−0.87	1.73	3.36	5.30	7.58	9.87	11.85	12.25	−1.10	1.01	2.66	5.04	7.06	8.48	11.38
13.75	−1.08	1.85	3.73	5.74	8.32	10.31	12.06	12.75	−1.47	0.67	2.52	5.05	7.03	8.47	11.31
14.25	−1.30	1.73	3.74	5.89	8.63	10.32	11.98	13.25	−1.88	0.20	2.23	4.74	6.72	8.29	11.04
14.75	−1.53	1.41	3.44	5.71	8.31	9.89	11.58	13.75	−2.32	−0.33	1.80	4.16	6.19	7.95	10.57
15.25	−1.76	0.99	2.95	5.20	7.47	9.06	10.86	14.25	−2.76	−0.86	1.28	3.41	5.48	7.48	9.94
15.50	−1.88	0.77	2.64	4.85	6.96	8.54	10.41	14.75	−3.22	−1.34	0.73	2.59	4.69	6.91	9.14
15.75	−2.00	0.54	2.31	4.44	6.44	7.97	9.92	15.25	−3.65	−1.75	0.23	1.89	3.91	6.29	8.22
16.25	−2.25	0.15	1.69	3.57	5.35	6.79	8.93	15.50	−3.86	−1.92	0.01	1.61	3.55	5.98	7.76
16.50	−2.38	−0.03	1.39	3.14	4.81	6.24	8.47	15.75	−4.06	−2.08	−0.17	1.37	3.24	5.67	7.32
16.75	−2.51	−0.21	1.11	2.75	4.29	5.74	8.06	16.50	−4.60	−2.44	−0.57	0.87	2.47	4.81	6.14
17.50	−2.90	−0.72	0.42	1.81	3.09	4.64	7.15	17.50	−5.06	−2.58	−0.74	0.51	1.74	3.80	4.98
18.50	−3.44	−1.29	0.04	1.05	2.46	3.92	6.41	18.50	−5.27	−2.33	−0.60	0.15	1.09	2.93	4.47
19.50	−3.99	−2.00	−0.04	0.51	2.10	3.31	5.53	19.50	−5.39	−1.85	−0.36	−0.05	0.30	2.10	4.39

of adult stature attained at a given age. Eruption and calcification of the teeth are occasionally used as maturity indicators, but they are independent of other maturity indicators. Dental maturation thus has limited utility in the sport sciences and will not be considered (see Demirjian, 1986).

Skeletal maturation

The bones of the hand and wrist provide the primary basis for assessing skeletal maturation, which is based upon changes in the developing skeleton which can be easily viewed and evaluated on a standardized radiograph. Traditionally, the left hand and wrist is used. It is placed flat on the X-ray plate with the fingers slightly apart. Hence, when a film is viewed, the hand–wrist skeleton is observed from the dorsal

(posterior) as opposed to the palmar (anterior) surface.

The changes which each bone goes through from initial ossification to adult morphology are fairly uniform and provide the basis for assessing skeletal maturation. These are referred to as maturity indicators, specific features of individual bones which can be noted on a hand–wrist X-ray and which occur regularly and in a definite, irreversible order (Greulich & Pyle, 1959).

Three methods are available for assessing skeletal maturity of the hand and wrist, the Greulich–Pyle (GP) (Greulich & Pyle, 1959), Tanner–Whitehouse (TW) (Tanner *et al.*, 1975, 1983) and Fels (Roche *et al.*, 1988) methods. The authors of each method define and describe specific maturity indicators used to make the assessments.

GREULICH—PYLE METHOD

The GP method is based on the original work of Todd (1937) and is sometimes called the atlas or inspectional method. It entails the matching of a hand—wrist X-ray of a specific child as closely as possible with a series of standard X-ray plates, which correspond to successive levels of skeletal maturation at specific CAs. The method is most often used as follows. The age identified as typical of the standard plate with which a given child's film coincides, represents the child's skeletal age (SA). Thus, if the hand—wrist X-ray of a 7-year-old child matches the standard plate for 8-year-old children, the child's SA is 8 years. However, the method was intended to and should be applied by rating the skeletal maturity of each individual bone. Each bone is matched to the standard plates in the atlas in the same manner as above, and the one with which the individual bone most closely coincides is noted. The SA of the standard plate is the assigned SA of the bone in question. The process is repeated for all bones that are present in the hand and wrist, and the child's SA is the median of the SAs of each individually rated bone.

TANNER—WHITEHOUSE METHOD

The TW method, sometimes called the bone-specific approach, entails matching features of 20 individual bones to a series of written criteria for stages through which each bone passes from initial appearance on a radiograph to the mature state. The 20 bones include seven carpals (excluding the pisiform) and 13 long bones (radius, ulna, and metacarpals and phalanges of the 1st, 3rd and 5th digits). Each stage is assigned a specific point score and the scores are summed to give a skeletal maturity score. The sum can be converted to an SA, which is referred to as the 20-bone SA. The revised TW method (TWII) provides a carpal SA based on the seven carpals and a radius, ulna and short bone (RUS) SA, in addition to the 20-bone SA.

FELS METHOD

The Fels method is based on the same 20 bones as the TW method plus the pisiform and adductor sesamoid. The authors defined their own maturity indicators and specific criteria for each. They are based on a variety of shape changes and several ratios between linear measurements of the long bones of the hand and wrist. Grades are assigned to the indicators for each bone by matching the film being assessed to the described criteria. The assigned grades and ratios are then entered into a microcomputer which calculates an SA and an SE.

Comparison of methods

Methods of skeletal maturity assessment are similar in principle. All entail matching a hand—wrist radiograph of a child to a set of criteria, pictorial, verbal or both. The methods vary, however, in maturity indicators and criteria for making assessments and in procedures used to construct a scale of skeletal maturity from which SAs are assigned. In the GP method, a child's hand—wrist film is matched to standard plates in the atlas, while in the TW and Fels methods, the child's film is matched to specific criteria for each bone. The Fels method also uses ratios between linear measurements of the long bones of the hand and wrist. The GP method uses all bones of the hand and wrist (30 bones). The TW and Fels methods use 20 bones; however, the Fels method also uses the pisiform and the adductor sesamoid of the 1st metacarpal.

The methods differ in scoring. The GP method assigns an SA based on either the standard plate to which the film of a child is most closely matched, or on the median of the SA assigned to each individual bone. The TW method results in a maturity point score which is based on the sum of the point scores for each of the 20 bones which are rated, or for the seven carpals, or for the 13 long bones. The specific score is then converted to an SA. The provision of carpal and RUS SAs is useful in adolescence since the carpals often attain maturity by 13 years of age or so, while the RUS continue to mature. The Fels method provides an SA with an SE; this is a unique feature which is not available with the GP and TW methods. The computation procedure for determining SA in the Fels method weights the contributions of specific indicators depending on the age of the child. For example, epiphyseal union of the radius may occur over several years while the appearance of a specific shape of another bone may be present only for a short period of time. Hence, the radius is given less statistical weight and the other bone more weight in calculating the SA.

Skeletal age

All of the methods for the estimation of skeletal maturity yield an SA which corresponds to the level of skeletal maturity attained by a child relative to the reference sample. In the GP method, the reference sample is American children in the Cleveland area of Ohio studied between 1931 and 1942; in the TW method, the reference sample is British children from several areas of the country studied between 1946 and 1972 (Beunen *et al.*, 1990 have reported more recent TWII reference data for Belgian youth); in the Fels method, the reference sample is the Fels longitudinal study which includes. American children from southern Ohio studied between 1932 and 1972. Given the differences in the methods as well as in the reference samples for each, the skeletal maturity status of a child rated by all three methods may be quite different. It is important that the method used to estimate SA be specified.

SA is expressed relative to a child's CA. It may simply be compared to CA, e.g. a child's CA is 10.5 years while his or her SA is 12.3 years. In this instance, the child has attained the skeletal maturity equivalent to that of a child of 12.3 years, and is advanced in skeletal maturity. Or, a child's CA may be 10.5 years but his or her SA is 9.0 years. The child is chronologically 10.5 years of age, while he or she has only attained the skeletal maturity of a 9.0-year-old child; this child is late in skeletal

maturity. SA may also be expressed as the difference between SA and CA, i.e. SA−CA. Thus, in the first example given above, 12.3−10.5 = +1.8 years, while in the second example, 9.0−10.5 = −1.5 years. Skeletal maturity is advanced in the former by 1.8 years and is late in the latter by 1.5 years relative to CA.

SA assessment is a method to estimate the level of maturity which a child has attained at a given point in time relative to reference data for healthy children. The three methods for assessing skeletal maturity have their strengths and limitations. It is important to note, however, that SAs derived from the GP, TW and Fels method are not equivalent. The methods differ in criteria, scoring and the reference samples upon which they are based. There are, in addition, apparent population differences in skeletal maturation. For example, skeletal maturation is somewhat advanced in American Black compared to American White girls (see Malina & Bouchard, 1991). The changes that each bone goes through from initial formation to epiphyseal union or adult morphology, however, are the same; the rate at which the process progresses varies among populations.

Each of the methods has advantages and disadvantages. The TW method is perhaps the more widely used method at present. The Fels method is relatively new, and as with other new procedures, acceptance and dissemination is a slow process. The GP method is widely used clinically and is good for identifying individuals who are very advanced or very delayed in skeletal maturation. It is not as finely tuned as the TW and Fels methods.

Sexual maturation

The assessment of sexual maturation is based upon the development of the secondary sex characteristics, i.e. breast development and menarche in girls, penis and testes (genital) development in boys, and pubic hair in both sexes. The use of secondary sex characteristics as indicators is obviously limited to the pubertal or adolescent phase of growth and maturation.

BREAST, GENITAL AND PUBIC HAIR DEVELOPMENT

The development of secondary sex characteristics is ordinarily summarized into scales of five stages or grades for each characteristic. The most commonly used criteria for pubic hair, breast and genital maturation are those described by Tanner (1962), which are based in part upon the criteria of earlier studies (e.g. Greulich et al., 1942; Reynolds & Wines, 1948, 1951). Stage 1 indicates the prepubertal state, i.e. the absence of development of each characteristic. Male genitalia, for example, are approximately the same size as in early childhood. Stage 2 indicates the initial development of each characteristic, i.e. the initial elevation of the breasts in girls, the initial enlargement of the genitals in boys, and the initial appearance of pubic hair in both sexes. Stages 3 and 4 indicate continued maturation of each characteristic, and are somewhat more difficult to evaluate. Stage 5 indicates the adult or mature state of development for each characteristic. Tanner's criteria for the evaluation of breast, genital and pubic hair development are readily available in textbooks of physical growth (Tanner, 1962; Malina & Bouchard, 1991). Excellent colour illustrations of the stages from the national survey of Dutch children are given in Roede and Van Wieringen (1985).

Ratings of the stages of sexual maturation are ordinarily made by direct observation at clinical examination. As such, these ratings may have limitations since the method requires invasion of the individual's privacy which is a matter of concern for many adolescents. At times, however, the development of secondary sex characteristics is made from standardized, nude photographs of high quality. As good as the photographs may be, it is often quite difficult to detect the initial appearance of pubic hair. For example, commonly used reference data from the Harpenden growth study of British youth (Marshall & Tanner, 1969, 1970) have somewhat later ages for stage 2 of pubic hair

development. This high value reflects the difficulty in detecting first appearance of pubic hair on photographs. Clinical observation gives better estimates.

There is a need for quality control in the assessment of secondary sex characteristics. How concordant are assessments made by two different examiners or by the same examiner on two independent occasions? Such data are rarely reported.

In practice ratings are used as follows. A girl, for example, may be rated at stage 2 of breast development (B2) and stage 1 for pubic hair (PH1). Thus, breast development has begun, while pubic hair has not yet appeared. This girl is just at the beginning of puberty, since the budding or initial elevation of the breasts (B2) is most often the first overt sign of sexual maturation in girls. Similarly in males, a boy may be rated at stage 2 of genital development (G2) and stage 1 for pubic hair (PH1). He is likewise just beginning puberty, since the initial enlargement of the testes (G2) is most often the first overt sign of sexual maturation in boys.

It should be noted that the development of secondary sex characteristics is a continuous process upon which the stages are superimposed. Thus, the five stages are somewhat arbitrary, as is the case for many developmental scales. For example, a boy just entering G3 of genital development is rated the same as a boy nearing the end of G3, i.e. they are both rated as being in G3. The latter boy is really more advanced in maturation than the former, but given the limitations of the procedure, both are rated as being in G3.

It is common in the paediatric literature to refer to the assessment of secondary sex characteristics as 'Tanner staging'. This is erroneous. Secondary sex characteristics are assessed using the criteria of Tanner. Further, the stages of pubertal development are specific to breasts, genitals and pubic hair. It is incorrect, for example, to take the average of breast and pubic hair stages to characterize the level of sexual maturation of a girl or group of girls.

As a related issue, individuals should not be assessed as being in 'puberty stage 2' or in 'Tanner stage 3'; the specific secondary sex characteristic and its stage should be noted, i.e. genital stage 4 (G4) or pubic hair stage 3 (PH3).

A more direct estimate of genital maturation in males is provided by measurements of testicular volume. It is estimated from the size of the testes using a series of models of known volume which have the shape of the testes (Prader orchidometer). Application of the models requires direct manipulation of the testes at clinical examination as the physician attempts to match the size of the testis with the ellipsoid model that most closely matches it. This procedure, though quite useful, has limited utility in surveys. It is most often used clinically to evaluate boys with extremely late maturation or disorders of growth and sexual maturation.

SELF-REPORTED ASSESSMENT OF SECONDARY SEX CHARACTERISTICS

Given the difficulty in direct assessment of sexual maturation status in non-medical settings, self-assessments by youth are often used (Duke et al., 1980; Kreipe & Gewanter, 1983; Brooks-Gunn et al., 1987; Hammer et al., 1991; Schlossberger et al., 1992). Youngsters are asked to rate their stage of sexual development relative to schematic drawings of stages prepared after the criteria of Tanner (1962). Note that the quality of schematic drawings varies among studies. Occasionally, photographs of the criteria and parental ratings are used. There are limited data on the concordance of self-ratings of youth and those of experienced assessors. In one study of 11–13-year-old girls, correlations between self-ratings and physician ratings of breast and pubic hair were moderate, ranging from 0.52 to 0.74 (Brooks-Gunn et al., 1987). In another study with small numbers, there was a tendency for youngsters to overestimate early stages and underestimate later stages of pubertal development (Schlossberger et al., 1992). The reproducibility of clinical assessments by physicians or other experienced raters is not generally reported, though in fact it should be.

If self-assessments are used, good quality photographs of the stages with simplified descriptions should be used. They should not be used in a group setting. Rather, they should be done individually in a quiet room after careful explanation of the purpose of the assessment.

MENARCHE

Menarche, the first menstrual period, is the most commonly reported indicator of female puberty. Significant value judgements are associated with the attainment of menarche in many cultures. There is no corresponding physiological event in the sexual maturation process of boys, although the psychological importance of puberty in boys cannot be overlooked.

AGES AT ATTAINING STAGES OF SEXUAL MATURATION

The ages at which individual children attain various stages of pubic hair, breast and genital development and attain menarche are ordinarily derived prospectively from longitudinal studies in which children are examined at close intervals during adolescence, usually every 3 months. The time of appearance of each stage and the duration of each stage of secondary sex characteristic development, i.e. how long the individual spends during a particular stage, can be estimated with a reasonable degree of accuracy. In the case of menarche, the girl is interviewed as to whether it has occurred and when. Given that the interval between examinations in most longitudinal studies is relatively short, age at menarche so derived is quite reliable.

Sample sizes in longitudinal studies, however, are not ordinarily large enough to derive population estimates and may not reflect the normal range of variation. Hence, a different method, the status quo method, is used to estimate ages at the attainment of specific secondary sex characteristic stages and of menarche. The resulting estimates apply only to the population and do not apply to individuals. A large sample of boys or girls, which spans the ages at which the particular developmental stage normally occurs, is surveyed. It is most often performed for menarche, but can be performed for the different stages of development of secondary sex characteristics. A representative sample of girls 9–17 years of age is surveyed. Two pieces of information are required: (i) the exact age of each girl; and (ii) whether or not she has attained menarche, i.e. simply yes or no. Status quo data for a nationally representative sample of Flemish girls are shown in Fig. 39.1. The figure shows the percentage of girls in each age class who attained menarche. Probits for each percentage are then plotted for each CA group, and a straight line is fitted to the points. The point at which the line intersects 50% of the points is the estimated median age at menarche for the sample.

Selected percentiles for ages at which specific stages of secondary sex characteristics are attained in a national sample of Dutch youths, based on status quo estimates, are given in

Table 39.7. Median ages at menarche in several samples of North American and European girls are summarized in Table 39.8. The menarcheal data are derived primarily from status quo surveys, but several ages from prospective (longitudinal) studies are also included.

In contrast to the status quo method for estimating the age at menarche, many studies use the retrospective method, which requires the girl to recall the age at which she attained menarche. If the interview is done at close intervals as in longitudinal studies, the method is quite accurate. If it is done some time after menarche, it is affected by error in recall. However, with careful interview procedures, e.g. attempting to place the event in the context of a season or event of the school year or holiday, reasonably accurate estimates of the age at menarche can be obtained from most adolescents and young adults.

Data on ages at menarche in athletes are largely obtained with the retrospective method, and as such, have a margin of error. There is a need for both prospective and status quo surveys of young athletes.

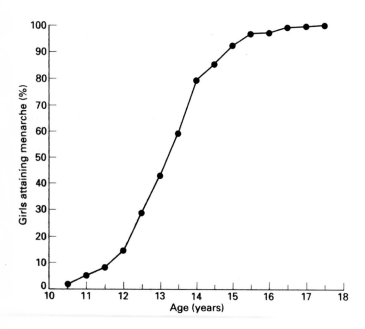

Fig. 39.1 Percentages of girls in each chronological age group who have attained menarche in the Leuven growth study of a national sample of Flemish girls. Redrawn from data in Wellens and Malina (1990).

Table 39.7 Selected percentiles for ages (years) at which stages of secondary sex characteristics are attained in a national sample of Dutch youth. Adapted from Roede and Van Wieringen (1985).

Sex characteristic stage		Percentiles		
		10	50	90
Females				
Breast	B2	9.1	10.5	12.3
	B3	10.2	11.7	13.1
	B4	11.4	12.9	14.5
	B5	12.5	14.2	—
Pubic hair	PH2	9.0	10.8	12.6
	PH3	10.2	11.7	13.1
	PH4	11.3	12.6	14.0
	PH5	12.2	14.0	16.4
Menarche		11.7	13.3	14.9
Males				
Genital	G2	9.3	11.3	13.3
	G3	11.6	13.1	14.5
	G4	12.7	14.0	15.6
	G5	13.5	15.3	18.6
Pubic hair	PH2	9.0	11.7	13.5
	PH3	11.7	13.1	14.5
	PH4	12.9	14.0	15.5
	PH5	13.5	15.0	18.4

B, breast; G, genitals; PH, pubic hair.

GONADOTROPHIC AND GONADAL HORMONES

The use of circulating levels of gonadotrophic (follicle-stimulating and luteinizing hormones) and gonadal (oestrogen in females and testosterone in males) hormones is occasionally suggested as a maturity indicator. Single serum samples have extremely limited utility in this regard since virtually all hormones are episodically secreted. Studies in which 24-h levels of hormones are monitored or in which actual pulses of the hormones are sampled every 20 min or so are needed to provide a more accurate indication of a child's hormonal status. Furthermore, the simple presence of a hormone does not necessarily imply that it is physiologically active. Variation in the responsiveness of hormone receptors at the tissue level is an additional factor.

Table 39.8 Median ages at menarche in several samples of North American and European girls. Adapted from Malina and Bouchard (1991) which contains the primary references.

North America	
Canada, Montreal	13.1
US, national	
White	12.8
Black	12.5
Europe	
Belgium, national, Flemish	13.2
Bulgaria, Plovdiv	13.0
Federal Republic of Germany, Bremen	13.3
France, Paris	12.8
German Democratic Republic, Gorlitz	13.0
Greece, Athens	12.6
Hungary	
Szeged	12.8
County Szeged	12.8
Italy	
Naples	12.5
Venetien	12.8
Netherlands, national	13.3
Norway, Oslo	13.2
Poland	
Warsaw	12.7
Wroclaw	13.0
Sweden, urban	13.0
Switzerland, Zurich	13.4
UK,	
Northumberland	13.3
Newcastle	13.4
Yugoslavia, Zagreb	12.7
Former USSR, Moscow	13.0

Somatic maturation

The use of stature as an indicator of maturity requires longitudinal data that span the adolescent years. This permits estimation of timing of the adolescent growth spurt. If adult stature is available, the percentage of adult size attained at different ages during growth can also be used as a maturity indicator.

AGE AT PEAK HEIGHT VELOCITY (PHV)

PHV refers to the maximum rate of growth in stature during the adolescent spurt, and the age when PHV occurs is an indicator of somatic maturity. Longitudinal data are necessary to estimate age at PHV and related parameters of the adolescent growth spurt.

The spurt in stature refers to the acceleration in stature which in boys begins at about 12 years, peaks at about 14 years and stops at about 18 years. In girls the spurt starts at about 10 years, peaks at about 12 years and stops at about 16 years. There is, however, an earlier midgrowth spurt in stature in many but not all children. It is usually observed between 6.5 and 8.5 years of age. This spurt is much smaller and some evidence suggests that it also occurs in other body dimensions (Tanner & Cameron, 1980; Meredith, 1981; Gasser et al., 1984).

Fitting growth curves to individual records is indicated for estimation of velocities and accelerations, and in turn, for calculation of the timing and magnitude of the spurt, although it is not the only approach to the analyses of longitudinal growth data (Goldstein, 1979). Several models have been described and new models are being proposed to quantify individual growth. Most models, however, have been developed for statural growth. In fitting mathematical models to growth curves a distinction has to be made between structural models and polynomials (Marubini, 1978). The former have a preselected form of the growth curve and the parameters or constants of the function have biological meaning. Structural models include the Gompertz function, single, double and triple logistic functions, the Preece–Baines family of growth functions, and a number of others. Although the use of polynomials has been severely criticized (see Marubini, 1978), several applications have been useful for describing growth over large age periods and characteristics with no uniform continuous increase. These applications include moving polynomials, cubic splines and kernel estimations. Regardless of the model used, curve fitting provides a convenient means of characterizing and comparing individual and/or group differences in adolescent growth in a biologically meaningful manner (see Beunen & Malina, 1988). It should also be noted that graphical smoothing has been used for the first published standards for height and weight velocity (Tanner et al., 1966).

TIMING OF THE ADOLESCENT SPURT

Several parameters of the adolescent growth spurt in stature for samples of North American and European children are summarized in Table 39.9. Double logistic parameters for the four major longitudinal studies of American children (the Berkeley growth study in California, the Child Research Council in Denver, the Fels Research Institute in Yellow Springs, Ohio and the Harvard School of Public Health in Boston) are not included in Table 39.9. El Lozy (1978) and Hauspie et al. (1980) have shown that the double logistic gives a poor fit of the adolescent growth period, an early age at take-off and age at PHV. Other samples were also not included because there was evidence that these samples included either a large group of late or early maturing girls (see Beunen & Malina, 1988; Malina et al., 1988).

Variation in the estimated parameters is considerable. Age at peak velocity in North American boys varies between 13.4 and 14.3 years. Much of the variation is related to the models and procedures used to derive them. There is, for example, good agreement in estimated ages at PHV in North American and European samples of girls when the Preece–Baines I model is used. The estimated ages at PHV vary between 11.6 and 11.9 years. This uniformity is of interest given the period over which the longitudinal studies have been made. The studies in California and Colorado were begun in the late 1920s, a number of European studies were begun in the mid-1950s, others in the 1960s or even 1970s.

Several features should be noted from Table 39.9. First, there is a clear sex difference. Girls are advanced, on average, about 2 years in ages at onset of the spurt and at PHV. In contrast, the magnitude of the spurt is generally smaller in girls than in boys, although the difference is not so large as compared to the differences in mean ages at take-off and PHV. Second, the SD around the mean ages are about 1 year or a bit more in most studies. This indicates considerable variation among individuals in the timing of the adolescent spurt and also in the magnitude. Within normal variation, an early maturing girl can experience her PHV at the age of 9.5 years whereas a late maturing girl can experience the same milestone at the age of 13.9. It has also been shown that adolescents with an early spurt tend to have a more intense spurt (Beunen & Malina, 1988; Beunen et al., 1988).

USES OF AGE AT PHV

Age at PHV is an indicator of when maximum growth occurs during the adolescent spurt. It also serves as a landmark against which attained sizes and velocities of other body dimensions, physical performance and the development of secondary sex characteristics can be expressed. Menarche, for example, occurs after PHV in girls, while peak strength development occurs after PHV in boys. The relationship of performance to PHV age is discussed in more detail in Chapter 1.

GROWTH SPURTS IN OTHER BODY DIMENSIONS

Some of the models that have been used to describe statural growth have also been applied to other body dimensions. Ages at peak velocity in other body dimensions are most often related to the age at PHV to demonstrate the sequence of changes occurring during the adolescent spurt. The available evidence for external body dimensions can be summarized as follows. Maximum velocity in body weight (peak weight velocity, PWV) generally occurs after PHV, and SDs of age at PWV are about 1 year. Among boys the differences between the ages at PWV and PHV range from 0.2 to 0.4 years, while among girls the differences vary between 0.3 and 0.9 years. Peak velocity for leg length occurs earlier than PHV (0.3−0.7 years in girls

and 0.2−0.5 years in boys), while peak velocity for trunk length or sitting height occurs after PHV (0.1−0.5 years in girls and 0.1−0.4 years in boys for sitting height). Rapid growth in the lower extremities is characteristic of the early part of the adolescent growth spurt. Only few studies report data for biacromial and bicristal breadths, and results are variable. Generally, peak velocity in biacromial breadth occurs after PHV and also after peak velocity in bicristal breadth (Beunen & Malina, 1988; Malina et al., 1988).

PERCENTAGE OF ADULT STATURE

Another indicator of somatic maturity is the percentage of adult stature attained at a given age. Children who are closer to their adult or mature stature compared to other children of the same CA are advanced in maturity status. For example, two 7-year-old boys have attained the same stature, 122 cm. For one of the boys this stature accounts for 72% of his adult stature, while for the other, it accounts for only 66% of his adult stature. The former is closer to the mature state and is, therefore, maturationally advanced in somatic growth compared to the latter.

Percentage of adult stature is based on size attained, and is thus the result of variation in tempo of growth and is not an indicator of tempo per se as is age at PHV. In other words, a child who reaches PHV early is also closer to adult size, while a child who reaches PHV later is also further from adult size.

Estimates of the percentage of adult stature attained at a given age during growth require longitudinal data. As such, this maturity indicator has limited utility. However, it may have some application if a child's stature at the time of examination is expressed as a percentage of his or her predicted adult stature. Such an approach may be useful in distinguishing youngsters who are tall at a given age because they are genetically tall or who are tall because they are maturationally advanced compared to their peers, i.e. they have attained a greater

Table 39.9 Means (M) and SDs (medians as indicated) for age at initiation of the spurt, age at peak height velocity (PHV) and PHV in North American and European youths. Adapted from Beunen and Malina (1988) and Malina et al. (1988) which contain the primary references with the exception of the following: Hägg and Taranger (1991), Hauspie and Wachholder (1986), Hauspie et al. (1991) and Karlberg (1987).

Sample	Method	Females							Males						
		n	Age at initiation (years) M	SD	Age at PHV (years) M	SD	PHV (cm·year⁻¹) M	SD	n	Age at initiation (years) M	SD	Age at PHV (years) M	SD	PHV (cm·year⁻¹) M	SD
North America															
California	Graphic	81			11.5	1.1			86			13.8	1.2		
California	Semi-annual increments	94			11.7	1.1			67			14.1	0.9		
California	Triple logistic	70			11.6	0.9			66			13.7	1.1		
Colorado	Gompertz	24			11.4	0.9	9.1	1.2	24			13.4	0.9	9.6	0.7
Colorado	Graphic	36	9.6	1.1	11.9	1.0			27	11.4	1.0	14.0	1.0		
Massachusetts	Preece–Baines I	332	8.7	1.6	11.6	1.2	7.8	1.7							
Quebec	Graphic	46			12.0	1.1									
Saskatchewan	Preece–Baines I	22	9.0	1.0	11.8	0.7	8.0	1.2	75	11.1	1.0	14.3	1.0	9.4	1.5
Europe															
Belgium, Brussels	Preece–Baines I	35	8.5	0.9	11.6	1.0	7.4	1.0							
Belgium, Brussels	Single logistic	35	9.9	1.1	11.4	1.0	7.8	1.1							
Belgium, Brussels	Graphic	35	9.9	1.1	11.7	1.0	7.8	0.9							
Belgium, Brussels	Preece–Baines I	50			11.6	0.9	7.5	1.1	48			14.0	1.0	9.1	1.4
Belgium, national	Non-smoothed polynomials								432			14.2	1.0	9.2	1.6

France, Paris	Graphic	80	9.3	1.1	12.0	0.9	8.4	0.9	68	11.0	1.3	13.8	0.9	9.7	1.1
Netherlands, Amsterdam	Moving polynomials								102/96			14.0*	0.9	9.6*	
Netherlands, Leiden	Graphic, 6-monthly increments								81			14.4			
Poland, Wroclaw	Graphic	234	9.7	1.1	11.7	0.9			111	11.8	1.2	13.9	1.1		
Poland, Wroclaw	Preece–Baines I								191	10.8	1.0	14.1	1.0		
Sweden, urban	Mid-year velocities	357/330			11.9	0.9	8.3	1.2	373/354			14.1	1.1	9.8	1.4
Sweden, Stockholm	3-month moving increments	90	10.0	1.3	12.0	1.0	8.6	1.1	122	12.1	1.2	14.1	1.1	9.9	1.1
Sweden, Stockholm	Graphic	80			12.0	1.0			103			14.0	1.2		
Sweden	Logistic	68			12.0	0.9			89			14.1	1.0		
Sweden, Umea	Midpoint	83			11.7	1.1	8.0	1.3							
Switzerland, Zürich	Splines†	110	9.6	1.1	12.2	1.0	7.1	1.0	112	11.0	1.2	13.9	0.8	9.0	1.1
Switzerland, Zürich	Kernel estimations	45	9.7	1.0	12.2	0.8	7.0	1.0	45	10.9	1.1	13.9	0.9	8.3	0.8
Switzerland, Zürich	Preece–Baines III	45	9.0	0.7	12.1	0.8	7.1	1.1	45	10.6	0.8	14.0	0.9	8.7	1.0
UK, Harpenden	Graphic	41			12.1	0.9	9.0	1.0	49			14.1	0.9	10.3	1.5
UK, Harpenden	Single logistic	35	10.3	0.9	11.9	0.9	8.1	0.8	55	12.1	0.9	13.9	0.8	8.8	1.1
UK, Harpenden	Preece–Baines I	23	9.0	0.7	11.9	0.7	7.5	0.8	35	10.7	0.9	14.2	0.9	8.2	1.2
UK, Harpenden and London	Preece–Baines I	38	8.7	0.6	11.9	0.7	7.5	0.7	61	10.3	0.9	13.9	1.0	8.5	1.1
UK, London	Preece–Baines I	42			12.2				50			13.9			
UK, Newcastle upon Tyne	Graphic	746/695			12.2	1.1	8.0	1.1	653/539			14.1	1.0	9.6	1.2

* Medians.

† Midpoint between the two consecutive height measurements during which growth was noted.

percentage of their predicted adult stature at a given CA.

There are three commonly used methods for predicting adult stature, the Bailey–Pinneau (BP; Bailey & Pinneau, 1952, see also Bayer & Bailey, 1959); Roche, Wainer and Thissen (RWT; Roche *et al.*, 1975a, b); and Tanner–Whitehouse stature prediction (TWSP; Tanner *et al.*, 1983). Note that all predictions have an associated error, and the range of error associated with a prediction should be recognized.

The BP method utilizes stature and GP SA, and provides an estimate of the percentage of adult stature attained at the time of the hand–wrist radiograph.

The RWT method uses CA, recumbent length (not stature), weight, mid-parent stature (stature of the mother and father divided by 2), and GP SA (based on median bone-specific SAs) to predict stature at 18 years of age. The RWT method has been modified to provide estimates of adult stature when SA is not available (Roche *et al.*, 1983). Parental statures provide a target range within which the adult stature of the child is likely to fall. The child's adult stature can be predicted from current stature and the statures of the parents. This modification of the RWT method has potential for application because it does not require an estimate of SA. However, the method needs to be evaluated in samples other than American middle-class children and youths.

The TWSP method includes several options to predict adult stature, e.g. CA, stature and RUS SA; CA, stature, RUS SA and the increment in stature during the previous year; and menarcheal status and age at menarche in addition to this.

Interrelationships among maturity indicators

Relationships between growth and maturation are discussed in Chapter 1. Two questions are especially important when using different maturity indicators. The first deals with relationships among indicators, i.e. do they measure the same kind of biological maturity? The second relates to the consistency of maturity ratings over time, i.e. is a child who is maturationally late at, for example, 6 years of age, also late at 11 years of age? The same question can be asked of those advanced and average in maturity status.

The issue of interrelationships is complex because only skeletal maturation spans the prepubertal and pubertal years, while indicators of sexual maturation and age at PHV are limited to the pubertal period. Furthermore, evidence suggests that the tempo of prepubertal growth and maturation may be somewhat independent of pubertal growth and maturation. For example, a cluster analysis of indicators of sexual (ages at attaining genital and pubic hair stages 2 and 4), skeletal (skeletal maturity at 11–15 years of age) and somatic (ages at peak velocity for stature, weight, leg length and trunk length, age at initiation of the stature spurt, ages at attaining 80, 90, 95 and 99% of adult stature) maturity among 111 Polish boys who were followed longitudinally from 8 to 18 years of age (Bielicki *et al.*, 1984) indicated two clusters. The first was a general maturity factor during adolescence. Ages at peak velocities and at attainment of stages of sexual maturation, SAs at 14 and 15 years, ages at attaining 90, 95 and 99% of mature stature, and age at initiation of the stature spurt all clustered together. Such a general maturity factor suggests that the tempo of maturation during adolescence is under common control. The second cluster concerned prepubertal growth and maturation. It included SAs at 11, 12 and 13 years and age at attaining 80% of mature stature, all of which are indices of prepubertal growth, and was independent of the other maturity indicators. Similar analyses of the patterns of relationships among maturity indicators in Polish girls and in other longitudinal studies have produced generally similar results (Nicolson & Hanley, 1953; Bielicki, 1975).

There is thus a general maturity factor which underlies the tempo of growth and maturation during adolescence. This factor discriminates among individuals who are early, average or late in the timing of adolescent events. There is, however, variation among maturity indicators, which suggests that no single system, sexual, skeletal or somatic, provides a complete description of the tempo of growth and maturation of an individual boy or girl during adolescence. This is related to the observation that there is no consistent relationship between the age at which a specific stage of a secondary sex characteristic develops and the rate of progress from one stage to the next. Some boys may pass from genital stages G2–G5 in about 2 years, while others may take about 5 years (Marshall & Tanner, 1969, 1970; Largo & Prader, 1983a,b).

Part of the variation in such analyses is due to the methods used to assess maturation. The five grade scales for rating secondary sex characteristics are somewhat arbitrary. Different intervals between observations among studies also contribute to the variable results. Methods of estimating ages at peak velocities and ages at attainment of specific stages of sexual and skeletal maturation also differ. Measurement variation is an additional contributing factor.

The independence of prepubertal growth from the events of adolescence raises the question of maturity indicators during childhood. Skeletal maturation is the primary indicator for the prepubertal years, and if longitudinal data are available, the percentage of adult stature may be useful. Relationships between skeletal maturity and the attained percentage of adult stature are moderately high and positive during the prepubertal years. Children advanced in SA are, on average, closer to adult stature at all ages during childhood and adolescence than those who are delayed in SA relative to CA. In late adolescence, catch-up of those later in skeletal maturation occurs. The child who is advanced in skeletal maturation attains adult stature earlier and thus stops growing earlier, while the child later in skeletal maturation

attains adult stature later and grows over a longer period of time. On average, both groups attain similar adult statures, but one attains it more rapidly than the other.

Although processes of maturation during prepuberty and puberty are somewhat independent, indicators of sexual and somatic maturity are positively related with each other during puberty (Table 39.10). All of the correlations are moderate to high, which suggests that youngsters early or late in sexual maturation are, respectively, early or late in the timing of the adolescent growth spurt in stature. Similarly, if the youngster is early or late in the appearance of one indicator of sexual maturation, he or she is early or late, respectively, in the appearance of the others. The correlations, though reasonably consistent across studies, are not perfect, which suggests variation in timing of somatic and sexual maturation.

Skeletal maturity is also related to the development of secondary sex characteristics and PHV. Variation in SA is considerably reduced at menarche and PHV in girls and boys, respectively. For example, mean CA and SA at menarche are 13.2 and 13.3 years, respectively, in girls from the Harpenden growth study (Marshall, 1974). However, SAs of about three-quarters of the girls cluster between 12.5 and 13.5 years, while less than half of the girls have CAs between 12.5 and 13.5 years. Thus, there is more variation in CA at the time of menarche than there is variation in SA. The same pattern is evident in boys at PHV (Fig. 39.2), i.e. there is more variation in CA at the time of PHV than there is variation in SA (Hauspie et al., 1991). It is important to note, however, that SA may vary as much as CA at the onset of sexual maturation in girls and the growth spurt in stature (take-off) in boys. As sexual maturation and the adolescent growth spurt proceed, skeletal maturity becomes more strongly related to these maturational events (Table 39.11). Correlations between SA and ages at attaining PHV, the later stages of breast, genital and pubic hair development, menarche and 95% of mature stature increase at successive ages. The corre-

Table 39.10 Correlations between ages at reaching several maturity indicators in North American and European youths. Adapted from Malina and Bochard (1991) which contains the primary references.

Area	Females PHV B2	PH2	M M	B2	PH2	B2 PH2	Males PHV G2	PH2	G2 PH2
North America									
California, Berkeley	0.80	0.75	0.71	0.74	0.74	0.75	0.67		
Colorado, Denver	0.78		0.93					0.56	
Ohio, Yellow Springs				0.86	0.70	0.66			
Massachusetts, Boston			0.71	0.86					
Quebec, Montreal			0.81						
Europe									
Poland, Wroclaw	0.76	0.77	0.76	0.72	0.73	0.77	0.87	0.84	0.85
Sweden, Stockholm	0.80	0.73	0.84	0.74	0.58	0.70	0.78	0.49	0.54
Sweden, Umea	0.63	0.68	0.63	0.51	0.52	0.70			
Sweden, urban			0.69						
Switzerland, Zürich	0.60	0.34	0.82	0.47	0.44	0.34	0.50	0.59	0.54
UK, Harpenden	0.82		0.91	0.64					
UK, Harpenden	0.78	0.77	0.84				0.47	0.84	
UK, Newcastle	0.69		0.80	0.62					

B2, breast stage 2; G2, genital state 2; M, menarche; PH2, pubic hair stage 2; PHV, peak height velocity.

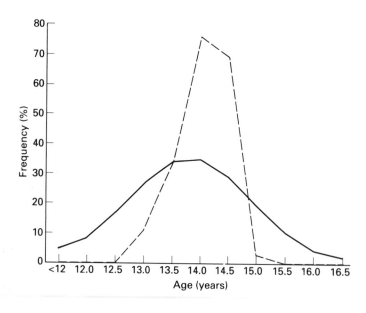

Fig. 39.2 Distribution of Gauss-adjusted expected frequencies of chronological ages (——) and observed frequencies of skeletal ages (---) (TWII 20 bones) at peak height velocity in boys from the Wroclaw growth study. Drawn from data in Hauspie *et al.* (1991).

Table 39.11 Correlations between skeletal maturity at successive ages and ages at attaining several indicators of sexual and somatic maturity in the Wroclaw growth study. Mean ages at reaching each maturity indicator are in parentheses. Adapted from Bielicki (1975) and Bielicki et al. (1984).

(a) Females

Skeletal maturity (years)	Breast 4 (13.5 years)	Pubic hair 4 (13.6 years)	PHV (11.7 years)	Menarche (13.1 years)
10	0.49	0.51	0.58	0.51
11	0.60	0.61	0.69	0.61
12	0.65	0.64	0.73	0.68
13	0.68	0.67	0.76	0.71
14	0.70	0.68	0.79	0.73

(b) Males

Skeletal maturity (years)	Genital 4 (14.5 years)	Pubic hair 4 (15 years)	PHV (13.9 years)	95% adult stature (14.8 years)
11	0.25	0.29	0.26	0.29
12	0.40	0.42	0.42	0.47
13	0.62	0.61	0.68	0.71
14	0.75	0.78	0.81	0.83
15	0.83	0.82	0.89	0.93

lations with SA are quite high near the mean
ages when these maturational stages or events
are attained. In boys, for example, the correlation between SA at 14 years and age at PHV
(13.9 years) is 0.81. Thus, the correlations between maturational events which occur closer
in time are higher than those separated in time.
In contrast, skeletal maturity in the early pubertal years, 9–10 years in girls and 11–12
years in boys, is not highly related to indices of
sexual and somatic maturation during adolescence. However, as adolescence progresses,
skeletal maturity is increasingly related to these
indices of sexual and somatic maturation. This
pattern reflects the observation that the tempo
of prepubertal growth and the events of puberty
are somewhat independent. Prepubertal growth
and skeletal maturation depend principally
upon the stimulation of growth hormone.
Conversely, sexual maturation, the growth
spurt and epiphyseal union are under the
influence of both growth and steroid hormones.
The latter are increasingly produced by the
gonads as they mature.

Challenges for future research

The following are suggested as areas which
need further study and application.
• Refinement of non-invasive methods for the
assessment of maturity status. Methods for
eliciting self-reports of sexual maturation and
the criteria need to be standardized.
• The use of predicted adult stature as an
indicator of maturity status needs to be further
explored. The RWT method which was modified for use without an assessment of SA needs
to be evaluated with different samples.
• Routine measurement of parental statures
and incorporation of these into the evaluation
of growth and maturity status. Reported statures, though useful, have limitations.

References

Baumgartner, R.N., Roche, A.F. & Himes, J.H. (1986)
Incremental growth tables: supplementary to pre-
viously published charts. *Am. J. Clin. Nutr.* **43**,
711–22.
Bayer, L.M. & Bayley, N. (1959) *Growth Diagnosis:
Selected Methods for Interpreting and Predicting
Development from One Year to Maturity.* University
of Chicago Press, Chicago.
Bayley, N. & Pinneau, S.R. (1952) Tables for predicting
adult height from skeletal age: revised for use with
the Greulich–Pyle hand standards. *J. Pediatr.* **4**,
423–41.
Beunen, G., Lefevre, J., Ostyn, M., Renson, R.,
Simons, J. & Van Gerven, D. (1990) Skeletal maturity
in Belgian youths assessed by the Tanner–Whitehouse method (TW2). *Ann. Hum. Biol.* **17**, 355–76.
Beunen, G. & Malina, R.M. (1988) Growth and physical performance relative to the timing of the adolescent spurt. *Exerc. Sport Sci. Rev.* **16**, 503–40.
Beunen, G.P., Malina, R.M., Van't Hof, M.A. *et al.*
(1988) *Adolescent Growth and Motor Performance: A
Longitudinal Study of Belgian Boys.* Human Kinetics,
Champaign, IL.
Bielicki, T. (1975) Interrelationships between various
measures of maturation rate in girls during ado-
lescence. *Stud. Phys. Anthropol.* **1**, 51–64.
Bielicki, T., Koniarek, J. & Malina, R.M. (1984) Inter-
relationships among certain measures of growth
and maturation rate in boys during adolescence.
Ann. Hum. Biol. **11**, 201–10.
Brooks-Gunn, J., Warren, M.P., Rosso, J. & Gargiulo,
J. (1987) Validity of self-report measures of girls'
pubertal status. *Child Dev.* **58**, 829–41.
Butler, G.E., McKie, M. & Ratcliffe, S.G. (1990) The
cyclical nature of prepubertal growth. *Ann. Hum.
Biol.* **17**, 177–98.
Demirjian, A. (1986) Dentition. In F. Falkner & J.M.
Tanner (eds) *Human Growth, Vol. 2. Postnatal
Growth, Neurobiology*, pp. 269–98. Plenum Press,
New York.
Duke, P.M., Litt, I.F. & Gross, R.T. (1980) Adolescents'
self-assessment of sexual maturation. *Pediatrics* **66**,
918–20.
El Lozy, M. (1978) A critical analysis of the double
and triple logistic growth curves. *Ann. Hum. Biol.* **5**,
389–94.
Gasser, T., Köhler, W., Müller, H.-G. *et al.* (1984)
Velocity and acceleration of height growth using
kernel estimation. *Ann. Hum. Biol.* **11**, 397–411.
Goldstein, H. (1979) *The Design and Analysis of Longi-
tudinal Studies.* Academic Press, London.
Greulich, W.W., Dorfman, R.I., Catchpole, H.R.,
Solomon, C.I. & Culotta, C.S. (1942) Somatic and
endocrine studies of pubertal and adolescent boys.
Monogr. Soc. Res. Child Dev. **7** (Serial No. 35).
Greulich, W.W. & Pyle, S.I. (1959) *Radiographic Atlas
of Skeletal Development of the Hand and Wrist*, 2nd
edn. Stanford University Press, Stanford, CA.

Hägg, U. & Taranger, J. (1991) Height and height velocity in early, average and late maturers followed to the age of 25: a prospective longitudinal study of Swedish urban children from birth to adulthood. *Ann. Hum. Biol.* **18**, 47–56.

Hamill, P.V.V., Drizd, R.A., Johnson, C.L., Reed, R.D. & Roche, A.F. (1977) NCHS growth charts for children, birth–18 years, United States. *Vital Health Stat. Ser. 11* **165**.

Hammer, L.D., Wilson, D.M., Litt, I.F. *et al.* (1991) Impact of pubertal development on body fat distribution among White, Hispanic, and Asian female adolescents. *J. Pediatr.* **118**, 975–80.

Hauspie, R., Bielicki, T. & Koniarek, J. (1991) Skeletal maturity at onset of the adolescent growth spurt and at peak velocity for growth in height: a threshold effect. *Ann. Hum. Biol.* **18**, 23–9.

Hauspie, R.C. & Wachholder, A. (1986) Clinical standards for growth velocity in height of Belgian boys and girls, aged 2 to 18 years. *Int. J. Anthropol.* **1**, 339–48.

Hauspie, R.C., Wachholder, A., Baron, G., Cantraine, F., Susanne, C. & Graffar, M. (1980) A comparative study of the fit of four different functions to longitudinal data of growth in height of Belgian girls. *Ann. Hum. Biol.* **7**, 347–58.

Karlberg, J. (1987) *Modelling of human growth.* Doctoral dissertation, Göteborg University, Göteborg, Sweden.

Kreipe, R.E. & Gewanter, H.L. (1983) Physical maturity screening for participation in sports. *Pediatrics* **75**, 1076–80.

Lampl, M., Veldhuis, J.D. & Johnson, M.L. (1992) Saltation and stasis: a model of human growth. *Science* **258**, 801–3.

Largo, R.H. & Prader, A. (1983a) Pubertal development in Swiss boys. *Helv. Paediatr. Acta* **38**, 211–28.

Largo, R.H. & Prader, A. (1983b) Pubertal development in Swiss girls. *Helv. Paediatr. Acta* **38**, 229–43.

Lohman, T.G., Roche, A.F. & Martorell, R. (eds) (1988) *Anthropometric Standardization Reference Manual.* Human Kinetics, Champaign, IL.

Malina, R.M. (1995) Anthropometry. In P.J. Maud & C. Foster (eds) *Physiological Assessment of Human Fitness.* Human Kinetics, Champaign, IL.

Malina, R.M. & Bouchard, C. (1991) *Growth, Maturation, and Physical Activity.* Human Kinetics, Champaign, IL.

Malina, R.M., Bouchard, C. & Beunen, G. (1988) Human growth: selected aspects of current research on well-nourished children. *Ann. Rev. Anthropol.* **17**, 187–219.

Malina, R.M., Hamill, P.V.V. & Lemeshow, S. (1973) Selected body measurements of children 6–11 years. *Vital Health Stat. Ser. 11* **123**.

Malina, R.M. & Roche, A.F. (1983) *Manual of Physical Status and Performance in Childhood*, Vol. 2. *Physical Performance.* Plenum Press, New York.

Marks, G.C., Habicht, J.-P. & Mueller, W.H. (1989) Reliability, dependability, and precision of anthropometric measurements: the second National Health and Nutrition Examination Survey 1976–1980. *Am. J. Epidemiol.* **130**, 578–87.

Marshall, W.A. (1974) Interrelationships of skeletal maturation, sexual development and somatic growth in man. *Ann. Hum. Biol.* **1**, 29–40.

Marshall, W.A. & Tanner, J.M. (1969) Variations in pattern of pubertal changes in girls. *Arch. Dis. Child.* **44**, 291–303.

Marshall, W.A. & Tanner, J.M. (1970) Variations in the pattern of pubertal changes in boys. *Arch. Dis. Child.* **45**, 13–23.

Marubini, E. (1978) Mathematical handling of long-term longitudinal data. In F. Falkner & J.M. Tanner (eds) *Human Growth*, Vol. 1. *Principles and Prenatal Growth*, pp. 209–25. Plenum Press, New York.

Meredith, H.V. (1981) An addendum on presence and absence of a mid-growth spurt in somatic dimensions. *Ann. Hum. Biol.* **8**, 473–6.

Mueller, W.H. & Martorell, R. (1988) Reliability and accuracy of measurement. In T.G. Lohman, A.R. Roche & R. Martorell (eds) *Anthropometric Standardization Reference Manual*, pp. 83–6. Human Kinetics, Champaign, IL.

Nicolson, A.B. & Hanley, C. (1953) Indices of physiological maturity: derivation and interrelationships. *Child Dev.* **24**, 3–38.

Prader, A., Largo, R.H., Molinari, L. & Issler, C. (1989) Physical growth of Swiss children from birth to 20 years of age. *Helv. Paediatr. Acta Suppl.* **52**.

Reynolds, E.L. & Wines, J.V. (1948) Individual differences in physical changes associated with adolescence in girls. *Am. J. Dis. Child.* **75**, 329–50.

Reynolds, E.L. & Wines, J.V. (1951) Physical changes associated with adolescence in boys. *Am. J. Dis. Child.* **82**, 529–47.

Roche, A.F., Chumlea, W.C. & Thissen, D. (1988) *Assessing the Skeletal Maturity of the Hand–Wrist: Fels Method.* C.C. Thomas, Springfield, IL.

Roche, A.F. & Malina, R.M. (1983) *Manual of Physical Status and Performance in Childhood*, Vol. 1. *Physical Status.* Plenum Press, New York.

Roche, A.F., Tyleshevski, F. & Rogers, E. (1983) Noninvasive measurement of physical maturity in children. *Res. Q. Exerc. Sport* **54**, 364–71.

Roche, A.F., Wainer, H. & Thissen, D. (1975a) *Predicting Adult Stature for Individuals.* Karger, Basel.

Roche, A.F., Wainer, H. & Thissen, D. (1975b) The RWT method for the prediction of adult stature. *Pediatrics* **56**, 1026–33.

Roede, M.J. & Van Wieringen, J.C. (1985) Growth

diagrams 1980: the Netherlands Third Nationwide Survey. *Tijdschr. Soc. Gezondheid. Suppl.* **63**.

Schlossberger, N.M., Turner, R.A. & Irwin, C.E. (1992) Validity of self-report of pubertal maturation in early adolescents. *J. Adolesc. Health* **13**, 109–13.

Tanner, J.M. (1962) *Growth at Adolescence*, 2nd edn. Blackwell Scientific Publications, Oxford.

Tanner, J.M. & Cameron, N. (1980) Investigation of the mid-growth spurt in height, weight and limb circumference in single-year velocity data from the London 1966–67 growth survey. *Ann. Hum. Biol.* **8**, 495–517.

Tanner, J.M., Whitehouse, R.H., Cameron, N., Marshall, W.A., Healy, M.J.R. & Goldstein, H. (1983) *Assessment of Skeletal Maturity and Prediction of Adult Height*, 2nd edn. Academic Press, New York.

Tanner, J.M., Whitehouse, R.H., Marshall, W.A., Healy, M.J.R. & Goldstein, H. (1975) *Assessment of Skeletal Maturity and Prediction of Adult Height*

(TW2 Method). Academic Press, New York.

Tanner, J.M., Whitehouse, R.H. & Takaishi, M. (1966) Standards from birth to maturity for height, weight, height velocity, and weight velocity. *Arch. Dis. Child.* **41**, 454–71, 613–35.

Todd, T.W. (1937) *Atlas of Skeletal Maturation*. C.V. Mosby, St Louis.

Van 't Hof, M.A., Roede, M.J., & Kowalski, C.J. (1976) Estimation of growth velocities from individual longitudinal data. *Growth* **40**, 217–40.

Waterlow, J.C., Buzina, R., Keller, W. *et al.* (1977) The presentation and use of height and weight data for comparing nutritional status of groups of children under the age of 10 years. *Bull. WHO* **55**, 489–98.

Wellens, R. & Malina, R.M. (1990) The age at menarche. In J. Simons, G.P. Beunen, R. Renson, A.L.M. Claessens & J.A.V. Lefevre (eds) *Growth and Fitness of Flemish Girls: The Leuven Growth Study*, pp. 119–25. Human Kinetics, Champaign, IL.

Chapter 40

Importance and Principles of Scaling for Size Differences

EDWARD M. WINTER

Introduction

It is clear that as children grow and develop their performance capabilities improve. What is less clear is the extent to which these improvements are attributable to increases in size or to qualitative changes in the distribution and properties of associated tissues and structures. To assess qualitative changes, differences in size have to be partitioned out and this partitioning is called scaling (Schmidt-Nielsen, 1984).

The principles which underpin scaling are well established and remarkably simple but intriguingly, they are all too frequently overlooked. As a consequence, there is an increasing body of evidence which suggests that traditional scaling techniques are incorrect and have misled our search for an understanding of how the body responds and adapts to exercise (Winter, 1992; Jakeman *et al.*, 1994). Whenever qualitative characteristics are compared in groups who differ in size, scaling is important. This is especially so when differences in size are marked, as is the case when children are compared with adults (Armstrong & Welsman, 1994).

The purpose of this chapter is to outline the basic principles which underlie scaling. This includes a historical background to the area, current approaches and suggestions for future research.

Ratio standards

Traditionally, the most common scaling technique involves the construction of a ratio standard (Tanner, 1949) in which either a physiological or performance variable is divided by an anthropometric characteristic. An example is oxygen uptake ($\dot{V}o_2$), either maximal or submaximal, which is expressed relative to body mass as $ml \cdot kg^{-1} \cdot min^{-1}$. This is probably the most used measure in the physiology of exercise in spite of the warnings made by Tanner (1949) who stated that ratio standards were, 'theoretically fallacious and, unless in exceptional circumstances, misleading'. Furthermore, he stated later (Tanner, 1964) that comparisons between groups based on mean ratios are also misleading because they, 'involve some statistical difficulties and are neither as simple nor as informative as they seem'. Curiously, in the 45 years or so that have intervened, Tanner's work in this area has been considered only rarely.

What are the 'special circumstances' and 'statistical difficulties' to which Tanner refers? A ratio standard is only valid when for an independent variable x and a dependent variable y:

$$v_x/v_y = r_{xy}$$

where v_x = coefficient of variation of x, v_y = coefficient of variation of y and r_{xy} = Pearson's product moment correlation coefficient. If this expression does not hold true, the ratio standard

673

y/x will distort the data under scrutiny by conferring an arithmetic advantage on small values of x and an arithmetic disadvantage on large values of x. If x is an index of body size, little people are treated preferentially in comparison with their larger peers. Figure 40.1 provides an illustration based on data for peak power output during cycle ergometry and lean leg volume in 11–13-year-old boys.

The lines which represent the ratio standard and linear regression are indicated in Fig. 40.1. Pearson's product moment correlation coefficient for these data was 0.694 ($P = 0.002$) whereas v_x/v_y was 1.266; clearly Tanner's special circumstance was not satisfied. If the ratio standard was to be used against which individuals were to be compared for diagnostic purposes, the distortion is self-evident when set against the 'true' relationship. Tanner (1949) gave an example in which patients had been ascribed the condition essential hyperkinaemia on the grounds that their ratio standard suggested that they had an abnormally high cardiac output for their body mass. He stated that the disease from which they were suffering, 'was no more formidable than statistical artifact'.

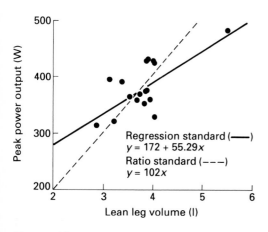

Fig. 40.1 The ratio standard (– – –) and regression standard (——) for peak power output during cycle ergometry and lean leg volume in 11–13-year-old boys. From Winter *et al.* (1993).

It is clear that the *a priori* use of ratio standards against which individuals can be compared should be avoided and their use should only occur when Tanner's special circumstance is satisfied. Similarly, when comparisons are made between groups, especially when the subjects across the groups differ markedly in size, 'statistical difficulties' will be introduced if ratio standards are the basis.

Regression standards

As a result of the imperfections of ratio standards, Tanner (1964) suggested that comparisons between groups should be based on analysis of covariance (ANCOVA) (Snedecor & Cochran, 1980). In ANCOVA, the effect of a covariate is partitioned out and an adjusted mean is calculated. The utility of this technique has been demonstrated. Winter *et al.* (1991) compared the abilities of men and women to perform maximal intensity exercise. Optimized peak power (OPP) output during cycle ergometry and lean upper leg volume (LULV) were assessed. Comparisons based on ratio standards OPP/LULV suggested that there were no qualitative differences between the sexes: values [mean (SEM)] were 204 (5) $W \cdot l^{-1}$ versus 204 (6) $W \cdot l^{-1}$ in men and women, respectively ($P > 0.05$). ANCOVA presented a different interpretation: adjusted means, standard error of the estimate (SEE) for men were 929 (120) W and 730 (101) W for women ($P < 0.001$). Differences in performance were not attributable simply to differences in size, there were distinct differences in the qualitative characteristics of the exercising segments, i.e. the legs.

A similar example was provided in a study which compared isometric strength of the quadriceps (Winter & Maughan, 1991). Strength per unit cross-sectional area was 9.49 (1.45) $N \cdot cm^{-2}$ in men and 8.95 (1.10) $N \cdot cm^{-2}$ in women ($P > 0.05$). Adjusted means were 688 (98) N and 541 (57) N, respectively ($P < 0.001$).

More recently the technique has been applied in studies on the effects of growth on performance and in comparisons of the physiological characteristics of children and adults. In both of these cases, there are distinct differences in the size of subjects. Williams *et al.* (1992) assessed $\dot{V}_{O_2 \, max}$ in pre- and postpubertal boys and noted that ratio standards suggested no change occurred according to chronological age 49 (0.4) ml·kg^{-1}·min^{-1} at age 10 versus 50 (1.3) ml·kg^{-1}·min^{-1} ($P > 0.05$) at age 15 years or physiological age 49 (0.7) ml·kg^{-1}·min^{-1} prepubertal versus 50 (1.3) ml·kg^{-1}·min^{-1} postpubertal ($P > 0.05$). Adjusted means were 2.20 (0.17) l·min^{-1} versus 2.32 (0.31) l·min^{-1} ($P < 0.01$) for 10 and 15 year olds and 1.93 (0.15) l·min^{-1} for prepubertals and 2.05 (0.32) l·min^{-1} postpubertals ($P < 0.01$). These data suggest that a maturational effect occurs which improves aerobic capabilities but that the effect is masked by the use of ratios. In another example, considered in Fig. 40.1, Winter *et al.* (1993) compared maximal exercise capabilities of boys aged 11−13 years and men via OPP and lean leg volume (LLV). Even though still less than men, ratio standards overestimated performance of the boys. Based on these standards the mean value of OPP/LLV in boys was 73% of the equivalent in men whereas the adjusted mean was 56%.

Allometric models

It would appear that ANCOVA solves scaling problems but this is not necessarily the case. Nevill *et al.* (1992) identified two major concerns over the use of this technique: (i) a linear model is not always appropriate; and (ii) error about regression is not necessarily constant, i.e. additive; it can be multiplicative, i.e. error increases as the magnitude of the independent variable increases.

The first of these concerns is well established in biology (Schmidt-Nielsen, 1984). For instance, the surface area of a body increases as the square of increases in linear dimensions. Similarly, volumetric increases are cubic. Indeed, Lilliputian mathematicians in Jonathan Swift's *Gulliver's Travels*, written more than 250 years ago in 1726, were aware of these relationships.

In calculating Gulliver's food requirement they surmised, not unreasonably, that because Gulliver was 12 times taller than a Lilliputian, he would need 1728 times as much food, i.e. 12^3. This calculation is based on Euclidean principles of geometric similarity and can be extended to consideration of the relationship between surface area and volume. In cubes:

surface area (SA) $\propto$ volume $(V)^{0.67}$;

but in fact

$SA = 6V^{0.67}$.

This relationship, known as the surface law is illustrated in Fig. 40.2 and it can be seen clearly that as a body increases in size, its volume increases proportionately more than its surface area. This observation has implications for thermoregulation. In comparison with adults, children have proportionately more surface for their size. As a consequence, because heat exchange occurs at the surface of a body, children are more susceptible to the effects of extremes of ambient conditions than adults; they will absorb heat more quickly if ambient temperatures are high and conversely, they will lose heat more quickly if ambient temperatures are low.

It must be emphasized that growing and

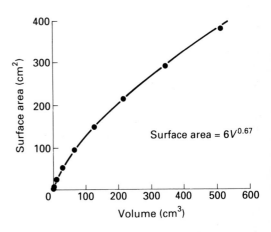

Fig. 40.2 The relationship between surface area and volume in cubes.

developing humans are not geometrically similar; growth is accompanied by changes in the relative sizes of the body's segments. These changes are said to be allometric, a term derived from the Greek *allios* which means to change, and the general equation that describes the non-linear allometric relationship between variables is as follows:

$$y = ax^b$$

where a = constant multiplier and b = exponent. The exponent in this expression is not necessarily an integer and it can have a numerical value greater or smaller than 1. The terms in the expression can be easily identified by taking logarithmic transformations of each variable and regressing ln y on ln x. This produces a linear relationship of the form:

$$\ln y = \ln a + b \ln x$$

which allows the identification of a and b in the allometric model. The known relationship in cubes between surface area and volume referred to earlier, can be used as an example to illustrate the principles. Table 40.1 shows the surface areas, volumes and their natural logarithmic (ln) equivalents for cubes of different side length. Figure 40.3 illustrates the relationship between ln area and ln volume. The slope, b, of the regression line is 0.666, i.e. 0.67, so b, the exponent in the allometric model, is identified.

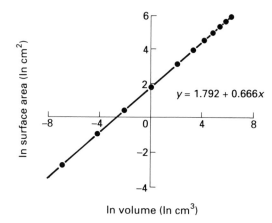

Fig. 40.3 The relationship between ln surface area and ln volume in cubes.

Similarly, the intercept ln a is 1.792 and the antilogue of this value identifies in turn a which is 6, the numerical value of the constant multiplier in the allometric model. These log–log transformations and accompanying manipulations are extraordinarily easy on modern microcomputers.

Nevill *et al.* (1992) demonstrated how error about the non-linear allometric model was usually multiplicative (technically hetero-scedastic) whereas an assumption in linear modelling is that error should be constant (technically homoscedastic). Conveniently, ANCOVA on the log–log transformations

Table 40.1 Length, surface area and volume in cubes.

Length (cm)	Surface area (cm^2)	ln surface area (ln cm^2)	Volume (cm^3)	ln volume (ln cm^3)
0.10	0.060	−2.813	0.0010	−6.908
0.25	0.375	−0.981	0.0156	−4.160
0.50	1.500	0.405	0.1250	−2.079
1	6	1.792	1	0
2	24	3.178	8	2.079
3	54	3.989	27	3.296
4	96	4.564	64	4.159
5	150	5.011	125	4.828
6	216	5.375	216	5.375
7	294	5.684	343	5.838
8	384	5.951	512	6.238

constrains error to be homoscedastic and in addition, allows comparisons between different groups. However, while the analyses are sound, it is not easy to ascribe qualitative characteristics to numerical values of adjusted means which are expressed as the natural log of the dependent variable. Clarity can be lost in this form of expression.

Power function ratios

A simple way to overcome potential lack of clarity is to construct power function ratios (Nevill et al., 1992; Welsman et al., 1993; Winter et al., 1993) which correctly scale a dependent physiological variable for an anthropometric-type independent variable. To do so, three simple steps have to be followed: (i) identify the exponent in the allometric equation (from logarithmic transformations of the data); (ii) raise the independent variable to this power; and (iii) divide this value into the dependent variable. For example, from the surface law $\dot{V}o_2$ relative to body mass would be expressed as $ml \cdot kg^{-0.67} \cdot min^{-1}$. Intergroup comparisons can be made using t-tests or analysis of variance as appropriate and depending on the outcome of ANCOVA on the logarithmic transformations, a common exponent can be applied to different groups. The power function ratio produced is a numerical value which is meaningful and can also be used as a standard against which physiological status can be assessed. As a safeguard, Nevill et al. (1992) suggested that the natural logarithm of the power function ratio should be used to ensure in the same way that ANCOVA on the log−log transformations ensured, homoscedasticity of error.

The application of these techniques has challenged our knowledge and understanding of children's responses and adaptations to exercise (Armstrong & Welsman, 1994). For instance, it has long been assumed that $\dot{V}o_{2\,max}$ relative to body mass deteriorates during puberty while corresponding performance capabilities improve; this contradiction is puzzling. However, the assumption is based on the use of ratio standards and where allometric modelling has been applied, it has been demonstrated clearly that there is a maturational effect on $\dot{V}o_{2\,max}$ and distinct improvements in aerobic capabilities accompany puberty which are independent of body mass (Welsman et al., 1993). Furthermore, the improvements continue later into puberty in boys rather than in girls. These findings are plausible because they are consistent with changes in performance.

It has been demonstrated that the surface law's exponent of 0.67 could be used when body mass is related to $\dot{V}o_{2\,max}$ in untrained adults (Nevill et al., 1992) whereas in children, higher values of 0.861 in girls and 0.917 in boys have been reported (Armstrong & Welsman, 1994). Nevill (1994) has addressed this apparent discrepancy and suggests that it is a feature of the non-isometric, i.e. disproportionate, growth that occurs in the body's segments. Furthermore, he offers a solution based on the study by Alexander et al. (1981) which demonstrates disproportionately large increase in leg volume compared with total body mass in a variety of species of mammal. Stature can be introduced either by classifying samples into discrete subgroups or as a continuous covariate. In both cases, the 'two-thirds' exponent is restored to body mass.

Multilevel modelling

Studies which investigate the effects of training are usually longitudinal and have a repeated measures design. When children and adolescents are the subjects, the effects of growth and development on performance have to be disentangled so that the effects of training can be assessed. A technique has been developed to meet this challenge. It is a multilevel regression modelling procedure (Goldstein, 1986) and it has been used to explore changes in cardiopulmonary function in élite standard child and adolescent athletes (Baxter-Jones et al., 1993) via the analysis program Multilevel Models Project ML3 (Prosser et al., 1990).

Age, anthropometric variables, pubertal stage

and sport were used as covariates to investigate the influence of training on $\dot{V}o_{2\,max}$. The study demonstrated size-independent increases in $\dot{V}o_{2\,max}$ towards the end of puberty in boys but not in girls. Furthermore, these increases were masked by the use of ratio standards. Strictly speaking this is not a scaling technique in the way that allometric modelling is and it is acknowledged that the technique 'is designed to study populations and not to predict individual values' (Baxter-Jones et al., 1993), but it is likely that this procedure will be used increasingly in longitudinal repeated measure-type studies.

The principles of scaling are well established and considerations of dimensions are included in a notable text (Åstrand & Rodahl, 1986). Furthermore, there are examples of allometric modelling (Sjödin & Svedenhag, 1992). Consequently, it is curious that sport and exercise scientists in general have been slow to recognize the imperfections of ratio standards and seemingly are unaware of the alternatives.

Challenges for future research

If research in the area of paediatric physiology of exercise is to develop, it is vital that the principles of scaling are embraced and applied. This will probably involve:
- Abandoning a priori use of ratio standards and restricting their use solely to when Tanner's (1949) special circumstance has been sought and verified.
- Restricting linear modelling via ANCOVA to comparisons of groups based on logarithmic transformations.
- Preferential use of allometric modelling to construct standards against which individuals can be compared and as a basis for comparisons between groups.
- The application of multilevel modelling to longitudinal repeated measures designs.

References

Alexander, R.McN., Jayes, A.S., Maloiy, G.M.O. & Wathuta, E.M. (1981) Allometry of the leg muscles of mammals. J. Zool. (London) 194, 539–52.

Armstrong, N. & Welsman, J.R. (1994) Assessment and interpretation of aerobic fitness in children and adolescents. In: J.O. Holloszy (ed.) Exercise and Sport Sciences Reviews, pp. 435–76. Williams & Wilkins, Baltimore.

Åstrand, P.-O. & Rodahl, K. (1986) Textbook of Work Physiology, 3rd edn. McGraw-Hill, New York.

Baxter-Jones, A., Goldstein, H. & Helms, P. (1993) The development of aerobic power in young athletes. J. Appl. Physiol. 75, 1160–7.

Goldstein, H. (1986) Efficient statistical modelling of longitudinal data. Ann. Hum. Biol. 13, 129–41.

Jakeman, P.M., Winter, E.M. & Doust, J. (1994) A review of research in sports physiology. J. Sports Sci. 12, 33–60.

Nevill, A.M. (1994) The need to scale for differences in body size and mass: an explanation of Kleiber's 0.75 mass exponent. J. Appl. Physiol. 77, 2870–3.

Nevill, A.M., Ramsbottom, R. & Williams, C. (1992) Scaling physiological measurements for individuals of different body size. Eur. J. Appl. Physiol. 65, 110–17.

Prosser, R., Rasbash, J. & Goldstein, H. (1990) ML3 Software for the Three-Level Analysis User's Guide. Institute of Education, University of London, London.

Schmidt-Nielsen, K. (1984) Scaling: Why is Animal Size so Important? Cambridge University Press, Cambridge.

Sjödin, B. & Svedenhag, J. (1992) Oxygen uptake during running as related to body mass in circum-pubertal boys. Eur. J. Appl. Phyiol. 65, 150–7.

Snedecor, G.W. & Cochran, W.G. (1980) Statistical Methods, 7th edn. Iowa State University Press, Ames.

Tanner, J.M. (1949) Fallacy of per-weight and per-surface area standards and their relation to spurious correlation. J. Appl. Physiol. 2, 1–15.

Tanner, J.M. (1964) The Physique of the Olympic Athlete. Allen & Unwin, London.

Welsman, J.R., Armstrong, N., Winter, E.M. & Kirby, B.J. (1993) The influence of various scaling techniques on the interpretation of developmental changes in peak $\dot{V}o_2$. Pediatr. Exerc. Sci. 5, 485.

Williams, J.R., Armstrong, N., Winter, E.M. & Crichton, N. (1992) Changes in peak oxygen uptake with age and sexual maturation in boys: physiological fact or statistical anamoly? In J. Coudert & E. Van Praagh (eds) Pediatric Work Physiology —

Children and Exercise, Vol. XVI, pp. 35–7. Masson, Paris.

Winter, E.M. (1992) Scaling: partitioning out differences in size. *Pediatr Exerc. Sci.* **4**, 296–301.

Winter, E.M., Brookes, F.B.C. & Hamley, E.J. (1991) Maximal exercise performance and lean leg volume in men and women. *J. Sports Sci.* **9**, 3–13.

Winter, E.M., Brookes, F.B.C. & Roberts, K.W. (1993) The effects of scaling on comparisons between maximal exercise performance in boys and men. *Pediatr. Exerc. Sci.* **5**, 488.

Winter, E.M. & Maughan, R.J. (1991) Strength and cross-sectional area of the quadriceps in men and women. *J. Physiol.* **43S**, 175P.

Index